Transcatheter Aortic Valve Implantation

Arturo Giordano
Giuseppe Biondi-Zoccai · Giacomo Frati
Editors

Transcatheter Aortic Valve Implantation

Clinical, Interventional and Surgical Perspectives

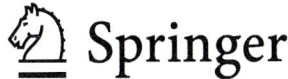 Springer

Editors
Arturo Giordano
Interventional Cardiology Unit
Pineta Grande Hospital
Castel Volturno
Caserta
Italy

Giuseppe Biondi-Zoccai
Department of Medico-Surgical
Sciences and Biotechnologies
Sapienza University of Rome
Latina
Italy

Giacomo Frati
Department of Medico-Surgical
Sciences and Biotechnologies
Sapienza University of Rome
Latina
Italy

ISBN 978-3-030-05911-8   ISBN 978-3-030-05912-5   (eBook)
https://doi.org/10.1007/978-3-030-05912-5

This Springer imprint is published by the registered company Springer Nature Switzerland AG
The registered company address is: Gewerbestrasse 11, 6330 Cham, Switzerland

To Salvatore and Celestina, my awesome parents

– A. Giordano

To Gianni, my father

– G. Biondi-Zoccai

To Greta, my love

– G. Frati

Foreword

The subspecialty of interventional cardiology was born out of the clinical need for lesser invasive approaches to serious cardiovascular disorders, initially coronary artery disease. The evolution of this subspecialty has been fostered by the relentless drive to recognize and overcome obstacles, propelled by creativity and ingenuity. This pattern is clearly evident in the progression from balloon angioplasty to bare metal stents to several generations of drug-eluting stents, aided by advances in intravascular imaging, physiologic lesion assessment, and adjunct pharmacotherapy. These developments over the last 4 decades have led to increasing success rates, reduced complications, and greater durability of outcomes such that percutaneous coronary intervention has become by far the most widely utilized revascularization modality for patients with coronary atherosclerosis and has been demonstrated to save lives and improve quality of life for millions of patients around the world.

As the subspecialty of coronary intervention matured, the spark of invention spread to other applications, most extraordinarily to the treatment of patients with severe aortic stenosis. Aortic stenosis is a "simple" but debilitating disease that affects 5% or more of elderly patients, robbing quality and years of life. Aortic stenosis is becoming an increasingly important societal issue given the aging of the general population. And 1–2% of younger patients have a congenitally bicuspid valve, which prematurely can fail. Fortunately, surgical aortic valve replacement (SAVR) is an excellent operation that is successful in most. However, SAVR is still a major surgery, and as such carries substantial perioperative risks and morbidity. Some patients are too high risk to undergo SAVR, while others would prefer a less invasive option, with fewer complications and faster recovery.

Transcatheter aortic valve implantation (TAVI, as it is most commonly called in Europe), also known as transcatheter aortic valve replacement (TAVR, the term more widely used in the USA), was born out of this clinical need. In hindsight a brilliant but simple concept, the TAVI device at its core consists of a stent frame with a bioprosthetic valve contained within. Delivered most commonly through femoral access, the crimped stent valve is typically passed retrogradely across the stenotic aortic valve and then either via balloon expansion or self-expanding properties is implanted in the aortic annulus, excluding the native diseased valve. The first procedure was performed by Alain Cribier in Rouen, France, on April 16th, 2002, in an inoperable and desperately ill 57-year-old man in refractory cardiogenic shock due to critical calcific aortic stenosis. The procedure was successful, igniting extraordinary enthusiasm, accelerated development efforts, and subsequent proof of clinical safety and efficacy of a new procedure to a degree heretofore not previously seen in medicine.

Initially TAVI was applied to very elderly patients at prohibitive surgical risk with severe aortic stenosis. A large-scale randomized trial demonstrated that a balloon-expandable device markedly improved quality of life and reduced mortality, with one life saved for every five patients treated—an almost unheard of magnitude of benefit. Similar outcomes were demonstrated with a self-expanding TAVI device in a similar patient population in a non-randomized study. TAVI with both balloon-expandable and self-expanding versions was subsequently shown in large randomized trials to have similar or even slightly higher rates of survival compared with SAVR in high-risk surgically eligible patients with severe aortic stenosis. But high complication rates with these early generation devices were evident, especially bleeding and vascular events, among others, and in some studies stroke tended to be more common than with surgery. In addition, severe peripheral vascular disease in some patients necessitated TAVI introduction through a transapical myocardial approach in some patients, a less desirable route fraught with more frequent complications.

Consistent with the history of interventional cardiology, once these issues were recognized they were addressed by improved technology and technique. Lower profile devices were developed translating to less bleeding and adverse vascular events, and fewer patients requiring transapical access. Paravalvular leaks in some devices were reduced by the addition of an external sealing cuff. An excessive rate of pacemakers with other devices was lowered with an optimal technique. Improved vascular closure approaches were developed. And so forth.

With these improvements large-scale randomized trials were progressively performed with each class of device first in intermediate-risk patients and then low-risk patients with severe aortic stenosis, demonstrating first comparable outcomes but most recently improved survival free from stroke and hospitalization compared with SAVR. Indeed, the rapidity with which a massive amount of high-quality randomized trial evidence was generated to support the safety and efficacy of these devices is unparalleled in the annals of medicine. And more is on the way, with ongoing studies in bicuspid aortic stenosis in younger patients, asymptomatic patients with severe aortic stenosis, moderate aortic stenosis with heart failure, predominant aortic regurgitation, treatment of failed surgically implanted valves and rings, and implants in diseased native mitral valves with heavy annular calcification. Additional studies are addressing the optimal periprocedural and long-term pharmacotherapy to prevent leaflet thrombosis after TAVI while minimizing bleeding. Novel approaches have been developed to prevent cerebral embolization, and avert or treat rare but serious complications such as coronary obstruction and aortic rupture. Large-bore closure devices have been introduced which promise to further reduce vascular complications and shorten time to ambulation and discharge. Dozens of novel TAVI designs have been developed to allow the device to be more easily repositioned or recaptured, to enhance tissue biocompatibility and longevity, treat patients with aortic insufficiency and dilated aortic roots, and further enhance the reproducibility and safety of the procedure.

An undeniable success story, the development, evolution, practice, and future of TAVI deserve documentation in a major textbook. In this regard *Transcatheter Aortic Valve Implantation: Clinical, Interventional and Surgical Perspectives*, edited by Arturo Giordano, Giuseppe Biondi-Zoccai, and Giacomo Frati, is an incredible effort in which the pathophysiology of aortic valve disease, diagnosis of severe aortic stenosis and patient selection for TAVI, alternative TAVI devices, techniques, outcomes, and adjunct technologies are thoroughly reviewed. The role of the heart team is emphasized, with the preferences of the informed patient at the center of clinical decision-making. The 48 chapters in this book contributed by more than 100 authors comprehensively describe the past, present, and future of this astonishing journey.

Gregg W. Stone
Columbia University Medical Center,
New York, NY, USA

Preface

The beginning is the most important part of the work

Plato

Cardiovascular disease represents one of the major causes of mortality, morbidity and resource use worldwide [1]. Rosy declines in the incidence of cardiovascular death in high-income countries have been partly offset by increased incidence and prevalence of several cardiovascular conditions in other countries, and a shift from coronary artery disease to other conditions. Accordingly, and also thanks to an overall increase in life expectancy, clinicians have seen an overall increase in the prevalence and burden of degenerative aortic valve stenosis [2, 3].

Such booming need for appropriate management of aortic valve disease poses several challenges [4]. First, the role of prevention and medical therapy is still very limited, if present at all, thus restricting the opportunity for simple, cheap, and large-scale approaches [5]. Second, aortic valve disease in general and degenerative aortic valve stenosis in particular often occur in elderly subjects fraught with major comorbidities, which heavily impact on treatment choices and subsequent management [6]. Third, surgical aortic valve replacement with a mechanical or biologic prosthesis has remained until recently the gold standard treatment for severe aortic disease in fit patients [7]. However, it represents major surgery requiring cardiopulmonary arrest and extracorporeal circulation, with substantial risk and cost implications.

Thanks to the pioneering efforts of Gruentzig, Labadibi and Cribier [8–10], among many others, severe aortic valve stenosis can now be managed with a minimally invasive technique: transcatheter aortic valve implantation (TAVI), also called transcatheter aortic valve replacement (TAVR). Despite its junior age, transcatheter aortic valve implantation has already managed to reach and overcome several important milestones. Indeed, devices have evolved dramatically from first-generation to more refined ones [11]. Accompanying clinical evidence has been accrued spanning from randomized trials to observational studies and case series, supporting the adoption of this technology in several settings, including prohibitive risk patients, intermediate risk patients, failed bioprostheses, highly selected cases of aortic regurgitation, and, most recently, low-risk subjects [12–15]. But the greatest driver of transcatheter aortic valve implantation successes is surely the team effort which has been sought from the beginning by all researchers, practitioners, and stakeholders involved. Indeed, transcatheter aortic valve implantation has proved as a landmark example of heart team involvement in device development, patient selection, procedural strategy, and subsequent management [16].

Several good books have been compiled on the topic of transcatheter aortic valve implantation or transcatheter valve repair at large, including the recent concise manual by Watkins et al. [17], as well as the leading textbooks by Ailawadi and Kron [18], and Tamburino et al. [19]. Yet, no work to date has explicitly aimed at capitalizing the successes of the heart team approach in the design and leadership of an authoritative textbook devoted to transcatheter aortic valve implantation.

Our aim was explicitly this. The editor team comprises a leading interventional cardiologist with hands-on transcatheter aortic valve implantation, an expert clinical cardiologist with established track record in evidence synthesis and non-structural cardiac interventions, and a pioneering cardiac surgeons with expertise in valve repair as well as translational research. Accordingly, chapters have been provided by leading clinicians, invasive cardiologists, and surgeons, with the shared belief that different perspectives may be integrated in a constructive fashion through the heart team approach, for the ultimate benefit of patients as well as everybody involved in their care.

More precisely, this textbook has been divided in five main sections. The first part of the work deals with the pathophysiology of aortic valve disease and most promising translational perspectives, including the role of inflammation and key hemodynamic issues. The second section focusing on clinical aspects of direct relevance for patient selection. Specifically, risk scores, imaging modalities, concomitant coronary artery disease, gender differences and implementation issues are all systematically analyzed. The third part includes chapters with an obvious interventional focus, including several chapters dedicated to the various available devices, individualized device choice, as well as ancillary management including antithrombotic therapy and renal protection. The fourth section maintains a direct surgical perspective, emphasing the role of the heart team, use of alternative accesses, and hybrid procedures. The last part of the textbook provides more thought-provoking contributions, for instance on medical therapy, pure aortic regurgitation, and bioresorbable valves.

In conclusion, we are confident that this comprehensive book on transcatheter aortic valve implantation will prove useful to clinicians, interventionists and surgeons by providing a plethora of important pieces of information, while emphasizing the need for heart team involvement and shared decision-making.

Acknowledgements

Funding: None.

Conflicts of interest: Dr. A. Giordano has consulted for Abbott Vascular and Medtronic. Prof. Biondi-Zoccai has consulted for Abbott Vascular and Bayer.

References

1. Atlas Writing Group, Timmis A, Townsend N, Gale C, Grobbee R, Maniadakis N, Flather M, Wilkins E, Wright L, Vos R, Bax J, Blum M, Pinto F, Vardas P. European Society of Cardiology: Cardiovascular disease statistics 2017. Eur Heart J 2018;39:508–79.
2. Domenech B, Pomar JL, Prat-González S, Vidal B, López-Soto A, Castella M, Sitges M. Valvular heart disease epidemics. J Heart Valve Dis 2016;25:1–7.
3. Iung B, Vahanian A. Epidemiology of acquired valvular heart disease. Can J Cardiol 2014;30:962–70.
4. Kanwar A, Thaden JJ, Nkomo VT. Management of Patients With Aortic Valve Stenosis. Mayo Clin Proc 2018;93:488–508.
5. Freeman PM, Protty MB, Aldalati O, Lacey A, King W, Anderson RA, Smith D. Severe symptomatic aortic stenosis: medical therapy and transcatheter aortic valve implantation (TAVI)-a real-world retrospective cohort analysis of outcomes and cost-effectiveness using national data. Open Heart 2016;3:e000414.
6. Kilic T, Yilmaz I. Transcatheter aortic valve implantation: a revolution in the therapy of elderly and high-risk patients with severe aortic stenosis. J Geriatr Cardiol 2017;14:204–17.
7. Li X, Kong M, Jiang D, Dong A. Comparison 30-day clinical complications between transfemoral versus transapical aortic valve replacement for aortic stenosis: a meta-analysis review. J Cardiothorac Surg 2013;8:168.
8. Gruntzig A. Transluminal dilatation of coronary-artery stenosis. Lancet 1978;1:263.
9. Lababidi Z, Wu JR, Walls JT. Percutaneous balloon aortic valvuloplasty: results in 23 patients. Am J Cardiol 1984;53:194–7.
10. Cribier A, Eltchaninoff H, Bash A, Borenstein N, Tron C, Bauer F, Derumeaux G, Anselme F, Laborde F, Leon MB. Percutaneous transcatheter implantation of an aortic valve prosthesis for calcific aortic stenosis: first human case description. Circulation 2002;106:3006–8.
11. Gatto L, Biondi-Zoccai G, Romagnoli E, Frati G, Prati F, Giordano A. New-generation devices for transcatheter aortic valve implantation. Minerva Cardioangiol 2018. https://doi.org/10.23736/S0026-4725.18.04707-2. [Epub ahead of print].
12. Lindman BR, Alexander KP, O'Gara PT, Afilalo J. Futility, benefit, and transcatheter aortic valve replacement. JACC Cardiovasc Interv 2014;7:707–16.
13. Rogers T, Thourani VH, Waksman R. Transcatheter aortic valve replacement in intermediate- and low-risk patients. J Am Heart Assoc 2018;7:e007147.
14. Dvir D, Webb JG, Bleiziffer S, Pasic M, Waksman R, Kodali S, Barbanti M, Latib A, Schaefer U, Rodés-Cabau J, Treede H, Piazza N, Hildick-Smith D, Himbert D, Walther T, Hengstenberg C, Nissen H, Bekeredjian R, Presbitero P, Ferrari E, Segev A, de Weger A, Windecker S, Moat NE, Napodano M, Wilbring M, Cerillo AG, Brecker S, Tchetche D, Lefèvre T, De Marco F, Fiorina C, Petronio AS, Teles RC, Testa L, Laborde JC, Leon MB, Kornowski R; Valve-in-Valve International Data Registry Investigators. Transcatheter aortic valve implantation in failed bioprosthetic surgical valves. JAMA 2014;312:162–70.
15. Abdelaziz HK, Wiper A, More RS, Bittar MN, Roberts DH. Successful transcatheter aortic valve replacement using balloon-expandable valve for pure native aortic valve regurgitation in the presence of ascending aortic dissection. J Invasive Cardiol 2018;30:E62–E63.
16. Sintek M, Zajarias A. Patient evaluation and selection for transcatheter aortic valve replacement: the heart team approach. Prog Cardiovasc Dis 2014;56:572–82.
17. Watkins AC, Gupta A, Griffith BP. Transcatheter aortic valve replacement: a how-to guide for cardiologists and cardiac surgeons. Cham, Switzerland: Springer International; 2018.
18. Ailawadi G, Kron IL, editors. Catheter based valve and aortic surgery. Cham, Switzerland: Springer International; 2016.
19. Tamburino C, Barbanti M, Capodanno D, editors. Percutaneous treatment of left side cardiac valves: a practical guide for the interventional cardiologist. 3rd ed. Cham, Switzerland: Springer International; 2018.

Acknowledgments

The common eye sees only the outside of things, and judges by that, but the seeing eye pierces through and reads the heart and soul

Mark Twain

When I try to think about the people who contributed to the realization of my professional life, I cannot really stop adding up names to the thank you list.

After a while, though, a clear sequence bumps into my mind. Indeed, at the first and foremost place, there is my family. Fiammetta, my wife, who is a passionate medical researcher, helped me discover my passions. She supported me in all the difficult moments and stimulated me culturally everyday. Furthermore, she owns the merit of raising our wonderful children: Celeste, Carolina and Salvatore, who are lovely and sympathetic, and have always been a strong motivation for me. My siblings. Then there is the person who introduced me to the world of invasive cardiology: Professor Carlo Vigorito. He was a true teacher and a distinguished connoisseur of cardiovascular physiopathology. I am infinitely grateful to him. Among his students, Paolo Ferraro, who has always been my partner in the catheterization laboratory. We spent all our professional careers side by side, thanks to his technical skills and human virtues, especially his patience. A great boost to our activity, for sure, began with Nicola Corcione. He is a great clinical cardiologist and an extraordinary interventional cardiologist, and indeed the catheterization laboratory is his natural habitat. Furthermore, Giuseppe Biondi-Zoccai highly contributed to the scientific aspects and elaboration of all the work that we have done. I must thank as well our lifetime cath lab collaborators, Pasquale and Riccardo, who have always been crucial to ensure the safety of our patients and the success of our procedures, as well as our secretaries Stefania, Eleonora and Raffaella, for constantly organizing our job and the latter for managing the scientific activities. A special thank goes to Vincenzo Schiavone, his wife Annamaria and his son Beniamino, who lead Pineta Grande Hospital and who believed in our job and supported, with great foresight, the structural interventional cardiology program.

Thanks also to all the people that work with me in the catheterization laboratory, who are fundamental for the best outcome of procedures and thus, most importantly, of patients.

Castel Volturno, Italy
April 25, 2019

Arturo Giordano

I am happy and honored to wholeheartedly thank by means of this opus my father, Gianni, who has always strived to do whatever it takes for the sake of his family, despite facing many adversities. His love and affection are unparalleled, as his ongoing support over the ups and downs of my professional and personal life. Indeed, I am really proud I named one of my sons, Giovanni Vincenzo, in his honor. Accordingly, on top of my father, I cannot forget the true love of my life, my children Attilio Nicola, Giuseppe Giulio and Giovanni Vincenzo, who continue to inspire and motivate me to humbly pursue excellence without ever discounting that what matters most is navigating life's journey together, rather than simply meeting its end alone. Finally, I wish to thank Barbara Antonazzo, who has lighted my path with her gifted caring eventually mending my troubled heart.

Besides my dear ones, I really wish to testify my gratitude to my many friends, colleagues and mentors (yes, only a true friend and colleague can be a nourishing mentor), but especially Enrico Romagnoli, Pierfrancesco Agostoni and Antonio Abbate. Whether close or at a distance, they have all supported enthusiastically my efforts in becoming a successful academic cardiologist (yes, it is possible despite appearing to some as a logical fallacy). And I also cannot stop thanking Arturo Giordano and Giacomo Frati, one leading interventional cardiologist and the other leading cardiac surgeon, for collaborating with me in coordinating this landmark textbook on structural cardiac interventions, as in many bread and butter activities or challenging fishing expeditions. Indeed, this work could not have seen the light if true friendship and mutual esteem had not preceded the careful planning and pursuing of this project.

Thanking my father and my loved ones brings to my mind also the many pioneers in interventional cardiology and cardiac surgery who have collaboratively led the field of transcatheter aortic valve implantation to its current successes. From Andreas Gruntzig and Julio Palmaz, whose inventive development of, respectively, angioplasty balloons and metallic stents cannot be overemphasized, the efforts of many have brought us to balloon aortic valvuloplasty up to first-generation transcatheter aortic valve implantation devices, and eventually, new-generation ones, as brilliantly highlighted in this book.

Latina, Italy   Giuseppe Biondi-Zoccai
April 25, 2019

I am proud to dedicate this textbook to the greatest love of my life, my daughter Greta.

Greta, you are the gift of my life.

This book is also dedicated to Giorgia, the love of my life, the mother of my princess.

A special mention should also be given to my beloved family: my father Luigi, source of inspiration and example of tenacity and persistency, my mother Luciana, woman of profound culture who gave me the passion for the investigation, my sister Paola, who was and is still always there for me, my worshiped niece Caterina, my second daughter.

I also really wish to testify my gratitude to many friends and colleagues ever helping me in becoming what I am: Elena "Walking" De Falco, Isotta "Pro-VAX" Chimenti, Mariangela "Chicca" Peruzzi, Elena "Elenuccia" Cavarretta, Sebastiano "Maschio" Sciarretta, Roberto "also platelets" Carnevale, Nino "Conte" Marullo.

Finally, I would like to express my very warm thanks to Arturo Giordano and Giuseppe Biondi-Zoccai for collaborating with me in this textbook on structural cardiac interventions.

Giuseppe, a special thank for you, your friendship, your continuous support, your valuable advices, the countless coffees and the weekend spent together with our families in the pool.

I should probably thank many others, but time and space induce me to stop here.

Latina, Italy   Giacomo Frati
April 25, 2019

Contents

Part I Pathophysiological and Translational Perspectives

1 History of Transcatheter Aortic Valve Implantation 3
Hans R. Figulla, Markus Ferrari, Marcus Franz,
and Alexander Lauten

2 Interventional Anatomy of Aortic Valve 11
Stefania Rizzo, Monica de Gaspari, Gaetano Thiene,
and Cristina Basso

3 Pathophysiology of Aortic Valve Stenosis 21
Gabriele Di Giammarco and Daniele Marinelli

**4 Predictive Computational Models of Transcatheter
Aortic Valve Implantation** 29
Simone Morganti, Michele Conti, Alessandro Reali,
and Ferdinando Auricchio

**5 Haemodynamic Issues with Transcatheter Aortic Valve
Implantation** 47
Jacob Salmonsmith, Anna Maria Tango, Andrea Ducci,
and Gaetano Burriesci

Part II Clinical Perspectives

6 Risk Scores for Aortic Valve Interventions 63
Tom Kai Ming Wang, Ralph Stewart, Mark Webster,
and Peter Ruygrok

**7 Role of Rest and Stress Echocardiography in
Transcatheter Aortic Valve Implantation** 75
Quirino Ciampi, Fiore Manganelli, and Bruno Villari

**8 Role of Computed Tomography in Transcatheter
Aortic Valve Implantation** 87
Zhen Qian

**9 Role of Magnetic Resonance Imaging in Transcatheter
Aortic Valve Implantation** 99
Giulia Pontecorboli, Silvia Pradella, Stefano Colagrande,
and Carlo Di Mario

10   **Concomitant Coronary Artery Disease
     and Aortic Stenosis** 115
     Carolina Espejo, Gabriela Tirado-Conte,
     Luis Nombela-Franco, and Pilar Jimenez-Quevedo

11   **Comparison of Transcatheter Aortic Valve Implantation
     to Medical Therapy in Prohibitive-Risk Patients**............. 127
     Gabriella Ricciardi, Piero Trabattoni, Maurizio Roberto,
     Marco Agrifoglio, and Giulio Pompilio

12   **Clinical and Imaging Follow-Up After Transcatheter
     Aortic Valve Implantation** 137
     Barbara D. Lawson, Mohammed Quader, Luis A. Guzman,
     and Zachary M. Gertz

13   **Cardiac Biomarkers in Transcatheter Aortic
     Valve Implantation** 147
     Paul L. Hermany and John K. Forrest

14   **Aortic Regurgitation After Transcatheter Aortic Valve
     Implantation** 165
     Bogdan Borz

15   **Leaflet Motion Abnormality Following Transcatheter
     Aortic Valve Implantation** 183
     Luca Testa, Matteo Casenghi, Antonio Popolo Rubbio,
     Magdalena Cuman, and Francesco Bedogni

16   **Gender-Related Differences in Transcatheter Aortic Valve
     Implantation** 189
     Brad Stair and John K. Forrest

17   **Implementation Issues for Transcatheter Aortic
     Valve Implantation: Access, Value, Affordability,
     and Wait Times** 201
     Harindra C. Wijeysundera, Gabby Elbaz-Greener,
     Derrick Y. Tam, and Stephen E. Fremes

Part III   Interventional Perspectives

18   **Access Management for Transfemoral Transcatheter
     Aortic Valve Implantation** 215
     Francesco Burzotta, Osama Shoeib, and Carlo Trani

19   **Challenging Anatomy in Transcatheter Aortic
     Valve Implantation** 229
     Antonio Colombo and Nicola Buzzatti

20   **Abbott Structural Heart Program for Transcatheter
     Aortic Valve Implantation** 243
     Vincent J. Nijenhuis, Jorn Brouwer, Pierfrancesco Agostoni,
     and Jurrien M. ten Berg

21 Boston Scientific Program for Transcatheter Aortic Valve Implantation 255
Mohammad Abdelghani and Mohamed Abdel-Wahab

22 Edwards Program for Transcatheter Aortic Valve Implantation 265
Grant W. Reed, Rachel Easterwood, and Samir R. Kapadia

23 The JenaValve Program for Transcatheter Aortic Valve Implantation 279
Hans R. Figulla, Markus Ferrari, Vicky Carr-Brendel, and Alexander Lauten

24 Medtronic Program for Transcatheter Aortic Valve Implantation 287
Yasuhiro Ichibori, Sandeep M. Patel, Ankur Kalra, and Guilherme F. Attizzani

25 New Valve Technology Program for Transcatheter Aortic Valve Implantation 301
Nicola Corcione, Salvatore Giordano, Alberto Morello, and Arturo Giordano

26 Self-Expanding vs. Balloon-Expandable Devices for Transcatheter Aortic Valve Implantation 305
Denise Todaro, Andrea Picci, Corrado Tamburino, and Marco Barbanti

27 Individualized Device Choice for Transcatheter Aortic Valve Implantation 329
Nicola Corcione, Salvatore Giordano, Alberto Morello, and Arturo Giordano

28 Predilation in Transcatheter Aortic Valve Implantation 339
Alexander Sedaghat, Eberhard Grube, and Jan-Malte Sinning

29 Balloon Post-dilation During Transcatheter Aortic Valve Implantation 351
Amit N. Vora, G. Chad Hughes IV, and J. Kevin Harrison

30 Embolic Protection Devices for Transcatheter Aortic Valve Implantation 363
Anna Franzone and Stefan Stortecky

31 Antithrombotic Therapy During and After Transcatheter Aortic Valve Implantation 377
Gennaro Sardella, Simone Calcagno, Nicolò Salvi, and Massimo Mancone

32 Contrast-Induced Acute Kidney Injury in Transcatheter Aortic Valve Implantation: Risk, Outcomes, Treatment, and Prevention 387
Andrew M. Goldsweig and J. Dawn Abbott

33   **Conduction Disorders and Permanent Pacemaker Implantation After Transcatheter Aortic Valve Implantation** 395
     Jorn Brouwer, Vincent J. Nijenhuis, Uday Sonker,
     and Jurrien M. ten Berg

34   **Radiation Exposure in Transcatheter Aortic Valve Implantation Procedure** 407
     Florian Stierlin, Nick Ryck, Stéphane Cook,
     and Jean-Jacques Goy

35   **Procedure Efficiency in Transcatheter Aortic Valve Implantation** 417
     Sandeep M. Patel, Yasuhiro Ichibori, Angela Davis,
     and Guilherme F. Attizzani

36   **Predictors of Success of Transcatheter Aortic Valve Implantation** 425
     Alessandro Maloberti, Domenico Sirico, Andrea Buono,
     and Giannattasio Cristina

37   **Learning Curve Characteristics and Relationship of Procedural Volumes with Clinical Outcomes for Transcatheter Aortic Valve Implantation** 445
     Anthony Wassef and Asim N. Cheema

38   **Role of Balloon Aortic Valvuloplasty in the Transcatheter Aortic Valve Implantation Era** 457
     Laura Gatto, Enrico Romagnoli, Vito Ramazzotti,
     and Francesco Prati

Part IV   Surgical Perspectives

39   **Role of the Heart Team in Decision-Making for Transcatheter Aortic Valve Implantation** 471
     Carlo Savini and Roberto Di Bartolomeo

40   **Comparison of Transcatheter Aortic Valve Implantation to Surgical Aortic Valve Replacement in Intermediate-Risk Patients** 479
     Anita W. Asgar and Nathan Messas

41   **New Approaches for Aortic Valve Disease: From Transcatheter Aortic Valve Implantation to Sutureless Aortic Valves** 487
     Giuseppe Santarpino, Renato Gregorini,
     and Theodor Fischlein

42   **Hybrid Procedures for Aortic Valve Disease: Transapical Aortic Valve Implantation Through Lower Left Anterior Mini-thoracotomy Versus Sutureless Valve Implantation Through Upper Right Anterior Mini-thoracotomy** 493
     Terézia B. Andrási

Part V   Future Perspectives

43   Medical Treatment for Aortic Valve Disease 507
Aydin Huseynov, Michael Behnes, and Ibrahim Akin

**44   Transcatheter Aortic Valve Implantation for
Pure Aortic Regurgitation** 515
Luca Testa, Matteo Casenghi, and Francesco Bedogni

**45   New Generation Devices for Transcatheter Aortic
Valve Implantation** 521
Iop Laura and Gerosa Gino

**46   Biorestorative Valve for Transcatheter Aortic Valve
Implantation: Tomorrow's World from Preclinical
to Clinical** 539
Rodrigo Modolo, Yosuke Miyazaki, Yoshinobu Onuma,
Osama I. Soliman, and Patrick W. Serruys

**47   Focus on Transcatheter Aortic Valve Implantation
in Low-Risk Patients** 549
A. K. Roy and B. Prendergast

48   Conclusion 557
Arturo Giordano, Giuseppe Biondi-Zoccai, and Giacomo Frati

Part I

Pathophysiological and Translational Perspectives

History of Transcatheter Aortic Valve Implantation

Hans R. Figulla, Markus Ferrari, Marcus Franz, and Alexander Lauten

Transcatheter valve technology (TVT) began with pulmonary valvuloplasty (1982), mitral valvuloplasty (1984), and later, aortic valve valvuloplasty (1986) [1–3]. Percutaneous aortic balloon valvotomy was first introduced into the therapeutic armamentarium in 1986 to treat for palliative purposes patients with aortic stenosis [4]. While mitral and pulmonary valvuloplasty have good long-term results, the high restenosis rate after aortic valvuloplasty initiated the development of percutaneous aortic valves, which began in the early 1990s to early 2000s; this was followed by the first human implants of a pulmonary valve, by Bonhoeffer et al., for the treatment of a stenosis in a pulmonary conduit, and an aortic valve replacement by Cribier et al. [5–9].

The pathway to these first successful human implants was paved with frustrations and drawbacks owing to the pessimistic views of our surgical colleagues, who exclusively dominated the field of valvular replacement at that time. The conservative view of valvular replacement was driven by the dogma that stenotic and sclerotic aortic valves had to be excised owing to their calcium burden and that a biological valve to be implanted should not be stressed by any compression, as is the case during the wrapping of catheter valves. Although this argumentation was never verified, it frequently pops up when the question of transcatheter aortic valve implantation (TAVI), also called transcatheter aortic valve replacement (TAVR), durability comes up. As cardiologists, we had the somehow naive but successful view that calcified aortic valves might not need to be excised, driven by our coronary angioplasty experience and by the indirect view of fluoroscopy, which showed that the calcified tissue would be sloughed off into the surrounding tissue without the need for removal and an extended lumen could be created.

We started our first in vitro experiments in 1995 after we had written a patent application for a self-expanding stent valve device, which extended in the ascending aorta to create friction on the stent, so the valve might not be dislodged

H. R. Figulla (✉)
Jena University Hospital, Jena, Germany
e-mail: figulla@figulla.org

M. Ferrari
Dr Horst Schmidt Kliniken, Klinik Innere MED I:
Kardiologie und Konservative Intensivmedizin,
Wiesbaden, Germany
e-mail: Markus.Ferrari@helios-gesundheit.de

M. Franz
Department of Cardiology, Clinic of Internal
Medicine I, Jena University Hospital, Jena, Germany
e-mail: marcus.franz@med.uni-jena.de

A. Lauten
Klinik für Kardiologie, Charité Campus Benjamin
Franklin, Universitätsmedizin Berlin,
Berlin, Germany
e-mail: alexander.lauten@charite.de

© Springer Nature Switzerland AG 2019
A. Giordano et al. (eds.), *Transcatheter Aortic Valve Implantation*,
https://doi.org/10.1007/978-3-030-05912-5_1

Fig. 1.1 Self-expanding 1996 valve prototypes from H.R. Figulla and M. Ferrari (Courtesy H.R. Figulla and M. Ferrari)

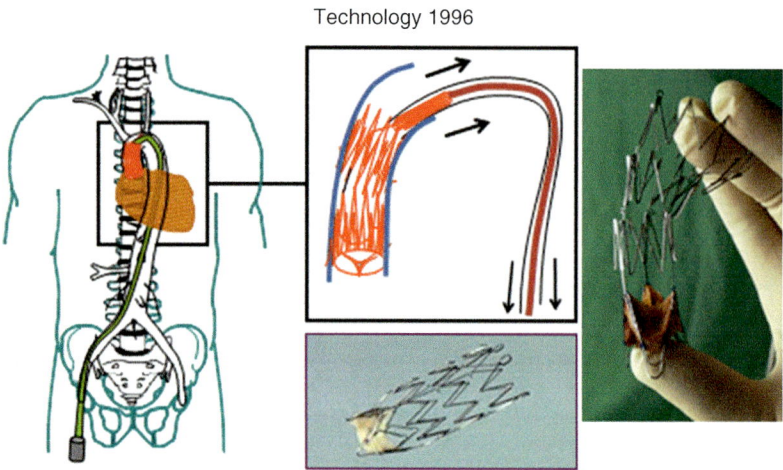

Fig. 1.2 First experiments measuring the dislocation forces on the stent in vitro and the hemodynamics of a valve fixed to the self-expanding stent, performed in 1995 by H.R. Figulla and M. Ferrari (Courtesy H.R. Figulla and M. Ferrari)

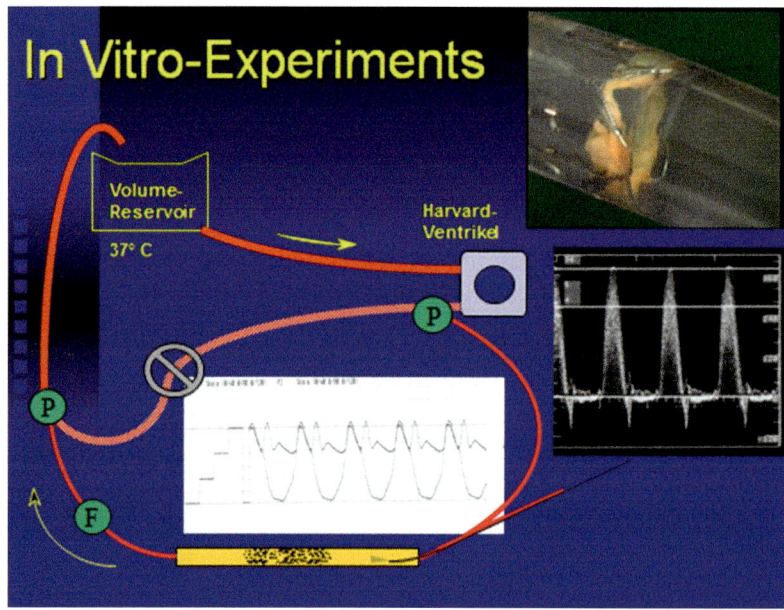

by the diastolic pressure into the left ventricle (Figs. 1.1 and 1.2).

At that time we were very skeptical that this would be sufficient, because so far all surgical valves had been fixed with multiple sutures, and even these sometimes broke. However, the in vitro experiments demonstrated that the valve stayed in position [10, 11]. Another concern was that the native leaflets left in place might obstruct the coronary ostia. In fact, in the case of a large annulus with large leaflets, low coronary takeoff, and a small sinus of Valsalva, this might happen.

1.1 The Development of Balloon-Expandable TAVI Devices

In the early 1990s, Alain Cribier began to work on a percutaneous aortic valve by means of a balloon-expandable stent. Cribier reported later, between 1995 and 1999, that a stent in a native aortic specimen could be fixed sufficiently to up to 2 kg, but the biomedical industry did not show any interest, an experience we also faced at that time period [12]. However, his idea was already protected by the patents of Anderson and Knudsen, which had to be bought if any commercialization of this idea might be successful [5]. The vision of the Percutaneous Valve Technologies (PVT, Fort Lee, NJ, USA) company founders in 1999, Stan Row, Stan Rabinowitch, and Martin Leon, allowed Cribier to acquire this patent and to finance further work, ending in the first human implant in 2002 [4]. The PVT company was acquired by Edwards Lifesciences (Irvine, CA, USA) (in December 2003) and then the Cribier-Edwards valve was developed; it was available in two sizes, for annulus diameters of 23 mm and 26 mm, with an introducer sheath size of 22 or 24 French. This valve was used in compassionate cases only, and had a 30-day mortality rate of 20% and frequent paravalular leaks (Revive Trial, Recast Trial 2005) [13, 14].

The procedure used in the first human implants by Alain Cribier was the antegrade transseptal route, with a venous arterial loop allowing in order to cross the large rigid valve covering the implant balloon, the atrial septum, and mitral valve antegrade into the stenotic aortic valve. The procedure was difficult and mitral leaflet damage was a risk.

The prostheses were available in two sizes (23 and 26 mm); the larger sizes were used in order to avoid the paravalvular leakage that was frequently observed in the first series. John Webb in Toronto, in cooperation with Edwards, developed the retrograde transarterial implantation technique with a deflectable pusher sheath to allow easy crossing of the aortic arch and the stenotic valve [15, 16].

Webb and colleagues also performed the first transapical valve implantations [17]. The Edwards transapical route was promoted by Walther et al. as an easier ("the front door approach") way to deploy the valve, reflecting the large size of the transfemoral introducer sheaths [18].

1.2 New Concepts and New Clinical Results

The transapical route created the need for close cooperation between cardiologists and heart surgeons, and the idea of the heart team approach was born. However, meanwhile, in all propensity scores for risk adjustments, the so-called front door approach demonstrated 30-day mortality almost double that of the arterial transfemoral route; therefore, at present, the transapical route is used only if no femoral arterial access is possible.

Following animal implants by Laborde in 2005 and the foundation of the CoreValve (Irvine, CA, USA) in 2001 by Jacques Seguin, Eberhard Grube carried out the first human implants of a CoreValve device in 2005 [19, 20]. The results were promising, and the concept of TAVI by means of a self-expanding valve could be demonstrated.

In 2006, at the American College of Cardiology (ACC) meeting, Grube reported on the first 14 patients treated with the self-expanding CoreValve device. At that time only 9 of these patients had an uneventful course during the first 14 days. The device could be introduced by the transarterial femoral route. The company was acquired by Medtronic (Minneapolis, MN, USA) in February 2009, after improvements of the device showed easy and uneventful deployments.

At that time the improvements of the technology focused on the development of smaller introducers, bigger valves to address larger annuli, and alternative access routes. While the development of transapical access in the CoreValve device was not successful, the development of an 18F device allowed more patients to be treated and greatly improved the success rate (Fig. 1.3). Other companies also reported the results of new-concept devices in animal trials in 2005, e.g., the JenaValve with clip technology, the Direct Flow (Santa Rosa, CA, USA) device with its hydrolic-ring fixation, and Sadra Medical (Los Gatos, CA, USA) with its mesh wire stent (Fig. 1.4).

Fig. 1.3 The CoreValve road of device evolution over patients with different surgical risk (Courtesy E. Grube, at Transcatheter Cardiovascular Therapeutics 2007)

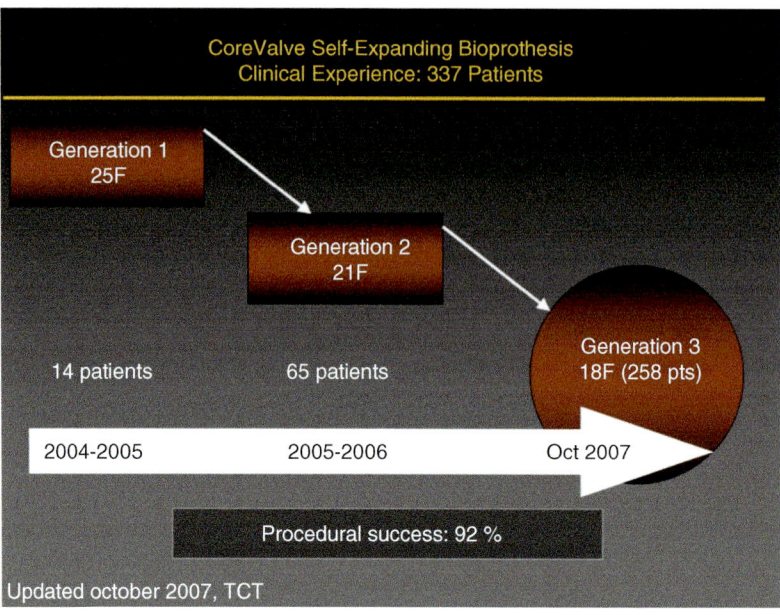

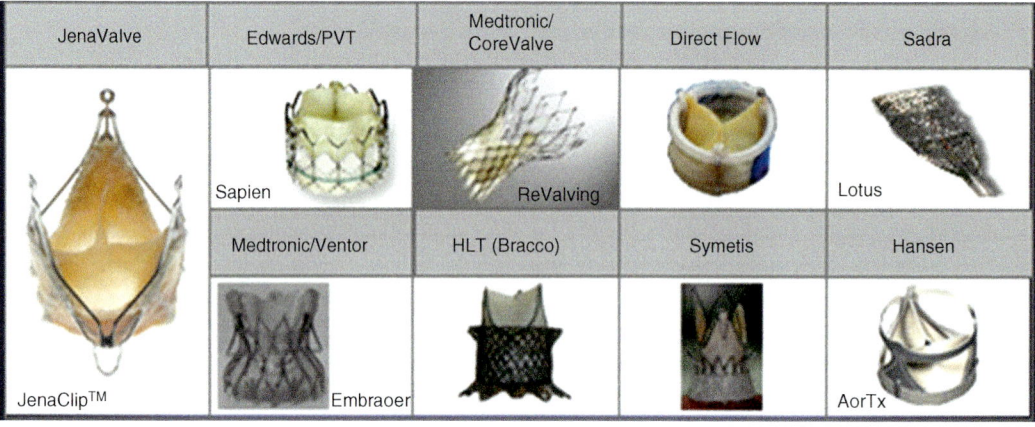

Fig. 1.4 Transcatheter aortic valve devices in 2005 (Courtesy of JenaValve)

1.3 Clinically Approved Devices and Future Developments

In 2007 the Edwards Sapien valve and CoreValve were the first to come onto the European market with a Conformité Européenne (CE) mark and since then the stage has been set for further improvement. The acceptance of these devices, especially in the German market, was huge, and all over Europe registries were installed to monitor the safety and efficiency of these new products [21–23].

In 2007 the PARTNER trials enrolled surgically inoperable patients for either TAVI or medical randomization. Within 1 year the medical group had an absolute mortality rate 20% higher than that in the TAVI group [24].

In the so-called PARTNER A trial, in high-surgical-risk patients, the results showed that TAVI was equivalent to surgical therapy, so the United States Food and Drug Administration (FDA) approved the marketing of the CoreValve and Sapien XT products from 2012 onwards in the United States for inoperable or very high-risk patients with a Society for Thoracic Surgery (STS) score above 10 [25].

Since 2007, several companies have brought devices to the market, while some companies

Fig. 1.5 CE-marked devices on the European market in 2018. The JenaValve and Lotus are temporarily unavailable

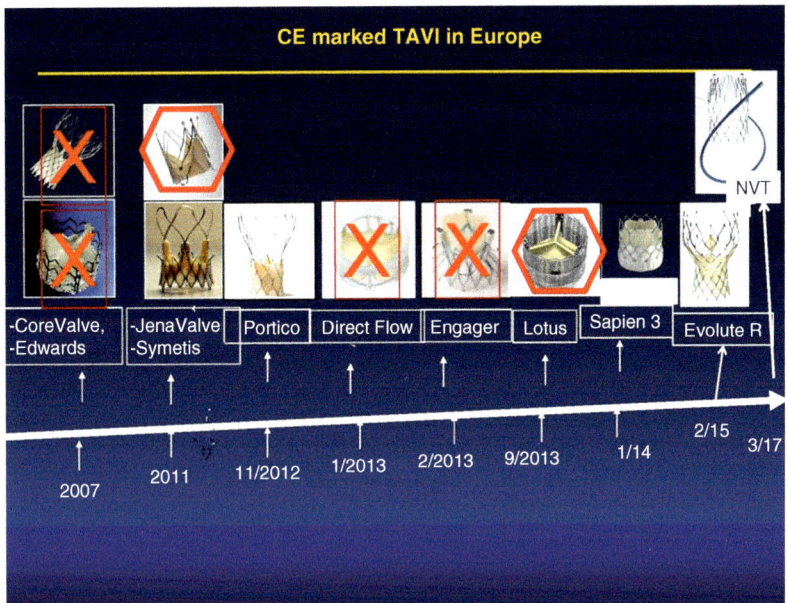

have even disappeared meanwhile, owing to technical or financial difficulties.

The JenaValve, with its transapical device, is the only device with CE approval for pure aortic regurgitation. However, the company subsequently withdrew the transapical device and meanwhile is working in clinical trials with its transfemoral device (see Chap. 6.1) (Fig. 1.5).

The high acceptance of TAVI by cardiologists and patients is possible, because even early in 2006, the audience at the meeting of the European Association for Percutaneous Cardiovascular Intervention (Euro PCR), in a poll at that meeting, foresaw that this technique would be used to replace a majority of surgical aortic valve implants (Fig. 1.6).

At present, in elderly patients above 75 years, TAVI is the preferred therapy irrespective of the individual risk [26].

New indications for TAVI are presently under study. As depicted in Table 1.1, there are investigations of TAVI in low-risk patient groups, as compared with surgical valve replacement, and TAVI investigations in asymptomatic patients with severe stenosis, in those with valve areas greater 1 cm² with congestive heart failure to reduce afterload, and in high-risk patients with aortic stenosis (Table 1.1).

In future, TAVI might completely replace surgical aortic valve replacement (SAVR) with

How long do you think will it take before it became standard of practic for percutaneous aortic valve replacement?

Presented at PCR Barcelona 2006

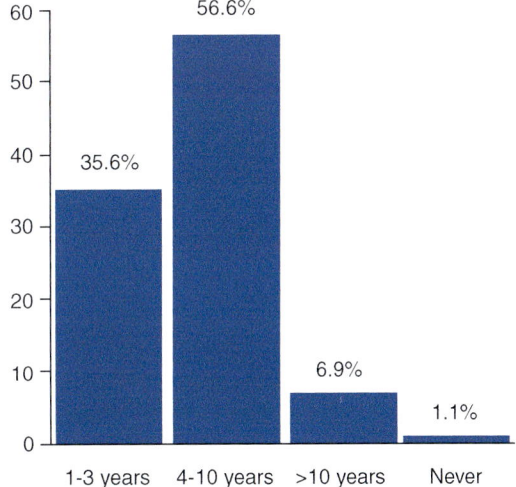

Fig. 1.6 Poll at the meeting of the European Association for Percutaneous Cardiovascular Intervention (Euro PCR) in 2006 about the future of transcatheter aortic valve implantation (Courtesy of H.R. Figulla)

Table 1.1 New indications for transcatheter aortic valve implantation (TAVI) presently under investigation

- Low-risk trials: PARTNER III, Medtronic: low risk
- Severe asymptomatic aortic stenosis (AS): EARLY trial
- Moderate AS + congestive heart failure (CHF): UNLOAD trial
- High-risk patients with aortic regurgitation (AR)

biological valves, and if the risk of TAVI is less than that of surgery, broader and earlier indications for the treatment of aortic stenosis might be warranted.

References

1. Buchanan JW, Anderson JH, White RI. The 1st balloon valvuloplasty: an historical note. J Vet Intern Med. 2002;16:116–7.
2. Inoue K, Owaki T, Nakamura T, Kitamura F, Miyamoto N. Clinical application of transvenous mitral commissurotomy by a new balloon catheter. J Thorac Cardiovasc Surg. 1984;87:394–402.
3. Lock JE, Khalilullah M, Shrivastava S, Bahl V, Keane JF. Percutaneous catheter commissurotomy in rheumatic mitral stenosis. N Engl J Med. 1985;313:1515–8.
4. Cribier A, Savin T, Saoudi N, Rocha P, Berland J, Letac B. Percutaneous transluminal valvuloplasty of acquired aortic stenosis in elderly patients: an alternative to valve replacement? Lancet. 1986;1:63–7.
5. Andersen HR, Knudsen LL, Hasenkam JM. Transluminal implantation of artificial heart valves. Description of a new expandable aortic valve and initial results with implantation by catheter technique in closed chest pigs. Eur Heart J. 1992;13:704–8.
6. Pavcnik D, Wright KC, Wallace S. Development and initial experimental evaluation of a prosthetic aortic valve for transcatheter placement. Work in progress. Radiology. 1992;183:151–4.
7. Ferrari M, Figulla HR, Schlosser M, Tenner I, Frerichs I, Damm C, Guyenot V, Werner GS, Hellige G. Transarterial aortic valve replacement with a self expanding stent in pigs. Heart. 2004;90:1326–31.
8. Bonhoeffer P, Boudjemline Y, Saliba Z, Merckx J, Aggoun Y, Bonnet D, Acar P, Le Bidois J, Sidi D, Kachaner J. Percutaneous replacement of pulmonary valve in a right-ventricle to pulmonary-artery prosthetic conduit with valve dysfunction. Lancet. 2000;356:1403–5.
9. Cribier A, Eltchaninoff H, Bash A, Borenstein N, Tron C, Bauer F, Derumeaux G, Anselme F, Laborde F, Leon MB. Percutaneous transcatheter implantation of an aortic valve prosthesis for calcific aortic stenosis: first human case description. Circulation. 2002;106:3006–8.
10. Ferrari M, Figulla HR. Selbstexpandierende Herzklappenprothese zur Implantation im menschlichen Körper über ein Kathetersystem (DGK Abstract 565). Z Kardiol. 1996;85(2):161.
11. Lauten A, Ferrari M, Petri A, Ensminger SM, Gummert JF, Boudjemline Y, Schubert H, Schumm J, Hekmat K, Schlosser M, Figulla HR. Experimental evaluation of the JenaClip transcatheter aortic valve. Catheter Cardiovasc Interv. 2009;74:514–9.
12. Cribier AG. The Odyssey of TAVR from concept to clinical reality. Tex Heart Inst J. 2014;41:125–30.
13. Cribier A, Eltchaninoff H, Tron C, Bauer F, Agatiello C, Sebagh L, Bash A, Nusimovici D, Litzler PY, Bessou JP, Leon MB. Early experience with percutaneous transcatheter implantation of heart valve prosthesis for the treatment of end-stage inoperable patients with calcific aortic stenosis. J Am Coll Cardiol. 2004;43:698–703.
14. Cribier A, Eltchaninoff H, Tron C, Bauer F, Agatiello C, Nercolini D, Tapiero S, Litzler PY, Bessou JP, Babaliaros V. Treatment of calcific aortic stenosis with the percutaneous heart valve: mid-term follow-up from the initial feasibility studies: the French experience. J Am Coll Cardiol. 2006;47:1214–23.
15. Webb JG, Chandavimol M, Thompson CR, Ricci DR, Carere RG, Munt BI, Buller CE, Pasupati S, Lichtenstein S. Percutaneous aortic valve implantation retrograde from the femoral artery. Circulation. 2006;113:842–50.
16. Webb JG, Pasupati S, Humphries K, Thompson C, Altwegg L, Moss R, Sinhal A, Carere RG, Munt B, Ricci D, Ye J, Cheung A, Lichtenstein SV. Percutaneous transarterial aortic valve replacement in selected high-risk patients with aortic stenosis. Circulation. 2007;116:755–63.
17. Lichtenstein SV, Cheung A, Ye J, Thompson CR, Carere RG, Pasupati S, Webb JG. Transapical transcatheter aortic valve implantation in humans: initial clinical experience. Circulation. 2006;114:591–6.
18. Walther T, Simon P, Dewey T, Wimmer-Greinecker G, Falk V, Kasimir MT, Doss M, Borger MA, Schuler G, Glogar D, Fehske W, Wolner E, Mohr FW, Mack M. Transapical minimally invasive aortic valve implantation: multicenter experience. Circulation. 2007;116:I240–5.
19. Grube E, Laborde JC, Zickmann B, Gerckens U, Felderhoff T, Sauren B, Bootsveld A, Buellesfeld L, Iversen S. First report on a human percutaneous transluminal implantation of a self-expanding valve prosthesis for interventional treatment of aortic valve stenosis. Catheter Cardiovasc Interv. 2005;66:465–9.
20. Laborde JC, Borenstein N, Behr L, Farah B, Fajadet J. Percutaneous implantation of an aortic valve prosthesis. Catheter Cardiovasc Interv. 2005;65:171–4; discussion 175
21. Thomas M, Schymik G, Walther T, Himbert D, Lefevre T, Treede H, Eggebrecht H, Rubino P, Colombo A, Lange R, Schwarz RR, Wendler O. One-year outcomes of cohort 1 in the Edwards SAPIEN Aortic Bioprosthesis European Outcome (SOURCE) registry: the European registry of transcatheter aortic valve implantation using the Edwards SAPIEN valve. Circulation. 2011;124:425–33.
22. Eltchaninoff H, Prat A, Gilard M, Leguerrier A, Blanchard D, Fournial G, Iung B, Donzeau-Gouge P, Tribouilloy C, Debrux JL, Pavie A, Gueret P, France Registry Investigators. Transcatheter aortic valve implantation: early results of the FRANCE (FRench Aortic National CoreValve and Edwards) registry. Eur Heart J. 2011;32:191–7.

23. Gilard M, Eltchaninoff H, Iung B, Donzeau-Gouge P, Chevreul K, Fajadet J, Leprince P, Leguerrier A, Lievre M, Prat A, Teiger E, Lefevre T, Himbert D, Tchetche D, Carrie D, Albat B, Cribier A, Rioufol G, Sudre A, Blanchard D, Collet F, Dos Santos P, Meneveau N, Tirouvanziam A, Caussin C, Guyon P, Boschat J, Le Breton H, Collart F, Houel R, Delpine S, Souteyrand G, Favereau X, Ohlmann P, Doisy V, Grollier G, Gommeaux A, Claudel JP, Bourlon F, Bertrand B, Van Belle E, Laskar M, France Registry Investigators. Registry of transcatheter aortic-valve implantation in high-risk patients. N Engl J Med. 2012;366:1705–15.

24. Leon MB, Smith CR, Mack M, Miller DC, Moses JW, Svensson LG, Tuzcu EM, Webb JG, Fontana GP, Makkar RR, Brown DL, Block PC, Guyton RA, Pichard AD, Bavaria JE, Herrmann HC, Douglas PS, Petersen JL, Akin JJ, Anderson WN, Wang D, Pocock S, PARTNER Trial Investigators. Transcatheter aortic-valve implantation for aortic stenosis in patients who cannot undergo surgery. N Engl J Med. 2010;363:1597–607.

25. Smith CR, Leon MB, Mack MJ, Miller DC, Moses JW, Svensson LG, Tuzcu EM, Webb JG, Fontana GP, Makkar RR, Williams M, Dewey T, Kapadia S, Babaliaros V, Thourani VH, Corso P, Pichard AD, Bavaria JE, Herrmann HC, Akin JJ, Anderson WN, Wang D, Pocock SJ, PARTNER Trial Investigators. Transcatheter versus surgical aortic-valve replacement in high-risk patients. N Engl J Med. 2011;364:2187–98.

26. Baumgartner H, Falk V, Bax JJ, De Bonis M, Hamm C, Holm PJ, Iung B, Lancellotti P, Lansac E, Rodriguez Munoz D, Rosenhek R, Sjogren J, Tornos Mas P, Vahanian A, Walther T, Wendler O, Windecker S, Zamorano JL, Group ESCSD. 2017 ESC/EACTS Guidelines for the management of valvular heart disease. Eur Heart J. 2017;38:2739–91.

Interventional Anatomy of Aortic Valve

2

Stefania Rizzo, Monica de Gaspari,
Gaetano Thiene, and Cristina Basso

2.1 Aortic Root Anatomy

The anatomy of the aortic root is complex, with morphological changes during the cardiac cycle. The aortic root extends from the basal attachment (nadir) of the aortic valve cusps to the sino-tubular junction. Aortic root components are the sinuses of Valsalva, which support the semilunar cusps, the fibrous interleaflet triangles, and the valve cusps themselves (Fig. 2.1). Proper functioning of the aortic valve depends on the proper relationship between the cusps within the aortic root. The tip of the semilunar cusp attachment, usually located between the sinus and tubular portions of the aorta, is the site of commissure, where adjacent cusps touch each other. The three commissures may be considered as the upper border of the semilunar valve attachment. At commissural level, in semilunar cuspshere is a sharp anatomical discontinuity, at difference from atrioventricular valves, where continuity is present between adjacent leaflets at commissural level. The space between the cusp attachment is called interleaflet triangle and represents the most distal component of the left ventricular outflow tract; on the other hand, some ventricular myocardium overcomes the ventricular arterial junction, becoming part of the Valsalva

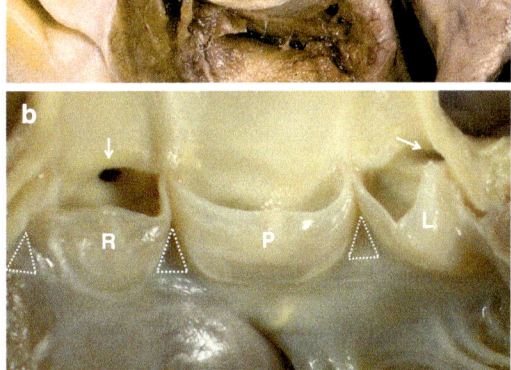

Fig. 2.1 (**a**) The aortic valve apparatus consists of three cusps ("semilunar valve") attached to the aortic sinusal wall; (**b**) The semilunar cusps are attached to the aortic sinusal wall with a crown-like shape. The tip of this attachment corresponds to the commissure, located between the sinus and tubular portions of the aorta (sinotubular junction). The spaces in between the cuspal attachment are called interleaflet triangles. Note the fibrous continuity of the posterior noncoronary cusps with the anterior ("aortic") leaflet of the mitral valve. Arrows indicate the origin of the coronary arteries. (*R* right, *L* left, *P* posterior) [2]

S. Rizzo · M. de Gaspari · G. Thiene · C. Basso (✉)
Cardiovascular Pathology, University of Padua,
Padua, Italy
e-mail: stefania.rizzo_01@aopd.veneto.it;
gaetano.thiene@unipd.it; cristina.basso@unipd.it

© Springer Nature Switzerland AG 2019
A. Giordano et al. (eds.), *Transcatheter Aortic Valve Implantation*,
https://doi.org/10.1007/978-3-030-05912-5_2

sinus, which means that the anatomic ventriculo-arterial junction does not necessarily correspond to the hemodynamic junction [1]. Each of the inter-leaflet triangle is in potential communication with the pericardial space or, in the case of the triangle between the two coronary sinuses, with the tissue plane between the back of the subpulmonary infundibulum and the front of the aorta. The triangle between the noncoronary and the right coronary sinuses incorporates the membranous septum.

Anatomic factors influencing a safe and proper device deployment during transcatheter aortic valve implantation (TAVI), also called transcatheter aortic valve replacement (TAVR) [2], relevant for interventional cardiologist to avoid risk of complications [3–6], include annular diameters, sinuses of Valsalva dimensions, and coronary ostia location; calcium deposits size (bulkiness) and location; subaortic septum thickness and morphology; and relationship with the membranous septum and the mitral valve.

2.2 Aortic Valve Stenosis

Three are the main causes of aortic valve stenosis in the adult: rheumatic valve disease, dystrophic calcification of a tricuspid valve, and dystrophic calcification of a congenitally unicuspid or bicuspid aortic valve [7, 8] (Fig. 2.2).

Rheumatic valve disease results from the fusion of the commissures between the cusps leading to a reduced central orifice with stenosis or steno-incompetence. Rheumatic aortic valve disease is often accompanied by concomitant rheumatic mitral valve disease.

Due to the dramatic decrease of rheumatic fever and increased life expectancy, aortic stenosis in Western countries is nowadays mostly due to dystrophic calcification of bicuspid or tricuspid aortic valves.

Dystrophic calcification of a tricuspid valve is characterized grossly by thickening of the cusps and calcification with coarse calcific nodules, on the aortic side of the cusps, which results in increased valve stiffness, reduced cusp excursion, and progressive valve orifice narrowing in the absence of commissural fusion. Microscopically, changes include increased fibrous tissue, lipid accumulation, and calcific deposits. Aortic root or ascending aorta dilatation is frequently observed in patients with degenerative calcific aortic valve diseases, due to increased aortic stiffness with age and atherosclerosis. Morphologically, the aneurysm is characterized by loss of elastic lamellae in the tunica media.

Bicuspid aortic valve is the most common congenital cardiovascular anomaly, with a prevalence of 1–2% in the general population [9]. It is characterized by two cusps instead of the normal three, most frequently due to fusion of the left and right cusps, with an antero-posterior disposition. The presence of a bicuspid aortic valve is associated with an increased incidence of complications such as stenosis, regurgitation, endocarditis, aneurysm of the ascending aorta, and risk of aortic dissection [10]. These complications tend to man-

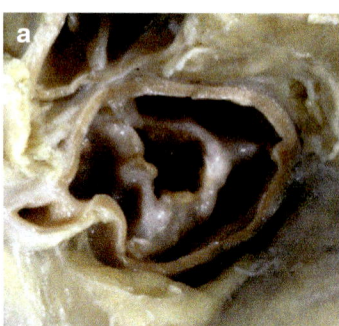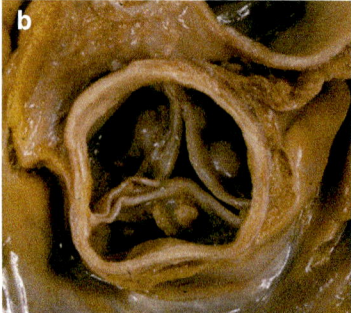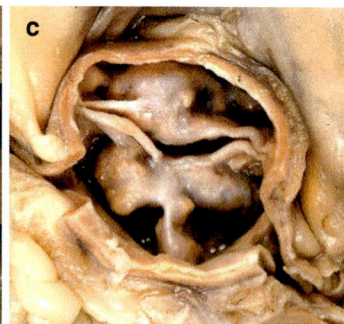

Fig. 2.2 Three are the main causes of aortic valve stenosis in the adult: (**a**) rheumatic valve disease with commissural fusion; (**b**) dystrophic calcification of a tricuspid valve, characterized by coarse calcific nodules on the aortic side of the cusps in the absence of commissural fusion; (**c**) dystrophic calcification of a congenitally bicuspid aortic valve, with fusion of the left and right cusps and an antero-posterior disposition

ifest at an earlier age in patients with a bicuspid valve. Moreover, other congenital cardiovascular abnormalities may be associated with a bicuspid aortic valve, in particular aortic coarctation.

2.3 Rings Within the Aortic Root

The aortic root presents three different annuli or rings, not all corresponding to discrete anatomic structures [11–13]:

- The virtual basal ring, the lowest attachment points of the cusps, representing the inlet from the left ventricular outflow tract into the aortic root;
- The anatomic ring, crown-shaped due to the semilunar cusp attachment to the aortic sinus wall;
- The commissural ring, corresponding to the sino-tubular junction, between the sinusal portion and the tubular ascending aorta. The sino-tubular junction is a true ring. It forms the outlet of the aortic root into the ascending aorta.

Marked variations exist in the shape and dimensions of the aortic root, even during the cardiac cycle. Measurements for TAVI are made in midsystole, when dimensions are at their maximum. The virtual basal ring may be not circular but elliptical in the majority of patients [14]. Eccentricity of the annulus is associated with a higher incidence of paravalvular aortic regurgitation and stent misdeployment, leading to prosthetic valve distortion and premature failure by leaflet tear or fibrosis.

When planning TAVI, accurate measurement of the aortic root dimensions is essential to determine eligibility for the procedure and the appropriate device size, reducing the risk of prosthesis mismatch. Patients with aortic dimensions outside the size range of available TAVI valves are not candidate for the procedure. An oversized prosthetic valve can result in folding of leaflet tissue, which may alter the function and reduce the durability of the valve. Moreover, valve oversizing is at increased risk of aortic root rupture, significant conduction disturbance requiring pacemaker implantation or device under expansion. On the contrary, if the valve prosthesis is too small for the patient, the prosthesis will be stenotic and may lead to paravalvular regurgitation or device embolization.

2.4 Semilunar Cusps

The semilunar cusps are usually three, two anterior and one posterior (Fig. 2.1). The anterior right is the one hosting the right coronary ostium (right coronary cusp), the anterior left is the one hosting the left coronary ostium (left coronary cusp), and finally the posterior is the noncoronary cusp. The latter is in fibrous continuity with the anterior ("aortic") leaflet of the mitral valve and in relationship (and potential communication) with the left atrium, the atrial septum, and the right atrium. The anterior right is attached at the base to the myocardium of the ventricular septum (Fig. 2.1b), whereas the anterior left is attached partially to the myocardium of the antero-lateral wall of the left ventricle and partially to the fibrous continuity of the anterior mitral leaflet. Therefore, approximately two thirds of the aortic root is connected to the muscular ventricular septum, with the remaining one third in fibrous continuity with the mitral valve, forming the so-called fibrous trigones.

The interleaflet triangle between the anterior right coronary cusp and posterior noncoronary cusp is in continuity with the membranous septum (Fig. 2.1); the postero-inferior border is the topographic landmark of the His bundle (Fig. 2.3).

The semilunar cusps touch each other during diastole, normally 1 mm below the free margin, thus ensuring orifice closure and avoiding blood regurgitation. In the middle of the closure line, a small fibrotic nodule (nodule of Arantius) may be present.

Microscopically, a semilunar cusp consists of three layers (Fig. 2.4): (a) ventricularis, facing the ventricular cavity and consisting of a thin fibroelastic layer; (b) fibrosa, facing the aortic wall (3–4 times thicker than the ventricularis), mostly consisting of collagen fibers, which are waived and allow an elongation during diastole, thus ensuring cusp pliability and "elasticity" [15]; (c) spongiosa, in the middle, made up of non-fibril-

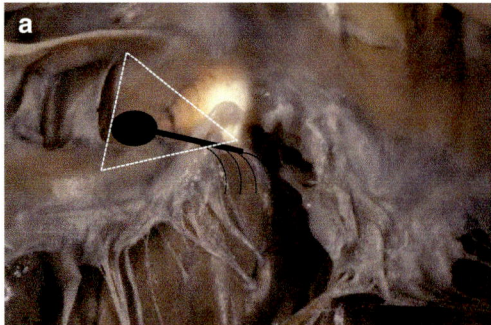
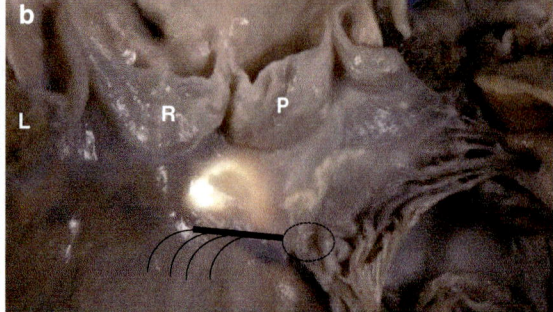

Fig. 2.3 Membranous septum and location of the atrio-ventricular conducting tissue on the right side (**a**) and left side (**b**). The postero-inferior border of the membranous septum is the topographic landmark of the His bundle, which is running under the commissure between the right coronary and posterior noncoronary cusps

Fig. 2.4 (**a**) Histology of the semilunar cusp three layers with the ventricularis (thin fibroelastic layer), the fibrosa, (mostly consisting of collagen fibers), and the spongiosa in the middle (non-fibrillar extracellular matrix with proteoglycans). (**b**) Schematic depiction of layered aortic valve cuspal structure and configuration of collagen and elastin during systole and diastole (modified from [8])

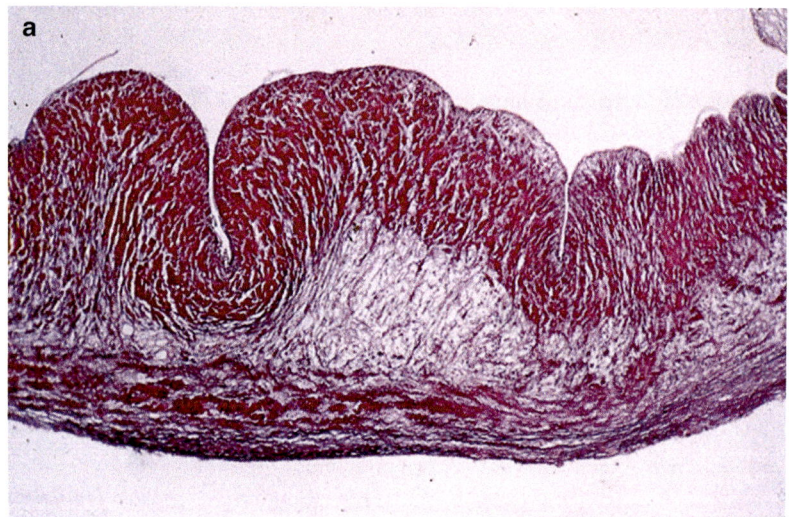
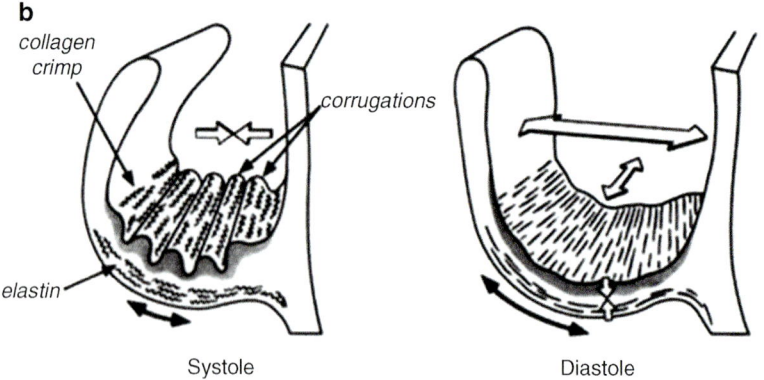

lar extracellular matrix (ground substance) with proteoglycans.

Interstitial cells are scattered within all the three layers and particularly abundant in the spongiosa. An endothelial lying covers both sides of the semilunar cusp.

Particular considerations before TAVI include valve cusps number and morphology and extent and distribution of calcifications, which may predict the patient's risk of paravalvular leak.

Bulky calcification of the aortic valve cusps facilitates positioning of the percutaneous valve but is a risk factor for embolization and for asymmetric expansion of the valve, with possible paravalvular leak [16].

Other significant risk factors for paravalvular leak following TAVI are annular calcification, calcification of the mitral-aortic fibrous continuity and bicuspid aortic valve [17]. Bicuspid aortic valve has long been considered a contraindication to TAVI procedure, due to the unfavorable anatomy including annular eccentricity, asymmetrical valve calcification, unequally sized leaflets, and concomitant aortopathy [10, 18, 19].

2.5   Coronary Artery Ostia

The coronary arteries usually arise from the two anterior sinuses of Valsalva with a distinct orifice, located just underneath the sino-tubular junction, at a distance of 10–15 mm from the basal attachment in adult hearts. The opening of the cusp during systole does not block the coronary ostia [20, 21] (Fig. 2.5). Origins of the coronary arteries above the sino-tubular junction are considered anatomical variations [22].

Variations in the location of the coronary ostia and measurement of the height of the coronary take-off in relationship to the length of the coronary cusps are important before TAVI to minimize the risk of myocardial ischemia. In case of a low coronary origin (<10 mm), the new guidelines recommend surgical aortic valve replacement [23]. The new valve prostheses are made by a skirt of tissue within the stent to create a seal and prevent paravalvular leak. When the coronary arteries take origin low within the sinuses of Valsalva and/or the prosthesis is placed too high, the skirt may obstruct their orifices [24]. Furthermore, when the valve is deployed, the native cusps may potentially obstruct the flow into the coronary arteries. Moreover, calcific fragments of the native valve may embolize, causing coronary occlusion. Delayed coronary obstruction is an uncommon complication occurring hours and days following TAVI, more commonly valve-in-valve procedures and use of self-expandable valves, requiring stent implantation [25]. It is probably due to the displacement of a calcified native valve cusp, previous surgical valve leaflet or bioprosthetic valve fibrous pannus, and embolization of a thrombus located on the TAVI valve.

Fig. 2.5 The coronary ostia are usually located just underneath the sino-tubular portion, at a distance of 10–15 mm from the basal attachment in adult hearts. (**a**) Gross view of the left ventricular outflow tract; (**b**) histology of the sino-tubular portion of the aorta, at the level of the coronary artery origin. (*LC*, left coronary)

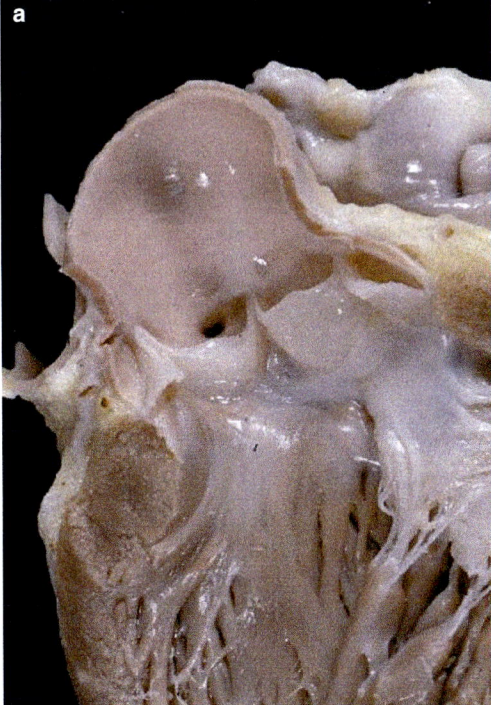
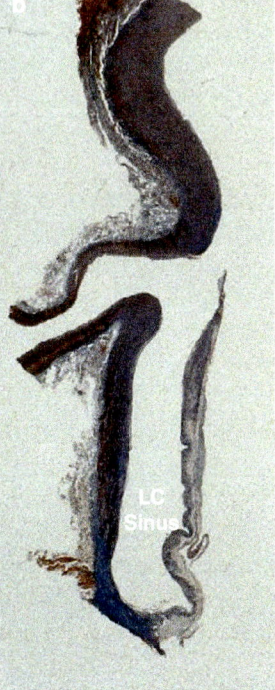

2.6 The Left Ventricular Outflow Tract and the Central Fibrous Body

The left ventricular outflow tract (LVOT) is composed of a muscular component (the muscular ventricular septum) and a fibrous component (the fibrous continuity between the aortic and mitral valves). The presence of a subaortic septal bulge and asymmetrical septal hypertrophy may be an obstacle for the proper seating of the aortic prosthesis within the left ventricular outflow tract, with paravalvular leak. The presence of calcific nodules along the mitro-aortic fibrous continuity can also account for paravalvular leak due to malapposition of the device.

As a result of the semilunar attachment of the aortic valve cusps, there are three triangular extensions of the left ventricular outflow tract to the level of the sino-tubular junction. These interleaflet triangles are formed of the aorta wall between the sinuses of Valsalva, with potential communication with the pericardial space. The two interleaflet triangles bordering the noncoronary cusp are also in fibrous continuity with the fibrous trigones, the mitral valve, and the membranous septum [12, 26].

The fibrous continuity is thickened to form the left and right fibrous trigones. The interleaflet triangle between the noncoronary and left coronary cusp is part of the fibrous continuity. Placement of the aortic valve prosthesis too low within the left ventricular outflow tract may impinge on the anterior leaflet of the mitral valve and impair its function. The interleaflet triangle between the right coronary and noncoronary aortic cusps is continuous with the membranous septum. The crest of the muscular ventricular septum, at the inferior border of the membranous septum, is the site of the atrioventricular conduction axis. Together, the membranous septum and the right fibrous trigone form the central fibrous body of the heart [26, 27].

Rupture of the "device landing zone" is a rare but severe complication of TAVI and mostly occurs in the subannular area of the left ventricular outflow tract [28] (Fig. 2.6).

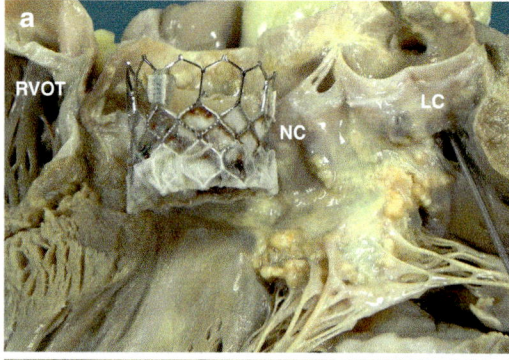

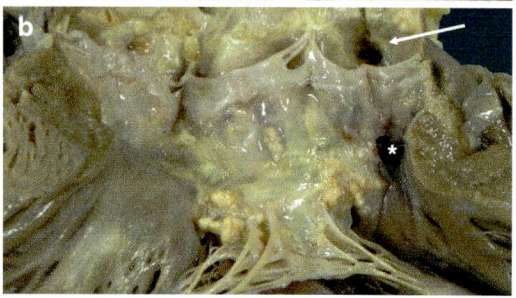

Fig. 2.6 Rupture of the landing zone after TAVI. (**a**) After opening of the LVOT, the prosthesis appears correctly implanted with no interference with the right and left coronary ostia, the anterior mitral valve leaflet, and the subaortic septum. Note the aortic annulus rupture (probe inside) at the nadir of the left coronary cusp (LC). (**b**) View of the LVOT after removal of the aortic valve prosthesis: note the amount of calcific nodules distributed along the mitro-aortic fibrous continuity and at the level of the right and left fibrous trigones. A perforation (*asterisk*) is visible at the nadir of the left coronary cusp, 1 cm below the ostium of the left main trunk (*arrow*), in correspondence of a calcific nodule which was outward displaced during the TAVI procedure. (*RVOT*, right ventricular outflow tract; *NC*, non coronary; *LC* left coronary)

2.7 The Conduction System

The atrioventricular node is located within the right atrium in the triangle of Koch, demarcated superiorly by the tendon of Todaro, inferiorly by the attachment of the septal leaflet of the tricuspid valve, and posteriorly by the orifice of the coronary sinus (Fig. 2.3a). The atrioventricular node is located just inferior to the apex of the interleaflet triangle adjacent to the membranous septum, separating the noncoronary and right coronary cusps of the aortic valve, and therefore the atrioventricular node is in close proximity to the subaortic region and membranous septum of the left ventricular outflow tract [29, 1] (Fig. 2.3b). Pathologies involving the aortic valve, in particular dystrophic calcification, can lead to heart block or intraventricular conduction abnormalities. The atrioventricular node continues as the bundle of His, penetrating to the left through the central fibrous body. On the left side, the conduction axis is located immediately beneath the membranous septum and runs superficially along the crest of the ventricular septum, giving rise to the fascicles of the left bundle branch [29].

The topographic anatomy can explain the onset of conduction abnormalities after TAVI [30–32].

An atrioventricular block requiring a permanent pacemaker implantation occurs in 10–50% of patients following TAVI, mostly with CoreValve due to deep valve implantation [31] (Fig. 2.7).

Figure 2.3 shows the anatomic relationship of the aortic annulus and its proximity to the conduction system.

2.8 The Mitral Valve

Dystrophic calcification of the mitral annulus is frequently associated with degenerative aortic valve stenosis. This condition seems to be associated with mitral regurgitation [33] and conduction abnormalities [34] after TAVI.

Mitral valve complications of the TAVI were first reported with the trans-septal approach. Injury may occur when the device passes through the anterior leaflet during delivery. Moreover, the ventricular portion of the TAVI prosthesis may contact the anterior leaflet of the mitral valve. In particular, when the placement of the device is too low into the left ventricle it may interfere with the movement of the anterior leaflet of the mitral valve [35].

2.9 Access Site

Among the various possible assess sites, trans-femoral access remains the most preferred option for TAVI. However, this approach is contraindi-

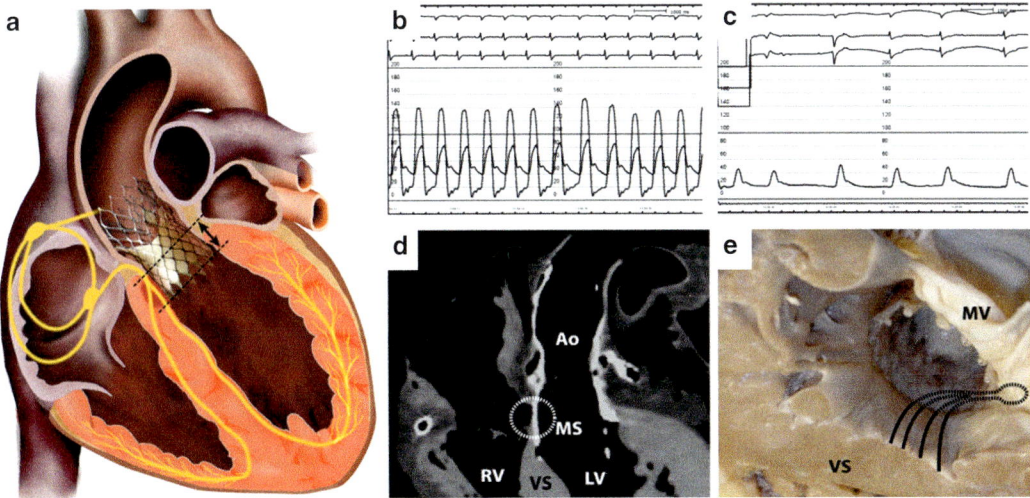

Fig. 2.7 Iatrogenic AV block after TAVI. (**a**) Diagram illustrating anatomic relation between a deep prosthesis implantation into left ventricular outflow tract affecting electrical conduction system; (**b**) electrocardiogram showing right bundle branch block and 60 mmHg trans-aortic gradient at baseline. (**c**) Electrocardiogram showing complete AV block immediately after TAVI. (**d**) Computed tomography scan of heart explanted at autopsy showing the deep positioning of CoreValve within left ventricular outflow tract, overlapping membranous septum (*dotted circle*), and crest of interventricular septum. (**e**) Gross anatomic view of left ventricular outflow seen from below: the expansion of prosthesis frames in subaortic region compresses the ventricular septum and overlapping proximal branching of left bundle branch (*dotted lines*). *Ao* aorta, *LV* left ventricle, *MS* membranous septum, *MV* mitral valve, *RV* right ventricle, *VS* ventricular septum

cated in patients with ileo-femoral atherosclerosis, porcelain aorta, calcifications, tortuosity, abdominal aneurysms, or previous vascular surgery. Alternative sites include transapical, transaortic, axillary/subclavian, and carotid access [36]. The transapical and transaortic approaches are more invasive, requiring a left minithoracotomy. These approaches are usually reserved for patients with severe peripheral vascular disease.

Stroke during or after TAVI may occur from thromboemboli [37], infective endocarditis [38], aortic injury (e.g., dissection or atheroemboli), hypotension, hemorrhage, or dislodgement of calcific fragments during valvuloplasty. No difference regarding cerebral complications is found related to the access site.

Vascular complications, in terms of bleeding at the insertion site, are the most common of the procedure and contribute to procedural mortality, particularly in patients with significant peripheral vascular disease. As smaller systems are developed, serious vascular injuries are expected to occur less frequently. Funding This work was supported by Registry of Cardio-Cerebro-Vascular Pathology, Veneto Region, Italy.

References

1. Cribier A, Eltchaninoff H, Bash A, Borenstein N, Tron C, Bauer F, Derumeaux G, Anselme F, Laborde F, Leon MB. Percutaneous transcatheter implantation of an aortic valve prosthesis for calcific aortic stenosis: first human case description. Circulation. 2002;106:3006–8.
2. Basso C, Rizzo S, Thiene G. Anatomy: the pathology of aortic incompetence. In: Schafers J, editor. Current treatment of aortic regurgitation. Bremen: Uni-Med Verlag; 2013. p. 15–31. ISBN: 9783837414066.
3. Roberts WC, Stoler RC, Grayburn PA, Hebeler RF Jr, Ko JM, Brown DL, Brinkman WT, Mack MJ, Guileyardo JM. Necropsy findings early after transcatheter aortic valve implantation for aortic stenosis. Am J Cardiol. 2013;111:448–52.
4. Loeser H, Wittersheim M, Puetz K, Friemann J, Buettner R, Fries JW. Potential complications of transcatheter aortic valve implantation (TAVI)-an autopsy perspective. Cardiovasc Pathol. 2013;22:319–23.
5. Fishbein GA, Schoen FJ, Fishbein MC. Transcatheter aortic valve implantation: status and challenges. Cardiovasc Pathol. 2014;23:65–70.
6. van Kesteren F, Wiegerinck EM, Rizzo S, Baan J Jr, Planken RN, von der Thüsen JH, Niessen HW, van Oosterhout MF, Pucci A, Thiene G, Basso C, Sheppard MN, Wassilew K, van der Wal AC. Autopsy after transcatheter aortic valve implantation. Virchows Arch. 2017;470:331–9.
7. Turri M, Thiene G, Bortolotti U, Milano A, Mazzucco A, Gallucci V. Surgical pathology of aortic valve disease. A study based on 602 specimens. Eur J Cardiothorac Surg. 1990;4:556–60.
8. Roberts WC, Janning KG, Ko JM, Filardo G, Matter GJ. Frequency of congenitally bicuspid aortic valves in patients ≥80 years of age undergoing aortic valve replacement for aortic stenosis (with or without aortic regurgitation) and implications for transcatheter aortic valve implantation. Am J Cardiol. 2012;109:1632–6.
9. Basso C, Boschello M, Perrone C, Mecenero A, Cera A, Bicego D, Thiene G, De Dominicis E. An echocardiographic survey of primary school children for bicuspid aortic valve. Am J Cardiol. 2004;93:661–3.
10. Nistri S, Grande-Allen J, Noale M, Basso C, Siviero P, Maggi S, Crepaldi G, Thiene G. Aortic elasticity and size in bicuspid aortic valve syndrome. Eur Heart J. 2008;29:472–9.
11. Piazza N, de Jaegere P, Schultz C, Becker AE, Serruys PW, Anderson RH. Anatomy of the aortic valvar complex and its implications for transcatheter implantation of the aortic valve. Circ Cardiovasc Interv. 2008;1:74–81.
12. Anderson RH. Anatomy: clinical anatomy of the aortic root. Heart. 2000;84:670–3.
13. Anderson RH, Devine WA, Ho SY, et al. The myth of the aortic annulus: the anatomy of the subaortic outflow tract. Ann Thorac Surg. 1991;52:640–6.
14. Doddamani S, Bello R, Friedman MA, et al. Demonstration of left ventricular outflow tract eccentricity by real time 3D echocardiography: implications for the determination of aortic valve area. Echocardiography. 2007;24:860–6.
15. Schoen FJ. Aortic valve structure-function correlations: role of elastic fibers no longer a stretch of the imagination. J Heart Valve Dis. 1997;6:1–6.
16. Razzolini R, Longhi S, Tarantini G, Rizzo S, Napodano M, Abate E, Fraccaro C, Thiene G, Iliceto S, Gerosa G, Basso C. Relation of aortic valve weight to severity of aortic stenosis. Am J Cardiol. 2011;107:741–6.
17. Tarantini G, Gasparetto V, Napodano M, Fraccaro C, Gerosa G, Isabella G. Valvular leak after transcatheter aortic valve implantation: a clinician update on epidemiology, pathophysiology and clinical implications. Am J Cardiovasc Dis. 2011;1:312–20.
18. Himbert D, Pontnau F, Messika-Zeitoun D, et al. Feasibility and outcomes of transcatheter aortic valve implantation in high-risk patients with stenotic bicuspid aortic valves. Am J Cardiol. 2012;110:877–83.
19. Zhao ZG, Jilaihawi H, Feng Y, Chen M. Transcatheter aortic valve implantation in bicuspid anatomy. Nat Rev Cardiol. 2015;12:123–8.
20. Muriago M, Sheppard MN, Ho SY, Anderson RH. Location of the coronary arterial orifices in the normal heart. Clin Anat. 1997;10:297–302.
21. Cavalcanti JS, de Melo NC, deVasconcelos RS. Morphometric and topographic study of coronary ostia. Arq Bras Cardiol. 2003;81:359–62.

22. Manghat NE, Morgan-Hughes GJ, Marshall AJ, et al. Multidetector row computed tomography: imaging congenital coronary artery anomalies in adults. Heart. 2005;91:1515–22.

23. Falk V, Baumgartner H, Bax JJ, et al. 2017 ESC/EACTS Guidelines for the management of valvular heart disease: the Task Force for the Management of Valvular Heart Disease of the European Society of Cardiology (ESC) and the European Association for Cardio-Thoracic Surgery (EACTS). Eur J Cardiothorac Surg. 2017;52:616–64.

24. Ribeiro HB, Nombela-Franco L, Urena M, Mok M, Pasian S, Doyle D, et al. Coronary obstruction following transcatheter aortic valve implantation: a systematic review. JACC Cardiovasc Interv. 2013;6:452–61.

25. Jabbour RJ, Tanaka A, Finkelstein A, et al. Delayed coronary obstruction after transcatheter aortic valve replacement. J Am Coll Cardiol. 2018;71:1513–24.

26. Sutton JPIII, Ho SY, Anderson RH. The forgotten interleaflet triangles: a review of the surgical anatomy of the aortic valve. Ann Thorac Surg. 1995;59:419–27.

27. Mori S, Tretter JT, Toba T, et al. Relationship between the membranous septum and the virtual basal ring of the aortic root in candidates for transcatheter implantation of the aortic valve. Clin Anat. 2018;31:525–34.

28. Tarantini G, Basso C, Fovino LN, Fraccaro C, Thiene G, Rizzo S. Left ventricular outflow tract rupture during transcatheter aortic valve implantation: anatomic evidence of the vulnerable area. Cardiovasc Pathol. 2017;29:7–10.

29. Basso C, Ho Y, Rizzo S, Thiene G. Anatomic and histopathologic characteristics of the conductive tissues of the heart. In: Gussak I, Antzelevitch C, editors. Electrical diseases of the heart. London: Springer; 2013. p. 1–25. ISBN: 9781447148814.

30. Auffret V, Puri R, Urena M, et al. Conduction disturbances after transcatheter aortic valve replacement: current status and future perspectives. Circulation. 2017;136:1049–69.

31. Fraccaro C, Buja G, Tarantini G, Gasparetto V, Leoni L, Razzolini R, Corrado D, Bonato R, Basso C, Thiene G, Gerosa G, Isabella G, Iliceto S, Napodano M. Incidence, predictors, and outcome of conduction disorders after transcatheter self-expandable aortic valve implantation. Am J Cardiol. 2011;107:747–54.

32. Roten L, Wenaweser P, Delacrtaz E, et al. Incidence and predictors of atrioventricular conduction impairment after transcatheter aortic valve implantation. Am J Cardiol. 2010;106:1473–80.

33. Cortés C, Amat-Santos IJ, Nombela-Franco N, Muñoz-Garcia AJ, Gutiérrez-Ibanes E, De La Torre Hernandez JM, et al. Mitral regurgitation after transcatheter aortic valve replacement. JACC Cardiovasc Interv. 2016;9:1603–14.

34. Abramowitz Y, Kazuno Y, Chakravarty T, Kawamori H, Maeno Y, Anderson D, et al. Concomitant mitral annular calcification and severe aortic stenosis: prevalence, characteristics and outcome following transcatheter aortic valve replacement. Eur Heart J. 2017;38:1194–203.

35. Wong DR, Boone RH, Thompson CR, Allard MF, Altwegg L, Carere RG, et al. Mitral valve injury late after transcatheter aortic valve implantation. J Thorac Cardiovasc Surg. 2009;137:1547–9.

36. Otto CM, Kumbhani DJ, Alexander KP, Calhoon JH, Desai MY, Kaul S, et al. 2017 ACC expert consensus decision pathway for transcatheter aortic valve replacement in the management of adults with aortic stenosis: a report of the American College of Cardiology Task Force on Clinical Expert Consensus Documents. J Am Coll Cardiol. 2017;69:1313–46.

37. D'Onofrio A, Rizzo S, Besola L, Isabella G, Rancitelli V, Randi ML, Campello E, Falasco G, Basso C, Thiene G, Gerosa G. Hyperacute valve thrombosis after transapical transcatheter aortic valve replacement in a patient with polycythemia vera. JACC Cardiovasc Interv. 2016;9:1746–7.

38. Santos M, Thiene G, Sievers HH, Basso C. Candida endocarditis complicating transapical aortic valve implantation. Eur Heart J. 2011;32:2265.

Pathophysiology of Aortic Valve Stenosis

3

Gabriele Di Giammarco and Daniele Marinelli

3.1 Introduction

Calcified aortic valve disease (CAVD) is the most common cause of heart valve disease in the western countries. EuroHeart Survey reports a prevalence in the general population of 43.1% with the most common cause being degenerative disease (81.9%). The prevalence of aortic valve stenosis in patients older than 70 years and candidate for intervention is 54.3% [1].

The process leading to aortic valve stenosis was considered in the past as isolated degeneration at valvular level. Recently, increasing evidence demonstrates a more complex process involving the left ventricular outflow tract beyond the valve itself, and this mechanism is responsible for the progression of the degree of stenosis.

G. Di Giammarco (✉)
Institute of Cardiac Surgery, Department of
Neurosciences, Imaging and Clinical Sciences,
University "G. D'Annunzio" Chieti & Pescara,
Chieti, Italy

Department of Cardiac Surgery,
Ospedale "S. S. Annunziata", Chieti, Italy

D. Marinelli
Department of Cardiac Surgery,
Ospedale "S. S. Annunziata", Chieti, Italy

3.2 Pathogenesis of CAVD

3.2.1 Anatomy of the Aortic Valve Leaflet

The aortic valve leaflet is less than 1 mm of thickness and its surface is covered by endothelium. The inner structure is composed of three layers:

– The *ventricularis*, in the ventricular face of the leaflet composed of fiber rich in elastin arranged radially and perpendicularly to leaflet margin;
– The *arterialis*, or *fibrosa*, in the aortic face of the leaflet made of strong collagen fibers oriented circumferentially;
– The *spongiosa*, between the *arterialis* and *ventricularis* made of loose connective tissue composed of mesenchymal cells, fibroblast, and mucopolysaccharide-rich matrix.

The organization of these three layers confers to the leaflets the characteristics of pliability and resistance to offer a very low obstacle to the left ventricle ejection during systole and the capacity to support the high aortic pressure during diastole.

© Springer Nature Switzerland AG 2019
A. Giordano et al. (eds.), *Transcatheter Aortic Valve Implantation*,
https://doi.org/10.1007/978-3-030-05912-5_3

3.2.2 The Initial Alteration of the Aortic Valve: The Sclerosis

Aortic valve sclerosis (AS) is defined as the presence at echocardiography of focal leaflet thickening with unmodified leaflet mobility preserving the commissures; its incidence is close to 25% in subjects of age 64–75 rising to 48% in patients older than 84 years [2–4].

The sclerosis of the valve does not cause hemodynamic alteration although it is possible on physical examination to catch a systolic murmur; echocardiography generally demonstrates an aortic valve flow velocity lower than 2.5 m/s.

The process of AS is complex and involves many different mechanisms as shown in Table 3.1.

In hypercholesterolemic rabbits, aortic valve sclerosis is related to a progressive accumulation of lipids, endothelial disruption, modification of the connective tissue, and presence of osteopontin and inflammatory cells [5]. Otto et al. demonstrated the presence of some similarities between atherosclerosis and AS. They found on human autoptic specimens of aortic valve (with different stages of disease progression) the presence of basal membrane disruption, thickening between the basal membrane and elastic lamina, and intra- and extracellular infiltration of lipids. At the same time they found important dissimilarities in the number of smooth muscular cells and the prominent mineralization process differentiating the two pathological processes [6].

Table 3.1 Mechanism and risk factors of aortic valve sclerosis and calcification

1. Age
2. Atherosclerosis risk factors:
   (a) Hypertension
   (b) Dyslipidemia
   (c) Smoking
   (d) Metabolic syndrome
3. Lipid accumulation
4. Inflammation
5. Oxidation process
6. Genetic mutations
7. Mechanical stress
8. Calcium metabolism alteration

Inflammation plays also a crucial role in the development of aortic valve sclerosis. In specimens of aortic valve some authors demonstrated T-lymphocyte infiltration and non-foam and foam cell macrophages [7, 8]. Soluble mediator of inflammation such as interleukin-1-beta and transforming growth factor beta-1 are overexpressed in AS and CAVD leading to extracellular matrix remodeling due to increased activity of matrix metalloproteinases-1 and calcification process associated with cell apoptosis [9, 10].

Angiotensin-converting enzyme and angiotensin II are also overexpressed at the level of the aortic valve lesion, suggesting that chronic inflammation process increased calcification with a positive feedback mechanism [11].

Another element that supports the inflammatory genesis of the lesions of aortic valve sclerosis is the overexpression of intercellular adhesion molecule 1 (ICAM-1), vascular cell adhesion molecule 1 (VCAM-1), and endothelial selectin (E-selectin) [12].

The role of mechanical stress on aortic valve leaflet in promoting the pathological changes is also supported by evidence of accelerated calcification of bicuspid aortic valve, a valve configuration characterized by higher shear stress on the leaflets, although patients with a bicuspid aortic valve may have also a genetic predisposition to calcification [13].

The association between aortic valve calcification, hypertension, and increased stiffness of the aortic root is reported in literature and this may lead to an increase of mechanical stress on the valve [14].

As previously suggested there is a partial overlapping in the pathogenesis of atherosclerosis and aortic valve sclerosis. Patients with CAVD often have the same risk factors for vascular atherosclerosis such as hypertension, dyslipidemia, smoking, diabetes, and metabolic syndrome [15–17]. On the other hand it is not uncommon in the clinical experience to observe patients affected by CAVD without any evidence of atherosclerosis on systemic and/or coronary arteries.

Miller et al. demonstrated that the oxidation process in aortic valve calcification is increased, and it is associated with uncoupled nitric oxide synthases activity. Consequently they showed that oxidation process differs greatly in aortic valve stenosis compared to arteries [18].

The influence of genetic factors in the development of AS and CAVD is demonstrated by the mutation in the signaling transcriptional regulator NOTCH-1 associated with bicuspid aortic valve calcification and different aortic valve abnormalities [19].

3.2.3 Progression to AS to CAVD

The rate of progression from AS to CAVD and severe aortic valve stenosis is reported in few prospective studies. In one of the largest studies enrolling more than 2000 patient, the rate of progression from AS to aortic stenosis was 16%, with mild stenosis in 10.5%, moderate stenosis in 3%, and severe stenosis in 2.5%. The average time from diagnosis of AS to valve stenosis was 8 years [20].

The most important determinant in evolution from valve sclerosis to valve stenosis is the calcium deposition. It leads to a decreased leaflet motion with consequent pressure gradient increase across the valve.

The accumulation of calcium in the leaflets is favored by an ossification-like mechanism mediated by osteogenic cells and a range of pro-calcific mediators; it ultimately leads to the presence in the valve of cartilaginous and bone tissue as showed in histological evaluation of surgical excised aortic valve leaflets [21].

3.2.4 Hemodynamic Progression of Aortic Valve Stenosis

The progression of aortic valve stenosis can be evaluated by means of velocity across the valve and the effective geometric area. According to the velocity follow-up the rate of hemodynamic progression of aortic valve stenosis is reported to be 0.3 m/s per year starting from the initial diagnosis with a reduction of 0.1 cm^2 of aortic valve area. The determinants of aortic valve stenosis progression are not well elucidated because many of the studies are retrospective. Older age, male sex, hypertension, high body mass index, chronic renal disease, calcium metabolism disorders, the initial aortic valve area, the presence of valve calcification at echocardiography, and CT scan are predictors of disease progression and incidence of adverse events as well [22, 23].

The progression of aortic valve stenosis is the key factor in induction of pressure overload on the left ventricle leading to hypertrophy and fibrosis.

3.3 Left Ventricle Hypertrophy

The pressure overload generated by aortic valve stenosis induces a concentric left ventricular hypertrophy characterized by a parallel replication of the sarcomere with the consequence of increased wall thickness. The main goal of this process is to maintain in the normal range the peak systolic wall stress of the myocardium preserving the left ventricular contractility [24].

However, there is a large amount of evidence demonstrating that myocardial hypertrophy determined by aortic valve stenosis is, at the end, a maladaptive process.

The Framingham Study was the first to demonstrate the association between myocardial hypertrophy and incidence of heart failure [25].

Patients affected by the same grade of left ventricular outflow obstruction show a different grade of hypertrophy.

This situation is probably responsible for the different clinical manifestations in presence of the same degree of left ventricular obstruction.

It is clearly demonstrated that there is no correlation between the degree of outflow obstruction and the amount of left ventricular hypertrophy. It may suggest that many other humoral, behavioral, and genetic factors are responsible for the extent of left ventricle response to the same degree of obstruction [26–28] (Table 3.2).

The lack of correlation between the degree of obstruction and left ventricular hypertrophy was firstly demonstrated with transthoracic echocardiography and recently confirmed by nuclear magnetic resonance. Dweck et al. analyzed 91

Table 3.2 Factors influencing the grade of left ventricle hypertrophy other than aortic valve stenosis

1. Age
2. Male sex
3. Obesity
4. ACE gene polymorphism
5. Systemic arterial hypertension
6. Increased arterial stiffness

patients with isolated aortic valve stenosis with magnetic resonance demonstrating that the degree of obstruction did not correlate with the extent and pattern of left ventricular hypertrophy. Moreover they were able to show that a large percentage of patients with aortic valve stenosis had a pattern of myocardial hypertrophy that is asymmetric and differs significantly from the typical concentric feature [29].

Some genetic factors play a significant role in the development and extent of myocardial hypertrophy. It is demonstrated that the presence of polymorphism of Angiotensin Converting Enzyme gene is responsible for more pronounced hypertrophy in the presence of the same degree of obstruction. The I/D polymorphism is reported to be be associated with variation of left ventricular mass [30].

The role of coexisting arterial hypertension and increased arterial afterload is crucial in the development of left ventricle hypertrophy.

The association of hypertension and left ventricle remodeling in asymptomatic patients affected by aortic valve stenosis was demonstrated by Riek et al. in a sub-study of the Simvastatin and Ezetimibe in Aortic Stenosis trial. The authors measured the left ventricle mass, diameters, wall thickness, degree of hypertrophy, and other functional parameters and demonstrated that the presence of hypertension is a factor influencing the left ventricular geometry, increasing left ventricular mass, wall thickness, and higher prevalence of hypertrophy [31].

The arterial compliance decrease in patients affected by aortic valve stenosis is a common finding as often these patients are old and affected by systemic arterial hypertension and diabetes, well-known factors of arterial stiffness increase.

Briand et al. investigated the impact of reduced arterial compliance in the development of left ventricle increased afterload in patients affected by aortic valve stenosis. To take in account both factors of increased afterload (aortic valve stenosis and reduced arterial compliance), they calculated the valvular-arterial impedance (Z_{va}). In the multivariate analysis the only hemodynamic predictive factor of increased afterload and left ventricle dysfunction, expressed by a reduction in ejection fraction, was the valvular-arterial impedance with an odds ratio of 4.2 (1.7–10.3) [32].

The increased valvular-arterial impedance has influence on the outcome of the patients affected by aortic valve stenosis. Hachicha et al. in a 4-year follow-up study demonstrated that, regardless of aortic valve replacement, patients with a value of Z_{va} greater than 3.5 had a poorer outcome compared with patients in whom Z_{va} was lower [33].

A high degree of left ventricular hypertrophy is a strong risk factor for poor patient outcome. Cioffi et al. clearly demonstrated that an inappropriate left ventricular hypertrophy (left ventricle mass greater than 10% of expected) in asymptomatic aortic valve stenosis is a strong predictor of adverse outcome (Exp b 3.08; CI 1.65–5.73) independently of diabetes, transaortic valve peak gradient, and extent of valvular calcification. Among patients with LV hypertrophy, those with inappropriate left ventricular hypertrophy had a risk of adverse events 4.5-fold higher than counterparts with appropriate left ventricle mass [34].

The worse outcome observed in patients with a greater left ventricle hypertrophy could be related to a high incidence of ventricular dilatation and failure.

In conclusion left ventricle remodeling in AS is only partially caused by the severity of valve stenosis and many other co-factors influence the response of the ventricle to an increased afterload.

3.4 The Evolution of Left Ventricular Function in Aortic Stenosis: From Hypertrophy to Dilatation

With the progression of the disease and the increased afterload of the left ventricle, the final evolution is the left ventricular dilation through a complex process involving cellular apoptosis, myocardial fibrosis, and ischemic events (Table 3.3).

Table 3.3 Determinants of progression from ventricle hypertrophy to dilatation

1. Apoptosis
2. Unbalanced oxygen supply
3. Myocardial ischemia
4. Myocardial fibrosis

This phase corresponds to the onset of symptoms of the aortic valve stenosis and is associated with a reduced prognosis and higher incidence of adverse events.

The apoptosis in hypertrophic myocardium is reported to cause the loss of 5–10% of myocardium per year; this condition will overcome the number of myocyte regeneration with a final net myocardium loss [35]. Cheng et al. demonstrated that increased stretching of cardiomyocytes determines an increased apoptotic rate by 21 times [36]. Moreover, they also showed that, in association with increased oxidative stress, the myocardium decreased its contractile force. Another important pro-apoptotic stimulus is the angiotensin II. Increased angiotensin II release can be directly stimulated by myocardium stretching; moreover, angiotensin II itself will increase myocyte apoptosis activating p53. The use of AT-1 receptor blocker blocks apoptosis process [37].

Another mechanism of left ventricle dysfunction is the presence of myocardial ischemia that is caused by increased wall tension, reduced capillary density, and increased oxygen demand.

It is well known that in physiologic hypertrophy there is a constant between the increased muscular mass and capillary network maintaining normal rate of perfusion of the myocardium. In pathological hypertrophy, as in case of aortic stenosis, the rate of capillary growth (with parallel increased distance between capillary network and cardiomyocytes) is inadequate to satisfy the increased myocardial oxygen demand contributing to myocardium loss [38].

The cellular loss related to apoptotic pathways and ischemic events is the cause of constant increase of fibrosis in the myocardium of the left ventricle in patients affected by aortic valve stenosis as reported by some authors who clearly demonstrated the increase of interstitial fibrous tissue in the myocardium [39, 40].

The mechanism on the base of increased fibrosis is based on a augmented synthesis of type I and III collagen by cardiac fibroblasts and myofibroblasts and unchanged or decreased collagen types I and III degradation by matrix metalloproteinases [41]. The mechanical overstretching of myocardium plays a role in the increased production of type I collagen and reduction of the activity of collagenase with a net balance towards fibrosis increase [42].

In a recent paper, Treibel et al. evaluated the myocardial fibrosis in 133 patients affected by severe aortic valve stenosis using intraoperative bioptic specimens of the left ventricle and nuclear magnetic resonance evaluating the late gadolinium enhancement and the extracellular volume fraction quantification. All the measurements demonstrated the presence of three types of myocardial fibrosis pattern: endocardial fibrosis, microscars (mainly in the subendomyocardium), and diffuse interstitial fibrosis. They were also able to demonstrate that the use of a multiparametric evaluation with late gadolinium enhancement and extracellular volume fraction can adequately predict a worse recovery of left ventricular function also after surgery [43].

3.5 Conclusion

The knowledge of the mechanism of aortic valve disease progression and calcification may represent a new start to discover novel therapeutic target with the aim to reduce the incidence of the disease and to optimize the timing of surgical or transcatheter aortic valve implantation improving the outcome of the patients.

Acknowledgement *Conflict of interest disclosure*: no disclosure

References

1. Iung B. A prospective survey of patients with valvular heart disease in Europe: The Euro Heart Survey on valvular heart disease. Eur Heart J [Internet]. 2003;24(13):1231–43. http://eurheartj.oxfordjournals.org/content/24/13/1231.long

2. Lindroos M, Kupari M, Heikkilä J, Tilvis R. Prevalence of aortic valve abnormalities in the elderly: an echocardiographic study of a random population sample. J Am Coll Cardiol. 1993;21(5):1220–5.

3. Stewart BF, Siscovick D, Lind BK, Gardin JM, Gottdiener JS, Smith VE, et al. Clinical factors associated with calcific aortic valve disease. J Am Coll Cardiol. 1997;29(3):630–4.

4. Otto CM, Lind BK, Kitzman DW, Gersh BJ, Siscovick DS. Association of aortic-valve sclerosis with cardiovascular mortality and morbidity in the elderly. N Engl J Med [Internet]. 1999;341(3):142–7. http://www.nejm.org/doi/abs/10.1056/NEJM199907153410302

5. Cimini M, Boughner DR, Ronald JA, Aldington L, Rogers KA. Development of aortic valve sclerosis in a rabbit model of atherosclerosis: an immunohistochemical and histological study. J Heart Valve Dis. 2005;14(3):365–75.

6. Otto CM, Kuusisto J, Reichenbach DD, Gown AM, O'Brien KD. Characterization of the early lesion of "degenerative" valvular aortic stenosis: histological and immunohistochemical studies. Circulation. 1994;90(2):844–53.

7. Wallby L, Janerot-Sjöberg B, Steffensen T, Broqvist M. T lymphocyte infiltration in non-rheumatic aortic stenosis: a comparative descriptive study between tricuspid and bicuspid aortic valves. Heart [Internet]. 2002;88(4):348–51. http://www.pubmedcentral.nih.gov/articlerender.fcgi?artid=1767380&tool=pmcentrez&rendertype=abstract

8. Olsson M, Rosenqvist M, Nilsson J. Expression of HLA-DR antigen and smooth muscle cell differentiation markers by valvular fibroblasts in degenerative aortic stenosis. J Am Coll Cardiol. 1994;24(7):1664–71.

9. Kaden JJ, Dempfle CE, Grobholz R, Tran HT, Kilic R, Sarikoc A, et al. Interleukin-1 beta promotes matrix metalloproteinase expression and cell proliferation in calcific aortic valve stenosis. Atherosclerosis [Internet]. 2003;170(2):205–11. http://www.ncbi.nlm.nih.gov/entrez/query.fcgi?cmd=Retrieve&db=PubMed&dopt=Citation&list_uids=14612199%5Cn http://www.sciencedirect.com/science/article/pii/S0021915003002843

10. Jian B, Narula N, Li QY, Mohler ER, Levy RJ. Progression of aortic valve stenosis: TGF-β1 is present in calcified aortic valve cusps and promotes aortic valve interstitial cell calcification via apoptosis. Ann Thorac Surg. 2003;75(2):457–65.

11. Helske S, Lindstedt KA, Laine M, Mäyränpää M, Werkkala K, Lommi J, et al. Induction of local angiotensin II-producing systems in stenotic aortic valves. J Am Coll Cardiol. 2004;44(9):1859–66.

12. Ghaisas NK, Foley JB, O'Briain DS, Crean P, Kelleher D, Walsh M. Adhesion molecules in non-rheumatic aortic valve disease: endothelial expression, serum levels and effects of valve replacement. J Am Coll Cardiol [Internet]. 2000;36(7):2257–62. http://www.sciencedirect.com/science/article/pii/S0735109700009980

13. Weinberg EJ, Kaazempur Mofrad MR. A multiscale computational comparison of the bicuspid and tricuspid aortic valves in relation to calcific aortic stenosis. J Biomech. 2008;41(16):3482–7.

14. Robicsek F, Thubrikar MJ, Fokin AA. Cause of degenerative disease of the trileaflet aortic valve: review of subject and presentation of a new theory. Ann Thorac Surg. 2002;73:1346–54.

15. Stritzke J, Linsel-Nitschke P, Markus MRP, Mayer B, Lieb W, Luchner A, et al. Association between degenerative aortic valve disease and long-term exposure to cardiovascular risk factors: results of the longitudinal population-based KORA/MONICA survey. Eur Heart J. 2009;30(16):2044–53.

16. Stewart BF, Siscovick D, Lind BK, Gardin JM, Gottdiener JS, Smith VE, et al. Clinical factors associated with calcific aortic valve disease. Cardiovascular Health Study. J Am Coll Cardiol [Internet]. 1997;29(3):630–4. http://www.ncbi.nlm.nih.gov/pubmed/9060903.

17. Olsen MH, Wachtell K, Bella JN, Gerdts E, Palmieri V, Nieminen MS, et al. Aortic valve sclerosis relates to cardiovascular events in patients with hypertension (a LIFE substudy). Am J Cardiol. 2005;95(1):132–6.

18. Miller JD, Chu Y, Brooks RM, Richenbacher WE, Peña-Silva R, Heistad DD. Dysregulation of antioxidant mechanisms contributes to increased oxidative stress in calcific aortic valvular stenosis in humans. J Am Coll Cardiol. 2008;52(10):843–50.

19. Garg V, Muth AN, Ransom JF, Schluterman MK, Barnes R, King IN, et al. Mutations in NOTCH1 cause aortic valve disease. Nature. 2005;437(7056):270–4.

20. Cosmi JE, Kort S, Tunick PA, Rosenzweig BP, Freedberg RS, Katz ES, et al. The risk of the development of aortic stenosis in patients with "benign" aortic valve thickening. Arch Intern Med [Internet]. 2002;162(20):2345. http://archinte.jamanetwork.com/article.aspx?doi=10.1001/archinte.162.20.2345

21. Mohler ER, Gannon F, Reynolds C, Zimmerman R, Keane MG, Kaplan FS. Bone formation and inflammation in cardiac valves. Circulation. 2001;103(11):1522–8.

22. Freeman RV, Otto CM. Spectrum of calcific aortic valve disease: pathogenesis, disease progression, and treatment strategies. Circulation. 2005;111:3316–26.

23. Clavel M-A, Pibarot P, Messika-Zeitoun D, Capoulade R, Malouf J, Aggarval S, et al. Impact of aortic valve calcification, as measured by MDCT,

on survival in patients with aortic stenosis results of an international registry study. J Am Coll Cardiol. 2014;64:1202–13.

24. Grossman W, Jones D, McLaurin LP. Wall stress and patterns of hypertrophy in the human left ventricle. J Clin Invest. 1975;56(1):56–64.

25. Levy D, Garrison RJ, Savage DD, Kannel WB, Castelli WP. Prognostic implications of echocardiographically determined left ventricular mass in the Framingham Heart Study. N Engl J Med [Internet]. 1990;322(22):1561–6. http://www.ncbi.nlm.nih.gov/pubmed/2139921

26. Salcedo EE, Korzick DH, Currie PJ, Stewart WJ, Lever HM, Goormastic M. Determinants of left ventricular hypertrophy in patients with aortic stenosis. Cleve Clin J Med. 1989;56(6):590–6.

27. Kupari M, Turto H, Lommi J. Left ventricular hypertrophy in aortic valve stenosis: preventive or promotive of systolic dysfunction and heart failure? Eur Heart J. 2005;26(17):1790–6.

28. Gunther S, Grossman W. Determinants of ventricular function in pressure-overload hypertrophy in man. Circulation. 1979;59(4):679–88.

29. Dweck MR, Joshi S, Murigu T, Gulati A, Alpendurada F, Jabbour A, et al. Left ventricular remodeling and hypertrophy in patients with aortic stenosis: insights from cardiovascular magnetic resonance. J Cardiovasc Magn Reson [Internet]. 2012;14(1):50. http://www.pubmedcentral.nih.gov/articlerender.fcgi?artid=3457907&tool=pmcentrez&rendertype=abstract

30. Orlowska-Baranowska E, Placha G, Gaciong Z, Baranowski R, Zakrzewski D, Michalek P, et al. Influence of ACE I/D genotypes on left ventricular hypertrophy in aortic stenosis: gender-related differences. J Heart Valve Dis [Internet]. 2004;13(4):574–81. http://www.ncbi.nlm.nih.gov/pubmed/15311863.

31. Rieck AE, Cramariuc D, Staal EM, Rossebø AB, Wachtell K, Gerdts E. Impact of hypertension on left ventricular structure in patients with asymptomatic aortic valve stenosis (a SEAS substudy). J Hypertens. 2010;28(2):377–83.

32. Briand M, Dumesnil JG, Kadem L, Tongue AG, Rieu R, Garcia D, et al. Reduced systemic arterial compliance impacts significantly on left ventricular afterload and function in aortic stenosis: implications for diagnosis and treatment. J Am Coll Cardiol. 2005;46(2):291–8.

33. Hachicha Z, Dumesnil JG, Pibarot P. Usefulness of the valvuloarterial impedance to predict adverse outcome in asymptomatic aortic stenosis. J Am Coll Cardiol. 2009;54(11):1003–11.

34. Cioffi G, Faggiano P, Vizzardi E, Tarantini L, Cramariuc D, Gerdts E, et al. Prognostic effect of inappropriately high left ventricular mass in asymptomatic severe aortic stenosis. Heart. 2011;97(4):301–7.

35. Bishopric NH, Andreka P, Slepak T, Webster KA. Molecular mechanisms of apoptosis in the cardiac myocyte. Curr Opin Pharmacol. 2001;1(2):141–50.

36. Cheng W, Li B, Kajstura J, Li P, Wolin MS, Sonnenblick EH, et al. Stretch-induced programmed myocyte cell death. J Clin Invest. 1995;96(5):2247–59.

37. Pierzchalski P, Reiss K, Cheng W, Cirielli C, Kajstura J, Nitahara JA, et al. p53 induces myocyte apoptosis via the activation of the renin-angiotensin system. Exp Cell Res. 1997;234(1):57–65.

38. Camici PG, Olivotto I, Rimoldi OE. The coronary circulation and blood flow in left ventricular hypertrophy. J Mol Cell Cardiol. 2012;52:857–64.

39. Anderson KR, Sutton MGSJ, Lie JT. Histopathological types of cardiac fibrosis in myocardial disease. J Pathol. 1979;128(2):79–85.

40. Krayenbuehl HP, Hess OM, Monrad ES, Schneider J, Mall G, Turina M. Left ventricular myocardial structure in aortic valve disease before, intermediate, and late after aortic valve replacement. Circulation. 1989;79(4):744–55.

41. Berk BC, Fujiwara K, Lehoux S. ECM remodeling in hypertensive heart disease. J Clin Investig. 2007;117:568–75.

42. Bishop JE, Lindahl G. Regulation of cardiovascular collagen synthesis by mechanical load. Cardiovasc Res. 1999;42(1):27–44.

43. Treibel TA, López B, González A, Menacho K, Schofield RS, Ravassa S, et al. Reappraising myocardial fibrosis in severe aortic stenosis: an invasive and non-invasive study in 133 patients. Eur Heart J [Internet]. 2017. https://academic.oup.com/eurheartj/article-lookup/doi/10.1093/eurheartj/ehx353

Predictive Computational Models of Transcatheter Aortic Valve Implantation

4

Simone Morganti, Michele Conti,
Alessandro Reali, and Ferdinando Auricchio

4.1 Introduction

In the last decade, computational tools have been increasingly and extensively used for the virtual simulation of transcatheter aortic valve implantation (TAVI), also called transcatheter aortic valve replacement (TAVR). The reason is twofold: on one side, from the medical point of view, TAVI is turning out to be not only a consolidated minimally invasive technique for inoperable patients but also a very promising solution even in high- or intermediate-risk patients [1–4]; on the other side, from the engineering point of view, computational tools and simulation technologies are becoming more and more powerful, allowing realistic virtual reproduction of real, even complex, procedures in short time.

Computer simulations of TAVI can in fact potentially produce a reliable prediction of the final configuration of the implanted device in a specific patient. This is the main reason of success of such innovative technologies. In particular, simulation results may let the medical team explore aspects and details that are not possible to observe in any other way, being the intervention minimally invasive (not open-chest) but, most importantly, simulation results represent possible predictions of the operation outcome. The real, tremendously high, potentiality of these tools indeed belongs to such an aspect. Obviously, computational models need to be accurate, reliable, and robust to appropriately represent reality and suggest correct scenarios to the interventional operators.

In order to satisfy such accuracy, reliability, and robustness requirements computational models have to take into account the patient-specific anatomical details, the characteristics of the patient's arteries (e.g., elasticity), the boundary conditions (i.e., how the considered model is kinematically linked to the surrounding structures), the loads acting on the anatomical structure, etc.

All these conditions can be translated into mathematical equations aiming at modeling the specific physical phenomenon. They are in general differential equations too complicated to be solved by classical analytical methods. Therefore, numerical methods have been introduced to let the computer solve such equations in an approximated fashion. Currently, the *finite element method* (FEM) is undoubtedly the most popular and utilized technique in this context [5–7].

In few and very simple words, FEM consists in subdividing the region under investigation into

S. Morganti (✉)
Department of Electrical, Computer, and Biomedical Engineering, University of Pavia, Pavia, Italy
e-mail: simone.morganti@unipv.it

M. Conti · A. Reali · F. Auricchio
Department of Civil Engineering and Architecture, University of Pavia, Pavia, Italy
e-mail: michele.conti@unipv.it;
alessandro.reali@unipv.it; auricchio@unipv.it

© Springer Nature Switzerland AG 2019
A. Giordano et al. (eds.), *Transcatheter Aortic Valve Implantation*,
https://doi.org/10.1007/978-3-030-05912-5_4

smaller parts (called finite elements) and then carrying out the approximation (usually a polynomial) over each single element. For the sake of clarity, Fig. 4.1 summarizes the main ingredients needed to predict with finite elements the diastolic performance of a (healthy or diseased) aortic valve taken as example.

With respect to such an example, TAVI computer models have to take into account further complexities (in addition to the abovementioned ingredients), such as, for example, the position and dimension of calcifications, that are known to strongly affect the final implantation outcome, and, of course, the geometry and material of the prosthetic device to be implanted. Moreover, the expansion procedure has to be realistically reproduced by applying appropriate boundary conditions and loading actions to the model.

If all these aspects are taken into account and are correctly modeled, as previously mentioned, computer FEM simulations represent possible predictors of future scenarios of transcatheter valve replacement.

In particular, there are several complications that may occur when performing the TAVI procedure that may be predicted and, hopefully, avoided using virtual simulation tools when they are used to support the operation planning procedure. In particular, also simpler structural analyses (as opposed to more complex fluid-structure interaction ones) are highly powerful for prediction purposes.

Paravalvular and *transvalvular leaks* that are purely hemodynamic complications associated with the presence of post-implant retrograde blood flow, for example, can be quite accurately predicted with simple structural simulations that

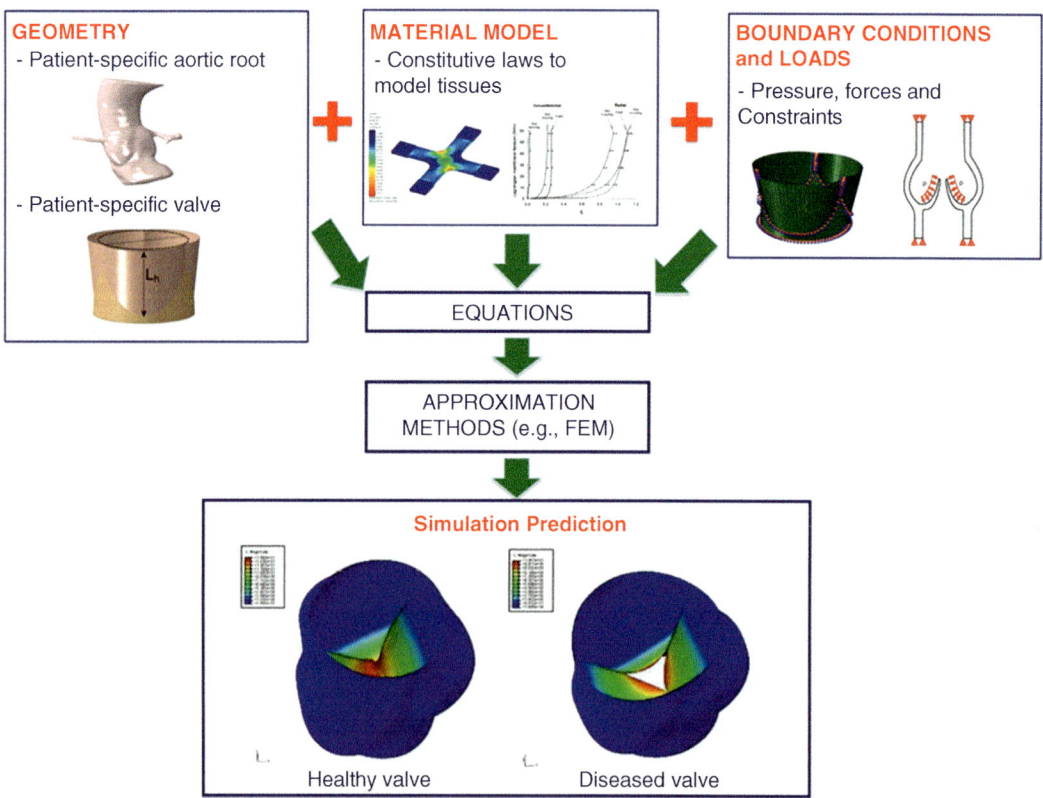

Fig. 4.1 Main ingredients needed to obtain a predictive approximated solution of aortic valve performance through the finite element method (FEM). Images of the simulation prediction for the healthy and diseased valves are adapted from [8]

allow evaluating the presence of possible orifices among the prosthetic leaflets during diastole (transvalvular leakage) or between the device skirt and the patient's root structure (paravalvular leakage).

Coronary occlusion and device deformation can be easily evaluated by simply observing the simulated configuration of the implanted device. At the same time, stress computations can be simply performed to measure the effects of prosthesis deployment onto the native patient's tissue (predicting possible injuries or inflammatory processes) or the risk of conduction impairments (by evaluating the combination of stress magnitude and location below the annular level).

In the present chapter, after proposing a synthetic literature review, we will mainly focus on two purely structural applications of finite element analysis to TAVI: one in case of balloon-expandable device, and one in case of self-expandable devices. The aim of the present chapter is thus to show in real cases what is the real current capability of computational tools to capture the real behavior of implanted devices and predict the postoperative performance of deployed prosthetic valve.

4.2 Computational Models: Literature Review

In the last decade, the number of publications dealing with finite element simulations of TAVI has constantly increased as depicted, for example, in Fig. 4.2. An exhaustive summary of the main publications on this topic can be found in [9].

From the first publication by Dwyer et al. [10] aiming at characterizing the blood ejection force able to induce a prosthesis migration, several other works have been published also using patient-specific data. We here recall the first study using patient's data (from a 68-year-old male), proposed by Sirois et al. [11]. The procedure of TAVI is quite complex and its main steps can be summarized in device crimping, positioning, and expansion.

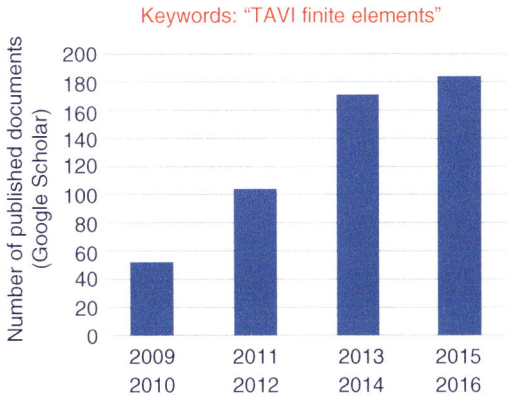

Fig. 4.2 Number of published documents (grouped in periods of 2 years) found using Google Scholar with the following keywords: "TAVI finite elements"

Additionally, each of the previously listed steps involves nontrivial physical phenomena, as the strong crimping of a complex-shape device made of materials exhibiting nonlinear behavior or the expansion of the same device that interacts with native tissues and calcifications. For this reason, many authors have focused their work on specific aspects of the entire TAVI procedure. Wang et al. [12], for example, focused only on the deployment of a balloon-expandable device within a patient-specific aortic root reconstructed from medical images. Analogously, Gunning et al. [13] analyzed in a patient-specific case the bioprosthetic leaflet deformation due to the deployment of a self-expanding valve. For simplicity, some authors considered only the stent for their numerical investigations: Schievano et al. [14] and Capelli et al. [15] proposed a FEA-based methodology to provide information and help clinicians during percutaneous pulmonary valve implantation planning. In these works, the implantation site has been simplified using rigid elements and, at the same time, the presence of the valve has been neglected. On the contrary, many other studies focus on the leaflets neglecting the stent: for example, Smuts et al. [16] developed new concepts for different percutaneous aortic leaflet geometries by means of FEA, while Sun et al. [17] have investigated the implications of asymmetric

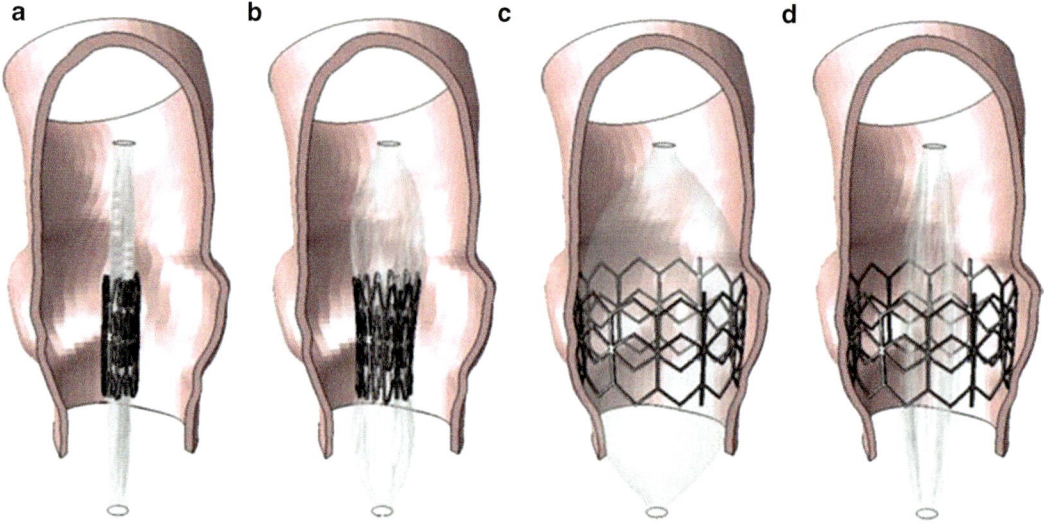

Fig. 4.3 Different frames of balloon expansion and stent apposition: (**a**) initial configuration; (**b**) the balloon starts to deploy the stent; (**c**) the balloon is fully expanded and the stent fully deployed; (**d**) final configuration after balloon deflation. The figure is adapted from [18]

transcatheter prosthesis deployment on the bioprosthetic valve. It is worth mentioning the other following works by Auricchio et al. [18] that proposed a step-by-step strategy to simulate the entire implantation procedure (from crimping to expansion) of a realistic prosthetic valve model made of both a metallic frame and biological leaflets (Fig. 4.3).

Capelli et al. [19] performed patient-specific analyses to explore the feasibility of TAVI in morphologies which are borderline cases for a minimally invasive approach. Tzamtzis et al. [20] compared the radial force produced by a self-expandable valve (i.e., the Medtronic Corevalve) and a balloon-expandable one (i.e., the Edwards Sapien valve). The radial force of a self-expanding valve was also investigated by Gessat et al. [21] who developed an innovative method for extracting such a force measure from images of an implanted device.

In the following two possible applications of the finite element method to simulate TAVI and obtain predictive indications potentially useful during the decision-making process are described in detail. The aim of the following sections is to prove the potentiality and capability of computational tools focusing on two different cases: a balloon-expandable valve and a self-expandable one.

4.3 An Application to Balloon-Expandable Devices

In this section we focus on one of the currently available percutaneous aortic valve prosthesis, probably the most famous one, i.e., the balloon-expandable Edwards Sapien, which is basically composed of three biological leaflets sutured within a cobalt-chromium alloy stent.[1] Details can be found in [22].

Two clinical cases of transcatheter aortic valve implantation will be investigated through structural finite element analysis. In particular, the impact of patient-specific anatomical features of the native aortic valve on the postoperative performance of the balloon-expandable Edwards Sapien XT device will be analyzed. Stress distributions, geometrical changes, coaptation values, and risk of paravalvular leakage will be computed and evaluated for both patients. Finally, comparison between the obtained numerical results

---

[1]In this section we take into consideration an Edwards Sapien XT valve, even if we know that currently also newer devices are available on the market. However, the ideas presented in the present section are definitely independent from the device model and specific details.

and in vivo postoperative measurements will be performed aiming at demonstrating that the proposed simulation strategy represents a valuable tool to predict clinically relevant aspects of TAVI. Realistic computer-based simulations are herein presented as a technology for virtual planning of TAVI procedures, which may improve the efficacy of the operation technique and support decision-making process.

4.3.1 Clinical Cases

Two patients who underwent TAVI were retrospectively selected. *Patient 1* had a positive outcome of TAVI, while Patient 2 presented a paravalvular leak at echocardiography and angiography performed after procedure. Two different patients allow testing the engineering model in two extremely different conditions. Patients were 83 and 84 years old, respectively, both males, suffering from severe comorbidities including extracardiac arteriopathy and coronary arteries disease for which they already underwent stenting and bypass grafting. Each patient selected to undergo TAVI was studied through echocardiography, CT scan, and coronary angiography. The two patients underwent TAVI in a hybrid room. For both patients transaortic access was chosen. General anesthesia was performed and ventricular tachycardia was induced (180–190 ppm) to have an almost static heart. Under angiographic view, valve pre-dilatation was performed using a 20 mm Edwards expandable balloon followed by valve delivery and catheter recovery (see Table 4.1).

Table 4.1 Procedure data

	Patient 1	Patient 2
Date of TAVI	25/01/2010	19/08/2011
Access	Transapical	Transapical
Anesthesia	General	General
Valve	Edwards Sapien XT 26	Edwards Sapien XT 26
Total procedure time (min)	140	90
Contrast agent used (mL)	430	130
Fluoroscopy (min)	8	9

TAVI procedure was successful. Angiography and echocardiography were performed in the operative room: both patients showed normal transaortic gradients, but *Patient 2* presented a mild paravalvular leak. *Patient 1* had regular staying and was discharged home on the ninth postoperative day. *Patient 2* had major stroke requiring longer ICU staying and was discharged to a rehab hospital on the 28th day after implantation.

Both patients underwent echocardiographic control before discharge from hospital. Only Patient 2 showed paravalvular leak.

Patient 1 underwent clinical and echocardiographic follow-up at 1, 6, 12, 24, 36, and 46 months after TAVI. Transvalvular gradients still decreased, intravalvular regurgitation did not worsen, and no paravalvular leak appeared. *Patient 2* was discharged to a rehab center where his neurological conditions improved, but he died of acute pneumonia 3 months after procedure. At 1 month echocardiographic follow-up transvalvular gradients kept stable and mild paravalvular leak remained.

4.3.2 Finite Element Analysis: Materials and Methods

The adopted computational framework to simulate transcatheter aortic valve implantation can be roughly divided into four main steps:

- Step 1: Processing of medical images.
- Step 2: Creation of analysis-suitable models.
- Step 3: Performance of all the required analyses to reproduce the entire clinical procedure.
- Step 4: Postprocessing of the simulation results and comparison with follow-up data.

Step 1: Medical image processing. Preoperative CT examinations were performed at IRCCS Policlinico San Matteo (Pavia, Italy) using a dual-source computed tomography scanner (Somatom Definition, Siemens Healthcare, Forchheim, Germany). To obtain contrast-enhanced images an iodinated contrast agent was injected. Scan main parameters for cardiac CT were as follows: scan direction, cranio-caudal;

slice thickness, 0.6 mm; spiral pitch factor, 0.2; tube voltage, 120 kV.

The CT data sets were processed using ITK-Snap v2.4 [23]. In particular, a confined region of interest (i.e., the aortic root from the left ventricular outflow to the sinotubular junction) was extracted from the whole reconstructed body exploiting the contrast enhancement, cropping, and segmentation capabilities of the software. Using different Hounsfield unit thresholds, it was possible to discern the calcific component from the surrounding healthy tissue and evaluate it in terms of both location and dimension. Once the segmented region was extracted, we exported the aortic lumen as well as the calcium deposits as stereolithographic (STL) files. With 2D ultrasound technique aortic valve leaflets resulted visible. Prosound Alpha 10 machine (ALOKA, Tokyo, Japan) was used to measure specific leaflet dimensions and, in particular, the leaflet free margin length.

Step 2: Analysis-suitable models. Herein we describe the procedure to obtain analysis-suitable models of both the native aortic valve including calcifications and the prosthetic device.

Native aortic valve model. The obtained STL file of the aortic root was processed implementing in Matlab (The Mathworks Inc., Natick, MA, USA) a procedure able to define a set of splines, resembling the cross-sectional contours of the aortic lumen. These curves were used to automatically generate a volume model of the aortic root wall, which was finally imported in Abaqus CAE software (Simulia, Dassáult Systems, Providence, RI, USA) for the finite element analysis setup. The geometrical model of the aortic root obtained by processing the STL file thus represented the starting point of the finite element analysis of TAVI. It is worth noting that we generated not only the aortic wall but also the native valve leaflets in order to get a complete and realistic model for the simulations (more details can be found in [22]).

Figure 4.4 shows the resulting aortic root model in the case of *Patient 1*; the model is composed of the vessel wall, the native leaflets, and calcific plaque. The superimposition of the model on the 3D reconstructions derived from medical images shows a good correspondence; in particular, in Fig. 4.4b, c the closed model of the native aortic valve, obtained through a simulation of valve closure, highlights a good agreement between the real patient's plaques and the position of calcific shell elements.

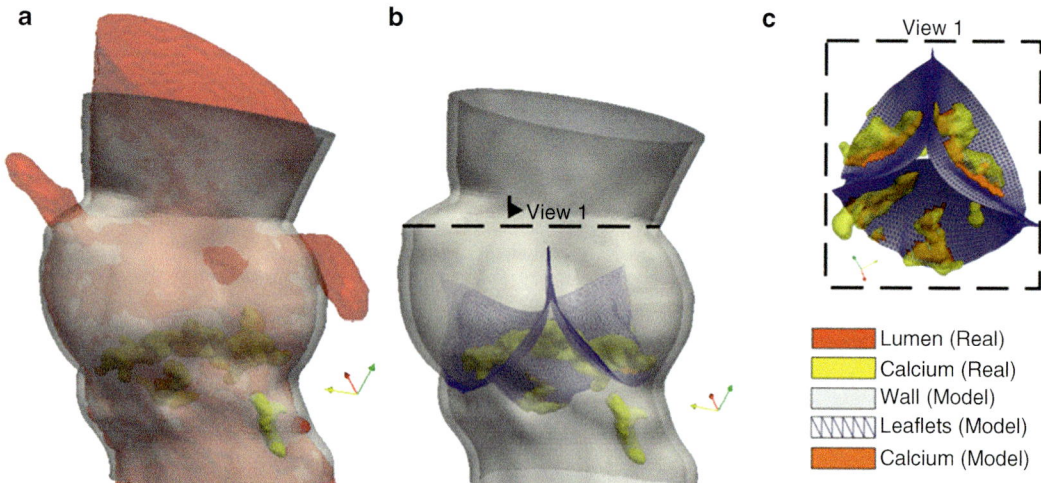

Fig. 4.4 Rendering of the STL file vs. aortic model created for simulations: (**a**) the real aortic root lumen (red) and calcifications (yellow) are overlapped to the aortic wall model (gray); (**b**) the closed native leaflets (blue mesh) of our model are perfectly matching with real calcifications obtained by processing CT images; (**c**) top view is shown. The figure is adapted from [22] (For interpretation of the references to color in this figure caption, the reader is referred to the web version of the book)

For the sake of simplicity, the material for the native aortic tissues is assumed to be isotropic and homogenous, as already assumed in [19, 24]. In particular, a nearly incompressible reduced polynomial form, calibrated on experimental data obtained from human samples for each single leaflet and sinus [25], was used to reproduce material behavior. Aortic wall and native valve leaflets are assumed to have a uniform thickness of 2.5 and 0.5 mm, respectively [18]. Following [19], calcified tissue is assumed to be characterized by an elastic modulus of 10 MPa, a Poisson ratio of 0.35, and a density of 2000 kg/m^3, while the thickness of calcific shell elements is chosen equal to 1.4 mm.

Prosthesis model. Both patients were treated with an Edwards Sapien XT size 26 device. A faithful geometrical model of the device is based on a high-resolution micro-CT scan (Skyscan 1172 with a resolution of 0.17 μm) of a real device sample. Regarding the prosthetic valve leaflets, there are different beliefs concerning the constitutive characteristics of bovine pericardium after the fixation process. In the present work, we model the leaflets as an isotropic material [26] and, in particular, an elastic modulus of 8 MPa, a Poisson coefficient of 0.45, and a density of 1100 kg/m^3 are used following [27].

Step 3: Finite element analyses. The TAVI procedure is a complex intervention composed of several steps; to realistically reproduce the whole procedure, we set up a simulation strategy consisting in the following two main stages:

- *Stent crimping and deployment:* In this step, the prosthesis stent model was crimped to achieve the catheter diameter which, for a transapical approach, is usually 24 French; then, the prosthetic stent was expanded within the patient-specific aortic root to reproduce the implantation due to balloon expansion.
- *Valve mapping and closure:* The prosthetic leaflets were mapped onto the implanted stent and a physiological pressure was applied to virtually recreate the diastolic behavior of the implanted device.

All the numerical analyses were nonlinear problems involving large deformation and contact. For this reason, Abaqus Explicit (Simulia, Providence, USA) solver was used to perform large deformation analyses.

Stent crimping and deployment. A cylindrical surface was gradually crimped from an initial diameter of 28 mm to a final diameter of 8 mm (24 French). For the setup of stent apposition simulation (see Fig. 4.5a), the deformed configuration of the stent was then reimported taking into account as initial state the tensional state resulting from the crimping analysis. To reproduce stent

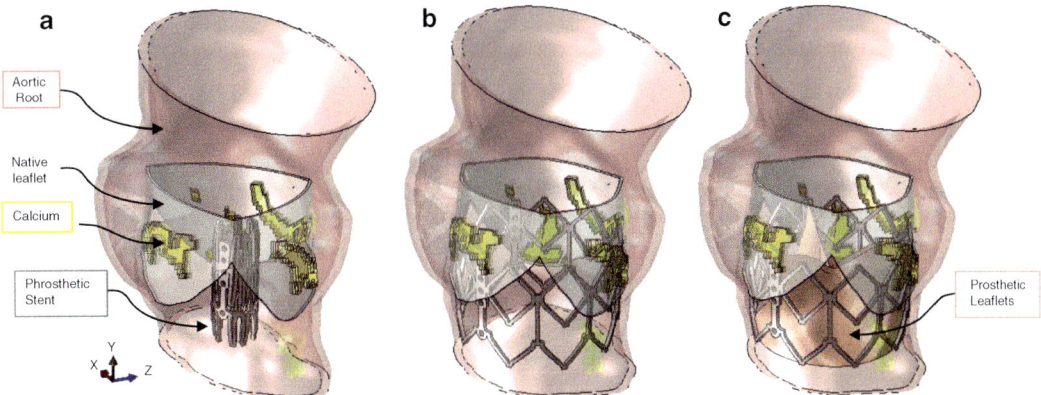

Fig. 4.5 Procedural steps of TAVI reproduced through a computer-based simulation strategy: (**a**) the crimped stent is properly placed inside the aortic root model; (**b**) the stent is expanded within the patient-specific aortic root; (**c**) prosthetic leaflet closure is reproduced to evaluate postoperative performance. The figure is adapted from [22]

expansion, a pure and uniform radial displacement was gradually applied to the nodes of a rigid cylindrical surface, which was assumed to represent the wall of the expanding balloon. The rigid cylinder was widened from an initial diameter of 6 mm to a final diameter of 26 mm. During stent expansion the balloon axis remained always fixed. This assumption could be accepted as observed through intraoperative angiography which showed negligible axis rotation and translation.

Valve mapping and closure. Following the procedure presented in [18], to reproduce the realistic behavior of the prosthetic device and evaluate the postoperative prosthesis performance, the prosthetic leaflets were mapped onto the implanted stent: precomputed displacements were assigned to the base of the valve and to the nodes of the leaflet commissures, which allowed to achieve a complete configuration of the

implanted prosthetic device, as shown in Fig. 4.5c. Consequently, given the complete model of the implanted prosthetic device, we are able to reproduce the patient-specific post-operative behavior of the Sapien XT valve in terms of cyclic valve opening/closing. To simulate valve behavior at the end of the diastolic phase, a uniform physiologic pressure of 0.01 MPa was applied to the prosthetic leaflets.

Step 4: Postprocessing and simulation outcomes. The results obtained with the developed computational tools can be classified into two main groups: (1) from the simulation of stent expansion we can evaluate the impact of the metallic frame of the stent on the native calcified aortic root wall; (2) from the simulation of valve closure, we can predict the postoperative device performance.

In Fig. 4.6 von Mises aortic wall stresses induced by stent expansion are shown from two

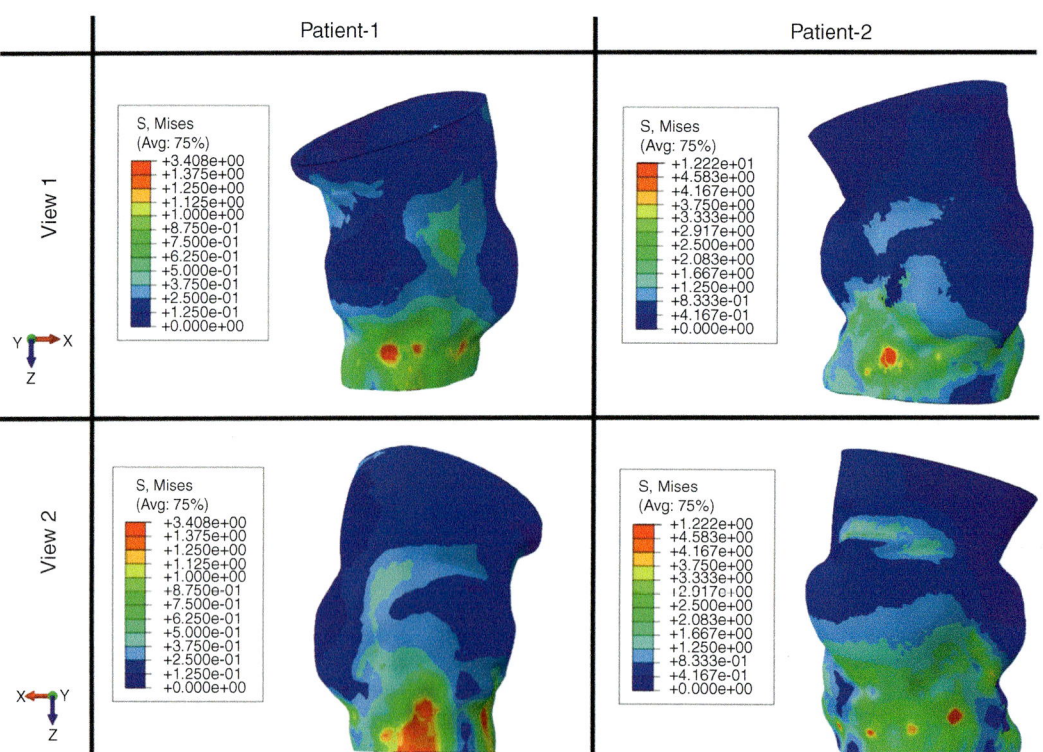

Fig. 4.6 Impact of the prosthesis implant on the aortic root: von Mises stress [MPa] distribution along the vessel is reported to evaluate the interaction between the prosthetic stent and the aortic root wall; a huge difference in terms of maximum stress values is observable. This is attributable to the position and extension of calcifications of the aortic root as well as to the preoperative configuration of the aortic annulus: for *Patient 2* a very irregular and elliptic shape has been extracted from CT images. The figure is adapted from [22]

different views for the two considered patients. Such a distribution should be ideally uniform, resembling a homogeneous interaction of the stent prosthesis with the aortic root base. The presented results suggest instead that the stresses are not uniformly distributed. In particular, in both cases, spots of concentrated stresses are visible in correspondence of the adhesion between the inner aortic wall and the metallic frame of the stent.

In Fig. 4.7a, a contour map representing the pointwise distance between the basal stent crown of the expanded stent and the inner aortic wall is shown. Higher values (up to 2 mm) are obtained for *Patient 2* while a good and uniform degree of adherence is achieved after stent expansion in *Patient 1*. Such results are also confirmed by Fig. 4.7b where two proximal cross sections of the implanted device are represented. Greater orifices (for a total area of 36.9 mm²) between the stent and the aortic root wall are found for *Patient 2* than for *Patient 1* whose area associated with paravalvular leakage is negligible being equal to 4.1 mm².

The native morphology of the aortic root and, in particular, the quantity and position of calcifications may induce a noncircular shape to the implanted device. In both cases, an elliptical shape of the device is obtained.

4.3.3   Discussion of the Obtained Results

It is well known and extensively reported in the literature that the selection of prosthetic device size and type is very important to avoid (or, at least, reduce) aortic regurgitation and/or other TAVI complications. Such a critical choice not only depends on annular dimensions but also on the complex native aortic root morphology, as well as on position and dimensions of calcifications [28]. Computational analyses, which take into account both the patient-specific structure of the native aortic valve and an accurate evaluation of calcifications, can be used to predict several parameters which, being of clinical interest, can support and guide device selection. In Sect. 4.3 of the present chapter, a complete framework to reproduce transcatheter aortic valve implantation has been developed and applied to two real clinical cases. Stress distribution is characterized by concentrated spots of higher stress values induced by the contact between the stent and the aortic wall (see Fig. 4.6). Additionally, in agreement with [12], high values of the maximum principal stress are obtained in the aortic regions close to calcifications. On one side,

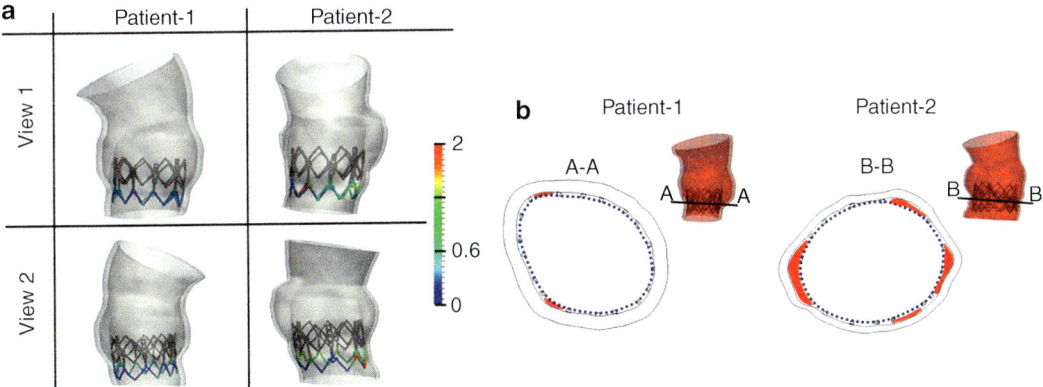

Fig. 4.7 Evaluation of the degree of apposition between the prosthesis stent and the patient-specific root anatomy: (**a**) the reconstructed model of the aortic root is represented in light gray, while the stent is shown in dark gray; on the basal crown of the stent, which, at the end of implantation, should completely adhere with the aortic annulus, a contour map of the radial distance [mm] between the inner aortic wall and the outer surface of the implanted stent is represented; (**b**) for both patients a cross section at the proximal side of the implanted device allows to highlight the holes between the stent and the aortic root wall, responsible for paravalvular leakage. Both figures are adapted from [22]

higher stress values can be related to higher force of adherence between stent and aortic wall; on the other side, high stress patterns concentrated in the annular region can indicate a major risk of aortic rupture [29] which is a possible TAVI complication leading to cardiac tamponade and subsequent fatal events. If aortic rupture is quite unusual, paravalvular leakage is one of the most frequent complications which may occur after TAVI due to incomplete adherence of the prosthetic stent to the aortic wall. For both considered patients, we can quantitatively evaluate the area of the perivalvular holes, which can be assumed to be proportional to the amount of retrograde perivalvular blood flow (i.e., perivalvular leakage). Interestingly, the obtained results are in agreement with postoperative medical data. Indeed, as reported in Fig. 4.8, quantitative postoperative Doppler echocardiography has highlighted a significantly higher regurgitant flow in *Patient 2* than in *Patient 1,* as observable by the diastolic recording. Also post-implant angiographic movies showed an agreement with our results since the postoperative retrograde flow, highlighted by a contrast agent, was qualitatively much more visible in *Patient 2* than in *Patient 1*. Finally, the computed eccentricity of the implanted stent indicated that for both patients the positioned stent assumed a noncircular shape. For *Patient 2* a slightly worst scenario was predicted. Eccentricity of the implanted stent directly influences valve

closure and, in particular, coaptation. In fact, the occurring nonsymmetric closure is attributed to the elliptical stent configuration, in agreement with results by [30] showing that one leaflet closes below the other two producing a small central gap responsible for a regurgitant flow (see Fig. 4.8b). Even though we think that the geometrical asymmetry of the stent is the main determinant of the central gap obtained during diastole, it is worth highlighting that the choice of the leaflet material model, which has been proven to have a strong impact on coaptation values [31], may alter the obtained results. However, the resulting intravalvular gap is in agreement with follow-up evaluations which, in both patients, have highlighted a central "*mild intraprosthetic leak*" (extraction from postoperative medical reports of *Patient 1* and *Patient 2*).

4.4 An Application to Self-Expandable Devices

In this section we present the predictive capabilities of the engineering models for the implantation of self-expandable transcatheter aortic valve device, again in patient-specific cases, with a special focus on the impact of prosthesis positioning on procedure outcomes. More details are reported in the paper by Morganti et al. [32]. The aim is to show that, through computational models and analyses, optimal positioning of the valve

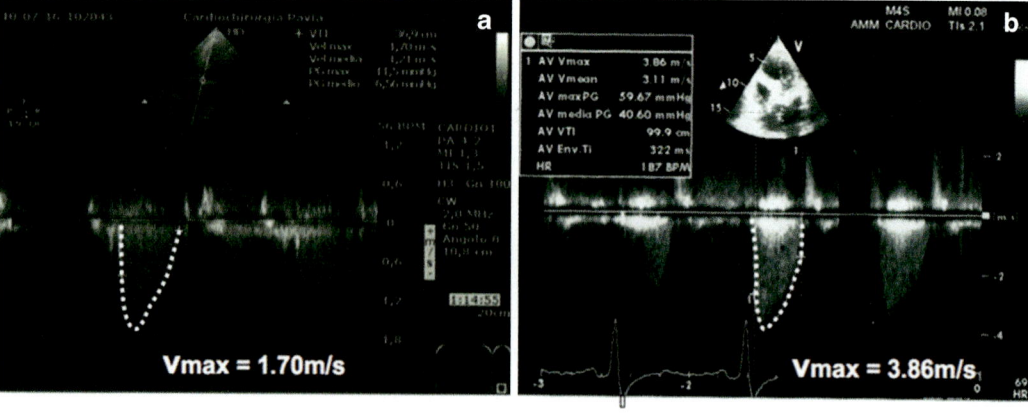

Fig. 4.8 Postoperative Doppler echocardiography records show a lower retrograde blood flow for (**a**) *Patient 1* than for (**b**) *Patient 2*. The figure is adapted from [22]

(that can be highly affected by patient-specific valve morphology and calcifications) can be a priori computed.

4.4.1   Finite Element Analysis: Materials and Methods

To set up the stent expansion analysis we followed the framework introduced in [22]. Accordingly, ITK-Snap v.2.4 was adopted to extract the STL representation of the aortic root and calcific deposits from CT images of a 75-year-old male patient. An in-house code was used to process the STL file and generate the finite element mesh of the aortic root (modeled with tetrahedral elements) including the native leaflets (modeled with shell elements under the assumption of a uniform). The lines of leaflet attachment and the leaflet free-margin lengths were obtained from the CT 3D reconstruction and from short-axis ultrasound images, respectively. The smaller calcific spots and, especially, those extracted at the ascending aorta level were not considered. The STL file of calcifications was then processed using VMTK (Vascular Modeling ToolKit, http://www.vmtk. org) to extract a regular tetrahedral mesh. Given the comparative nature of the present study focused on the prosthetic device postoperative configuration and performance, simplified elastic properties were adopted to model the aortic tissue, the native leaflets, and the calcifications.

The Abaqus Explicit solver was used for all the simulations presented in this chapter section.

A kinematic constraint was defined to couple the motion of the calcific deposits on the leaflets and the leaflets themselves. The Corevalve model (size 29) was generated from a micro-CT scan of the actual device that allowed a very accurate geometrical reconstruction. The Abaqus built-in constitutive model able to reproduce the super-elastic effect was used, with material properties assigned to the hexahedral elements of the structured stent mesh according to [33]. The simulation of prosthesis implantation was performed in two steps: first, as sketched in Fig. 4.9c, the stress-free open configuration of the device is crimped within a rigid cylinder modeled with surface elements to a diameter of 6 mm (18F), then the rigid catheter is gradually removed with a sliding upwards movement to let the stent expand exploiting the Nitinol super-elastic effect (as depicted in Fig. 4.9d). Finally, the prosthetic valve was mapped inside the implanted stent and physiologic uniform pressure applied to the leaflets to reproduce the diastolic behavior (Fig. 4.9e). In Fig. 4.10 the main simulation steps are shown.

The simulation strategy described above was implemented and repeatedly used to evaluate the impact of different positioning choices on prosthesis postoperative configuration and performance. In particular, three different implantation depths and angles were analyzed, as summarized in Fig. 4.11. The implantation depth d is defined as the distance between the lower end of the prosthesis metallic frame and the aortic annulus level (corresponding to the plane passing through the

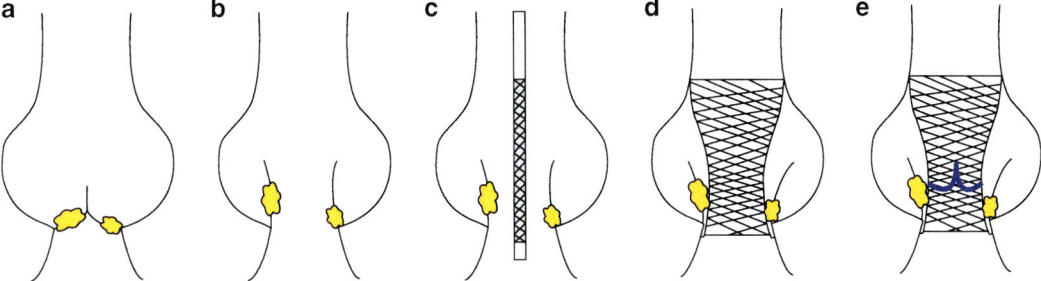

Fig. 4.9 Sketch of the simulation workflow. (**a**) Native aortic valve model reconstructed in the diastolic phase from CT images and ultrasound measures; (**b**) native valve opening; (**c**) Corevalve stent configuration after crimping; (**d**) Corevalve stent expansion; (**e**) prosthetic leaflets mapping inside the stent and valve closure. The figure is adapted from [32]

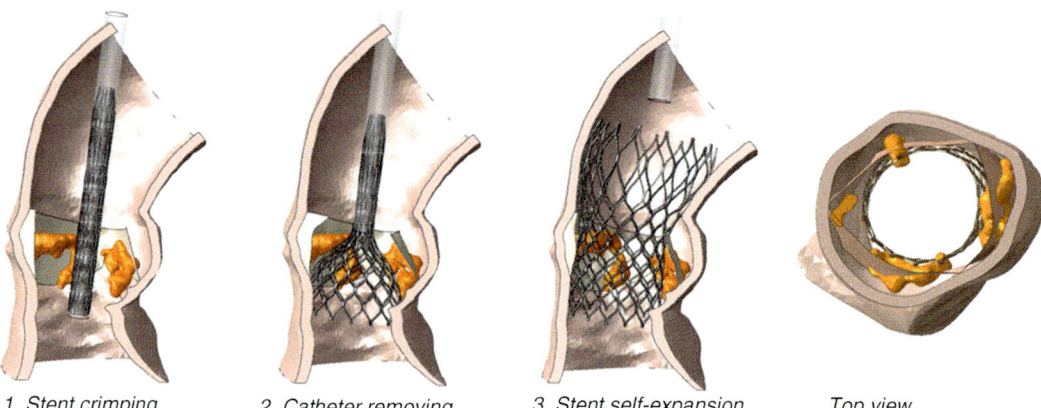

1. Stent crimping   2. Catheter removing   3. Stent self-expansion   Top view

Fig. 4.10 Procedural steps of Corevalve implantation reproduced through a computer-based simulation strategy

ID	description	d [mm]
T0	high	1
T1	medium	4
T2	low	8

ID	description	φ [deg]
T1_R-10	left	-10°
T1	vertical	0°
T1_R+10	right	+10°

Fig. 4.11 Summary of the simulated device configurations within the patient's aortic valve model; we name each configuration as follows: T0, the device is implanted with its lower end 1 mm below the annulus level; T1, the device is implanted with its lower end 4 mm below the annulus level; T2, the device is implanted with its lower end 8 mm below the annulus level; T1_R−10, the axis of the crimped device forms an angle of −10° with the axis of the aortic root; T1_R+10, the axis of the crimped device forms an angle of +10° with the axis of the aortic root. Figure adapted from [32]

three nadirs of the sinuses). The implantation angle φ is defined as the angle between the tangent of the aortic root centerline at the annulus level and the axis of the crimped device (i.e., before expansion).

4.4.2 Postprocessing and Simulation Outcomes

Each simulated configuration was post-processed to extract quantitative measures of (1) prosthetic stent deformation, (2) grade of device apposition, and (3) prosthetic valve performance. In particular, stent deformation was evaluated by measuring the eccentricity of the device cross section. In Fig. 4.12 an example of eccentricity measurement is reported for the configuration named T2 (see Fig. 4.11): On the left, three representative cross sections (at the bottom, middle,

and top of the stent) are shown. The nodes of the stent corresponding to the specific cross section were extracted (red dots in Fig. 4.12a) and used to fit an ellipse (blue line) from which the minor (a) and major (b) axes are highlighted. The eccentricity was evaluated as the ratio between the two axes: $e = b/a$. As an example, the curve representing the eccentricity along the device height is shown in Fig. 4.12b.

The grade of device apposition and, consequently, a correspondent measure of device anchoring could be evaluated by measuring the area of the contact surface between the stent and the aortic root (that we call *stent-root interaction area*). In particular, we considered only the elements of the aortic root whose contact pressure after stent expansion simulation was greater than zero and, then, we summed the areas of all the considered element faces belonging to the internal surface of the root. Such a "contact" measure could

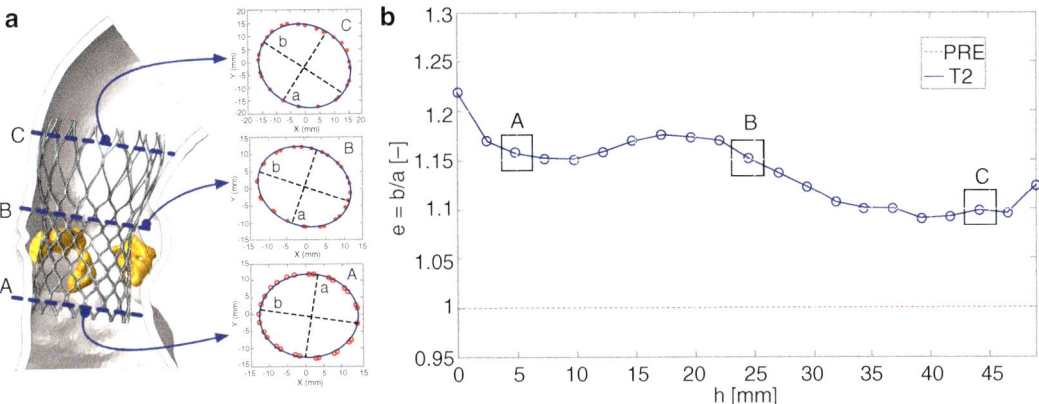

Fig. 4.12 Postprocessing of simulation outcomes: measure of post-implant stent eccentricity. (**a**) Three representative cross sections of the implanted device are shown; (**b**) the obtained eccentricity is plotted for 21 equally spaced stent sections. Figure adapted from [32]

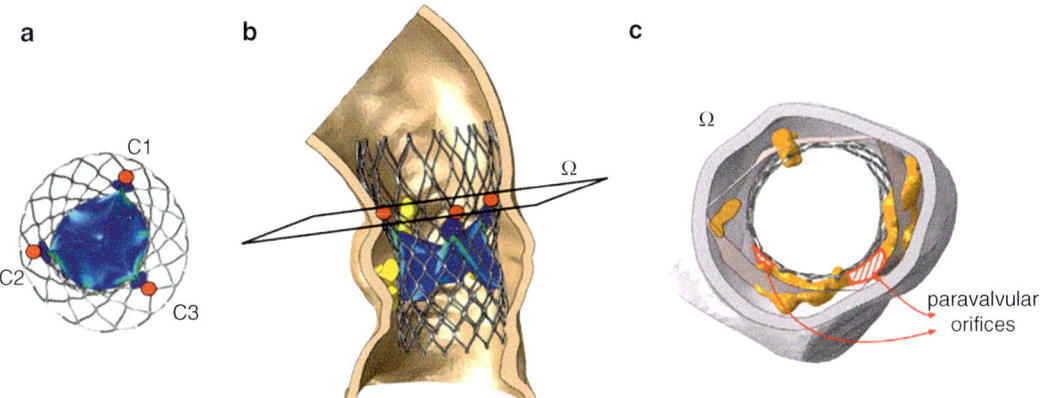

Fig. 4.13 Measure of the risk of paravalvular leakage: (**a**) top view of the prosthetic device; the three end points of the prosthetic leaflet commissures (C1, C2, and C3) are highlighted; (**b**) the plane Ω passes through the points C1, C2, and C3; (**c**) the cross section of the valve at the level of the plane Ω is taken into account to identify eventual paravalvular orifices and compute their area. The figure is adapted from [32]

be improved and completed by a measure of the stress induced in the aortic root due to stent contact after expansion. The risk of paravalvular leakage could be associated with the mismatch (i.e., missed adhesion) between the implanted Corevalve stent, on one side, and the aortic valve structure (including calcifications), on the other side. Following the strategy proposed in [22], the index of potential paravalvular leakage was related to the total area of such mismatch generating paravalvular orifices (highlighted by a red line in Fig. 4.13) measured taking a cross section of the whole model in the plane (Ω in Fig. 4.13b, c) through the three end points of the prosthetic leaflet commissures (C1, C2, and C3 in Fig. 4.13a). Finally, the coaptation area, measured as the total area of the leaflet elements in contact with each other, was computed to evaluate prosthetic leaflet performance.

4.4.3 Discussion of the Obtained Results

In this case, computational tools allowed to evaluate the impact of the positioning on the postoperative configuration and performance of the prosthetic device used for percutaneous aortic valve replacement. Finite element models were developed to achieve this goal starting from medical images of a real case, allowing to obtain the following results:

- *Postoperative prosthetic valve configuration* (in terms of stent deformation and leaflet coaptation): Measurements of the elliptic shape of the implanted device were used to evaluate stent deformation. In Fig. 4.14a the eccentricity (measured as described in Sect. 4.4.2 of the present chapter) is plotted versus the stent height for configurations T0, T1, and T2, highlighting the impact of the positioning depth d, and in Fig. 4.14b for configurations T1, T1_R−10, and T1_R+10, highlighting the impact of the positioning angle Φ. The maximum distorsion ($e = 1.32$) was obtained for the T1_R−10 configuration, while the most regular post-implant geometry was observed in the T1_R+10 configuration.

It is well known that the performance of the implanted valve is strongly affected by device deformation [34, 35] and results show that the device implantation strategy (i.e., the combination of implantation depth and angle) significantly affects stent distortion. In particular, Fig. 4.14a shows that the lower the valve is implanted, the worse is the situation in terms of postoperative stent regularity and symmetry, even if only one configuration (i.e., T2) leads to very poor results with an eccentricity higher than 10%, highlighting an incomplete expansion of the metallic frame at almost all levels. The implantation angle

also affects device deformation inducing, in one case (i.e., T1_R+10), a significant improvement in terms of regularity and, in the other case (i.e., T1_R−10), a relevant worsening (see Fig. 4.14b).

It is interesting to observe that such a measure of post-implant stent distortion is related to the measure of valve coaptation (Fig. 4.15): configurations T2 and T1_R−10, which show a higher stent distortion, as reported in Fig. 4.14, are characterized by lower values of coaptation area (54.8 and 60.3 mm²) while the other three configurations, which show similar distortion level, are associated with similar values of coaptation area. This result confirms that the deformation of the metallic frame of the prosthetic device affects the configuration of the leaflets, as already demonstrated by [35].

- *Measure of paravalvular leakage*: The grade of mismatch (in terms of paravalvular orifice area) between the expanded stent and the internal aortic root surface was measured in the plane passing through the three commissural points of the prosthetic valve, as already mentioned and shown in Fig. 4.13. The obtained values are reported for each configuration in Table 4.2.

Table 4.2 Measures of prosthetic valve paravalvular leakage for each simulated configuration

Configuration	Paravalvular orifice area [mm²]
T0	6.8
T1	12.9
T2	18.6
T1_R−10	5.3
T1_R+10	8.7

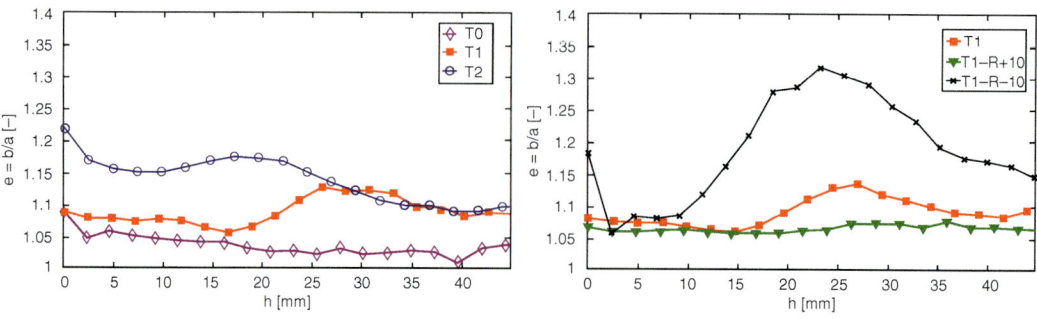

Fig. 4.14 Measure of stent cross-section eccentricity for each simulated configuration. The figure is adapted from [32]

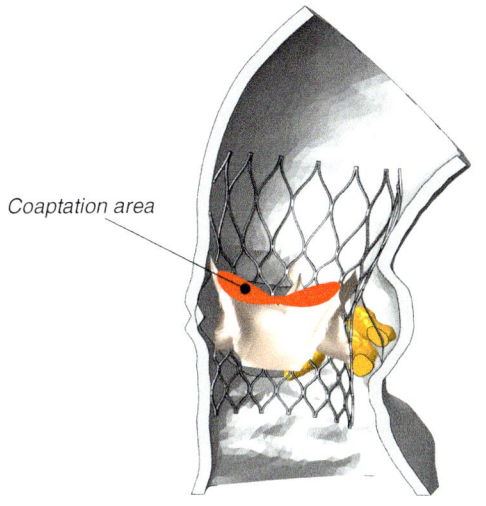

Configuration	Coaptation area [mm²]
T0	91.6
T1	91.5
T2	54.8
T1_R-10	89.8
T1_R+10	60.3

Fig. 4.15   Measure of prosthetic valve coaptation for each simulated configuration. Figure adapted from [32]

As reported by [36], the performance of the percutaneous procedure and, in particular, the occurrence of aortic regurgitation are affected not only by stent deformation but are also related to the size of the patient's annulus and to the degree of native valve calcifications. The model here presented included both these ingredients, which were accurately reconstructed from patient-specific images, thus allowing a quantitative evaluation of the lack of congruence between the native calcified valve and the device. Such a prosthesis-host mismatch, possibly due to inappropriate sizing or nonuniform expansion related to extensive calcifications, was measured in terms of paravalvular orifice dimension. As summarized in Table 4.2, the lower-implanted device (T2) leads to the worst scenario with an associated mismatch area of 18.6 mm². It is worth noting that the obtained values could be reduced by device adjustment (which may occur some days after treatment) or by post-valve implant re-ballooning, which are both complex phenomena not included in our simulations. However, the medical operators can consider the simulation result itself as a prediction of the potential need of re-ballooning.

- *The measure of the stent-root contact area* as well as the measure of the *average and maximum root wall stress* may represent an

indication of the grade of stent apposition and device anchoring; they are thus measured for each simulated configuration and reported in Fig. 4.16a, b.

The device anchoring and, from the opposite point of view, the risk of device migration can be quantitatively evaluated both from the average stress σ_{av} induced by the prosthesis expansion in the aortic root (also associated with the radial forces of the metallic frame which tends to recover its expanded configuration once extracted from the catheter) and from the stent-root interaction area. As expected, the two measures are related: in fact, higher values of σ_{av} are associated with higher values of contact area between the frame and the native aortic structure (see configurations T1, T1_R+10, and T1_R−10), which could highlight a superior anchoring of the prosthesis. On the contrary, lower values of σ_{av} are associated with lower values of interaction area (configurations T0 and T2), which could reveal a higher risk of device migration. Our results thus show that the stent-root interaction can be largely affected by implantation depth. All these information and data can be conveniently shared and discussed to the surgeon, and used to optimally plan the intervention or at least to predict (and avoid) possible complications.

a

CPRESS
+5.566e+00
+1.000e-02
+9.167e-03
+8.333e-03
+7.500e-03
+6.667e-03
+5.833e-03
+5.000e-03
+4.167e-03
+3.333e-03
+2.500e-03
+1.667e-03
+8.333e-04
+0.000e+00

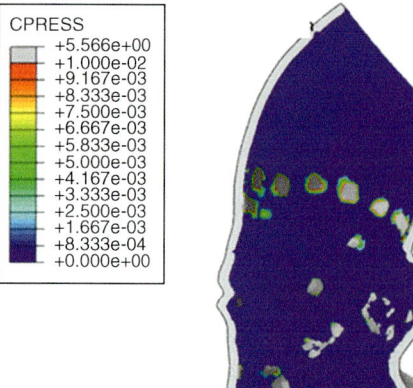

Configuration	Stent-root interaction area
T0	131.1 mm²
T1	222.8 mm²
T2	130.9 mm²
T1_R-10	168.1 mm²
T1_R+10	166.1 mm²

b

S, Mises
(Avg: 75%)
+2.896e+03
+2.000e-01
+1.833e-01
+1.667e-01
+1.500e-01
+1.333e-01
+1.167e-01
+1.000e-01
+8.333e-02
+6.667e-02
+5.000e-02
+3.333e-02
+1.667e-02
+0.000e+00

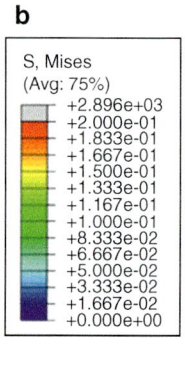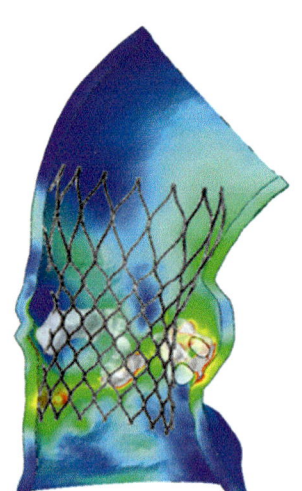

$$\sigma_{av} = \frac{\sum_{i=1}^{N} \sigma_i V_i}{\sum_{i=1}^{N} V_i}$$

Configuration	σ_{av}/σ_{max} [kPa/kPa]
T0	33.9/173
T1	44.1/168
T2	38.4/151
T1_R-10	40.0/165
T1_R+10	46.2/169

Fig. 4.16 Measures of: (**a**) postoperative stent-root interaction area (gray spots) and (**b**) average and maximum stress induced by device expansion on the aortic wall (details about the computation of the average stress can be found in [32]). Measures are reported for each simulated configuration. The figures are adapted from [32]

4.5 Conclusions

In the present chapter, the potential of computer-based simulations as a supporting tool for medical operators during TAVI has been presented and discussed. The predictive capabilities of numerical analyses can really guide the decision-making process for very critical cases, when deciding the prosthetic device (and its size) providing the best possible performance, as well as the optimal placement strategy, is not a trivial task for different reasons (LVOT morphology, amount and distributions of calcifications, etc.).

We have demonstrated that the outcomes of TAVI for both balloon-expandable and self-expandable devices can be preoperatively evaluated based on high-resolution CT scans (routinely performed). In particular, treatment outcomes are predicted in terms of device deformation after implantation and consequent prosthetic valve performance and coaptation, potential presence of paravalvular leaks, anchoring conditions (to avoid migration), and stress distributions within the aortic and cardiac wall (to predict possible local tissue damages or bundle branch impairment).

In the future, such results may be even improved by including fluid-structure interaction analyses providing an estimation of the postoperative hemodynamic conditions. A more extensive validation study including a consistent number of patients has still to be performed. However, at present, the premises of computer-based predictive simulations have shown to be more than bright.

Acknowledgments The presented results are extracted from papers published by our group in collaboration with medical equipes. We wish to acknowledge all medical operators that provided support to the computational studies; in particular we would like to thank Dr. Nedy Brambilla and Dr. Francesco Bedogni of IRCCS Policlinico San Donato and Dr. Marco Aiello and Dr. Eliana Raviola of IRCCS Policlinico San Matteo of Pavia.

Conflict of Interest Statement None declared.

References

1. Adams DH, et al. Transcatheter aortic-valve replacement with a self-expanding prosthesis. N Engl J Med. 2014;370(19):1790–8.
2. Smith CR, et al. Transcatheter versus surgical aortic-valve replacement in high-risk patients. N Engl J Med. 2011;364(23):2187–98.
3. Leon MB, et al. Transcatheter aortic-valve implantation for aortic stenosis in patients who cannot undergo surgery. N Engl J Med. 2010;363(17):1597–607.
4. Leon MB, et al. Transcatheter or surgical aortic-valve replacement in intermediate-risk patients. N Engl J Med. 2016;374:1609–20.
5. Zienkiewicz OC, et al. The finite element method, vol. 3. London: McGraw-Hill; 1977.
6. Hughes TJR. The finite element method: linear static and dynamic finite element analysis. Chelmsford: Courier Corporation; 2012.
7. Bathe KJ. Finite element method. New York: Wiley; 2008.
8. Auricchio F, et al. Finite element analysis of aortic root dilation: a new procedure to reproduce pathology based on experimental data. Comput Method Biomech Biomed Eng. 2011;14(10):875–82. https://doi.org/10.1080/10255842.2010.499867.
9. Vy P, et al. Review of patient-specific simulations of transcatheter aortic valve implantation. Int J Adv Eng Sci Appl Math. 2016;8(1):2–24.
10. Dwyer HA, et al. Computational fluid dynamics simulation of transcatheter aortic valve degeneration. Interact Cardiovasc Thorac Surg. 2009;9(2):301–8.
11. Sirois E, Wang Q, Sun W. Fluid simulation of a transcatheter aortic valve deployment into a patient-specific aortic root. Cardiovasc Eng Technol. 2011;2(3):186–95.
12. Wang Q, Sirois E, Sun W. Patient-specific modeling of biomechanical interaction in transcatheter aortic valve deployment. J Biomech. 2012;45(11):1965–71.
13. Gunning PS, Vaughan TJ, McNamara LM. Simulation of self expanding transcatheter aortic valve in a realistic aortic root: implications of deployment geometry on leaflet deformation. Ann Biomed Eng. 2014;42(9):1989–2001.
14. Schievano S, et al. Patient specific finite element analysis results in more accurate prediction of stent fractures: application to percutaneous pulmonary valve implantation. J Biomech. 2010;43(4):687–93.
15. Capelli C, et al. Patient-specific reconstructed anatomies and computer simulations are fundamental for selecting medical device treatment: application to a new percutaneous pulmonary valve. Philos Trans R Soc. 2010;368:3027–38.
16. Smuts AN, et al. Application of finite element analysis to the design of tissue leaflets for a percutaneous aortic valve. J Mech Behav Biomed Mater. 2011;4(1):85–98.
17. Sun W, Li K, Sirois E. Simulated elliptical bioprosthetic valve deformation: implications for asymmetric transcatheter valve deployment. J Biomech. 2010;43(16):3085–90.
18. Auricchio F, et al. Simulation of transcatheter aortic valve implantation: a patient-specific finite element approach. Comput Method Biomech Biomed Eng. 2014;17(12):1347–57.
19. Capelli C, et al. Patient-specific simulations of transcatheter aortic valve stent implantation. Med Biol Eng Comput. 2012;50(2):183–92.
20. Tzamtzis S, et al. Numerical analysis of the radial force produced by the Medtronic-CoreValve and Edwards-SAPIEN after transcatheter aortic valve implantation (TAVI). Med Eng Phys. 2013;35(1):125–30.
21. Gessat M, et al. Image-based mechanical analysis of stent deformation: concept and exemplary implementation for aortic valve stents. IEEE Trans Biomed Eng. 2014;61(1):4–15.
22. Morganti S, et al. Simulation of transcatheter aortic valve implantation through patient-specific finite element analysis: two clinical cases. J Biomech. 2014;47(11):2547–55.
23. Yushkevich PA, et al. User-guided 3D active contour segmentation of anatomical structures: significantly improved efficiency and reliability. NeuroImage. 2006;31(3):1116–28.
24. Gnyaneshwar R, Kumar RK, Balakrishnan KR. Dynamic analysis of the aortic valve using a finite element model. Ann Thorac Surg. 2002;73(4):1122–9.
25. Martin C, Pham T, Sun W. Significant differences in the material properties between aged human and

porcine aortic tissues. Eur J Cardiothorac Surg. 2011;40(1):28–34.

26. Trowbridge EA, Black MM, Daniel CL. The mechanical response of glutaraldehyde-fixed bovine pericardium to uniaxial load. J Mater Sci. 1985;20(1): 114–40.

27. Xiong FL, et al. Finite element investigation of stentless pericardial aortic valves: relevance of leaflet geometry. Ann Biomed Eng. 2010;38(5): 1908–18.

28. Feuchtner G, et al. Prediction of paravalvular regurgitation after transcatheter aortic valve implantation by computed tomography: value of aortic valve and annular calcification. Ann Thorac Surg. 2013;96(5):1574–80.

29. Eker A, et al. Aortic annulus rupture during transcatheter aortic valve implantation: safe aortic root replacement. Eur J Cardiothorac Surg. 2012;41(5):1205.

30. Auricchio F, et al. A computational tool to support pre-operative planning of stentless aortic valve implant. Med Eng Phys. 2011;33(10):1183–92.

31. Auricchio F, et al. Patient-specific simulation of a stentless aortic valve implant: the impact of fibres on leaflet performance. Comput Method Biomech Biomed Eng. 2014;17(3):277–85.

32. Morganti S, et al. Prediction of patient-specific postoperative outcomes of TAVI procedure: the impact of the positioning strategy on valve performance. J Biomech. 2016;49(12):2513–9.

33. Auricchio F, et al. Shape memory alloy: from constitutive modeling to finite element analysis of stent deployment. Comput Model Eng Sci (CMES). 2010;57(3):225–43.

34. Schultz CJ, et al. Geometry and degree of apposition of the CoreValve ReValving system with multislice computed tomography after implantation in patients with aortic stenosis. J Am Coll Cardiol. 2009;54(10):911–8.

35. Zegdi R, et al. Is it reasonable to treat all calcified stenotic aortic valves with a valved stent?: Results from a human anatomic study in adults. J Am Coll Cardiol. 2008;51(5):579–84.

36. Iqbal J, Serruys PW. Comparison of Medtronic CoreValve and Edwards Sapien XT for transcatheter aortic valve implantation. JACC Cardiovasc Interv. 2014;7:293–5.

Haemodynamic Issues with Transcatheter Aortic Valve Implantation

5

Jacob Salmonsmith, Anna Maria Tango, Andrea Ducci, and Gaetano Burriesci

Abbreviations

ΔP	Change in pressure (i.e. aortic transvalvular pressure gradient)
EOA	Effective orifice area
GOA	Geometric orifice area
PVL	Paravalvular leakage
RBC	Red blood cell
SAV	Surgical aortic valve
SAVR	Surgical aortic valve replacement
SCLT	Subclinical leaflet thrombosis
STJ	Sinotubular junction
TAV	Transcatheter aortic valve
TAVI	Transcatheter aortic valve implantation
ViV	Valve-in-valve
WSS	Wall shear stress

J. Salmonsmith · A. M. Tango
Cardiovascular Engineering Laboratory,
UCL Mechanical Engineering, University College
London, Torrington Place, London, UK
e-mail: ucemjas@ucl.ac.uk; a.tango@ucl.ac.uk

A. Ducci
UCL Mechanical Engineering, University College
London, Torrington Place, London, UK
e-mail: a.ducci@ucl.ac.uk

G. Burriesci (✉)
Cardiovascular Engineering Laboratory,
UCL Mechanical Engineering, University College
London, Torrington Place, London, UK

Bioengineering Group, Ri.MED Foundation,
Palermo, Italy
e-mail: g.burriesci@ucl.ac.uk

5.1 Introduction

Heart valves ensure unidirectional blood flow throughout the cardiac cycle, and their operation is directly controlled by the pressure difference and local flow dynamics upstream and downstream of the valve. This passive mechanism implies that the interaction between the valve components and their surrounding fluid environment is critical to optimal valve function. As a consequence, the haemodynamics, or blood motion, within the aortic root provides crucial information and indicators about the performance and prognostication of heart valves. Analyses of these haemodynamics enable improved design of prosthetic replacement heart valves by enhancing the valve performance. Taking inspiration from the flow dynamics observed in healthy, physiological valves, such as vortex generation patterns, may aid the improvement of the valve performance as well as improving less quantifiable flow properties such as turbulence levels or stagnation zones. In fact, non-physiologically high blood shear can result in blood damage in the form of haemolysis and/or platelet activation, whilst at the other extreme, low shear can lead to blood stagnation and thrombosis, with coagulation occurring more quickly on artificial surfaces [1].

Native valve pathologies, such as senile calcification, can severely alter the local flow downstream of the aortic valve, impairing its function. When the haemodynamic performance

© Springer Nature Switzerland AG 2019
A. Giordano et al. (eds.), *Transcatheter Aortic Valve Implantation*,
https://doi.org/10.1007/978-3-030-05912-5_5

is deemed to be insufficient and the native valve is replaced with a prosthetic valve, the haemodynamics of the region would ideally be returned to the healthy physiological state, but the current level of clinical intervention does not allow a full recovery of the optimum valve haemodynamics and results in increased peak blood flow velocity, formation of stagnant regions within the Valsalva sinuses, and/or local flow characteristics that increase the risk of haemolysis.

The non-invasive nature of transcatheter aortic valve implantation (TAVI), also called transcatheter aortic valve replacement (TAVR), provides treatment for patients who would be too weak for surgery, but also results in the calcified native leaflets being kept in the aortic region, left in a forced open position between the prosthetic valve and the sinuses of Valsalva. As a consequence, besides the non-optimum haemodynamics comparable to those of a surgical aortic valve (SAV) procedure, TAVI results in further changes to the local flow dynamics. In order to fully clarify and interpret these changes, some basic review of the critical haemodynamic factors affecting the valve safety and performance is necessary, as well as a summary of the haemodynamic conditions occurring in healthy and pathological native valves and after correction with bioprosthetic SAVs and TAVs.

5.2   Haemodynamic Considerations

The pulsatile nature of blood flow results in four distinct stages of the cardiac cycle for the aortic valve: opening, open, closing, and closed.

As valve opening is initiated, it is important that the valve provides minimal resistance, promptly reconfiguring to offer the largest possible orifice area of the valve and, hence, conserve as much of the energy and pressure of the flow as possible [2]. In this stage, the valve resistance is related to the energy needed to reverse the leaflet curvature between the shut and open configurations. A prompt opening, requiring lower pressure differences across the valve leaflets, results in minimum flow energy

loss, and lower levels of strain and stress in the leaflets [2].

During the ejection phase, the widest valve opening is desirable, as it would utilise as much of the aortic lumen as possible, reducing the energetic losses. The valve opening is quantified by the geometric orifice area (GOA), defined as the smallest transversal section encompassed within the open leaflets at the maximum systolic pressure. However, this parameter is difficult to measure in clinical environments and is not directly related to the systolic performance of the valve. In fact, the effective dimension of the ejected flow does not only depend on the area of the valve passage, but also on the downstream jet contraction due to leaflet profile and the extension and location of the vortices generated at the valve exit. Hence, a more indicative quantification of the haemodynamic efficiency during valve opening is provided by the effective orifice area (EOA), which corresponds to the cross-sectional area of the blood streamtube (a tubular region of fluid delimited by streamlines, i.e. lines locally parallel to the flow) ejected through the valve during systole, at the downstream point of its maximum contraction (*vena contracta*) [3, 4]. The EOA is directly proportional to the systolic flow rate and inversely proportional to the transvalvular pressure drop (ΔP) across the valve and can be easily estimated *in vivo* and *in vitro*. GOA and EOA are directly related to the cross-section geometry of the jet flow contraction. Another factor that may introduce fluid energy losses, concurring to increased ΔP, is the presence of turbulence generated by non-physiological peak blood velocities [5].

Valve closure is determined by a combination of reverse transvalvular pressure, associated with the drop in pressure in the left ventricle due to diastolic relaxation, and the action of the vortices in the sinuses, which guide the leaflets profile before and during closure [6]. The synergy between these two mechanisms reduces the closing regurgitant volume and the loss of flow energy. Similar to valve opening, a reduced resistance to the change in leaflets' curvature also contributes to reduce the stresses in the leaflets and minimise the energy consumed during closing.

Once the valve is fully closed, the main factor responsible for the loss of performance is the leakage of blood from the aorta to the ventricle. In the case of native valves, this is typically due to valvular incompetency (intra-valvular leakage). For prosthetic valves and, in particular, TAVI devices, paravalvular leakage (PVL) external to the functional leaflets, occurring through potential gaps between the implanted valve and the surrounding host tissues, can be a major contributor to the regurgitant volume.

In summary, the overall left ventricular energy loss during the valve function is primarily associated with the ΔP across the aortic valve during systole, also related to the EOA, and with regurgitation during diastole [7].

However, other fluid dynamic parameters acting at a more local scale need to be taken into account, in order to evaluate the safety and efficacy of heart valves. As mentioned above, alteration of the physiological flow may induce turbulence, which is related to chaotic velocity fluctuations, and leads to increased aortic wall and leaflet stresses and an elevated risk of haemolysis. Also, during the cardiac cycle the levels of shear rate and shear stress experienced by the blood vary greatly, with undesirable phenomena resulting at both non-physiologically high and low shear rates [1], promoting red blood cell (RBC) damage [8]. High blood shear rate results into haemolysis, especially when exacerbated by prolonged exposure, with the rupture of RBCs releasing their contents, and increasing the platelet activation levels and thrombogenicity of the blood [1, 9]. Activated platelets are complementary to the aggregation of RBCs and have been identified as the primary cells involved in cardio-embolism, via haemostasis and thrombosis [10, 11]. As the flow has a significant role in platelet activation, any deviation from the healthy, physiological behaviour is of clinical concern [10]. Although there is no consensus on the magnitude of turbulent viscous shear stress (calculated as the viscous dissipation of turbulent energy) or Reynolds shear stress (derived from the effect of convective acceleration upon the mean velocity profile) to be identified for the threshold of haemolysis, it is agreed that the higher the shear stress and the longer the exposure, the greater the amount of haemolysis [9, 12, 13]. In addition, the presence of turbulent blood flow, with associated high levels of turbulent stress, can also result in platelet activation and endothelial cell damage to the vessel walls [14, 15].

On the other end of the scale, shear stresses below a threshold of 0.4 Pa increase the likelihood of thrombosis and cell aggregation, with platelets adhering to the surfaces leading to the formation of thrombi in sizes inversely proportional to the shear forces produced in static and low-flow conditions [1, 16–18]. As well as the amount of flow stasis, thrombogenicity is affected by the amount and type of non-native material in contact with the blood, and the blood coagulability, dependent upon blood properties such as haematocrit and protein levels and any anti-coagulation regimen [18]. Washout of a region will decrease the risk of thrombosis, with a RBC residence time less than 10 s significantly reducing the chance of cell aggregation, and blood flow speeds higher than 0.05 m/s drastically reducing any persistent stagnation [18, 19]. The washout effect associated with the vortices shed from the aortic leaflets during systole reduces the prolonged presence of activated platelets in the sinuses of Valsalva [18]. Once thrombi form and grow, portions may break away from the primary site and block cardiovascular vessels, causing downstream areas of the body to become starved of oxygen and other nutrients, with potentially fatal consequences, such as a stroke or myocardial infarction [20]. Even if not detached, thrombus formation upon the bioprosthetic leaflets has been identified as the primary event resulting in reduced leaflet motion [21], potentially causing suboptimal valve performance and flow separation downstream of the valve.

5.3 Physiological Haemodynamics

5.3.1 Healthy

The proper operating function of the native healthy valve is directly controlled by the interaction between the leaflets and the structural/fluid

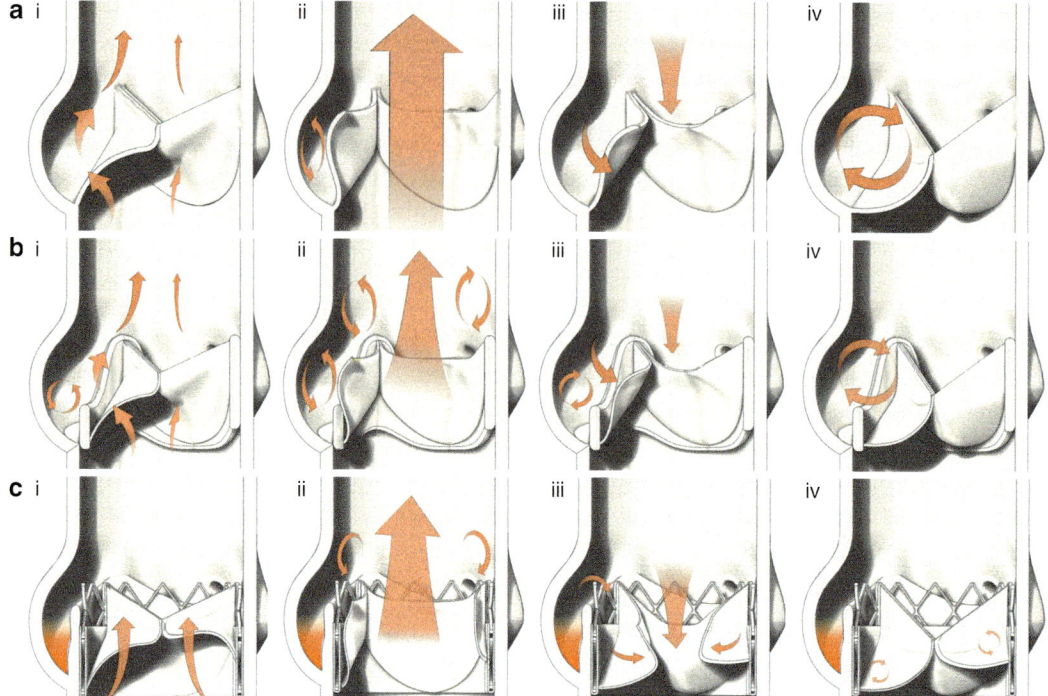

Fig. 5.1 Schematics of fluid flow within the aortic root throughout the cardiac cycle for physiological (**a**), post-surgical (**b**), and post-transcatheter valve implantation (**c**) configurations. (**a**) (**i**) As the valve opens, radial flow directed towards the sinuses from the valve inflow supports leaflet motion towards the open configuration; (**ii**) the leaflets assume an approximately circular orifice shape, as a jet is ejected through the valve, and vortices are generated at the leaflets' edge - these vortices are subsequently captured within the Valsalva sinuses; (**iii**) at the end of systole, the pressure difference inversion and reverse flow generate a vortex ring with the opposite rotation, aiding valve closure; (**iv**) the vortex fills the whole sinus in diastole, washing out the region. (**b**) (**i**) The flow is similar to that in (**a**), although the presence of the sewing ring and covered stent reduces the orifice area and results in a vortex at the base of the sinus; (**ii**) a non-physiological vortex forms above the commissure stent post, impinging the jet flow, whilst the sinus vortex either remains in the sinus or migrates into the aortic root, depending on the relative size of the surgical valve. If the vortex migrates, a second vortex forms in its stead, with opposite rotation direction; (**iii**) this counter vortex is still effective in washing out the sinus and supporting valve closure; (**iv**) similar to A, during diastole, the vortex fills the whole sinus and washes out the region. (**c**) (**i**) the native leaflets form a permanent pseudo-cylindrical structure around the prosthesis, decreasing the sinus volume, reducing flow in the lower regions of the sinus throughout the cycle, and potentially preventing the prosthetic valve from fully expanding to its designed geometry, thus narrowing the geometric orifice; (**ii**) the vortices generated by the opening of the valve do not remain at the bioprosthetic's leaflets' edges, but rather at the tip of the stationary native leaflets, delaying the opening of the valve and reducing sinus washout; (**iii**) during valve closure, the vortical structures observed in the physiological configuration are not present, reducing washout of the sinuses and delaying valve closure; (**iv**) the sinus filling vortex observed in (**a**) and (**b**) is not present, reducing washout during diastole

dynamics established in the aortic root (Fig. 5.1a) [6, 22, 23]. The valve opens under the effect of an essentially radial flow, directed from the valve inflow towards the Valsalva's sinuses and following the root wall so as to realign with the root axis towards the sinotubular junction (STJ) [24]. This mechanism supports a prompt leaflet motion towards the open configuration, with the leaflets pushed into the sinuses until they assume an approximately circular orifice shape [25]. During this stage, a jet with a nearly flat velocity profile is ejected into the aortic root, with very little reverse flow through the aortic annulus during systole [25, 26]. At the beginning of systole, the interaction between this fast jet and the low inertial flow in the developing boundary layer of the root results in the formation of vortices at the valve exit [26, 27]. These vortices are captured in the sinuses throughout the forward flow phase, up to the early stages of diastole, disappearing only after complete valve closure [26]. As the vortices are confined, the central jet flow is unrestricted as it spreads out across the aortic root at the STJ, occupying most of the root section [26]. The presence of the vortices in the sinuses also contributes to stabilise the leaflets' position during the forward flow phase, keeping them away from the aortic lumen [27]. The flow becomes more complex further downstream in the aortic arch [25, 26].

In late systole and early diastole, the pressure difference inversion and reverse flow generate a vortex ring spinning in the opposite direction to that observed after valve opening. Though axial pressure alone is sufficient to close the valve, this vortical structure promotes a swift and efficient closure [27, 28], minimising the closing regurgitation. The location and size of these vortices affect the pressure within the sinuses, with optimal position aiding the coronary flow and pressure gradient across the coronary ostia [28]. The closing vortex fills the whole sinus throughout diastole, providing continuous washout of the region, even when the overall blood velocity is zero.

Physiological flow conditions are also essential in maintaining the healthy mechanical properties and function of the tissues of the leaflets and root. In fact, together with the annulus expansion and contraction during the cycle, the physiological opening and closing mechanisms described above minimise the levels of shear and bending stresses in the leaflets, high levels of which would typically result in tissue degradation [29]. Moreover, it has been reported that the majority of aortic valve diseases occur on the aortic side of the valve, which might be directly linked with the more unstable flow conditions and shear rate present on the downstream side of the valve, as opposed to the comparably more uniform and regular ventricular flow [27]. Altered velocity gradients (i.e. shear rate) leading to abnormal viscous forces at the root wall have been shown to potentially change gene expres-sions, resulting in endothelial remodelling and alterations of the root geometry [30]. Healthy aortic root regions experience an average wall shear stress (WSS) of 13.3 Pa at peak systole, with an increase in WSS towards the leaflet tips [31]. Oscillating shear stress at a magnitude lower than that experienced physiologically is associated with regions prone to atherosclerosis, resulting in a far more aggressive and proliferative phenotype [17].

5.3.2 Pathological and Surgically Corrected

Various pathologies can affect the performance of the aortic valve, with degenerative aortic valve stenosis due to senile calcification currently the most prevalent valvular disease, affecting about 3% of individuals over the age of 65 [32] and more than 10% of adults over the age of 75 [33]. Treatment of calcific aortic stenosis via pharmacological therapies is currently limited and palliative, being unable to reverse or prevent the progression of aortic stenosis [34]. As a result of the increased leaflet stiffness due to calcification, the resultant haemodynamics are altered, with a reduction in EOA and less complete closing of the valve [27]. As the main jet cross section reduces in size, the peak velocity correspondingly increases — for example, a mildly stenotic valve of orifice area 1.5 cm^2 (for a reference STJ diameter of 2.5 cm) can result in a ΔP of 20 mmHg and peak jet velocities up to 70% faster than in the healthy condition [35, 36]. Consequentially, the elevated levels of shear stress and turbulence intensity increase the likelihood of damage to the root walls and blood, whilst the jet itself is typically angulated and off-centred [36]. Combined with commonly asymmetrical leaflet calcification across the aortic valve leaflets, this can result in very complex patient-specific conditions, especially when surface irregularities of calcified leaflets are taken into account [27].

For a more severe stenosis, the ΔP may rise above 40 mmHg and the EOA may drop beneath 1 cm^2, with the outflow jet diameter significantly decreased at the base of the aorta, reducing the size of the central jet and increasing the flow's peak velocity by up to four times that of the physiological condition [27, 35]. This is accompanied by increased flow separation and highly turbulent shear layers between the central jet and the walls of the aortic root, enough to cause damage to RBCs and platelets within the flow, and to the endothelial cells on the aortic walls [27]. In addition to the elevated risk of thrombosis and thromboembolism, the altered wall shear stress can lead to dilation of the ascending aorta, whilst the increased force of the faster jet can weaken the distal portion of the ascending arch [36].

Valve stenosis can also significantly alter the flow in the Valsalva sinus, with the systolic vortices becoming larger and more distorted, and located further from the leaflet tips soon after generation [31]. As a result, rather than being confined within the sinuses during valve closure and enhance the efficiency of this phase, the vortices leave the sinus region during late systole [26, 31], causing further deterioration to the cardiovascular performance. In addition, the reduced recirculation in the sinus might be linked to the decrease in coronary flow, which has been encountered alongside an increase in leaflet stiffness [37].

Surgical valve replacement via bioprosthetic substitutes aims to restore healthy functional conditions and physiological haemodynamics. However, whilst biological tissue valves are more biomechanically compatible than their mechanical counterparts, they are still not able to reproduce the healthy physiological state (Fig. 5.1b) [2, 26]. In fact, the presence of the supporting stent and the implantation strategy determine a mismatch between the aortic root and the shape and position of the prosthetic leaflets. The presence of the sewing ring and pledget-armed sutures used to fix the valve into place at the basal annulus, together with the restriction due to the stent thickness, result in a reduction of the GOA [38]. Similarly, the structures of the man-made commissures and the increased stiffness of the crosslinked tissue determine the formation of a non-physiological vortex above the commissures, which expands as the flow rate decreases in

late systole. This impinges upon the central jet flow [26] and affects the flow in the sinus [39]. Depending on the proportion between the bioprosthetis and the host root, the start-up vortex generated in early systole remains in the sinus, as in the physiological case, or migrates into the aortic root, narrowing the flow and decreasing the potential performance of the valve [26]. In its stead, a second vortex forms in the sinus, with a direction of rotation opposite to that of the initial vortex, which is still effective in providing washout of the sinuses and supporting valve closure — the configuration produces similar levels of regurgitation to a larger surgical valve with vortical structures more closely aligned to those observed physiologically [26].

All these factors contribute towards producing a slightly stenotic valve performance, characterised by an increase of peak jet velocity and ΔP of 70% and 60% respectively, whilst the EOA reduces by 30%, when compared to that of a native valve in the same size aortic root [26, 40]. The smaller leaflet lengths appear to reduce the closing regurgitant volume, mitigating some of the loss due to the smaller EOA [26]. Bioprosthetic valve performance can be improved by using stentless configurations, which give less forward flow obstruction and improved haemodynamic performance compared to their stented equivalents [40]. However, their production and implantation procedure are more complex, and their performance can be affected by the irregularity of the host anatomy, and by procedural inaccuracies. In fact, the leaflets are normally designed to operate properly in a regular circular configuration, which is difficult to attain in the absence of a supporting stent. Generally, stentless valves are reported to restore flow velocities closed to the physiological ones, and better coronary flow than their stented equivalents, due to the resultant lower transvalvular pressure drop and the decreased turbulence downstream of the valve [41].

The leaflets of bioprosthetic valves are usually constructed out of porcine or bovine tissue [42], which makes them vulnerable to calcification, resulting in valve stenosis and associated higher ΔP and peak blood flow velocity [40]. Leaflets have been constructed from polymeric materials to prevent calcification, but these tend to have more constricted flow orifices, reducing valve performance, decreasing the central jet diameter, and increasing the shear stresses experienced by the blood flow [43].

5.3.3 TAVI Haemodynamics

Transcatheter valves merge some of the features of stented and stentless bioprosthetic valves, maintaining the presence of a frame which supports and leads the prosthetic leaflets' attachment line, but minimising its thickness to about 0.5 mm [44, 45]. Due to the presence of the pathological native leaflets, the functional orifice area of the transcatheter aortic valve (TAV) may be limited by the irregularly calcified native valve leaflets, and operate at a configuration that is suboptimal, normally smaller than the fully expanded design geometry [46, 47]. In fact, the nature of the implantation procedure, whether trans-femoral, trans-apical, or otherwise, implies an inherently increased level of variability of prosthetic valve positioning than in an equivalent surgical aortic valve replacement (SAVR) procedure [48]. Deviation from the ideal position by a few millimetres can potentially result in alteration of valvular haemodynamics, decreased ventricular performance, decreased TAV durability, seal zone mismatch leading to severe PVL, coronary artery obstruction, conduction abnormalities, and/or increased wall stress potentially resulting in valve embolization or annulus rupture [48, 49]. Moreover, implanting the TAV into an annulus with a relatively high degree of ovality, exacerbated by heavy calcification or an inhomogeneous implantation layer, can result in the TAV itself being warped and/or deployed with an oval shape, without the possibility to correct this imperfection [46, 50]. High level of eccentricity may lead to large increase in regurgitation, probably due to the lack of leaflet apposition [46, 51]. Oversizing is commonly used to overcome this issue and attain more secure valve anchoring, but it can adversely affect the valve haemodynamics [52, 53]. In fact, excess leaflet tissue relative to the stent orifice area results in severe/moderate stenosis of the TAV, increasing ΔP by up to three times [54].

Despite the mentioned limitations, transcatheter valves still result in reduced patient prosthesis mismatch compared to SAV, as the valve expands to fit into an annulus which, in turn, distends to an extent, accommodating a better valve fit [45]. As a result, the procedure is normally characterised by a larger increase in the systolic performance, with ΔP below 10 mmHg and EOA up to 2.0 cm^2, for a reference STJ diameter of 2.5 cm, with this performance maintained at follow-up [45, 55].

Nevertheless, the fluid dynamics of the region after TAVI are different to both the healthy native aortic region and a post-SAVR aortic region (Fig. 5.1c), with some of the prominent complications observed being flow separation regions downstream of the valve, energy losses across the valve, non-physiological coronary flow, and PVL [42]. Further complications can also occur downstream of the valve, and TAVI is associated with an increased risk of stroke, cerebral embolism, and silent ischaemic lesions post-implantation [56–59].

The difference in flow pattern is mainly due to the fact that the calcified leaflets are not removed during the implantation, but rather radially displaced into the Valsalva's sinuses, in a permanently open position. As a result, the volume of these sinuses is reduced by the presence of the displaced native leaflets, and radial flow during systole is confined to the upper regions of the sinus, around the free edges of the native leaflets [60]. Consequently, average flow velocity in the sinuses of Valsalva is reduced to a quarter of the physiological velocity, and the peak velocity in the region is halved [61]. This reduction in the fluid velocity and shear rate increases the chance of formation of thrombi [24, 62], whose fracture and downstream transportation can eventually lead to neurological pathologies [56–59].

The space between the native leaflets and the TAV stent can be regarded as a neo-sinus, with a size dependent upon not only the geometry of the native region and the prosthesis, but also the angular orientation of the TAV — non-alignment of the TAV with the commissures may further reduce the flow within sinuses [63]. Flow in the neo-sinuses may be particularly prone to stagnation and associated thrombosis; so lowering the heart rate whilst increasing the stroke volume maintains the cardiac output but improves the flow in this region, reducing the chance of leaflet thrombosis [63]. As previously mentioned, the flow within the Valsalva sinuses plays a key role in blood supply to the coronary arteries and sinus washout [6, 22, 64].

The described configuration of the implant also determines major variations in both the fluid mechanics and operating mechanisms of the valve [24]. In the case of TAVI devices, the start-up vortices generated during opening do not hold in position at the tip of the dynamic leaflets inside the upper part of the sinus, but form further downstream at the edge of the native leaflets, which act as a continuous wall [24]. This is associated with reduced washout of the sinuses [24, 51] and some delay of around 10 ms in the opening of the valve [61, 65].

During systole, in most designs the valve stent prevents the operating leaflets from opening beyond $90°$, resulting in a narrower, centrally located systolic jet [61, 65], characterised by higher peak velocities, up to double that in healthy native valves [5, 25, 64]. The raised central jet velocities produce higher viscous shear stresses, up to 6 Pa [51], which, however, is still below the haemolytic threshold [60].

During valve closing, the return of fluid in the axial direction is not accompanied by the vortical structures observed in the physiological configuration, reducing washout of the sinuses [24]. The presence of the static native leaflets also alters the effect of the fluid suction generated by the closing leaflets upon the fluid within the sinuses [60]. Consequently, valve closure is delayed by about 10 ms [61, 65], and extended and prolonged stagnation zones develop between each sinus and its corresponding native leaflet throughout the entire cardiac cycle, with a shear rate below $100 \, s^{-1}$ [24, 48].

During the closed stage, PVL is far more common than in SAV, due to the elliptical shape of the native annulus combined with heavy calcification of the region, which can lead to a reduction of annular sealing [41, 75–77]. Asymmetrical deployment may also result in intra-valvular leakage, as full closure of the leaflets is inhibited by the deployed frame shape [46, 66]. The high level of PVL is mitigated to an extent by redilation of the prosthesis and, in more recent devices, by the use of external skirts around the upstream base of the valve frame [65, 67]. Despite these improvements, moderate and severe PVL is still frequent in TAVI and is associated with increased mortality [66]. In fcat, PVL produces substantial energy losses in diastole, imposing a higher workload upon the left ventricle [54]. This form of leakage may be reduced in the months post-procedure by tissue overgrowth from the surrounding physiology and/or coagulation of blood filling in the gaps between the prosthesis and host tissue. However, mild leakages are reported as remaining constants, and the statistics indicating decreases in severe or moderate PVL over time may be biased by the increased mortality associated with higher levels of PVL [66, 68].

The regions of flow stagnation described as a result of TAV implantation can lead to thrombo-embolic complications [60, 64]. In particular, the regions of permanent low level of shear rate observed at the base of the Valsalva's sinuses, associated with the rheology of blood, lead to a substantial increase in the local dynamic viscosity, thus prolonging residence time and producing thrombogenic conditions [24]. This effect is mitigated in the coronary sinuses, as the flow accessing the coronary arteries slightly increases the shear stress in the sinus [39]. The sinus flow alterations can have a detrimental effect upon the coronary reserve, with reductions of up to 20% of the coronary flow [22, 69, 70]. This is not necessarily a critical problem, as myocardial demand typically reduces as a result of improved left ventricular performance, but this may depend on the long-term myocardial needs of the individual patient [41].

The effect of TAV on coronary artery flow is not agreed upon in the literature. There are reports that the post-TAV implantation flow of some coronary arteries is increased from the pathological level, thanks to decreased central flow velocity, reducing the resultant Venturi effect during systole, and improved coronary bed pressure gradients [41]. However, there are also reports that sinus flow alterations resulting from TAVI in aortic roots with low positioned coronary ostia may have a reduction in coronary flow by up to 20% [68]. Coronary ostia have an increased risk of being obstructed when in the vicinity of native leaflets thickened due to calcification, a problem exacerbated by using an oversized TAV relative to the native region [62, 71]. The implantation procedure itself can also cause obstruction, whether due to fragmentation of the calcified native leaflet during TAV insertion, high implantation of the TAV, or as a consequence of a balloon expansion method [55].

Non-ideal positioning of the TAV also increases the risk of coronary ischaemia and conduction abnormalities of the heart, with atrioventricular block occurring after 16% of procedures, compared to 1% of SAVR [44, 72–74].

Increased blood residence times have also been observed close to the leaflets and around the non-physiological neo-sinus zone in general, resulting in more thrombotic conditions [75]. As a result, risk of clinical thrombotic events is not insignificant after TAVI, particularly in the first 3 months following the implant, with most cases occurring within 6 months; although the variance in manifestation is large, with some events occurring within 2 weeks of the procedure and others not becoming present for over 9 months [76, 77]. If the thrombosis does not directly affect the valve performance, this may be undetected for some time, as subclinical leaflet thrombosis (SCLT) results in the presence of lesions and reduced leaflet motion, but not to the extent that the valve performance is noticeably affected [78, 79]. Though the performance of the valve is not affected, SCLT can be associated with transient ischaemic attacks and strokes, so prevention may improve long-term clinical outcomes [78]. Clinical thrombotic behaviour is observed when the thrombosis reduces the mobility of the prosthetic leaflets, thus increasing the transvalvular pressure drop [76, 77]. Clinical thrombosis is treatable by oral anti-coagulation, such as

Heparin or Warfarin, which restores both TAV function and, correspondingly, haemodynamic performance for 75% of patients, although this anti-coagulation treatment is not a viable option for all patients [64, 76]. The increased level of co-morbidities of the older patients who require TAVI is possibly an important contributing factor to thrombosis [79], though it is plausible that the valve thrombosis is caused by the leaflets themselves, due to the high levels of inflammatory cells in the thrombus. In fact, leaflet damage occurring during balloon expansion can result in native leaflet fissuring, perforation, and endothelial denudation [76, 77], increasing the likelihood of thrombosis [78, 79]. It is still debated if the metallic frame of TAVs may act as a nidus for thrombi until endothelialization occurs, although it is plausible that the level of turbulent shear stresses in the region should provide sufficient washout [64, 76, 79]. Folding or geometric confinement of the leaflets may increase the blood residence time, indicated as a permissive factor in TAV leaflet thrombosis, with no preference to occurrence on the leaflet associated with the non-coronary sinus [75]. The lower rate of thrombosis in bioprostheses when the native valve is excised suggests that the lack of native leaflet ablation for TAVI may be another source of thrombosis, as their presence causes a reduction of sinus washout during systole [24, 63].

5.3.4 Valve-In-Valve

Another relevant application of TAVI is their use for the treatment of dysfunctional or underperforming bioprosthetic valves [55, 66, 71], by expanding the device inside a previously implanted prosthesis, in a valve-in-valve (ViV) configuration.

The approach further narrows the orifice area, and therefore it may not be indicated for patients requiring small prostheses, as this additional reduction may result in critically reduced valve performance [66, 80, 81]. Supra-annular positioning can help to reduce this negative effect, allowing the transvalvular pressure drop to halve, but increase the risk of further reduction of the flow in the sinuses [82]. In fact, as the flexibility of the stent posts of the host prosthetic valve is greater than the annulus, they tend to splay outwards, resulting in a 'flower pot' arrangement [53] which results in a less constrained operating configuration for the operating leaflets, especially at their free margin. Moreover, this provides a wedge effect which improves the securing of the valve, especially in the case of balloon-expandable devices, where the post-ballooning recoil results in the radial forces being reduced as the prosthesis is fitted into the rigid section at the base of the host stent [83].

Though effective in dropping the energetic losses during systole, the 'flower pot' arrangement narrows the available access to the Valsalva's sinuses, resulting in further reduction of the sinus washout [80]. However, the increase in stagnation is less severe in the coronary sinuses, as the flow towards the ostia generates some motion in the region [39]. Still, the chance of coronary obstruction is raised after ViV treatment, especially when the original prosthesis had badly calcified leaflets, the ostia are located close to the annulus, the aortic region and STJ have a narrow diameter, and/or the sinuses themselves are particularly narrow [41, 68, 71, 80].

Blood residence time is reported to increase also in the neo-sinuses, in proximity of the TAV leaflets, with a longer residence time during systole (about 40% longer) and higher mean value of residence time from the end of systole until mid-diastole (about 150% longer), elevating the thromboembolic risk of the valve [75]. In addition, other ViV issues include bad positioning of the TAV (15% of procedures), leaflet thrombosis (4%), coronary artery obstruction (3.5%), and increased conduction issues for ViV configurations than for TAVI within a native valve [66, 80].

5.4   Conclusion

Being able to circumvent the necessity of surgery when replacing the aortic valve is the vital value of TAVI, enabling weak patients who would be at high risk of morbidity from surgery to receive life changing improvements to their cardiac function. However, this primary benefit necessarily comes with some drawbacks, which need to be fully understood, appreciated, and assessed when pondering the opportunity to expand the crucial advantages of TAVI to lower risk patients and devising new generation valves.

The presence of the native leaflets reduces the sinus volume [60], restricting the flow in the Valsalva sinus chambers [61] and minimising the development of vortical structures and associated flow, especially at the basal end of the sinuses [24]. Coronary arteries with particularly low ostia seem to be at higher risk of reduced flow or blockage by either the native leaflet or a detached thrombus from the basal portion of the sinus [62, 71]. Similarly, the region between the native and the bioprosthetic leaflets is also particularly prone to stagnation and thrombus formation [75]. In the case of valve-in-valve procedures, the functional orifice area is further reduced, whilst blood residence time in the sinuses is increased again due to even more diminished sinus washout [66, 80, 81]. These thrombogenic conditions could be linked to the increased rates of strokes and transient ischaemic attacks [56–59], as well as the more recent concern of subclinical leaflets thrombosis [78, 79]. Anti-coagulation treatment can be used to control these thrombotic concerns, although this comes with the inherent risks and management of the anticoagulant drugs themselves [64, 76].

In terms of orifice area, the TAV's design and method of expansion enables a better fit into the annulus than the rigid SAV [45]. However, the positioning of transcatheter devices is currently less precise and affected by the asymmetries of the host region [46, 50], and these factors have been linked to increased leakage of the bioprosthesis [46, 51].

Despite these drawbacks, the resultant blood flow through a TAV after implantation is much improved from that of a moderately stenotic valve — blood velocity is decreased [5, 64], and the shear stress of the aortic region is normally maintained below the haemolytic threshold [51, 60]. The bioprosthetis produces good pressure gradients, generally below 10 mmHg [45, 55], and these benefits normally outweigh the disadvantages highlighted above, especially in high-risk patients.

References

1. Corbett SC, Ajdari A, Coskun AU, N-Hashemi H. In vitro and computational thrombosis on artificial surfaces with shear stress. Artif Organs. 2010;34(7):561–9.

2. Burriesci G, Marincola FC, Zervides C. Design of a novel polymeric heart valve. J Med Eng Technol. 2010;34(1):7–22.

3. Gorlin R, Gorlin SG. Hydraulic formula for calculation of the area of the stenotic mitral valve, other cardiac valves, and central circulatory shunts. I. Am Heart J. 1951;41(1):1–29.

4. Akins CW, Travis B, Yoganathan AP. Energy loss for evaluating heart valve performance. J Thorac Cardiovasc Surg [Internet]. 2008;136(4):820–33. https://doi.org/10.1016/j.jtcvs.2007.12.059

5. Saikrishnan N, Gupta S, Yoganathan AP. Hemodynamics of the Boston Scientific Lotus™ valve: an in vitro study. Cardiovasc Eng Technol. 2013;4(4):427–39.

6. Bellhouse BJ, Bellhouse FH. Mechanism of closure of the aortic valve. Nature. 1968;217:86–7.

7. Rahmani B, Tzamtzis S, Sheridan R, Mullen MJ, Yap J, Seifalian AM, et al. In vitro hydrodynamic assessment of a new transcatheter heart valve concept (the TRISKELE). J Cardiovasc Transl Res. 2017;10(2):104–15.

8. Dasi LP, Simon HA, Sucosky P, Yoganathan AP. Fluid mechanics of artificial heart valves. Clin Exp Pharmacol Physiol. 2009;36(2):225–37.

9. Leverett LB, Hellums JD, Alfrey CP, Lynch EC. Red blood cell damage by shear stress. Biophys J. 1972;12(3):257–73.

10. Morbiducci U, Ponzini R, Nobili M, Massai D, Montevecchi FM, Bluestein D, et al. Blood damage safety of prosthetic heart valves. Shear-induced platelet activation and local flow dynamics: a fluid-structure interaction approach. J Biomech. 2009;42(12):1952–60.

11. Heemskerk JWM, Bevers EM, Lindhout T. Platelet activation and blood coagulation. Thromb Haemost. 2002;88(2):186–93.

12. Caro CG, Pedley TJ, Schroter RC, Seed WA. The mechanics of circulation. 2nd ed. Cambridge: Oxford University Press; 2012.

13. Yen JH, Chen SF, Chern MK, Lu PC. The effect of turbulent viscous shear stress on red blood cell hemolysis. J Artif Organs. 2014;17(2):178–85.

14. Bluestein D, Chandran KB, Manning KB. Towards non-thrombogenic performance of blood recirculation devices. Ann Biomed Eng. 2010;38(3):1236–56.

15. Hope MD, Sedlic T, Dyverfeldt P. Cardiothoracic magnetic resonance flow imaging. J Thorac Imaging. 2013;28(4):217–30.

16. Baskurt OK, Meiselman HJ. Blood rheology and hemodynamics. Semin Thromb Hemost. 2003;29(5):435–50.

17. Malek AM, Alper SL, Izumo S. Hemodynamic shear stress and its role in atherosclerosis. J Am Med Assoc [Internet]. 1999;282(21):2035–42. http://jama.jamanetwork.com/article.aspx?doi=10.1001/jama.282.21.2035

18. Corbett SC, Ajdari A, Coskun AU, Nayeb-Hashemi H. Effect of pulsatile blood flow on thrombosis potential with a step wall transition. ASAIO J. 2010;56(4):290–5.

19. Wootton DM, Ku DN. Fluid mechanics of vascular systems, diseases, and thrombosis. Annu Rev Biomed Eng. 1999;1(1):299–329.

20. Chandran KB, Rittgers SE, Yoganathan AP. Biofluid mechanics—the human circulation. 2nd ed. Boca Raton: CRC Press; 2012.

21. Makkar RR, Fontana G, Jilaihawi H, Chakravarty T, Kofoed KF, De Backer O, et al. Possible subclinical leaflet thrombosis in bioprosthetic aortic valves. N Engl J Med. 2015;373(21):2015–24.

22. Van Steenhoven AA, Van Dongen MEH. Model studies of the closing behaviour of the aortic valve. J Fluid Mech. 1978;90:21–32.

23. Leyh RG, Schmidtke C, Sievers HH, Yacoub MH. Opening and closing characteristics of the aortic valve after different types of valve-preserving surgery. Circulation. 1999;100(21):2153–60.

24. Ducci A, Pirisi F, Tzamtzis S, Burriesci G. Transcatheter aortic valves produce unphysiological flows which may contribute to thromboembolic events: An in-vitro study. J Biomech. 2016;49(16):4080–9.

25. Sacks MS, David Merryman W, Schmidt DE. On the biomechanics of heart valve function. J Biomech. 2009;42(12):1804–24.

26. Toninato R, Salmon J, Susin FM, Ducci A, Burriesci G. Physiological vortices in the sinuses of Valsalva: an in vitro approach for bio-prosthetic valves. J Biomech. 2016;49(13):2635–43.

27. Sacks MS, Yoganathan AP. Heart valve function: a biomechanical perspective. Philos Trans R Soc B Biol Sci. 2007;362(1484):1369–91.

28. Korakianitis T, Shi Y. Numerical simulation of cardiovascular dynamics with healthy and diseased heart valves. J Biomech. 2006;39(11):1964–82.

29. Balachandran K, Sucosky P, Yoganathan AP. Hemodynamics and mechanobiology of aortic valve inflammation and calcification. Int J Inflam [Internet]. 2011;2011:263870. http://www.pubmedcentral.nih.gov/articlerender.fcgi?artid=3133012&tool=pmcentrez&rendertype=abstract

30. Barker AJ, Markl M. Editorial. The role of hemodynamics in bicuspid aortic valve disease. Eur J Cardiothorac Surg. 2011;39(6):805–6.

31. Amindari A, Saltik L, Kirkkopru K, Yacoub M, Yalcin HC. Assessment of calcified aortic valve leaflet deformations and blood flow dynamics using fluid-structure interaction modeling. Informatics Med Unlocked. 2017;9(September):191–9.

32. Otto CM, Lind BK, Kitzman DW, Gersh BJ, Siscovick DS. Association of aortic valve sclerosis

with cardiovascular mortality and morbidity in the elderly. N Engl J Med. 1999;341:142–7.

33. Lindroos M, Kupari M, Heikkilä J, Tilvis R. Prevalence of aortic valve abnormalities in the elderly: an echocardiographic study of a random population sample. J Am Coll Cardiol. 1993;21(5):1220–5.

34. Díez JG. Transcatheter aortic valve implantation (TAVI): the hype and the hope. Tex Heart Inst J [Internet]. 2013;40(3):298–301. http://www.pubmedcentral.nih.gov/articlerender.fcgi?artid=3709202&tool=pmcentrez&rendertype=abstract

35. Ostadfar A. Biofluid mechanics—principles and applications. 1st ed. London: Academic Press; 2016.

36. Yoganathan AP. Fluid mechanics of aortic stenosis. Eur Heart J. 1988;9(Suppl E):13–7.

37. Nobari S, Mongrain R, Gaillard E, Leask R, Cartier R. Therapeutic vascular compliance change may cause significant variation in coronary perfusion: a numerical study. Comput Math Methods Med [Internet]. 2012;2012:791686. http://www.pubmedcentral.nih.gov/articlerender.fcgi?artid=3303727&tool=pmcentrez&rendertype=abstract

38. Capelli C, Corsini C, Biscarini D, Ruffini F, Migliavacca F, Kocher A, et al. Pledget-armed sutures affect the haemodynamic performance of biologic aortic valve substitutes: a preliminary experimental and computational study. Cardiovasc Eng Technol. 2017;8(1):17–29.

39. Hatoum H, Moore BL, Maureira P, Dollery J, Crestanello JA, Dasi LP. Aortic sinus flow stasis likely in valve-in-valve transcatheter aortic valve implantation. J Thorac Cardiovasc Surg [Internet]. 2017;154(1):32–43.e1. https://doi.org/10.1016/j.jtcvs.2017.03.053

40. Yoganathan AP, He Z, Casey Jones S. Fluid mechanics of heart valves. Annu Rev Biomed Eng. 2004;6:331–62.

41. Ben-Dor I, Malik R, Minha S, Goldstein SA, Wang Z, Magalhaes MA, et al. Coronary blood flow in patients with severe aortic stenosis before and after transcatheter aortic valve implantation. Am J Cardiol. 2014;114(8):1264–8.

42. Padala M, Sarin EL, Willis P, Babaliaros V, Block P, Guyton RA, et al. An engineering review of transcatheter aortic valve technologies. Cardiovasc Eng Technol. 2010;1(1):77–87.

43. Leo HL, Dasi LP, Carberry J, Simon HA, Yoganathan AP. Fluid dynamic assessment of three polymeric heart valves using particle image velocimetry. Ann Biomed Eng. 2006;34(6):936–52.

44. D'Errigo P, Barbanti M, Ranucci M, Onorati F, Covello RD, Rosato S, et al. Transcatheter aortic valve implantation versus surgical aortic valve replacement for severe aortic stenosis: Results from an intermediate risk propensity-matched population of the Italian OBSERVANT study. Int J Cardiol [Internet]. 2013;167(5):1945–52. https://doi.org/10.1016/j.ijcard.2012.05.028

45. Clavel MA, Webb JG, Pibarot P, Altwegg L, Dumont E, Thompson C, et al. Comparison of the hemodynamic performance of percutaneous and surgical bio-prostheses for the treatment of severe aortic stenosis. J Am Coll Cardiol. 2009;53(20):1883–91.

46. Kuetting M, Sedaghat A, Utzenrath M, Sinning JM, Schmitz C, Roggenkamp J, et al. In vitro assessment of the influence of aortic annulus ovality on the hydrodynamic performance of self-expanding transcatheter heart valve prostheses. J Biomech [Internet]. 2014;47(5):957–65. https://doi.org/10.1016/j.jbiomech.2014.01.024

47. Tang GHL, Lansman SL, Cohen M, Spielvogel D, Cuomo L, Ahmad H, et al. Transcatheter aortic valve replacement: current developments, ongoing issues, future outlook. Cardiol Rev. 2013;21(2):2944–8.

48. Groves EM, Falahatpisheh A, Su JL, Kheradvar A. The effects of positioning of transcatheter aortic valve on fluid dynamics of the aortic root. ASAIO J. 2014;60(5):545–52.

49. Vahl TP, Kodali SK, Leon MB. Transcatheter aortic valve replacement 2016—a modern-day "through the looking-glass" adventure. J Am Coll Cardiol [Internet]. 2016;67(12):1472–87. https://doi.org/10.1016/j.jacc.2015.12.059

50. Stuhle S, Wendt D, Houl G, Wendt H, Schlamann M, Thielmann M, et al. In-vitro investigation of the hemodynamics of the Edwards Sapien transcatheter heart valve. J Heart Valve Dis. 2011;20(1):53–63.

51. Gunning PS, Saikrishnan N, Mcnamara LM, Yoganathan AP. An in vitro evaluation of the impact of eccentric deployment on transcatheter aortic valve hemodynamics. Ann Biomed Eng. 2014;42(6):1195–206.

52. Piazza N, de Jaegere P, Schultz C, Becker AE, Serruys PW, Anderson RH. Anatomy of the aortic valvar complex and its implications for transcatheter implantation of the aortic valve. Circ Cardiovasc Interv. 2008;1:74–81.

53. Tseng EE, Wisneski A, Azadani AN, Ge L. Engineering perspective on transcatheter aortic valve implantation. Interv Cardiol [Internet]. 2013;5(1):53–70. http://www.futuremedicine.com/doi/abs/10.2217/ica.12.73

54. Azadani AN, Jaussaud N, Matthews PB, Ge L, Guy TS, Chuter TAM, et al. Energy loss due to paravalvular leak with transcatheter aortic valve implantation. Ann Thorac Surg. 2009;88(6):1857–63.

55. Fishbein GA, Schoen FJ, Fishbein MC. Transcatheter aortic valve implantation: status and challenges. Cardiovasc Pathol [Internet]. 2014;23(2):65–70. https://doi.org/10.1016/j.carpath.2013.10.001

56. Kahlert P, Knipp SC, Schlamann M, Thielmann M, Al-Rashid F, Weber M, et al. Silent and apparent cerebral ischemia after percutaneous transfemoral aortic valve implantation: a diffusion-weighted magnetic resonance imaging study. Circulation. 2010;121(7):870–8.

57. Astarci P, Glineur D, Kefer J, D'Hoore W, Renkin J, Vanoverschelde JL, et al. Magnetic resonance imaging evaluation of cerebral embolization during percutaneous aortic valve implantation: comparison of transfemoral and trans-apical approaches using Edwards Sapiens valve. Eur J Cardiothorac Surg. 2011;40(2):475–9.

58. Schaff HV. Transcatheter aortic-valve implantation—at what price? N Engl J Med. 2011;364(23):2256–8.

59. Rodes-Cabau J, Webb JG, Cheung A, Ye J, Dumont E, Feindel CM, et al. Transcatheter aortic valve implantation for the treatment of severe symptomatic aortic stenosis in patients at very high or prohibitive surgical risk. Acute and late outcomes of the multicenter Canadian experience. J Am Coll Cardiol. 2010;55(11):1080–90.

60. Ducci A, Tzamtzis S, Mullen MJ, Burriesci G Phase-resolved velocity measurements in the Valsalva sinus downstream of a Transcatheter Aortic Valve. In: 16th int symposium on applications of laser techniques to fluid mechanics, July. 2012. p. 9–12.

61. Ducci A, Tzamtzis S, Mullen MJ, Burriesci G. Hemodynamics in the Valsalva sinuses after transcatheter aortic valve implantation (TAVI). J Heart Valve Dis. 2013;22(5):688–96.

62. Horne A, Reineck EA, Hasan RK, Resar JR, Chacko M. Transcatheter aortic valve replacement: historical perspectives, current evidence, and future directions. Am Heart J [Internet]. 2014;168(4):414–23. http://linkinghub.elsevier.com/retrieve/pii/S0002870314004372

63. Kapadia S, Tuzcu EM, Svensson LG. Anatomy and flow characteristics of neosinus: important consideration for thrombosis of transcatheter aortic valves. Circulation. 2017;136:1610–2.

64. Saikrishnan N, Yoganathan A. Transcatheter valve implantation can alter the fluid flow fields in the aortic sinuses and ascending aorta: an in vitro study. J Am Coll Cardiol [Internet]. 2013;61(10):E1957. http://content.onlinejacc.org/article.aspx?articleid=1666166%5Cn http://linkinghub.elsevier.com/retrieve/pii/S0735109713619579

65. Kumar G, Raghav V, Lerakis S, Yoganathan AP. High transcatheter valve replacement may reduce washout in the aortic sinuses: an in-vitro study. J Heart Valve Dis [Internet]. 2015;24(1):22–9. http://www.ncbi.nlm.nih.gov/pubmed/26182616

66. Lerakis S, Hayek SS, Douglas PS. Paravalvular aortic leak after transcatheter aortic valve replacement: current knowledge. Circulation. 2013;127(3):397–407.

67. Davies WR, Thomas MR. European experience and perspectives on transcatheter aortic valve replacement. Prog Cardiovasc Dis [Internet]. 2014;56(6):625–34. https://doi.org/10.1016/j.pcad.2014.02.002

68. Azadani AN, Jaussaud N, Ge L, Chitsaz S, TAM C, Tseng EE. Valve-in-valve hemodynamics of 20-mm transcatheter aortic valves in small bioprostheses. Ann Thorac Surg. 2011;92(2):548–55.

69. Bellhouse BJ, Bellhouse FH, Reid KG. Fluid mechanics of the aortic root with application to coronary flow. Nature. 1968;219:1059–61.

70. Sirois E, Wang Q, Sun W. Fluid simulation of a transcatheter aortic valve deployment into a patient-specific aortic root. Cardiovasc Eng Technol. 2011;2(3):186–95.

71. Stock S, Scharfschwerdt M, Meyer-Saraei R, Richardt D, Charitos EI, Sievers HH, et al. In vitro coronary flow after transcatheter aortic valve-in-valve implantation: a comparison of 2 valves. J Thorac Cardiovasc Surg [Internet]. 2016;153(2):255–63. https://doi.org/10.1016/j.jtcvs.2016.09.086

72. Piazza N, Onuma Y, Jesserun E, Kint PP, Maugenest AM, Anderson RH, et al. Early and persistent intraventricular conduction abnormalities and requirements for pacemaking after percutaneous replacement of the aortic valve. JACC Cardiovasc Interv. 2008;1(3):310–6.

73. van der Boon RM, Nuis R-J, Van Mieghem NM, Jordaens L, Rodés-Cabau J, van Domburg RT, et al. New conduction abnormalities after TAVI—frequency and causes. Nat Rev Cardiol. 2012;9(8):v454–63.

74. Rubín JM, Avanzas P, Del Valle R, Renilla A, Ríos E, Calvo D, et al. Atrioventricular conduction disturbance characterization in transcatheter aortic valve implantation with the corevalve prosthesis. Circ Cardiovasc Interv. 2011;4(3):280–6.

75. Vahidkhah K, Javani S, Abbasi M, Azadani PN, Tandar A, Dvir D, et al. Blood stasis on transcatheter valve leaflets and implications for valve-in-valve leaflet thrombosis. Ann Thorac Surg [Internet]. 2017;104(3):751–9. https://doi.org/10.1016/j.athoracsur.2017.02.052

76. Córdoba-Soriano JG, Puri R, Amat-Santos I, Ribeiro HB, Abdul-Jawad Altisent O, del Trigo M, et al. Valve thrombosis following transcatheter aortic valve implantation: a systematic review. Rev Esp Cardiol (Engl Ed). 2015;68(3):198–204.

77. De Marchena E, Mesa J, Pomenti S, Marin Y Kall C, Marincic X, Yahagi K, et al. Thrombus formation following transcatheter aortic valve replacement. JACC Cardiovasc Interv [Internet]. 2015;8(5):728–39. https://doi.org/10.1016/j.jcin.2015.03.005

78. Chakravarty T, Søndergaard L, Friedman J, De Backer O, Berman D, Kofoed KF, et al. Subclinical leaflet thrombosis in surgical and transcatheter bioprosthetic aortic valves: an observational study. Lancet. 2017;389(10087):2383–92.

79. Trantalis G, Toutouzas K, Latsios G, Synetos A, Brili S, Logitsi D, et al. TAVR and thrombosis. JACC Cardiovasc Imaging. 2017;10(1):86–7.

80. Midha PA, Raghav V, Okafor I, Yoganathan AP. The effect of valve-in-valve implantation height on sinus flow. Ann Biomed Eng. 2017;45(2):405–12.

81. Dvir D, Lavi I, Eltchaninoff H, Himbert D, Almagor Y, Descoutures F, et al. Multicenter evaluation of Edwards SAPIEN positioning during transcatheter aortic valve implantation with correlates for device movement during final deployment. JACC Cardiovasc Interv [Internet]. 2012;5(5):563–70. https://doi.org/10.1016/j.jcin.2012.03.005

82. Midha PA, Raghav V, Sharma R, Condado JF, Okafor IU, Rami T, et al. The fluid mechanics of transcatheter heart valve leaflet thrombosis in the neo-sinus. Circulation. 2017;136(17):1598–609.

83. Azadani AN, Jaussaud N, Matthews PB, Ge L, Chuter TAM, Tseng EE. Transcatheter aortic valves inadequately relieve stenosis in small degenerated bioprostheses. Interact Cardiovasc Thorac Surg. 2010;11(1):70–7.

Part II

Clinical Perspectives

Risk Scores for Aortic Valve Interventions

6

Tom Kai Ming Wang, Ralph Stewart,
Mark Webster, and Peter Ruygrok

6.1 Introduction

Transcatheter aortic valve implantation (TAVI), also called transcatheter aortic valve replacement (TAVR), has expanded rapidly over the last decade as a proven treatment for severe aortic valve disease and as an alternative to aortic valve replacement (AVR) [1, 2]. Randomised trials to date have evaluated the efficacy and safety of TAVI in high-risk [3, 4] and intermediate-risk [5, 6] surgical candidates comparable to AVR, and low-risk patient trials are underway. Amongst a multitude of factors in the preoperative evaluation of patients by the clinician and multidisciplinary heart team, as well as in research and guidelines, risk models play a central role [1–6]. Accurate prediction and stratification by risk models are therefore critical in the decision-making and management of possible TAVI candidates, as they have been in many forms of cardiac interventions and surgeries.

This chapter aims to provide an overview regarding risk modelling pertinent to aortic valve interventions. It begins with statistics, then contemporary surgical risk scores and their performance for AVR and TAVI, the development of novel TAVI-specific risk models, followed by clinical implications and future direction of this important field.

6.2 Statistics of Risk Modelling

Risk models have been developed and used in all areas of diagnostic, prognostic and therapeutic medicine [7, 8]. The constituents of any risk model include a number of independent variables (also known as predictors, factors or parameters), the dependent variable (which can be a disease, event or outcome) and the equation connecting these. Each variable may be quantitative or categorical, and the dependent variable may be cross-sectional or longitudinal.

In cardiac surgery and interventions, operative mortality in-hospital or within 30 days is the commonest endpoint in the construction of a risk model. Other outcomes of interest include long-term mortality from 1 year onwards, stroke, myocardial infarction, bleeding, renal failure, redo operations, intensive care or hospital stay or composite endpoints. The parameters range even more widely, including demographics, presentation, past history, investigation and procedural characteristics. Risk models are developed from a cohort of patients which may be different in

T. K. M. Wang (✉) · R. Stewart · M. Webster
P. Ruygrok
Green Lane Cardiovascular Service, Auckland City Hospital, Auckland, New Zealand

Department of Medicine, University of Auckland, Auckland, New Zealand
e-mail: Twang@adhb.govt.nz; RStewart@adhb.govt.nz; MWebster@adhb.govt.nz; PRuygrok@adhb.govt.nz

© Springer Nature Switzerland AG 2019
A. Giordano et al. (eds.), *Transcatheter Aortic Valve Implantation*,
https://doi.org/10.1007/978-3-030-05912-5_6

place (such as multicentre cohorts) or time (such as several years apart), from which these variables have been collected for multivariate analysis. In general risk models perform best in the cohorts they were derived from. Sometimes the cohort is randomly split into a development cohort to construct the risk model and a validation cohort to test the performance of the developed risk model. As both groups come from the same original cohort, the validation cohort is not a truly external and independent sample [9]. Validation should be performed in foreign cohorts before wider clinical utility.

The commonest way to develop a multivariate risk model is using logistic regression, based on binary cross-sectional outcomes such as operative mortality. Selection of variables to be analysed in logistic regression is not always straightforward as there is no standardised strategy [7, 8]. Full model approach, univariate testing for significance and backward elimination approach are the methods used [9]. The estimated risk formula from logistic regression is $1/(1 + e^{-(\beta_0 + \Sigma\beta_i X_i)})$, where each variable X_i is the number predefined for the presence of an independent variable, β_i is their corresponding coefficient, and β_0 is the constant which calibrates the equation. For each X_i, the odds ratio is calculated by e^{β_i}. Online calculators are frequently designed to enable clinicians to more rapidly calculate the formula. Apart from logistic scores, additive scores are also used regularly in clinical practice, although these are also typically developed from logistic regression. The score is then a sum of coefficients which are usually the odds ratio of each parameter rounded to the nearest whole number. Of note, calibration cannot be assessed for the additive model as the score does not represent the predicted risk.

The two main measures of risk model accuracy are discrimination and calibration. Discrimination reflects how strongly a higher score for a patient equates to a higher chance of having the outcome. It is assessed using the area under the receiver-operative characteristic curve, also known as the c-statistic when applied to binary outcomes. The curve plots true positive or sensitivity against false positive or 1-specificity,

and a straight line or c-statistic 0.5 means no discrimination, with stronger discrimination the further from 0.5 the c-statistic. The plot also allows the determination of the optimal sensitivity × specificity cutpoint which may have clinical relevance. Discrimination slope is another technique calculated by differences in the mean scores of patients with and without outcomes [10–12].

Calibration assesses whether the predicted risk is an accurate estimate of the observed risk for patients and cohorts. The observed-to-expected ratio directly compares the mean score and observed event rate of a cohort, where <1.0 and > 1.0 implies over- and underestimation of the score. The Hosmer-Lemeshow test is another measure of calibration, where $P < 0.05$ indicates discordance and poor calibration between outcome and the score [11]. Finally, calibration plots graphically evaluate with observed and predicted risk, with the slope measuring strength of association and intercept measuring degree of systematic bias [8].

Other accuracy measures of risk scores include the Brier score, coefficient of determination R^2 and reclassification [8]. The Brier score is a quadratic equation of the mean-squared difference between the score and observed outcome of all patients in the cohort. A higher number means relatively lower accuracy, although the range of values is also determined by the observed rate. The R^2 is also the correlation coefficient squared with range of 0 to 1, examining the strength of association between two continuous measures, and therefore only applies to quantitative outcomes. Reclassification is the concept of the proportion of patients reclassified appropriately or not when adding another parameter or risk model for prediction [13]. The net reclassification index, reclassification statistic and tables can be used to examine this novel measure.

6.3   Surgical Risk Scores and Aortic Valve Surgery

Cardiac surgery carries one of the highest risks amongst all medical procedures, and risk models play a critical role in the decision-making of treatment modality and have guided perioperative care for at least the last two decades. A number of risk models have been developed for cardiac surgery, including the EuroSCOREs, the Society of Thoracic Surgeons' (STS) Score, Northern New England Cardiovascular Disease Study Group Score, New York's cardiac surgery reporting system, Ambler Score, ACEF Score and so on [14–23]. The EuroSCOREs and STS Score are by far the most widely used, detailed in Table 9.1 for AVR, and both have online calculators [15, 16, 18]. They are also the guideline-recommended risk models for both AVR and TAVI pre-procedural assessment [1, 2].

The original EuroSCORE was based on 19,030 consecutive patients having all types of cardiac surgery across 8 European countries during September–November 1995. It was initially published as an additive model in 1999 [14] and then logistic model in 2003 [15]. It was designed to estimate operative mortality within 30 days or during the same hospital admission, which occurred in 4.8%, and was internally validated. The commonest form of surgery was isolated CABG in 64% followed by valve surgery in 30%. It was the only widely used cardiac surgery risk score for many years. Over time however it began to consistenly overestimate operative mortality, seen in many studies and two meta-analyses one specific for valve surgery, although discrimination remained adequate with c-statistic of 0.73–0.77 [24, 25]. This is due to improving surgical outcomes from evolving surgical technique, selection of patients and perioperative management over time. A new risk model was therefore warranted at this time around 10 years ago.

The EuroSCORE II was based on 22,381 consecutive patients undergoing cardiac surgery across 43 countries around the world beyond Europe during May–July 2010 [16], with operative mortality of 3.9% and a slightly different set of parameters in the final model. In this cohort, isolated CABG and valve surgery numbers were similar at 47% and 46% respectively. The goal was for improved calibration which it achieved in external validation of recent studies and meta-analyses, although discrimination is not dissimilar to EuroSCORE with c-statistic of 0.73–0.79 [26–28].

Guidelines followed suit replacing EuroSCORE with EuroSCORE II in its recommendations for clinical use in coronary and valve surgery [2].

The Society of Thoracic Surgeons database is a United States cardiothoracic surgery database established in 1998 [29] and by 2008 included 90% of cardiac surgery providers in the United States and is amongst the largest registry in the world [17–19]. The STS scores were published in 2009, based on their 2002–2006 cardiac surgery experience, and have two unique features. The first is that there are separate models for different types of cardiac surgery, for which the two that are relevant here are the isolated AVR model and the isolated AVR and coronary artery bypass grafting (CABG) models [18, 19]. There were 67,292 and 66,074 patients, respectively, in the developmental cohort of these two models, with operative mortality of 3.2 and 5.6%.

The second feature is that STS scores have separate logistic models for a range of outcomes beyond operative mortality [17–19]. These include defined morbidity outcomes of stroke, renal failure, prolonged ventilation >24 h, mediastinitis and reoperation in-hospital, composite morbidity or mortality and short or long length of hospital stay. The STS Score appears to have a more complex calculation with more parameters than the EuroSCOREs, but that is solely due to the greater number of outcomes it can predict. It also has good discrimination and calibration in contemporary cohorts of cardiac surgery similar to EuroSCORE II with c-statistic of 0.75–0.76 [27, 28]. The STS Score has gained popular use, especially in the United States, and is the other main risk model suggested by guidelines for clinical practice [2]. Notably all these surgical risk models are developed using logistic regression, and none predict long-term outcomes such as mortality [14–23].

6.4   Applying Surgical Risk Scores to TAVI

Prior to surgical risk scores being validated for TAVI, they had already been readily used in the workup of TAVI patients. This was because TAVI

Table 9.1 Characteristics of risk models for cardiac surgery

Score	Cardiac surgery	Cohort date	Countries	Cohort Size	Endpoint	Rate (%)	Parameters	C-statistic development	C-statistic validation
EuroSCOREs									
EuroSCORE (additive)	All	1995 Sep–Nov	Europe (8)	19,030	Operative mortality	4.8	17	0.79	N/A
EuroSCORE (logistic)	All	1995 Sep–Nov	Europe (8)	19,030	Operative mortality	4.8	17	0.79	0.76
EuroSCORE II	All	2010 May–July	World (43)	22,381	Operative mortality	3.9	18	N/A	0.81
STS Scores									
STS-AVR	AVR	2002–2007	USA	67,292	Operative mortality	3.2	10	0.78	0.76
				67,292	Stroke	1.5	6	0.68	0.69
				65,828	Renal failure	4.1	8	0.77	0.75
				67,292	Ventilation > 24 h	10.9	10	0.75	0.74
				67,292	Mediastinitis	0.3	5	0.71	0.64
				67,292	Reoperation	8.0	10	0.63	0.62
				67,292	Composite morbidity and mortality	17.4	10	0.70	0.69
				67,292	Prolonged length of stay	7.9	10	0.75	0.76
				67,292	Short length of stay	38.9	9	0.71	0.71
STS-AVR + CABG	AVR + CABG	2002–2010	USA	66,074	Operative mortality	5.6	12	0.74	0.74
				66,074	Stroke	2.7	8	0.65	0.61
				64,710	Renal failure	7.6	11	0.72	0.72
				66,074	Ventilation > 24 h	17.6	12	0.71	0.70
				66,074	Mediastinitis	0.6	3	0.64	0.66
				66,074	Reoperation	10.7	11	0.61	0.60
				66,074	Composite morbidity and mortality	26.3	12	0.68	0.67
				66,074	Prolonged length of stay	12.7	12	0.71	0.70
				66,074	Short length of stay	25.7	11	0.70	0.70

was introduced as an alternative to AVR for severe aortic valve disease patients in both clinical trials and practice. The exception is patients recruited for the original PARTNER IB trial comparing TAVI to medical therapy in the so-called "inoperable" patients; however as TAVI indications have widened into intermediate- and lower-risk patients, these patients who sometimes have futile prognosis constitute a diminishing proportion of all TAVI patients [30]. Therefore, the risk scores are mainly used to predict the mortality risk of AVR in such patients to then decide whether TAVI should be considered, rather than predicting the mortality risk of TAVI. This is important to understand, for the reason that AVR is traditionally the gold standard for management of such patients and that the surgical risk scores had not been formally evaluated in TAVI at the time.

The TAVI randomised trials, perhaps because most were undertaken in the United States, generally used the STS Score as guideline for patient selection. The PARTNER I trials suggested STS Score >10% to be deemed high surgical risk and then used the surgeon's judgement of whether to be included in the PARTNER IA TAVI versus AVR in high-risk "operable" trial or the PARTNER IB "inoperable" trial mentioned previously [3, 30]. In fact, the mean STS scores in the four arms of the two trials were similar at 11.2–12.1%. The CoreValve trial was different in that patient selection relied on "consensus" judgement that individuals' 30-day risk of death was >15% and complication risk <50% without specifying use of a particular risk model. The mean STS Scores of the TAVI and AVR arm in this study were 7.3–7.5%, highlighting discrepancy between clinical judgement and risk scores [4]. The PARTNER II study used an STS Score of 4–8% as a selection criterion for intermediate-risk patients, with the mean STS Score being 5.8% [5]. Finally, the SURTAVI trial, another study of intermediate-risk patients, had wider STS Score eligibility of 3–15%, and had the lowest mean STS Score of 4.4–4.5% amongst all trials [6].

What is also fascinating in the randomised trials were the 30-day mortality rates reported. In general they were significantly lower than their corresponding STS Score suggesting significant overestimation by the score and poor calibration [3–6, 30]. This was not just for TAVI but for AVR as well, with observed/expected ratio of 0.38–0.71. However, the STS Score still had some discriminative ability, where subgroups with a higher STS Score mostly had higher observed 30-day mortality for the same procedure, either TAVI or AVR, even with the poor calibration. Discrimination was not formally evaluated in these trials.

The performance of surgical risk scores to predict outcomes after TAVI, particularly their discriminative ability, has only been evaluated very recently, and observational study findings are summarised well in a meta-analysis [31]. This meta-analysis pooled 24 studies during 2011–2015, totalling 12,346 TAVI patients to evaluate the discrimination and calibration of the EuroSCORE, EuroSCORE II and STS Scores for mortality after TAVI. Importantly, the discrimination of 30-day mortality was only modest for all three scores with c-statistic of 0.62, as well as of 1-year mortality c-statistic of 0.58–0.66. In terms of calibration, the Peto odds ratio indicated significant overestimation at 0.31 for EuroSCORE, slight underestimation of 1.26 for EuroSCORE II and adequate at 0.95 for STS Score. In the Labbe plots, whereas EuroSCORE II somewhat underestimated operative mortality in all studies, the STS Score appeared to underestimate in lower-risk studies and over-estimate in higher-risk studies.

There are several reasons for why surgical risk scores perform suboptimally in the TAVI studies. Firstly, the surgical risk models were designed for cardiac surgery including AVR rather than TAVI; however, this would not explain why they also had poor calibration for the AVR arm of the randomised trials. Secondly, to a certain extent, surgical outcomes may have improved further in recent years when the later trials were published in 2014–2017 compared to when the STS Score was published based on 2002–2006 cohorts a decade ago. TAVI outcomes are also expected to improve with time, experience and newer technology. Thirdly, and perhaps the most important reason, is that risk models generally don't perform as well at the extreme ends of risk, for which patients considered for TAVI are mostly on the higher-risk end of the spectrum, only a small proportion of patients in the developmental cohort of risk scores are high risk. This observation has been reported elsewhere for high-risk cardiac surgery patients, although the STS Score may perform better than EuroSCORE II in this subgroup [31–33]. Finally, there may be other important predictors of TAVI not incorporated in surgical risk scores, which will be discussed later.

6.5   TAVI-Specific Risk Models

Due to the inadequate performance of conventional surgical risk models for TAVI, a number of risk models developed from TAVI cohorts have recently been published, including the OBSERVANT, post-TAVI, FRANCE-2, TAVI2-SCORe, CoreValve and STS/ACC/TVT scores, listed in Table 9.2 [34–39]. The OBSERVANT, FRANCE-2, CoreValve and STS/ACC/TVT scores were for 30-day or in-hospital mortality, while the postTAVI, TAVI2-SCORe and CoreValve score again were for 1-year mortality. Whereas logistic regression is used to construct the multivariate model for 30-day mortality, Cox proportional hazard regression is used to construct the multivariate model for a longitudinal or survival outcome such as 1-year mortality. Where reported, the 30-day or in-hospital mortality was 5.3–7% [35, 37–39] and 1-year mortality 15–23%, which are higher than 30-day mortality of 2–5% but similar 1-year mortality of 7–31% of the TAVI arms of randomised trials (2–5%) [34–39].

The size of these cohorts are small, despite the longer duration of patient selection at 1.5–5 years, with the only model with comparable developmental cohort size to surgical risk models being the STS/ACC/TVT score. As a result, a smaller number of independent predictors were identified in multivariate analysis and therefore less parameters in the risk model than surgical scores. Furthermore, the parameters of some of these scores have not been used before in surgical risk scores such as low albumin, assisted living, home oxygen and falls of the CoreValve score [38], porcelain aorta and aortic valve gradient of the

TAVI2-SCORe [37] and the TAVI approach of the FRANCE-2 and STS/ACC/TVT scores [36, 39]. These unique predictors can also partly explain why surgical risk models don't perform well in TAVI patients.

From Table 9.2 we can see that the c-statistics of TAVI-specific scores for its developmental cohort were 0.67–0.79, ranging from modest to moderate discrimination and lower for their respective TAVI validation cohort from the same publication [34–39]. These c-statistics are at best similar if not slightly lower than internal validation results of surgical risk models described previously and perhaps suggest a higher complexity in the modelling of TAVI patients. Despite this, the early results of discrimination are promising for TAVI-specific scores compared to using surgical risk scores in TAVI. Somewhat disappointingly, only the STS/ACC/TVT score reported the constant of its risk model formula so that the logistic score could be calculated [39], whereas the other scores reported their multivariate analysis results without the constant, and usually publishes an additive score, which then doesn't allow the assessment of calibration [34–38]. True external validation studies comparing the performance of TAVI-specific risk scores in other cohorts unrelated to any of the development cohorts are eagerly awaited.

6.6   Clinical Implications and Future Directions

The EuroSCORE II and STS Score continue to be the risk model of choice in the management of severe aortic valve disease in international guidelines [1, 2, 40]. They have moderate discrimination and adequate calibration for AVR; however as noted previously, caution needs to be taken in the higher-risk patients considered for TAVI where the scores could be less accurate. The figure calculated from these two logistic risk models should only be used to estimate operative mortality if the patient underwent AVR, rather than TAVI, which may not be the same [4, 5]. The American guidelines propose STS Score >8% for operative mortality as high risk, 4–8% as inter-

Table 9.2 TAVI-specific risk models

Score	Cohort date	Country	Cohort Size	Dependent variable	30-day mortality (%)	1-year mortality (%)	Parameters	C-statistic development	C-statistic validation
OBSERVANT	2010 Dec–2012 Jun	Italy	1256	30-day mortality	6.1	N/A	7	0.73	0.71
postTAVI	2007–2012	Italy	1064	1-year mortality	7.0	15	3	0.68	0.67
FRANCE-2	2010–2011	France	2552	30-day or in-hospital mortality	10.0	N/A	9	0.67	0.59
TAVI2-SCORe	2007 Nov–2012 Nov	The Netherlands	511	1-year mortality	5.7	17	8	0.72	
CoreValve	2011 Feb–2012 Sep	USA	2482	30-day and 1-year mortality	5.8	23	4, 5	0.75, 0.79	
STS/ACC/TVT	2011 Nov–2014 Feb	USA	13,718	In-hospital mortality	5.3	N/A	7	0.67	0.66

mediate risk and <4% as low risk, and these were considered in TAVI randomised trials and reasonable benchmarks in clinical practice [1]. An estimated risk of >50% for composite mortality or major morbidity at 1 year was deemed prohibitive risk, although how this is assessed wasn't described, relying on clinical judgement. TAVI-specific scores as discussed earlier show some early promise in improving discrimination for TAVI outcomes into the moderate range compared to surgical risk scores.

Beyond the risk models above, there are other important predictors and factors to take into account [1, 2, 40]. An important one is the concept of frailty, and these indices encompass many aspects of function including independence in activities of daily living such as feeding, bathing, dressing and toileting, grip strength, cognition, mobility and speed, with both subjective and objective measures [41–43]. Several studies and one meta-analysis found frailty to be associated with increased early and late mortality as well as morbidities after TAVI [44–47]. It has been a challenge to attempt to incorporate this into an overall risk model with other predictors of TAVI outcomes, although the CoreValve score did manage to do that [38]. As stand-alone criteria, guidelines recommend frailty indices to be divided into low risk (no frailty), intermediate risk (mild frailty) or high risk (moderate or severe frailty) so that it can be more easily applied [1].

Two other important groups of determinants to consider are severe organ compromise and procedure-specific issues [1]. Severe organ compromise is often overlooked in risk models because they are usually uncommon and individual variables not powered to be divided into levels of severity. This can include severe right ventricular systolic dysfunction, severe lung disease or oxygen requirement, severe neurological impairment such as disabling stroke, dementia and Parkinson Disease, active and especially metastatic malignancy, liver cirrhosis and severe malnourishment. The presence of any one or more of these may put patients at higher and at times prohibitive risk for a procedure. Procedural-specific issues which could make TAVI both risky and technically difficult to perform include porcelain or heavily calcified aorta or aortic annulus, severe vascular disease, tortuous arterial anatomy and chest deformities. Again these may automatically put patients at higher risk.

Clearly further research is required in this important field. In terms of TAVI-specific scores, external validation studies are required and pending, but also publication of full logistic risk models is crucial for calibration and clinical use, rather than just additive risk models. Incorporation of other predictors not found in conventional risk models will also be important, either directly as part of the development of newer risk models or like the guidelines be used as a combination of criteria or algorithm. The importance of accurate risk stratification will continue as TAVI is expanded into lower-risk patients and newer technologies emerge, where clinicians will have even more difficult decisions to make regarding treatment modality for patients in front of them and the options available in different settings and countries.

6.7 Conclusion

Risk modelling plays an important role in the management of patients in clinical practice, including cardiac surgery and interventions. Risk models are commonly created using logistic regression, and their accuracy is assessed in terms of discrimination and calibration. The most widely used contemporary cardiac surgery risk scores are the EuroSCORE II and STS Scores, with good performance in estimating operative mortality risk for patients undergoing cardiac surgery, and could influence the decision-making of their treatment modality. The scores perform less well in TAVI, and therefore, TAVI-specific scores are in development and appear to have improved accuracy. Other factors especially frailty and severe organ dysfunction are also important determinants. It is critical for the clinician and multidisciplinary heart team to take all these factors into account to make the optimal decision in the treatment of patients with severe aortic valve disease.

Acknowledgement No conflicts of interests or funding to disclose for all authors.

References

1. Nishimura RA, Otto CM, Bonow RO, Carabello BA, Erwin JP 3rd, Fleisher LA, Jneid H, Mack MJ, McLeod CJ, O'Gara PT, Rigolin VH, Sundt TM 3rd, Thompson A. 2017 AHA/ACC Focused Update of the 2014 AHA/ACC Guideline for the management of patients with valvular heart disease: a report of the American College of Cardiology/American Heart Association Task Force on Clinical Practice Guidelines. Circulation. 2017;135:e1159–95.

2. Baumgartner H, Falk V, Bax JJ, De Bonis M, Hamm C, Holm PJ, Iung B, Lancellotti P, Lansac E, Rodriguez Muñoz D, Rosenhek R, Sjögren J, Tornos Mas P, Vahanian A, Walther T, Wendler O, Windecker S, Zamorano JL, ESC Scientific Document Group. 2017 ESC/EACTS Guidelines for the management of valvular heart disease. Eur Heart J. 2017;38:2739–91.

3. Smith CR, Leon MB, Mack MJ, Miller DC, Moses JW, Svensson LG, Tuzcu EM, Webb JG, Fontana GP, Makkar RR, Williams M, Dewey T, Kapadia S, Babaliaros V, Thourani VH, Corso P, Pichard AD, Bavaria JE, Herrmann HC, Akin JJ, Anderson WN, Wang D, Pocock SJ, PARTNER Trial Investigators. Transcatheter versus surgical aortic-valve replacement in high-risk patients. N Engl J Med. 2011;364:2187–98.

4. Adams DH, Popma JJ, Reardon MJ, Yakubov SJ, Coselli JS, Deeb GM, Gleason TG, Buchbinder M, Hermiller J Jr, Kleiman NS, Chetcuti S, Heiser J, Merhi W, Zorn G, Tadros P, Robinson N, Petrossian G, Hughes GC, Harrison JK, Conte J, Maini B, Mumtaz M, Chenoweth S, Oh JK, U.S. CoreValve Clinical Investigators. Transcatheter aortic-valve replacement with a self-expanding prosthesis. N Engl J Med. 2014;370:1790–8.

5. Leon MB, Smith CR, Mack MJ, Makkar RR, Svensson LG, Kodali SK, Thourani VH, Tuzcu EM, Miller DC, Herrmann HC, Doshi D, Cohen DJ, Pichard AD, Kapadia S, Dewey T, Babaliaros V, Szeto WY, Williams MR, Kereiakes D, Zajarias A, Greason KL, Whisenant BK, Hodson RW, Moses JW, Trento A, Brown DL, Fearon WF, Pibarot P, Hahn RT, Jaber WA, Anderson WN, Alu MC, Webb JG, PARTNER 2 Investigators. Transcatheter or surgical aortic-valve replacement in intermediate-risk patients. N Engl J Med. 2016;374:1609–20.

6. Reardon MJ, Van Mieghem NM, Popma JJ, Kleiman NS, Søndergaard L, Mumtaz M, Adams DH, Deeb GM, Maini B, Gada H, Chetcuti S, Gleason T, Heiser J, Lange R, Merhi W, Oh JK, Olsen PS, Piazza N, Williams M, Windecker S, Yakubov SJ, Grube E, Makkar R, Lee JS, Conte J, Vang E, Nguyen H, Chang Y, Mugglin AS, Serruys PW, Kappetein AP, SURTAVI Investigators. Surgical or transcatheter aortic-valve replacement in intermediate-risk patients. N Engl J Med. 2017;376:1321–31.

7. Collins GS, Reitsma JB, Altman DG, Moons KG, TRIPOD Group. Transparent reporting of a multivariable prediction model for individual prognosis or diagnosis (TRIPOD): the TRIPOD statement. The TRIPOD Group Circulation. BMJ. 2015;131:211–9.

8. Steyerberg EW, Vickers AJ, Cook NR, Gerds T, Gonen M, Obuchowski N, Pencina MJ, Kattan MW. Assessing the performance of prediction models: a framework for traditional and novel measures. Epidemiology. 2010;21:128–38.

9. Royston P, Moons KG, Altman DG, Vergouwe Y. Prognosis and prognostic research: developing a prognostic model. BMJ. 2009;338:b604.

10. Yates JF. External correspondence: decomposition of the mean probability score. Organ Behav Hum Perform. 1982;30:132–56.

11. Miller ME, Langefeld CD, Tierney WM, Hui SL, McDonald CJ. Validation of probabilistic predictions. Med Decis Mak. 1993;13:49–58.

12. Cook NR. Use and misuse of the receiver operating characteristic curve in risk prediction. Circulation. 2007;115:928–35.

13. Pencina MJ, D'Agostino RB Sr, D'Agostino RB Jr, Vasan RS. Evaluating the added predictive ability of a new marker: from area under the ROC curve to reclassification and beyond. Stat Med. 2008;27:157–72.

14. Nashef SA, Roques F, Michel P, Gauducheau E, Lemeshow S, Salamon R. European system for cardiac operative risk evaluation (EuroSCORE). Eur J Cardiothorac Surg. 1999;16:9–13.

15. Roques F, Michel P, Goldstone AR, Nashef SA. The logistic EuroSCORE. Eur Heart J. 2003;24:882–3.

16. Nashef SA, Roques F, Sharples LD, Nilsson J, Smith C, Goldstone AR, Lockowandt U. EuroSCORE II. Eur J Cardiothorac Surg. 2012;41:734–44.

17. Shahian DM, O'Brien SM, Filardo G, Ferraris VA, Haan CK, Rich JB, Normand SL, DeLong ER, Shewan CM, Dokholyan RS, Peterson ED, Edwards FH, Anderson RP. Society of Thoracic Surgeons Quality Measurement Task Force. The Society of Thoracic Surgeons 2008 cardiac surgery risk models: part 1--coronary artery bypass grafting surgery. Ann Thorac Surg. 2009;88(1 Suppl):S2–22.

18. O'Brien SM, Shahian DM, Filardo G, Ferraris VA, Haan CK, Rich JB, Normand SL, DeLong ER, Shewan CM, Dokholyan RS, Peterson ED, Edwards FH, Anderson RP. Society of Thoracic Surgeons Quality Measurement Task Force. The Society of Thoracic Surgeons 2008 cardiac surgery risk models: part 2—isolated valve surgery. Ann Thorac Surg. 2009;88:S23–42.

19. Shahian DM, O'Brien SM, Filardo G, Ferraris VA, Haan CK, Rich JB, Normand SL, DeLong ER, Shewan CM, Dokholyan RS, Peterson ED, Edwards FH, Anderson RP. Society of Thoracic Surgeons Quality Measurement Task Force. The Society of Thoracic Surgeons 2008 cardiac surgery risk models: Part 3—valve plus coronary artery bypass grafting surgery. Ann Thorac Surg. 2009;88:S43–62.

20. Nowicki ER, Birkmeyer NJ, Weintraub RW, Leavitt BJ, Sanders JH, Dacey LJ, Clough RA, Quinn RD, Charlesworth DC, Sisto DA, Uhlig PN, Olmstead EM, O'Connor GT. Northern New England Cardiovascular Disease Study Group and the Center for Evaluative Clinical Sciences, Dartmouth Medical School. Multivariable prediction of in-hospital mortality associated with aortic and mitral valve surgery in Northern New England. Ann Thorac Surg. 2004;77:1966–77.

21. Hannan EL, Racz M, Culliford AT, Lahey SJ, Wechsler A, Jordan D, Gold JP, Higgins RS, Smith CR. Risk score for predicting in-hospital/30-day mortality for patients undergoing valve and valve/coronary artery bypass graft surgery. Ann Thorac Surg. 2013;95:1282–90.

22. Ambler G, Omar RZ, Royston P, Kinsman R, Keogh BE, Taylor KM. Generic, simple risk stratification model for heart valve surgery. Circulation. 2005;112:224–31.

23. Ranucci M, Castelvecchio S, Menicanti L, Frigiola A, Pelissero G. Risk of assessing mortality risk in elective cardiac operations: age, creatinine, ejection fraction, and the law of parsimony. Circulation. 2009;119:3053–61.

24. Parolari A, Pesce LL, Trezzi M, Cavallotti L, Kassem S, Loardi C, Pacini D, Tremoli E, Alamanni F. EuroSCORE performance in valve surgery: a meta-analysis. Ann Thorac Surg. 2010;89:787–93.

25. Siregar S, Groenwold RH, de Heer F, Bots ML, van der Graaf Y, van Herwerden LA. Performance of the original EuroSCORE. Eur J Cardiothorac Surg. 2012;41:746–54.

26. Guida P, Mastro F, Scrascia G, Whitlock R, Paparella D. Performance of the European System for Cardiac Operative Risk Evaluation II: a meta-analysis of 22 studies involving 145,592 cardiac surgery procedures. J Thorac Cardiovasc Surg. 2014;148:3049–57.

27. Sullivan PG, Wallach JD, Ioannidis JP. Meta-Analysis Comparing Established Risk Prediction Models (EuroSCORE II, STS Score, and ACEF Score) for perioperative mortality during cardiac surgery. Am J Cardiol. 2016;118:1574–82.

28. Biancari F, Juvonen T, Onorati F, Faggian G, Heikkinen J, Airaksinen J, Mariscalco G. Meta-analysis on the performance of the EuroSCORE II and the Society of Thoracic Surgeons scores in patients undergoing aortic valve replacement. J Cardiothorac Vasc Anesth. 2014;28:1533–9.

29. Edwards FH. Evolution of the Society of Thoracic Surgeons National Cardiac Surgery Database. J Invasive Cardiol. 1998;10:485–8.

30. Leon MB, Smith CR, Mack M, Miller DC, Moses JW, Svensson LG, Tuzcu EM, Webb JG, Fontana GP, Makkar RR, Brown DL, Block PC, Guyton RA, Pichard AD, Bavaria JE, Herrmann HC, Douglas PS, Petersen JL, Akin JJ, Anderson WN, Wang D, Pocock S, PARTNER Trial Investigators. Transcatheter aortic-valve implantation for aortic stenosis in patients who cannot undergo surgery. N Engl J Med. 2010;363:1597–607.

31. Wang TKM, Wang MTM, Gamble GD, Webster M, Ruygrok PN. Performance of contemporary surgical risk scores for transcatheter aortic valve implantation: a meta-analysis. Int J Cardiol. 2017;236:350–5.

32. Wendt D, Osswald BR, Kayser K, Thielmann M, Tossios P, Massoudy P, Kamler M, Jakob H. Society of Thoracic Surgeons score is superior to the EuroSCORE determining mortality in high risk patients undergoing isolated aortic valve replacement. Ann Thorac Surg. 2009;88:468–74.

33. Frilling B, von Renteln-Kruse W, Riess FC. Evaluation of operative risk in elderly patients undergoing aortic valve replacement: the predictive value of operative risk scores. Cardiology. 2010;116:213–8.

34. Capodanno D, Barbanti M, Tamburino C, D'Errigo P, Ranucci M, Santoro G, Santini F, Onorati F, Grossi C, Covello RD, Capranzano P, Rosato S, Seccareccia F, OBSERVANT Research Group. A simple risk tool (the OBSERVANT score) for prediction of 30-day mortality after transcatheter aortic valve replacement. Am J Cardiol. 2014;113:1851–8.

35. D'Ascenzo F, Capodanno D, Tarantini G, Nijhoff F, Ciuca C, Rossi ML, Brambilla N, Barbanti M, Napodano M, Stella P, Saia F, Ferrante G, Tamburino C, Gasparetto V, Agostoni P, Marzocchi A, Presbitero P, Bedogni F, Cerrato E, Omedè P, Conrotto F, Salizzoni S, Biondi Zoccai G, Marra S, Rinaldi M, Gaita F, D'Amico M, Moretti C. Usefulness and validation of the survival posT TAVI score for survival after transcatheter aortic valve implantation for aortic stenosis. Am J Cardiol. 2014;114:1867–74.

36. Iung B, Laouenan C, Himbert D, et al. Predictive factors of early mortality after transcatheter aortic valve implantation: individual risk assessment using a simple score. Heart. 2014;100:1016–23.

37. Debonnaire P, Fusini L, Wolterbeek R, Kamperidis V, van Rosendael P, van der Kley F, Katsanos S, Joyce E, Tamborini G, Muratori M, Gripari P, Bax JJ, Marsan NA, Pepi M, Delgado V. Value of the "TAVI2-SCORe" versus surgical risk scores for prediction of one year mortality in 511 patients who underwent transcatheter aortic valve implantation. Am J Cardiol. 2015;115:234–42.

38. Hermiller JB Jr, Yakubov SJ, Reardon MJ, Deeb GM, Adams DH, Afilalo J, Huang J, Popma JJ, CoreValve United States Clinical Investigators. Predicting early and late mortality after transcatheter aortic valve replacement. J Am Coll Cardiol. 2016;68:343–52.

39. Edwards FH, Cohen DJ, O'Brien SM, Peterson ED, Mack MJ, Shahian DM, Grover FL, Tuzcu EM, Thourani VH, Carroll J, Brennan JM, Brindis RG, Rumsfeld J, Holmes DR Jr, Steering Committee of the Society of Thoracic Surgeons/American College of Cardiology Transcatheter Valve Therapy Registry. Development and validation of a risk prediction model for in-hospital mortality after transcatheter aortic valve replacement. JAMA Cardiol. 2016;1:46–52.

40. Otto CM, Kumbhani DJ, Alexander KP, Calhoon JH, Desai MY, Kaul S, Lee JC, Ruiz CE, Vassileva CM. 2017 ACC expert consensus decision pathway for

transcatheter aortic valve replacement in the management of adults with aortic stenosis: a report of the American College of Cardiology Task Force on Clinical Expert Consensus Documents. J Am Coll Cardiol. 2017;69:1313–46.

41. Katz S, Ford AB, Moskowitz RW, Jackson BA, Jaffe MW. Studies of illness in the aged. The index of ADL: a standardized measure of biological and psychosocial function. JAMA. 1963;185:914–9.

42. Rockwood K, Song X, MacKnight C, Bergman H, Hogan DB, McDowell I, Mitnitski A. A global clinical measure of fitness and frailty in elderly people. CMAJ. 2005;173:489–95.

43. J MC, Bellavance F, Cardin S, Trépanier S, Verdon J, Ardman O. Detection of older people at increased risk of adverse health outcomes after an emergency visit: the ISAR screening tool. J Am Geriatr Soc. 1999;47:1229–37.

44. Puls M, Sobisiak B, Bleckmann A, Jacobshagen C, Danner BC, Hünlich M, Beißbarth T, Schöndube F, Hasenfuß G, Seipelt R, Schillinger W. Impact of frailty on short- and long-term morbidity and mortality after transcatheter aortic valve implantation: risk assessment by Katz Index of activities of daily living. EuroIntervention. 2014;10:609–19.

45. Kleczynski P, Dziewierz A, Bagienski M, Rzeszutko L, Sorysz D, Trebacz J, Sobczynski R, Tomala M, Stapor M, Dudek D. Impact of frailty on mortality after transcatheter aortic valve implantation. Am Heart J. 2017;185:52–8.

46. Shimura T, Yamamoto M, Kano S, Kagase A, Kodama A, Koyama Y, Tsuchikane E, Suzuki T, Otsuka T, Kohsaka S, Tada N, Yamanaka F, Naganuma T, Araki M, Shirai S, Watanabe Y, Hayashida K, OCEAN-TAVI Investigators. Impact of the clinical frailty scale on outcomes after transcatheter aortic valve replacement. Circulation. 2017;135:2013–24.

47. Anand A, Harley C, Visvanathan A, Shah ASV, Cowell J, MacLullich A, Shenkin S, Mills NL. The relationship between preoperative frailty and outcomes following transcatheter aortic valve implantation: a systematic review and meta-analysis. Eur Heart J Qual Care Clin Outcomes. 2017;3:123–32.

Role of Rest and Stress Echocardiography in Transcatheter Aortic Valve Implantation

Quirino Ciampi, Fiore Manganelli, and Bruno Villari

7.1 Rest Echocardiography in Aortic Stenosis

7.1.1 Echocardiographic Criteria of Severity

Aortic stenosis (AS) is the most common valvular disease, and echocardiography is the key tool for the diagnosis and evaluation of AS and is the primary noninvasive imaging method for AS assessment [1].

In the echocardiographic evaluation of AS severity, we should use a stepwise integrated approach, according to the European Society of Cardiology (ESC) guidelines [2].

The first step is the evaluation of valve morphology suspicious of AS: transthoracic imaging is usually adequate, although transesophageal echocardiography is superior in assessing aortic valve morphology and it may be helpful when image quality is suboptimal. The most common cause of valvular AS is calcific aortic stenosis of a tricuspid valve in elderly patients and bicuspid aortic valve in younger patients (age <65 years) [3].

Two-dimensional (2D) echocardiography allows to identify a number of cusps in systole, to assess cusp mobility and commissural fusion and the presence, extension, and severity of aortic valve calcification. Additional remarkable findings are the presence of left ventricular (LV) hypertrophy and the evaluation of LV systolic function.

The second step is to quantify the severity of AS by trans-aortic valve velocities measured using continuous-wave Doppler [4, 5]. Mean transvalvular aortic gradient, i.e., the pressure difference between the LV and aorta in systole, is the standard measure of stenosis severity [1, 2, 4, 5]. A mean transvalvular pressure gradient ≥40 mmHg or peak jet velocity ≥4 m/s identifies a severe AS [2]. For an accurate measurement of the trans-aortic jet velocity, multiple acoustic windows should be used in order to determine the highest velocity: in fact, alignment errors in Doppler beam lead to an underestimation of the true velocity and, consequently, of the calculated gradients resulting in an underestimation of AS severity.

Different pathophysiological conditions may be associated with significant pressure difference between the LV and aorta in systole, such as hypertrophic obstructive cardiomyopathy or subvalvular aortic stenosis (Fig. 7.1). The shape of continuous-wave Doppler velocity curve may be helpful in distinguishing the level and severity of obstruction.

Q. Ciampi (✉) · B. Villari
Division of Cardiology, Fatebenefratelli Hospital, Benevento, Italy

F. Manganelli
Division of Cardiology, San Giuseppe Moscati Hospital, Avellino, Italy

© Springer Nature Switzerland AG 2019
A. Giordano et al. (eds.), *Transcatheter Aortic Valve Implantation*,
https://doi.org/10.1007/978-3-030-05912-5_7

Aortic
stenosis

HOCM

Subvalvular
Aortic stenosis

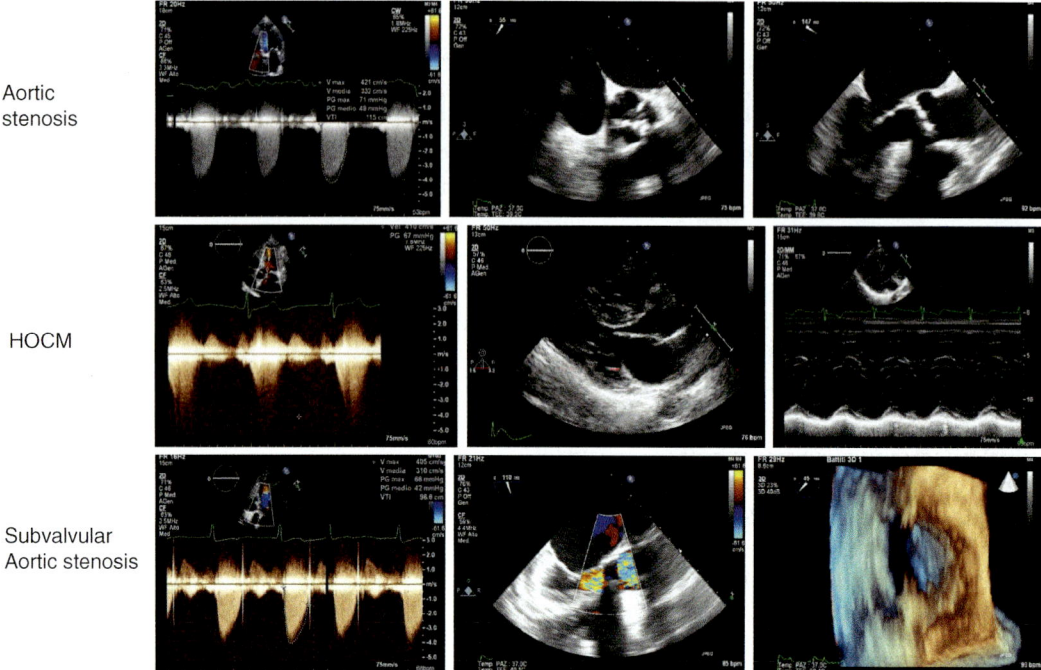

Fig. 7.1 Differential diagnosis of different pathophysiological conditions with high aortic valve peak velocity. *HOCM* hypertrophic obstructive cardiomyopathy

Trans-aortic jet velocities and gradients are flow dependent: in the presence of associated aortic regurgitation, high cardiac output states, such as anemia, hyperthyroidism, or arterial-venous shunts, may result in an increase in trans-aortic flow velocities, while a low cardiac output may result in relatively low velocities.

Therefore, in the presence of severe trans-aortic valve gradient (i.e., peak jet velocity is ≥ 4 m/s and mean transvalvular pressure gradient ≥ 40 mmHg), with high-flow status excluded, we can confirm the diagnosis of severe AS.

On the other hand, in the presence of low-flow condition (i.e., peak jet velocity is <4 m/s and mean transvalvular pressure gradient <40 mmHg), we have to search for other echo-cardiographic parameters to exclude a severe AS.

Aortic valve area (AVA) is a relatively flow-independent variable that is calculated using the continuity equation. It is based on the principle of the conservation of mass: flows through the LVOT and through the stenotic aortic valve are equal (Fig. 7.2) [6]. Even if carefully performed, one major limitation of the method remains the LVOT area calculation from its diameter. Another source of error ensues from geometrical assump-

tion of a circular shape of the LVOT that is somewhat elliptical, rather than circular, resulting in an underestimation of LVOT area and, as a consequence, of SV and eventually of AVA [6–9].

Planimetric evaluation of AVA, primarily by 2D echocardiography, has also been proposed; however, the presence of valvular calcification causes shadows or reverberations limiting identification and accurate delineation of the aortic valve orifice.

The presence of AVA <1 cm^2 is diagnostic for severe AS [2].

Any of the three criteria, a valve area <1.0 cm^2, a peak velocity ≥ 4.0 m/s, or a mean gradient ≥ 40 mmHg, can be considered to suggest severe AS. Ideally, all the criteria must be consistent with each other. In the case of conflicting criteria, it is important to integrate these criteria with additional imaging findings and clinical data before a final judgment.

In the presence of a valve area ≥ 1.0 cm^2 despite a peak velocity ≥ 4 m/s and mean gradient ≥ 40 mmHg, high cardiac output state should be excluded.

More challenging is the discordant finding of a valve area <1.0 cm^2 with a peak velocity <4 m/s

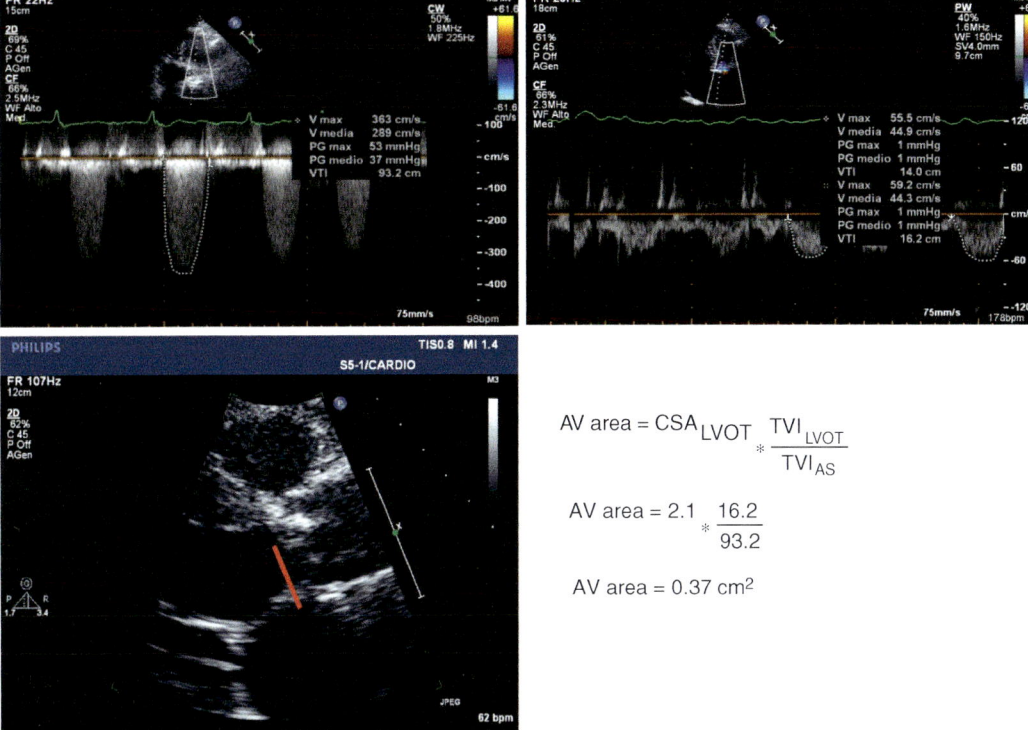

$$AV\ area = CSA_{LVOT} * \frac{TVI_{LVOT}}{TVI_{AS}}$$

$$AV\ area = 2.1 * \frac{16.2}{93.2}$$

$$AV\ area = 0.37\ cm^2$$

Fig. 7.2 Aortic valve area (AVA) calculated using continuity equation: *SV* stroke volume, *CSA_LVOT* cross-sectional area at the level of the left ventricular outflow tract (LVOT). *TVI_LVOT* velocity time integral at the level of LVOT measured with pulsed-wave Doppler proximally to the aortic valve. *TVI_AS* velocity time integral at the level of aortic valve determined from the continuous-wave Doppler peak trans-aortic velocity signal

and mean gradient <40 mmHg. In this situation, measurement errors for all components (trans-aortic velocity, LVOT velocity, LVOT area) need to be carefully excluded.

7.1.2 Low-Flow Low-Gradient Aortic Stenosis with Reduced LVEF

When LV systolic dysfunction with reduced SV coexists with severe AS, the AS velocity and gradient may be low, despite a small valve area [10]. A widely used definition of low-flow low-gradient (LF-LG) "classical" AS with reduced ejection fraction requires the following parameters and includes the following conditions [10]:

- Effective AVA <1.0 cm².
- Mean aortic transvalvular pressure gradient <40 mmHg.
- LVEF <50%.
- SVi (stroke volume index) <35 mL/m².

One reason for the confirmed combination of an AVA less than 1 cm² in the presence of a peak velocity lower than 4 m/s and a mean gradient less than 40 mmHg is a reduced flow in the presence of LV dysfunction (LVEF < 50%). As definition of low flow, a SVi of 35 mL/m² or less has been commonly used and was included in the current ESC guidelines [2].

7.1.3 Aortic Stenosis Low-Flow Low Gradient with Preserved LVEF

The most challenging finding in clinical practice is a valve area <1 cm² with a peak velocity <4 m/s and a mean pressure gradient <40 mmHg despite normal LVEF. The entity of "paradoxical" low-flow low-gradient AS with preserved LVEF [11] has been introduced in this setting and appears to be typical of elderly patients, with small left ventricular cavities, marked hypertrophy, and history of hypertension, resulting in reduced transvalvular flow (for which SVi <35 mL/m² is a surrogate) despite normal LVEF. However, this entity has to be diagnosed with particular care because other more frequent reasons for the finding of a small valve area and low gradient in the presence of normal LVEF may be more likely such as technical factors in AVA calculation and have to be carefully excluded.

"Paradoxical" LF-LG AS with preserved systolic function is characterized by:

- AVA <1 cm².
- AV mean gradient <40 mmHg.
- Normal LVEF (>50%).
- Stroke volume index <35 mL/m².
- Zva (valvuloarterial impedance) ≥5.5 mmHg/mL m².

The Zva is defined as the ratio of the estimated LV systolic pressure to the stroke volume indexed [12].

Lastly, in LF-LG AS patients, the projected AVA (AVA$_{Proj}$) [1, 13] is an important echocardiographic parameter. AVA$_{Proj}$ is calculated using AVA, assessed with continuity equation, at rest and at peak stress, and transvalvular flow rate (Q) obtained by dividing stroke volume by the LV ejection time measured on the continuous-wave Doppler spectral envelope of aortic flow. The projected AVA at a normal transvalvular flow rate (250 mL/min) was calculated using the equation:

$$AVA_{proj} = AVA_{rest} - \frac{AVA_{rest} - AVA_{peak}}{Q_{peak} - Q_{rest}} \times \left(250 - Q_{rest}\right)$$

7.2 Rest Echocardiography in Transcatheter Aortic Valve Implantation

7.2.1 Selection of AS Patients

As the number of patients undergoing transcatheter aortic valve implantation (TAVI), also called transcatheter aortic valve replacement (TAVR),

continues to increase, echocardiographic study plays an important role throughout all stages of the procedure [14–16]. Many echocardiographic parameters should be assessed, including evaluation of left and right ventricular size and function, associated aortic regurgitation, or other valvular diseases. Once the diagnosis of severe AS has been confirmed (see previous paragraph), further evaluation of the aortic valve and the aortic root is required.

Detailed anatomic characteristics of the aortic valve including leaflet mobility, thickness, and degree of calcification should be described. Patients with a bicuspid aortic valve have been excluded from major trials for TAVI [17]. Bicuspid aortic valves present various problems for TAVI: very elliptical aortic valve orifice and asymmetric calcifications are frequently associated, may preclude full expansion of prosthesis with resulting paravalvular leak, and increased shear stress on the valve, thereby contributing to early degeneration. Nevertheless, reports of TAVI in patients with bicuspid aortic valve have been documented [17, 18].

Accurate sizing of the aortic annular dimension is critical to the success of TAVI, as it will guide the selection of valve type and size [14–16]. Annular anteroposterior diameter is measured in the parasternal long-axis view (Fig. 7.3). The measurement should be made at the lowest hinge point of insertion of the aortic valve cusps. As the annulus is usually elliptical, further measurements in an orthogonal plane should be performed, using parasternal short-axis view (Fig. 7.3). When transthoracic two-dimensional echocardiographic measurements of the annulus are uncertain, transesophageal echocardiographic evaluation may be necessary (Fig. 7.3) [14, 19]. Transesophageal echocardiography is superior because it allows better image quality and more accurate measurement of the aortic annular diameter.

Measurement of the distance between the aortic annulus and ostia of the coronary arteries will help appropriate valve selection. During TAVI, the native aortic valve leaflets are crushed against the walls of the aortic root. This can cause aortic rupture and/or coronary ostial obstruction with

Transthoracic echocardiography

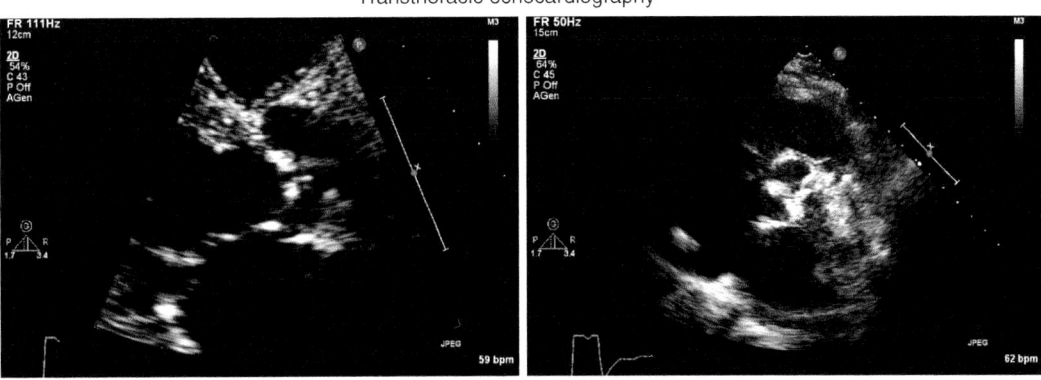

Transesophageal echocardiography

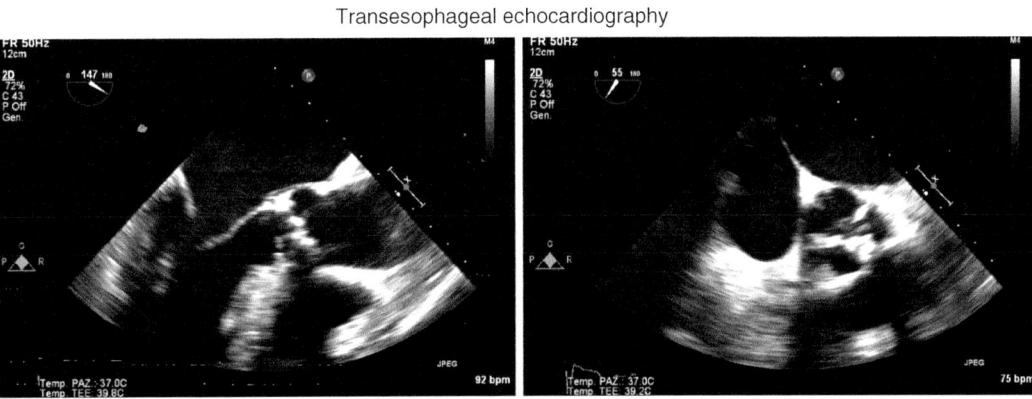

Fig. 7.3 *Top panel*: transthoracic echocardiography, annular anteroposterior diameter in AS patient in parasternal long-axis view zoomed on the left ventricular outflow tract (LVOT) and in parasternal short-axis view. *Bottom* *panel*: transesophageal echocardiography in AS patient on the left ventricular outflow tract (LVOT) in lower transesophageal view and in short-axis upper transesophageal view

potentially life-threatening complications [14, 16]. Measurement of right coronary ostial distance can be made on 2D transesophageal echocardiographic imaging modality for annulus sizing, but identification of left coronary ostium requires 3D transesophageal echocardiography or CT examination [14].

It is important to assess the characteristics of the ascending aorta, the aortic arch, and the descending thoracic aorta since the presence of aortic arch atheromas may increase the risk of periprocedural embolization. It is also necessary to exclude significant mitral valve disease, thrombus in left atrium or in left atrial appendance or in left ventricle, and to assess baseline LV function. Furthermore, a significant LVOT obstruction due to septal hypertrophy should be ruled out [14, 15].

7.2.2 Intraprocedural Monitoring

Transesophageal echocardiography may be used during TAVI to confirm the echocardiographic findings during work-up and to assist monitoring during different stages of the procedure [14]. However, the need of general anesthesia and the potential obstruction of the fluoroscopic view by the transesophageal probe are clear disadvantages of periprocedural transesophageal echocardiography that reduce its use.

Both 2D and 3D techniques have a complementary role during TAVI [16]. 3D transesophageal echocardiography provides better spatial visualization than 2D; therefore, it allows better appreciation of the guidewire path and evaluation of the prosthesis position on the balloon, relative to the native valve annulus and surrounding structures [20].

Immediately after prosthesis deployment, echocardiographic evaluation is used to confirm satisfactory positioning and function of the prosthesis: when the prosthesis is positioned too low, it may impinge on the mitral valve apparatus, or it may be difficult to stabilize in patients with marked subaortic septal hypertrophy. If the prosthesis is implanted too high, it may migrate up the aorta, obstruct the coronary ostia, or be associated with significant paravalvular leak.

Echocardiography is capable to verify that all the prosthetic cusps are moving well and that the valve stent has assumed a circular configuration. Some mild regurgitation through the prosthesis may be transiently observed when the delivery system has not yet been pulled back and/or guide wire is still across the valve. Trace or mild paravalvular leaks usually have a benign course [15]: a transverse (short-axis) view across the LVOT, just beneath the prosthesis, is very helpful in differentiating transvalvular from paravalvular leaks (Fig. 7.4). In addition, the circumferential extent of regurgitant jets from this view appears to be a practical method for preliminary evaluation of the degree of paravalvular leak and to decide if post-dilatation is necessary; in fact, paravalvular leak may occur secondary to undersizing of the prosthesis, restricted cusp motion, incomplete expansion, or incorrect positioning of the device [14, 20, 21].

A complete echocardiography assessment should include pericardium, LV function, and the mitral valve [14, 15] during the procedure. An enlarging pericardial effusion, due to wire perforation of the left or right ventricle, may cause sudden cardiac tamponade and acute hemody-namic compromise that must be promptly recognized. Acute LV dysfunction with regional wall motion abnormalities may be secondary to ostial occlusion by fragment embolization or by an obstructive portion of the valve frame. Although this complication may be fatal, successful management of ostial occlusions with percutaneous angioplasty or bypass surgery has been reported [21]. Sudden worsening of mitral regurgitation may occur as a consequence of ventricular pacing or by direct damage or distortion of the subvalvular apparatus (i.e., implantation of the device too low within the LVOT): this may cause temporary or, in the case of chordal or leaflet rupture, permanent distortion and severe mitral regurgitation [14].

Imaging of the aortic root after TAVI is mandatory to detect tear or rupture, and the integrity of the ascending aortic wall should also be assessed.

7.2.3 Post-TAVI Follow-Up

Echocardiographic post-TAVI follow-up is similar to that of postsurgical aortic valve replacement [2]. Calculation of gradients across the valve and effective orifice area should be performed and other indices of valve opening, with awareness that the gradients tend to be lower than the equivalent aortic valve size by surgical replacement.

A second area of difficulty arises with the accurate quantification of aortic regurgitation which may consist of central regurgitation and paravalvular leak, the latter not infrequently including

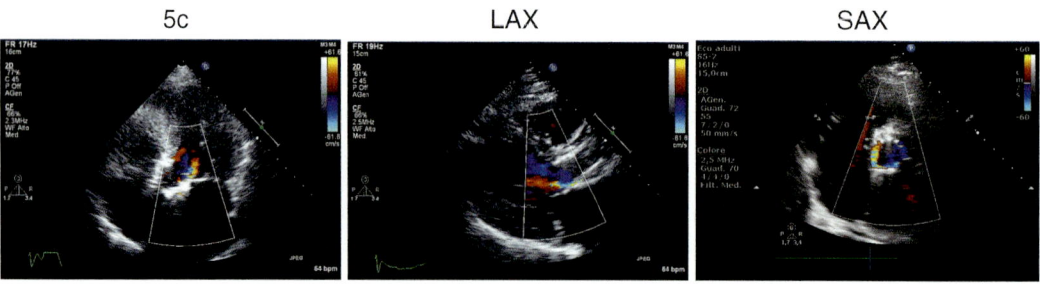

Fig. 7.4 2D color Doppler in showing regurgitation (paravalvular leak) post-TAVI in apical five-chamber view (5C), in parasternal long-axis view (LAX), and in parasternal short-axis view (SAX)

multiple small jets [21]. Accurate assessment of the severity of post-TAVI aortic regurgitation is difficult in the absence of validated methods to quantify paravalvular leak (Fig. 7.4) [13].

The ESC appropriateness criteria for the use of cardiovascular imaging in heart valve disease in adults suggest annual echocardiographic surveillance after TAVI procedure [22].

7.3   Stress Echocardiography in AS

Stress echocardiography (SE) has an established role in the evaluation of patients with valvular heart disease and can significantly aid in clinical decision-making. The evaluation of LF-LG AS with reduced LVEF is the first indication for SE in valvular heart disease [23].

Patients with severe AS and left ventricular systolic dysfunction (LVEF <40%) often have a low mean aortic transvalvular gradient (<40 mmHg). This entity represents a diagnostic challenge because it is difficult to distinguish patients who have severe AS from those with pseudo-severe AS [1, 24, 25]. In truly severe AS, the small area of the aortic valve contributes to an increase in afterload, a reduction in LVEF, and cardiac output. In pseudo-severe AS, the severity of AS is overestimated since the reduction of the opening force generated by the underlying

LV systolic dysfunction results in an incomplete opening of the valve and, as a consequence, to a reduced AVA [25]. In patients with LF-LG AS with LV dysfunction, it may be helpful to determine the transvalvular gradient and the AVA both in resting conditions and during low-dose dobutamine stress echocardiography (up to 20 mcg/kg/min), to differentiate severe (true AS) from pseudo-severe AS [24–28]. Patients who have pseudo-severe AS will show an increase in the aortic valve area and little change in gradient in response to the increase in transvalvular flow rate, while those with severe aortic stenosis will have a fixed valve area with an increase in stroke volume and in gradient [24–27].

The main goal of dobutamine stress is to increase the transvalvular flow rate while not inducing myocardial ischemia (low-dose). The key element in "classical" LF-LG AS with reduced LVEF is the evaluation of the LV contractile reserve: patients with reduced LV contractile reserve show an increased risk of adverse events [24–26]. The imaging assessment relies on the evaluation of LV systolic function (changes in ejection fraction or global longitudinal strain) and flow reserve (increase in stroke volume ≥20%) [24–26] and analysis of changes in pressure gradients and in AVA (Fig. 7.5). The increase in stroke volume >20% is indicative of significant LV contractile reserve [27, 28]. The lack of stroke volume increase during dobutamine SE

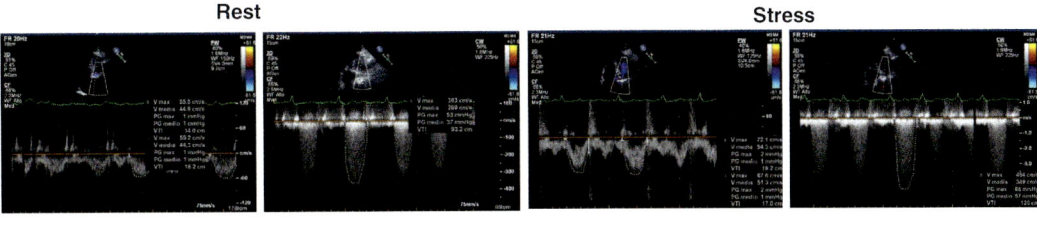

Rest	Stress
AV peak gradient: 53 mmHg	AV peak gradient: 86 mmHg
AV mean gradient: 37 mmHg	AV mean gradient: 57 mmHg
SVi: 22 ml/m^2	SVi: 29 ml/m^2
COi: 1.9 l/min/m^2	COi: 2.8 l/min/m^2
AVA: 0.37 cm^2	AVA: 0.36 cm^2

Fig. 7.5 Low dose of dobutamine stress echocardiography with evaluation at rest and at peak stress of *AV* aortic valve peak and mean gradient, *SVi* stroke volume index, *COi* cardiac output index, and *AVA* aortic valve area

can result from (1) afterload mismatch due to an imbalance between the severity of the stenosis and myocardial reserve, (2) inadequate increase of myocardial blood flow due to associated coronary artery disease, and/or (3) irreversible myocardial damage due to previous myocardial infarction or extensive myocardial fibrosis [29]. Further modality can be achieved by a noninvasive assessment of LV contractile reserve through changes in LV force, a load-independent index of left ventricular contractility [30, 31].

LV contractile reserve is usually evaluated through the improvement in LVEF, but under some circumstances, it may even be misleading, due to its dependence not only on myocardial contractility but also on preload and afterload, as well as heart rate and synchronicity of contraction [30]. However, the LV contractile reserve assessed by LV force is profoundly different from LVEF from the conceptual, methodological, and clinical viewpoint. It is independent from preload and afterload changes [31], which affect LVEF, and requires only the measurement of systolic blood pressure by cuff sphygmomanometer and end-systolic volume by 2D echocardiography, rather than end-diastolic and end-systolic volume (Fig. 7.6). Moreover, LV contractile reserve is more prognostically powerful than ejection fraction changes in identifying patients at higher risk, both in patients with normal and in those with

markedly abnormal resting left ventricular function, with all forms of stress echocardiography—exercise, dobutamine, and dipyridamole [31–34]. In AS patients, for the evaluation of LV force, it should add to systolic blood pressure the peak AV gradient (Fig. 7.6). This parameter will be tested in Stress Echo 2020, a prospective, multicenter study aimed to obtain original safety, feasibility, and outcome data of multiparametric approach in different subsets of pathophysiological conditions beyond coronary artery disease, such as valvular heart disease [35].

Preliminary papers suggest a potential role for SE in the correct evaluation of the severity of LF-LG "paradoxical" AS with preserved LVEF [36]. Dobutamine stress echocardiography has been proposed in this setting. The same dobutamine stress echocardiographic parameters and criteria described for classical LF-LG AS can be applied to paradoxical LF-LG AS in order to identify true-severe stenosis. Approximately, one-third of patients with paradoxical LF-LG AS has pseudo-severe AS, which is similar to that observed in classical LF-LG AS [36]. Dobutamine stress echocardiography should not be performed in patients with restrictive LV physiology pattern, which is frequently found in the paradoxical LF-LG AS population. Exercise stress echocardiography may be useful in patients with paradoxical LF-LG who claim to be asymptomatic or

Rest   **Stress**

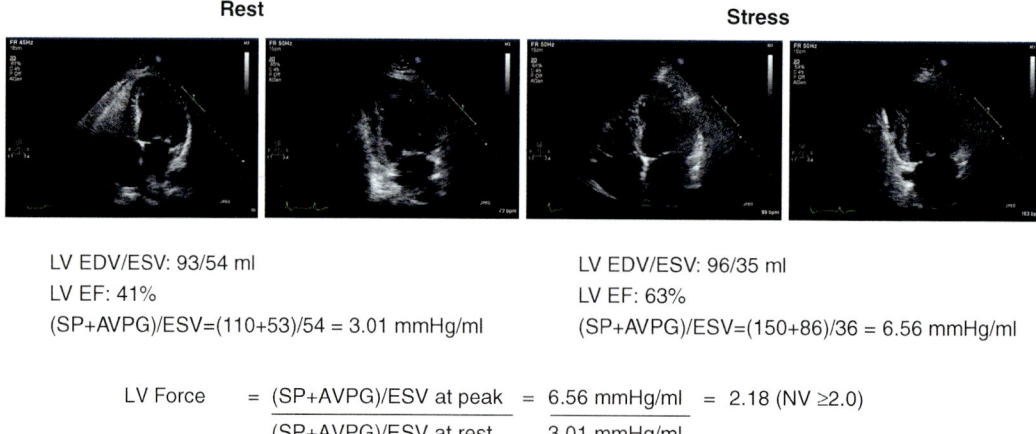

LV EDV/ESV: 93/54 ml
LV EF: 41%
(SP+AVPG)/ESV=(110+53)/54 = 3.01 mmHg/ml

LV EDV/ESV: 96/35 ml
LV EF: 63%
(SP+AVPG)/ESV=(150+86)/36 = 6.56 mmHg/ml

$$\text{LV Force} = \frac{(SP+AVPG)/ESV \text{ at peak}}{(SP+AVPG)/ESV \text{ at rest}} = \frac{6.56 \text{ mmHg/ml}}{3.01 \text{ mmHg/ml}} = 2.18 \ (NV \geq 2.0)$$

Fig. 7.6 Low dose of dobutamine stress echocardiography with evaluation at rest and at peak stress of *EDV* end-diastolic volume, *ESV* end-systolic volume, *LVEF* left ventricular ejection fraction, *SP* systolic blood pressure, *AVPG* aortic valve peak gradient, and *NV* normal value

have equivocal symptoms to ascertain the symptomatic status and to differentiate true- vs. pseudo-severe AS [36]. Data are very interesting but they require further confirmation on larger populations.

7.4 Stress Echocardiography in TAVI

The main factors that have been associated with increased risk of mortality under conservative management as well as after aortic valve replacement in patients with classical LF-LG AS include (1) very low LVEF (<35%) at rest or at dobutamine stress echocardiography, (2) severe impairment of LV longitudinal systolic function at rest or at dobutamine stress echocardiography, and (3) absence of LV contractile reserve [24–29, 37, 38].

In LF-LG classical severe AS, patients with LV contractile reserve have a much better outcome with aortic valve replacement (percutaneous or surgical technique) than with medical therapy [28, 29]: absence of LV contractile reserve during dobutamine SE is observed in approximately one-third of patients and is associated with high operative mortality (6–33%) with surgical aortic valve replacement [29, 37, 38]. However, this factor does not predict lack in LV function improvement and in symptomatic status improvement and late survival after surgery [37, 38]. Thus, the absence of LV contractile reserve should not preclude consideration for surgical or transcatheter aortic valve replacement [38], but it is associated with high intra- and perioperative mortality [37].

The recent ESC guidelines suggest that the management of patients with low-gradient aortic stenosis is more challenging: in the setting of LF-LG classical AS with reduced LVEF, intervention is indicated in symptomatic patients with severe low-flow, low-gradient (<40 mmHg) aortic stenosis with reduced ejection fraction and evidence of LV contractile reserve (class I), in symptomatic patients with LF-LG classical AS with reduced LVEF without LV contractile reserve (class IIa), excluding pseudo-severe aortic stenosis [2].

In patients with LF-LG classical AS without LV contractile reserve during low-dose dobutamine stress echocardiography, TAVI may provide a good alternative to surgery [39–41]. In patients in whom recovery of LV function and the regression of symptoms after procedure are uncertain (e.g., patients with extensive myocardial fibrosis, severe frailty, and/or severe comorbidities, such as oxygen-dependent chronic obstructive pulmonary disease), a staged approach with balloon valvuloplasty first followed by surgical or transcatheter aortic valve replacement (if LV function/symptoms improve) may be the preferred strategy [42]. The PARTNER I trial cohort A (high risk) showed no significant difference between transcatheter and surgical aortic valve replacement in the subset of patients with classical LF-LG AS [43]. However, patients without LV contractile reserve (i.e., patients with higher surgical risk) were excluded from this trial, therefore introducing a selection bias. In a nonrandomized study including LF-LG patients with and those without LV contractile reserve, TAVI was associated with better and faster recovery of LVEF [39].

The recent ESC guidelines suggest that patients with low-flow, low-gradient aortic stenosis and preserved LVEF are the most challenging subgroup. Data on their natural history and outcome after surgical or catheter intervention remain controversial [44–46]. In such cases, intervention should only be performed when symptoms are present and if a comprehensive evaluation suggests significant valve obstruction.

References

1. Baumgartner H, Hung J, Bermejo J, Chambers JB, Edvardsen T, Goldstein S, Lancellotti P, LeFevre M, Miller F Jr, Otto CM. Recommendations on the echocardiographic assessment of aortic valve stenosis: a focused update from the European Association of Cardiovascular Imaging and the American Society of Echocardiography. Eur Heart J Cardiovasc Imaging. 2017;18:254–75.
2. Baumgartner H, Falk V, Bax JJ, De Bonis M, Hamm C, Holm PJ, Iung B, Lancellotti P, Lansac E, Rodriguez Muñoz D, Rosenhek R, Sjögren J, Tornos Mas P, Vahanian A, Walther T, Wendler O, Windecker S, Zamorano JL. 2017 ESC/EACTS Guidelines for the management of valvular heart disease. ESC Scientific Document Group. Eur Heart J. 2017;38:2739–91.

3. Roberts WC, Ko JM. Frequency by decades of unicuspid, bicuspid, and tricuspid aortic valves in adults having isolated aortic valve replacement for aortic stenosis, with or without associated aortic regurgitation. Circulation. 2005;111:920–5.

4. Currie PJ, Seward JB, Reeder GS, Vlietstra RE, Bresnahan DR, Bresnahan JF, et al. Continuous-wave Doppler echocardiographic assessment of severity of calcific aortic stenosis: a simultaneous Doppler-catheter correlative study in 100 adult patients. Circulation. 1985;71:1162–9.

5. Smith MD, Kwan OL, DeMaria AN. Value and limitations of continuous-wave Doppler echocardiography in estimating severity of valvular stenosis. JAMA. 1986;255:3145–51.

6. Baumgartner H, Kratzer H, Helmreich G, Kuehn P. Determination of aortic valve area by Doppler echocardiography using the continuity equation: a critical evaluation. Cardiology. 1990;77: 101–11.

7. Otto CM, Pearlman AS, Comess KA, et al. Determination of the stenotic aortic valve area in adults using Doppler echocardiography. J Am Coll Cardiol. 1986;7:509–17.

8. Rosenhek R, Klaar U, Schemper M, et al. Mild and moderate aortic stenosis. Natural history and risk stratification by echocardiography. Eur Heart J. 2004;25:199–205.

9. Gaspar T, Adawi S, Sachner R, Asmer I, Ganaeem M, Rubinshtein R, et al. Three-dimensional imaging of the left ventricular outflow tract: impact on aortic valve area estimation by the continuity equation. J Am Soc Echocardiogr. 2012;25:749–57.

10. Pibarot P, Dumesnil JG. Aortic stenosis suspected to be severe despite low gradients. Circ Cardiovasc Imaging. 2014;7:545–51.

11. Dumesnil JG, Pibarot P, Carabello B. Paradoxical low flow and/or low gradient severe aortic stenosis despite preserved left ventricular ejection fraction: implications for diagnosis and treatment. Eur Heart J. 2010;31:281–9.

12. Lancellotti P, Magne J. Valvuloarterial impedance in aortic stenosis: look at the load, but do not forget the flow. Eur J Echocardiogr. 2011;12:354–7.

13. Clavel M-A, Burwash IG, Mundigler G, Dumesnil JG, Baumgartner H, Bergler- Klein J, et al. Validation of conventional and simplified methods to calculate projected valve area at normal flow rate in patients with low flow, low gradient aortic stenosis: the multicenter TOPAS (True or Pseudo Severe Aortic Stenosis) study. J Am Soc Echocardiogr. 2010;23:380–6.

14. Zamorano JL, Badano LP, Bruce C, Chan KL, Goncalves A, Hahn RT, Keane MG, La Canna G, Monaghan MJ, Nihoyannopoulos P, Silvestry FE, Vanoverschelde JL, Gillam LD. EAE/ASE recommendations for the use of echocardiography in new transcatheter interventions for valvular heart disease. Eur Heart J. 2011;32:2189–214.

15. DeMarco DC, Monaghan MJ. The role of echocardiography in transcatheter aortic valve implantation. Interv Cardiol. 2014;6:547–55.

16. Moss RR, Ivens E, Pasupati S, Humphries K, Thompson CR, Munt B, et al. Role of echocardiography in percutaneous aortic valve implantation. JACC Cardiovasc Imaging. 2008;1:15–24.

17. Wijesinghe N, Ye J, Rodés-Cabau J, et al. Transcatheter aortic valve implantation in patients with bicuspid aortic valve stenosis. J Am Coll Cardiol Intv. 2010;3:1122–5.

18. Himbert D, Pontnau F, Messika-Zeitoun D, et al. Feasibility and outcomes of transcatheter aortic valve implantation in high-risk patient with stenotic bicuspid aortic valves. Am J Cardiol. 2012;110: 877–33.

19. Moss RR, Ivens E, Pasupati S, et al. Role of echocardiography in percutaneous valve intervention. J Am Coll Cardiol Img. 2008;1:15–24.

20. Smith LA, Dworakowski R, Bhan A, et al. Real-time three-dimensional transesophageal echocardiography adds value to transcatheter aortic valve implantation. J Am Soc Echocardiogr. 2013;26:359–69.

21. Messika-Zeitoun D, Serfaty JM, Brochet E, Ducrocq G, Lepage L, Detaint D, et al. Multimodal assessment of the aortic annulus diameter: implications for transcatheter aortic valve implantation. J Am Coll Cardiol. 2010;55:186–94.

22. Chambers JB, Garbi M, Nieman K, Myerson S, Pierard LA, Habib G, Zamorano JL, Edvardsen T, Lancellotti P. This document was reviewed by members of the 2014—16 EACVI Scientific Documents Committee:, Delgado V, Cosyns B, Donal E, Dulgheru R, Galderisi M, Lombardi M, Muraru D, Kauffmann P, Cardim N, Haugaa K, Rosenhek R. Appropriateness criteria for the use of cardiovascular imaging in heart valve disease in adults: a European Association of Cardiovascular Imaging report of literature review and current practice. Eur Heart J Cardiovasc Imaging. 2017;18:489–98.

23. Bhattacharyya S, Chehab O, Khattar R, Lloyd G, Senior R. Stress echocardiography in clinical practice: a United Kingdom National Health Service Survey on behalf of the British Society of Echocardiography. Eur Heart J Cardiovasc Imaging. 2014;15: 158–63.

24. Lancellotti P, Pellikka PA, Budts W, Chaudhry FA, Donal E, Dulgheru R, Edvardsen T, Garbi M, Ha JW, Kane GC, Kreeger J, Mertens L, Pibarot P, Picano E, Ryan T, Tsutsui JM, Varga A. The clinical use of stress echocardiography in non-ischaemic heart disease: recommendations from the European Association of Cardiovascular Imaging and the American Society of Echocardiography. Eur Heart J Cardiovasc Imaging. 2016;17:1191–229.

25. Picano E, Pibarot P, Lancellotti P, Monin JL, Bonow RO. The emerging role of exercise testing and stress echocardiography in valvular heart disease. J Am Coll Cardiol. 2009;54:2251–60.

26. Picano E, Pellikka PA. Stress echo applications beyond coronary artery disease. Eur Heart J. 2014;35:1033–40.

27. Nishimura RA, Grantham JA, Connolly HM, Schaff HV, Higano ST, Holmes DR Jr. Low-output, low-gradient aortic stenosis in patients with depressed left ventricular systolic function: the clinical utility of the dobutamine challenge in the catheterization laboratory. Circulation. 2002;106:809–13.

28. Monin JL, Monchi M, Gest V, Duval-Moulin AM, Dubois-Rande JL, Gueret P. Aortic stenosis with severe left ventricular dysfunction and low transvalvular pressure gradients: risk stratification by low dose dobutamine echocardiography. J Am Coll Cardiol. 2001;37:2101–7.

29. Monin JL, Quere JP, Monchi M, et al. Low-gradient aortic stenosis: operative risk stratification and predictors for long-term outcome: a multicenter study using dobutamine stress hemodynamics. Circulation. 2003;108:319–24.

30. Cikes M, Solomon SD. Beyond ejection fraction: an integrative approach for assessment of cardiac structure and function in heart failure. Eur Heart J. 2016;37:1642–50.

31. Bombardini T, Costantino MF, Sicari R, Ciampi Q, Pratali L, Picano E. End-systolic elastance and ventricular-arterial coupling reserve predict cardiac events in patients with negative stress echocardiography. Biomed Res Int. 2013;2013:235194.

32. Bombardini T, Gherardi S, Marraccini P, Schlueter MC, Sicari R, Picano E. The incremental diagnostic value of coronary flow reserve and left ventricular elastance during high-dose dipyridamole stress echocardiography in patients with normal wall motion at rest. Int J Cardiol. 2013;168:1683–4.

33. Grosu A, Bombardini T, Senni M, Duino V, Gori M, Picano E. End-systolic pressure/volume relationship during dobutamine stress echo: a prognostically useful non-invasive index of left ventricular contractility. Eur Heart J. 2005;26:2404–12.

34. Cortigiani L, Huqi A, Ciampi Q, Bombardini T, Picano E. The prognostic value of triple functional assessment vasodilator stress echocardiography in diabetic patients: integration of wall motion, coronary flow velocity and left ventricular contractile reserve in a single test. J Am Soc Echocardiogr 2018;31:692-701.

35. Picano E, Ciampi Q, Citro R, D'Aandrea A, Scali MC, Cortigiani L, Olivotto I, Mori F, Galderisi M, Costantino MF, Pratali L, Di Salvo G, Bossone E, Ferrara F, Gargani L, Rigo F, Gaibazzi N, Limongelli G, Pacileo G, Andreassi MG, Pinamonti B, Massa L, Torres MA, Miglioranza MH, Daros CB, de Castro E Silva Pretto JL, Beleslin B, Djordjevic-Dikic A, Varga A, Palinkas A, Agoston G, Gregori D, Trambaiolo P, Severino S, Arystan A, Paterni M, Carpeggiani C, Colonna P. Stress echo 2020: the international stress echo study in ischemic and non-ischemic heart disease. Cardiovasc Ultrasound. 2017;15(18):3.

36. Clavel M, Ennezat P, Marechaux S, et al. Stress echocardiography to assess stenosis severity and predict outcome in patients with paradoxical low-flow, low-gradient aortic stenosis and preserved LVEF. J Am Coll Cardiol Imaging. 2013;6:175–83.

37. Quere JP, Monin JL, Levy F, Petit H, Baleynaud S, Chauvel C, Pop C, Ohlmann P, Lelguen C, Dehant P, Gueret P, Tribouilloy C. Influence of preoperative left ventricular contractile reserve on postoperative ejection fraction in low-gradient aortic stenosis. Circulation. 2006;113:1738–44.

38. Tribouilloy C, Levy F, Rusinaru D, Guéret P, Petit-Eisenmann H, Baleynaud S, et al. Outcome after aortic valve replacement for low-flow/low-gradient aortic stenosis without contractile reserve on dobutamine stress echocardiography. J Am Coll Cardiol. 2009;53(20):1865–73.

39. Clavel MA, Webb JG, Rodés-Cabau J, Masson JB, Dumont E, De Larochellière R, Doyle D, Bergeron S, Baumgartner H, Burwash IG, Dumesnil JG, Mundigler G, Moss R, Kempny A, Bagur R, Bergler-Klein J, Gurvitch R, Mathieu P, Pibarot P. Comparison between transcatheter and surgical prosthetic valve implantation in patients with severe aortic stenosis and reduced left ventricular ejection fraction. Circulation. 2010;122:1928–36.

40. Gotzmann M, Lindstaedt M, Bojara W, Ewers A, Mugge A. Clinical outcome of transcatheter aortic valve implantation in patients with low-flow, low gradient aortic stenosis. Catheter Cardiovasc Interv. 2012;79:693–701.

41. Bauer F, Coutant V, Bernard M, Stepowski D, Tron C, Cribier A, Bessou JP, Eltchaninoff H. Patients with severe aortic stenosis and reduced ejection fraction: earlier recovery of left ventricular systolic function after transcatheter aortic valve implantation compared with surgical valve replacement. Echocardiography. 2013;30:865–70.

42. O'Sullivan CJ, Wenaweser P. Low-flow, low-gradient aortic stenosis: should TAVI be the default therapeutic option? EuroIntervention. 2014;10:775–7.

43. Pibarot P, Weissman NJ, Stewart WJ, Hahn RT, Lindman BR, McAndrew T, Kodali SK, Mack MJ, Thourani VH, Miller DC, Svensson LG, Herrmann HC, Smith CR, Rodés-Cabau J, Webb J, Lim S, Xu K, Hueter I, Douglas PS, Leon MB. Incidence and sequelae of prosthesis-patient mismatch in transcatheter versus surgical valve replacement in high-risk patients with severe aortic stenosis—a PARTNER Trial Cohort A analysis. J Am Coll Cardiol. 2014;30:1323–34.

44. Clavel MA, Dumesnil JG, Capoulade R, Mathieu P, Senechal M, Pibarot P. Outcome of patients with aortic stenosis, small valve area, and low-flow, low-gradient despite preserved left ventricular ejection fraction. J Am Coll Cardiol. 2012;60:1259–67.

45. Tribouilloy C, Rusinaru D, Marechaux S, Castel AL, Debry N, Maizel J, Mentaverri R, Kamel S, Slama M,

Levy F. Low-gradient, low-flow severe aortic stenosis with preserved left ventricular ejection fraction: characteristics, outcome, and implications for surgery. J Am Coll Cardiol. 2015;65:55–66.

46. Jander N, Minners J, Holme I, Gerdts E, Boman K, Brudi P, Chambers JB, Egstrup K, Kesaniemi YA, Malbecq W, Nienaber CA, Ray S, Rossebo A, Pedersen TR, Skjaerpe T, Willenheimer R, Wachtell K, Neumann FJ, Gohlke-Barwolf C. Outcome of patients with low-gradient "severe" aortic stenosis and preserved ejection fraction. Circulation. 2011;123:887–95.

Role of Computed Tomography in Transcatheter Aortic Valve Implantation

8

Zhen Qian

8.1 Introduction

Computed tomography (CT) plays a critical role in appropriate patient selection and procedural planning for transcatheter aortic valve implantation (TAVI), also called transcatheter aortic valve replacement (TAVR). Contrary to surgical aortic valve replacement, in which the size of the valve can be directly measured using a sizing probe, the catheter-based TAVI procedure heavily relies on the preprocedural imaging for a comprehensive assessment of the aortic root, the aorta, and the peripheral access vessels [1]. Pre-TAVI imaging of high quality has been shown to be crucial for achieving optimal outcomes of TAVI [2, 3]. The dimensions of the aortic annulus and the aortic root need to be measured before the TAVI procedure using an imaging approach for proper selection and sizing of the transcatheter heart valve (THV). Peripheral vessels, including the iliofemoral and subclavian arteries, and the aorta also need to be imaged before TAVI to assess the potential risks of the occurrence of periprocedural vascular complications that are associated with variant TAVI access routes. Furthermore, preprocedural imaging can also be utilized to evaluate the extent of valvular calcification in the aortic root and the left ventricular outflow tract (LVOT). The amount and spatial distribution of the aortic valve calcification are believed to be associated with complications such as the occurrence of post-TAVI paravalvular leak (PVL) and the needs of installing permanent pacemakers (PPM). Imaging may provide quantitative information of the calcification to improve the strategy of the THV selection and optimize the deployment technique accordingly. Finally, imaging can also be used post TAVI to assess the position and frame deformation of the THV and evaluate the mobility of the THV leaflets and diagnose subclinical leaflet thrombosis.

Imaging in TAVI was historically done using two-dimensional (2D) imaging techniques, such as the transthoracic echocardiography (TTE), transesophageal echocardiography (TEE), and angiography. Compared to these 2D imaging modalities, CT imaging has unique advantages [4]. The aortic root has a double-oblique orientation with an oval-shaped annulus, which makes it difficult to be viewed and accurately assessed using a 2D imaging technique [5]. CT is intrinsically a noninvasive three-dimensional (3D) imaging technology. Modern multi-detector row CT (MDCT) scanners (64-detector row and/or higher) achieve a submillimeter isotropic resolution and a good balance between the spatial and temporal resolving power. CT imaging in TAVI typically provides a full volumetric coverage of the region from the supraclavicular level

Part of the work was done at Piedmont Heart Institute, Atlanta, GA, USA

Z. Qian (✉)
Medical AI Lab, Tencent America, Palo Alto, CA, USA
e-mail: zhen.qian@piedmont.org

to below the common femoral artery, which makes it possible to retrospectively select the 2D double-oblique image slices or 3D subregions for a detailed assessment of the targeted anatomies. Compared to other 3D imaging techniques, such as the 3D TEE and cardiac magnetic resonance (CMR) imaging, CT is superior in terms of the spatial resolution and the capability of imaging calcifications. However, on the other hand, CT imaging in TAVI requires the administration of an iodinated contrast media to enhance the differentiability between the soft tissue and the blood pool. Because of the average patients' advanced age, renal disease is a common comorbidity among the TAVI patients, which is in need of special cautions to prevent the occurrence of contrast-induced nephropathy (CIN). In patients with severe renal dysfunction, alternative imaging modalities, such as CMR and 3D TEE, could be performed as a replacement of the contrast-enhanced CT.

Currently, several types of THVs are available for the TAVI procedure. In this chapter, we will focus on the two types of THVs that are most commonly used: the balloon-expandable Edwards Sapien series (Edwards Lifesciences, Irvine, CA), including the Sapien, Sapien XT, and Sapien 3 valves, and the self-expandable CoreValve series (Medtronic, Minneapolis, MN), including the CoreValve Classic, Evolut R, and Evolut Pro valves. We will review the role of CT imaging in TAVI using those two types of THVs as examples and discuss the data acquisition protocols and the image processing and evaluation techniques of the CT images.

8.2 Preprocedural CT for TAVI

8.2.1 CT Imaging Protocols

CT imaging in TAVI can be generally performed on a modern multi-detector row CT scanner that is capable of acquiring coronary CT angiography (CTA). The minimum hardware requirement includes a 64-detector row or higher CT scanner with electrocardiography (ECG)-gating capacity and a dual-head power injector for contrast media

administration. Patient preparation is similar to that of conventional coronary CTA, in which the patient remains in supine position and is asked to hold breath during image acquisition. Beta-blocker is not typically used because it may worsen symptoms of aortic stenosis.

The scan range should be determined by the diagnostic question and the patient's condition, specifically the renal function. In patients with impaired renal function, the scan range can be shortened to focus on the aortic root only to reduce the dose of contrast media. However, in the majority of TAVI patients, evaluation of the peripheral access arteries is often required, in which the scan range needs to cover a large area from the neck base to below the common femoral artery. In order to reduce the radiation dose and the use of contrast media, a two-step imaging strategy is often implemented. As shown in Fig. 8.1, first, a prospective ECG-triggered or a retrospective ECG-gated acquisition is performed to cover the cardiac region, which is similar to the acquisition of a conventional coronary CTA. Then, it is followed by a non-gated acquisition to cover the full scan range from the supra-clavicular level to the groin level. The ranges and timing of the two steps should be adjusted based on the available CT hardware. For example, for CT scanners with a wide detector, the scan range of step one can be expanded to the neck base, followed by an immediate step two with a contiguous scan range from the diaphragm to the groin level. On the other hand, for high-speed CT scanners, such as the dual-source MDCT, it may be possible to omit step two and scan the whole range using a single prospective ECG-triggered high-pitch spiral acquisition.

ECG gating is a prerequisite of CT imaging of the aortic root. The dimension of the aortic annulus varies in cardiac phases. In most cases, it reaches the maximum annular diameter in peak systole [6]. To avoid selecting an undersized THV, it is recommended to image the aortic root in the systolic phase to capture the largest annular dimension. Another important rationale of using an ECG-gated acquisition for the cardiac region is to freeze the motion of the aortic root as much as possible in order to improve the CT image

Fig. 8.1 The scan range of TAVI CT. The two scan ranges are selected based on the scout image of the patient. The scan range of the first step that covers the cardiac region is depicted in the red box. The scan range of the second step that covers from the supraclavicular level to the groin level is depicted in the green box

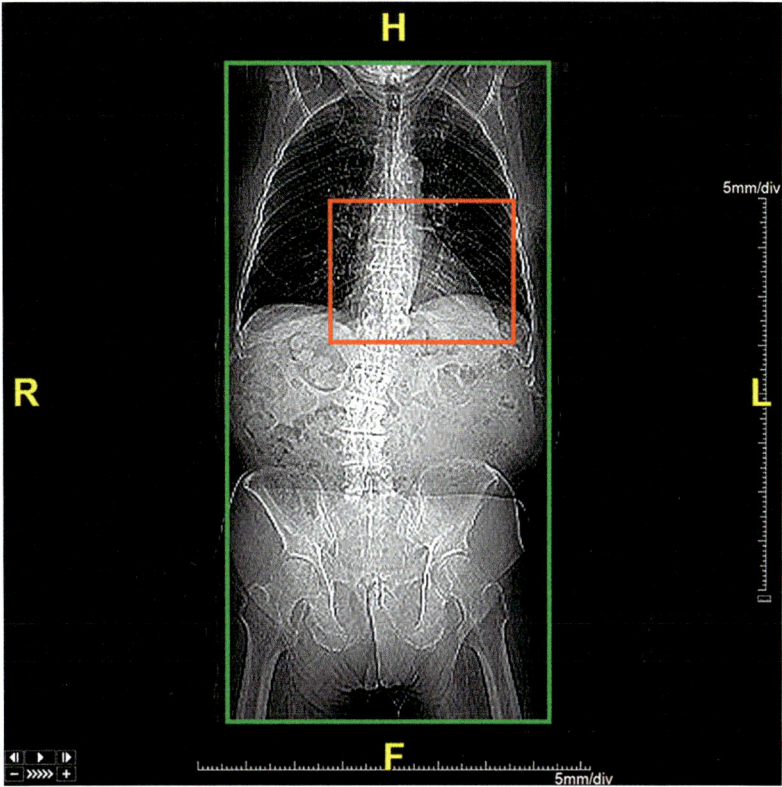

quality. Compared to prospective ECG-triggering, retrospective ECG-gated acquisition is typically associated with a higher dose of radiation exposure, but a better tolerance to irregular and/or fast heart rhythm. Depending on the patient's condition and the hardware of the CT scanner, the prospective ECG-triggered technique or the retrospective ECG-gated technique with a tube current modulation can be elected at the physician's or CT technician's discretion. The systolic phase (30–40% R-R interval) is usually targeted for data acquisition and reconstruction.

The choice of CT imaging parameters in TAVI greatly depends on the CT hardware. For centers with prior experiences of performing coronary CTA, it is recommended to start with the parameters of the coronary CTA protocol and adjust accordingly based on the clinical needs. The reconstruction slice thickness should be <1 mm to allow accurate geometric assessment of the aortic root. The tube voltage of TAVI CT can be set to lower than that of coronary CTA because image noise does not affect the assessment of the

aortic root to the same extent as to coronary CTA. More importantly, a lower tube voltage may increase the attenuation of the contrast-enhanced aortic root and, therefore, reduce the necessary dose of the contrast media. In CT scanners with high tube current capacities, imaging with a high tube current and a low tube voltage has been implemented to greatly reduce the dose of the contrast media [7]. Spectral imaging-enabled CT scanners have also been used to cut the contrast dose [8].

To ensure the presence of adequate contrast in the aortic root and the peripheral arteries, image acquisition should be initiated by using a Hounsfield unit (HU)-based bolus tracking method or using a test bolus. However, the latter induces the use of an additional contrast dose (typically 20 mL). In the bolus tracking method, the region of interest (ROI) can be placed in an area close to the aortic root but with less motion, such as in the left atrium or in the proximal descending aorta. The attenuation threshold and the time intervals between the triggering time, the first-step imaging of the heart, and the second-step imaging of the peripheral arteries should be adjusted based on the considerations of a number of factors, including the CT hardware, the contrast media injection rate and duration, the patient size, the severity of the aortic stenosis, and the patient's cardiac function. In some slower CT systems, an additional contrast injection may be needed in between the first and second steps. As stated previously, renal insufficiency is not a rare comorbidity in TAVI patients, which requires special considerations to reduce the dose of the contrast media. A common practice is to use a lower contrast injection rate, such as 3–4 mL/s, as compared to the 5 mL/s in conventional coronary CTA protocols. The pre-TAVI CT imaging and the TAVI procedure should also be performed on different days to reduce the burden of impaired renal function.

8.2.2 Evaluation of Pre-TAVI CT

Accurate assessment of the aortic annular dimension is critical for the selection of the optimal THV size. Aortic annulus is a virtual fibrous ring connecting the left ventricle and the aortic root. Some TAVI CT post-processing software provides automated functions for aortic annulus detection and measurement. However, manual assessment is also straightforward to perform. The aortic annulus can be found by rotating the 3D CT image in a double-oblique fashion and looking for the three hinge points of the aortic cusps, i.e., the three lowest insertion points of the aortic leaflets to the aortic root. As shown in Fig. 8.2, these three hinge points define the aortic annulus plane, in which the aortic annulus can be delineated. Because CT is an isotropic 3D imaging technique with a submillimeter resolution, studies have shown it is superior to 2D echocardiography in predicting post-TAVI complications, such as PVL, and determining the ideal THV size [9, 10]. A number of different measurements of the annular dimension have been proposed. The mean diameter of the annulus can be calculated as the average of the longest and shortest diameters of the oval-shaped annulus. The perimeter-derived diameter D_p and

the area-derived diameter D_A can be calculated assuming a circular annulus: $D_p = P/\pi$ and $D_p = 2\sqrt{A/\pi}$, respectively, where P is the annular perimeter and A is the annular area.

The selection of the THV size should be guided by the measurements of the aortic annulus. THV manufacturers, including Edwards Lifesciences and Medtronic, provide guidelines for THV size selections based on the annular dimensions derived from preprocedural imaging. Because of the systematic measurement discrepancy between different imaging modalities, the sizing scales are usually technique specific. In the early generations of the THVs, the manufacturer-provided sizing scale was derived from 2D echocardiography due to the lack of CT imaging data. Therefore, caution must be exercised when interpreting those guidelines. Modified sizing scales for CT-derived annular dimension have been proposed and have been validated for improving the outcome of TAVI [11]. It is recommended to use those modified sizing scales that are tailored to CT imaging. In the newer generations of THVs, the sizing scales for echocardiography and CT are usually both provided by the manufacturers. In the self-expandable valves, the mean diameter and the perimeter-derived diameter are mostly used to determine the THV size, mainly because of the elliptical shape of the self-expandable valve post valve deployment. On the contrary, in the balloon-expandable valves, the annular area and/or the area-derived annular diameter is mostly used for valve sizing because of the more circular shape of the balloon-expandable valve post valve deployment. Generally, the size of the selected THV should be larger than the native aortic annulus to prevent PVL. The oversizing of the annular area can be set to about 10% in the balloon-expandable valves [12], and the oversizing of the annular perimeter can be set to about 10–25% in the self-expandable valves [13]. The presence and the severity of aortic calcification should also be considered for determining the degree of THV oversizing, specifically for annulus with a borderline dimension. In patients with a heavily calcified aortic root, a lower oversizing degree should be considered.

In addition to the annulus dimension, a number of other geometric parameters of the aortic

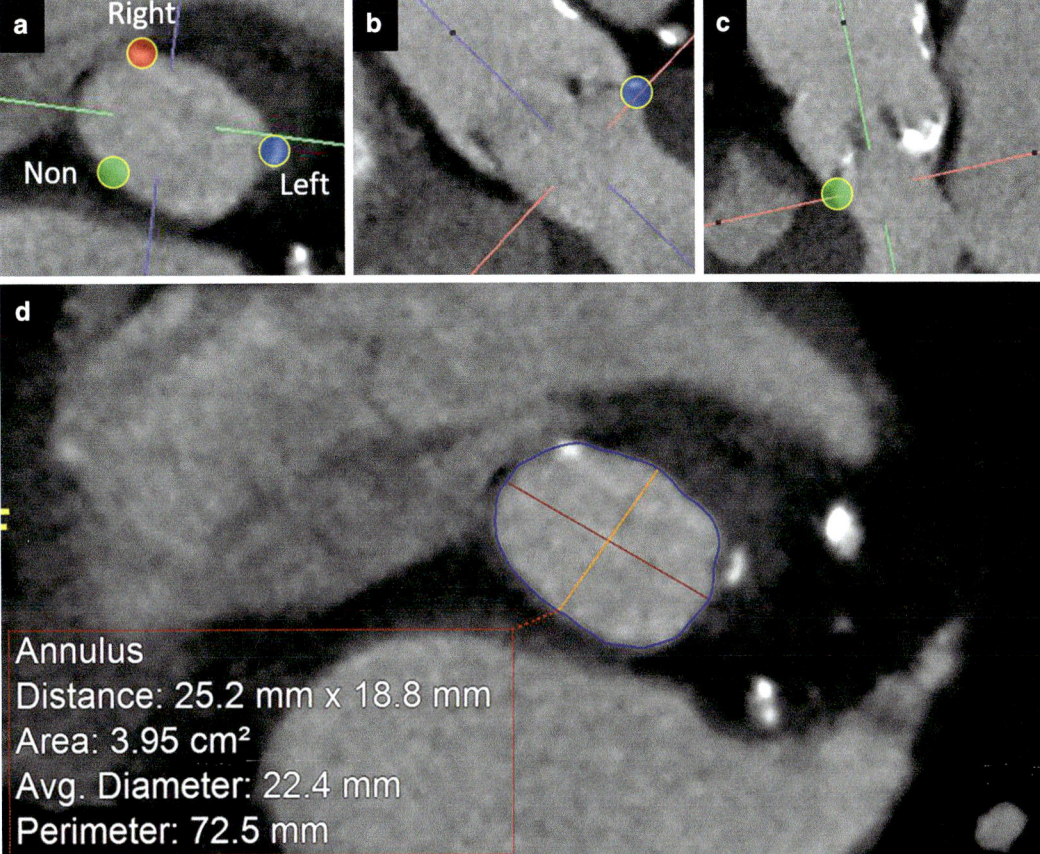

Fig. 8.2 Assessment of the aortic annulus. (**a**) The annular plane is defined by the three hinge points, i.e., the right coronary hinge point (red), the left coronary hinge point (blue), and the noncoronary hinge point (green). (**b, c**) In the longitudinal views, the hinge points are the lowest insertion points of the aortic leaflets to the aortic root. (**d**) The aortic annulus can be delineated in the cross-sectional view of the annular plane. Annular size can be measured as the maximum and minimum diameters, the annular area, the average diameter, and the annular perimeter

root should be measured from the CT image for the selection of the THV types and sizes. Because the balloon-expandable valves and the self-expandable valves are two very different designs, the required measurements by the two systems are also different. As shown in Fig. 8.3a, b, in balloon-expandable valves, it is required by the manufacturer to measure the distances from the coronary ostia to the annular plane to assess the risk of coronary obstruction. In addition, the length of the aortic leaflets and the presence of severe leaflet calcification may also be reported, because they have been shown to contribute to coronary obstruction in balloon-expandable valves [14], too. As shown in Fig. 8.3c–e, manufacturer's guideline of the self-expandable valve requires the assessment of the diameter of the ascending aorta, which is measured at 4 cm above the annular plane, and the diameter and height of the sinus of Valsalva. Because the self-expandable valve has a taller profile that extends into the ascending aorta after deployment, such measurements are needed to ensure the appropriate anchoring and apposition of the self-expandable valve in the aortic root.

CT imaging has a unique strength in assessing the extent and morphology of calcium depositions in the aortic root, which have been shown to be related to various complications post TAVI [15–17]. Excessive aortic root calcification is considered a risk factor of device landing-zone rupture. Calcification in the sinus of Valsalva,

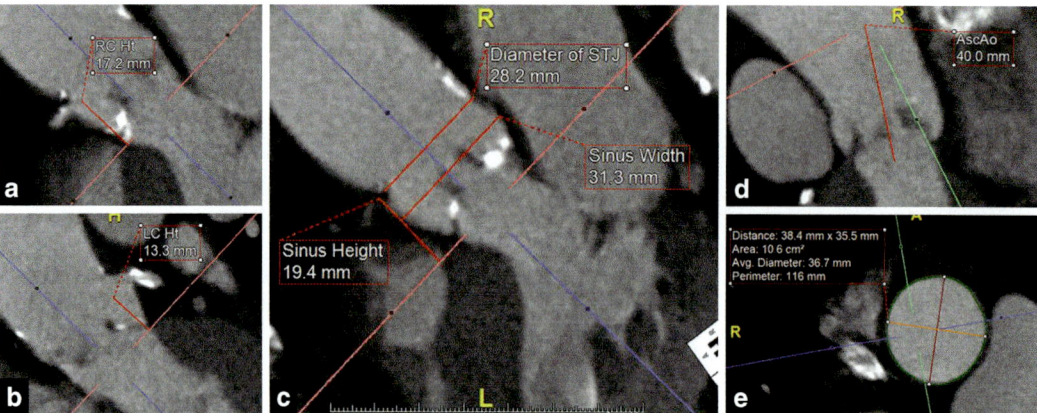

Fig. 8.3 Measurements of the aortic root. (**a**) and (**b**) show the measurements of the left and right coronary heights, respectively, which are defined as the distances from the coronary ostia to the annular plane. (**c**) shows the measurement of the sinus height, the sinus width, and the diameter of the sinotubular junction (STJ). (**d, e**) show the measurement of the diameter of the ascending aorta 4 cm above the annular plane

specifically on the leaflets, may also increase the risk of coronary obstruction. Moreover, landing-zone calcification could lead to an incomplete sealing between the THV and the native aortic root, which is believed to be an important cause of the occurrence of PVL post TAVI. Aortic root calcification may also interfere with the THV deployment and result in valve malapposition, requiring a post-dilation after the initial valve deployment. In addition, recent development in the design of THVs, such as adding a sealing cuff to the Sapien 3 [18] and an outer wrap to the Evolut Pro [19], has significantly reduced the rate of PVL occurrence post TAVI. However, the rates of needing new permanent pacemaker (PPM) implantations in both types of THVs remain high. Calcifications in the LVOT, specifically in the areas below the left and right coronary cusps, have been shown to be associated with increased risks of the use of PPM [20].

Calcification in the vicinity of the aortic root should be qualitatively graded and reported. The morphology and spatial distribution of the calcium depositions, such as the presences of large nodular calcifications in the annulus and streaks of calcification protruding into the LVOT, may also be reported for their clinical significances. Quantitative assessment of calcification is traditionally performed on non-enhanced CT images using the conventional Agatston score [21], volume score [22], or mass score [23] method. It is optional to perform a non-enhanced CT acquisition of the aortic root region before the contrast administration for the purpose of calcium quantification at the physician's discretion. However, this will also lead to an increased radiation exposure to the patient. Caution must also be exercised when using a lower tube voltage (<120 kV) in the non-enhanced CT acquisition, where the conventional calcium cutoff (130 HU) should be adjusted. Methods that use a higher attenuation threshold to derive calcium volume and calcium mass in contrast-enhanced CT images have been proposed [24]. However, there is currently no large studies that support the accuracy and effectiveness of these quantitative calcium analysis methods in enhanced CT images.

8.2.3 Angiographic Projection Angles

During the TAVI procedure, the interventionist relies on the 2D fluoroscopic projection image of the aortic root to guide the THV deployment. The 2D projection angle needs to be adjusted to be perpendicular to the center line of the aortic root and parallel to the aortic annulus plane, which is, as previously stated, defined by the three lowest insertion points of the aortic valve leaflets. If the pre-TAVI CT imaging had not been performed, the interventionist would be required to manually find the 2D projection angle by performing repeated aortograms to fine-tune the fluoroscopy orientation. This would lead to increased radiation and contrast doses administered to the patient and lengthen the procedural time. Assuming the positioning of the patient during the pre-TAVI CT acquisition is the same as during the actual TAVI procedure, a series of 2D projection angles can be derived from the pre-TAVI CT image to predict the appropriate fluoroscopic projection angles in the TAVI procedure. Although the assumption of the unchanged patient positioning does not always hold true, such a prediction before TAVI could reduce the need for the multiple aortograms and more importantly, reduce the contrast media volume, which is often a critical issue in the elderly population of the TAVI patients [25, 26].

The angiographic projection angle can be automatically calculated using a designated TAVI CT post-processing software based on the three leaflet insertion points [27]. As shown in Fig. 8.4, the projection angle can also be manually derived by rotating the 3D rendering of the heart and searching for a viewing angle that aligns the three insertion points to form a straight line. Once a projection angle is determined, theoretically an infinite number of projection angles can be obtained by revolving the projection around the center line of the aortic root. However, such angles are often restricted by the physical environment. The setup of the catheterization laboratory and the configuration of the angiography equipment need to be considered for the selection of the appropriate projection angles.

8.2.4 Evaluation of Vascular Access

The delivery system of TAVI is designed to transport the THV to the aortic root for deployment without an open-chest surgery. The delivery of the TAVI valve can be done via different access routes. For the commonly used CoreValve and Sapien valves, the most frequently used access route is the iliofemoral axis. Other less frequently used routes may include the transaxillary, transaortic, and transapical accesses. The selection of the access route of TAVI should be made based on a comprehensive consideration of the characteristics of the THV valve, the delivery system, and the vascular anatomy/pathology of the patient. Because of the isotropic 3D imaging capability, preprocedural CT angiography plays a

Fig. 8.4 Method of finding the angiographic projection angle. The angiographic projection angle can be derived by rotating the 3D-rendered reconstruction of the heart and aligning the left (L), right (R), and noncoronary (N) hinge points to form a straight line

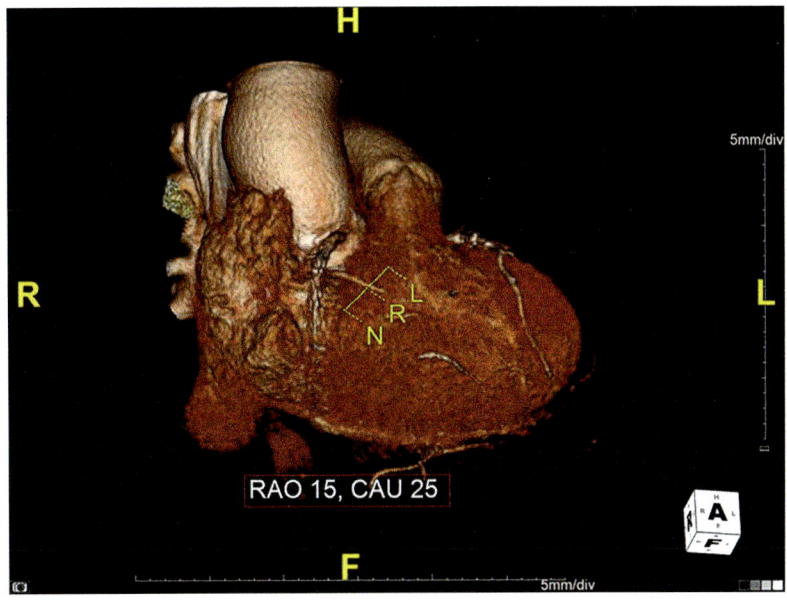

critical role in finding the optimal access route to minimize the potential risks of vascular complications, which have been defined by the Valve Academic Research Consortium [28].

To assess the appropriateness of the potential transfemoral access route using a peripheral CT angiography, starting from the access site of the transfemoral route, the complete endovascular delivery pathway, including the common femoral, the external iliac, the common iliac, the descending aorta, the aortic arch, the ascending aorta, and the aortic root, should be evaluated. Ideally, the luminal diameter of the endovascular pathway should be always larger than the sheath size of the THV delivery system to ensure a smooth passage of the transcatheter device. However, the sheath size and the introducer pro-

file vary in type and size of the TAVI valve. Moreover, the development of a delivery system with a smaller sheath size and a lower profile introducer has been actively carried out by both TAVI vendors. A continuous improvement of the delivery system has been witnessed over the generations of the TAVI valves. Therefore, the evaluation of the delivery pathway should be performed on a THV-specific basis. The ratio of the sheath size to the femoral artery size (SFAR) has been proposed recently [6], in which a threshold of 1.05 has been shown to be predictive of periprocedural vascular injuries. Depending on the type and size of the valves, the minimum luminal diameters have also been recommended [29].

As shown in Fig. 8.5a, for the measurement of the minimum luminal diameter, the peripheral

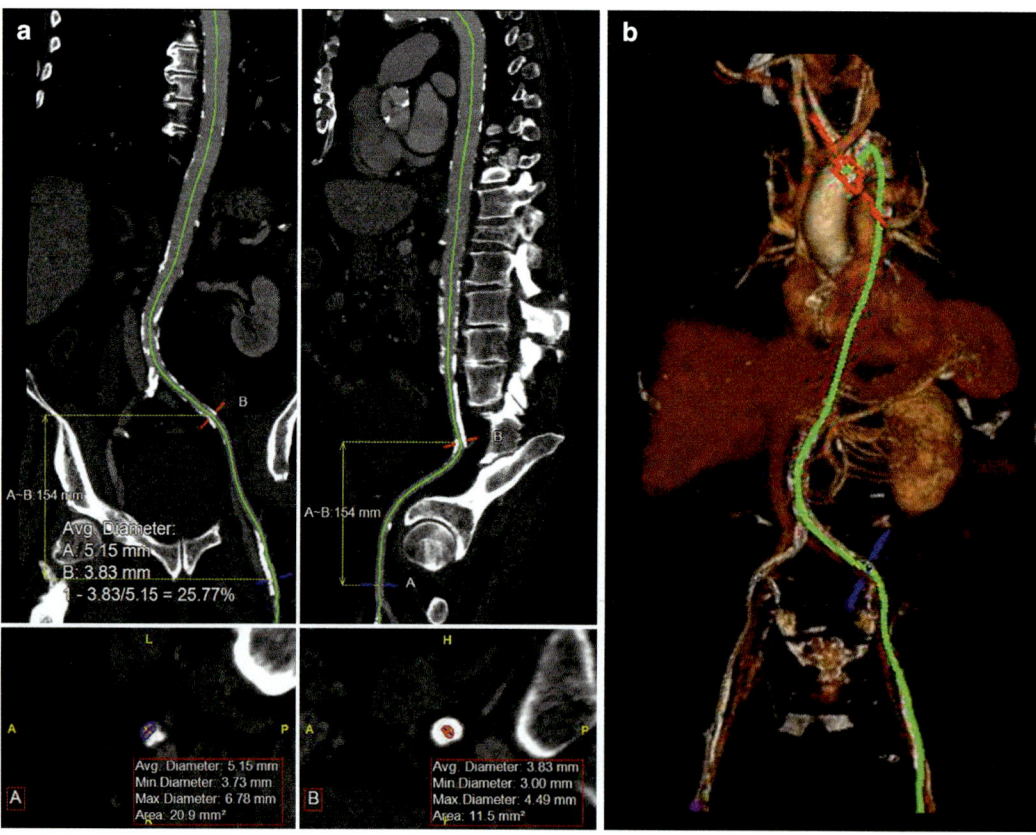

Fig. 8.5 Analysis of the CT angiography for the evaluation of the vascular access. (**a**) The peripheral CT angiography is typically depicted using a curved multiplanar reformation. Minimum luminal diameter is measured in the potentially most stenotic segments. The degree and morphology of calcification can also be visualized. (**b**) The 3D-rendered volumetric reconstruction of the iliofemoral axis can be used for the evaluation of vessel tortuosity

CT angiography is usually depicted using a curved multiplanar reformation for an initial visual assessment of the iliofemoral axis. Both the left and right iliofemoral pathways should be analyzed. Along the center line of the pathway, the most stenotic locations that may potentially lead to delivery failures can be annotated for further inspection. The luminal areas and diameters at those locations can be measured in the cross-sectional views of the artery. It must be noted that the minimum luminal diameter is not the only factor that determines the appropriateness of the access route. It has been shown that in relatively compliant arteries without excessive calcification, a short segment with a minimum luminal diameter 1–2 mm smaller than the sheath size may still allow a successful TAVI deployment [30, 31].

In addition to the luminal diameters, a number of other variables, such as the regional calcium burdens and calcium morphologies, the degrees of the arterial tortuosities, and any vascular anomalies, should also be reported for full consideration. Atherosclerosis and calcium burdens should be qualitatively graded. The extent and morphology of the atherosclerotic calcification, which are important for the interpretation of the CT angiography, should be reported. The partial volume artifact associated with severe calcifications may overestimate the stenosis degree of the target vessel and result in a lower estimation of the luminal diameters. On the other hand, if the morphology of the calcification exhibits a circumferential or horseshoe pattern, it may more likely restrict the expansion of the artery when the delivery sheath passes. Moreover, the arterial tortuosity is also a risk factor when atherosclerosis and calcification are presented. As shown in Fig. 8.5b, the 3D-rendered volumetric reconstruction of the iliofemoral axis is often used for the evaluation of vessel tortuosity.

If the transfemoral access route is deemed not suitable for the TAVI procedure, the potential transaxillary, transaortic, and transapical access routes should also be assessed. The aforementioned CT analysis technique of the transfemoral access can be similarly applied to the transaxillary approach. For the evaluation of the transaor-tic access, CT image can be used to identify the aortic access site and select the optimal delivery trajectory. In the preparation of the transapical approach, the location of the left ventricular apex can also be identified in the CT image to facilitate the transapical puncture.

8.3   Postprocedural Imaging

Postprocedural follow-up CT imaging is not recommended for routine clinical use in TAVI patients. The exact clinical role of post-TAVI CT remains unclear. However, CT has been used as a valuable tool to evaluate the position and the shape of the valve post TAVI in the aortic root. CT has been successfully used to reveal THV migration and strut fractures and degenerations [32]. Moreover, subclinical leaflet thrombosis post TAVI has been found using CT imaging, which is believed to be associated with increased risks of strokes and/or transient ischemic attacks [33]. Subclinical leaflet thrombosis can be identified as hypoattenuating lesions adjacent to the bioprosthetic leaflets with reduced leaflet motions using 4D CT acquisitions [34, 35].

8.4   Conclusion

CT imaging has emerged as the standard of care to be routinely performed before the TAVI procedure for patient screening, THV selection, and access route evaluation. Evidences from recent trials showed that it may be appropriate to expand the indication of TAVI to patients with intermediate or even low risk of surgery [36]. Given such an emerging expansion of the TAVI indication, preprocedural planning of TAVI has become even more critical for the prevention of post-TAVI complications. CT-based annular sizing has been shown to be superior to 2D echocardiography in reducing the occurrence of PVL post TAVI [2, 10]. CT allows a more accurate and more reproducible 3D assessment of the aortic root and the endovascular pathway than the other 2D imaging modalities. Moreover, CT has a unique ability of imaging calcification and vessel tortuosity. In this chapter, we have reviewed the role of CT imaging in TAVI and discussed the data acquisition protocols and the image processing and evaluation techniques. CT imaging may also potentially play an important role in the postprocedural evaluation of TAVI.

Acknowledgments *Conflict of Interest*: None.

References

1. Blanke P, Schoepf UJ, Leipsic JA. CT in transcatheter aortic valve replacement. Radiology. 2013;269(3):650–69.
2. Jilaihawi H, Kashif M, Fontana G, Furugen A, Shiota T, Friede G, et al. Cross-sectional computed tomographic assessment improves accuracy of aortic annular sizing for transcatheter aortic valve replacement and reduces the incidence of paravalvular aortic regurgitation. J Am Coll Cardiol. 2012;59(14):1275–86.
3. Schultz CJ, Tzikas A, Moelker A, Rossi A, Nuis R-J, Geleijnse MM, et al. Correlates on MSCT of paravalvular aortic regurgitation after transcatheter aortic valve implantation using the Medtronic CoreValve prosthesis. Catheter Cardiovasc Interv. 2011;78(3):446–55.
4. Gurvitch R, Webb JG, Yuan R, Johnson M, Hague C, Willson AB, et al. Aortic annulus diameter determination by multidetector computed tomography: reproducibility, applicability, and implications for transcatheter aortic valve implantation. JACC Cardiovasc Interv. 2011;4(11):1235–45.
5. Ng ACT, Delgado V, van der Kley F, Shanks M, van de Veire NRL, Bertini M, et al. Comparison of aortic root dimensions and geometries before and after transcatheter aortic valve implantation by 2- and 3-dimensional transesophageal echocardiography and multislice computed tomography. Circ Cardiovasc Imaging. 2010;3(1):94–102.
6. Hayashida K, Lefèvre T, Chevalier B, Hovasse T, Romano M, Garot P, et al. Transfemoral aortic valve implantation new criteria to predict vascular complications. JACC Cardiovasc Interv. 2011;4(8):851–8.
7. Felmly LM, De Cecco CN, Schoepf UJ, Varga-Szemes A, Mangold S, McQuiston AD, et al. Low contrast medium-volume third-generation dual-source computed tomography angiography for transcatheter aortic valve replacement planning. Eur Radiol. 2017;27(5):1944–53.
8. Yuan R, Shuman WP, Earls JP, Hague CJ, Mumtaz HA, Scott-Moncrieff A, et al. Reduced iodine load at CT pulmonary angiography with dual-energy monochromatic imaging: comparison with standard CT pulmonary angiography—a prospective randomized trial. Radiology. 2012;262(1):290–7.
9. Schoenhagen P, Kapadia SR, Halliburton SS, Svensson LG, Murat Tuzcu E. Computed tomography evaluation for transcatheter aortic valve implantation (TAVI): imaging of the aortic root and iliac arteries. J Cardiovasc Comput Tomogr. 2011;5(5):293–300.
10. Willson AB, Webb JG, Labounty TM, Achenbach S, Moss R, Wheeler M, et al. 3-Dimensional aortic annular assessment by multidetector computed tomography predicts moderate or severe paravalvular regurgitation after transcatheter aortic valve replacement: a multicenter retrospective analysis. J Am Coll Cardiol. 2012;59(14):1287–94.
11. Binder RK, Webb JG, Willson AB, Urena M, Hansson NC, Norgaard BL, et al. The impact of integration of a multidetector computed tomography annulus area sizing algorithm on outcomes of transcatheter aortic valve replacement: a prospective, multicenter, controlled trial. J Am Coll Cardiol. 2013;62(5):431–8.
12. Willson AB, Webb JG, Freeman M, Wood DA, Gurvitch R, Thompson CR, et al. Computed tomography-based sizing recommendations for transcatheter aortic valve replacement with balloon-expandable valves: comparison with transesophageal echocardiography and rationale for implementation in a prospective trial. J Cardiovasc Comput Tomogr. 2012;6(6):406–14.
13. Schultz CJ, Moelker A, Piazza N, Tzikas A, Otten A, Nuis RJ, et al. Three dimensional evaluation of the aortic annulus using multislice computer tomography: are manufacturer's guidelines for sizing for percutaneous aortic valve replacement helpful? Eur Heart J. 2010;31(7):849–56.
14. Webb JG, Chandavimol M, Thompson CR, Ricci DR, Carere RG, Munt BI, et al. Percutaneous aortic valve implantation retrograde from the femoral artery. Circulation. 2006;113(6):842–50.
15. Delgado V, Ng ACT, van de Veire NR, van der Kley F, Schuijf JD, Tops LF, et al. Transcatheter aortic valve implantation: role of multi-detector row computed tomography to evaluate prosthesis positioning and deployment in relation to valve function. Eur Heart J. 2010;31(9):1114–23.
16. Koos R, Mahnken AH, Dohmen G, Brehmer K, Günther RW, Autschbach R, et al. Association of aortic valve calcification severity with the degree of aortic regurgitation after transcatheter aortic valve implantation. Int J Cardiol. 2011;150(2):142–5.
17. John D, Bullesfeld L, Yuecel S, Mueller R, Latsios G, Beucher H, et al. Correlation of device landing zone calcification and acute procedural success in patients undergoing transcatheter aortic valve implantations with the self-expanding CoreValve prosthesis. JACC Cardiovasc Interv. 2010;3(2):233–43.
18. Herrmann HC, Thourani VH, Kodali SK, Makkar RR, Szeto WY, Anwaruddin S, et al. One-year clinical outcomes with SAPIEN 3 transcatheter aortic valve replacement in high-risk and inoperable patients with severe aortic stenosis. Circulation. 2016;134(2):130–40.

19. Forrest JK, Mangi AA, Popma JJ, Khabbaz K, Reardon MJ, Kleiman NS, et al. Early outcomes with the Evolut PRO repositionable self-expanding transcatheter aortic valve with pericardial wrap. JACC Cardiovasc Interv. 2018;11(2):160–8.

20. Mauri V, Reimann A, Stern D, Scherner M, Kuhn E, Rudolph V, et al. Predictors of permanent pacemaker implantation after transcatheter aortic valve replacement with the SAPIEN 3. JACC Cardiovasc Interv. 2016;9(21):2200–9.

21. Agatston AS, Janowitz WR, Hildner FJ, Zusmer NR, Viamonte M, Detrano R. Quantification of coronary artery calcium using ultrafast computed tomography. J Am Coll Cardiol. 1990;15(4):827–32.

22. Callister TQ, Cooil B, Raya SP, Lippolis NJ, Russo DJ, Raggi P. Coronary artery disease: improved reproducibility of calcium scoring with an electron-beam CT volumetric method. Radiology. 1998;208(3):807–14.

23. Hong C, Becker CR, Joseph Schoepf U, Ohnesorge B, Bruening R, Reiser MF. Coronary artery calcium: absolute quantification in nonenhanced and contrast-enhanced multi-detector row CT studies. Radiology. 2002;223(2):474–80.

24. Schultz C, Rossi A, van Mieghem N, van der Boon R, Papadopoulou S-L, van Domburg R, et al. Aortic annulus dimensions and leaflet calcification from contrast MSCT predict the need for balloon post-dilatation after TAVI with the Medtronic CoreValve prosthesis. EuroIntervention. 2011;7(5):564–72.

25. Kurra V, Kapadia SR, Tuzcu EM, Halliburton SS, Svensson L, Roselli EE, et al. Pre-procedural imaging of aortic root orientation and dimensions: comparison between X-ray angiographic planar imaging and 3-dimensional multidetector row computed tomography. JACC Cardiovasc Interv. 2010;3(1):105–13.

26. Gurvitch R, Wood DA, Leipsic J, Tay E, Johnson M, Ye J, et al. Multislice computed tomography for prediction of optimal angiographic deployment projections during transcatheter aortic valve implantation. JACC Cardiovasc Interv. 2010;3(11):1157–65.

27. Binder RK, Leipsic J, Wood D, Moore T, Toggweiler S, Willson A, et al. Prediction of optimal deployment projection for transcatheter aortic valve replacement: angiographic 3-dimensional reconstruction of the aortic root versus multidetector computed tomography. Circ Cardiovasc Interv. 2012;5(2):247–52.

28. Kappetein AP, Head SJ, Généreux P, Piazza N, van Mieghem NM, Blackstone EH, et al. Updated standardized endpoint definitions for transcatheter aortic valve implantation: the Valve Academic Research Consortium-2 consensus document. Eur Heart J. 2012;33(19):2403–18.

29. Achenbach S, Delgado V, Hausleiter J, Schoenhagen P, Min JK, Leipsic JA. SCCT expert consensus document on computed tomography imaging before transcatheter aortic valve implantation (TAVI)/transcatheter aortic valve replacement (TAVR). J Cardiovasc Comput Tomogr. 2012;6(6):366–80.

30. Leipsic J, Hague CJ, Gurvitch R, Ajlan AM, Labounty TM, Min JK. MDCT to guide transcatheter aortic valve replacement and mitral valve repair. Cardiol Clin. 2012;30(1):147–60.

31. Masson J-B, Kovac J, Schuler G, Ye J, Cheung A, Kapadia S, et al. Transcatheter aortic valve implantation: review of the nature, management, and avoidance of procedural complications. JACC Cardiovasc Interv. 2009;2(9):811–20.

32. Tay ELW, Gurvitch R, Wijeysinghe N, Nietlispach F, Leipsic J, Wood DA, et al. Outcome of patients after transcatheter aortic valve embolization. JACC Cardiovasc Interv. 2011;4(2):228–34.

33. Chakravarty T, Søndergaard L, Friedman J, De Backer O, Berman D, Kofoed KF, et al. Subclinical leaflet thrombosis in surgical and transcatheter bioprosthetic aortic valves: an observational study. Lancet. 2017;389(10087):2383–92.

34. Pislaru SV, Nkomo VT, Sandhu GS. Assessment of prosthetic valve function after TAVR. JACC Cardiovasc Imaging. 2016;9(2):193–206.

35. Jilaihawi H, Asch FM, Manasse E, Ruiz CE, Jelnin V, Kashif M, et al. Systematic CT methodology for the evaluation of subclinical leaflet thrombosis. JACC Cardiovasc Imaging. 2017;10(4):461–70.

36. Moat NE. Will TAVR become the predominant method for treating severe aortic stenosis? N Engl J Med. 2016;374(17):1682–3.

Role of Magnetic Resonance Imaging in Transcatheter Aortic Valve Implantation

Giulia Pontecorboli, Silvia Pradella, Stefano Colagrande, and Carlo Di Mario

9.1 Introduction

Magnetic resonance imaging (MRI) is a noninvasive imaging technique that combines a powerful magnetic field with radiofrequencies in order to produce three-dimensional detailed anatomical images without the use of ionizing radiation. Cardiovascular MR (CMR) imaging is gaining importance in clinical and interventional cardiology as an emerging diagnostic tool to evaluate a wide spectrum of cardiovascular diseases. In a single exam, in fact, it can provide detailed information on cardiac and aortic anatomy, myocardial tissue characterization, and valve morphology and function. CMR is considered the gold standard imaging modality to assess cardiac volumes and function and to quantify myocardial mass

[1]. Valve pathology can be accurately evaluated through the use of different CMR sequences such as cine imaging and phase-contrast (PC) velocity mapping.

Computed tomography (CT) and echocardiography play a pivotal role in the setting of transcatheter aortic valve implantation (TAVI), also called transcatheter aortic valve replacement (TAVR), thanks to the excellent spatial resolution of CT and the wide availability and optimal temporal resolution of echocardiography. However, MRI is a noninvasive, radiation-free emergent alternative for both preoperative assessment and postoperative surveillance in patients undergoing TAVI, and there is increasing evidence that it can offer equivalent information to the other imaging modalities. In addition, MRI can provide incremental diagnostic and prognostic information, thanks to its unique properties, such as detailed anatomic assessment and advanced tissue characterization.

In current clinical practice of preoperative evaluation for TAVI, non-contrast MRI is commonly performed in patients with contraindications to CT such as severe renal function impairment (GFR < 30 mL/min/m²) or history of allergic reactions to iodinated contrast media. Furthermore, it has an important role in the evaluation of patients with inadequate acoustic window or in the event of discrepancy between echocardiographic parameters and symptoms, particularly in the context of low-gradient aortic stenosis (AS) and/or left ventricular systolic dysfunction [2, 3].

G. Pontecorboli
Department of Clinical and Experimental Medicine, AOU Careggi, University of Florence, Florence, Italy

S. Pradella
Department of Radiology, AOU Careggi, University of Florence, Florence, Italy

S. Colagrande
Radiodiagnostic Unit n. 2, AOU Careggi, University of Florence, Florence, Italy
e-mail: stefano.colagrande@unifi.it

C. Di Carlo (✉)
Structural Interventional Cardiology, Department of Clinical and Experimental Medicine, AOU Careggi, University of Florence, Florence, Italy
e-mail: carlo.dimario@unifi.it

© Springer Nature Switzerland AG 2019
A. Giordano et al. (eds.), *Transcatheter Aortic Valve Implantation*,
https://doi.org/10.1007/978-3-030-05912-5_9

There is a growing evidence base to suggest that tissue characterization using post-contrast CMR sequences such as late gadolinium enhancement (LGE) or novel non-contrast sequence (T1 mapping) provides prognostic information in patients with AS, and its incremental value is increasingly recognized in the clinical decision-making of patients who are potential candidates for valve correction [4–7].

MRI is also feasible and safe in the postoperative setting because the most widely implanted TAVI prostheses (Medtronic CoreValve® and Edward Sapien®) are MRI conditional in the static fields of 1.5 or 3.0 Tesla scanners [8]. One of the major determinants of procedural success, i.e., the degree of paravalvular aortic regurgitation, can be easily assessed with PC sequence, regardless of the presence of image artifacts around the prosthesis.

This chapter will explore the current role of MRI in the evaluation and management of patients undergoing TAVI and will offer a perspective on its future potential.

9.2 Pre-procedural Planning

9.2.1 Patient Selection: Determination of Severity of Aortic Stenosis

Transthoracic echocardiography (TTE) is the standard method for the evaluation of the severity of AS [9]. However, 20% of the TTE examinations result to be nondiagnostic due to suboptimal image quality [10]. In the setting of AS assessment in potential TAVI candidates, when echocardiography is not feasible or anatomical and functional measurements are inconsistent or even discordant, CMR may be a reliable alternative using either direct planimetry of the aortic valve orifice or velocity-encoded CMR techniques and assessing the hemodynamic status, which is particularly relevant in low-flow-low-gradient AS [3].

Two principal sequences are used for the assessment of the aortic stenosis: (1) cine imaging, which produces short movies showing heart and valve motion throughout the cardiac cycle, obtained with ECG triggering, and (2) velocity-encoded PC imaging, which is able to visualize moving fluid and analyze flows and velocities through a plane. Both sequences do not need contrast administration and thus can be performed safely in patients with renal failure.

Aortic valve area and morphology: CMR is a reliable technique to evaluate the morphology and function of the aortic valve. High-quality images can be acquired in any plane or phase of the cardiac cycle without limitations of acoustic windows, allowing for correct alignment and accurate measurements of the aortic valve orifice either with direct planimetry or continuity equation-based measurement. Direct planimetry is the most used technique and is achieved by placing a cine imaging plane through the valve tips in systole, starting from the left ventricular outflow tract (LVOT) views. Image slice must be thin (4–5 mm) and precisely at the valve tips. Acquisition of multiple thin slices in the aortic root parallel to the valve orifice is advisable in order to identify the true orifice, which is the smallest area between the aortic valve cusps at the time of maximal opening in ventricular systole (Fig. 9.1). This technique had shown a good agreement with transesophageal echocardiography in previous studies [11, 12] but can be limited by the difficult visualization of the aortic leaflets due to the presence of heavy calcifications, flow turbulence artifacts, and respiratory artifacts. Alternatively, the aortic valve area (AVA) can be computed from PC images using the continuity equation. Peak velocities are computed in regions of interest drawn in the transvalvular and LVOT plane, approximately 1 cm below the aortic annulus, and the LVOT dimensions are measured at the same level from cine images. By using the modified Bernoulli equation, peak and mean gradients are obtained.

Flow quantification: CMR enables direct flow quantification using through-plane PC velocity mapping [13] and allows for direct quantification of important parameters such as stroke volume, peak aortic valve velocity, peak and mean aortic gradient using the modified Bernoulli equation, and aortic regurgitant volume and fraction, with

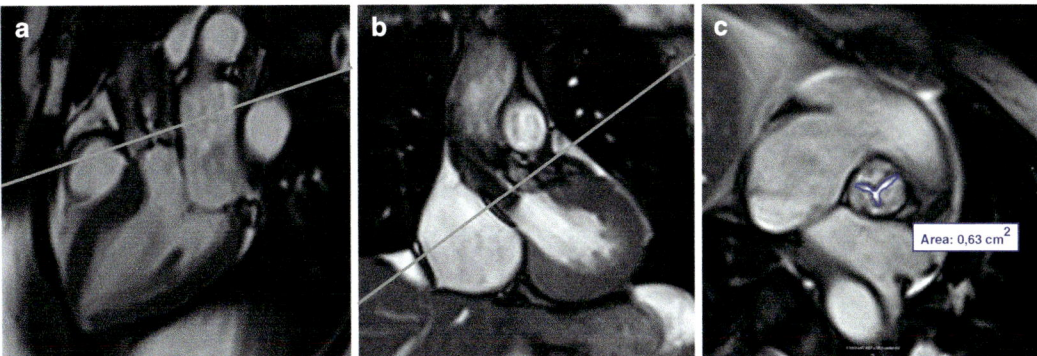

Fig. 9.1 Determination of severity of aortic stenosis by planimetry method. Starting from the two orthogonal views of the left ventricle outflow tract ((**a**) 3-chamber view and (**b**) coronal view), a cine imaging plane is placed through the aortic valve tips in systole. The planimetric area can be calculated on the short axis plane (**c**) manually drawing the anatomical aortic valve orifice area at the time of maximal opening of the valve during systole. The derived calculated area of 0.63 cm^2 is consistent with severe aortic stenosis

high reproducibility [14]. The imaging plane should be positioned in the aortic root, a few millimeters distal to the tips of the aortic valve leaflets, and must be orthogonal to the aortic flow jet (Fig. 9.2). CMR presents advantages over echocardiography in those cases where aortic roots are angulated or when the stenotic jets are not parallel to the LVOT resulting in difficult echo beam alignment. Nevertheless, one of the major drawbacks of the technique in this setting is that temporal resolution of CMR is lower than that of continuous-wave Doppler echocardiography (25–50 ms vs. 2 ms), and this often leads to the underestimation of aortic valve velocity measurements, especially when peak velocities exceed 3.5 m/s [15]. Additionally, a wrong slice positioning, i.e., not perpendicular to flow, inhomogeneous magnetic field, arrhythmias and turbulent post-stenotic flow can cause inaccuracies in measurements.

Hemodynamic assessment: Accurate measurement of left and right ventricular volumes, function, and mass are crucial for assessing the impact of valve lesions on the ventricles. CMR is the gold standard technique for this purpose as it does not rely on geometrical assumption for volume biplane calculation as echocardiography but is based on the Simpson's method of disks summation, whereby the sum of cross-sectional areas is multiplied by slice thickness (usually 8 mm) leading to precise volumetric assessment

(Fig. 9.3). In the setting of low-flow-low-gradient AS, which accounts approximately for 5–10% of patients with severe AS [16], CMR can diagnose a low-flow state by deriving the stroke volume index (SVI) either from the aortic flow data or from the volumetric analysis of the left ventricle (low-flow state is defined when SVI <35 mL/m^2) [17]. Moreover, adding a stress perfusion sequence to the protocol, LV function assessment can be repeated during administration of low-dose dobutamine in order to evaluate the contractile reserve and differentiate pseudo-aortic stenosis from real aortic stenosis [9].

9.3 Valve Sizing

Accurate measurement of the aortic annulus is essential for appropriate valve sizing in TAVI. Although this was initially performed using TTE or TEE, there is growing evidence that 3D techniques such as multidetector CT (MDCT) or CMR can provide more precise measurements, avoiding potential complications of over- and under-sizing such as aortic annular rupture and/or paravalvular aortic regurgitation (PAR). MDCT has become the reference standard for aortic root measurements, thanks to its excellent spatial resolution, but it requires ionizing radiation and the administration of iodinated contrast agents. It has been reported that approximately

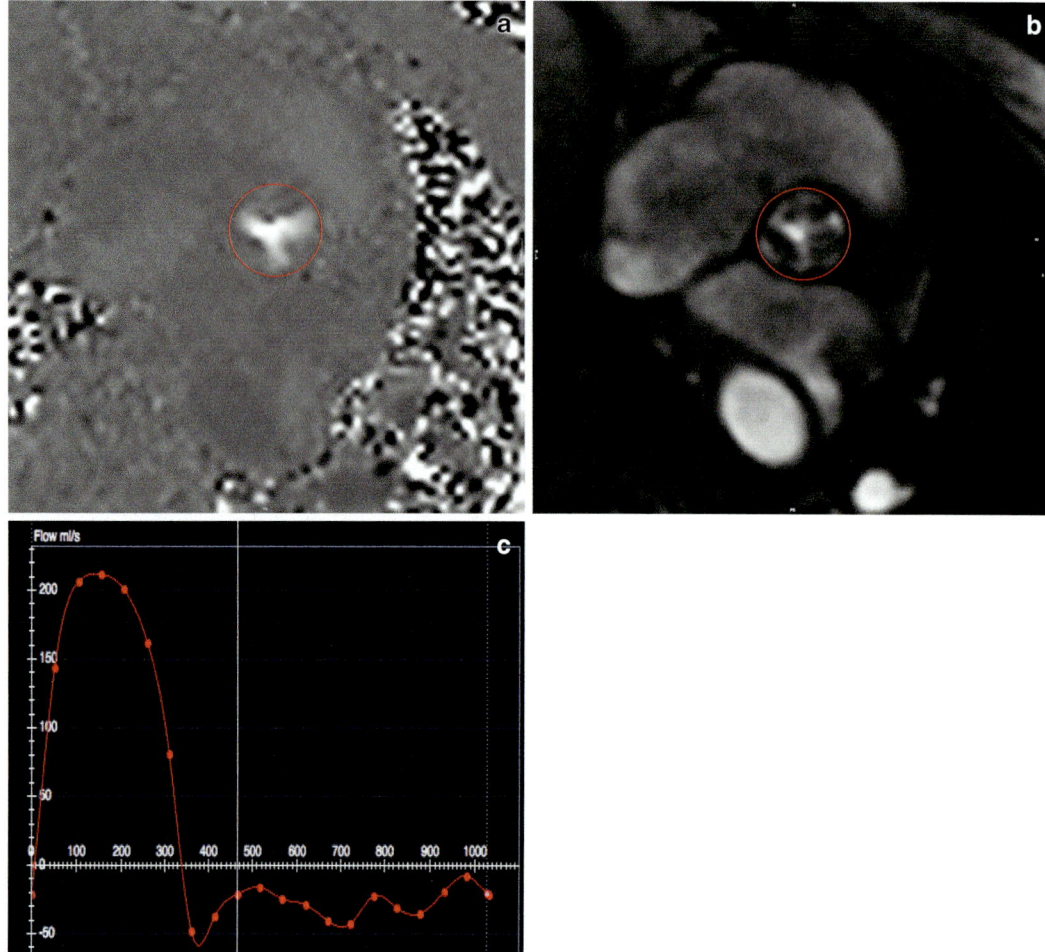

Fig. 9.2 Example of CMR assessment of aortic valve severity using through-plane phase contrast velocity mapping: from phase (**a**) and magnitude (**b**) images flow mea- surements of peak aortic valve velocity, peak and mean aortic gradient, stroke volume, regurgitant volume and regurgitant fraction can be derived (**c**)

20% of patients undergoing TAVI present contra- indication to MDCT due to renal failure, high heart rate, or arrhythmias [18]. CMR can be a contrast-free, noninvasive valuable alternative, thanks to its high spatial resolution and multipla- nar imaging reconstruction capabilities, and can provide comprehensive and accurate pre-proce- dural measurements of the aortic annulus, of the dimensions of the aortic valve leaflets, and of the height of the coronary ostia.

Precise measurement of the annulus is neces- sary to avoid mismatch between annulus and prosthesis. The aortic annulus has an ellipsoid shape, with larger coronal than sagittal diame- ters. Measurement of the annulus by CMR is performed meticulously at the plane of the vir- tual basal ring, identified by joining the basal attachments of aortic valve leaflets and is feasi- ble both with multiplanar 2D and 3D sequences. Sagittal and coronal 2D cine imaging of the LVOT can be used to measure annulus diame- ters, while a short-axis cine stack can be used to calculate the annular area, which is the most reproducible value (Fig. 9.4). 3D reconstruction performed by using non-contrast-enhanced nav- igator-gated 3D whole-heart sequence has been shown to give accurate measurements of the annulus perimeter, area, and diameters, thanks

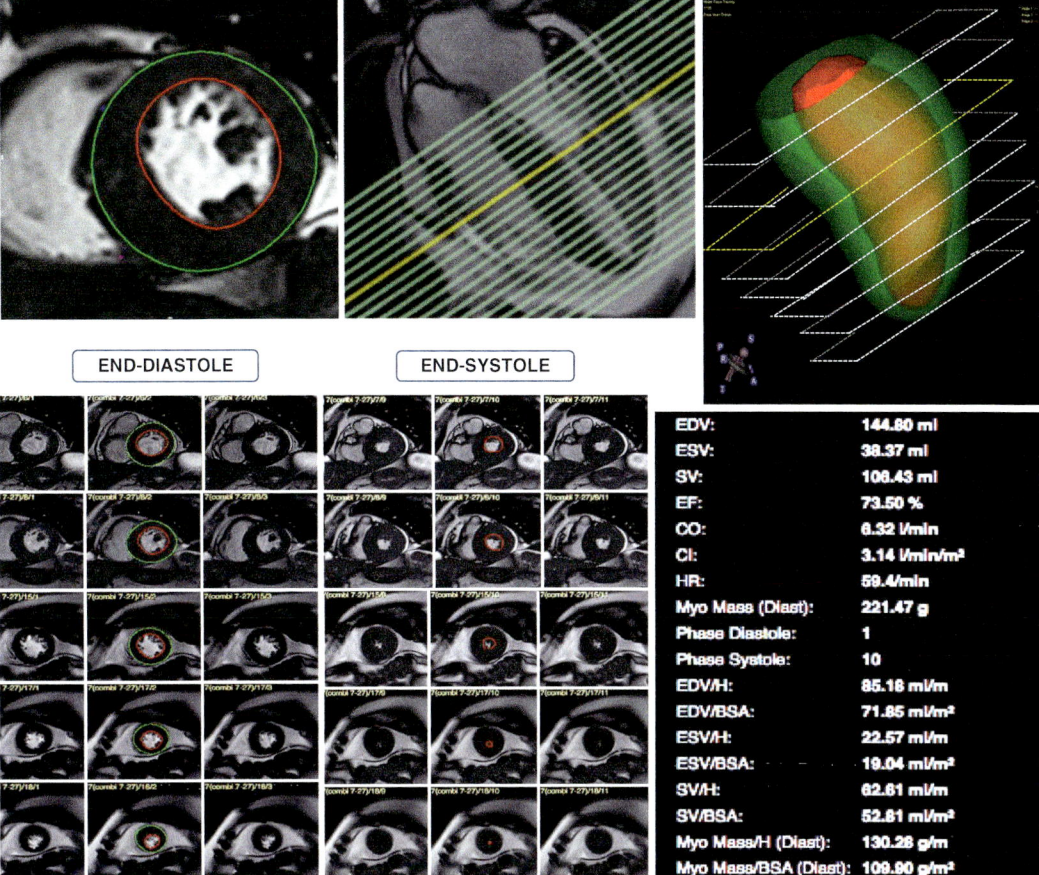

END-DIASTOLE	END-SYSTOLE

EDV:	144.80 ml
ESV:	38.37 ml
SV:	106.43 ml
EF:	73.50 %
CO:	6.32 l/min
CI:	3.14 l/min/m²
HR:	59.4/min
Myo Mass (Diast):	221.47 g
Phase Diastole:	1
Phase Systole:	10
EDV/H:	85.18 ml/m
EDV/BSA:	71.85 ml/m²
ESV/H:	22.57 ml/m
ESV/BSA:	19.04 ml/m²
SV/H:	62.61 ml/m
SV/BSA:	52.81 ml/m²
Myo Mass/H (Diast):	130.28 g/m
Myo Mass/BSA (Diast):	109.90 g/m²

Fig. 9.3 Morphological and functional MRI analysis of the left ventricle. Endocardial borders are outlined manually in both the end-diastolic and end-systolic phase in all short-axis cine images. Epicardial borders are contoured in end-diastole in order to measure LV mass. LV volumes, ejection fraction, stroke volume, cardiac output are calculated by the software (Circle Medical Imaging) using Simpson's method of disks summation, whereby the sum of the ventricular cavity areas is multiplied by slice thickness

to its submillimeter resolution [19]. From the same 2D and 3D CMR images, reliable measurements of the coronary ostia height and aortic valve leaflets length can also be obtained, which are of fundamental importance to prevent the occlusion of the coronary arteries caused by the displacement of the native aortic leaflets toward the aortic wall following prosthesis implantation.

CMR has demonstrated excellent correlation with CT-based measurements related to aortic root dimension, with a low intra- and interobserver variability [20], even in the setting of valve-in-valve TAVI planning, despite the presence of image artifacts generated by the metal components of the original aortic prosthesis [21].

9.4   Choice of Access

The evaluation of the best access route for TAVI is commonly performed using CT, which can accurately image the aorta and the peripheral vessel and evaluate caliber, tortuosity, and calcification. MRI could represent an alternative for access planning, but the suboptimal visualization of calcifications, which are often present and abundant in elderly patients' peripheral vasculature, limits the use of the

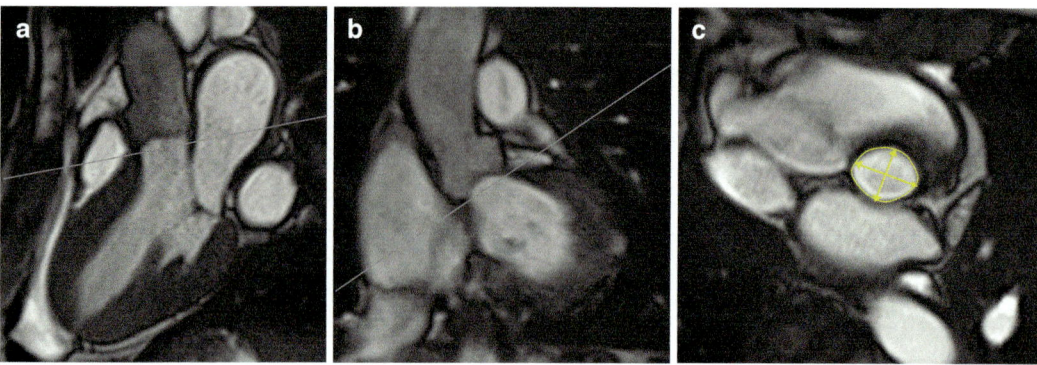

Fig. 9.4 Aortic annulus measurement by MRI. Starting from the two orthogonal views of the left ventricle outflow tract ((**a**) 3-chamber view; (**b**) coronal view), a cine imaging plane is placed in the virtual basal ring. Maximum and minimum diameter and annulus area can be measured at this level (**c**)

technique in the assessment of aortoiliac access, which represents more than 90% of the current implants. MRI angiography (or MRA) could overcome this shortcoming, but it requires contrast administration, which can cause nephrogenic systemic fibrosis in patients with preexisting severe renal dysfunction [22] and as such is not a valid alternative to CT in these patients. Conversely, when transfemoral access is contraindicated due to severe peripheral artery disease, MRI can be useful for preprocedural planning of alternative access, measuring the distance from the ascending aorta access site to the skin and to the aortic valve plane in case of transaortic access or the distance between LV apex from the sternum and skin surface in case of transapical access, similar to CTA but without using ionizing radiation and contrast agent [23]. In patients with socalled porcelain aortas, CMR is considered a second-line image modality, and CT remains the standard of choice not only because it permits better visualization of calcium but also because in this instance contrast agent administration is not required.

9.5 Predicting Prognosis

9.5.1 Myocardial Fibrosis

Myocardial fibrosis is the hallmark of the myocardial adaptation to the chronic pressure overload due to aortic stenosis. The increased LV wall stress secondary to the valve disease is initially compensated by LV hypertrophy to maintain good systolic function. However, the persistence of the increased afterload may lead to cellular apoptosis, myofibroblast activation, and changes in the extracellular matrix, with deposition of collagen I and loss of myofibers. Chronic ischemia caused by oxygen supply-demand mismatch and impaired coronary flow reserve may also play a role [24]. This structural remodeling, characterized by the transition from myocardial hypertrophy to myocardial fibrosis, results in adverse effects on systolic and diastolic LV function and can lead to heart failure, affecting prognosis.

The greatest advantage of MRI over other imaging modalities is its unique ability to perform tissue characterization, providing "in vivo histology" based on the inherent different magnetic properties of human tissues. CMR is the gold standard noninvasive imaging modality to visualize and quantify myocardial fibrosis, by using (1) late gadolinium enhancement (LGE) sequence for the evaluation of focal replacement fibrosis and (2) T1 mapping sequence, for assessing more diffuse patterns of interstitial fibrosis.

Late gadolinium enhancement (LGE): LGE sequence involves the intravenous administration of gadolinium-based contrast agents and is considered the reference method to quantify focal replacement fibrosis by MRI [25]. The technique relies on the altered washout of the contrast agents within damaged myocardial tissue, with fibrotic myocardium appearing bright, while normal myocardium appears as black on late inversion recovery T1-weighted imaging. The strong correlation between histologic findings of myocardial biopsy reported in previous studies [26] has confirmed the accuracy and reliability of this method, which has become the technique of choice to assess and quantify myocardial replacement fibrosis. LGE is detected in up to 62% of patients with severe aortic stenosis [5, 6, 27, 28], both with ischemic and non-ischemic patterns. While the ischemic LGE pattern involves the subendocardium along a coronary artery perfusion territory, the nonischemic pattern is mid-wall or epicardial and can be either diffuse, patchy, focal, or linear but typically spares the endocardium and does not follow a coronary distribution territory. In patients with moderate to severe AS, the presence of LGE has been reported as an independent predictor of mortality, increasing the risk of death of 6–8 times, being of incremental value to ejection fraction alone in the risk stratification of these patients [5]. In patients undergoing AVR and TAVI, the presence and extent of myocardial fibrosis detected by LGE predict increased perioperative risk and worse all-cause and cardiovascular disease-related survival, mainly due to an increased risk of sudden cardiac death [6]. Therefore, it has been suggested that fibrosis could serve as a substrate for life-threatening arrhythmias, raising the possibility that prophylactic implantable cardioverter defibrillators may improve long-term survival in this population. Moreover, previous studies reported that myocardial fibrosis does not regress significantly after surgery, and it correlates with incomplete LV functional recovery and worse New York Heart Association functional class [4, 6, 29]. Therefore, although the current clinical management of patients with AS is based mainly on the assessment of valvular parameters, EF, and symptoms [17], LGE has all the potential to improve patient selection, timing of intervention, operative approach, and primary prevention of sudden cardiac death.

T1 mapping: T1 mapping has recently emerged as a novel MRI technique to assess noninvasively the presence of diffuse interstitial fibrosis that may go undetected on LGE imaging (Fig. 9.5). This technique relies on T1 relaxation time of tissues, a measure of how fast the nuclear spin magnetization returns to its equilibrium state after a radiofrequency pulse. The myocardial T1 time can be measured without contrast (native T1 mapping) or following the administration of intravenous gado-

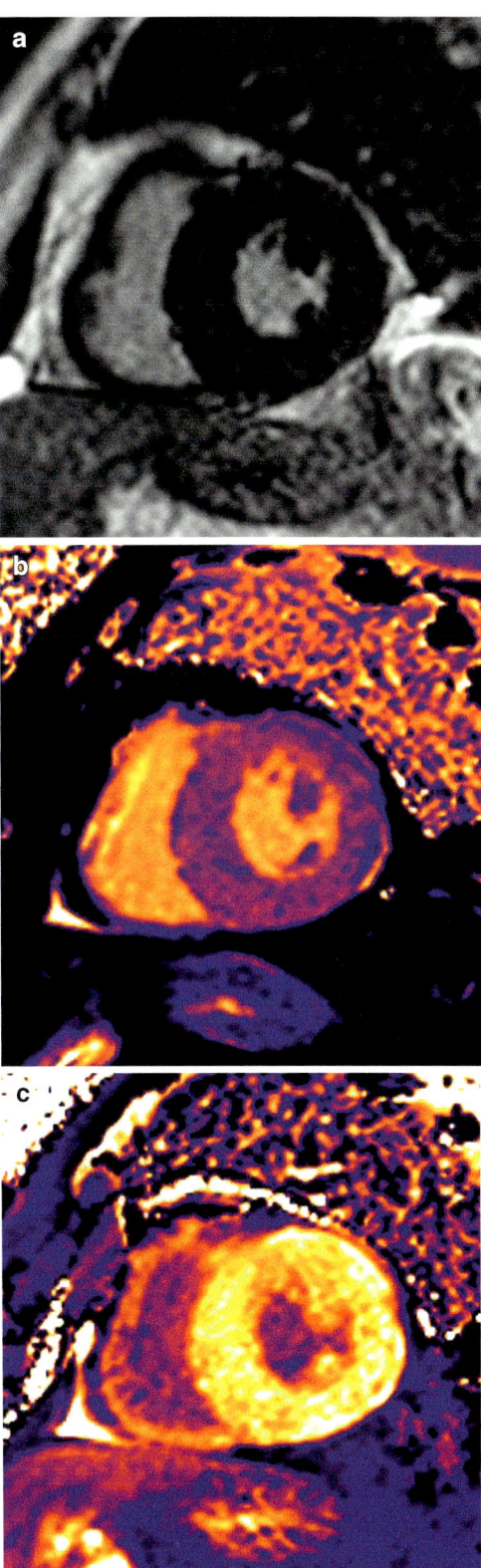

Fig. 9.5 Characterization of myocardial fibrosis by LGE (**a**), native T1 mapping (**b**) and post-contrast T1 mapping (**c**)

linium-based contrast agent (post-contrast T1). By combining both measures, the myocardial extracellular volume (ECV) fraction can be calculated. Since myocardial fibrosis has different relaxation properties compared to the normal myocardium and the ECV is expanded in the damaged tissue, even subtle changes can be detected and quantified. Native T1 mapping values are higher in patients with aortic stenosis and further increase in symptomatic compared with asymptomatic patients [7, 30]. Albeit not performed routinely, native T1 values and myocardial ECV fraction have been found to be predictors of poor prognosis in patients with aortic stenosis [7, 31] and thus hold promise to improve risk stratification in patients undergoing AVR and TAVI by detecting early and potentially reversible myocardial changes.

9.6   Aortic Stiffness

Arterial stiffness is an early marker of adverse morphological and functional vessel changes. A reduced compliance of the aortic wall is associated with aging and has been shown to be an independent predictor of cardiovascular events and mortality in general population and in patients with arterial hypertension, diabetes, and severe renal failure [32, 33]. In patients with aortic stenosis, valve dynamics and the combination of multiple risk factors can lead to aortic stiffening [34]. Previous studies have shown that aortic stiffness improves after both AVR and TAVI [35, 36], likely due to the recovery of the damaged aortic root endothelium, which has an important role in the production of vasorelaxant factors. Moreover, aortic biomechanics have been proposed as a predictor of outcome in patients undergoing TAVI, which can help in the risk stratification of patients undergoing the procedure [36]. Aortic distensibility and pulse wave velocity are the two main parameters to assess aortic stiffness and can be accurately calculated by CMR. Aortic distensibility is measured from two-dimensional cine images acquired in the transverse plane perpendicular to the aortic lumen at different levels of the vessel. It is calculated as follows:

$$\text{Aortic distensibility} = \frac{\text{maximum area} - \text{minimum area}}{\text{minimum area} \times \Delta P}$$

where ΔP is the pulse pressure in mmHg [37]. Pulse wave velocity (PWV) is the most reproducible and validated parameter to assess aortic stiffness. It is calculated from axial phase-contrast images by dividing the distance between the ascending and descending thoracic aorta by the transit time of the flow wave. PWV values are higher in stiffened arteries because they conduct the pulse wave faster compared to more distensible arteries [38]. Another method based on CMR analysis allows to estimate PWV and hence distensibility based on fractional changes in aortic area and changes in aortic flow velocity [39].

9.6.1   Post-procedure Assessment

9.6.1.1 Assessment of Paravalvular Aortic Regurgitation

Paravalvular aortic regurgitation (PAR) is the most common complication following TAVI and, when moderate to severe, affects negatively the prognosis [40]. Although TTE is the first-line test for PAR quantification, the presence of poor acoustic window, turbulent flows, multiple and eccentric regurgitant jets, and irregular regurgitant orifices can affect both accuracy and consistency of the echocardiographic measurement. TEE is a possible alternative and easily quantifies the arc of the paravalvular leak, but its use during TAVI has been reduced by the general switch to conscious sedation, and the procedure is cumbersome and not well accepted. CMR overcomes these limitations by offering a direct quantification of retrograde diastolic flow in the proximal aorta through PC velocity mapping imaging, regardless of the visualization of location and direction of PAR jets. The scan plane is placed perpendicular to the long axis of the proximal ascending aorta, 2–3 mm above the valve prosthesis, avoiding regions of flow turbulence, aliasing, and susceptibility artifacts. By using dedicated software, the cross-sectional area of the aorta is contoured throughout the cardiac cycle to define regions of interest (ROI), and the volume of blood moving in an anterograde and retrograde direction through the ROI is determined, allowing calculation of forward and reversal flow volumes (Fig. 9.6). The aortic regurgitant fraction is calculated as reverse flow volume/forward flow volume × 100. The same PC analysis can be

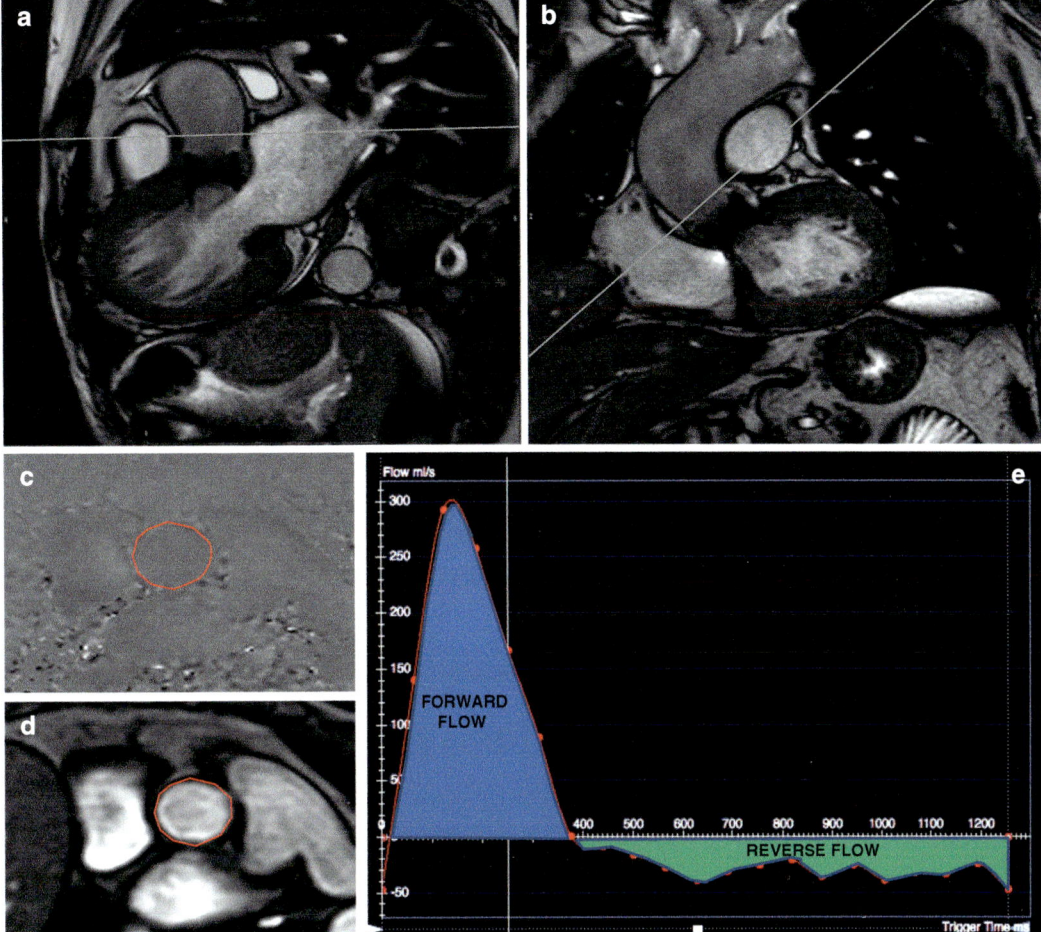

Fig. 9.6 Quantification of paravalvular aortic regurgitation in a patient post-TAVI using through-Plane Phase-Contrast Imaging. The scan plane is placed perpendicular to the long-axis of the proximal ascending aorta above the valve prosthesis (**a, b**). The volume of blood moving in an anterograde and retrograde direction the cross sectional area of the aorta (**c, d**) is analyzed by the software and the calculation of forward and reverse flow volumes is automatically performed (**e**)

repeated selecting a plane in the descending aorta: the presence of holodiastolic flow reversal at this level is a supportive element of the severity of aortic regurgitation.

At present, there is no general agreement about the cutoffs to define the degree of PAR with CMR. Most of the current published data has used the values of regurgitant fraction previously identified for native aortic regurgitation (mild ≤20%, moderate 21–39%, severe ≥40%), but these have not been validated in the setting of PAR after TAVI [41]. The lack of consensus is partially due to the modest correlation between 2D echocardiography and CMR in the grading of PAR, where in general 2D echocardiography underestimates

its entity compared to CMR and patients who are diagnosed with mild PAR by echocardiography often show CMR-derived regurgitation fractions >20% [42–44]. By using the VARC-2 criteria (mild<10%, moderate 10–29%, severe >30%), it was demonstrated that the cutoff of severe PAR was better at identifying patients at greater risk of 2-year all-cause mortality and mortality and hospitalization for heart failure [44, 45]. Importantly, compared to 2D TTE and 3D TTE, CMR has shown dramatically lower intraobserver and interobserver variability (intraobserver variability 73% by 2D TTE, 16% by 3D TTE vs. 2.2% by CMR; interobserver variability 108% by 2D TTE, 24% by 3D TTE vs. 1.5% by CMR) [42].

9.6.1.2 Assessment of Myocardial Injury: LGE Analysis

CMR with LGE is the gold standard technique for detection and quantification of myocardial injury, as it is able to detect myocardial necrosis of size <1 g, thanks to its high spatial resolution. Although cardiac biomarkers are ubiquitously elevated after TAVI, not all patients present signs of new myocardial injury on CMR images. It is estimated that only approximately 20% of patients develop new areas of LGE after the procedure, and this is commonly associated with an impairment of LV systolic function [46]. The pattern of LGE is mostly ischemic, with subendocardial or transmural localization, usually of small size (average 1.8% of the LV mass) and multifocal distribution, suggesting that the leading cause of myocardial damage may be coronary embolism. However, other LGE patterns have been described, such as that of extensive myocardial infarction secondary to coronary ostia occlusion or the apical scarring following a transapical access procedure [47]. While troponin elevation after TAVI appears to correlate with short-term and long-term outcomes [48], the prognostic importance of CMR-detected new myocardial injury after the intervention has still to be clarified.

9.6.1.3 Assessment of Reverse Ventricular Remodeling: Volumetric Analysis and Strain

The elimination of pressure overload by TAVI leads to a reduction of LV size and mass, improvement in LV systolic function and LV strain. Such favorable reverse remodeling is affected by the presence of PAR and correlates with clinical outcomes [49]. Reverse remodeling of the right ventricle is also observed, with a similar reduction of volumes and improvement of systolic function, and this appears to be more favorable after TAVI than after SAVR [50].

CMR is considered the ideal technique to monitor reverse remodeling of both left and right ventricles after TAVI due to its accurate volumetric estimation of cardiac chambers. Recently, new sophisticated CMR techniques of strain imaging have been introduced to study myocardial deformation and to detect more subtle contractile changes compared to EF. The most widely used technique is called feature-tracking CMR, and it is based on post-processing of standard cine images, similar to the strain analysis performed by echocardiographic speckle tracking, but with a lower observer variability [51]. After the manual contouring of the endocardial border in long- and short-axis cine imaging, the software identifies features along the cavity-myocardial tissue boundary and tracks them throughout the cardiac cycle, calculating global and regional radial, circumferential, longitudinal strain (Fig. 9.7). Patients with AS show impaired LV mechanics in relation to the extent of LV hypertrophy and fibrosis and cardiac surgery risk profile of the patient; after TAVI, a significant improvement of myocardial deformation parameters is observed in all three directions, with a later additional change due to the reduction of LV hypertrophy observed in the long term [52].

9.6.1.4 Cerebral Microembolism

Diffusion-weighted MRI (DW-MRI) is nowadays the most powerful tool for diagnosing acute ischemic brain injury, being more sensitive and specific than CT and conventional MRI [53, 54]. DW-MRI is able to detect the restriction of water diffusion from extracellular to intracellular compartment in cerebral tissue caused by hypoxic edema within minutes of the onset of ischemia. The regional decrease of diffusion is visible as hyperintensity on DW-MRI images and as hypointensity on quantitative maps of the apparent diffusion coefficient (ADC). Lesions can be quantified in number, size, and location using this modality. Although the incidence of stroke within 30 days of the TAVI procedure is low (approximately 5% [55], with very few truly disabling strokes), cerebral microemboli detected by DW-MRI are frequent, occurring in 58–91% of patients. They are usually clinically silent and their impact on prognosis is still unclear [56, 57]. Furthermore, 80% of new brain lesions demonstrate reversal during the 3-month follow-up, without leaving any residual signal change [58]. The use of cerebral protection devices during TAVI procedure has shown to reduce the frequency and the size of ischemic cerebral lesions, but its clinical benefit remains to be demonstrated [59].

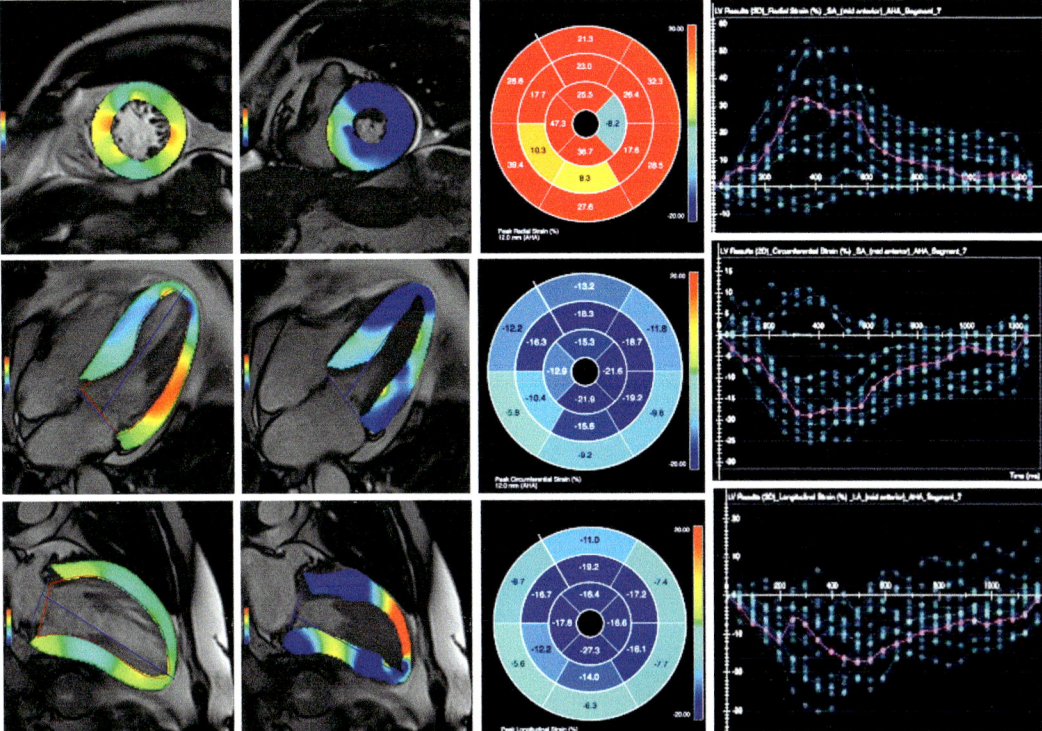

Fig. 9.7 Myocardial deformation analysis by CMR-Feature Tracking. After the manual countouring of the LV endocardial and epicardial borders in long- and short- axis cine images in end-diastole, radial, circumferential and longitudinal strain measurements are calculated by a dedicated software (Circle Medical imaging) in the 17 LV segments

9.7   Limitations of the Technique

CMR presents potential drawbacks in patients undergoing TAVI. The first is the limitation of the technique in detection of calcification of cardiac structures, which are well imaged with CT. As mentioned before, the suboptimal temporal resolution of CMR and other specific technical limitations can cause underestimation of peak trans-stenotic velocities, potentially leading to the underestimation of the degree of the aortic valve severity in the pre-procedural planning of TAVI. Cine images are susceptible to variability of the heart rate, and image quality can be compromised in patients with arrhythmias. Additionally, MRI is contraindicated in patients with conventional permanent pacemakers and intracardiac defibrillators, which are common in patients undergoing TAVI. The recent introduction of MRI-conditional devices has opened this tech-nology also for patients with these devices but they can still produce prominent imaging artifacts, which might reduce image quality and limit the study inter-pretation. Finally, not only the CMR examination is substantially longer than CT acquisition or echocar-diography, but it also requires multiple breath holds, which can be problematic for elderly patients.

9.8   Future Perspectives

9.8.1   4D Flow

Advances in MRI technology are leading to the development of new sequences that may provide additional insight into the pathophysi-ology of cardiac diseases. The 4D flow MRI technique is one of the most valuable and visu-ally appealing examples of a new tool with great clinical potential as it allows for a sophisticated evaluation of the hemodynamics of the cardiovascular system both qualitatively and quantitatively [60]. The technique provides a three-dimensional representation of blood flow over time, thanks to a complete spatial and temporal coverage of a volume of interest by using the intrinsic magnetic properties of blood flow, without the use of a contrast agent. This technique provides a noninvasive in vivo assessment of blood flow dynamics, enabling the analysis of parameters such as wall shear stress, turbulent kinetic energy, pressure difference, and pulse wave velocity throughout the heart and major vessels of the cardiovascular system (Fig. 9.8)

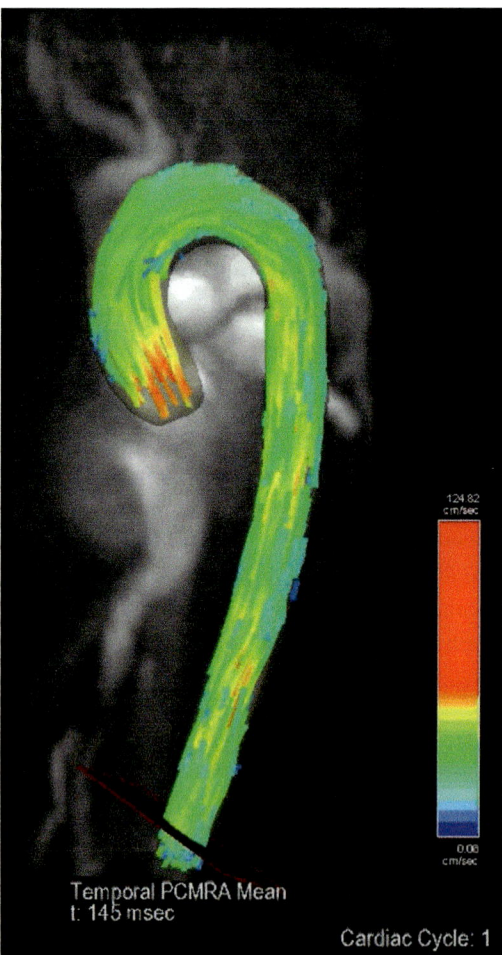

Fig. 9.8 Example of aortic 4D-flow CMR showing velocity streamlines in the aorta. Image courtesy of Giovanni Biglino, Bristol Heart Institute, Bristol, UK (unpublished data)

[61, 62]. Clinical applications of 4D flow are still in the early stage but are likely to expand in the near future. Previous studies have demonstrated that changes in the morphology of the aortic valve such as bicuspid valves result in altered blood flow dynamic [63]. Both TAVI and AVR lead to altered blood flow parameters in the ascending aorta, with more intense flow eccentricity and regional elevation of wall shear stress when compared to healthy controls, but further research is needed to understand their significance in terms of prognosis [64], especially if TAVI is going to be performed in an increasingly younger patient population. The development of faster acquisition sequences along with user-friendly image processing software is overcoming the main limitations of the techniques, which are the long acquisition time and the difficult processing and interpretation of data, contributing to the implementation of the technique in daily clinical practice.

9.8.2 MRI-Guided Procedure

MRI is considered an attractive and promising tool for guiding TAVI, since it potentially overcomes inherent shortcomings of X-ray fluoroscopy and angiography, which are currently used for the procedure guidance. Compared to these imaging modalities, a real-time CMR approach offers an image acquisition with unlimited plane orientation with superior soft-tissue contrast, without ionizing radiations and contrast agent. In a single session, MRI may provide comprehensive pre-interventional assessment (as previously described in this chapter), optimal guidance through the vasculature and during valve delivery, the possibility to evaluate immediately procedure-related complication, and, after the procedure, the validation of the procedural success. This approach has been shown to be feasible in preclinical studies in animal models using modified CMR-compatible delivery catheter without ferromagnetic components [65, 66], but at present, further studies for validation and clinical use assessment are still needed.

9.9 Conclusion

MRI is emerging as a robust noninvasive, radiation-free imaging modality for assessing patients undergoing TAVI. Thanks to its high spatial resolution and the unique strength of tissue characterization, it offers the possibility of a comprehensive pre- and postoperative assessment and supports the clinician in the decision-making process. In view of the fast development of the technique, MRI holds promise to overcome its current limitations and to play a central role in the field of structural interventional cardiology.

References

1. Pennell DJ, Sechtem UP, Higgins CB, Manning WJ, Pohost GM, Rademakers FE, van Rossum AC, Shaw LJ, Yucel EK. Clinical indications for cardiovascular magnetic resonance (CMR): consensus panel report. Eur Heart J. 2004;25:1940–65.
2. Pellikka PA, Nagueh SF, Elhendy AA, Kuehl CA, Sawada SG. American society of echocardiography recommendations for performance, interpretation, and application of stress echocardiography. J Am Soc Echocardiogr. 2007;20:1021–41.
3. Chahal N, Vieira MS, Mohiaddin R. Assessment of aortic stenosis severity by rest CMR correlates well with stress echocardiography in the setting of low left ventricular flow states. J Cardiovasc Magn Reson. 2014;16(Suppl 1):P264.
4. Weidemann F, Herrmann S, Stork S, Niemann M, Frantz S, Lange V, Beer M, Gattenlohner S, Voelker W, Ertl G, Strotmann JM. Impact of myocardial fibrosis in patients with symptomatic severe aortic stenosis. Circulation. 2009;120:577–84.
5. Dweck MR, Joshi S, Murigu T, Alpendurada F, Jabbour A, Melina G, Banya W, Gulati A, Roussin I, Raza S, Prasad NA, Wage R, Quarto C, Angeloni E, Refice S, Sheppard M, Cook SA, Kilner PJ, Pennell DJ, Newby DE, Mohiaddin RH, Pepper J, Prasad SK. Midwall fibrosis is an independent predictor of mortality in patients with aortic stenosis. J Am Coll Cardiol. 2011;58:1271–9.
6. Barone-Rochette G, Piérard S, De Meester de Ravenstein C, Seldrum S, Melchior J, Maes F, Pouleur AC, Vancraeynest D, Pasquet A, Vanoverschelde JL, Gerber BL. Prognostic significance of LGE by CMR in aortic stenosis patients undergoing valve replacement. J Am Coll Cardiol. 2014;64:144–54.
7. Lee H, Park JB, Yoon YE, Park EA, Kim HK, Lee W, Kim YJ, Cho GY, Sohn DW, Greiser A, Lee SP. Noncontrast myocardial T1 mapping by cardiac magnetic resonance predicts outcome in patients with aortic stenosis. JACC Cardiovasc Imaging. 2018;11(7):974–83.
8. Saeedi M, Thomas A, Shellock FG. Evaluation of MRI issues at 3-Tesla for a transcatheter aortic valve replacement (TAVR) bioprosthesis. Magn Reson Imaging. 2015;33:497–501.
9. Bonow RO, Carabello BA, Chatterjee K, de Leon AC Jr, Faxon DP, Freed MD, Gaasch WH, Lytle BW, Nishimura RA, O'Gara PT, O'Rourke RA, Otto CM, Shah PM, Shanewise JS. Focused update incorporated into the ACC/AHA 2006 guidelines for the management of patients with valvular heart disease: a report of the American College of Cardiology/American Heart Association Task Force on Practice Guidelines (Writing Committee to Revise the 1998 Guidelines for the Management of Patients With Valvular Heart Disease): endorsed by the Society of Cardiovascular Anesthesiologists, Society for Cardiovascular Angiography and Interventions, and Society of Thoracic Surgeons. Circulation. 2008;118(15):e523–661.
10. Yu EH, Sloggett CE, Iwanochko M. Feasibility and accuracy or left ventricular volumes and ejection fraction determination by fundamental, tissue harmonic, and intravenous contrast imaging in difficult-to-image patients. J Am Soc Echocardiogr. 2000;13:216–24.
11. Reant P, Lederlin M, Lafitte S, Serri K, Montaudon M, Corneloup O, Roudaut R, Laurent F. Absolute assessment of aortic valve stenosis by planimetry using cardiovascular magnetic resonance imaging: comparison with transesophageal echocardiography, transthoracic echocardiography, and cardiac catheterisation. Eur J Radiol. 2006;59:276–83. https://doi.org/10.1016/j.ejrad.2006.02.011.
12. John AS, Dill T, Brandt RR, Rau M, Ricken W, Bachmann G, Hamm CW. Magnetic resonance to assess the aortic valve area in aortic stenosis: how does it compare to current diagnostic standards? J Am Coll Cardiol. 2003;42:519–26.
13. Gatehouse PD, Keegan J, Crowe LA, Masood S, Mohiaddin RH, Kreitner KF, Firmin DN. Applications of phase-contrast flow and velocity imaging in cardiovascular MRI. Eur Radiol. 2005;15:2172–84.
14. Caruthers SD, Lin SJ, Brown P, Lin SJ, Brown P, Watkins MP, Williams TA, Lehr KA, Wickline SA. Practical value of cardiac magnetic resonance imaging for clinical quantification of aortic valve stenosis: comparison with echocardiography. Circulation. 2003;108:2236–43.
15. O'Brien KR, Cowan BR, Jain M, Stewart RA, Kerr AJ, Young AA. MRI phase contrast velocity and flow errors in turbulent stenotic jets. J Magn Reson Imaging. 2008;28:210–8. https://doi.org/10.1002/jmri.21395.
16. Pibarot P, Dumesnil JG. Low-flow, low-gradient aortic stenosis with normal and depressed left ventricular ejection fraction. J Am Coll Cardiol. 2012;60:1845–53.
17. 2017 ESC/EACTS Guidelines for the management of valvular heart disease. Eur Heart J. 2017;38(36):2739–86.

18. Pontone G, Andreini D, Bartorelli AL, Annoni A, Mushtaq S, Bertella E, Formenti A, Cortinovis S, Alamanni F, Fusari M, Bona V, Tamborini G, Muratori M, Ballerini G, Fiorentini C, Biglioli P, Pepi M. Feasibility and accuracy of a comprehensive multidetector computed tomography acquisition for patients referred for balloon-expandable transcatheter aortic valve implantation. Am Heart J. 2011;161:1106–13.

19. Gopal A, Grayburn PA, Mack M, Chacon I, Kim R, Montenegro D, Phan T, Rudolph J, Filardo G, Mack MJ, Gopalakrishnan D. Noncontrast 3D CMR imaging for aortic valve annulus sizing in TAVR. J Am Coll Cardiol Img. 2015;8:375–8.

20. Koos R, Altiok E, Mahnken AH, Neizel M, Dohmen G, Marx N, Kühl H, Hoffmann R. Evaluation of aortic root for definition of prosthesis size by magnetic resonance imaging and cardiac computed tomography: implications for transcatheter aortic valve implantation. Int J Cardiol. 2012;158(3):353–8.

21. Quail MA, Nordmeyer J, Schievano S, Reinthaler M, Mullen MJ, Taylor AM. Use of cardiovascular magnetic resonance imaging for TAVR assessment in patients with bioprosthetic aortic valves: comparison with computed tomography. Eur J Radiol. 2012;81(12):3912–7.

22. Ledneva E, Karie S, Launa-Vacher V, Janus N, Deray G. Renal safety of gadolinium-based contrast media in patients with chronic renal insufficiency. Radiology. 2009;250:618–28.

23. Chaturvedi A, Hobbs SK, Ling FS, Chaturvedi A, Knight P. MRI evaluation prior to Transcatheter Aortic Valve Implantation (TAVI): when to acquire and how to interpret. Insights into Imaging. 2016;7(2):245–54.

24. Krayenbuehl HP, Hess OM, Monrad ES, Schneider J, Mall G, Turina M. Left ventricular myocardial structure in aortic valve disease before, intermediate, and late after aortic valve replacement. Circulation. 1989;79:744–55.

25. Kim RJ, Fieno DS, Parrish TB, Harris K, Chen EL, Simonetti O, Bundy J, Finn JP, Klocke FJ, Judd RM. Relationship of MRI delayed contrast enhancement to irreversible injury, infarct age, and contractile function. Circulation. 1999;100:1992–2002.

26. Schelbert EB, Hsu LY, Anderson SA, Mohanty BD, Karim SM, Kellman P, Aletras AH, Arai AE. Late gadolinium-enhancement cardiac magnetic resonance identifies postinfarction myocardial fibrosis and the border zone at the near cellular level in ex vivo rat heart. Circ Cardiovasc Imaging. 2010;3:743–52.

27. Debl K, Djavidani B, Buchner S, Lipke C, Nitz W, Feuerbach S, Riegger G, Luchner A. Delayed hyperenhancement in magnetic resonance imaging of left ventricular hypertrophy caused by aortic stenosis and hypertrophic cardiomyopathy: visualisation of focal fibrosis. Heart. 2006;92:1447–51.

28. Rudolph A, Abdel-Aty H, Bohl S, Boyé P, Zagrosek A, Dietz R, Schulz-Menger J. Noninvasive detection of fibrosis applying contrast-enhanced cardiac magnetic resonance in different forms of left ventricular hypertrophy relation to remodeling. J Am Coll Cardiol. 2009;53:284–91.

29. Azevedo CF, Nigri M, Higuchi ML, Pomerantzeff PM, Spina GS, Sampaio RO, Tarasoutchi F, Grinberg M, Rochitte CE. Prognostic significance of myocardial fibrosis quantification by histopathology and magnetic resonance imaging in patients with severe aortic valve disease. J Am Coll Cardiol. 2010;56:278–87.

30. Bull S, White SK, Piechnik SK, Flett AS, Ferreira VM, Loudon M, Francis JM, Karamitsos TD, Prendergast BD, Robson MD, Neubauer S, Moon JC, Myerson SG. Human non-contrast T1 values and correlation with histology in diffuse fibrosis. Heart. 2013;99:932–7.

31. Chin CW, Everett RJ, Kwiecinski J, Vesey AT, Yeung E, Esson G, Jenkins W, Koo M, Mirsadraee S, White AC, Japp AG, Prasad SK, Semple S, Newby DE, Dweck MR. Myocardial fibrosis and cardiac decompensation in aortic stenosis. JACC Cardiovasc Imaging. 2017;10(11):1320–33.

32. Mitchell GF, Hwang SJ, Vasan RS, Larson MG, Pencina MJ, Hamburg NM, Vita JA, Levy D, Benjamin EJ. Arterial stiffness and cardiovascular events: the Framingham Heart Study. Circulation. 2010;121(4):505–11.

33. C V, Aznaouridis K, Stefanadis C. Prediction of cardiovascular events and all-cause mortality with arterial stiffness: a systematic review and meta-analysis. J Am Coll Cardiol. 2010;55(13):1318–27.

34. Nemes A, Forster T, Csanady M. Decreased aortic distensibility and coronary flow velocity reserve in patients with significant aortic valve stenosis with normal epicardial coronary arteries. J Heart Valve Dis. 2004;13:567–73.

35. Nemes A, Galema TW, Geleijnse ML, Soliman OI, Yap SC, Anwar AM. Aortic valve replacement for aortic stenosis is associated with improved aortic distensibility at long-term follow-up. Am Heart J. 2007;153:147–51.

36. Harbaoui B, Montoy M, Charles P, Boussel L, Liebgott H, Girerd N, Courand PY, Lantelme P. Aorta calcification burden: towards an integrative predictor of cardiac outcome after transcatheter aortic valve implantation. Atherosclerosis. 2016;246:161–8. https://doi.org/10.1016/j.atherosclerosis.2016.01.013.

37. Herment A, Kachenoura N, Lefort M, Bensalah M, Dogui A, Frouin F, Mousseaux E, De Cesare A. Automated segmentation of the aorta from phase contrast MR images: validation against expert tracing in healthy volunteers and in patients with a dilated aorta. J Magn Reson Imaging. 2010;31:881–8.

38. Redheuil A, Yu WC, Wu CO, Mousseaux E, de Cesare A, Yan R, Kachenoura N, Bluemke D, Lima JA. Reduced ascending aortic strain and distensibility: earliest manifestations of vascular aging in humans. Hypertension. 2010;55:319–26.

39. Biglino G, Steeden JA, Baker C, Schievano S, Taylor AM, Parker KH, Muthurangu V. A non-invasive clinical application of wave intensity analysis based on ultrahigh temporal resolution phase-contrast

cardiovascular magnetic resonance. J Cardiovasc Magn Reson. 2012 Aug 9;14:57. https://doi.org/10.1186/1532-429X-14-57.

40. Sinning JM, Hammerstingl C, Vasa-Nicotera M, Adenauer V, Lema Cachiguango SJ, Scheer AC, Hausen S, Sedaghat A, Ghanem A, Müller C, Grube E, Nickenig G, Werner N. Aortic regurgitation index defines severity of peri-prosthetic regurgitation and predicts outcome in patients after transcatheter aortic valve implantation. J Am Coll Cardiol. 2012;59:1134–41.

41. Gabriel RS, Renapurkar R, Bolen MA, Verhaert D, Leiber M, Flamm SD, Griffin BP, Desai MY, et al. Comparison of severity of aortic regurgitation by cardiovascular magnetic resonance versus transthoracic echocardiography. Am J Cardiol. 2011;108:1014–20.

42. Altiok E, Frick M, Meyer CG, Al Ateah G, Napp A, Kirschfink A, Almalla M, Lotfi S, Becker M, Herich L, Lehmacher W, Hoffmann R. Comparison of two- and three-dimensional transthoracic echocardiography to cardiac magnetic resonance imaging for assessment of paravalvular regurgitation after transcatheter aortic valve implantation. Am J Cardiol. 2014;113:1859–66.

43. Salaun E, Jacquier A, Theron A, Giorgi R, Lambert M, Jaussaud N, Hubert S, Collart F, Bonnet JL, Habib G, Cuisset T, Grisoli D. Value of CMR in quantification of paravalvular aortic regurgitation after TAVI. Eur Heart J Cardiovasc Imaging. 2016;17:41–50.

44. Ribeiro HB, Orwat S, Hayek SS, Larose É, Babaliaros V, Dahou A, Le Ven F, Pasian S, Puri R, Abdul-Jawad Altisent O, Campelo-Parada F, Clavel MA, Pibarot P, Lerakis S, Baumgartner H, Rodés-Cabau J. Cardiovascular magnetic resonance to evaluate aortic regurgitation after transcatheter aortic valve replacement. J Am Coll Cardiol. 2016;68:577–85.

45. Kappetein AP, Head SJ, Généreux P, Piazza N, van Mieghem NM, Blackstone EH, Brott TG, Cohen DJ, Cutlip DE, van Es GA, Hahn RT, Kirtane AJ, Krucoff MW, Kodali S, Mack MJ, Mehran R, Rodés-Cabau J, Vranckx P, Webb JG, Windecker S, Serruys PW, Leon MB, Valve Academic Research Consortium-2. Updated standardized endpoint definitions for transcatheter aortic valve implantation: the Valve Academic Research Consortium-2 consensus document (VARC-2). Eur J Cardiothorac Surg. 2012;42:S45–60. https://doi.org/10.1093/ejcts/ezs533.

46. Kim W-K, Rolf A, Liebetrau C, Van Linden A, Blumenstein J, Kempfert J, Bachmann G, Nef H, Hamm C, Walther T, Möllmann H. Detection of myocardial injury by CMR after transcatheter aortic valve replacement. J Am Coll Cardiol. 2014;64:349–57.

47. Ribeiro HB, Larose E, de la Paz RM, Le Ven F, Nombela-Franco L, Urena M, Allende R, Amat-Santos I, Dahou A, Capoulade R, Clavel MA, Mohammadi S, Paradis JM, De Larochellière R, Doyle D, Dumont É, Pibarot P, Rodés-Cabau J. Myocardial injury following transcatheter aortic valve implantation: insights from delayed enhancement cardiovascular magnetic resonance. EuroIntervention. 2015;11:205–13.

48. Koskinas KC, Stortecky S, Franzone A, O'Sullivan CJ, Praz F, Zuk K, Räber L, Pilgrim T, Moschovitis A, Fiedler GM, Jüni P, Heg D, Wenaweser P, Windecker S. Post-procedural troponin elevation and clinical outcomes following transcatheter aortic valve implantation. J Am Heart Assoc. 2016;5(2). pii: e002430. https://doi.org/10.1161/JAHA.115.002430.

49. Sato K, Kumar A, Jones BM, Mick SL, Krishnaswamy A, Grimm RA, Desai MY, Griffin BP, Rodriguez LL, Kapadia SR, Obuchowski NA, Popović ZB. Reversibility of cardiac function predicts outcome after transcatheter aortic valve replacement in patients with severe aortic stenosis. J Am Heart Assoc. 2017;6(7). pii: e005798. https://doi.org/10.1161/JAHA.117.005798.

50. Fairbairn TA, Steadman CD, Mather AN, Motwani M, Blackman DJ, Plein S, McCann GP, Greenwood JP. Assessment of valve haemodynamics, reverse ventricular remodelling and myocardial fibrosis following transcatheter aortic valve implantation compared to surgical aortic valve replacement: a cardiovascular magnetic resonance study. Heart. 2013;99:1185–91.

51. Obokata M, Nagata Y, Wu VC, Kado Y, Kurabayashi M, Otsuji Y, Takeuchi M. Direct comparison of cardiac magnetic resonance feature tracking and 2D/3D echocardiography speckle tracking for evaluation of global left ventricular strain. Eur Heart J Cardiovasc Imaging. 2016;17(5):525–32.

52. Nucifora G, Tantiongco JP, Crouch G, Bennetts J, Sinhal A, Tully PJ, Bradbrook C, Baker RA, Selvanayagam JB. Changes of left ventricular mechanics after trans-catheter aortic valve implantation and surgical aortic valve replacement for severe aortic stenosis: a tissue-tracking cardiac magnetic resonance study. Int J Cardiol. 2017;228:184–90. https://doi.org/10.1016/j.ijcard.2016.11.200.. Epub 2016 Nov 9

53. Lansberg MG, Albers GW, Beaulieu C, Marks MP. Comparison of diffusion-weighted MRI and CT in acute stroke. Neurology. 2000;54:1557–61.

54. Fiebach J, Jansen O, Schellinger P, Knauth M, Hartmann M, Heiland S, Ryssel H, Pohlers O, Hacke W, Sartor K. Comparison of CT with diffusion-weighted MRI in patients with hyperacute stroke. Neuroradiology. 2001;43:628–32.

55. Leon MB, Smith CR, Mack M, Miller DC, Moses JW, Svensson LG, Tuzcu EM, Webb JG, Fontana GP, Makkar RR, Brown DL, Block PC, Guyton RA, Pichard AD, Bavaria JE, Herrmann HC, Douglas PS, Petersen JL, Akin JJ, Anderson WN, Wang D, Pocock S, Investigators PT. Transcatheter aortic-valve implantation for aortic stenosis in patients who cannot undergo surgery. N Engl J Med. 2010;363(17):1597–607.

56. Astarci P, Glineur D, Kefer J, D'Hoore W, Renkin J, Vanoverschelde JL, El Khoury G, Grandin C. Magnetic resonance imaging evaluation of cerebral embolization during percutaneous aortic valve implantation: comparison of transfemoral and trans-

apical approaches using Edwards Sapiens valve. Eur J Cardiothorac Surg. 2011;40(2):475–9.

57. Ghanem A, Müller A, Nähle CP Kocurek J, Werner N, Hammerstingl C, Schild HH, Schwab JO, Mellert F, Fimmers R, Nickenig G, Thomas D. Risk and fate of cerebral embolism after transfemoral aortic valve implantation: A prospective pilot study with diffusion-weighted magnetic resonance imaging. J Am Coll Cardiol. 2010;55:1427–32.

58. Kahlert P, Knipp SC, Schlamann M, Thielmann M, Al-Rashid F, Weber M, Johansson U, Wendt D, Jakob HG, Forsting M, Sack S, Erbel R, Eggebrecht H. Silent and apparent cerebral ischemia after percutaneous transfemoral aortic valve implantation: a diffusion-weighted magnetic resonance imaging study. Circulation. 2010;121:870–8.

59. Haussig S, Mangner N, Dwyer MG, Lehmkuhl L, Lücke C, Woitek F, Holzhey DM, Mohr FW, Gutberlet M, Zivadinov R, Schuler G, Linke A. Effect of a cerebral protection device on brain lesions following transcatheter aortic valve implantation in patients with severe aortic stenosis the CLEAN-TAVI randomized clinical trial. JAMA. 2016;316(6):592–601. https://doi.org/10.1001/jama.2016.10302.

60. Dyverfeldt P, Bissell M, Barker AJ, Bolger AF, Carlhäll CJ, Ebbers T, Francios CJ, Frydrychowicz A, Geiger J, Giese D, Hope MD, Kilner PJ, Kozerke S, Myerson S, Neubauer S, Wiehen O, Markl M. 4D flow cardiovascular magnetic resonance consensus statement. J Cardiovasc Magn Reson. 2015;17:72.

61. Rodriguez Munoz D, Markl M, Moya Mur JL, Barker A, Fernandez-Golfin C, Lancellotti P, Zamorano Gomez JL. Intracardiac flow visualization: current status and future directions. Eur Heart J Cardiovasc Imaging. 2013;14:1029–38.

62. Von Knobelsdorff-Brenkenhoff F, Karunaharamoorthy A, Trauzeddel RF, Barker AJ, Blaszczyk E, Markl M, Schulz-Menger J. Evaluation of aortic blood flow and wall shear stress in aortic stenosis and its association with left ventricular remodeling. Circ Cardiovasc Imaging. 2016;9(3):e004038.

63. Barker AJ, Markl M, Burk J, Lorenz R, Bock J, Bauer S, Schulz-Menger J, von Knobelsdorff-Brenkenhoff F. Bicuspid aortic valve is associated with altered wall shear stress in the ascending aorta. Circ Cardiovasc Imaging. 2012;5(4):457–66. https://doi.org/10.1161/CIRCIMAGING.112.973370.

64. Trauzeddel RF, Löbe U, Barker AJ, Gelsinger C, Butter C, Markl M, Schulz-Menger J, von Knobelsdorff-Brenkenhoff F. Blood flow characteristics in the ascending aorta after tavi compared to surgical aortic valve replacement. Int J Card Imaging. 2016;32(3):461–7.

65. Kahlert P, Parohl N, Albert J, Schafer L, Reinhardt R, Kaiser GM, McDougall I, Decker B, Plicht B, Erbel R, Eggebrecht H, Ladd ME, Quick HH. Towards real-time cardiovascular magnetic resonance guided transarterial CoreValve implantation: in vivo evaluation in swine. J Cardiovasc Magn Reson. 2012;14:21.

66. Miller JG, Li M, Mazilu D, Hunt T, Horvath KA. Real-time magnetic resonance imaging-guided transcatheter aortic valve replacement. J Thorac Cardiovasc Surg. 2016;151:1269–77.

Concomitant Coronary Artery Disease and Aortic Stenosis

10

Carolina Espejo, Gabriela Tirado-Conte,
Luis Nombela-Franco, and Pilar Jimenez-Quevedo

10.1 Introduction

Transcatheter aortic valve implantation (TAVI), also called transcatheter aortic valve replacement (TAVR), has been established worldwide as the standard of care in nonsurgical candidates and high-surgical-risk patients with symptomatic severe aortic stenosis (AS). Following the latest results of randomized trials [1, 2], TAVI is becoming more frequently used to treat AS in patient at lower-risk. The TAVI procedure can lead to a clinical and functional improvement in high-risk aortic stenosis patients; nevertheless, long-term outcomes are determined primarily by comorbidities beyond aortic valve disease. As risk factors for AS are similar to atherosclerosis risk factors, coronary artery disease (CAD) is a common finding in patients with AS [3–5].

The presence of CAD, variously identified as angina, reduced left ventricular function, previous myocardial infarction, or surgical revascularization, negatively affects prognosis in patients undergoing surgical valve replacement [6, 7] (SAVR) and is consequently evaluated in the most commonly used surgical risk scores. In addition, combining coronary artery bypass grafting (CABG) and SAVR increases risk compared with CABG alone [8]. The recommendation for patients with a primary indication for aortic/mitral valve surgery and coronary artery diameter stenosis ≥70% is to perform CABG (class Ic) [9]. Conversely, the prognostic implications of CAD in patients with severe AS undergoing TAVI and also the need of PCI are subject to ongoing debate. The European guidelines on myocardial revascularization, recommend, PCI in patients with a primary indication to undergo TAVI and a coronary artery diameter stenosis >70% in proximal segments (IIa) [9]. In contrast, current valvular guidelines [10] state that combined PCI and TAVI is feasible but more data are required before a firm recommendation can be made. In this chapter we will review the information available to date on coronary disease in patients with severe AS susceptible to TAVI.

10.2 Assessing the Severity of Coronary Artery Disease in Patients Undergoing TAVI

Currently, the literature shows no consensus on the importance of CAD in patients undergoing TAVI. The variability in the definition of CAD used to evaluate the prognostic implications in these patients makes it difficult to know the true effect of the disease on short- and long-term clinical outcomes [11].

C. Espejo · G. Tirado-Conte · L. Nombela-Franco
P. Jimenez-Quevedo (✉)
Interventional Cardiology Department, Hospital
Clinico San Carlos, Madrid, Spain

© Springer Nature Switzerland AG 2019
A. Giordano et al. (eds.), *Transcatheter Aortic Valve Implantation*,
https://doi.org/10.1007/978-3-030-05912-5_10

Another challenge in evaluating CAD in patients with AS is the classification of lesion severity. Noninvasive functional testing in the presence of AS is difficult, given the global subendocardial ischemia which is often present. Myocardial perfusion scans can be falsely positive in up to 20% of cases, mainly due to the presence of ventricular hypertrophy, fibrosis or scar formation in the myocardium, and dilation of the left ventricle. In addition, myocardial perfusion has been shown to be abnormal in the absence of coronary disease in severe AS on cardiac magnetic resonance imaging [12, 13]. For this reason, the use of stress tests to detect CAD associated with severe valvular disease is discouraged because of their low diagnostic value and potential risks [11]. In patients without AS, the use of invasive functional test such as fractional flow reserve (FFR) to assess the severity of the coronary lesions and to guide revascularization reduces major adverse cardiac events (MACE), compared with angiography-guided revascularization [10]. Regarding functional invasive techniques, AS may influence coronary hemodynamics and functional indexes may vary in this clinical and physiological context. In this regard, Pesarini et al. [14] evaluated the functional relevance of 133 coronary lesions assessed by FFR in 54 patients with severe AS during the TAVI procedure before and after the valve implantation. Although overall FFR values did not differ before and after the aortic valve stenosis removal (0.89 ± 0.10 versus 0.89 ± 0.13; $P = 0.73$), different trends were found after TAVI. Positive FFR values (FFR $\leq$ 0.8) worsened after TAVI (0.71 ± 0.11 versus 0.66 ± 0.14). Conversely, negative FFR values (FFR > 0.8) improved after TAVI (0.92 ± 0.06 versus 0.93 ± 0.07). Similarly, FFR values in coronary arteries with lesions presenting percent diameter stenosis >50 worsened after TAVI (0.84 ± 0.12 versus 0.82 ± 0.16; $P = 0.02$), whereas FFR values in arteries with mild lesions (percent diameter stenosis <50) trended toward improvement after TAVI (0.90 ± 0.07 versus 0.91 ± 0.09; $P = 0.69$). Despite these variations in the FFR value before and after TAVI, the indication to treat the lesions only changed in the 6% of the cases. On the other hand, the use of the non-hyperemic index instantaneous wave-free ratio (iFR) [15] in patients with AS showed significant and mostly erratic individual variations after valve treatment. In fact, the delta iFR was influenced by the extent of the transaortic gradient drop induced by TAVI. Compare to iFR, it seems that FFR assessment in patients with severe AS undergoing TAVI provides more reliable information about the functional relevance of coronary lesions.

One important aspect that may affect the outcome of patients who undergo TAVI is the extension and complexity of the CAD according to the SYNTAX score (SS) [16]. In this published study, the preoperative SS, determined from baseline coronary angiograms, showed that patients with high SS (SS >22) compared with low SS (SS < 22) or not CAD had a significant increase in the composite endpoint of cardiovascular death, stroke, or myocardial infarction (MI) at 1 year. This increase was driven by differences in cardiovascular mortality, whereas the risk of stroke and MI was similar across the three groups. In addition, after revascularization, the residual SS was also associated with poor clinical outcome at 1 year in this patients [16]. Recently, the value of the SS-II in predicting outcomes in patients undergoing TAVI has been evaluated. The SS-II is a clinical tool that combines the anatomical SS and some clinical characteristics for risk assessment. This study showed that an increase in SS-II was associated with higher 30-day mortality and major bleeding. Moreover, patients with SS-II scores in the 3rd tertile had an increased 1-year risk of death and MACE compared with patients in the 1st and 2nd tertile. The highest SS-II tertile was an independent predictor of long-term mortality and MACE [17].

In summary, the standard noninvasive functional tests are not useful to assess the severity or impact on prognosis of CAD in patients undergoing TAVI. However, the use of specific risk scores (SS and SS II) that consider the extension and complexity of CAD and, the invasive functional evaluation of individual lesions with FFR may contribute to predicting CAD impact in long-term clinical outcome and can guide revascularization and clinical decision-making, especially if lower-risk patients are to be treated with TAVI.

10.3 Indication for Revascularization in Patients Referred to TAVI

Although the prevalence of CAD is high, ranging from 44.3% to 77.6% (Fig. 10.1) [5, 18, 19] the optimal treatment of the disease in patients undergoing TAVI remains to be elucidated. Many of these patients may require percutaneous coronary intervention (PCI), and the key question is the identification of patients with both diseases are amenable to perform a coronary revascularization in addition to TAVI implantation.

First, it is essential to know the prognostic role of CAD in patients undergoing TAVI. Second, it is important to define highly significant CAD among these elderly patients with multiple comorbidities in order to identify patients who can be referred for combined procedure of TAVI implantation and PCI.

The prognostic role of CAD in patients undergoing TAVI remains unknown. Whereas the presence of CAD negatively affects prognosis in patients undergoing SAVR [7], results obtained in those undergoing TAVI are controversial. The risk scores applied in patients with severe AS were validated for surgical patients, and might have low accuracy in the TAVI population [20], which limits evaluation and risk classification in these patients.

There is no consensus on the optimal approach in treating concomitant CAD in patients scheduled to TAVI. On the one hand, some studies have shown that CAD associated with severe AS was related to a greater mortality [20, 21]. Others have found that patients with critical ostial disease without revascularization more frequently had myocardial infarction within 1 year than those with revascularization prior to TAVI [22]. In another trial, 3-year-survival rates were similar in patients with significant CAD undergoing both procedures, TAVI and PCI, and in those patients without CAD who received only TAVI [23], pointing to a potential benefit of revascularization in patients with both diseases.

Nevertheless, limited reports in the literature (mostly observational studies) demonstrate higher mortality rates in patients with CAD who receives only TAVI [20, 23]. On the other hand, several studies have found that CAD has no effect upon outcomes [18, 24], calling into question a mixed approach with both PCI and TAVI. One of the studies that found no advantage in a combined management approach compared major cardiovascular events and mortality in patients with CAD undergoing TAVI alone versus the combined procedure. No significant differences were found in the rate of MACE and mortality at 1 year; however, the incidence of MI was higher when PCI was not performed [22]. In addition, Griese et al. found a increased cardiovascular

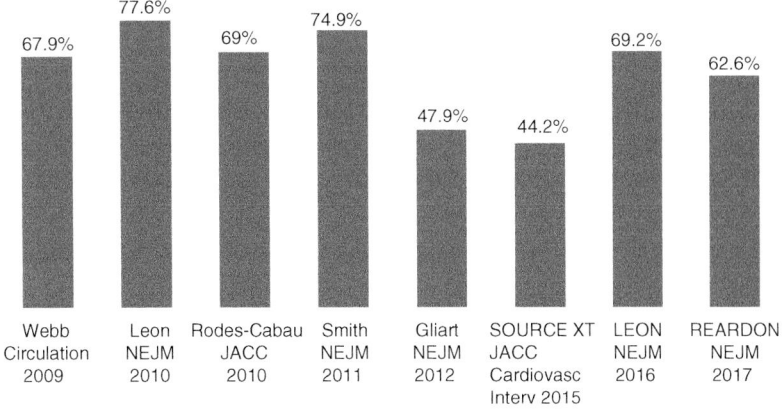

Fig. 10.1 Prevalence of coronary artery disease in patients undergoing TAVI

mortality and 30-day myocardial infarction in patients who underwent PCI and TAVI than in patients receiving TAVI alone [25]. D'Ascenzo et al. presented the first pooled analysis on the prognostic role of CAD in TAVI; involving 2472 patients that were treated with Edwards SAPIEN or CoreValve prosthesis. Although CAD was a common anamnestic finding in these patients, it did not affect midterm outcome of the studied procedures after adjustment for several confounding factors [18]. Finally, the ongoing ACTIVATION study will be the first randomized trial to compare no PCI strategy versus PCI prior to TAVI. This study will shed a light on the optimum treatment approach in these patients [11].

Considering the available data, an individualized approach should be used in order to select the best strategy in each patient. In addition a clear definition of highly significant CAD must be established in each patient. Usually, coronary artery stenosis is regarded as highly significant if the stenotic artery vascularizes a large myocardial territory which affects a large myocardial area [23]. According to the most recent European guidelines on myocardial revascularization, percutaneous revascularization along with TAVI, must be considered in patients with stenosis >70% in proximal coronary segments of the main vessels, including left anterior descending coronary artery, right coronary, or circumflex coronary artery (class IIa, level of evidence C) [10]. Likewise, coronary lesions should be amenable to PCI with a high likelihood of successful PCI. Thus, candidates for a mixed procedure must be selected from among symptomatic patients with significant and technically approachable flow-limiting stenosis [20].

Once patients amenable to a mixed procedure are identified, it is important to balance risks and benefits according to each patient's individual medical profile.

Potential benefits of PCI strategy could be amelioration of left ventricular ejection fraction owing to an improvement in coronary flow [11, 18, 19, 23]. In this way, patients may better withstand the TAVI procedure [20].

Nonetheless, potential PCI risks should be taken into account in those patients undergoing TAVI. Risk of death, myocardial infarction, CABG or stroke, as well as vascular access complication or renal failure, may limit a combined approach in some frailty and elderly patients. For instance, up to 1% may experience stent thrombosis, which is also favored by periods of marked hypotension during the TAVI procedure especially, during the rapid ventricular pacing [11]. The antiplatelet therapy used after stenting may have an impact on the risk of bleeding during TAVI procedures [24, 26, 27]. In addition, angiography performed from 5 days to 24 hours before the TAVI procedure is associated with increased risk of renal failure, which is also observed in a hybrid procedure that lasts longer and used more contrast than the single procedure [11, 28].

In summary, the lack of definitive data on preprocedural revascularization has led to some variability between centers regarding indication and timing. Current guidelines do not provide specific directions, and the management must be individualized and multidisciplinary in patients having both significant CAD and severe AS. Concurrent coronary revascularization may be needed, particularly if multivessel or left main coronary disease is present, although it is unclear if 30-day mortality is influenced by revascularization status [19]. Until more definitive randomized data are available from randomized trials, the Heart Valve Team should decide on a case-by-case basis whether to revascularize before TAVI or simultaneously, according to the individual patient's anatomic, clinical, and physiological characteristics.

10.4 Timing for Revascularization: Concomitant vs. a Staged Approach

There is no consensus on optimal timing for treating CAD in patients with severe AS. Once a patient's clinical condition and risks have been evaluated, the patient can be referred to a mixed strategy, which combines PCI and TAVI [19, 23]. The chronology of interventions remains controversial, and has been the subject of discussions about the most appropriated strategy [9, 10]. Two options are currently under discussion: performing PCI and TAVI simultaneously or carrying out a staged intervention with PCI prior to TAVI. There are examples in the literature for each of these two choices, reporting on attempts to answer the question about choosing the most feasible and safe management approach (Fig. 10.2).

10.4.1 Staged PCI and TAVI

Some authors promote a staged procedure, which consists of revascularization in the first place followed by a second stage with TAVI procedure

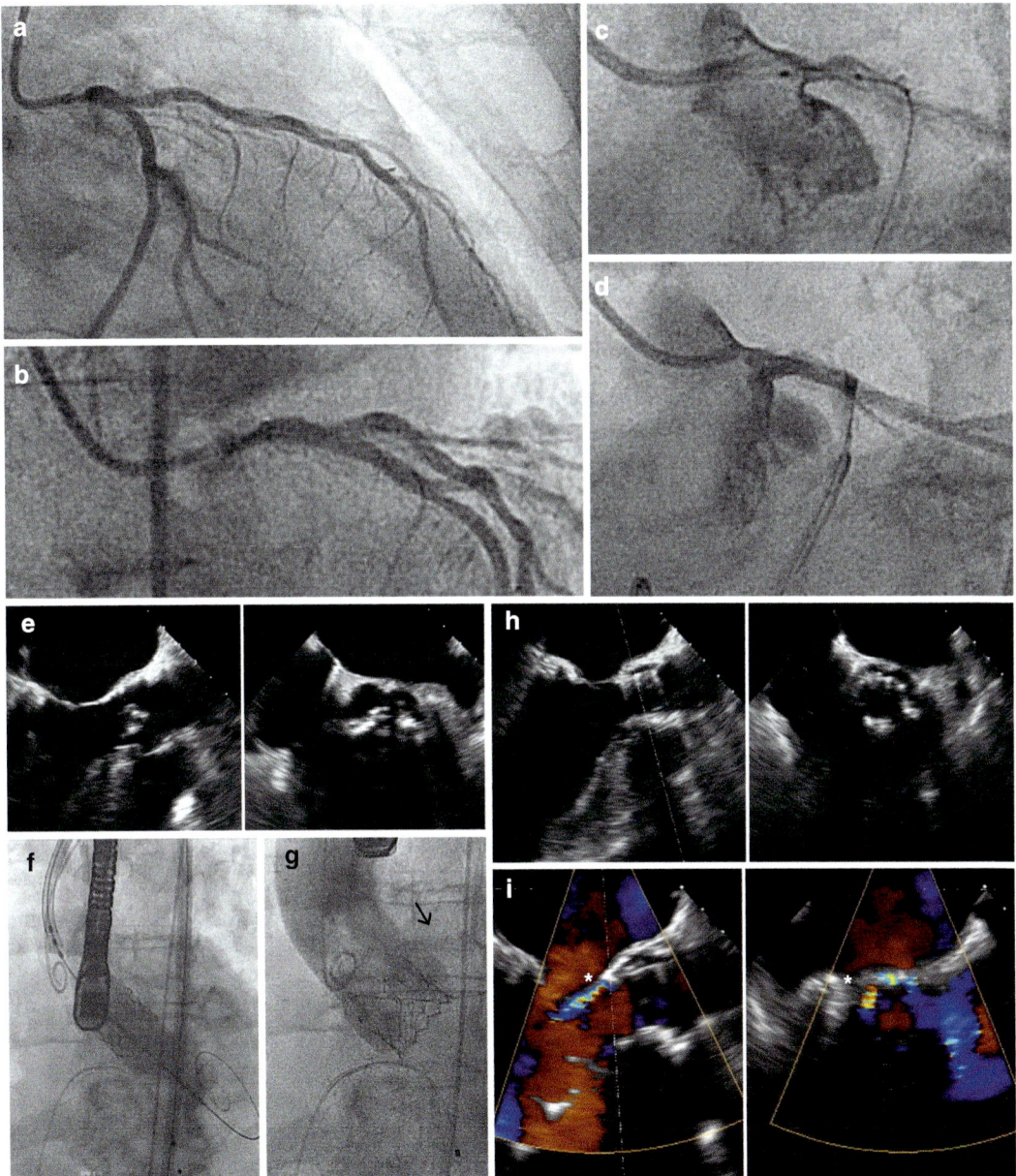

Fig. 10.2 Combined elective percutaneous coronary intervention (PCI) and transfemoral transcatheter aortic valve implantation (TAVI). (**a**, **b**) Coronary angiograms in RAO/caudal and AP projections revealing severe left main coronary artery (LMCA) ostial stenosis in a patient with severe aortic stenosis and cardiogenic shock. (**c**, **d**) Successful PCI of LMCA stenosis with drug-eluting stent (3.5 × 8 mm). (**e**) Transesophageal echocardiography (TEE) showing left ventricular outflow tract and severe calcific aortic valve stenosis. (**f**) Transfemoral TAVI with 23-mm Edwards SAPIEN 3 valve in a concomitant procedure. Final result in the aortography (**g**) and TEE (**h**, **i**) showing LMCA patency (black arrow) and mild paravalvular leak (asterisk). After TAVI patient was discharged without any complication

[21, 29]. Performing revascularization before TAVI implantation could have benefits in terms of limiting radiation or preserving renal function, as well as some technical advantages, since complex anatomies and difficult procedures should be carefully addressed. A prior PCI allows focusing on a more specific treatment of technically difficult stenosis [19, 21, 23] and a protective effect against the ischemic burden of the TAVI procedure may be achieved. Furthermore, left ventricular systolic function might be improved helping patients to better endure the TAVI procedure [11, 19]. Finally, procedural risks during the TAVI performance would be reduced, since both the complexity and duration of the TAVI intervention would decrease. A shorter procedural time also lowers radiation exposure and the amount of contrast required; thereby, preserving renal function [19, 23]. In fact, as much of the available literature shows, there is no definitive evidence of increased complications when PCI is performed prior to TAVI, compared to standard management. For instance, Abdel-Wahab and Jaffe have reported that a PCI procedure staged prior to TAVI had a rate of adverse events comparable to the group of patients undergoing only TAVI [21].

On the other hand, reasons against this approach are mainly concentrated on the risk of bleeding owing to antiaggregant therapy and risk of stent thrombosis. Regarding stent thrombosis, hypotension during the rapid right ventricular pacing could play a role increasing the risk of thrombosis beyond discontinuation of medication intake [11]. Likewise, performing PCI before TAVI may increase the risk of bleeding complications during later TAVI due to antiplatelet therapy [24, 26, 27]. In this regard, Pilgrim et al. performed a prospective study to investigate predictors of periprocedural bleeding in TAVI patients. Paradoxically, against the odds, rates of life-threatening and major bleeding according to therapeutic regimen (dual antiplatelet therapy, single antiplatelet therapy, vitamin K antagonist only, or antiplatelet therapy in combination with vitamin K antagonist) did not present significant differences. Moreover, there were no significant differences in bleeding for both approaches, staged and simultaneous TAVI and revascularization [24].

Among other potential complications, renal failure must be contemplated despite the staged approach, since angiographies performed from 5 days to 24 hours before the procedure may be related with an increased risk of renal failure owing to cumulative dose of contrast. Moreover, carrying out this strategy, patients would require two hospital admissions with additional costs [11, 19, 23].

Despite theses arguments against the staged procedure, two studies observed no valve-related complications when PCI was performed prior to TAVI [21, 29]. Considering differences in patient's profiles and vascular anatomies, revascularization prior to TAVI can be considered when greater PCI complexity is anticipated, in order to reduce periprocedural complications and optimize revascularization outcomes.

10.4.2 Concomitant PCI and TAVI

The second therapeutic option is a simultaneous approach with concomitant PCI and TAVI. The strength of this method is that it might eliminate potential complications associated with not treating one of both diseases at the same time [19]. Several studies have shown that a combined treatment of severe AS and significant coronary lesions is a safe and feasible procedure [19, 30]. A concomitant approach may reduce hospital admissions as well as risk of bleeding related to DAPT [19]. Penkalla et al. analyzed a cohort of 389 patients undergoing TAVI combined with PCI, and reported that early survival and 3-year survival were comparable between patients undergoing the combined procedure and those without CAD who received only TAVI, even though simultaneous treatment is expected to have greater procedural complexity than a conventional method [23].

On the other hand, the main drawbacks of concomitant PCI and TAVI are the amount of radiation and of contrast involved, as well as a longer procedural time. An increased risk of renal failure also might be observed, due to a large amount of contrast used [11, 19, 23]. It should not be forgotten that complex CAD may add unacceptable risk for intervention in certain difficult cases, so the global procedural and personal risks must be balanced according to each patient's profile. A simultaneous mixed method should be considered as long as procedural complexity allows it.

In conclusion, each approach could be adopted in compliance with the patient's characteristics and needs. Some authors suggest that revascularization prior to TAVI could be more desirable than performing both procedures at once in terms of safety or procedural time, offering the advantage of treating more severe CAD in a focused procedure, when a complex PCI is foreseen. This might reduce subsequently complications during the TAVI procedure and might improve left ventricular ejection fraction before the TAVI intervention, and may decrease procedural time or the amount of contrast [11, 21, 29]. Conversely, both CAD and AS can be resolved at once, by applying a combined method, which reduces further complications associated with an additional invasive procedure. This approach should be strongly considered if PCI complexity is expected to be low (Table 10.1) [19, 30].

10.4.3 Therapy After Revascularization in TAVI

There is no robust evidence about the optimal antiplatelet regimen after TAVI. Current European guidelines establish recommendations in the standard isolated TAVI procedure, which consist in low-dose aspirin and a thienopyridine after TAVI, followed by ASA or a thienopyridine alone [10]. The American Heart Association (AHA) guidelines recommend ASA 75–100 mg daily and clopidogrel 75 mg daily for 6 months after TAVI,

Table 10.1 Advantages and drawbacks in combined procedures considering timing

	Staged procedures	Concomitant procedures
Advantages	– Lower radiation exposure – Smaller amount of contrast – Decrease in the complexity of the TAVI procedure √ **Complex coronary stenosis**	– Both problems at once, less further complications – One admission – Less risk of bleeding √ **Complexity expected low**
Drawbacks	– Risk of bleeding in 2nd step – Risk of stent thrombosis – More than one admission	– Higher radiation rate – Larger amount of contrast – Not recommended for complex anatomies

followed by monotherapy with aspirin 75–100 mg to lifelong. The dosage and duration of DAPT are not further specified [31]. These recommendations are based on expert opinion; owing to the limited studies to date, heterogeneity in therapies between centers has been reported [32].

In this regard, specific recommendations for combined treatment with PCI and TAVI have not been established. In order to define the optimal antiplatelet regimen, bleeding risk factors and coronary stent choice must be considered.

- *Risk of bleeding*
  Despite its clinical benefits, TAVI is associated with the risk of hemorrhagic events, both periprocedural and postprocedural. The risk of bleeding could be increased in patients who take antiplatelet therapy, especially those ones undergoing dual antiplatelet therapy [32].
  The incidence of periprocedural life-threatening and major bleedings in patients undergoing TAVI ranges from 5 to 38% [32, 33]. As mentioned above, Pilgrim et al. analyzed predictors of periprocedural bleeding in TAVI patients identifying renal

impairment, diabetes, and transapical approach (TA) as independent risk factors for life-threatening bleeding events. Moreover, patients with periprocedural bleeding events had a higher logistic EuroSCORE, more advanced renal disease, and a greater New York Heart Association functional class. Significant differences in bleeding events according to therapeutic regimen (DAPT or SAPT, anticoagulant alone, or in combination with antiplatelet agents) or concomitant revascularization procedures were not found [24]. Additionally, Bogdan Borz et al. performed a multivariate analysis and found that TA access was the only independent predictor of life-threatening bleeding (OR 3.7, 95% CI 1.73–7.9, $p = 0.001$). The presence of carotid stenosis (OR 7.86, 95% CI 1.2–51.55, $p = 0.032$) and TA route (OR 5.2, 95% CI 1.02–26.53, $p = 0.047$) were independent predictors of major bleeding [34].

Among patients undergoing combined procedures with PCI and TAVI, antiplatelet regimen should be accurately addressed so as to prevent bleeding events as much as possible, especially, in those who receive a staged intervention.

- *Coronary stent choice to treat CAD in TAVI patients*
  Bleeding risk and stent thrombosis risk should be balanced in order to choose the most suitable type of stent in each patient. Drug-eluting stents reduce the risk of restenosis as well as the risk of stent thrombosis, while the main advantage in bare metal stents is the reduced lengh of DAPT. In addition, the type of stent selection is especially relevant in patients with atrial fibrillation (AF) who require anticoagulant therapy [26, 27, 32].

- *Antiplatelet regimen in patients undergoing TAVI and PCI*
  Different antiplatelet regimens have been heterogeneously applied since specific guidelines have not been defined in patients undergoing TAVI. Hassell et al. performed an analysis including 672 patients receiving dual ($n = 257$) or single ($n = 415$) antiplatelet therapy, and did not observe significant differences in 30-day net adverse clinical and cerebral events

(NACE), between aspirin-only and DAPT after TAVI (pooled OR 0.83, 95% CI 0.48–1.43, $p = 0.50$). Moreover, a trend toward less life-threatening and major bleeding was observed in favour of ASA (pooled OR 0.56, 95% CI 0.28–1.11, $p = 0.09$) [32]. Similarly, in the ARTE randomized trial [35], SAPT reduced the risk for major or life-threatening events while not increasing the risk for MI or stroke. Consequently, the additive value of clopidogrel warrants further investigation since DAPT fails to reduce stroke rates, while simultaneously increasing bleeding rates in patient undergoing TAVI.

There is limited evidence to support decision-making on antiplatelet therapy following TAVI and PCI. Abdel Wahab et al. propose preloading with clopidogrel 600 mg + ASA 500 mg and continuing clopidogrel 75 mg for 6 months and aspirin indefinitely. For those patients who have indication for oral anticoagulation, treatment with oral vitamin K antagonist and clopidogrel has been suggested [21]. Pasic et al. and Penkalla et al. recommend the same strategy based on preloading with 600 mg clopidogrel and 100 mg aspirin followed by 75 mg clopidogrel daily for 6 months for bare-metal stents and for 12 months for drug-eluting stents, together with a daily 100 mg aspirin permanently [19, 23].

In patients with AF, balancing risk and benefits of additional antithrombotic treatment is challenging, and limited evidence is available to support this decision. The recommended regimen consists of triple therapy (dual antiplatelet therapy + anticoagulant therapy) for 3 or 12 months (depending on the bleeding risk), followed by anticoagulant + antiplatelet monotherapy [32].

In conclusion, a regimen with dual antiplatelet therapy (aspirin + clopidogrel) for 6 or 12 months according to each type of stent, followed by lifelong antiplatelet in monotherapy, is the most extended strategy in patients undergoing both PCI and TAVI [19, 21, 23]. The presence of AF complicates the therapeutic choice, pushing toward a regimen based on triple therapy during the early-period after

Table 10.2 Recommendations for treatment in combined procedures, short term, and lifelong

Indication for antiplatelets/antithrombotics before TAVI	TAVI ± PCI 6 months after (BMS) 12 months after (DES)	lifelong
Neither	DAPT/clopidogrel[b]	Aspirin
CAD	DAPT/clopidogrel[b]	Aspirin
Prior PCI	DAPT/clopidogrel[b]	Aspirin
Patients with atrial fibrillation (AF)	**3–6 months**	**lifelong**
AF	Triple therapy[a]/VKA + aspirin[b]	VKA + aspirin/VKA
AF + CAD	Triple therapy/VKA + clopidogrel[b]	VKA + aspirin/VKA
AF + PCI	Triple therapy/VKA + clopidogrel[b]	VKA + aspirin/VKA

CAD coronary artery disease, *PCI* percutaneous coronary intervention, *VKA* vitamin-K antagonist, *DAPT* dual antiplatelet therapy, *BMS* bar-metal stent, *DES* drug-eluting stent
[a]Triple therapy: VKA + aspirin+clopidogrel
[b]In patients at high risk of bleeding

TAVI [26]. The revascularization leads to prolonged duration of DAPT increasing the period of bleeding risks (Table 10.2) [19, 23, 32].

References

1. Leon MB, Smith CR, Mack MJ, et al. PARTNER 2 Investigators. Transcatheter or surgical aortic-valve replacement in intermediate-risk patients. N Engl J Med. 2016;374:1609–20.
2. Reardon MJ, Van Mieghem NM, Popma JJ, Kleiman NS, Søndergaard L, Mumtaz M, Adams DH, Deeb GM, Maini B, Gada H, Chetcuti S, Gleason T, Heiser J, Lange R, Merhi W, Oh JK, Olsen PS, Piazza N, Williams M, Windecker S, Yakubov SJ, Grube E, Makkar R, Lee JS, Conte J, Vang E, Nguyen H, Chang Y, Mugglin AS, Serruys PW, Kappetein AP, SURTAVI Investigators. Surgical or transcatheter aortic-valve replacement in intermediate-risk patients. N Engl J Med. 2017;376:1321–31.
3. Ramsdale DR, Bennett DH, Bray CL, et al. Angina, coronary risk factors and coronary artery disease in patients with valvular disease. A prospective study. Eur Heart J. 1984;5:716–26.
4. Vandeplas A, Willems JL, Piessens J, de Geest H. Frequency of angina pectoris and coronary artery disease in severe isolated valvular aortic stenosis. Am J Cardiol. 1988;62:117–20.
5. Mohler ER, Sheridan MJ, Nichols R, Harvey WP, Waller BF. Development and progression of aortic valve stenosis: atherosclerosis risk factorsDOUBLE-HYPHENa causal relationship? A clinical morphologic study. Clin Cardiol. 1991;14(12):995–9.
6. Beach JM, Mihaljevic T, Svensson LG, Rajeswaran J, Marwick T, Griffin B, Johnston DR, Sabik JF 3rd, Blackstone EH. Coronary artery disease and outcomes of aortic valve replacement for severe aortic stenosis. J Am Coll Cardiol. 2013;61:837–48.
7. Leon MB, Kodali S, Williams M, Oz M, Smith C, Stewart A, Schwartz A, Collins M, Moses JW. Transcatheter aortic valve replacement in patients with critical aortic stenosis: rationale, device descriptions, early clinical experiences, and perspectives. Semin Thorac Cardiovasc Surg. 2006;18(2):165–74.
8. Alexander KP, Anstrom KJ, Muhlbaier LH, Grosswald RD, Smith PK, Jones RH, Peterson ED. Outcomes of cardiac surgery in patients > or = 80 years: results from the National Cardiovascular Network. J Am Coll Cardiol. 2000;35(3):731–8.
9. Windecker S, Kolh P, Alfonso F, Collet JP, Cremer J, Falk V, Filippatos G, Hamm C, Head SJ, Juni P, Kappetein AP, Kastrati A, Knuuti J, Landmesser U, Laufer G, Neumann FJ, Richter DJ, Schauerte P, Sousa Uva M, Stefanini GG, Taggart DP, Torracca L, Valgimigli M, Wijns W, Witkowski A. 2014 ESC/EACTS Guidelines on myocardial revascularization: the Task Force on Myocardial Revascularization of the European Society of Cardiology (ESC) and the European Association for Cardio-Thoracic Surgery (EACTS). Developed with the special contribution of the European Association of Percutaneous Cardiovascular Interventions (EAPCI). Eur Heart J. 2014;35:2541–619.
10. Baumgartner H, Falk V, Bax JJ, De Bonis M, Hamm C, Holm PJ, Iung B, Lancellotti P, Lansac E, Rodriguez Muñoz D, Rosenhek R, Sjögren J, Tornos Mas P, Vahanian A, Walther T, Wendler O, Windecker S, Zamorano JL, ESC Scientific Document Group. 2017 ESC/EACTS Guidelines for the management of valvular heart disease. Eur Heart J. 2017;38(36):2739–279.
11. Khawaja MZ, Wang D, Pocock S, Redwood SR, Thomas MR. The percutaneous coronary intervention prior to transcatheter aortic valve implantation (ACTIVATION) trial: study protocol for a randomized controlled trial. Trials. 2014;15:300.
12. Steadman CD, Jerosch-Herold M, Grundy B, Rafelt S, Ng LL, Squire IB, Samani NJ, McCann GP. Determinants and functional significance of

myocardial perfusion reserve in severe aortic stenosis. JACC Cardiovasc Imaging. 2012;5:182–9.

13. Tonino PAL, De Bruyne B, Pijls NHJ, Siebert U, Ikeno F, van't Veer M, Klauss V, Manoharan G, Engstrøm T, Oldroyd KG, Ver Lee PN, MacCarthy PA, Fearon WF. Fractional flow reserve versus angiography for guiding percutaneous coronary intervention. N Engl J Med. 2009;360(3):213–24.

14. Pesarini G, Scarsini R, Zivelonghi C, Piccoli A, Gambaro A, Gottin L, Rossi A, Ferrero V, Vassanelli C, Ribichini F. Functional assessment of coronary artery disease in patients undergoing transcatheter aortic valve implantation: influence of pressure overload on the evaluation of lesions severity. Circ Cardiovasc Interv 2016;9(11). pii: e004088.

15. Scarsini R, Pesarini G, Zivelonghi C, Piccoli A, Ferrero V, Lunardi M, Gottin L, Zanetti C, Faggian G, Ribichini F. Physiologic evaluation of coronary lesions using instantaneous wave-free ratio (iFR) in patients with severe aortic stenosis undergoing transcatheter aortic valve implantation. EuroIntervention. 2018;13:1512–9.

16. Stefanini GG, Stortecky S, Cao D, Rat-Wirtzler J, O'Sullivan CJ, Gloekler S, Buellesfeld L, Khattab AA, Nietlispach F, Pilgrim T, Huber C, Carrel T, Meier B, Jüni P, Wenaweser P, Windecker S. Coronary artery disease severity and aortic. stenosis: clinical outcomes according to SYNTAX score in patients undergoing. transcatheter aortic valve implantation. Eur Heart J. 2014;35(37):2530–40.

17. Ryan N, Nombela-Franco L, Jiménez-Quevedo P, Biagioni C, Salinas P, Aldazábal A, Cerrato E, Gonzalo N, Del Trigo M, Núñez-Gil I, Fernández-Ortiz A, Macaya C, Escaned J. The value of the SYNTAX Score II in predicting clinical outcomes in patients undergoing transcatheter aortic valve implantation. Rev Esp Cardiol (Engl Ed). 2018;71(8):628–37.

18. D'Ascenzo F, Conrotto F, Giordana F, Moretti C, D'Amico M, Salizzoni S, Omedè P, La Torre M, Thomas M, Khawaja Z, Hildick-Smith D, Ussia G, Barbanti M, Tamburino C, Webb J, Schnabel RB, Seiffert M, Wilde S, Treede H, Gasparetto V, Napodano M, Tarantini G, Presbitero P, Mennuni M, Rossi ML, Gasparini M, Biondi Zoccai G, Lupo M, Rinaldi M, Gaita F, Marra S. Mid-term prognostic value of coronary artery disease in patients undergoing transcatheter aortic valve implantation: a meta-analysis of adjusted observational results. Int J Cardiol. 2013;168(3):2528–32.

19. Pasic M, Dreysse S, Unbehaun A, Buz S, Drews T, Klein C, et al. Combined elective percutaneous coronary intervention and transapical transcatheter aortic valve implantation. Interact Cardiovasc Thorac Surg. 2012;14:463–8.

20. Dewey TM, Brown DL, Herbert MA, Culica D, Smith CR, Leon MB, et al. Effect of concomitant coronary artery disease on procedural and late outcomes of transcatheter aortic valve implantation. Ann Thorac Surg. 2010;89:758–67.

21. Abdel-Wahab M, Zahn R, Horack M, Gerckens U, Schuler G, Sievert H, Naber C, Voehringer M, Schäfer U, Senges J, Richardt G. Transcatheter aortic valve implantation in patients with and without concomitant coronary artery disease: comparison of characteristics and early outcome in the German multicenter TAVI registry. Clin Res Cardiol. 2012;101(12):973–81.

22. Ussia GP, Barbanti M, Colombo A, Tarantini G, Petronio AS, Ettori F, Ramondo A, Santoro G, Klugmann S, Bedogni F, Antoniucci D, Maisano F, Marzocchi A, Poli A, De Carlo M, Fiorina C, De Marco F, Napodano M, Violini R, Bortone AS, Tamburino C, CoreValve Italian Registry Investigators. Impact of coronary artery disease in elderly patients undergoing transcatheter aortic valve implantation: insight from the Italian CoreValve Registry. Int J Cardiol. 2013;167(3):943–50.

23. Penkalla A, Pasic M, Drews T, Buz S, Dreysse S, Kukucka M, Mladenow A, Hetzer R, Unbehaun A. Transcatheter aortic valve implantation combined with elective coronary artery stenting: a simultaneous approach. Eur J Cardiothorac Surg. 2015;47(6):1083–9.

24. Pilgrim T, Stortecky S, Luterbacher F, Windecker S, Wenaweser P. Transcatheter aortic valve implantation and bleeding: incidence, predictors and prognosis. J Thromb Thrombolysis. 2013;35(4):456–62.

25. Griese DP, Reents W, Tóth A, Kerber S, Diegeler A, Babin-Ebell J. Concomitant coronary intervention is associated with poorer early and late clinical outcomes in selected elderly patients receiving transcatheter aortic valve implantation. Eur J Cardiothorac Surg. 2014;46(1):e1–7.

26. Czerwińska-Jelonkiewicz K, Witkowski A, Dąbrowski M, Banaszewski M, Księżycka-Majczyńska E, Chmielak Z, Kuśmierski K, Hryniewiecki T, Demkow M, Orłowska-Baranowska E, Stępińska J. Antithrombotic therapy - predictor of early and long-term bleeding complications after transcatheter aortic valve implantation. Arch Med Sci. 2013;9(6):1062–70.

27. Rodés-Cabau J, Dauerman HL, Cohen MG, Mehran R, Small EM, Smyth SS, Costa MA, Mega JL, O'Donoghue ML, Ohman EM, Becker RC. Antithrombotic treatment in transcatheter aortic valve implantation: insights for cerebrovascular and bleeding events. J Am Coll Cardiol. 2013;62(25):2349–59.

28. Ranucci M, Ballotta A, Kunkl A, De Benedetti D, Kandil H, Conti D, Mollichelli N, Bossone E, Mehta RH. Influence of the timing of cardiac catheterization and the amount of contrast media on acute renal failure after cardiac surgery. Am J Cardiol. 2008;101(8):1112–8.

29. Gasparetto V, Fraccaro C, Tarantini G, Buja P, D'Onofrio A, Yzeiraj E, et al. Safety and effectiveness of a selective strategy for coronary artery revascularization before transcatheter aortic valve implantation. Catheter Cardiovasc Interv. 2013;81:376–83.

30. Wenaweser P, Pilgrim T, Guerios E, Stortecky S, Huber C, Khattab AA, et al. Impact of coronary artery disease and percutaneous coronary intervention on outcomes in patients with severe aortic stenosis undergoing transcatheter aortic valve implantation. EuroIntervention. 2011;7:541–8.

31. Nishimura RA, Otto CM, Bonow RO, Carabello BA, Erwin JP 3rd, Guyton RA, O'Gara PT, Ruiz CE, Skubas NJ, Sorajja P, Sundt TM 3rd, Thomas JD, American College of Cardiology/American Heart Association Task Force on Practice Guidelines. 2014 AHA/ACC guideline for the management of patients with valvular heart disease: executive summary: a report of the American College of Cardiology/American Heart Association Task Force on Practice Guidelines. J Am Coll Cardiol. 2014;63(22):2438–88.

32. Hassell ME, Hildick-Smith D, Durand E, Kikkert WJ, Wiegerinck EM, Stabile E, Ussia GP, Sharma S, Baan J Jr, Eltchaninoff H, Rubino P, Barbanti M, Tamburino C, Poliacikova P, Blanchard D, Piek JJ, Delewi R. Antiplatelet therapy following transcatheter aortic valve implantation. Heart. 2015;101(14):1118–25.

33. Généreux P, Head SJ, Van Mieghem NM, et al. Clinical outcomes after transcatheter aortic valve replacement using valve academic research consortium definitions: a weighted meta-analysis of 3,519 patients from 16 studies. J Am Coll Cardiol. 2012;59:2317–26.

34. Borz B, Durand E, Godin M, Tron C, Canville A, Litzler PY, Bessou JP, Cribier A, Eltchaninoff H. Incidence, predictors and impact of bleeding after transcatheter aortic valve implantation using the balloon-expandable Edwards prosthesis. Heart. 2013;99(12):860–5.

35. Rodés-Cabau J, Masson JB, Welsh RC, Garcia Del Blanco B, Pelletier M, Webb JG, Al-Qoofi F, Généreux P, Maluenda G, Thoenes M, Paradis JM, Chamandi C, Serra V, Dumont E, Côté M. Aspirin versus aspirin plus clopidogrel as antithrombotic treatment following transcatheter aortic valve replacement with a balloon-expandable valve: the ARTE (aspirin versus aspirin + clopidogrel following transcatheter aortic valve implantation) randomized clinical trial. JACC Cardiovasc Interv. 2017;10(13):1357–65.

Comparison of Transcatheter Aortic Valve Implantation to Medical Therapy in Prohibitive-Risk Patients

11

Gabriella Ricciardi, Piero Trabattoni, Maurizio Roberto, Marco Agrifoglio, and Giulio Pompilio

11.1 Introduction

Epidemiology of aortic stenosis (AS) is today pandemic in industrialized countries. Recent studies highlight that the prevalence of AS in the elderly (age ≥ 75 years) is as high as 12.4%. Moreover, severe AS is detected in about 3.4% of these patients, of which approximately 75.6% have symptoms [1].

The current management of patients with severe AS includes three options: medical therapy; surgical treatment, which is still considered the gold standard [2]; and the rapidly emerging technology of transcatheter aortic valve implantation (TAVI), also called transcatheter aortic valve replacement (TAVR). Among symptomatic patients with severe AS, 40.3% can potentially be today TAVR candidates, being this number expected to grow consistently in the near future.

G. Ricciardi · P. Trabattoni · M. Roberto
Cardiovascular Surgery Department, Centro Cardiologico Monzino IRCCS, Milan, Italy

M. Agrifoglio · G. Pompilio (✉)
Cardiovascular Surgery Department, Centro Cardiologico Monzino IRCCS, Milan, Italy

Department of Clinical Sciences and Community Health, Cardiovascular Section, University of Milano, Milan, Italy
e-mail: giulio.pompilio@ccfm.it;
Giulio.Pompilio@cardiologicomonzino.it

In the absence of contraindications, a patient is deemed "TAVR-eligible" in case of severe symptomatic AS and high surgical risk [3]. Within this population, the so-called prohibitive risk patient (PRP) subset, which includes patients who are not suitable for conventional surgery, accounts for the considerable amount of 12.3% [1]. These numbers could potentially increase in the near future.

As TAVR may offer a real therapeutic option to PRPs on top of medical therapy, the focus on this particular patient population deserves today more consideration. It is worth, however, to mention that overtreatment in patients who derive little long-term benefit due to irreversible and severe coexisting conditions must be avoided and that TAVR risk/benefit ratio in these patients has to be carefully assessed. Therefore, the delicate balance between feasibility and appropriateness is emerging in this particular patient cohort as an evolving challenge.

The aim of this chapter is to compare, analyzing available literature, the outcome of such a challenging prohibitive population whether medically managed or undergoing TAVR.

11.2 TAVR as a Game Changer

Given its association with ageing, by the time AS becomes clinically apparent, patients who require treatment often develop severe comor-

© Springer Nature Switzerland AG 2019
A. Giordano et al. (eds.), *Transcatheter Aortic Valve Implantation*,
https://doi.org/10.1007/978-3-030-05912-5_11

bidities. Historically, as high as 30% of elderly patients with symptomatic severe AS are at excessive perioperative procedural risk not allowing corrective surgery for a number of different reasons [4].

Chronological age is certainly a risk factor for morbidity and mortality after cardiac surgery, although number and severity of pathology-related comorbidities are important additional factors for the perioperative and long-term prognosis of these high-risk patients. PRP population shows in fact a greater prevalence of cerebrovascular disease, left ventricular dysfunction, diabetes mellitus, chronic obstructive pulmonary disease, renal impairment, and peripheral arterial disease [5].

Retrospective studies have shown that the overall operative mortality in octogenarians undergoing AVR is about 6% [6] and that 1- and 5-year survivals are up to 90% and 70%, respectively. Predictors of 6-month postoperative mortality in this cohort of patients include female gender, preoperative renal failure, severe chronic obstructive pulmonary disorder (COPD) requiring oral steroid treatment, and postoperative stroke [7].

Up to the recent past, patients who were considered to be at excessive risk for traditional surgery were considered for medical therapy only [2]. With the advent of TAVR, this paradigm has changed. Specifically, it has been demonstrated that TAVR is an effective method to improve quality of life and decrease mortality for high-risk patients with severe symptomatic AS [8]. Therefore, TAVR can be viewed as a real "game changer" in PRPs, although medical therapy remains an available option that must be carefully evaluated in managing of this fragile patient population.

11.3 Randomized Controlled Studies

Useful information in this regard can be drawn from pivotal TAVR randomized controlled trials. In this context, the Placement of Aortic Transcatheter Valves (PARTNER) [9] and the CoreValve [10] studies represent the most important breakthrough in the field of transcatheter treatment of AS for high-risk patients. Table 11.1 shows the mean characteristics of these trials.

In the PARTNER trial, patients enrolled showed severe aortic stenosis (aortic valve area [AVA] less than 0.8 cm^2, mean gradient >40 mmHg, or jet velocity >4 m/s) with NYHA class II symptoms. They were divided into two cohorts: cohorts A, including patients considered to be candidates for surgery despite a high surgical risk, as defined by a Society of Thoracic

Table 11.1 TAVR randomized controlled trials

Definition	Trial design	Control	N° pts	Primary endpoints
Extreme risk or inoperable patients				
PARTNER I-B: >50% risk of death or irreversible morbidity at 30 days	Prospective, randomized 1:1	Medical therapy, including BAV	358	Rate of death from any cause over the duration of the trial. Co-primary endpoint was the rate of a hierarchical composite of the time to death from any cause or the time to the first occurrence of repeat
US CoreValve: >50% risk of death or irreversible morbidity at 30 days	Registry	Performance goal	487	1-year all-cause mortality and major stroke (versus performance goal)
High-risk surgical patients				
PARTNER I-A: >15% risk of 30-day death (with STS >8)	Prospective, randomized 1:1	AVR	699	1-year all-cause mortality
US CoreValve: >15% risk of 30-day death	Prospective, randomized 1:1	AVR	790	1-year all-cause mortality

Surgeons (STS) risk score of 10% or higher or by the presence of coexisting conditions that predict a risk of death by 30 days after surgery of 15% or higher; cohort B, including patients who were not considered to be suitable candidates for surgery because of coexisting conditions with a predicted probability of 50% or more of either death by 30 days after surgery or a serious irreversible condition.

Pertinent exclusion criteria were bicuspid or non-calcified aortic valve, acute myocardial infarction, substantial coronary artery disease requiring revascularization, a left ventricular ejection fraction of less than 20%, a diameter of the aortic annulus of less than 18 mm or more than 25 mm, severe (>3+) mitral or aortic regurgitation, a transient ischemic attack or stroke within the previous 6 months, and severe renal insufficiency. Notably, mean age was 83 years.

The PARTNER cohort A trial showed for the first time that in high-risk patients with severe AS both surgery and TAVR were associated with similar rates of survival at 1 year. In this patient cohort, 358 patients with severe AS who were not eligible for AVR were randomly assigned to either medical care (including balloon aortic valvulotomy) or TAVR with an Edwards SAPIEN valve via transfemoral approach.

The PARTNER cohort B trial specifically provided for the first time the evidence of a benefit of TAVR versus standard medical therapy in prohibitive-risk patients [11–14]. The 1-year mortality rate was reduced in TAVR group compared with medical therapy, including balloon aortic valvulotomy (30.7 vs. 50.7%). Of note, this outcome remained stable up to 2, 3, and 5 years. NYHA functional class was also better for TAVR patients (86 vs. 60% in NYHA I or II at 5 years). In the TAVR group, authors found moderate or severe paravalvular aortic regurgitation in 12.4% of patients at 30 days, which was reduced at 8.8% at 1 year and at 4.5% at 3 years.

Although the stroke rate was significantly higher in TAVR rather than medical therapy group at 30 days, at 2 and 3 years, such neurologic complication was similar in both groups at 5 years [9].

The CoreValve Extreme Risk United States Pivotal Trial was a prospective single-arm study, comparing TAVR with the self-expanding CoreValve to a pre-specified estimate of 12-month mortality or major stroke versus medical therapy (43%, based upon the results of a meta-analysis and data from the PARTNER cohort B) [10]. The inclusion criteria included severe AS and functional impairment in an AS high-risk population with life expectancy exceeding 1 year.

The results of this study indicated consistent mortality benefit with TAVR in comparison with standard therapy, as well as improved NYHA functional status and fewer hospitalizations over the 3-year follow-up. Moreover, authors found a durable valve function improvement with minimal signs of deterioration over the follow-up. However, it has to be mentioned that mortality in the TAVR-treated patients was high at 3 years (about 50%), suggesting the need for accurate patient selection in such a fragile patient population.

The following table summarizes these main studies.

11.4 Registries

TAVR registries represent another important source to have insights on outcomes and benefits in the real-world context.

The first European consensus document on TAVR, called Valve Academic Research Consortium (VARC), with standardized definitions on clinical endpoints, was published in October 2011. The goals of VARC are combining the expertise to reach a consensus for selecting appropriate clinical endpoints and standardizing definitions for single and composite clinical endpoints [15]. The VARC-2 definition [16] is an updated version from the first VARC definition. For the major complications, the VARC-2 refines the selection and definitions of TAVR-related clinical endpoints and stresses the understanding of patient risk stratification and case selection, using Logistic EuroSCORE and STS-Score to select suitable patients. The VARC-2 definitions for TAVR registry study was published in 2013

[17]. In a large report, 20 TAVR registries are listed according to VARC-2 definitions [18]. Overall, the take-home message is that mortality and complication rates are reduced over time despite an unchanged risk of patient profile. This feature appears to be not dependent on valve type or access site and is part of practice of evenly experienced centers [19, 20].

The recent published UK TAVI registry represents to date the largest country-based long-term experience with up to 6-year follow-up [21]. In agreement with US Transcatheter Valve Therapy (TVT) registry report, UK TAVI registry provides a model of patient selection and is reflective of a "real world" clinical experience in the management of very sick patients with severe comorbidities. Along the same line in the setting of high-risk-profile patients, the FRANCE-2 (FRench Aortic National CoreValve and Edwards) registry, including all patients from all centers in France, was set to analyze late clinical outcome and its determinants in all high-risk patients who underwent TAVR in France during a 2-year period [22]. This prospective registry included all symptomatic adults (NYHA functional class ≥ II) requiring TAVR for severe AS, with contraindications to AVR or considered at high risk by a multidisciplinary team. The primary endpoint was death from any cause at 1 month, 6 months, or 1, 2, 3, 4, or 5 years. Secondary safety endpoints were major adverse cardiovascular or cerebrovascular events, cardiac events, cardiac or vascular surgery, bleeding or stroke during follow-up, and NYHA functional class. Secondary efficacy endpoints were success rate and complications on the VARC criteria. The overall 30-day mortality was 9.2% (388 patients). For patients suitable for a transfemoral approach, all-cause mortality at 3 years was 39.6% and cardiovascular mortality 15.9%; for those suitable for a transapical approach, all-cause mortality was 47.7% and cardiovascular mortality 21.2%. All-cause and cardiovascular mortality rates were significantly lower with the femoral approach at all assessment time points: 1, 2, 3, and 4 years. Multivariate predictive factors of 3-year all-cause mortality comprised male sex, low BMI, atrial fibrillation, dialysis, NYHA functional class III or IV, higher logistic EuroSCORE, transapical and subclavian approaches, need for permanent pacemaker implantation, and post-implant periprosthetic AR grade ≥2 of 4. The majority of severe events according to VARC criteria occurred during the first month, and the incidence was subsequently below 2% per year. Hospital readmission for any reason occurred in 1032 (28.1%) patients between 30 days and 1 year, 557 (21.5%) patients during the second year, and 515 (25.6%) patients during the third year. At 3 years, 90.0% of surviving patients were asymptomatic or only not particularly symptomatic (NYHA functional class I or II).

Taken together, the sustained clinical improvement and acceptable rate of clinical events after the first month from implantation strengthen current guidelines for TAVR in high-risk patients on top of medical therapy alone. It has to be highlighted that in such a risky subset, particular attention may be deserved for those cases in which the transfemoral approach is not suitable.

11.5 Patient Stratification

According to the current practice, a patient is deemed at low risk for surgical treatment if the estimated 30-day mortality is <4%, at intermediate risk if 4–10%, high risk if >10%, and very high risk if >15% [23]. Such a risk assessment is imperative to identify patients who are likely not to benefit from AVR and may be TAVR candidates. In this evaluation, an expected improvement in quality of life (QoL) has also its importance to discriminate between responder and non-responder patients. Moreover, prognostic indices of life expectancy may also play a central role in moving beyond arbitrary age-based cutoffs.

As for the sicker PRP population, stratification is crucial to identify appropriate TAVR candidates. The main risk scores today available are the Society of Thoracic Surgeon (STS) and the EuroSCORE II scores. Although they both have the capacity to reliably predict operative mortality in AVR, their usefulness for TAVR is not yet confirmed. In a study by Rosa et al. [24], STS is shown to often overestimate the in-hospital and 30-day mortality TAVR rates, while the EuroSCORE II underestimates such outcomes. This divergence is probably due to the fact that STS score is composed of 40 clinical parameters for calculation, while the EuroSCORE II only requires 18 items. Despite that, the STS score has not proven to be able to predict mortality better than EuroSCORE in the TAVR patient population. For this reason, the STS has released a specific TAVR calculator, which is a risk-adjusted mortality estimate recommended to use as guidance in the overall conversation about the TAVR procedure (http://tools.acc.org/tavrrisk/#!/content/evaluate/). Interestingly, the adjusted TAVR in-hospital mortality risk includes a stratification for access site and a careful evaluation of prior acuity of cardiac events.

On the base of the large body of evidence about patient risk profile in TAVR, besides ordinary contraindications related to anatomic features and critical clinical conditions, absolute contraindications to candidate a patient for TAVR treatment must include the following clinical issues:

– Estimated life expectancy <12 months due to non-cardiac conditions
– Unexpected improvement of QoL after treatment because of severe comorbidities
– Severe concomitant mitral or tricuspid valve disease with a major impact on patient's symptoms

It is worth to note that, particularly for a prohibitive risk assessment going beyond the classical parameters, the capability of a reliable prediction both of life expectancy and of quality of life will be in the future increasingly important, since the main goal of TAVR in PRPs who are likely to survive beyond 1 year must be a relevant improvement of symptoms and related functional status.

11.6 The Heart Team

The Heart Team (HT) plays a further important part of the decision-making of the best management option for high-risk patients with severe AS. HT should consist of at least interventional cardiologists, cardiovascular surgeons, imaging specialists, and anesthesiologists. The discussion within HT members allows for a careful decision-making process, taking into an account the local experience. The decision to classify a patient at high risk despite low or intermediate STS score, in fact, is often based on other factors or comorbidities, such as cancer history and frailty, that are not included in the standard risk scores. Moreover, within the PRPs are included other variables surgery-wise technically extremely challenging, such as porcelain aorta, a hostile chest wall, or redo-surgery with the presence of bypass grafts in proximity to the sternum [25].

11.7 Toward a Consensus for Risk Definition for the Sicker Patients

In an effort to identify best candidates to TAVR, the elegant study by Brecker and Aldea [26] reviewed therapy options for PRPs with severe AS, taking into account risks, benefits, and possible complications. For patients with prohibitive surgical risk (defined as ≥50% probability of death or serious irreversible complications) or with an absolute contraindication to AVR, they recommended TAVR over medical therapy for those individuals in which a transfemoral TAVR is feasible. The transfemoral access for TAVR is commonly preferred to alternative sites, because of the greater experience gained with this approach and the reported superior outcomes. For those patients in which transfemoral TAVR is technically demanding or not feasible, authors suggest to perform an individualized risk-benefit assessment of medical therapy versus alternative access TAVR by the Heart Team. This evaluation should take into consideration important variables such as life expectancy, frailty, comorbidities, specific anatomy, and, finally, patient's preferences. In the PARTNER 2 Trial and United States Pivotal Trial, the benefits of TAVR over surgery were higher in the transfemoral cohort of patients. However, it is unclear how much the increased mortality observed in patients undergoing alternative strategies is due to procedural access per se and how much is dependent on the excessive risk associated with the presence of a severe peripheral vasculopathy.

In a study by Freeman et al. [27], authors conducted a retrospective analysis to determine mortality rate differences, admission profiles, and associated healthcare costs in a real-world setting of two groups of high-risk patients with severe symptomatic AS medically vs. TAVR managed. Survival analysis demonstrated that patients treated with TAVR are more likely to survive compared with the medical therapy group and that TAVR patients experience significantly less hospital admissions per year.

Interestingly, a recent study by Barbash et al. shows that procedural TAVR success rates are high irrespective of the patient's risk without significant differences in most of the periprocedural complications as well as mortality [23]. Of importance, the difference between low-, intermediate-, and high-risk patient is almost found in terms of short- and long-term mortality. Assessment of the specific complications according to the mechanism by which they occur may provide some insights to clarify this finding. In fact, vascular complications are typically associated with anatomic and technical aspects and are not affected by patients' comorbidities. For the same reason, tamponade and other procedural complications (i.e., conversion to open heart surgery and need for permanent PM) remain stable across risk categories. Instead, some baseline comorbidities can influence the result of the TAVR procedure. Among these, the higher prevalence of peripheral vascular disease and previous stroke and the higher rate of renal failure explain the higher stroke rates and the higher acute kidney injury rates in the high-risk group of patients.

Another important consideration emerging from this study is that the mortality curves of low-, intermediate-, and high-risk patients diverge early, with significantly higher in-hospital mortality rate in intermediate- and high-risk patients [23]. This mortality difference is stable also after adjustment for multiple covariants that may affect the outcome. In addition, comorbidities exhibited by this group of patients may contribute especially to higher non-cardiovascular deaths, which may be an important driver for its poor long-term survival.

Finally, the selection of transcatheter heart valve is not influenced by patient's risk; nevertheless, high-risk patients often receive smaller-sized valves, whereas low-risk patients receive larger-sized valves. In addition, high-risk patients show higher rate of valve-in-valve procedure. Generally speaking, the access for TAVR is more frequently transfemoral in low-risk patients when compared to intermediate- and high-risk patients (95% vs. 88% vs. 81%, respectively), with lower rates of general anesthesia (19% vs. 28% vs. 31%, respectively). Instead, patient's risk does not influence the procedure fluoroscopy time, contrast use, or the procedural success, which are comparable between patient groups.

Taking these data together, it can be assumed that TAVR has now gained widespread acceptance as an alternative treatment modality for high surgical risk patients with symptomatic severe AS and represents today the preferred treatment modality for appropriately selected PRPs [28]. It has however to be highlighted that high priority of caring physicians must be in the future the development of better clinical research models to assess TAVR futility from a patient's perspective. The final decision to proceed or withhold therapy must be carefully individualized and should take into consideration a careful assessment of the patient's expectations by means of a patient-centric approach [29].

11.8   Future Directions

The extraordinary evolution of TAVR technology since the early proof-of-concept cases has importantly contributed to the widespread clinical acceptance of this new, less-invasive therapy. Looking ahead, future directions are meant to further reduce the interventional trauma, in an attempt to widen indications for those patients who are at higher risk, including the PRP population.

TAVR standardization has undoubtedly resulted into a high procedural success and less complication rates. The focus has today shifted toward the simplification of the procedure. This strategy is known as the "minimalist" approach. The components of a minimalist TAVR strategy include percutaneous transfemoral vascular access, monitored anesthesia control (i.e., conscious sedation) without general anesthesia, reduction or elimination of intra-procedural TEE guidance, reduction or elimination of balloon pre-dilation before valve implantation, and pre-specified care plans to encourage rapid ambulation and early hospital discharge [30]. Some high-volume centers are already promoting a minimalistic strategy with conscious sedation and without routine use of TEE as the standard approach for most TAVR patients [31].

The adoption of minimalist periprocedural approaches is nowadays gaining interest [32]. In 2014, the European Society of Cardiology Transcatheter Valve Treatment Sentinel Registry described the rapid increase in the adoption of local anesthesia, moving from 37.5% of all procedures in the early 2011 to 57% a year later, without any alert for deleterious effects on outcomes [33].

Another option for patient triaging is the so-called "hybrid" strategy, which encourages a minimalist approach in straightforward cases with adequate imaging windows for transthoracic echocardiography and a more conventional approach in either high-risk or ambiguous cases, wherein the virtues of TEE guidance would be especially advantageous. This hybrid strategy requires careful preoperative assessment of comorbidities and identification of high-risk anatomic features with CT angiography to optimally risk-stratify patients.

As for available devices, it seems that the majority of patients with AS who are candidates for TAVR can be treated with similar excellent clinical outcomes by using either Sapien or CoreValve devices. Nevertheless, in the prohibitive-risk subset of patients, it is necessary to pay attention to specific anatomic factors or clinical circumstances in the choice of the optimal valve to minimize procedural complications. As an example, CoreValve technology can be more challenging to implant in horizontal aortas

and, due to the higher rates of pacemaker implantation, may be less favorable in patients with heart failure and reduced left ventricular function. Conversely, in patients with considerably high risk of annulus rupture due to severe calcification and frailty of the aortic valve apparatus, the self-expanding CoreValve may be a viable option.

Currently, three large randomized trials in the United States (each including approximately 1000 patients) are on-going comparing new TAVR devices versus devices already approved by the US Food and Drug Administration (CoreValve and Sapien). These studies should provide in the future further interesting head-to-head comparisons among novel TAVR technologies [34].

TAVR has also emerged as a novel, less-invasive therapy for failed bioprosthetic surgical valves [35] with the so-called "valve-in-valve" procedure. Based on clinical registry data, the self-expanding CoreValve and the balloon-expandable Sapien XT valve have been approved for use in high-risk patients with aortic bioprosthetic valve failure. In the largest international registry of transcatheter aortic valve-in-valve implantations [36], using both balloon-expandable and self-expanding transcatheter valves, early hemodynamic findings were encouraging, and 1-year survival was 83.2%. Of note, in this multicenter report, stenotic degeneration of the surgical bioprosthesis and small valve implant size (usually resulting in higher post-procedural gradients) were associated with worse clinical outcomes. From a technical standpoint, compared with native valve TAVR, transcatheter valve-in-valve therapy results in less frequent PVR and new pacemakers but more common coronary occlusions, particularly in surgical valves, in which the leaflets are sutured outside the stent frame [35]. This option is particularly appealing in the PRP population with bioprosthetic valve degeneration/failure in which conventional surgery is deemed at high risk. Further controlled studies, currently lacking, are required to define the advantage of TAVR vs. surgery for PRP patients in this context.

An interesting recently emerged additional topic is the possibility to perform TAVR procedure in nonagenarians. Since the prevalence of severe symptomatic AS increases with age, the management of nonagenarians has nowadays gained consideration. Even if this population is often composed of frail patients who suffer from severe comorbidities, some are in such good health conditions, without relevant concomitant diseases, and still enjoy a good quality of life with a low level of disability. Indeed, according to Fries' theory [37], the age at which disease and functional impairment appear is progressively postponed, resulting in the phenomenon of "compression of morbidity," which in parallel influences the important concept of "healthy life expectancy."

According to this statement, TAVR may offer a valid therapeutic alternative to selected nonagenarian patients with symptomatic severe AS [38, 39]. A recent study by Noble et al. [40] shows that TAVR in selected nonagenarians is safe and effective. It was previously reported in a single-center experience that TAVR outcome in 26 nonagenarians showed a 30-day overall mortality of 15% [41]. In Noble's work the 30-day mortality rate was 8.7%. Importantly, approaches other than TF accounted for more than half of the 30-day overall mortality. This is probably one factor that may be a discriminant in the decision-making process in nonagenarians.

The results from these experiences are encouraging and compare favorably with 8–20% of 30-day mortality rate reported for cardiac surgery in selected nonagenarians [42–45]. Indeed, in the recent multicenter study of eight Italian centers, cardiac surgery in nonagenarians represented only 1.2% of their cardiac surgery activity [43]. Interestingly, the oldest patient in Noble's single-center experience, 99 years at the time of the procedure, was still alive at 20 months of post-TAVR implant with an excellent quality of life [46].

Some important lessons can be learned at this point about age and interventional risk. The first notion is that age itself should not preclude the possibility of performing TAVR in accurately selected patients; conversely, it should be highlighted that the absence of comorbidities has to be carefully assessed in patients with very advanced age.

11.9 Conclusions

Given the potential impact of TAVR in AS, we believe that the balance in the decision-making process for TAVR in the high- and prohibitive-risk population will be one of those relevant issues to be solved to make the economic burden of the National Health Systems sustainable. As long as the mean age of TAVR patients will increase, physicians will face more and more AS patients with very high and prohibitive risk. The triage will be a hard task to operate in the absence of strict guidelines.

The explosive demographics of aortic stenosis will then eventually force payers and physicians to set guidelines for TAVR especially for the older and frail patients, in order to discriminate those individuals in which the procedure can be really effective.

Ultimately, we believe that such a difficult balance will be only reached if all players involved will take full responsibility in the single interest of patients and caregivers.

References

1. Osnabrugge RL, et al. Aortic stenosis in the elderly: disease prevalence and number of candidates for transcatheter aortic valve replacement: a meta-analysis and modeling study. J Am Coll Cardiol. 2013;62(11):1002–12.
2. Baumgartner H, Falk V, Bax JJ, De Bonis M, Hamm C, Johan P, Iung HB, Lancellotti P, Lansac E, Muñoz DR, Rosenhek R, Sjögren J, Tornos P, Alec M, Thomas V, Wendler WO, Windecker S, Zamorano JL, ESC Scientific Document Group. Valvular heart disease (management of) ESC Clinical Practice Guidelines. Eur Heart J. 2017;38(36):2739–91.
3. Holmes DR Jr, Mack MJ, Kaul S, et al. 2012 ACCF/AATS/SCAI/STS Expert Consensus Document on Transcatheter Aortic Valve Replacement: developed in collaboration with the American Heart Association, American Society of Echocardiography, European Association for Cardio-Thoracic Surgery, Heart Failure Society of America, Mended Hearts, Society of Cardiovascular Anesthesiologists, Society of Cardiovascular Computed Tomography, and Society for Cardiovascular Magnetic Resonance. Ann Thorac Surg. 2012;93:1340–95.
4. Iung B, Cachier A, Baron G, Messika-Zeitoun D, Delahaye F, Tornos P, et al. Decision-making in elderly patients with severe aortic stenosis: why are so many denied surgery? Eur Heart J. 2005;26(24):2714–20.

5. Nicolini F, Agostinelli A, Vezzani A, et al. The evolution of cardiovascular surgery in elderly patient: a review of current options and outcomes. Biomed Res Int. 2014;2014:736298.

6. Florath I, Albert A, Boening A, Ennker IC, Ennker J. Aortic valve replacement in octogenarians: identification of high-risk patients. Eur J Cardiothorac Surg. 2010;37:1304–10.

7. ElBardissi AW, et al. Minimally invasive aortic valve replacement in octogenarian, high-risk, transcatheter aortic valve implantation candidates. J Thorac Cardiovasc Surg. 2011;141(2):328–35.

8. Freeman PM, Protty MB, Aldalati O, et al. Severe symptomatic aortic stenosis: medical therapy and transcatheter aortic valve implantation (TAVI)—a real world retrospective cohort analysis of outcomes and cost-effectiveness using national data. Open Heart. 2016;3:e000414.

9. Smith CR, Leon MB, Mack MJ, Miller DC, Moses JW, Svensson LG, Tuzcu EM, Webb JG, Fontana GP, Makkar RR, Williams M, Dewey T, Kapadia S, Babaliaros V, Thourani VH, Corso P, Pichard AD, Bavaria JE, Herrmann HC, Akin JJ, Anderson WN, Wang D, Pocock SJ. PARTNER Trial Investigators. Transcatheter versus surgical aortic-valve replacement in high-risk patients. N Engl J Med. 2011;364:2187–98.

10. Adams DH, Popma JJ, Reardon MJ. Transcatheter aortic-valve replacement with a self-expanding prosthesis. N Engl J Med. 2014;371(10):967–8.

11. Holmes DR Jr, Mack MJ, Kaul S, et al. 2012 ACCF/AATS/SCAI/STS expert consensus document on transcatheter aortic valve replacement. J Am Coll Cardiol. 2012;59:1200.

12. Kodali SK, Williams MR, Smith CR, Svensson LG, Webb JG, Makkar RR, Fontana GP, Deweytm TM, Thourani VH, Pichard AD, Fischbein M, Szeto WY, Lim S, Greason KL, Teirstein PS, Malaisrie SC, Douglas PS, Hahn RT, Whisenant B, Zajarias A, Wang D, Akin JJ, Anderson WN, Leon MB, Partner Trial Investigators. Two-year outcomes after transcatheter or surgical aortic-valve replacement. N Engl J Med. 2012;366:1686–95.

13. Leon MB, Smith CR, Mack M, Miller DC, Moses JW, Svensson LG, Tuzcu EM, Webb JG, Fontana GP, Makkar RR, Brown DL, Block PC, Guyton RA, Pichard AD, Bavaria JE, Herrmann HC, Douglas PS, Petersen JL, Akin JJ, Anderson WN, Wang D, Pocock S, Partner Trial Investigators. Transcatheter aortic-valve implantation for aortic stenosis in patients who cannot undergo surgery. N Engl J Med. 2010;363:1597–607.

14. Makkar RR, Fontana GP, Jilaihawi H, Kapadia S, Pichard AD, Douglas PS, Thourani VH, Babaliaros VC, Webb JG, Herrmann HC, Bavaria JE, Kodali S, Brown DL, Bowers B, Dewey TM, Svensson LG, Tuzcu M, Moses JW, Williams MR, Siegel RJ, Akin JJ, Anderson WN, Pocock S, Smith CR, Leon MB, PARTNER Trial Investigators. Transcatheter aortic-valve replacement for inoperable severe aortic stenosis. N Engl J Med. 2012;366:1696–704.

15. Leon MB, Piazza N, Nikolsky E, Blackstone EH, Cutlip DE, et al. Standardized endpoint definitions for Transcatheter Aortic Valve Implantation clinical trials: a consensus report from the Valve Academic Research Consortium. J Am Coll Cardiol. 2011;57:253–69.

16. Kappetein AP, Head SJ, Genereux P, Piazza N, van Mieghem NM, et al. Updated standardized endpoint definitions for transcatheter aortic valve implantation: the Valve Academic Research Consortium-2 consensus document. J Thorac Cardiovasc Surg. 2013;145:6–23.

17. Tarantini G, Gasparetto V, Napodano M, Frigo AC, Fraccaro C, et al. Transcatheter aortic valve implantation and bleeding: focus on Valve Academic Research Consortium-2 classification. Int J Cardiol. 2013;168:5001–3.

18. Haussig S, Schuler G, Linke A. Worldwide TAVI registries: what have we learned? Clin Res Cardiol. 2014;103(8):603–12.

19. Wendler O, Walther T, Schroefel H, et al. The SOURCE Registry: what is the learning curve in transapical aortic valve implantation? Eur J Cardiothorac Surg. 2011;39:853–9.

20. Gilard M, Eltchaninoff H, Iung B, et al. Registry of transcatheter aortic-valve implantation in high-risk patients. N Engl J Med. 2012;366:1705–15.

21. Suradi HS, Hijazi ZM. TAVR update: contemporary data from UK TAVI and US TVT registries. Glob Cardiol Sci Pract. 2015;2015:21.

22. Gilard M, Eltchaninoff H, Donzeau-Gouge P, Chevreul K, Fajadet J, Leprince P, Leguerrier A, Lievre M, Prat A, Teiger E, Lefevre T, Tchetche D, Carrié D, Himbert D, Albat B, Cribier A, Sudre A, Blanchard D, Rioufol G, Collet F, Houel R, Santos PD, Meneveau N, Ghostine S, Manigold T, Guyon P, Grisoli D, Le Breton H, Delpine S, Didier R, Favereau X, Souteyrand G, Ohlmann P, Doisy V, Grollier G, Gommeaux A, Claudel J-P, Bourlon F, Bertrand B, Laskar M, Iung B, for the FRANCE 2 Investigators. Late outcomes of transcatheter aortic valve replacement in high-risk patients. The FRANCE-2 Registry. J Am Coll Cardiol. 2016;68(15):1637–47.

23. Barbash IM, Finkelstein A, Barsheshet A, Segev A, Steinvil A, Assali A, Gal YB, Assa HV, Fefer P, Sagie A, Guetta V, Kornowski R. Outcomes of patients at estimated low, intermediate, and high risk undergoing transcatheter aortic valve implantation for aortic stenosis. Am J Cardiol. 2015;116:1916–22.

24. Rosa VEE, Lopes AS d SA, Accorsi TAD, Fernandes JRC, Spina GS, Sampaio RO, Paixão MR, Pomerantzeff PM, Lemos Neto PA, Tarasoutchi F. EuroSCORE II and STS as mortality predictors in patients undergoing TAVI. Rev Assoc Med Bras. 2016;62(1):32–7.

25. Yourman LC, Lee SJ, Schonberg MA, Widera EW, Smith AK. Prognostic indices for older adults: a systematic review. JAMA. 2012;307:182–92.

26. Brecker SJD, Aldea GS. Choice of therapy for symptomatic aortic stenosis. UptoDate Jan 2017.

27. Freeman PM, Protty MB, Aldalati O, Lacey A, King W, Anderson RA, Smith D. Severe symptomatic aortic stenosis: medical therapy and transcatheter aortic valve implantation (TAVI)—a real-world retrospective cohort analysis of outcomes and cost-effectiveness using national data. Open Heart. 2016;3: e000414.

28. Gooley R, et al. Transcatheter aortic valve implantation—yesterday, today and tomorrow. Heart Lung Circ. 2015;24:1149–61.

29. Kapadia SR, Murat Tuzcu E, Makkar RR, Svensson LG, Agarwal S, Kodali S, Fontana GP, Webb JG, Mack M, Thourani VH, Babaliaros VC, Herrmann HC, Szeto WY, Pichard A, Williams MR, Anderson WN, Akin JJ, Craig Miller D, Smith CR, Leon MB. Response to letter regarding article, "long-term outcomes of inoperable patients with aortic stenosis randomly assigned to transcatheter aortic valve replacement or standard therapy". Circulation. 2015;132:e118–9.

30. Durand E, Borz B, Godin M, et al. Transfemoral aortic valve replacement with the Edwards SAPIEN and Edwards SAPIEN XT prosthesis using exclusively local anesthesia and fluoroscopic guidance: feasibility and 30-day outcomes. J Am Coll Cardiol Intv. 2012;5:461–7.

31. Barbanti M, Capranzano P, Ohno Y, et al. Early discharge after transfemoral transcatheter aortic valve implantation. Heart. 2015;101:1485.

32. Wiegerinck EMA, Dijk K B-v, Koch KT, Yong ZY, Vis MM, Planken RN, Eberl S, de Mol BA, Piek JJ, Tijssen JG, Baan J Jr. Towards minimally invasiveness: transcatheter aortic valve implantation under local analgesia exclusively. Int J Cardiol. 2014;176:1050–2.

33. Dall'Ara G, Eltchaninoff H, Moat N, Laroche C, Goicolea J, Ussia GP, Kala P, Wenaweser P, Zembala M, Nickenig G, Snow T, Price S, Barrero EA, Estevez-Loureiro R, Iung B, Zamorano JL, Schuler G, Alfieri O, Prendergast B, Ludman P, Windecker S, Sabate M, Gilard M, Witkowski A, Danenberg H, Schroeder E, Romeo F, Macaya C, Derumeaux G, Mattesini A, Tavazzi L, DiMario C, Transcatheter Valve Treatment Sentinel Registry (TCVT) Investigators of the EurObservational Research Programme (EORP) of the European Society of Cardiology. Local and general anaesthesia do not influence outcome of transfemoral aortic valve implantation. Int J Cardiol. 2014;177:448–54.

34. Vahl TP, Kodali SK, Leon MB. Transcatheter aortic valve replacement 2016: a modern-day "through the looking-glass" adventure. J Am Coll Cardiol. 2016;67(12):1472–87.

35. Webb JG, Wood DA, Ye J, et al. Transcatheter valve-in-valve implantation for failed bioprosthetic heart valves. Circulation. 2010;121:1848–57.

36. Dvir D, Webb JG, Bleiziffer S, For the Valve-in-Valve International Data Registry Investigators, et al. Transcatheter aortic valve implantation in failed bioprosthetic surgical valve. JAMA. 2014;312:162–70.

37. Fries JF. Aging, cumulative disability, and the compression of morbidity. Compr Ther. 2001;27:322–9.

38. Leon MB, Smith CR, Mack M, Miller DC, Moses JW, Svensson LG, et al. Transcatheter aortic-valve implantation for aortic stenosis in patients who cannot undergo surgery. N Engl J Med. 2010;363:1597–607.

39. Wenaweser P, Pilgrim T, Kadner A, Huber C, Stortecky S, Buellesfeld L, et al. Clinical outcomes of patients with severe aortic stenosis at increased surgical risk according to treatment modality. J Am Coll Cardiol. 2011;58:2151–62.

40. Noble S, Frangos E, Samaras N, Ellenberge C, Frangos C, Cikirikcioglu M, Bendjelid K, Frei A, Myers P, Licker M, Roffi M. Transcatheter aortic valve implantation in nonagenarians: effective and safe. Eur J Intern Med. 2013;24:750–5.

41. Moreno R, Salazar A, Banuelos C, Hernandez R, Alfonso F, Sabate M, et al. Effectiveness of percutaneous coronary interventions in nonagenarians. Am J Cardiol. 2004;94:1058–60.

42. Speziale G, Nasso G, Barattoni MC, Bonifazi R, Esposito G, Coppola R, et al. Operative and middle-term results of cardiac surgery in nonagenarians: a bridge toward routine practice. Circulation. 2010;121:208–13.

43. Guilfoyle MR, Drain AJ, Khan A, Ferguson J, Large SR, Nashef SA. Cardiac surgery in nonagenarians: single-centre series and review. Gerontology. 2010;56:378–84.

44. Bridges CR, Edwards FH, Peterson ED, Coombs LP, Ferguson TB. Cardiac surgery in nonagenarians and centenarians. J Am Coll Surg. 2003;197:347–56.

45. Edwards M-B, Taylor KM. Outcomes in nonagenarians after heart valve replacement operation. Ann Thorac Surg. 2003;75:830–4.

46. Noble S, Frangos E, Frei A, Roffi M. Transcatheter aortic valve implantation in a 99-year-old woman: are we going too far? J Am Geriatr Soc. 2012;60:1774–5.

Clinical and Imaging Follow-Up After Transcatheter Aortic Valve Implantation

12

Barbara D. Lawson, Mohammed Quader,
Luis A. Guzman, and Zachary M. Gertz

12.1 Introduction

Although follow-up after transcatheter aortic valve implantation (TAVI), also called transcatheter aortic valve replacement (TAVR), is variable across programs, it is widely accepted that patients require close monitoring, as they are often elderly and have many comorbid conditions [1]. Procedural complications are most common in the first 30 days following TAVI [2], and follow-up in that time frame should be with the Heart Valve Team. After the first month, patient care can be transitioned back to the referring cardiologist and primary care provider. Current recommendations from the American College of Cardiology Expert Consensus [3] are for initial primary care follow-up within 3 months of the procedure and for primary cardiology follow-up at 6 months and then annually. Such close monitoring is important because readmission rates approach 50% in the first year following TAVI, and readmission is associated with poorer clinical outcomes [4]. More than half of these readmissions are related to noncardiac causes such as infection (often access

site), bleeding, and respiratory failure. Among the cardiac causes for readmission, heart failure and arrhythmias are the most common [2, 4].

Immediately following valve implantation, the valve should be assessed with any or all of the following methods: measurement of hemodynamics, echocardiogram, and ascending aortogram (Fig. 12.1). The purpose of this evaluation is to determine, intraprocedurally, the degree of paravalvular regurgitation and to guide further interventions, such as valvuloplasty. In addition, the underlying rhythm and the presence of any conduction disturbances should be evaluated, in case backup pacing is needed (Table 12.1).

The Valve Academic Research Consortium-2 (VARC-2) recommends that the first clinical, electrocardiographic, and echocardiographic exam following TAVI should be performed prior to discharge, followed by 1 month, 6 months, 1 year, and yearly thereafter [5].

12.2 Clinical Follow-Up

12.2.1 Antithrombotic Therapy

While it is generally agreed upon that antiplatelet or antithrombotic agents are needed following TAVI, the optimal regimen and duration are still unknown. Current recommendations include aspirin 75–100 mg daily indefinitely and clopidogrel 75 mg daily for 3–6 months, which is based upon the initial clinical trials investigating

B. D. Lawson · M. Quader · L. A. Guzman (✉)
Z. M. Gertz
VCU School of Medicine, VCU Pauley Heart Center,
Richmond, VA, USA
e-mail: barbara.lawson@vcuhealth.org;
mohammed.quader@vcuhealth.org;
luis.guzman@vcuhealth.org;
zachary.gertz@vcuhealth.org

© Springer Nature Switzerland AG 2019
A. Giordano et al. (eds.), *Transcatheter Aortic Valve Implantation*,
https://doi.org/10.1007/978-3-030-05912-5_12

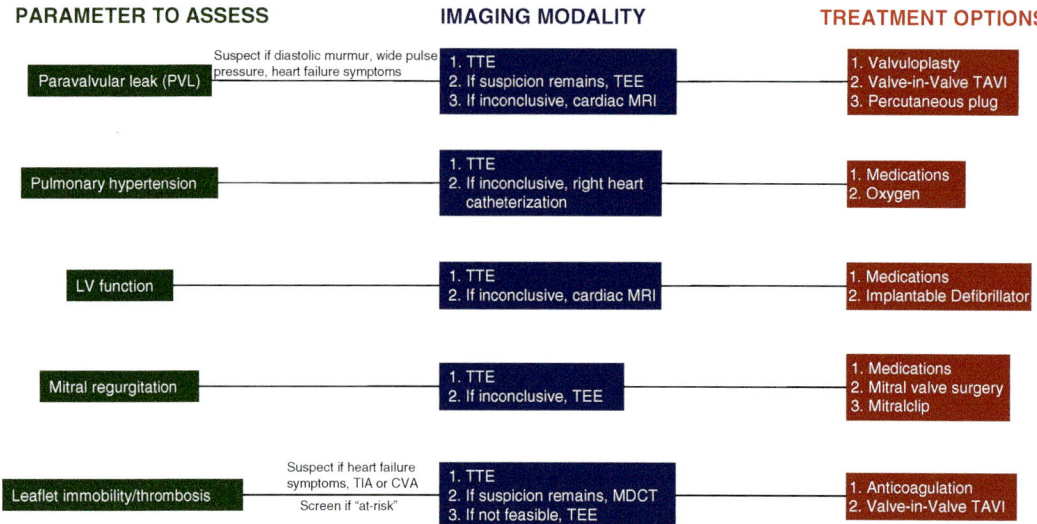

Fig. 12.1 Evaluation of cardiac parameters following TAVI, and their potential management

Table 12.1 Clinical considerations and their timing following TAVI

Clinical considerations	Timing
Antiplatelet/anticoagulant	Initiate prior to discharge Continue 3–6 months Longer based on comorbid disease
Electrocardiogram (heart rhythm)	Immediately post-procedure Prior to discharge 1 month As clinically indicated
Echocardiogram (valve function)	Prior to discharge 1 month Yearly
Quality of life	1 month 1 year Possibly yearly
Cerebrovascular event	CT/MRI as clinical indicated Possibly neurocognitive testing
Exercise training	Following recovery from procedure

balloon-expandable and self-expanding transcatheter valves [6–8]. If patients are already taking dual antiplatelet therapy for another condition (i.e., coronary stents), then no change is needed. Patients who have an indication for systemic anticoagulation (atrial fibrillation, deep vein thrombosis, mechanical valve, etc.) should be treated according to the guidelines for their respective condition (novel oral anticoagulant or vitamin K antagonist). In these patients, it is generally agreed upon that aspirin or clopidogrel be added to the regimen. Because the incidence of leaflet thrombosis is higher than once realized (7–15% on computed tomography studies) [9–13], there are ongoing trials investigating the use of systemic anticoagulation in addition to antiplatelet therapy.

12.2.2 Conduction/Rhythm Disorders

A large Transcatheter Valve Therapies (TVT) Registry assessing more than 26,000 patients undergoing TAVI demonstrated a 10% incidence of permanent pacemaker (PPM) implantation and 7% incidence of new atrial fibrillation [14]. In addition, although the incidence of new left bundle branch block (LBBB) has decreased with the newer-generation valves, it still develops in nearly one quarter of patients [15]. An electrocardiogram (ECG) should be performed in recovery to determine any immediate conduction or rhythm changes and again before discharge, as some changes resolve within the first 24 h. Routine ECG monitoring is also necessary in follow-up, as the risk of heart block requiring PPM implantation extends beyond the time of discharge [16, 17], and the persistence of LBBB can affect left ventricular ejection fraction (EF) and may alter treatment decisions (resynchronization therapy). Our practice is to perform ECG at 1-month follow-up and regularly as indicated by the patient's symptoms and/or comorbid conditions.

Early data reported new-onset atrial fibrillation in approximately one third of patients undergoing TAVI [18], whereas more recent data show less than 10% of patients with this complication [14]. The timing of onset is most often during or within 48 h of the procedure (~60%) and often resolves within 24 h (~75%) of onset [18]. However, it can develop even after discharge and sometimes becomes persistent [18]. Predictors of atrial fibrillation include age, left atrial size, non-transfemoral access, and post-implant valvuloplasty [18, 19]. New-onset atrial fibrillation is associated with higher risk of stroke [18], making early identification important as it may change the anticoagulation strategy. If ECG does not show atrial fibrillation, but there is clinical suspicion, a heart monitor should be prescribed.

12.2.3 Cerebrovascular Events

Clinically evident cerebrovascular events occur in 2–5% of patients within 30 days post-TAVI [14, 20, 21], but subclinical events are much more common. New ischemic brain lesions are found by diffusion-weighted magnetic resonance imaging (MRI) [22–24] in 65–85% of patients, and high-intensity transient signals are notable on transcranial Doppler in nearly all patients undergoing TAVI [25]. These findings do not correlate with clinical events, however, and their role in routine post-TAVI care remains questionable. The long-term impact of subclinical embolism in this elderly population is unknown, although neurologic studies show they cause subtle deficits in physical and cognitive function and portend a twofold increase in the risk of subsequent dementia [26]. Neurocognitive testing can be used to detect changes in higher-order cerebral func-

tion, but there are a number of different tests that assess different factors (memory, learning, attention, language), and the results depend on which test is used. The surgical literature has used auditory evoked potentials to assess neurocognitive function, a test which is objective and reproducible [27, 28], but this has not been studied in TAVI. The few studies investigating cognitive function after TAVI have used more subjective scales and have shown some improvements in cognitive function, possibly related to improved cardiac output and cerebral perfusion, but also some cognitive decline [25, 29]. At this point, the neurologic follow-up after TAVI is driven by clinical presentation, and brain imaging with CT or MRI should be pursued when there is suspicion for an acute event.

12.2.4 Quality of Life

Aortic valve replacement is known to alter the natural history of severe aortic stenosis as well as improve quality of life (QOL) to age-adjusted population norms [30, 31]. There are numerous ways to assess for improvement in patients' QOL following TAVI, both general and disease-specific. The Kansas City Cardiomyopathy Questionnaire (KCCQ) has been validated as a reliable assessment of symptoms, functional status, and quality of life in severe aortic stenosis [32]. The landmark TAVI trials (PARTNER and CoreValve) showed improved health-related QOL [33, 34] using both the KCCQ and two general health questionnaires, more so in those patients treated via the transfemoral versus transapical approach. This improvement has been repeatedly demonstrated in "real-life cohorts" as TAVI has become more widespread, but not all patients derive the same benefit [35, 36].

The largest improvement in health status occurs within 30 days of TAVI, with some additional improvement appreciable out to 1 year in the majority of patients [36]. Factors associated with worse health status at 1 year include worse health status at baseline, slow gait speed, nonfemoral access, lower mean aortic valve gradients, and comorbid conditions such as lung disease, stroke, diabetes mellitus, atrial fibrillation, and PPM [36]. Health status should be assessed with the KCCQ at minimum of 1 month and 1 year following TAVI and possibly yearly thereafter.

The four domains assessed by the KCCQ include physical limitation, symptom frequency, QOL, and social limitation. Following TAVI, the greatest improvements are noted in the QOL domain, with the smallest increase noted in the physical limitation domain [36]. Lack of improvement in exercise capacity is associated with increased rehospitalization and mortality [37], whereas exercise after TAVI has been shown to be safe and effective as measured by muscle strength, peak oxygen consumption, and QOL [38]. Exercise training should be recommended to patients following recovery from their procedure, either in the form of cardiac rehabilitation or other less formal activities.

12.3 Imaging Follow-Up

The mainstay of imaging follow-up after TAVI is echocardiography. This should be focused on hemodynamic assessment (valvular gradients, valve area), quantification of regurgitation, and other cardiac parameters affected by valve replacement (chamber size and function, other valvular pathologies).

Echocardiography prior to discharge establishes baseline transcatheter valve function, including peak velocity across the valve, mean gradient across the valve, valve area, and assessment of paravalvular regurgitation [39]. Many patients who undergo TAVI have other concomitant cardiac disease, including coronary disease [40], systolic dysfunction, mitral valve disease, or pulmonary hypertension. Routine echocardiography is equally important in following these factors, as they can be positively and negatively affected by the hemodynamic changes that accompany aortic valve replacement. Tracking these changes can help to ensure the patient is receiving guideline-directed medical therapy. As the durability of transcatheter prosthetic valves is still unknown [41], annual evaluation is needed for the detection of long-term complications

(device migration, thrombus formation, endocarditis, valve degeneration). Many definitions have been suggested for structural valve degeneration in TAVI, but none has been agreed upon [42]. Monitoring the abovementioned parameters (regurgitation, stenosis, calcification) is therefore important, as changes over time may indicate degeneration of the prosthesis and warrant further investigation or intervention.

12.3.1 Paravalvular Regurgitation

The incidence of paravalvular regurgitation following TAVI has decreased with the advent of newer-generation prostheses. A meta-analysis looking at patients treated with first-generation CoreValve and Sapien valves between 2002 and 2012 estimated moderate to severe regurgitation in 11.7% of patients [43], whereas the newer-generation valves are reported to have 1–5% incidence [44–46]. Factors associated with paravalvular regurgitation include a heavily calcified annulus [44], undersized prosthesis [45], and malpositioning of the prosthesis [46].

As mentioned above, aortography can be used intraprocedurally to assess the degree of paravalvular regurgitation and is accomplished by grading the density of contrast opacification of the left ventricle [47]. This method is highly subjective and also dependent on the volume of contrast used, the position of the catheter, and the strength of fluoroscopy used and is therefore not ideal.

The mainstay of detecting paravalvular regurgitation following TAVI is echocardiography, either transesophageal (during the procedure, if general anesthesia is used) or transthoracic (during the procedure, if moderate sedation is used, and in long-term follow-up). Current experts in echocardiography recommend a grading scheme that relies on various parameters, including prosthesis position and shape, left ventricular size and function, and data from color Doppler images in multiple views [48]. Regurgitation is more severe in valves that are too low or too high in the annulus and have irregular shapes, and in which there is space visible between the native and prosthetic valves. Deterioration in ventricular size and/or function over time suggests significant paravalvular regurgitation. In transesophageal echocardiography (TEE), the midesophageal long-axis and short-axis views and the transgastric view are best to visualize paravalvular jets with color Doppler. In transthoracic echocardiography (TTE), color Doppler assessment in the parasternal long and short axis and the apical five-chamber and three-chamber views are most helpful and should be performed in both traditional and off-axis views. Using these views, in both modalities, the severity of regurgitation is based on the number and location of jets, the size of the jet, the circumferential extent of the jet, and more quantitative measures including regurgitant volume and fraction and effective regurgitant orifice area. The presence of multiple, eccentric, and irregularly shaped jets as well as acoustic shadowing from calcium or the prosthesis itself can limit the ability of TTE to accurately quantify paravalvular regurgitation [48]. As higher degrees of regurgitation correlate with worse outcomes, including mortality and heart failure rehospitalization [49], accurate quantification is important to identify patients who may benefit from additional treatment such as valvuloplasty, second valve implant, or paravalvular leak closure.

Cardiac MRI (CMR) has emerged as the preferred imaging modality to determine the extent of paravalvular regurgitation when echocardiographic findings are inconclusive. CMR accurately and reproducibly quantifies the regurgitant volume and fraction [50] independent of the number or shape of the jets [48] and reclassifies the severity in approximately 50% of patients [51, 52].

12.3.2 Structural Valve Degeneration

Valvular degeneration is most common in the form of valvular stenosis, although transvalvular regurgitation and mixed stenosis/regurgitation are also possible [42]. Stenosis can result from leaflet immobility or leaflet thrombosis, terms which are not interchangeable as immobility can result for a number of reasons (pannus, incom-

plete stent deployment, etc.). Leaflet immobility has been defined as diffuse thickening of one or more transcatheter heart valve cusps identifiable in multiple views [53, 54], whereas leaflet thrombosis is any thrombus attached to or near the valve, resulting in some degree of blood flow obstruction and interference with valve function, or large enough to warrant treatment [55]. A large registry demonstrated that 4.5% of patients develop valve hemodynamic deterioration, defined as greater than 10 mmHg increase in mean transprosthetic gradient between discharge and follow-up [56]. Several studies have shown that higher aortic valve gradients are present in most (~90%) patients with leaflet thrombosis [57–59], but leaflet immobility is not always associated with elevated aortic valve gradients. TTE is not sensitive enough to visualize within the stent frame and assess leaflet motion [9].

While there are no randomized controlled trials comparing imaging modalities for leaflet immobility, small series and anecdotal experience have indicated the superiority of both multidetector computed tomography (MDCT) and TEE over TTE [9, 53, 60]. The most common findings on TEE are thickened leaflets, immobile or restricted leaflets, and thrombotic apposition of leaflets, whereas a thrombotic mass is less often visualized [54, 57]. Despite its superiority over TTE, up to 10% of patients with leaflet immobility or thrombosis will have no abnormal findings on TEE [10]. Findings on MDCT include hypoattenuated masses attached to the aortic cusp, leaflet thickening, or reduced leaflet motion [11, 53, 54]. Hypo-attenuating lesions always involve the base of the leaflet and extend toward the center, and reduced leaflet motion is identified by the presence of wedge-shaped or semilunar opacities in both systole and diastole (normal leaflets only seen on diastole) [9].

Leaflet immobility and thrombosis can present clinically as exertional dyspnea or congestive heart failure [57], and thrombosis has been associated with increased incidence of transient ischemic attack (TIA) and stroke [9, 59]. However, a large portion (30%) present subclinically and are diagnosed based on imaging findings alone [57]. TTE can act as an initial screening tool, and the presence of rising aortic valve gradients should prompt either empiric treatment with systemic anticoagulation or further imaging investigation. However, normal TTE findings should not rule out the presence of leaflet immobility/thrombosis when the suspicion is high. MDCT should be performed in symptomatic patients and those with stroke or TIA [61]. TEE is a reasonable alternative in patients in whom MDCT is not feasible (renal failure, availability, etc.). In addition, MDCT or TEE should be considered in asymptomatic patients who are considered at-risk for leaflet immobility or thrombosis [61]. Risk factors include male gender, absence of systemic anticoagulation, larger sinuses of Valsalva, larger bioprosthetic valve size, balloon-expandable prosthesis, and valve-in-valve procedures [10, 11, 54]. Numerous studies have shown restoration of leaflet function with systemic anticoagulation [9, 10, 12], with both novel oral anticoagulants and vitamin K antagonists considered reasonable options. Either aspirin or clopidogrel should be continued even if anticoagulation is initiated, and repeat imaging should be considered after 3–6 months of treatment.

12.3.3 Other Cardiac Parameters

Many cardiac parameters are affected by the hemodynamic changes that accompany aortic valve replacement, including systolic function, mitral regurgitation (MR), and pulmonary hypertension. In patients with left ventricular dysfunction, an improvement in EF is often detectable prior to discharge [62, 63]. In fact, reverse remodeling begins to occur even before changes in EF are noticeable, as measured by speckle tracking and strain imaging [64, 65]. Significant MR is associated with increased early and late mortality in patient undergoing TAVI [65–67], and worsening MR after TAVI portends even worse survival [68]. The degree of MR improves in 50–60% of patients following TAVI, whereas it remains stable in approximately 40% and deteriorates in less than 10% [66, 67, 69, 70]. Improvement is more likely to occur in functional MR as opposed to degenerative MR [71]

and is related to improved left ventricular hemodynamics and decreased leaflet tethering following aortic valve replacement [69]. Predictors of persistent or worsening mitral regurgitation include degenerative valve findings on echocardiography and calcified mitral apparatus or mitral annular diameter greater than 35.5 mm on MDCT [67]. Lastly, pulmonary hypertension (PHTN) has been shown to improve in 32–57% of patients after TAVI, as assessed by TTE [72–74]. Echocardiographic factors associated with persistent PHTN following TAVI include greater than moderate mitral or tricuspid regurgitation, atrial fibrillation/flutter, early (E) to late (A) ventricular filling velocities (E/A ratio), and left atrial volume index [74]. The severity of PHTN pre- and post-TAVI predicts mortality, and improvement in pulmonary artery pressures is associated with better prognosis [75].

Routine echocardiography is important in following all of these factors to ensure the patient is receiving optimal treatment. Accurate assessment of left ventricular function can help guide medical and device therapy, and persistent or worsening severe mitral regurgitation can often be treated with percutaneous mitral valve repair or replacement. Higher pulmonary pressures are associated with more frequent heart failure hospitalizations [73] and may identify patients who would benefit from closer follow-up. CMR can be helpful in measuring left ventricular function and mass when TTE findings are uncertain and in quantifying mitral regurgitation when TTE and/or TEE is equivocal.

12.4   Conclusion

Close follow-up after TAVI involves not only careful attention to clinical variables but also to specific cardiac parameters. Beginning immediately after valve implantation and continuing at regular intervals, the functional and general health status of patients should be monitored and further imaging pursued when clinically indicated. Such care can help optimize quality of life as well as guide therapy for comorbid conditions or valve degeneration.

References

1. Holmes DR, Nishmura RA, Grover FL, Brindis RG, Carroll JD, Edwards FH, et al. Annual outcomes with transcatheter valve therapy: from the STS/ACC TVT Registry. J Am Coll Cardiol. 2015;66:2813–23.

2. Kolte D, Khera S, Sardar R, Gheewala N, Gupta T, Chatterjee S, et al. Thirty-day readmissions after transcatheter aortic valve replacement in the United States: insights from the nationwide readmissions database. Circ Cardiovasc Interv. 2017;10:e004472. https://doi.org/10.1161/CIRCINTERVENTIONS.116.004472.

3. Otto CM, Kumbhani DJ, Alexander KP, Calhoon JH, Desai MY, Kaul S, Lee JC, Ruiz CE, Vassileva CM. 2017 ACC expert consensus decision pathway for transcatheter aortic valve replacement in the management of adults with aortic stenosis. J Am Coll Cardiol. 2017;69:1313–46.

4. Nombela-Franco L, del Trigo M, Morrison-Polo G, Veiga G, Jimenez-Quevedo P, Altisent OA, et al. Incidence, causes, and predictors of early (≤ 30 days) and late unplanned hospital readmissions after transcatheter aortic valve replacement. J Am Coll Cardiol Intv. 2015;8:1748–57.

5. Kappetein AP, Head SJ, Généreux P, Piazza N, van Mieghem NM, Blackstone EH, et al. Updated standardized endpoint definitions for transcatheter aortic valve implantation: the Valve Academic Research Consortium-2 consensus document. J Thorac Cardiovasc Surg. 2013;145:6–23.

6. Leon MB, Smith CR, Mack M, Miller DC, Moses JW, Svensson LG, et al. Transcatehter aortic-valve implantation for aortic stenosis in patients who cannot undergo surgery. N Engl J Med. 2010;363:1597–607.

7. Smith CR, Leon MB, Mack MJ, Miller DC, Moses JW, Svensson LG, et al. Transcatheter versus surgical aortic-valve replacement in high-risk patients. N Engl J Med. 2011;364:2187–98.

8. Popma JJ, Adams DH, Reardon MJ, Yakuboc SJ, Kleiman NS, Heimansohn D, et al. Transcatheter aortic valve replacement using a self-expanding bioprosthesis in patients with severe aortic stenosis at extreme risk for surgery. J Am Coll Cardiol. 2014;63:1972–81.

9. Makkar RR, Fontana G, Jilaihawi H, Chakravarty T, Kofoed KF, De Backer O, et al. Possible subclinical leaflet thrombosis in bioprosthetic aortic valves. N Engl J Med. 2015;373:2015–24.

10. Hansson NC, Grove EL, Andersen HR, Leipsic J, Mathiassen ON, Jensen JM, et al. Transcatheter aortic valve thrombosis: incidence, predisposing factors, and clinical implications. J Am Coll Cardiol. 2016;68:2059–69.

11. Yanagisawa R, Hayashida K, Yamada Y, Tanaka M, Yashima F, Inohara T, et al. Incidence, predictors, and mid-term outcomes of possible leaflet thrombosis after TAVR. J Am Coll Cardiol Img. 2017;10:1–11.

12. Pache G, Schoechlin S, Blanke P, Dorfs S, Jander N, Arepalli CD, et al. Early hypo-attenuated leaflet thickening in balloon-expandable transcatheter aortic heart valves. Eur Heart J. 2016;37:2263–71.

13. Vollema EM, Kong WKF, Katsanos S, Kamperidis V, van Rosendael PJ, ver der Kley F, et al. Transcatheter aortic valve thrombosis: the relation between hypo-attenuated leaflet thickening, abnormal valve hemodynamics, and stroke. Eur Heart J. 2017;38:1207–17.

14. Holmes DR, Nishimura RA, Grover FL, Brindis RG, Carroll JD, Edwards FH, et al. Annual outcomes with transcatheter valve therapy: from the STS/ACC TVT registry. Ann Thorac Surg. 2016;101:789–800.

15. Auffret V, Puri R, Urena M, Chamandi C, Rodriguez-Gabella T, Phillippon F, Rodes-Cabau J. Conduction disturbances after transcatheter aortic valve replacement: current status and future perspectives. Circulation. 2017;136:1049–69.

16. Nazij TM, Dizon JM, Hahn RT, Babaliaros V, Douglas PS, El-Chami MF, et al. Predictors and clinical outcomes of permanent pacemaker implantation after transcatheter aortic valve replacement: the PARTNER (Placement of AoRtic TraNscathetER Valves) Trial and Registry. J Am Coll Cardiol Intv. 2015;8:60–9.

17. Urena M, Webb JG, Tamburino C, Munoz-Garcia AJ, Cheema A, Dager AE, et al. Permanent pacemaker implantation after transcatheter aortic valve implantation: impact on late clinical outcomes and left ventricular function. Circulation. 2014;129:1233–43.

18. Amat-Santos IJ, Rodes-Cabau J, Urena M, DeLarochelliere R, Doyle D, Bagur R, et al. Incidence, predictive factors, and prognostic value of new-onset atrial fibrillation following transcatheter aortic valve implantation. J Am Coll Cardiol. 2012;59:178–88.

19. Tarantini G, Mojoli M, Windecker S, Wendler O, Lefevre T, Saia F, et al. Prevalence and impact of atrial fibrillation in patients with severe aortic stenosis undergoing transcatheter aortic valve replacement: An analysis from the SOURCE XT prospective multicenter registry. JACC Cardiovasc Interv. 2016;9:937–46.

20. Leon MB, Smith CR, Mack MJ, Makkar RR, Svensson LG, Kodali SK, et al. Transcatheter or surgical aortic valve replacement in intermediate-risk patients. N Engl J Med. 2016;374:1609–20.

21. Reardon MJ, Van Mieghem NM, Popma JJ, Kleiman NS, Sondergaard L, Mumtaz M, et al. Surgical or transcatheter aortic valve replacement in intermediate-risk patients. N Engl J Med. 2017;376:1321–31.

22. Kahlert P, Knipp SC, Schlamann M, Thielmann M, Al-Rashid F, Weber M, et al. Silent and apparent cerebral ischemia after percutaneous transfemoral aortic valve implantation: a diffusion-weighted magnetic resonance imaging study. Circulation. 2010;121:870–8.

23. Fairbairn TA, Mather AN, Bijsterveld P, Worthy G, Currie S, Goddard AJ, et al. Diffusion-weighted MRI determined cerebral embolic infarction following transcatheter aortic valve implantation: assessment of predictive risk factors and the relationship to subsequent health status. Heart. 2012;98:18–23.

24. Van Belle E, Hengstenberg C, Lefevre T, Kupatt C, Debry N, Husser O, et al. Cerebral embolism during transcatheter aortic valve replacement: the BRAVO-3 MRI study. J Am Coll Cardiol. 2016;68:589–99.

25. Spaziano M, Francese D, Leon MB, Genereux P. Imaging and functional testing to assess clinical and subclinical neurological events after transcatheter or surgical aortic valve replacement: a comprehensive review. J Am Coll Cardiol. 2014;64:1950–63.

26. Vermeer SE, Longstreth WT Jr, Koudstaal PJ. Silent brain infarcts: a systematic review. Lancet Neurol. 2007;6:611–9.

27. Zimpfer D, Czerny M, Kilo J, Kasimir MT, Madl C, Kramer L, et al. Cognitive deficit after aortic valve replacement. Ann Thorac Surg. 2002;75:407–12.

28. Zimpfer D, Kilo J, Czerny M, Kasimir MT, Madl C, Bauer E, et al. Neurocognitive deficit following aortic valve replacement with biological/mechanical prosthesis. Eur J Cardiothorac Surg. 2003;23:544–51.

29. Auffret V, Campelo-Parada F, Regueiro A, del Trigo M, Chiche O, Chamandi C, et al. Serial changes in cognitive function following transcatheter aortic valve replacement. J Am Coll Cardiol. 2016;68:2129–41.

30. Schwartz F, Bauman P, Manthey J, Hoffmann M, Schuler G, Mehmel HC, et al. The effect of aortic valve replacement on survival. Circulation. 1982;66:1105–10.

31. Sundt TM, Bailey MS, Moon MR, Mendeloff EN, Huddleston CB, Pasque MK, et al. Quality of life after aortic valve replacement at the age of >80 years. Circulation. 2000;102(Suppl 3):70–4.

32. Arnold SV, Spertus JA, Lei Y, Allen KB, Chhatriwalla AK, Leon MB, et al. Use of the Kansas City Cardiomyopathy Questionnaire for monitoring health status in patients with aortic stenosis. Circ Heart Fail. 2013;6:61–7.

33. Reynolds MR, Magnuson EA, Wang K, Thourani VH, Williams M, Zajarias A, et al. Health-related quality of life after transcatheter or surgical aortic valve replacement in high-risk patients with severe aortic stenosis: results from the PARTNER (Placement of AoRTic TraNscatheteER Valve) trial (Cohort A). J Am Coll Cardiol. 2012;60:548–58.

34. Arnold SV, Reynolds MR, Wang K, Magnuson EA, Baron SJ, Chinnakondepalli KM, et al. Health status after transcatheter or surgical aortic valve replacement in patients with severe aortic stenosis at increased surgical risk: results from the CoreValve US Pivotal Trial. J Am Coll Cardiol Intv. 2015;8:1207–17.

35. Lange R, Beckmann A, Neumann T, Krane M, Deutsch MA, Landwehr S, et al. Quality of life after transcatheter aortic valve replacement: prospective data from GARY (German Aortic Valve Registry). J Am Coll Cardiol Intv. 2016;9:2541–54.

36. Arnold SV, Spertus JA, Vemulapalli S, Li Z, Matsouaka RA, Baron SJ, et al. Quality-of-life outcomes after transcatheter aortic valve replacement in an unselected population: a report from the STS/ACC transcatheter valve therapy registry. JAMA Cardiol. 2017;2:409–16.

37. Altisent OA, Puri R, Regueiro A, Chamandi C, Rodriguez-Gabella T, del Trigo M, et al. Predictors and association with clinical outcomes of the changes in exercise capacity after transcatheter aortic valve replacement. Circulation. 2017;136:632–43.

38. Pressler A, Christle JW, Lechner B, Grabs V, Haller B, Hettich I, et al. Exercise training improves exercise capacity and quality of life after transcatheter aortic valve implantation: a randomized pilot trial. Am Heart J. 2016;182:44–53.

39. Arsalan M, Walther T. Durability of prostheses for transcatheter aortic valve implantation. Nat Rev Cardiol. 2016;13:360–7.

40. Rodriguez-Gabella T, Voisine P, Puri R, Pibarot P, Rodes-Cabau J. Aortic bioprosthetic valve durability: incidence, mechanisms, predictors, and management of surgical and transcatheter valve degeneration. J Am Coll Cardiol. 2017;70:1013–28.

41. Zoghbi WA, Chambers JB, Dumesnil JG, Foster E, Gottdiener JS, Grayburn PA, et al. Recommendations for evaluation of prosthetic valves with echocardiography and Doppler ultrasound. J Am Soc Echocardiogr. 2009;22:975–1014.

42. Goel SS, Ige M, Tuzcu EM, Ellis SG, Stewart WJ, Svensson LG, et al. Severe aortic stenosis and coronary artery disease—implications for management in the transcatheter aortic valve replacement era: a comprehensive review. J Am Coll Cardiol. 2013;62:1–10.

43. Genereux P, Head SJ, Hahn R, Deneault B, Kodali S, Williams MR, et al. Paravalvular leak after transcatheter aortic valve replacement: the new Achilles' heel? A comprehensive review of the literature. J Am Coll Cardiol. 2013;61:1125–36.

44. Sorajja P, Kodali S, Reardon MJ, Szeto WY, Chetcuti SJ, Hermiller J, et al. Outcomes for the commercial use of self-expanding prostheses in transcatheter aortic valve replacement: a report from the STS/ACC TVT Registry. J Am Coll Cardiol Intv. 2017;10:2090–8.

45. Thourani VH, Kodali S, Makkar RR, Hermann HC, Williams M, Babaliaros V, et al. Transcatheter aortic valve replacement versus surgical valve replacement in intermediate-risk patients: a propensity score analysis. Lancet. 2016;387:2218–25.

46. Meredith IT, Walters DL, Dumonteil N, Worthley SG, Tchetche D, Manoharan G, et al. 1-Year outcomes with the fully repositionable and retrievable Lotus transcatheter aortic replacement valve in 120 high-risk surgical patients with severe aortic stenosis: results of the REPRISE II study. J Am Coll Cardiol Intv. 2016;9:376–84.

47. Sinning JM, Vasa-Nicotera M, Chin D, Hammerstingl C, Ghanem A, Bence J, et al. Evaluation and management of paravalvular aortic regurgitation after transcatheter aortic valve replacement. J Am Coll Cardiol. 2013;62:11–20.

48. Pibarot P, Hahn RT, Weissman NJ, Monagham MJ. Assessment of paravalvular regurgitation following TAVR: a proposal of unifying grading scheme. J Am Coll Cardiol Img. 2015;8:340–60.

49. Ribeiro HB, Orwat S, Hayek SS, Larose E, Babaliaros V, Abdellaziz D, et al. Cardiovascular magnetic resonance to evaluate aortic regurgitation after transcatheter aortic valve replacement. J Am Coll Cardiol. 2016;68:577–85.

50. Rogers T, Waksman R. Role of CMR in TAVR. J Am Coll Cardiol Img. 2016;9:593–602.

51. Hartlage GR, Babaliaros VC, Thourani VH, Hayek S, Ghasemzadeh N, Stillman AE, et al. The role of cardiovascular magnetic resonance in stratifying paravalvular leak severity after transcatheter aortic valve replacement: an observational outcome study. J Cardiovasc Magn Reson. 2014;16:93–103.

52. Crouch G, Tully PJ, Bennetts J, Sinhal A, Bradbrook C, Penhall AL, et al. Quantitative assessment of paravalvular regurgitation following transcatheter aortic valve replacement. J Cardiovasc Magn Reson. 2015;17:32–7.

53. Leetmaa T, Hansson NC, Leipsic J, Jensen K, Poulsen SH, Andersen HR, et al. Early aortic transcatheter heart valve thrombosis: diagnostic value of contrast enhanced multidetector computed tomography. Circ Cardiovasc Interv. 2015;8:e001596. https://doi.org/10.1161/Circinterventiontions.114.001596.

54. Jose J, Sulimov DS, El-Mawardy M, Sato T, Allali A, Holy EW, et al. Clinical bioprosthetic heart valve thrombosis after transcatheter aortic valve replacement: incidence, characteristics, and treatment outcomes. J Am Coll Cardiol Intv. 2017;10:686–97.

55. Akins CW, Miller DC, Turina MI, Kouchoukos NT, Blackstone EH, Grunkemeier GL, Takkenberg JJ, David TE, Butchart EG, Adams DH, Shahian DM, Hagl S, Mayer JE, Lytle BW, Councils of the American Association for Thoracic Surgery; Society of Thoracic Surgeons; European Association for Cardio-Thoracic Surgery; Ad Hoc Liaison Committee for Standardizing Definitions of Prosthetic Heart Valve Morbidity. Guidelines for reporting mortality and morbidity after cardiac valve interventions. J Thorac Cardiovasc Surg. 2008;135:732–8.

56. Del Trigo M, Munoz-Garcia AJ, Wijeysundera HC, Nombela-Franco L, Cheema AN, Gutierrez E, et al. Incidence, timing, and predictors of valve hemodynamic deterioration after transcatheter aortic valve replacement: multicenter registry. J Am Coll Cardiol. 2016;67:644–55.

57. Latib A, Naganuma T, Abdel-Wahab M, Danenberg H, Cota L, Barbanti M, et al. Treatment and clinical outcomes of transcatheter heart valve thrombosis. Circ Cardiovasc Interv. 2015;8:e001779. https://doi.org/10.1161/CircInterventions.114.001779.

58. De Marchena E, Mesa J, Pomenti S, Marin y Kall C, Marincic X, Yahagi K, et al. Thrombus formation following transcatheter aortic valve replacement. J Am Coll Cardiol Intv. 2015;8:728–39.

59. Chakravarty T, Sondergaard L, Friedman J, De Backer O, Berman D, Kofoed KF, et al. Subclinical leaflet thrombosis in surgical and transcatheter bioprosthetic aortic valves: an observational study. Lancet. 2017;389:2383–92.

60. Egbe AC, Pislaru SV, Pellikka PA, Poterucha JT, Schaff HV, Maleszewski JJ, Connolly HM. Bioprosthetic valve thrombosis versus structural failure: clinical and echocardiographic predictors. J Am Coll Cardiol. 2015;66:2285–94.

61. Holmes DR, Mack MJ. Aortic valve bioprostheses: leaflet immobility and valve thrombosis. Circulation. 2017;135:1749–56.

62. Fraccaro C, Al-Lamee R, Tarantini G, Maisano F, Napodano M, Montorfano M, et al. Transcatheter aortic valve implantation in patients with severe left ventricular dysfunction: intermediate and mid-term results, a multicenter study. Circ Cardiovasc Interv. 2012;5:253–60.

63. Clavel MA, Webb JG, Rodes-Cabau J, Masson JB, Dumont E, De Larochelliere R, et al. Comparison between transcatheter and surgical prosthetic valve implantation in patients with severe aortic stenosis and reduced left ventricular ejection fraction. Circulation. 2010;122:1928–36.

64. Schattke S, Baldenhofer G, Prauka I, Zhang K, Laule M, Stangl V, et al. Acute regional improvement of myocardial function after interventional transfemoral aortic valve replacement in aortic stenosis: a speckle tracking echocardiography study. Cardiovasc Ultrasound. 2012;10:15–22.

65. Giannini C, Petronio AS, Talini E, De Carlo M, Guarracino F, Delle Donne MG, et al. Early and late improvement of global and regional left ventricular function after transcatheter aortic valve implantation in patients with severe aortic stenosis: an echocardiographic study. Am J Cardiovasc Dis. 2011;1:264–73.

66. Nombela-Franco L, Eltchaninoff H, Zahn R, Testa L, Leon MB, Trillo-Nouche R, et al. Clinical impact and evolution of mitral regurgitation following transcatheter aortic valve replacement: a meta-analysis. Heart. 2015;101:1395–405.

67. Cortes C, Amat-Santos IJ, Nombela-Franco L, Munoz-Garcia AJ, Gutierrez-Ibanes E, De La Torre Hernandez JM, et al. Mitral regurgitation after transcatheter aortic valve replacement: prognosis, imaging predictors, and potential management. J Am Coll Cardiol Intv. 2016;9:1603–14.

68. Szymanski P, Hryniewiecki T, Dabrowski M, Sorysz KJ, Jastrzebski J, et al. Mitral and aortic regurgitation following transcatheter aortic valve replacement. Heart. 2016;102:701–6.

69. Shibayama K, Harada K, Berdejo J, Mihara H, Tanaka J, Gurudevan SV, et al. Effect of transcatheter aortic valve replacement on the mitral valve apparatus and mitral regurgitation: real-time three-dimensional transesophageal echocardiography study. Circ Cardiovasc Imaging. 2014;7:344–51.

70. Barbanti M, Webb JG, Hahn RT, Feldman T, Boone RH, Smith CR, et al. Impact of preoperative moderate/severe mitral regurgitation on 2-year outcome after transcatheter and surgical aortic valve replacement: insight from the Placement of Aortic Transcatheter Valve (PARTNER) trial cohort A. Circulation. 2013;128:2776–84.

71. Kiramijyan S, Koifman E, Asch FM, Magalhaes MA, Didier R, Escarcega RO, et al. Impact of functional versus organic baseline mitral regurgitation on short- and long-term outcomes after transcatheter aortic valve replacement. Am J Cardiol. 2016;117:839–46.

72. Medvedofsky D, Klempfner R, Fefer P, Chernomordik F, Hamdan A, Hay I, et al. The significance of pulmonary arterial hypertension pre- and post-transfemoral aortic valve implantation for severe aortic stenosis. J Cardiol. 2015;65:337–42.

73. Testa L, Latib A, De Marco F, De Carlo M, Fiorina C, Montone R, et al. Persistence of severe pulmonary hypertension after transcatheter aortic valve replacement: incidence and prognostic impact. Cir Cardiovasc Interv. 2016;9:e003563. https://doi.org/10.1161/CircInterventions.115.003563.

74. Masri A, Abdelkarim I, Sharbaugh MS, Althouse AD, Xu J, Han W, et al. Outcomes of persistent pulmonary hypertension following transcatheter aortic valve replacement. Heart. 2018;104:821–7. https://doi.org/10.1136/heartjnl.2017.311978.

75. Sinning JM, Hammerstingl C, Chin D, Ghanem A, Schueler R, Sedaghat A, et al. Decrease of pulmonary hypertension impacts prognosis after transcatheter aortic valve replacement. EuroIntervention. 2014;9:1042–9.

Cardiac Biomarkers in Transcatheter Aortic Valve Implantation

13

Paul L. Hermany and John K. Forrest

13.1 Introduction

Transcatheter aortic valve implantation (TAVI), also called transcatheter aortic valve replacement (TAVR), has become the standard of care for patients with severe symptomatic aortic stenosis or severe aortic stenosis with evidence of worsening left ventricular function who are at increased risk for surgical aortic valve replacement (SAVR) [1–4]. This indication has recently been expanded to patients at an intermediate surgical risk [5, 6] and is currently being investigated in low-risk patients. The approach to and appropriateness of AVR in many patients with severe aortic stenosis must be met with clinical equipoise and a careful consideration of the merits and risks of a transcatheter versus surgical strategy. Part of this consideration, in addition to a detailed conversation with the patient regarding goals of care and expectations and careful review of valvular and vascular anatomy, is an accurate risk assessment. Historically, a surgical risk calculation has been made by evaluating the patient and utilizing risk scoring models. Risk scores serve two main purposes in the evaluation of patients for TAVR. Firstly, they ascribe a degree of risk to a patient to better help guide the decision to pursue a percutaneous versus surgical approach to AVR (or medical management). Secondly, they better help the clinician identify, upfront, patients who may respond suboptimally to TAVR. Risk score models such as Society of Thoracic Surgeons (STS) score, logistic EuroSCORE, and EuroSCORE II have been derived in cardiac surgery patients, and thus extrapolation to predicting outcomes in patients undergoing TAVR must be exercised with caution. Alternative methods, therefore, with higher accuracy and prognostic value must be developed for assessing patients with aortic stenosis.

One of the growing areas of interest in risk assessment and risk model development is the role of cardiac biomarkers. Cardiac biomarker levels have been studied in both preoperative risk assessment and in guiding the postoperative management and predicting the postoperative outcomes of patients undergoing both percutaneous and surgical aortic valve replacement since the first TAVR studies. There is expanding evidence that cardiac biomarkers may help predict adverse outcomes in higher-risk patients, which may influence the decision of how to manage their aortic stenosis and how to best optimize the patient's clinical condition prior to valve replacement.

In this chapter, we review the commonly used cardiac biomarkers and discuss their relationship to myocardial injury as well as adverse cardiac physiology and hemodynamics. We consider the

P. L. Hermany · J. K. Forrest (✉)
Yale University School of Medicine,
Yale New Haven Hospital,
New Haven, CT, USA
e-mail: Paul.hermany@yale.edu;
John.k.forrest@yale.edu

© Springer Nature Switzerland AG 2019
A. Giordano et al. (eds.), *Transcatheter Aortic Valve Implantation*,
https://doi.org/10.1007/978-3-030-05912-5_13

standardized definitions of myocardial injury and infarction and debate the prognostic and predictive value of the biomarkers with regard to post-procedural morbidity and mortality. Lastly, we examine novel biomarkers which may prove useful in the management of patients with aortic stenosis who are undergoing TAVR.

13.2 Standardized Definitions of Myocardial Injury

The Valve Academic Research Consortium (VARC) consists of representatives of a collection of academic research organizations, sur-

gery and cardiology societies, members of the US Food and Drug Administration, and select independent experts. This group was tasked with creating a consensus statement identifying and defining various clinical endpoints to provide uniformity in data collection for trials evaluating TAVR. The most recently published consensus document from this group (VARC-2) provides definitions for both periprocedural and spontaneous myocardial infarction in the setting of TAVR (Fig. 13.1). Periprocedural myocardial infarction occurs ≤72 h from valve implantation and is associated with new ischemic signs or symptoms *and* elevated cardiac biomarkers. Elevated biomarkers [preferably creatine kinase-

Fig. 13.1 Definition of myocardial infarction by VARC-2 criteria

Peri-procedural MI (≤72 h after the index procedure)
  New ischaemic symptoms (e.g. chest pain or shortness of breath), or new ischaemic signs (e.g. ventricular arrhythmias, new or worsening heart failure, new ST-segment changes, haemodynamic instability, new pathological Q-waves in at least two contiguous leads, imaging evidence of new loss of viable myocardium or new wall motion abnormality) AND
  Elevated cardiac biomarkers (preferable CK-MB) within 72 h after the index procedure, consisting of at least one sample post-procedure with a peak value exceeding 15× as the upper reference limit for troponin or 5× for CK-MB.[a] If cardiac biomarkers are increased at baseline (>99th percentile), a furhter increase in at least 50% post-procedure is required AND the peak value must exceed the previously stated limit
Spontaneous MI (>72 h after the index procedure)
  Any one of the following criteria
  Detection of rise and/or fall of cardiac biomarkers (preferably troponin) with at least one value above the 99th percentile URL, together with the evidence of myocardial ischaemia with at least one of the following:
  Symtoms of ischaemia
  ECG changes indicative of new ischaemia [new ST-T changes or new left bundle branch block (LBBB)]
  New pathological Q-waves in at least two contiguous leads
  Imaging evidence of a new loss of viable myocardium or new wall motion abnormality
Sudden, unexpected cardiac death, involving cardiac arrest, often with symptoms suggestive of myocardial ischaemia, and accompanied by presumably new ST elevation, or new LBBB, and/or evidence of fresh thrombus by coronary angiography and/or at autopsy but death occurring before blood samples could be obtained, or at a time before the appearance of cardiac biomarkers in the blood.
Pathological findings of an acute myocardial infarction

[a]Previously in the original VARC it was 10× and 5× for troponin and CK-MB, respectively.

MB (CK-MB)] in this setting occurred within 72 h and consist of at least one sample post-procedure with a peak value exceeding 15× the upper reference limit (URL) for troponin or 5× for CK-MB (previously defined as 10× URL for troponin and 5× URL for CK-MB) [7]. If cardiac biomarkers are increased at baseline (>99th percentile), a further increase in at least 50% post-procedure is required, *and* the peak value must exceed the previously stated limit.

A spontaneous myocardial infarction in the setting of TAVR as defined by the VARC-2 consensus document occurs 72 h or later following valve replacement and is defined as a rise and/or fall of cardiac biomarkers (in this case, preferably a troponin assay is used) with at least one value above the 99th percentile of the upper reference limit, which is coupled with evidence of myocardial ischemia. Such evidence may include at least one of the following: symptoms, ECG changes suggesting new ischemia (e.g., new ST-T changes or new left bundle branch block), new pathological Q waves in at least two contiguous leads,

imaging evidence of a new loss of viable myocardium or new wall motion abnormalities, sudden cardiac death involving cardiac arrest (often with symptoms suggesting myocardial ischemia and accompanied by new ST elevation or new LBBB and/or evidence of fresh thrombus by coronary angiography and/or at autopsy), and pathological findings of an acute myocardial infarction [7].

By comparison, criteria for defining an acute myocardial infarction in certain clinical scenarios were proscribed in the Third Universal Definition of Myocardial Infarction consensus document published in 2012 by a Joint ESC/ACCF/AHA/WHF Task Force [8]. Similar to the VARC-2 criteria, this document considered *clinical* (presence of biomarker elevation, ECG evidence, and symptoms), *imaging* (including evidence on invasive testing of coronary thrombosis and loss of myocardial viability or new wall motion abnormality by noninvasive testing), and *pathologic* features. Five subtypes of MI (Fig. 13.2) were defined in this document two of which considered MI in the setting of recent cardiac procedures. In the set-

Type 1: Spontaneous myocardial infarction
Spontaneous myocardial infarction related to atherosclerotic plaque rupture, ulceration, fissuring, erosion, or dissection with resulting intraluminal thrombus in one or more of the coronary arteries leading to decreased myocardial blood flow or distal platelet emboli with ensuing myocyte necrosis. The patient may have underlying severe CAD but on occasion non-obstructive or no CAD.
Type 2: Myocardial infarction secondary to an ischaemic imbalance
In instances of myocardial injury with necrosis where a condition other than CAD contributes to an imbalance between myocardial oxygen supply and/or demand, e.g. coronary endothelial dysfunction, coronary artery spasm, coronary embolism, tachy-/brady-arrhythmias, anaemia, respiratory failure, hypotension, and hypertension with or without LVH.
Type 3: Myocardial infarction resulting in death when biomarker values are unavailable
Cardiac death with symptoms suggestive of myocardial ischaemia and presumed new ischaemic ECG changes or new LBBB, but death occurring before blood samples could be obtained, before cardiac biomarker could rise, or in rare cases cardiac biomarkers were not collected.
Type 4a: Myocardial infarction related to percutaneous coronary intervention (PCI)
Myocardial infarction associated with PCI is arbitrarily defined by elevation of cTn values >5 × 99th percentile URL in patients with normal baseline values (≤99th percentile URL) or a rise of cTn values > 20% if the baseline values are elevated and are stable or falling. In addition, either (i) symptoms suggestive of myocardial ischaemia, or (ii) new ischaemia ECG changes or new LBBB, or (iii) angiographic loss of patency of a major coronary artery or a side branch or persistent slow or no-flow or embolization, or (iv) imaging demonsration of new loss of viable myocardium or new regional wall motion abnormality are required.
Type 4b: Myocardial infarction related to stent thrombosis
Myocardial infarction associated with stent thrombosis is detected by coronary angiography or autopsy in the setting of myocardial ischaemia and with a rise and/or fall of cardiac biomarkers values with at least one value above the 99th percentile URL.
Type 5: Myocardial infarction related to coronary artery bypass grafting (CABG)
Myocardial infarction associated with CABG is arbitrarily defined by elevation of cardiac biomarker values >10 × 99th percentile URL in patients with normal baseline cTn values ((≤99th percentile URL). In addition, either (i) new pathological Q waves or new LBBB, or (ii) angiographic documented new graft or new native coronary artery occlusion, or (iii) imaging eveidence of new loss of viable myocardium or new regional wall motion abnormality.

Fig. 13.2 Third universal definition of myocardial infarction. Adopted from consensus documented put forth by Joint ESC/ACCF/AHA/WHF Task Force

ting of percutaneous coronary intervention (PCI), biomarker elevation of 5× the URL (or >20% rise above baseline if baseline levels were elevated) was considered suggestive of MI. For coronary artery bypass grafting (CABG), biomarker elevation >10× URL corresponded with new infarction in patients with normal (≤99th percentile URL) baseline levels. These cutoffs were arbitrarily defined, and no criteria were provided for abnormal biomarker elevation in the setting of aortic valve replacement.

Exploration into the association of abnormal levels of circulating cardiac biomarkers and TAVR outcomes has been limited, to a degree, by inconsistency in the definition of myocardial injury and infarction. These are important clinical endpoints in such research, and thus consistent nomenclature is crucial for the comparison and interpretation of data across studies aiming to answer similar questions. The VARC-2 definition of MI in the setting of TAVR is not without criticism as some data has suggested overestimation of MI rates when using troponin cutoffs as particularized by the VARC-2 criteria and a possible underestimation when employing CK-MB cutoffs. In one series looking at 515 patients undergoing TF and TA-TAVR, 88.1% of patients undergoing TF-TAVR had VARC-2-defined MI versus 9% by CK-MB thresholds in the same cohort [9]. There is certainly difficulty in interpreting the clinical significance of these elevations, but a standardized definition provides the uniformity and consistency necessary for higher-quality research and analysis. For this reason, we endorse following the VARC-2 criteria when evaluating patients for possible myocardial infarction following TAVR and encourage its standardized use in future TAVR research.

13.3 Biomarker Types

A variety of cardiac biomarkers have been studied over the years, and laboratory assays have made use of varying biomarker kinetics to help guide the appropriate blood testing and test interpretation in the hours and days following myocardial injury.

13.3.1 Causes of Elevation

While the detection of cardiac biomarkers in the blood stream suggests myocardial breakdown, the mechanism by which these proteins are released requires further clinical investigation. Elevations in biomarker assays may be seen in the setting of *acute cardiac thrombosis*, *demand ischemia* in the setting of underlying nonocclusive but flow-limiting coronary disease (where oxygen demand of the myocardium outweighs supply provided by coronary flow as seen in a number of clinical conditions), *myocardial/pericardial inflammation* (pericarditis, myocarditis, infiltrative disease, auto-inflammatory, viral/bacterial disease, etc.), *high-intensity activity* (e.g., high-intensity aerobic and anaerobic exercise and/or prolonged periods of exercise), *poor clearance* (i.e., renal disease and reduced glomerular filtration rate), and *false-positivity* as induced by cross-reactive antibodies.

Cardiac biomarker elevation following TAVR is commonly observed. In one series, 67% of patients were found to have elevated biomarker levels relative to their pre-procedure baseline [10]. The approach to TAVR is an important factor in defining this rate as roughly one-half of patients undergoing transfemoral TAVR experience a significant rise in CK-MB levels, whereas up to 97% of patients undergoing transapical TAVR have abnormally high levels of circulating CK-MB in the postoperative period [10]. These differences reflect the invasiveness of the transapical approach with direct myocardial injury inherent to the procedure as well as patient selection. Transapical (TA) access is most often reserved for patients with significant vascular disease whose iliofemoral system is not amenable to a transfemoral (TF) approach. Concurrent with their peripheral vascular disease, patients undergoing TA-TAVR have an increased incidence of comorbid conditions placing them at a higher perioperative risk for cardiac ischemia. The first-generation transcatheter heart valve systems were associated with near universal myocardial injury by troponin I assay with 97% of TF cases and 100% of TA cases demonstrating elevated post-procedural levels. In the same patients, only 47%

Fig. 13.3 Cardiac biomarker kinetics demonstrated by serum marker concentration following onset of chest pain. Adapted from Yang et al. Unstable angina. Emedicine.medscape. com

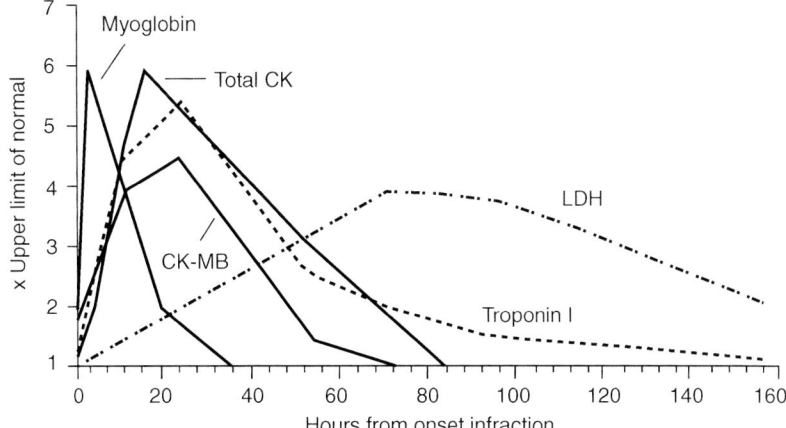

Time course of elevations of serum markers after acute myocardial infarction.
CK = creatine kinase;
CK-MB = creatine kinase MB fraction;
LDH = lactate dehydrogenase.

of TF cases demonstrated myocardial injury by CK-MB levels (95% by CK-MB for TA cases) [11]. In another cohort of 150 patients undergoing TAVR, elevated troponin I levels were observed in 90% of patients and elevated CK-MB elevations in 50% [12]. This disparity reflects differences in biomarker kinetics (Fig. 13.3) and assay sensitivity. As discussed below, there are also significant differences in specificity of these assays as they pertain to clinically significant myocardial injury, ventricular function, and cardiovascular mortality. As such, it is important to note that not all biomarker elevations correlate with clinically significant myocardial injury.

With regard to TAVR, there are several mechanisms for biomarker release into the systemic circulation. Access considerations and patient selection, discussed above, certainly influence the presence and degree of biomarker elevation, but, ultimately, it is the development of biomechanical stress leading to cardiac myocyte apoptosis that results in the release of cardiac biomarkers. Factors which trigger this cascade include *transient global ischemia* in the setting of anesthesia induction, valve deployment, pre- or post-deployment balloon valvuloplasty, ventricular and atrial tachyarrhythmia, sudden heart block, and rapid ventricular pacing; *acute changes in preload conditions* as may be seen

with severe aortic insufficiency; *acute coronary occlusion* as a result of embolic phenomena or direct flow impedance by the native valve leaflets or the implanted valve itself; and *direct myocardial injury*. Both early and more recent data have suggested that mechanically expanding systems and, to a lesser extent, self-expanding systems result in more frequent and sizeable increases in biomarker elevation relative to baseline than balloon-expandable systems [13]. Interestingly, a deeper depth of implantation has been associated with higher circulating biomarkers presumably due to contact with the muscular septum, and the absence of periprocedural beta-blocker therapy has been linked to increased rate of myocardial injury following TAVR [14]. Beta-blocker use may help mitigate acute upregulation of sympathetic nervous system in patients with systolic dysfunction during TAVR and temper some of the above physiologic stressors triggered during TAVR leading to myocardial injury. The clinical role of beta-blockers in TAVR, though currently, has yet to be well-defined.

13.3.2 Troponins

Cardiac troponins I (24 kDa) and T (37 kDa) are large proteins that, along with cardiac troponin

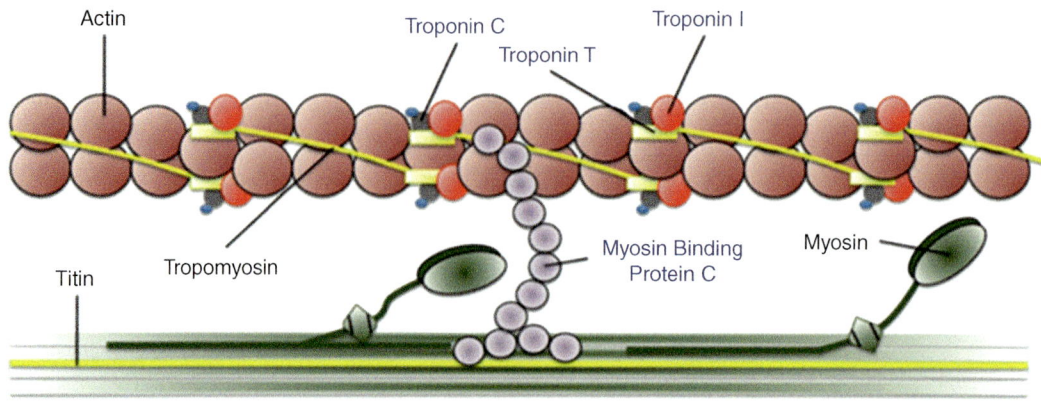

Fig. 13.4 Troponin within actin-myosin binding complex. Reproduced from Chin et al. [15]

C, are found in the contractile structure of myocardial cells and make up the troponin complex, a thin filament that regulates calcium-modulated striated muscle actomyosin ATPase activity (Fig. 13.4). Troponins I and T are exclusively found in cardiac muscle (troponin C is found in both skeletal and cardiac muscle), and their clinical utility in the detection of myocardial injury and necrosis is predicated on wide commercial availability and well-validated data correlating troponin elevation with myocardial damage. More recently high-sensitivity (Hs) troponin assays have been used in the screening of patients presenting with a chest pain syndrome helping to guide and triage their care in the acute setting. The interpretation of low-level, mild troponin elevation or discordant biomarker data especially when coupled with a complicated medical history or, conversely, a lack of other clinical features (i.e., ECG changes, symptoms, evidence of cardiac dysfunction, etc.) can be challenging and often requires input from an appropriately trained cardiac consultant.

In the natural progression of aortic valve stenosis, where gradual narrowing of the aortic valve leads to increased afterload and left ventricular wall stress, decreased coronary perfusion, and reduced cardiac output with concomitant left ventricular remodeling, troponin elevation has had some modest utility in predicting outcomes and identifying patients at higher risk of mortality prior to intervention. Baseline Hs-TnT abnormalities in such patients who are observed with medical management correlated with poorer clinical outcomes over a 5- to 7-year follow-up period [16].

In the setting of surgical aortic valve replacement (SAVR), troponin levels have been evaluated in the pre-, peri-, and post-procedural period to better predict outcomes following valve replacement. Recent data published evaluating 3-year outcomes in Norwegian patients undergoing SAVR found that elevated baseline Hs-TnT levels were associated with increased all-cause mortality regardless of treatment type assigned; however after adjusted analysis, elevated preoperative Hs-TnT provided no significant prognostic information in patients who underwent SAVR [17]. Another study of 57 patients with moderate to severe aortic stenosis demonstrated that detectable levels of troponin in the pre-AVR evaluation period were independently associated with increased mortality [18].

As the clinical experience with TAVR has grown, increasing evidence has become available examining the impact of troponin elevations on short- and long-term clinical outcomes following valve replacement. Pre-procedural troponin elevations have been associated with poorer 1-year mortality despite subsequent successful TAVR [19]. This speaks to the importance of early identification of patients with severe aortic stenosis preferably prior to symptom onset for close observation and identification of early symptoms before echocardiographic left ventricular dysfunction is detected. Identification of biomarker abnormalities in the pre-procedural period allows the clinician to identify higher-risk, decompensated patients who would benefit from optimization prior to undergoing TAVR.

While data supporting the prognostic utility of troponin elevation following TAVR is provocative, there are some data tempering the enthusiasm for troponins as a predictive marker in TAVR patients. In post hoc analysis of the PARTNER trial, which evaluated high (cohort A) or extreme (cohort B) surgical risk patients with severe symptomatic AS, those who underwent TF-TAVR with the early-generation Sapien valve system (Edwards Lifesciences) were stratified into three groups based on elevations in cardiac biomarkers on postoperative day 1. Those at the highest tertile of troponin elevation had a nearly 100-fold increase in all-cause mortality and cardiovascular mortality at 30 days when compared to those in the lowest tertile [20]. In the same analysis, the degree of biomarker elevation was not predictive of 30-day and 1-year outcomes in patients who underwent transapical (TA)-TAVR. TA- and transaortic (TAo)-TAVR have demonstrated the near ubiquitous presence of VARC-2 significant troponin elevation in the post-procedural period; however a transapical approach correlates with a greater magnitude of rise, and this translated to poorer left ventricular function and poorer survival in mid- and long-term follow-up [10, 21]. Such an effect most likely applies, as well, to transfemoral patients where a greater magnitude in troponin rise does seem to correlate with more significant decline in LV function. Clinically significant decline (>5% drop from baseline LVEF) though often occurs when troponin levels exceed 0.8 µg/L [11]. Another study evaluating only TF-TAVR in 201 patients using early-generation valve systems found that both elevated baseline and post-procedural hsTnT were predictive of 1-year mortality [22]. In contrast, a series of 474 patients who underwent TF-TAVR showed that troponin elevations >15 ULN had no impact on 1-year survival, although troponin elevation was associated with post-procedural conduction abnormalities [23]. Similarly, another early TAVR series showed uniform myocardial injury post-TAVR by troponin elevation; however the degree of troponin elevation did not correlate with increased 1-year mortality [24].

Ultimately, cardiac troponins appear to demonstrate some prognostic utility in predicating poorer short- and long-term outcomes following TAVR. This conclusion is tempered by a handful of data showing no prognosticative role for cardiac troponin elevations. In patients undergoing TF-TAVR, this discordance likely reflects the sensitivity of troponin assays for detection of myocardial injury and necrosis which may often be trivial and subclinical in its magnitude. Indeed, the magnitude of troponin release is certainly influential to its predictive power. In TA-TAVR patients, the near ubiquity of troponin elevation in the immediate post-procedural period makes a dichotomous comparison of outcomes difficult. Troponin assays are relatively rapid and widely available making their use practical in the clinical setting. The routine assessment of post-TAVR troponin levels, especially in patients without clinical evidence of myocardial ischemia, does not seem to provide any additive benefit to patient management. In the pre-AVR evaluation period, elevated troponin levels may be useful in identifying patients (in the absence of obstructive coronary disease) earlier in the progression of their disease possibly prior to symptom onset. This may better guide follow-up strategy and timing of valve replacement, although there are no data to suggest that earlier intervention based on the appearance of abnormal troponin levels in the absence of symptoms confers any significant long-term mortality benefit over a traditional strategy of replacement at time of symptom onset or LV dysfunction (EF <50%).

13.3.3 Creatine Kinase-MB

Creatine kinase (CK) is a dimer composed of some combination of two (M and B) subunits. CK, therefore, exists in the bloodstream as isoenzymes CK-MM, CK-BB, or CK-MB. Total CK measurements reflect the total concentration of these circulating isoenzymes. CK regulates high-energy phosphate production and use in contractile proteins and is involved in the cleavage and shuttling of high-energy phosphate bonds from the mitochondria where ATP is produced to the cytoplasm for cellular use [25]. While CK-MM is the predominant isoform found in striated muscle (97% of CK), CK-MB is clinically relevant as it comprises only 3% of CK found in striated muscle but 15–40% of CK activity found in cardiac muscle. CK-BB, meanwhile, is found in the bladder, gastrointestinal tract, and brain. The disproportionate concentration of the CK-MB isoenzyme in cardiac muscle makes it a useful clinical marker for myocardial injury and cardiac myocyte necrosis. That CK-MB is found in non-cardiac muscle may confound the interpretation of elevated CK-MB levels especially in the setting of total CK level elevation (as may be seen, e.g., with skeletal muscle trauma or rhabdomyolysis). The fraction, or *relative index*, of CK-MB to CK is a useful adjunctive indicator of myocardial injury with a value greater than 5% consistent with myocardial injury especially in the setting of an elevated total CK level. When properly timed, direct immunologic assay for CK-MB has an excellent specificity for acute myocardial infarction approaching 100% in some reports [26].

Several studies looking at the clinical relevance of elevated cardiac biomarkers in the setting of TAVR have suggested that post-procedural CK-MB elevation corresponds with poorer long-term clinical outcomes. CK-MB elevations >5× ULN appear to have a higher positive predictive value for post-procedural mortality than troponin elevations >15× ULN, an observation that reflects the higher specificity of CK-MB assays potentially at the expense of sensitivity. Elevated CK-MB levels have been associated with an increase in 30 day and 1-year mortality as well as increased rates of AKI [12]. CK-MB elevations have been predictive of poorer post-procedural left ventricular function [10, 11], and the magnitude of CK-MB elevation has also been shown to be a critical predictor of mortality as patients with >5-fold increases had significantly higher rates of death than those patients with no or lesser increase relative to baseline [10]. In a post hoc analysis of the PARTNER trial, Paradis and colleagues found that cardiac biomarker elevation in patients undergoing TF-TAVR predicted 30-day all-cause and cardiovascular mortality and that post-procedural CK-MB elevation predicted 1-year mortality [20]. CK-MB levels >5× ULN have been associated with higher bleeding rates and higher rates of stroke [23].

When compared to troponin, CK-MB demonstrates higher specificity for myocardial necrosis at the expense of sensitivity. In the setting of TAVR, significant CK-MB elevation appears to correlate better with clinically significant myocardial injury as evidenced by an association with poorer subsequent cardiac function and prognosticates increased morbidity and mortality in the short- and long-term follow-up period.

13.3.4 B-Type Natriuretic Peptide (BNP) and NT-proBNP

Brain (B-type) natriuretic peptide (BNP) is a 32-amino acid protein found in cardiac myocytes and brain tissue (where it was first identified). In healthy individuals, BNP concentrations are highest in the atria; however, in response to alterations in left ventricular loading conditions, the protein is synthesized in and released from the left ventricle. In the production of BNP, preproBNP is first proteolyzed to proBNP (a 108-amino acid protein) which is subsequently cleaved to form BNP and N-terminal proBNP. Natriuretic peptides act as vasodilatory and, as their name suggests, diuretic agents in reaction to upregulation of the neurohormonal response (activation of the renin-angiotensin-aldosterone axis and sympathetic nervous system) seen in acute heart failure (Fig. 13.5). BNP is a well-validated marker of left ventricular wall stress induced by a variety of adverse cardiac conditions affecting normal left ventricular hemodynamics. BNP is particularly sensitive to acute alterations in preload and/or afterload and, as such, is a biomarker of both systolic and diastolic dysfunction. It is believed that in heart failure conditions, natriuretic peptide metabolism is dysregulated resulting in a disproportionately high level of biologically inactive proteins (viz., intact proBNP, BNP by-products, and NT-proBNP). These inactive compounds

Fig. 13.5 Properties and functions of B-type natriuretic peptide. Reproduced from Chin et al. [15]

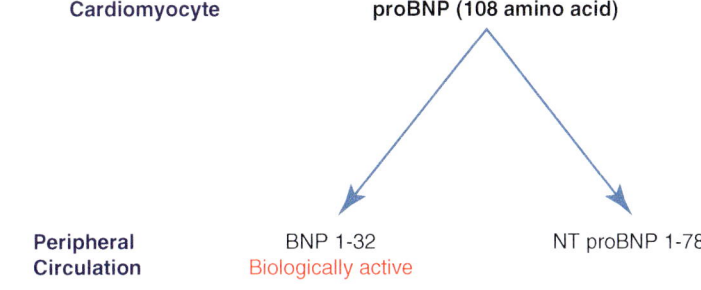

	BNP	**NT-proBNP**
Half life	20 mins	60 to 120 mins NT-proBNP has higher values compared to BNP
Clearance	1. Endocytosis by natriuretic peptide receptors 2. Neutral endopeptidase degradation 3. Renal excretion	Organs with high metabolic rates: kidneys, liver, muscles In renal failure, there are greater increases in NT-proBNP than BNP levels
In vitro stability	+ Samples should be analyzed preferably < 4 hours of collection at room temperature	++
Psysiological effects	1. Promote natriuresis and diuresis 2. Inhibition of sympathetic activity 3. Inhibition of rennin-angiotensin aldosterone system 4. Promote vasodilatation 5. Inhibition of adverse cardiac remodeling	Biologically inert

may cross-react with BNP assays, explaining higher laboratory measurements in acute heart failure despite an ineffective counter response to neurohormonal activation [15].

For years, the literature on the natural course of aortic stenosis has highlighted the importance of natriuretic peptide evaluation in patients with aortic stenosis. Natriuretic peptides have been associated with mortality and the extent of myocardial remodeling and have aided in predicting the transition from asymptomatic to symptomatic AS, as well as identification of high-risk patients [16, 17, 27]. In a large clinical series of over 1900 patients with at least moderate aortic stenosis, BNP clinical activation (defined as a ratio of the subject's BNP to the maximum normal values of age- and sex-matched controls greater than 1) was associated with higher mortality regardless of symptomatology, and the hazard ratio for mortality incrementally increased as the degree of clinical activation increased [28]. This ratio allows for patient-specific normalization of BNP values and may be a more clinically useful measurement especially when comparing BNP levels in a spectrum of patients. BNP elevation also correlates with degree of diastolic dysfunction in patients with severe aortic stenosis with higher levels demonstrating greater specificity for moderate or severe diastolic impairment [29] and has been shown to be predictive of adverse outcomes in patient with low-flow, low-gradient severe aortic stenosis [30]. The utility of BNP measurement in asymptomatic patient with severe AS to better perform risk stratification has prompted its recommendation in the European guidelines on the management of valvular heart disease [31, 32].

In the surgical and transcatheter management of aortic stenosis, pre-procedural BNP has been useful in predicting long-term outcomes. In one series examining patients who underwent balloon aortic valvuloplasty (BAV), SAVR, and TAVR, patients with the lowest levels of pre-intervention BNP had significantly lower 10-month mortality than those with the highest levels regardless of intervention strategy. Interestingly, those who underwent SAVR and those who underwent TAVR both had significant absolute declines in their BNP levels at 1 year with gradual decline during that timeframe. Those patients who underwent BAV had an initial decline in their BNP during the first 30 days with a subsequent uptrend to their pre-procedural baseline at 1 year [33]. This mimics with the general course of patients who have undergone BAV and have initial symptomatic relief but achieve no significant long-

term mortality benefit and frequently become symptomatic again within months. TAVR and SAVR, on the other hand, have consistently demonstrated a sustained clinical and mortality benefit over medical management. High baseline BNP levels confer a three- to fivefold risk in short-term, 6-month, and 2-year all-cause mortality (ACM) and 2-year cardiovascular mortality when compared to low baseline levels in patients undergoing TAVR [34, 35]. Additionally, persistently high BNP levels confer the highest risk of cardiovascular and all-cause mortality following TAVR (Fig. 13.6) [34], and high pre-procedural BNP has been associated with lower device deployment success rates during TAVR.

In addition to BNP, NT-proBNP—the biologically inactive by-product of proBNP proteolysis—is a well-validated prognosticator in patients with AS and those undergoing TAVR. Not surprisingly, elevations in NT-proBNP levels correlate with increasing transaortic valvular gradients [36, 37]—a corollary of disease severity, onset of symptoms, and timing of valve replacement. NT-proBNP has been shown to be independently predictive of 1-year mortality in TAVR patients [38]. NT-proBNP ratio (measured level/maximum normal level for age- and gender-matched controls) is an alternative method to measure and interpret natriuretic peptide levels akin to

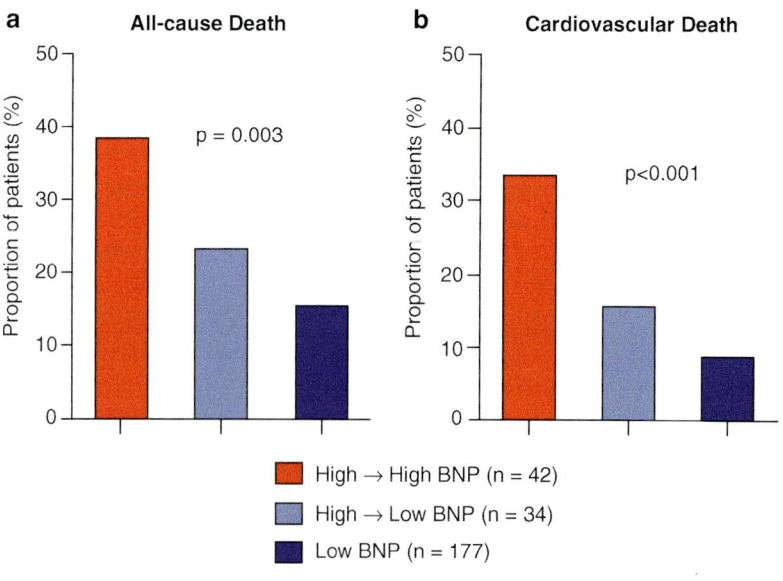

Fig. 13.6 Correlation between pre- and post-TAVR BNP levels and all-cause death (**a**) and cardiovascular death (**b**). Reproduced from Koskinas et al. [34]

the previously discussed BNP clinical activation ratio. The NT-proBNP ratio has been evaluated in post-TAVR patients and strongly correlates with short- and long-term outcomes following valve implantation. In a series of 244 patients who underwent TAVR, the group with a ratio <4.2 had an 8.5% 1-year all-cause mortality, whereas those with a ratio >4.2 had a 32.1% all-cause mortality at 1 year. Interesting, there were no deaths in the group of patients with a post-procedural ratio of <1.5 [39]. The predictive value of proBNP in one study was found to outperform the logistic EuroSCORE which has been used routinely, in conjunction with the STS score, in the perioperative risk assessment of patients with severe aortic stenosis [40].

Measuring natriuretic peptides to diagnose heart failure and stratify patients according to their short- and long-term mortality risk may have limitations in some select patient populations. BNP levels are known to be lower in obese patients. This paradox has been incompletely explained but may be a consequence of increased clearance of active natriuretic peptides by increased expression of clearance receptors on adipocytes. Increased lipid deposition in the heart has been hypothesized to result in a lipotoxic cardiac effect secreting adipokines and cytokines which may inhibit the cardiac endocrine system and reduce production of natriuretic peptides. On a systemic level, abnormalities in endocrine function and hormonal concentrations in obese patients may also inhibit cardiac endocrine function [41]. Measurement of BNP and interpretation of normal or only modestly elevated absolute values in this group must be done so cautiously with careful consideration of and evaluation for other clinical signs and symptoms of heart failure. A few studies in elderly patients with severe aortic stenosis have shown a tempered or no predictive value of BNP in predicting long-term outcomes [33, 42]. However, there are data to support the prognostic utility of natriuretic peptides in patients at extreme age. Patients over the age of 90 years who had elevated NT-proBNP levels demonstrated a >2.5-fold increase in cardiovascular mortality (2.3-fold increase in all-cause mortality) [43].

Natriuretic peptides have proven to be a useful marker in both the pre- and post-AVR period. Their presence in the circulation reflects a different cellular process than that suggested by the release of cardiac troponins and creatine kinase-MB although there is often overlap in the presence of these biomarkers. Circulating BNP and the by-products of its metabolism can be a sensitive and powerful surrogate for acute changes in left ventricular loading conditions and may serve as an additional data point in the pre-procedural evaluation period to hasten the course to valve replacement. Additionally, the ability to identify high-risk patients in the post-AVR setting is quite useful to the clinician and can better inform surveillance strategy and medical management of these patients.

13.4 Novel Biomarkers

There are a number of novel biomarkers currently being studied in patients with aortic stenosis with varying degrees of success in predicting outcomes and comorbidity associated with aortic stenosis itself and TAVR. Most of the markers discussed below are used routinely in clinical practice although a few are measured in the evaluation of other medical conditions and could be potentially employed in the clinical realm for aortic stenosis.

13.4.1 microRNAs

microRNAs (miRNAs) are small (~21 nucleotides in length), noncoding RNA molecules that help regulate gene expression at the post-transcriptional level. Circulating signatures of miRNA have been shown to differentiate subtypes of cardiac hypertrophy [44], implicated in cardiac remodeling and heart failure [45], and identified in various myotonic and muscular dystrophies affecting cardiac tissue [46, 47].

In patients with severe aortic stenosis undergoing TAVR evaluation in Hannover, Germany, miRNA molecules found in higher concentrations in cardiac muscle (including miRNA-1, miRNA-21, miRNA-30e, miRNA-33, miRNA-133a, miRNA-155, and miRNA-206) were measured via PCR assay. Of these markers, miRNA-206 was negatively associated with LVEF following TAVR, suggesting higher circulating levels of miRNA-206 may reflect active cardiac conditions following valve implantation. Interestingly in murine models, low levels of circulating miRNA-206 had an inhibitory effect on cardiomyocyte hypertrophy [48].

Another study looking at myocardial fibrosis and abnormalities in global longitudinal strain (GLS) by echocardiography in patients with severe aortic stenosis examined circulating levels of miRNA-21 which has been associated with myocardial fibrosis. miRNA-21 levels were high in these patients with severe AS when compared to expected circulating levels. Furthermore, abnormalities in GLS were observed in these patients. Such findings suggest a correlation between AV stenosis and echocardiographic abnormalities in GLS and elevated levels of circulating miRNA as surrogates for myocardial fibrosis [49]. Similarly, Villar et al. [50] demonstrated elevated miRNA-21 levels in AS patient when compared to controls.

Data on miRNA role in predicting cardiac outcomes are limited by small sample sizes. Additionally, the role miRNA plays in observed cardiac dysfunction is unclear and may be causative or simply a downstream marker of cardiac dysfunction. There are some data to suggest these miRNA molecules may target and upregulate TGF-B1, a key agent in the pathologic remodeling of the heart in response to pressure overload by inducing cardiac myocyte hypertrophy and interstitial fibrosis [51].

13.4.2 Acylcarnitines

Long-chain acylcarnitines have been associated with maladaptive left ventricular remodeling, and circulating levels were reduced following transcatheter AVR, suggesting a potential role in assessment of acylcarnitines as a biomarker for abnormalities in LV function and LV mass index [52]. To date, there is no evidence to sup-

port the prognostic role of acylcarnitines in short- and long-term outcomes following TAVR, but these early data provide a foundation for further research.

13.4.3 GDF-15

Growth differentiating factor (GDF)-15 is another protein which may prove to be a useful biomarker in the evaluation and risk stratification of patient with aortic stenosis. GDF-15 a cytokine within the family of TGF-B expressed in cardiac myocytes, macrophages, vascular smooth muscle cells, and endothelial cells. It is induced by stress specifically related to tissue injury and inflammatory states. There is evidence to suggest that GDF-15 may predict a lack of reverse remodeling and correlates strongly with 1-year all-cause mortality in patients following TAVR. When added to STS score along with the marker CRP, GDF-15 improves the score's c-index and provided a net reclassification improvement. Furthermore, GDF-15 levels were inversely related to improvement in global longitudinal strain at 1 year suggesting that lower GDF-15 levels correlate with the reversal of myocardial fibrosis and LV dysfunction following TAVR [53]. Another study evaluating predictors of 1-year mortality following TAVR identified GDF-15, in addition to logistic EuroSCORE and EuroSCORE II, as the strongest predictors of outcomes among a number of cardiac biomarkers and scoring systems [54]. As with many novel biomarkers discussed in this section, the clinical application of GDF-15 will hinge upon more robust data supporting its use.

13.4.4 Soluble ST2

Soluble ST2 is a cytokine found in the interleukin-1 receptor class of immunomodulatory compounds and shows a modest correlation with adverse outcomes in patient following TAVR. Elevated circulating levels of sST2 are associated with poorer 1- and 2-year survival in patients with aortic stenosis undergoing

TAVR. Adding sST2 to STS score has been shown to improve prediction of 2-year survival; however sST2 is a less robust prognosticator than NT-proBNP and standard surgical risk scores [55, 56]. A larger series of 345 patients with AS referred for AVR evaluated a panel of novel biomarkers including GDF15, sST2, NT-proBNP, galectin-3, high-sensitivity cardiac troponin T, myeloperoxidase, high-sensitivity CRP, and monocyte chemotactic protein-1. Of these markers, sST2 along with the presence of GDF15 and NT-proBNP was predictive of poorer outcomes following AVR with similar prognostic power in both the transcatheter and surgical cohorts. When adjusted for STS score, the presence of all three of these markers conferred a >4.5-fold increase in 1-year mortality [57]. Given the limited standalone predictive power of sST2, its role in the management of patients with aortic stenosis remains uncertain, but it may be useful as a component of a panel of markers employed in the evaluation of AS patients prior to AVR to better identify their peri- and post-procedural risk.

13.4.5 Blood Cell Markers

Neutrophil-to-lymphocyte ratio (NLR), as a marker of inflammation, has been evaluated in patients with severe calcific aortic stenosis. NLR was shown predictive of MACE defined as a composite of all-cause mortality, cardiac death, and nonfatal myocardial infarction. Furthermore, 5-year survival rates differed significantly among groups stratified by low (84.6% for NLR ≤ 2), intermediate (67.7% for NLR of 2–9), and high (42.6% for NLR >9) ratios [58]. This is an appealing marker as this ratio can be easily and affordably obtained from routine complete blood counts. At this time, the clinical utility of NLR is limited by a lack of comprehensive supportive data.

Alterations in distribution of monocyte subsets, which are defined by the expression profiles of surface molecules CD14 and CD16, have been observed in various cardiovascular disease states [59–61]. Flow cytometry performed in 57 patients undergoing TF-TAVR showed a decline in inter-

mediate subtype (CD14++CD16+) monocytes shortly after valve replacement despite no absolute change in monocyte counts. This suggests a shift in monocyte distribution due to modulation of the cardiac disease state by AVR. Lower levels of intermediate monocytes corresponded with better cardiac function and improvement in NYHA class [62].

13.4.6 Cellular Microparticles

Endothelial cell microparticles (EMPs) are a collection of small phospholipid vesicles released from endothelial cells. Elevated concentration of EMP reflects endothelial dysfunction and may be seen in a variety of conditions often as a marker of inflammation or shear stress. Compared to production of endogenous inflammatory proteins such as CRP, EMP release is more rapid occurring just after endothelial injury [63]. Following TAVR, EMP levels have been shown to decrease due to improved endothelial function and wall shear stress [64, 65].

13.4.7 Galectin-3

In both heart failure with reduced ejection fraction and heart failure with preserved ejection fraction, galectin-3 has emerged as a novel potential prognostic marker [66–68]. Galectin-3 is a proinflammatory molecule implicated in the process of vascular osteogenesis characteristic of atherosclerosis. In vitro studies of galectin-3 have shown induction of inflammatory, osteogenic, and fibrotic markers. Spontaneous galectin-3 expression has also been demonstrated in valvular interstitial cells, and thus it is hypothesized that galectin-3 plays an active role in progression of calcification seen in senile aortic stenosis [69]. Such cells sampled from patients with advanced aortic stenosis have higher levels of galectin-3 than those cells from controls without aortic stenosis. Baldenhofer et al. [70] prospectively observed 101 patients undergoing TAVR and used a dichotomous cutoff of 17.8 ng/mL to define groups with low versus high levels of circulating serum galectin-3. Those in the higher group had a 4.5-fold increase in 1-year cardiovascular event rates and a >5-fold increase in 1-year all-cause mortality. This data suggests a strong correlation between adverse clinical events and elevated circulating levels of galectin-3 in patients undergoing TAVR. Galectin-3 shows promise as a cardiac biomarker with validated utility in heart failure and with more clinical research may have a clinical role in post-TAVR risk stratification.

13.4.8 Mid-Regional Pro-Adrenomedullin

Adrenomedullin is a natriuretic and vasodilatory agent and is expressed in a wide spectrum of clinical conditions including cardiovascular and non-cardiovascular diseases such as sepsis, pneumonia, chronic renal insufficiency, and chronic obstructive pulmonary disease [71–73]. Mid-regional pro-adrenomedullin (MR-proADM) is a marker of cardiac hemodynamic stress and has been shown to have prognostic utility in patients with heart failure [74]. With the aim to predict all-cause mortality, this novel marker was evaluated in 153 patients who underwent TAVR and subsequently compared to an external validation cohort of 205 patients undergoing TAVR. In patients with MR-proADM levels above the 75th percentile, mortality was 31% at 9 months versus 4% in those with levels below that threshold. When added to EuroSCORE II, MR-proADM significantly improved the model's net reclassification index [75].

13.4.9 Novel Markers for Prediction of Acute Kidney Injury After TAVR

Acute kidney injury (AKI) is one of the more commonly realized complications following TAVR, owing to contrast exposure; transient alterations in hemodynamics including decreases in cardiac output and arterial pressures; and patient risk factors including underlying renal disease, advanced age, diabetes, and heart failure. Early detection of AKI relies on serial measurement of serum creatinine levels, calculation of estimated glomerular filtration rate (eGFR), and close monitoring of changes in urinary output. Such prompt detection is crucial for the early initial medical management to optimize renal perfusion. Early detection of AKI is hindered; however, by limitations inherent to serum creatinine, changes in which are often delayed 1–2 days after injury has occurred. Additionally, eGFR calculations are often inaccurate in the setting of acute alterations in renal function. Ideally, renal injury would be detected prior to a decline in urine output which is often a downstream consequence of progressive renal dysfunction. To this end, several novel biomarkers have been proposed in the setting of TAVR, to more powerfully and rapidly identify patients at risk of AKI and long-term renal impairment.

Cystatin C, an alternative marker for renal function, has previously been suggested to more accurately reflect renal function following cardiac surgery when compared to s-creatinine levels [76]. In patients undergoing TAVR, post-procedural cystatin C levels may identify a larger cohort of patients at risk for late-onset AKI than s-creatinine levels [77]. Routine clinical use of cystatin C in post-TAVR management of patients is hindered by a paucity of supportive data and lack of widespread assay availability.

Urinary G1 cell cycle arrest biomarkers, tissue inhibitor of metalloproteinases-2 (TIMP-2), and insulin-like growth factor binding protein 7 (IFGBP7) have been implicated as key markers of AKI. In a small series of patients undergoing TAVR, in the post-procedural period, urinary cell cycle arrest biomarkers demonstrated superior diagnostic accuracy for the prediction of AKI than serum creatinine [78].

Serum B2-microglobulin has been shown to be a possible predictor of end-stage kidney disease and was evaluated along with several other potential biomarkers, including cystatin C and neutrophil gelatinase-associated lipocalin (NGAL), in 80 patients undergoing either SAVR or TAVR. In the cohort of 40 patients who underwent TAVR, serum B2-microglobulin and cystatin C were the strongest predictors of early detection of acute kidney injury with serum B2-microglobulin demonstrating the highest area under the curve (AUC) of the novel markers studied [79]. In this study, NGAL was not shown to be a powerful predictor of AKI; however following cardiac surgery, NGAL has been shown to be an early and significant predictor of AKI [80]. NGAL concentration in renal proximal tubules increases rapidly in response to renal hypoperfusion injury, and these increases can be detected much earlier than rises in serum creatinine—often within 1 h [81]. Given these unique qualities of NGAL, there may yet be some clinical utility for its measurement in patients following aortic valve replacement; however supportive data is lacking at this time.

13.5 Conclusion

Degree of myocardial injury and left ventricle wall stress appears to be the common dominator in the ability to predict long-term outcomes in patients undergoing TAVR. In clinical practice, the markers by which these conditions are measured include biomarkers for cardiac necrosis and injury (troponin, CK-MB as the principle proteins) and b-type natriuretic protein (as marker of acute left ventricular systolic and diastolic dysfunction in response to changes in loading conditions). The utility of these individual markers, especially in the case of myocardial injury detection, relates to the sensitivity of their assays and the definitions laid out in such guidelines as the VARC-2 consensus document. Markers that are highly sensitive for such injury may overestimate events and identify subclinical injury not particularly helpful in the management of patients with aortic stenosis undergoing TAVR. It is important, therefore, not just to consider whether abnormal levels of circulating biomarkers are present or not but to consider the magnitude of elevation as a correlate of extent of myocardial injury. The highest levels of circulating biomarkers which are more powerfully associated with increases in complication, morbidity, left ventricular dysfunction, and mortality rates may be more useful in the postprocedural management of TAVR patients.

In addition to the commonly used biomarkers in clinical practice today, there is exciting research into novel markers that may help to better predict clinical outcomes following TAVR and identify patients in the preoperative setting who may be at higher risk for adverse events. Continued evaluation of these emerging biomarkers as well as refinement of procedural risk prediction models will hopefully improve our ability to care for an ever-growing patient population with severe aortic stenosis.

Conflict of Interest None.

References

1. Smith CR, Leon MB, Mack MJ, Miller DC, Moses JW, Svensson LG, et al. Transcatheter versus surgical aortic-valve replacement in high-risk patients. N Engl J Med. 2011;364(23):2187–98.
2. Kodali SK, Williams MR, Smith CR, Svensson LG, Webb JG, Makkar RR, et al. Two-year outcomes after transcatheter or surgical aortic-valve replacement. N Engl J Med. 2012;366(18):1686–95.
3. Thomopoulou S, Vavuranakis M, Karyofyllis P, Kariori M, Karavolias G, Balanika M, et al. Four-year clinical results of transcatheter self-expanding Medtronic CoreValve implantation in high-risk patients with severe aortic stenosis. Age Ageing. 2016;45(3):427–30.
4. Adams DH, Popma JJ, Reardon MJ, Yakubov SJ, Coselli JS, Deeb GM, et al. Transcatheter aortic-valve replacement with a self-expanding prosthesis. N Engl J Med. 2014;370(19):1790–8.
5. Leon MB, Smith CR, Mack MJ, Makkar RR, Svensson LG, Kodali SK, et al. Transcatheter or surgical aortic-valve replacement in intermediate-risk patients. N Engl J Med. 2016;374(17):1609–20.
6. Reardon MJ, Van Mieghem NM, Popma JJ, Kleiman NS, Sondergaard L, Mumtaz M, et al. Surgical or transcatheter aortic-valve replacement in intermediate-risk patients. N Engl J Med. 2017;376(14):1321–31.
7. Kappetein AP, Head SJ, Genereux P, Piazza N, van Mieghem NM, Blackstone EH, et al. Updated standardized endpoint definitions for transcatheter aortic valve implantation: the Valve Academic Research Consortium-2 consensus document (VARC-2). Eur J Cardiothorac Surg. 2012;42(5):S45–60.
8. Thygesen K, Alpert JS, Jaffe AS, Simoons ML, Chaitman BR, White HD, et al. Third universal definition of myocardial infarction. Circulation. 2012;126(16):2020–35.
9. Liebetrau C, Kim WK, Meyer A, Arsalan M, Gaede L, Blumenstein JM, et al. Identification of periprocedural myocardial infarction using a high-sensitivity troponin I assay in patients who underwent transcatheter aortic valve implantation. Am J Cardiol. 2017;120(7):1180–6.

10. Ribeiro HB, Nombela-Franco L, Munoz-Garcia AJ, Lemos PA, Amat-Santos I, Serra V, et al. Predictors and impact of myocardial injury after transcatheter aortic valve replacement: a multicenter registry. J Am Coll Cardiol. 2015;66(19):2075–88.

11. Rodes-Cabau J, Gutierrez M, Bagur R, De Larochelliere R, Doyle D, Cote M, et al. Incidence, predictive factors, and prognostic value of myocardial injury following uncomplicated transcatheter aortic valve implantation. J Am Coll Cardiol. 2011;57(20):1988–99.

12. Barbash IM, Dvir D, Ben-Dor I, Badr S, Okubagzi P, Torguson R, et al. Prevalence and effect of myocardial injury after transcatheter aortic valve replacement. Am J Cardiol. 2013;111(9):1337–43.

13. Stundl A, Schulte R, Lucht H, Weber M, Sedaghat A, Shamekhi J, et al. Periprocedural myocardial injury depends on transcatheter heart valve type but does not predict mortality in patients after transcatheter aortic valve replacement. JACC Cardiovasc Interv. 2017;10(15):1550–60.

14. Yong ZY, Wiegerinck EM, Boerlage-van Dijk K, Koch KT, Vis MM, Bouma BJ, et al. Predictors and prognostic value of myocardial injury during transcatheter aortic valve implantation. Circ Cardiovasc Interv. 2012;5(3):415–23.

15. Chin CW, Djohan AH, Lang CC. The role of cardiac biochemical markers in aortic stenosis. Biomarkers. 2016;21(4):316–27.

16. Solberg OG, Ueland T, Wergeland R, Dahl CP, Aakhus S, Aukrust P, et al. High-sensitive troponin T and N-terminal-brain-natriuretic-peptide predict outcome in symptomatic aortic stenosis. Scand Cardiovasc J. 2012;46(5):278–85.

17. Auensen A, Hussain AI, Falk RS, Walle-Hansen MM, Bye J, Pettersen KI, et al. Associations of brain-natriuretic peptide, high-sensitive troponin T, and high-sensitive C-reactive protein with outcomes in severe aortic stenosis. PLoS One. 2017;12(6):e0179304.

18. Rosjo H, Andreassen J, Edvardsen T, Omland T. Prognostic usefulness of circulating high-sensitivity troponin T in aortic stenosis and relation to echocardiographic indexes of cardiac function and anatomy. Am J Cardiol. 2011;108(1):88–91.

19. Frank D, Stark S, Lutz M, Weissbrodt A, Freitag-Wolf S, Petzina R, et al. Preprocedural high-sensitive troponin predicts survival after transcatheter aortic valve implantation (TAVI). Int J Cardiol. 2013;169(3):e38–9.

20. Paradis JM, Maniar HS, Lasala JM, Kodali S, Williams M, Lindman BR, et al. Clinical and functional outcomes associated with myocardial injury after transfemoral and transapical transcatheter aortic valve replacement: a subanalysis from the PARTNER Trial (Placement of Aortic transcatheter Valves). JACC Cardiovasc Interv. 2015;8(11):1468–79.

21. Ribeiro HB, Dahou A, Urena M, Carrasco JL, Mohammadi S, Doyle D, et al. Myocardial injury after transaortic versus transapical transcatheter aortic valve replacement. Ann Thorac Surg. 2015;99(6):2001–9.

22. Chorianopoulos E, Krumsdorf U, Geis N, Pleger ST, Giannitsis E, Katus HA, et al. Preserved prognostic value of preinterventional troponin T levels despite successful TAVI in patients with severe aortic stenosis. Clin Res Cardiol. 2014;103(1):65–72.

23. Koifman E, Garcia-Garcia HM, Alraies MC, Buchanan K, Hideo-Kajita A, Steinvil A, et al. Correlates and significance of elevation of cardiac biomarkers elevation following transcatheter aortic valve implantation. Am J Cardiol. 2017;120(5):850–6.

24. Carrabba N, Valenti R, Migliorini A, Vergara R, Parodi G, Antoniucci D. Prognostic value of myocardial injury following transcatheter aortic valve implantation. Am J Cardiol. 2013;111(10):1475–81.

25. Kemp M, Donovan J, Higham H, Hooper J. Biochemical markers of myocardial injury. Br J Anaesth. 2004;93(1):63–73.

26. Collinson PO, Stubbs PJ, Kessler AC, Multicentre Evaluation of Routine Immunoassay of Troponin TS. Multicentre evaluation of the diagnostic value of cardiac troponin T, CK-MB mass, and myoglobin for assessing patients with suspected acute coronary syndromes in routine clinical practice. Heart. 2003;89(3):280–6.

27. Weber M, Arnold R, Rau M, Elsaesser A, Brandt R, Mitrovic V, et al. Relation of N-terminal pro B-type natriuretic peptide to progression of aortic valve disease. Eur Heart J. 2005;26(10):1023–30.

28. Clavel MA, Malouf J, Michelena HI, Suri RM, Jaffe AS, Mahoney DW, et al. B-type natriuretic peptide clinical activation in aortic stenosis: impact on long-term survival. J Am Coll Cardiol. 2014;63(19):2016–25.

29. Mannacio V, Antignano A, De Amicis V, Di Tommaso L, Giordano R, Iannelli G, et al. B-type natriuretic peptide as a biochemical marker of left ventricular diastolic function: assessment in asymptomatic patients 1 year after valve replacement for aortic stenosis. Interact Cardiovasc Thorac Surg. 2013;17(2):371–7.

30. Dahou A, Clavel MA, Capoulade R, O'Connor K, Ribeiro HB, Cote N, et al. B-type natriuretic peptide and high-sensitivity cardiac troponin for risk stratification in low-flow, low-gradient aortic stenosis: a substudy of the TOPAS study. JACC Cardiovasc Imaging. 2018;11:939–47.

31. Baumgartner H, Falk V, Bax JJ, De Bonis M, Hamm C, Holm PJ, et al. 2017 ESC/EACTS guidelines for the management of valvular heart disease. Eur Heart J. 2017;38(36):2739–91.

32. Vahanian A, Alfieri O, Andreotti F, Antunes MJ, Baron-Esquivias G, Baumgartner H, et al. Guidelines on the management of valvular heart disease (version 2012): the Joint Task Force on the Management of Valvular Heart Disease of the European Society of Cardiology (ESC) and the European Association for Cardio-Thoracic Surgery (EACTS). Eur J Cardiothorac Surg. 2012;42(4):S1–44.

33. Ben-Dor I, Minha S, Barbash IM, Aly O, Dvir D, Deksissa T, et al. Correlation of brain natriuretic peptide levels in patients with severe aortic stenosis undergoing operative valve replacement or percutane-

ous transcatheter intervention with clinical, echocardiographic, and hemodynamic factors and prognosis. Am J Cardiol. 2013;112(4):574–9.

34. Koskinas KC, O'Sullivan CJ, Heg D, Praz F, Stortecky S, Pilgrim T, et al. Effect of B-type natriuretic peptides on long-term outcomes after transcatheter aortic valve implantation. Am J Cardiol. 2015;116(10):1560–5.

35. Abramowitz Y, Chakravarty T, Jilaihawi H, Lee C, Cox J, Sharma RP, et al. Impact of preprocedural B-type natriuretic peptide levels on the outcomes after transcatheter aortic valve implantation. Am J Cardiol. 2015;116(12):1904–9.

36. Neverdal NO, Knudsen CW, Husebye T, Vengen OA, Pepper J, Lie M, et al. The effect of aortic valve replacement on plasma B-type natriuretic peptide in patients with severe aortic stenosis—one year follow-up. Eur J Heart Fail. 2006;8(3):257–62.

37. Georges A, Forestier F, Valli N, Plogin A, Janvier G, Bordenave L. Changes in type B natriuretic peptide (BNP) concentrations during cardiac valve replacement. Eur J Cardiothorac Surg. 2004;25(6):941–5.

38. Elhmidi Y, Bleiziffer S, Piazza N, Ruge H, Krane M, Deutsch MA, et al. The evolution and prognostic value of N-terminal brain natriuretic peptide in predicting 1-year mortality in patients following transcatheter aortic valve implantation. J Invasive Cardiol. 2013;25(1):38–44.

39. Stahli BE, Gebhard C, Saleh L, Falk V, Landmesser U, Nietlispach F, et al. N-terminal pro-B-type natriuretic peptide-ratio predicts mortality after transcatheter aortic valve replacement. Catheter Cardiovasc Interv. 2015;85(7):1240–7.

40. Lopez-Otero D, Trillo-Nouche R, Gude F, Cid-Alvarez B, Ocaranza-Sanchez R, Alvarez MS, et al. Pro B-type natriuretic peptide plasma value: a new criterion for the prediction of short- and long-term outcomes after transcatheter aortic valve implantation. Int J Cardiol. 2013;168(2):1264–8.

41. Clerico A, Giannoni A, Vittorini S, Emdin M. The paradox of low BNP levels in obesity. Heart Fail Rev. 2012;17(1):81–96.

42. Cimadevilla C, Cueff C, Hekimian G, Dehoux M, Lepage L, Iung B, et al. Prognostic value of B-type natriuretic peptide in elderly patients with aortic valve stenosis: the COFRASA-GENERAC study. Heart. 2013;99(7):461–7.

43. Raposeiras-Roubin S, Abu-Assi E, Lopez-Rodriguez E, Agra-Bermejo R, Pereira-Lopez EM, Calvo-Iglesias F, et al. NT-proBNP for risk stratification of nonagenarian patients with severe symptomatic aortic stenosis. Int J Cardiol. 2016;223:785–6.

44. Derda AA, Thum S, Lorenzen JM, Bavendiek U, Heineke J, Keyser B, et al. Blood-based microRNA signatures differentiate various forms of cardiac hypertrophy. Int J Cardiol. 2015;196:115–22.

45. Kumarswamy R, Thum T. Non-coding RNAs in cardiac remodeling and heart failure. Circ Res. 2013;113(6):676–89.

46. Perfetti A, Greco S, Cardani R, Fossati B, Cuomo G, Valaperta R, et al. Validation of plasma microRNAs as biomarkers for myotonic dystrophy type 1. Sci Rep. 2016;6:38174.

47. Matsuzaka Y, Kishi S, Aoki Y, Komaki H, Oya Y, Takeda S, et al. Three novel serum biomarkers, miR-1, miR-133a, and miR-206 for Limb-girdle muscular dystrophy, Facioscapulohumeral muscular dystrophy, and Becker muscular dystrophy. Environ Health Prev Med. 2014;19(6):452–8.

48. Yang Y, Del Re DP, Nakano N, Sciarretta S, Zhai P, Park J, et al. miR-206 mediates YAP-induced cardiac hypertrophy and survival. Circ Res. 2015;117(10):891–904.

49. Fabiani I, Scatena C, Mazzanti CM, Conte L, Pugliese NR, Franceschi S, et al. Micro-RNA-21 (biomarker) and global longitudinal strain (functional marker) in detection of myocardial fibrotic burden in severe aortic valve stenosis: a pilot study. J Transl Med. 2016;14(1):248.

50. Villar AV, Garcia R, Merino D, Llano M, Cobo M, Montalvo C, et al. Myocardial and circulating levels of microRNA-21 reflect left ventricular fibrosis in aortic stenosis patients. Int J Cardiol. 2013;167(6):2875–81.

51. Creemers EE, Pinto YM. Molecular mechanisms that control interstitial fibrosis in the pressure-overloaded heart. Cardiovasc Res. 2011;89(2):265–72.

52. Elmariah S, Farrell LA, Furman D, Lindman BR, Shi X, Morningstar JE, et al. Association of acylcarnitines with left ventricular remodeling in patients with severe aortic stenosis undergoing transcatheter aortic valve replacement. JAMA Cardiol. 2018;3(3):242–6.

53. Kim JB, Kobayashi Y, Moneghetti KJ, Brenner DA, O'Malley R, Schnittger I, et al. GDF-15 (growth differentiation factor 15) is associated with lack of ventricular recovery and mortality after transcatheter aortic valve replacement. Circ Cardiovasc Interv. 2017;10(12):e005594.

54. Sinning JM, Wollert KC, Sedaghat A, Widera C, Radermacher MC, Descoups C, et al. Risk scores and biomarkers for the prediction of 1-year outcome after transcatheter aortic valve replacement. Am Heart J. 2015;170(4):821–9.

55. Stundl A, Lunstedt NS, Courtz F, Freitag-Wolf S, Frey N, Holdenrieder S, et al. Soluble ST2 for risk stratification and the prediction of mortality in patients undergoing transcatheter aortic valve implantation. Am J Cardiol. 2017;120(6):986–93.

56. Schmid J, Stojakovic T, Zweiker D, Scharnagl H, Maderthaner RD, Scherr D, et al. ST2 predicts survival in patients undergoing transcatheter aortic valve implantation. Int J Cardiol. 2017;244:87–92.

57. Lindman BR, Breyley JG, Schilling JD, Vatterott AM, Zajarias A, Maniar HS, et al. Prognostic utility of novel biomarkers of cardiovascular stress in patients with aortic stenosis undergoing valve replacement. Heart. 2015;101(17):1382–8.

58. Cho KI, Cho SH, Her AY, Singh GB, Shin ES. Prognostic utility of neutrophil-to-lymphocyte ratio on adverse clinical outcomes in patients with severe calcific aortic stenosis. PLoS One. 2016;11(8):e0161530.

59. Berg KE, Ljungcrantz I, Andersson L, Bryngelsson C, Hedblad B, Fredrikson GN, et al. Elevated CD14++CD16− monocytes predict cardiovascular events. Circ Cardiovasc Genet. 2012;5(1):122–31.

60. Rogacev KS, Cremers B, Zawada AM, Seiler S, Binder N, Ege P, et al. CD14++CD16+ monocytes independently predict cardiovascular events: a cohort study of 951 patients referred for elective coronary angiography. J Am Coll Cardiol. 2012;60(16):1512–20.

61. Passlick B, Flieger D, Ziegler-Heitbrock HW. Identification and characterization of a novel monocyte subpopulation in human peripheral blood. Blood. 1989;74(7):2527–34.

62. Neuser J, Galuppo P, Fraccarollo D, Willig J, Kempf T, Berliner D, et al. Intermediate CD14++CD16+ monocytes decline after transcatheter aortic valve replacement and correlate with functional capacity and left ventricular systolic function. PLoS One. 2017;12(8):e0183670.

63. Jansen F, Rohwer K, Vasa-Nicotera M, Mellert F, Grube E, Nickenig G, et al. CD-144 positive endothelial microparticles are increased in patients with systemic inflammatory response syndrome after TAVI. Int J Cardiol. 2016;204:172–4.

64. Horn P, Stern D, Veulemans V, Heiss C, Zeus T, Merx MW, et al. Improved endothelial function and decreased levels of endothelium-derived microparticles after transcatheter aortic valve implantation. EuroIntervention. 2015;10(12):1456–63.

65. Jung C, Lichtenauer M, Figulla HR, Wernly B, Goebel B, Foerster M, et al. Microparticles in patients undergoing transcatheter aortic valve implantation (TAVI). Heart Vessel. 2017;32(4):458–66.

66. Tang WH, Shrestha K, Shao Z, Borowski AG, Troughton RW, Thomas JD, et al. Usefulness of plasma galectin-3 levels in systolic heart failure to predict renal insufficiency and survival. Am J Cardiol. 2011;108(3):385–90.

67. de Boer RA, Lok DJ, Jaarsma T, van der Meer P, Voors AA, Hillege HL, et al. Predictive value of plasma galectin-3 levels in heart failure with reduced and preserved ejection fraction. Ann Med. 2011;43(1):60–8.

68. de Boer RA, Edelmann F, Cohen-Solal A, Mamas MA, Maisel A, Pieske B. Galectin-3 in heart failure with preserved ejection fraction. Eur J Heart Fail. 2013;15(10):1095–101.

69. Sadaba JR, Martinez-Martinez E, Arrieta V, Alvarez V, Fernandez-Celis A, Ibarrola J, et al. Role for galectin-3 in calcific aortic valve stenosis. J Am Heart Assoc. 2016;5(11):e004360.

70. Baldenhofer G, Zhang K, Spethmann S, Laule M, Eilers B, Leonhardt F, et al. Galectin-3 predicts short- and long-term outcome in patients undergoing transcatheter aortic valve implantation (TAVI). Int J Cardiol. 2014;177(3):912–7.

71. Albrich WC, Dusemund F, Ruegger K, Christ-Crain M, Zimmerli W, Bregenzer T, et al. Enhancement of CURB65 score with proadrenomedullin (CURB65-A) for outcome prediction in lower respiratory tract infections: derivation of a clinical algorithm. BMC Infect Dis. 2011;11:112.

72. O'Malley RG, Bonaca MP, Scirica BM, Murphy SA, Jarolim P, Sabatine MS, et al. Prognostic performance of multiple biomarkers in patients with non-ST-segment elevation acute coronary syndrome: analysis from the MERLIN-TIMI 36 trial (Metabolic Efficiency With Ranolazine for Less Ischemia in Non-ST-Elevation Acute Coronary Syndromes-Thrombolysis In Myocardial Infarction 36). J Am Coll Cardiol. 2014;63(16):1644–53.

73. Schuetz P, Marlowe RJ, Mueller B. The prognostic blood biomarker proadrenomedullin for outcome prediction in patients with chronic obstructive pulmonary disease (COPD): a qualitative clinical review. Clin Chem Lab Med. 2015;53(4):521–39.

74. Pousset F, Masson F, Chavirovskaia O, Isnard R, Carayon A, Golmard JL, et al. Plasma adrenomedullin, a new independent predictor of prognosis in patients with chronic heart failure. Eur Heart J. 2000;21(12):1009–14.

75. Csordas A, Nietlispach F, Schuetz P, Huber A, Muller B, Maisano F, et al. Midregional proadrenomedullin improves risk stratification beyond surgical risk scores in patients undergoing transcatheter aortic valve replacement. PLoS One. 2015;10(12):e0143761.

76. Bronden B, Eyjolfsson A, Blomquist S, Dardashti A, Ederoth P, Bjursten H. Evaluation of cystatin C with iohexol clearance in cardiac surgery. Acta Anaesthesiol Scand. 2011;55(2):196–202.

77. Johansson M, Nozohoor S, Bjursten H, Kimblad PO, Sjogren J. Acute kidney injury assessed by cystatin C after transcatheter aortic valve implantation and late renal dysfunction. J Cardiothorac Vasc Anesth. 2014;28(4):960–5.

78. Dusse F, Edayadiyil-Dudasova M, Thielmann M, Wendt D, Kahlert P, Demircioglu E, et al. Early prediction of acute kidney injury after transapical and transaortic aortic valve implantation with urinary G1 cell cycle arrest biomarkers. BMC Anesthesiol. 2016;16:76.

79. Zaleska-Kociecka M, Skrobisz A, Wojtkowska I, Grabowski M, Dabrowski M, Kusmierski K, et al. Serum beta-2 microglobulin levels for predicting acute kidney injury complicating aortic valve replacement. Interact Cardiovasc Thorac Surg. 2017;25(4):533–40.

80. Kidher E, Harling L, Ashrafian H, Naase H, Chukwuemeka A, Anderson J, et al. Pulse wave velocity and neutrophil gelatinase-associated lipocalin as predictors of acute kidney injury following aortic valve replacement. J Cardiothorac Surg. 2014;9:89.

81. Wagener G, Jan M, Kim M, Mori K, Barasch JM, Sladen RN, et al. Association between increases in urinary neutrophil gelatinase-associated lipocalin and acute renal dysfunction after adult cardiac surgery. Anesthesiology. 2006;105(3):485–91.

Aortic Regurgitation After Transcatheter Aortic Valve Implantation

14

Bogdan Borz

Abbreviations

AR	Aortic regurgitation
BE	Balloon-expandable
CMR	Cardiovascular magnetic resonance imaging
DBP	Diastolic blood pressure
LV	Left ventricle
LVEDP	Left ventricular end-diastolic pressure
LVOT	Left ventricular outflow tract
MRI	Magnetic resonance imaging
PAR	Paravalvular aortic regurgitation
SAVR	Surgical valve replacement
SE	Self-expandable
TAVI	Transcatheter aortic valve implantation
TEE	Transesophageal echocardiography
THV	Transcatheter heart valve
TTE	Transthoracic echocardiography
VARC	Valve Academic Research Consortium

14.1 Introduction

Transcatheter aortic valve implantation (TAVI), also called transcatheter aortic valve replacement (TAVR), has become standard therapy for high-risk and inoperable patients. The major particu-

B. Borz (✉)
Clinique de l'Union, Saint-Jean, France

Rangueil University Hospital, Toulouse, France

larity of the technique, which differentiates it from classical surgical valve replacement (SAVR), is that the native valve is preserved, and the prosthesis is implanted and fixed in the native annulus via mechanical constraint. The apposition to the native, calcified leaflets and annulus can be imperfect, and the incomplete sealing can lead to paravalvular aortic regurgitation (PAR). PAR has been dubbed the "Achilles' heel" of TAVI, being one the significant complications of the technique [1].

This chapter reviews the incidence, mechanisms, and clinical impact of PAR, with an emphasis on the relationship with transcatheter heart valve (THV) design, its prevention, and treatment.

14.2 Incidence

PAR is a frequent complication of TAVI, and the majority of patients have some degree of PAR (Table 14.1). This contrasts with the low incidence of PAR after SAVR illustrated by an incidence of more than mild aortic regurgitation (AR) of 4.2% in a large Canadian cohort of 3201 patients [2]. The recent meta-analysis performed by Villablanca et al. [3] which included 46 observational studies and 4 randomized controlled trials enrolling a total of 44,247 patients found an incidence of moderate or severe AR of 6.7% after TAVI compared to only 0.8% in patients treated with SAVR. The relative risk of

© Springer Nature Switzerland AG 2019
A. Giordano et al. (eds.), *Transcatheter Aortic Valve Implantation*,
https://doi.org/10.1007/978-3-030-05912-5_14

Table 14.1 Selected studies reporting the incidence of PAR after TAVI

Study author	Study title	N	Year	Valve type	Imaging	Moment of evaluation	None/trace PAR (%)	Mild PAR (%)	Moderate (%)	Severe (%)	TF access route (%)	Corelab
Leon et al. [80]	PARTNER B	358	2010	Sapien	Echo	30 days	14.0	68.0	12.0		100	Yes
Eltchaninoff et al. [81]	France	244	2011	Sapien and CoreValve	TTE/TEE	N/A	90.5		9.0	0.5	65.6	No
Thomas et al. [82]	SOURCE	1038	2010	Sapien	N/A	30 days	N/A	N/A	N/A	1.9	47.0	No
Smith et al. [83]	PARTNER A	699	2011	Sapien	Echo	30 days	22.6	65.2	12.2		70.1	Yes
Tamburino et al. [84]	Italian registry	663	2011	CoreValve	Echo	Through 30 days	N/A	N/A	21	N/A	90.3	No
Abdel-wahab et al. [85]	German registry	690	2011	Sapien and CoreValve	Angio	Post-procedure	27.7	55.1	14.9 (2 moderate to severe)	0.3	93.0	No
Moat et al. [86].	UK	870	2011	Sapien and CoreValve	Angio	Post-procedure	39.0	47.4	13.6 moderate to severe		69.0	No
Gilard et al. [50]	France 2	3195	2012	Sapien/XT and CoreValve	Echo	30 days	37.8	45.7	15.7	0.8	74.6	No
Webb et al. [87]	Registry	150	2014	Sapien 3	Echo	30 days	74.3	22.1	3.5	None	64.0	Yes
Adams et al. [88]	US CoreValve	795	2014	CoreValve	Echo	30 days	55.4	35.7	7.3	1.7	82.8	Yes
Meredith et al. [7]	REPRISE II	120	2014	Lotus	Echo	30 days	78.1 (none) 5.2 (trivial)	15.6	1	None	100	Yes

Study	Trial/Registry	n	Year	Valve	Modality	Timing						
Schofer et al. [89]	Direct Flow Medical	100	2014	Direct flow	Echo	Through 30 days	70.3	28.4	1.4	None	100	N/A
Linke et al. [90]	ADVANCE registry	996	2014	CoreValve	Echo	Discharge	19.2	62.5	15.4	0.2	87.8	No
Thyregod et al. [91]	NOTION	280	2015	CoreValve	Echo	3 months	23.4	61.3	14.5	0.8	96.5	N/A
Herrmann et al. [92]	PARTNER II US	583	2016	Sapien 3	Echo	30 days	64.3	33.2	2.5	None	84.2	Yes
Vahanian et al. [93]	Registry	101	2016	Sapien 3	Echo	30 days	23.0	26.4	2.3	None	100	Yes
Kodali et al. [94]	Registry	1661	2016	Sapien 3	Echo	30 days	55.9	40.7	3.4	None	86.9	Yes
Popma et al. [95]	Evolut R US	241	2017	Evolut R	Echo	30 days	62.6	32.2	5.3	None	89.5	Yes
Reardon et al. [96]	SURTAVI	1746	2017	CoreValve 84% Evolut R 16%	Echo	Discharge	63.0	33.7	3.3	0.1	N/A	Yes
Wendler et al. [97]	SOURCE 3	1947	2017	Sapien 3	Echo	30 days	73.7	23.3	3	0.1	87.1	No

Studies reporting the incidence of none and trace PAR or of moderate and severe PAR under one category are represented in a single cell

Echo echocardiography, *Angio* angiography, *TTE* transthoracic echocardiography, *TEE* transesophageal echocardiography

residual AR was seven times higher after TAVI than after SAVR. This finding was confirmed in a separate analysis of observational and randomized trials, with a stronger signal in randomized trials, which were more likely to use a core laboratory. The effect was similar in high-risk and in low-risk patients. Another meta-analysis [4], which included four randomized trials, two with the self-expandable (SE) CoreValve (Medtronic, Minneapolis, Minnesota) and two with the Edwards Sapien valve (Edwards Lifesciences, Irvine, California), found that moderate or severe AR was six times more likely to occur after TAVI when compared to SAVR. However, there was significant statistical heterogeneity between trials.

Even if these meta-analyses give a clear signal in favor of an increased risk of PAR after TAVI, the precise assessment of PAR incidence after TAVI is difficult due to the high variability between studies and the differences in the reported severity of AR. This heterogeneity is caused by several factors: (1) use of various methods of imagery for evaluating PAR, like transthoracic echocardiography (TTE), transesophageal echocardiography (TEE), and aortic angiography; (2) frequent absence of a core laboratory, especially in the early period of the technique; (3) variability in the moment of assessment of PAR (periprocedural, at discharge or at 30 days); (4) use of different grading schemes; and (5) the evolution of various TAVI devices and improvement in technique. The publication of the Valve Academic Research Consortium (VARC) consensus report in 2011 overcomes the inherent limitations of the initial publications of TAVI outcomes, including the evaluation of PAR [5]. An update version appeared in 2012 [6].

The interventional community and the industry responded to the issue of PAR by improving the technique and the devices used. Last-generation THV were conceived with the goal of decreasing the risk of PAR. The impact of valve design can be seen with the reduction of PAR obtained with the Sapien 3 THV (Edwards Lifesciences, Irvine, California) when compared with previous models and in the very low rate of moderate or severe residual PAR obtained with the Lotus Valve (Boston Scientific, Natick, MA,

USA), of 1% [7], or the Direct Flow valve (Direct Flow Medical, Santa Rosa, CA, USA), 1.2% [8].

Moderate to severe PAR was observed in 1.6% after Sapien 3 implantation compared to 6.9% after Sapien XT, according to the meta-analysis performed by Ando et al. [9]. Another meta-analysis confirmed these findings, with a lower incidence of PAR with the Sapien 3 valve: 5.58% vs. 19.35%, OR: 0.27 [10]. The improvement with the Evolut-R THV as compared to the previous CoreValve is less spectacular: the Swiss registry, using VARC-2 definitions, found no significant difference in PAR ≥ 2 between the two devices (8.5% vs. 10.6%) [11]. However, the analysis of SE devices from the TVT registry found a significant reduction of moderate or severe PAR in favor of Evolut-R: 4.4% vs. 6.2%, $p < 0.001$ [12]. The latest generation of Evolut PRO valve showed no moderate or severe regurgitation in the pilot study including 60 patients [13]. The majority of patients, 72.4%, showed absent or trace PAR. While the interpretation of these results is of course limited by the small sample size and non-randomized selection of patients, the data suggest a significant improvement in annular sealing added by the presence of the external pericardial wrap on the distal portion of the metallic frame.

Various comparisons of the balloon-expandable (BE) and SE THV exist in the literature, but the majority are observational [14–18]. The CHOICE trial was the first trial to perform a randomized comparison of the Sapien XT and CoreValve THV [19]. The incidence of more than mild PAR was significantly lower with the Sapien XT valve, 4.1% vs. 18.3%, RR 0.23; 95% CI 0.09–0.58; $p < 0.01$. These findings were confirmed in a recent analysis of the French registry [20], where the use of the self-expanding THV was associated with a higher risk of significant PAR: OR 2.03 [1.46–2.83], $P < 0.0001$. The comparative meta-analysis by Agarwal et al. [21], which included 35,347 patients from 5 randomized trials and 28 multicenter registries, reported a higher incidence of moderate or severe PAR with the CoreValve THV, 15.5% vs. 8.9%. The difference between the next generation of BE and SE devices, the Sapien 3 and the Evolut R, is less important, but the statistical power of the available studies is limited [15, 17, 18]. Two of these studies found comparable rates of moderate or severe PAR, while one found a higher rate with the Evolut R device.

A novel SE device, the Symetis Acurate Neo TF™, presented a statistically nonsignificant difference in moderate or severe PAR, when compared to the Sapien 3 THV [22].

14.3 Causes and Predictors

The presence of a residual PAR after TAVI logically depends on the presence of a free space between the prosthesis and the native annular complex, including the native leaflets, the aortic annulus, and the left ventricular outflow tract (LVOT). Secondly, the annular sealing is generally performed by a tissue skirt attached to the stent frame, which has an external component in the last generation Sapien 3 and Evolut Pro THV. The Lotus Valve System comes with an external adaptive seal, and the Direct flow THV presents an inflatable aortic and ventricular ring designed to minimize the risk of PAR.

Taking these two factors into account, it can be deduced that all situation that will tend to decrease the contact between the sealing part of the prosthesis and the native annular complex will lead to residual PAR. Several factors have been described in the literature [23–28]. The meta-analysis by Athappan et al. [29] found three major predictors of PAR: (1) valve undersizing, (2) aortic valve calcification, and (3) implantation depth.

14.3.1 Undersizing

Undersizing of the prosthesis will fail to generate a good apposition on the native annulus, increasing the risk of PAR. Various studies have confirmed this hypothesis [23, 30, 31]. Détaint et al. [23] first introduced the "cover index," defined as [(prosthesis diameter − TEE annulus diameter)/prosthesis diameter] × 100. Residual AR ≥ 2 was not observed in patients with a cover index >8%, which actually represents an oversize over 8%.

While the initial studies of the cover index reported 2D diameters generally measured using TEE, it has been observed that 3D measurements are superior in predicting the occurrence of PAR [26, 32–34]. The use of 3D MSCT measures leads to a decrease in the incidence of PAR, as compared to 2D TEE measurements [33, 35]. It is widely accepted based on comparative studies that echocardiography tends to underestimate the annulus diameter and it is highly influenced by the oval shape of the annulus [26]. MSCT measurements are highly reproducible, and an oversize calculation based on annular area seems optimal as it is less influenced by the eccentricity of the annulus. An area oversize of 10% or more is associated with a significant reduction in PAR [34, 36]. It is important to underline that the majority of these studies were performed using the Edwards THV system.

14.3.2 Aortic Valve Calcification

Aortic valve calcification has been reported as a predictor of PAR in multiple studies [27, 36–40]. Interestingly, an analysis of the German registry did not find an association between the severity of the annular calcification and PAR, but it used a subjective visual assessment of the degree of calcification [41]. The degree of calcification can be quantified using the Agatston score or calcium volume scoring. The location of the calcification is important in anticipating significant residual PAR, as is its asymmetrical distribution [36]. Presence of LVOT calcium seems to have a particular importance. The presence of any amount of LVOT calcification was the only independent predictor of more than mild PAR in a study with the Sapien THV [26]. It was also found to be an independent predictor of PAR after Lotus valve implantation, while the volume of the aortic valvar complex did not reach statistical significance [27]. In a study including multiple devices, increasing annular complex calcification was associated with AR only if more than 10 mm^3 of LVOT calcium was present [25]. Location of calcium at the commissures is another significant predictor of residual PAR [38].

14.3.3 Implantation Depth

Implantation depth is a particular issue especially for the CoreValve THV, as this device is longer and allows for a higher range of implantation depths compared with the BE THV. The depth of implantation is a predictor of PAR after CoreValve implantation [28, 30, 42–44]. A deep implantation leads to PAR because it reduces the sealing provided by the tissue skirt and leaks are possible above the skirt through the stent struts. A high implantation will not assure a good and complete contact between the valve and the annulus or the LVOT. A small pilot study found an optimal implantation depth of 10 mm [42], which deep by current standards. A larger study reported a mean implantation depth of 6.7 mm in patients having less than moderate PAR [28]. The optimal depth has to minimize the risk of pacemaker implantation (recommended depth <6 mm [45]), and the final target implantation depth is the best trade-off between the risk of pacemaker implantation and significant PAR. The target implant depth actually recommended by the manufacturer is between 3 and 5 mm.

14.3.4 Aortic Root Angulation

Another problem which seems to be specific to the SE THV due to its length and interaction with the aortic root is that of aortic angulation [24, 42]. Greater angle between the LVOT and the aortic root has been associated with an increased risk of PAR in a pilot study [42]. Abramowitz et al. confirmed this finding in a larger cohort and found that an angle between the horizontal and annular planes greater than 48° best predicts the risk of significant PAR [24]. In contrast, aortic angulation did not impact the success of BE valve implantation.

14.4 Assessment

Multiple methods can be used to assess PAR, and a multiparametric approach is generally recommended. The imaging techniques are (1) aortic angiography; (2) invasive hemodynamic pressure measurement (e.g., aortic regurgitation index); (3) echocardiography: TTE and TEE, the latter requiring general anesthesia; and (4) cardiovascular magnetic resonance imaging (CMR). Natriuretic peptides can give an estimation of the importance of the PAR.

14.4.1 Aortic Angiography

Aortic angiography is performed by injecting 20–40 mL of contrast medium in the ascending aorta generally at 15 mL/s via a pigtail catheter. The angiography is performed in the right anterior oblique 30° projection or in the left anterior oblique projection 20° to 30°. The pigtail should be place 2 cm above the valve. It is best to perform the injection once the hemodynamics have normalized after implantation. Some protocols required a delay of 10 min after SE TAVI in order to allow full expansion of the device [30].

The Sellers classification [46] includes four grades of aortic regurgitation: grade 0, absence of aortic regurgitation; grade 1, small amount of contrast entering the left ventricle (LV) during diastole without filling the entire cavity and clearing with each cardiac cycle; grade 2, contrast filling of the entire LV in diastole, but with less density as compared to contrast opacification of the ascending aorta; grade 3, contrast filling of the entire LV in diastole equal in density to the contrast opacification of the ascending aorta; and grade 4, contrast filling of the entire LV in diastole on the first beat with greater density as compared to the contrast opacification of the ascending aorta.

The angiographic method represents a semi-quantitative assessment of aortic regurgitation and is subject to various limitations. It is characterized by possible inter-operator variability since it is a subjective visual evaluation. Position of the pigtail catheter and the quantity of contrast will influence the apparent AR severity. Angiography characterizes total AR, including transvalvular and PAR. Since operators need to quantify the severity of PAR in order to see if further intervention is needed, sometimes the angiography is performed with the LV guidewire across the valve which can cause additional, artificial AR, due to incomplete valve closure. While performing the aortography without the guidewire across the valve will solve this problem, recrossing the valve if post-dilatation is needed can create the risk of passing in the paravalvular space in some cases. Hemodynamic parameters, like high blood pressure, can lead to overestimation of the grade of AR, while elevated heart rate can provoke an underestimation due to a shorter diastole.

The new angiographic technique using videodensitometry correlates well with CMR grading and has a low interobserver variability [47].

14.4.2 Hemodynamic Indices

Hemodynamic indices for evaluating PAR are an attractive idea since they are independent of the various echocardiographic limitations which characterize paravalvular jets. Sinning et al. [30] proposed a dimensionless AR index defined as $[(DBP - LVEDP)/SBP] \times 100$ where DBP is the diastolic blood pressure, LVEDP is the left ventricular end-diastolic pressure, and SBP is the systolic blood pressure. The pressure measurement was made 10–15 min after implantation, and all patients received the CoreValve THV. The AR index decreased proportionally to the increase in echocardiographic severity of PAR. They found that an AR index <25 predicted a significant increase in 1-year mortality: HR: 2.9, 95% CI: 1.3–6.4; $p < 0.009$. Since the AR index can be evaluated periprocedurally, it allows the operator to decide if further intervention for reducing PAR is needed. Several factors can render the AR index imprecise. An elevated LVDEP before implantation, from causes independent of the presence of PAR, will tend to underestimate the AR index and therefore overestimate PAR severity. A rapid heart will increase DBP and the AR index, underestimating the real PAR severity.

The discriminating value of the AR index has not been confirmed in two other studies that assessed the impact of PAR on mortality. In a larger German cohort of 723 patients implanted with both types of valves, 1-year mortality was similar in patients with an AR index >25 and those with an AR index <25 [48]. Höllriegel et al. found that the AR index did not predict 1-year mortality in the univariate analysis, in a population implanted with SE and BE valves [49].

Another proposed hemodynamic index is the diastolic pressure time (DPT) index [49]. It was formulated in order to account for the duration of the diastole and the variation in SBP. It is calculated as the ratio between the area between the aortic and left ventricular pressure-time curves and diastolic duration. It is then adjusted by accounting for the SBP: DPT index adjusted = (DPT index/SBP) × 100. It was significantly higher in patients with less than moderate angiographic AR and an independent predictor of 1-year mortality. It was also superior to the AR index in predicting mortality and had a significantly higher area under the ROC curve. Further studies are needed to confirm its value. An important limitation of this index is its relative complexity.

14.4.3 Echocardiography

Echocardiography, including TTE, TEE, and 3D echocardiography (3D TTE), is the most used method for evaluating PAR. TEE is usually used during periprocedural assessment and requires general anesthesia. Due to a gradual shift toward a minimalist approach to TAVI and increased use of conscious sedation [50], TEE is used less often during the TAVI procedure. 3D TTE had better concordance with CMR grading of PAR than TTE, in a study comparing the three techniques and using VARC-2 definitions. Correlation between regurgitation fraction (RF) assessed by 3D TTE and CMR imaging was superior to correlation between RF by 2D TTE and CMR imaging [32]. 3D TTE also has lower interobserver variability, but it is of course subject to the same limitations of echogenicity.

The severity of aortic regurgitation can be evaluated using semiquantitative measures and quantitative measures. The semiquantitative measures include vena contracta width, pressure halftime, jet width in the left ventricular outflow tract, diastolic flow reversal in the descending aorta, and the more recently introduced circum-

Table 14.2 Comparative echocardiographic criteria for PAR evaluation according to the VARC-2 definitions and the new unifying 5-class grading scheme

VARC-2	Mild		Moderate		Severe
Unifying 5-class grading scheme	Mild	Mild to moderate	Moderate	Moderate to severe	Severe
Semi-quantitative parameters					
Diastolic flow reversal in the descending aorta	Absent or brief early diastolic		Intermediate		Prominent, holodiastolic
	Absent or brief early diastolic	Intermediate	Intermediate	Holodiastolic (end-diastolic velocity >20 and <30 cm/s)	Holodiastolic (end-diastolic velocity ≥30 cm/s)
Circumferential extent of prosthetic valve paravalvular regurgitation (%)	<10		10 to 20		≥30
	<5	5 to <10	10 to <20	20 to <30	≥30
Quantitative parameters					
Regurgitant volume (mL/beat)		<30		30–59	≥60
	<15	15 to <30	30 to <45	45 to <60	≥60
Regurgitant fraction (%)	<30		30–49		≥50
	<15	<15 to 30	30 to <40	40 to <50	≥50
EROA (cm²)	0.10		0.10 to 0.29		≥0.30
	<5	5 to <10	10 to <20	20 to <30	≥0.30

EROA effective regurgitant orifice area, *PAR* paravalvular aortic regurgitation. Adapted from Kappetein et al. [6] and Ruiz et al. [52]

ferential extent of prosthetic valve paravalvular regurgitation. The used quantitative measures are regurgitation volume, regurgitation fraction, and the regurgitant orifice area. Echocardiographic criteria for PAR evaluation according to the VARC-2 consensus and the new 5-class grading scheme are presented in Table 14.2.

Precise assessment of PAR is challenging due to multiple factors. PAR can present multiple jets, and global quantification can be difficult. Since echocardiographic criteria having been developed for native valves and central jets, their application to eccentric, paravalvular leaks that do not fulfill the same hemodynamic assumptions can lead to imprecise grading. The paravalvular leak is generated by an irregular orifice that will provoke an eccentric, usually high velocity jet with a wide spray that can be overestimated by visual Doppler assessment. The quantitative PISA method assumes a hemispherical isovelocity area and a regular regurgitation jet that applies best for central valvular regurgitation.

The last guidelines for grading PAR use three grades, divided in mild, moderate, and severe, while the previous ones used a 4-grade classification, grade 3 being considered moderate to severe [51]. The difference in grading adds to the difficulty of a uniform assessment of PAR between studies. The latest expert statement defining paravalvular leaks in surgical prosthesis adopted a 5-grade classification Scheme [52], previously proposed by Pibarot et al. [53]. It grades PAR in (1) mild, (2) mild to moderate, (3) moderate, (4) moderate to severe, and (5) severe.

A particular method of quantifying PAR, found in the VARC criteria and in the 2009 ASE recommendations for prosthetic valve evaluation [51], is the circumferential extent of the jet. However, the cutoff for severe PAR is different in the two documents, being 30% in the VARC-2 document and 20% in the ASE recommendations. The circumferential extent is evaluated in the parasternal short-axis view, by carefully sweeping the probe toward the cranial end of the prosthesis in order to find the origin and the narrowest portion of the jet. In case of multiple jets, the evaluation becomes difficult, since the jet origins are not always at the same level. An addition is performed, and the jet is located using a clocklike orientation in a horizontal plane. The location of the jets is usually at the level of valve commissures or at the level of a calcific nodule, due to malapposition of the stent [53]. A footnote in the VARC-2 consensus warns that this criterion is not well-validated and may overestimate the severity compared with the quantitative Doppler.

14.4.4 Magnetic Resonance Imaging

Magnetic resonance imaging (MRI) is an emerging valuable method for evaluating aortic regurgitation in native and prosthetic valves. It is based on the velocity-encoded cardiovascular magnetic resonance imaging (CMR), also known as phase-contrast flow quantification, as a way of measuring blood flow [54]. CMR is considered as the "gold standard" for measuring LV mass, function, and volumes [55]. It requires an 8- to 16-s breath hold [55]. An image slice perpendicular to the flow direction is chosen, and an encoding velocity is chosen, higher than flow velocity in order to avoid aliasing. Forward and regurgitant flow through the defined aortic region of interest, usually at the sino-tubular junction [54, 56] or proximal to the prosthesis [57] in case of PAR, is used to calculate regurgitant volumes and the regurgitant fraction (RF) [55]. CMR quantification of AR is characterized by excellent intraobserver and interobserver agreement, being superior to TTE in this regard [58]. It is limited by the presence of metallic implants, claustrophobia, breath-holding issues, metallic artifacts, and arrhythmias. CMR quantification cannot discriminate between central and paravalvular regurgitation, and it also includes the coronary blood flow, which can overestimate the degree of PAR.

The first study that assessed PAR after TAVI using CMR, published in 2011 by Sherif et al., included only 16 patients, all implanted with the Medtronic CoreValve [59]. It did not study the circumferential extent of the regurgitant jet, and the echographic evaluation was based mainly on jet with in the LVOT assessed in the parasternal long-axis view. A CMR RF less than 15% was graded mild, and a RF > 50% was graded severe, while 31–50% was classified as moderate to severe. It included aortic angiography as standard evaluation, which adds interesting information. The correlation between echocardiographic and CMR grading of PAR was very low, with a weighted kappa of 0.2. The agreement between angiography and CMR, however, had a kappa value of 0.72. When compared to CMR, TTE underestimated PAR severity in half of the patients.

In the comparative study of Ribeiro et al., the authors assessed AR before and after TAVI with TTE and CMR in 50 patients, the circumferential jet extent being included in the echocardiographic criteria [54]. Over 95% of THV were BE. There were three categories of PAR, the second category being categorized as "mild" instead of moderate, and the third collapsed moderate and severe into "moderate/severe." CMR cut point for severe AR was ≥30% and for mild AR < 20%. The agreement between TTE and CMR was higher before TAVI, becoming poor after TAVI, with a weighted kappa of 0.3. Post-TAVI AR was underestimated by multiparametric TTE in two-thirds of patients when compared to CMR. The circumferential extent of AR was poorly correlated with CMR grading, leading mostly to overestimation but also to underestimation of PAR grade (Fig. 14.1). The same tendency of overestimation when using the circumferential extent of AR was reported by Hartlage et al. [60], albeit this was a small sample study and used a RF of ≥40% for severe PAR.

Other authors sought the CMR cutoff for predicting more than mild PAR as evaluated by TTE and found the best discriminating value at 14% of RF, lower than the VARC-2 criterion. However, it is unclear which technique was considered the gold standard, and probably the cutoff is best determined by assessing the value that best predicts an impact on survival. Moderate to severe PAR, defined by a CMR RF ≥ 30%, had a negative impact on survival in a multicenter study of 135 patients, the evaluation being performed at 40 days post-TAVI [57].

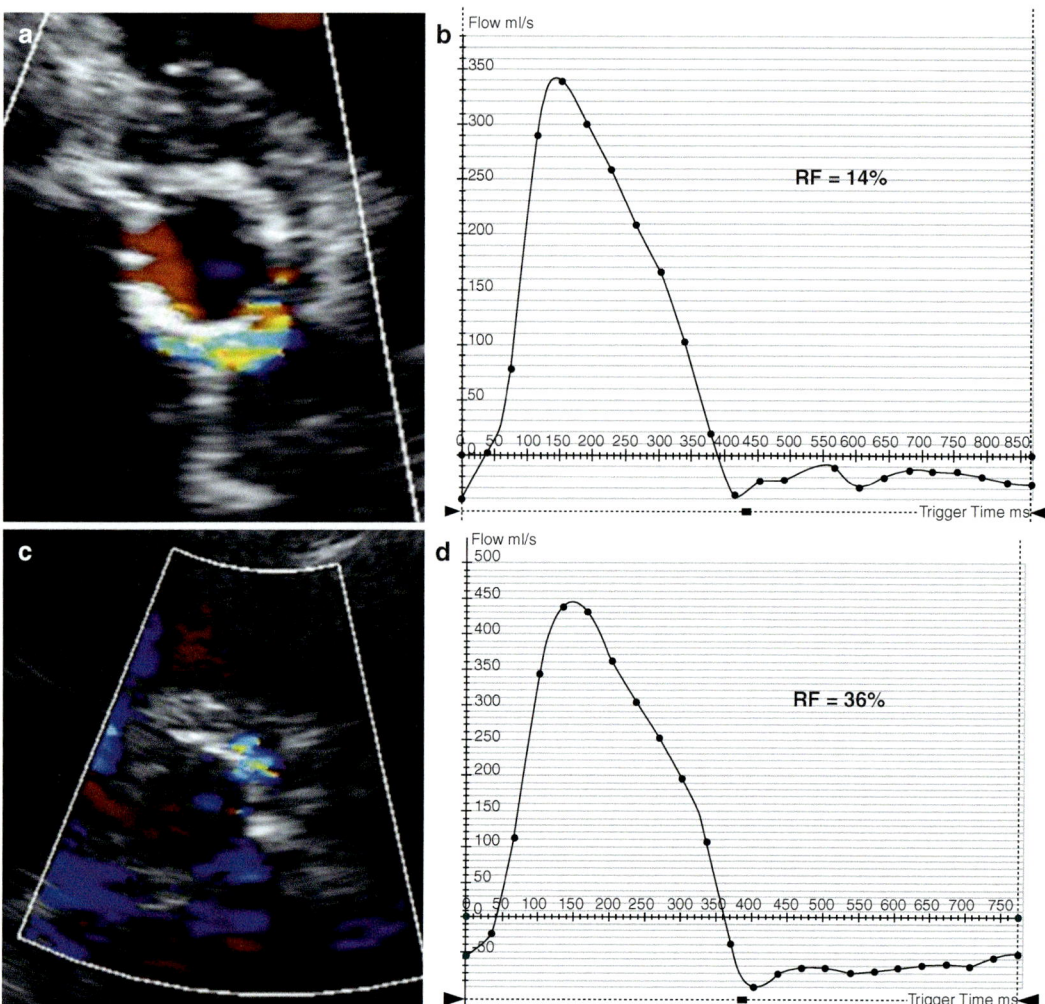

Fig. 14.1 Examples of discrepancies between echocardiographic and cardiac magnetic resonance (CMR) quantification of aortic regurgitation (AR). Example 1: transthoracic echocardiography showing jet arc length in the short-axis view that covers >30% of circumference (**a**) consistent with severe AR, whereas CMR shows a regurgitant fraction (RF) of 14% (**b**), which is consistent with mild AR by CMR. Example 2: transthoracic echocardiography showing jet arc length in the short-axis view that covers 10–20% of circumference (**c**) consistent with moderate AR, while CMR showed a RF of 36%, which is consistent with severe AR (**d**). From Ribeiro et al. [54] with permission

14.5 Impact on Mortality and Mechanisms

14.5.1 Impact

More than mild residual PAR after surgical valve replacement is associated with an almost double risk of mid-term mortality [2]. Given the much higher frequency of PAR after TAVI, its impact on mortality has been extensively studied. Various studies have confirmed an independent association between moderate or severe PAR and increased 1-year mortality, after multivariate analysis (Table 14.3). A meta-analysis of 45 studies, including 12,296 patients, has found a HR of 2.27 for increased 1-year mortality in patients with moderate or severe PAR [29]. Mild residual PAR was also associated with a higher risk of 1-year mortality, with a HR of 1.83, but it was no longer significant after sensitivity analysis. A more recent meta-analysis including 15,131 patients confirmed the negative impact on sur-

Table 14.3 Selected studies reporting the impact of PAR on mortality

Study author	Study title	N	Year	Valve type	Imaging	PAR grade	Impact on mortality	Time point
Tamburino et al. [84]	Italian registry	663	2011	CoreValve	Echo	Moderate or severe	HR 3.78; 95% CI: 1.57–9.10	1 year
Abdel-Wahab et al. [85]	German registry	690	2011	Sapien and CoreValve	Angio	Moderate or severe	OR 2.43, 95% CI: 1.22–4.85	Inhospital
Moat et al. [86]	UK	870	2011	Sapien and CoreValve	Angio	Moderate or severe	HR 1.66; 95% CI: 1.10–2.51	1 year
Gilard et al. [50]	France 2	3195	2012	Sapien/XT and CoreValve	Echo	Moderate or severe	HR 2.49; 95% CI: 1.91–3.25	1 year
Hayashida et al. [98]	Registry	400	2012	Edwards and CoreValve	Echo	Moderate or severe	HR 1.7; 95% CI: 1.13–2.56	Median 297 days
Kodali et al. [62]	PARTNER	699	2012	Sapien	Echo	Mild to severe	HR 2.11; 95% CI: 1.43–3.10	2 years
Zahn et al. [99]	GARY	1391	2013	Sapien and CoreValve	Angio	Moderate or severe	HR 2.43; 95% CI: 1.36–4.32	Inhospital
Linke et al. [90]	ADVANCE registry	996	2014	CoreValve	Echo	Moderate or severe	HR 1.63; 95% CI: 1.03–2.59 d	1 year
Van Belle et al. [20]	France 2	3195	2014	Edwards and CoreValve	Echo	Moderate or severe	HR 2.43; 95% CI: 1.83–3.25	Median 306 days
Kodali et al. [63]	PARTNER pooled	2434	2015	Sapien	Echo	Mild	HR 1.37; 95% CI: 1.14–1.90	1 year
Kodali et al. [63]	PARTNER pooled	2434	2015	Sapien	Echo	Moderate or severe	HR 2.18; 95% CI: 1.69–3.35	1 year
Herrmann et al. [92]	PARTNER II US	583	2016	Sapien 3	Echo	Moderate	HR 3.75; 95% CI: 1.57–8.96	1 year

PAR paravalvular aortic regurgitation, *HR* hazard ratio, *OR* odds ratio

vival of moderate or severe PAR, which doubles the risk of death at 1 year [61].

While the mortality risk associated with moderate or severe PAR is clearly established, the signals concerning a possible association of mild residual PAR and mortality should be interpreted carefully. The first study that reported an association between mild PAR and mortality was the 2-year follow-up analysis of the PARTNER A trial [62]. The authors later quantified the impact of mild PAR on mortality in a multivariate analysis of the PARTNER studies and ongoing registries, finding a moderate but significant effect: HR 1.37, $p = 0.012$ [63]. However, this effect was not confirmed in the US registry of the CoreValve THV [64]. The large real-life French registry, which included 3195 consecutive patients, found no association between post-procedural mild PAR and total cardiovascular mortality [65]. Another multicentric study using VARC-2 definitions, including 1735 patients implanted

with SE and BE THV, found no impact of mild PAR on mortality after a median follow-up of 21 ± 17 months.

A recent analysis of the PARTNER II SAPIEN 3 trial used a 5-class grading scheme to assess the impact of PAR on 1-year outcomes [66]. It included 1592 patients implanted with the Sapien 3 THV at 51 centers in the United States and Canada. Mild and even mild to moderate PAR, representing 32.6% and 8.2%, had no effect on 1-year mortality. This trial adds important information, addressing specifically the issue of PAR classification, which has been hypothesized as one explanation of finding a mortality impact for mild residual PAR after TAVI.

14.5.2 Mechanisms

Native moderate AR does not have an impact on mortality, and only patients with chronic severe AR present a possible indication for valvular replacement, when certain conditions are met [67]. Residual PAR after TAVI represents a volume overload on a ventricle adapted to a pressure overload, concentrically hypertrophied and non-compliant. The supplementary volume overload leads to elevated diastolic pressures, which is the pathophysiological basis of the AR index as an indicator of PAR severity [30]. However, an elevated diastolic pressure could be due to other factors, like diastolic dysfunction, which lowers the specificity of the index. Various data indicate that the impact of residual PAR after TAVI depends on the pre-existing hemodynamic conditions and previous adaptation of the left ventricle to a volume overload. The increase in LV end-diastolic volume provides hemodynamic compensation in AR.

The impact of moderate or severe PAR was dependent on the baseline level of NT-proBNP in a TAVI population implanted with the Edwards THV [68]. Patients with baseline NT-proBNP over the median were not affected by the presence of moderate or severe PAR, while patients with a low NT-proBNP had a significant higher risk of 2-year mortality, with a HR of 4.6. Natriuretic peptides were associated with larger LV diameters, pre-existing AR ≥ 2 and mitral regurgitation, indicating a previous adaptation to volume overload. The same mechanism is suggested by the strong interaction between the impact of moderate or severe PAR and the presence of AR at baseline in the FRANCE2 Registry [20]. In patients with baseline AR ≥ 2, residual AR ≥ 2 was not associated with increased 1-year mortality. A multicenter study taking into account the change in degree of AR after TAVI found that only acute moderate or severe AR (increase of at least 1 grade vs. baseline) had a negative impact on mortality, chronic moderate or severe AR after TAVI being mortality neutral [69]. One analysis of the Italian registry did not confirm the protective role of pre-existing AR [70]. It is found that LV dilation was protective in patients having a mixed, stenotic, and regurgitant disease at baseline. These data underline the thesis that it is the volumetric and hemodynamic baseline conditions that will influence how a patient will be affected by the residual PAR after implantation.

14.6 Treatment

Various measures have been described as useful for reducing residual PAR after TAVI implantation. Their indication and efficacy can be optimized by using a systematic approach after TAVI in (1) grading the severity of PAR and (2) identifying the mechanism responsible for PAR. While corrective measures should be envisaged in case of moderate or severe PAR, treatment of mild PAR should be reserved for patients in whom one anticipates poor tolerance of the AR (small ventricles, pure aortic stenosis, low pre-procedural level of natriuretic peptides). One also has to keep in mind a possible spontaneous reduction in PAR degree with the SE THV, as the nitinol frame continues to expand, a phenomenon suggested by the findings from the CoreValve US Pivotal Trial [71].

Grading of the PAR is usually performed immediately after deployment via aortography. TTE can also be used and can locate the site of the AR (e.g., paravalvular vs. transvalvular, at the level of a calcific nodule, etc.). The operator usually has two practical solutions, depending on the mechanism: (1) perform post-dilation or (2) implant a second valve. Snaring of a too deep SE THV has been described [72] but is less needed with the current recapturable generation and high implantation target zones.

14.6.1 Post-dilation

If the valve is implanted in a correct position, the presence of PAR can be reduced using post-dilation. The presence of severe calcium in a multicenter study using the BE THV post-dilation was needed in 28% of patients and reduced PAR by at least 1° in 71% of patients [73]. This analysis found that the volume of calcium and the transfemoral approach was independent predictors of the need of post-dilation, while severe calcification over 3874 mm^3 was the only predictor of unsuccessful post-dilation. The frequency of post-dilation seems to differ between types of valves in the large clinical randomized trials and registries. The analysis of PARTNER I randomized trial and registry reported a frequency of 12% [74], lower than the 22% found in the CoreValve US Clinical Trials [75], which is coherent with the higher frequency of PAR described after the SE THV implantation. The post-dilation after CoreValve implantation was highly efficacious, reducing the incidence of moderate or severe PAR by 75%. While the first study by Nombela-Franco et al. [73] reported an excess of cerebrovascular event in case of post-dilation, this was not confirmed by the larger trials with the BE and SE THV. Post-dilation appears to be a safe procedure, without an increased risk of neurological events or central AR. However, careful assessment of the position of the valve should be performed, since post-dilating a prosthesis implanted too high will increase the risk of embolization. The balloon should be adapted to the measured native aortic annulus and the size of the prosthesis in case of the SE THV, while generally 1 mL of volume is added in the balloon initially used to implant the BE THV. Massive calcification in the LVOT could expose the patient to the catastrophic risk of annular rupture, and the benefit of post-dilation should be assessed in function of PAR severity (Fig. 14.2).

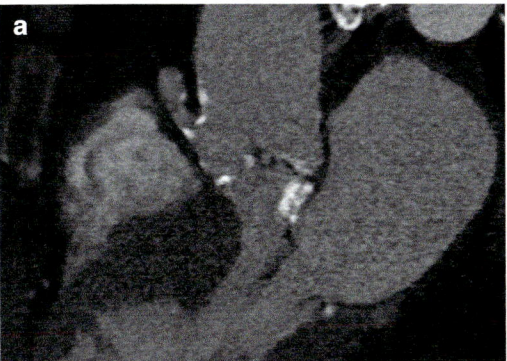

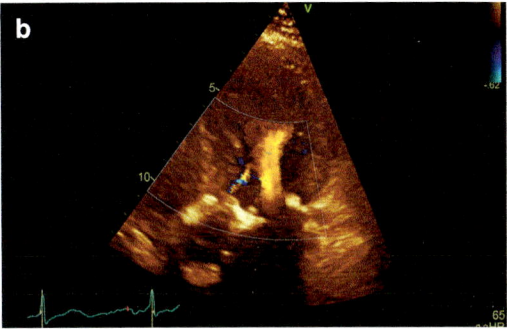

Fig. 14.2 Severe calcifications of the left ventricular outflow tract in patient implanted with a Sapien 3 valve (Panel **a**). In spite of intentional undersizing in order to avoid annular rupture, the final PAR was mild, illustrating the usefulness of the outer skirt (Panel **b**)

14.6.2 Implantation of a Second Valve: Valve-in-Valve Procedure

This technique represents an option in case of incorrect height of implantation, too ventricular or too aortic. The second valve is placed in order to seal the perivalvular space which was "missed" by the first valve. In case of a lower position of the first BE valve, the risk of ventricular migration should be kept in mind, especially if the valve was undersized, and coaxiality should be maintained at all times. In the Italian CoreValve registry, the need for a second valve was due to a too ventricular deployment in 75% of patients [76]. Interestingly in the PARTNER trial and registries with the Sapien valve, half of indications for a second prosthesis were due to a transvalvular AR with leaflet malfunction [77]. The risk of pacemaker implantation was increased, while the incidence of stroke and mortality was not statistically significant.

14.6.3 Percutaneous Paravalvular Leak Closure

This technique represents a later option of PAR reduction that is performed for significant symptoms associated with moderate or severe PAR. The device used is generally the Amplatzer Vascular Plug III (AVP III, AGA Medical Corp., Plymouth, Minnesota). It can be performed successfully [78], but the results are less favorable than with paravalvular closure after surgical valve replacement. The rate of success was only 60%, compared to 100% for surgical valve in a single-center series [79]. Various explanations for this finding are available. Since the native valve is in place, calcific nodules can impede the advancement of the material. Frequently, PAR post-TAVI presents multiple jets, and placement of a plug represents an incomplete solution. Another potential issue is interference with coronary flow. Cases selected for percutaneous closure should be carefully screened with pre-procedural imagery.

14.7 Conclusion

PAR is one of the major complications after TAVI, being significantly more frequent than after surgical valve replacement. However, the technical evolution in the field has been spectacular, and current devices have reduced the incidence of significant PAR to less than 5%. The assessment of PAR is complex and should be an integrative multimodal process. Standardized definitions and expert consensus are now available and should clarify the problem of grading and improve the coherence between various reports. MRI presents various advantages over classical echocardiographic evaluation. While a clear impact on mortality has been observed for moderate or severe PAR, the association of mild PAR and decreased survival observed in the PARTNER trial has not been confirmed in subsequent studies. PAR should be evaluated immediately after the procedure along with its mechanism, which allows for several corrective measures to be applied.

References

1. Généreux P, Head SJ, Hahn R, et al. Paravalvular leak after transcatheter aortic valve replacement: the new achilles' heel? A comprehensive review of the literature. J Am Coll Cardiol. 2013;61:1125–36.
2. Sponga S, Perron J, Dagenais F, Mohammadi S, Baillot R, Doyle D, Nalli C, Voisine P. Impact of residual regurgitation after aortic valve replacement. Eur J Cardiothorac Surg. 2012;42:486–92.
3. Villablanca PA, Mathew V, Thourani VH, et al. A meta-analysis and meta-regression of long-term outcomes of transcatheter versus surgical aortic valve replacement for severe aortic stenosis. Int J Cardiol. 2016;225:234–43.
4. Siontis GCM, Praz F, Pilgrim T, Mavridis D, Verma S, Salanti G, Søndergaard L, Jü Ni P, Windecker S. Transcatheter aortic valve implantation vs. surgical aortic valve replacement for treatment of severe aortic stenosis: a meta-analysis of randomized trials aortic stenosis transcatheter aortic valve replacement transcatheter aortic valve implantation Surg. Eur Heart J. 2016;37:3503–12.
5. Leon MB, Piazza N, Nikolsky E, et al. Standardized endpoint definitions for transcatheter aortic valve implantation clinical trials: a consensus report from the Valve Academic Research Consortium. Eur Heart J. 2011;32:205–17.
6. Kappetein AP, Head SJ, Généreux P, et al. Updated standardized endpoint definitions for transcatheter aortic valve implantation: the Valve Academic Research Consortium-2 consensus document. Eur Heart J. 2012;33:2403–18.
7. Am Meredith IT, Walters DL, Dumonteil N, et al. Transcatheter aortic valve replacement for severe symptomatic aortic stenosis using a repositionable valve system 30-day primary endpoint results from the REPRISE II study. J Am Coll Cardiol. 2014;64:1339–48.
8. Schofer J, Colombo A, Klugmann S, et al. Prospective multicenter evaluation of the direct flow medical® transcatheter aortic valve. J Am Coll Cardiol. 2013;63:763–8.
9. Ando T, Briasoulis A, Holmes AA, Taub CC, Takagi H, Afonso L. Sapien 3 versus Sapien XT prosthetic valves in transcatheter aortic valve implantation: a meta-analysis. Int J Cardiol. 2016;220:472–8.
10. Tummala R, Banerjee K, Sankaramangalam K, et al. Clinical and procedural outcomes with the SAPIEN 3 versus the SAPIEN XT prosthetic valves in transcatheter aortic valve replacement: a systematic review and meta-analysis. Catheter Cardiovasc Interv. 2017;92:E149–58. https://doi.org/10.1002/ccd.27398.
11. Noble S, Stortecky S, Heg D, et al. Comparison of procedural and clinical outcomes with Evolut R versus Medtronic CoreValve: a Swiss TAVI registry analysis. EuroIntervention. 2017;12:e2170–6.
12. Sorajja P, Kodali S, Reardon MJ, Szeto WY, Chetcuti SJ, Hermiller J, Chenoweth S, Adams DH, Popma JJ. Outcomes for the commercial use of self-expanding prostheses in transcatheter aortic valve replacement: a report from the STS/ACC TVT Registry. JACC Cardiovasc Interv. 2017;10:2090–8.
13. Forrest JK, Mangi AA, Popma JJ, et al. Early outcomes with the Evolut PRO repositionable self-expanding transcatheter aortic valve with pericardial wrap. JACC Cardiovasc Interv. 2018;11:181–91.
14. Chieffo A, Buchanan GL, Van Mieghem NM, et al. Transcatheter aortic valve implantation with the Edwards SAPIEN versus the medtronic corevalve revalving system devices: a multicenter collaborative study: the PRAGMATIC plus initiative (Pooled-RotterdAm-Milano-Toulouse in Collaboration). J Am Coll Cardiol. 2013;61:830–6.
15. Enríquez-Rodríguez E, Amat-Santos IJ, Jiménez-Quevedo P, et al. Comparison of the hemodynamic performance of the balloon-expandable SAPIEN 3 versus self-expandable Evolut R transcatheter valve: a case-matched study. Rev Esp Cardiol (Engl Ed). 2017;71:735–42. https://doi.org/10.1016/j.rec.2017.10.025.
16. Jatene T, Castro-Filho A, Meneguz-Moreno RA, et al. Prospective comparison between three TAVR devices: ACURATE neo vs. CoreValve vs. SAPIEN XT. A single heart team experience in patients with severe aortic stenosis. Catheter Cardiovasc Interv. 2017;90:139–46.

17. Rogers T, Steinvil A, Buchanan K, et al. Contemporary transcatheter aortic valve replacement with third-generation balloon-expandable versus self-expanding devices. J Interv Cardiol. 2017;30:356–61.

18. Ben-Shoshan J, Konigstein M, Zahler D, et al. Comparison of the Edwards SAPIEN S3 versus Medtronic Evolut-R devices for transcatheter aortic valve implantation. Am J Cardiol. 2017;119:302–7.

19. Abdel-Wahab M, Mehilli J, Frerker C, et al. Comparison of balloon-expandable vs self-expandable valves in patients undergoing transcatheter aortic valve replacement. JAMA. 2014;311:1503.

20. Van Belle E, Juthier F, Susen S, et al. Postprocedural aortic regurgitation in balloon-expandable and self-expandable transcatheter aortic valve replacement procedures: analysis of predictors and impact on long-term mortality: insights from the France2 registry. Circulation. 2014;129:1415–27.

21. Agarwal S, Parashar A, Kumbhani DJ, Svensson LG, Krishnaswamy A, Tuzcu EM, Kapadia SR. Comparative meta-analysis of balloon-expandable and self-expandable valves for transcatheter aortic valve replacement. Int J Cardiol. 2015;197:87–97.

22. Schaefer A, Linder M, Seiffert M, et al. Comparison of latest generation transfemoral self-expandable and balloon-expandable transcatheter heart valves. Interact Cardiovasc Thorac Surg. 2017;25:905–11.

23. Détaint D, Lepage L, Himbert D, Brochet E, Messika-Zeitoun D, Iung B, Vahanian A. Determinants of significant paravalvular regurgitation after transcatheter aortic valve implantation. Impact of device and annulus discongruence. JACC Cardiovasc Interv. 2009;2:821–7.

24. Abramowitz Y, Maeno Y, Chakravarty T, Kazuno Y, Takahashi N, Kawamori H, Mangat G, Cheng W, Jilaihawi H, Makkar RR. Aortic angulation attenuates procedural success following self-expandable but not balloon-expandable TAVR. JACC Cardiovasc Imaging. 2016;9:964–72.

25. Seiffert M, Fujita B, Avanesov M, et al. Device landing zone calcification and its impact on residual regurgitation after transcatheter aortic valve implantation with different devices. Eur Heart J Cardiovasc Imaging. 2016;17:576–84.

26. Jilaihawi H, Kashif M, Fontana G, Furugen A, Shiota T, Friede G, Makhija R, Doctor N, Leon MB, Makkar RR. Cross-sectional computed tomographic assessment improves accuracy of aortic annular sizing for transcatheter aortic valve replacement and reduces the incidence of paravalvular aortic regurgitation. J Am Coll Cardiol. 2012;59:1275–86.

27. Blackman DJ, Meredith IT, Dumonteil N, et al. Predictors of paravalvular regurgitation after implantation of the fully repositionable and retrievable lotus transcatheter aortic valve (from the REPRISE II Trial Extended Cohort). Am J Cardiol. 2017;120:292–9.

28. Ali OF, Schultz C, Jabbour A, et al. Predictors of paravalvular aortic regurgitation following self-expanding Medtronic CoreValve implantation: the role of annulus size, degree of calcification, and balloon size during pre-implantation valvuloplasty and implant depth. Int J Cardiol. 2015;179:539–45.

29. Athappan G, Patvardhan E, Tuzcu EM, et al. Incidence, predictors, and outcomes of aortic regurgitation after transcatheter aortic valve replacement: meta-analysis and systematic review of literature. J Am Coll Cardiol. 2013;61:1585–95.

30. Sinning JM, Hammerstingl C, Vasa-Nicotera M, et al. Aortic regurgitation index defines severity of peri-prosthetic regurgitation and predicts outcome in patients after transcatheter aortic valve implantation. J Am Coll Cardiol. 2012;59:1134–41.

31. Husser O, Rauch S, Endemann DH, et al. Impact of three-dimensional transesophageal echocardiography on prosthesis sizing for transcatheter aortic valve implantation. Catheter Cardiovasc Interv. 2012;80:956–63.

32. Altiok E, Frick M, Meyer CG, et al. Comparison of two- and three-dimensional transthoracic echocardiography to cardiac magnetic resonance imaging for assessment of paravalvular regurgitation after transcatheter aortic valve implantation. Am J Cardiol. 2014;113:1859–66.

33. Binder RK, Webb JG, Willson AB, et al. The impact of integration of a multidetector computed tomography annulus area sizing algorithm on outcomes of transcatheter aortic valve replacement: a prospective, multicenter, controlled trial. J Am Coll Cardiol. 2013;62:431–8.

34. Willson AB, Webb JG, Labounty TM, et al. 3-dimensional aortic annular assessment by multidetector computed tomography predicts moderate or severe paravalvular regurgitation after transcatheter aortic valve replacement: a multicenter retrospective analysis. J Am Coll Cardiol. 2012;59:1287–94.

35. Hansson NC, Thuesen L, Hjortdal VE, et al. Three-dimensional multidetector computed tomography versus conventional 2-dimensional transesophageal echocardiography for annular sizing in transcatheter aortic valve replacement: influence on postprocedural paravalvular aortic regurgitation. Catheter Cardiovasc Interv. 2013;82:977–86.

36. Kaneko H, Hoelschermann F, Tambor G, Yoon SH, Neuss M, Butter C. Predictors of paravalvular regurgitation after transcatheter aortic valve implantation for aortic stenosis using new-generation balloon-expandable SAPIEN 3. Am J Cardiol. 2017;119:618–22.

37. Ewe SH, Ng AC, Schuijf JD, et al. Location and severity of aortic valve calcium and implications for aortic regurgitation after transcatheter aortic valve implantation. Am J Cardiol. 2011;108:1470–7.

38. Delgado V, Ng ACT, van de Veire NR, et al. Transcatheter aortic valve implantation: role of multidetector row computed tomography to evaluate prosthesis positioning and deployment in relation to valve function. Eur Heart J. 2010;31:1114–23.

39. Blanke P, Pibarot P, Hahn R, et al. Computed tomography–based oversizing degrees and incidence of paravalvular regurgitation of a new generation

transcatheter heart valve. JACC Cardiovasc Interv. 2017;10:810–20.

40. Khalique OK, Hahn RT, Gada H, et al. Quantity and location of aortic valve complex calcification predicts severity and location of paravalvular regurgitation and frequency of post-dilation after balloon-expandable transcatheter aortic valve replacement. JACC Cardiovasc Interv. 2014;7:885–94.

41. Staubach S, Franke J, Gerckens U, et al. Impact of aortic valve calcification on the outcome of transcatheter aortic valve implantation: results from the prospective multicenter German TAVI registry. Catheter Cardiovasc Interv. 2013;81:348–55.

42. Sherif MA, Abdel-Wahab M, Stöcker B, Geist V, Richardt D, Tölg R, Richardt G. Anatomic and procedural predictors of paravalvular aortic regurgitation after implantation of the medtronic CoreValve bioprosthesis. J Am Coll Cardiol. 2010;56:1623–9.

43. Jilaihawi H, Chin D, Spyt T, Jeilan M, Vasa-nicotera M, Bence J, Logtens E, Kovac J. Prosthesis-patient mismatch after transcatheter aortic valve implantation with the Medtronic-Corevalve bioprosthesis. Eur Heart J. 2010;31:857–64.

44. Takagi K, Latib A, Al-Lamee R, Mussardo M, Montorfano M, Maisano F, Godino C, Chieffo A, Alfieri O, Colombo A. Predictors of moderate-to-severe paravalvular aortic regurgitation immediately after corevalve implantation and the impact of postdilatation. Catheter Cardiovasc Interv. 2011;45:432–43.

45. Petronio AS, Sinning J-M, Van Mieghem N, et al. Optimal implantation depth and adherence to guidelines on permanent pacing to improve the results of transcatheter aortic valve replacement with the Medtronic CoreValve System: The CoreValve Prospective, International, Post-Market ADVANCE-II Study. JACC Cardiovasc Interv. 2015;8: 837–46.

46. Sellers RD, Levy MJ, Amplatz K, Lillehei CW. Left retrograde cardioangiography in acquired cardiac disease: technic, indications and interpretations in 700 cases. Am J Cardiol. 1964;14:437–47.

47. Abdel-Wahab M, Abdelghani M, Miyazaki Y, et al. A novel angiographic quantification of aortic regurgitation after TAVR provides an accurate estimation of regurgitation fraction derived from cardiac magnetic resonance imaging. JACC Cardiovasc Interv. 2018;11:287–97.

48. Schoechlin S, Brennemann T, Allali A, Ruile P, Jander N, Allgeier M, Gick M, Richardt G, Neumann F-J, Abdel-Wahab M. Hemodynamic classification of paravalvular leakage after transcatheter aortic valve implantation compared with angiographic or echocardiographic classification for prediction of 1-year mortality. Catheter Cardiovasc Interv. 2017;91:E56–63. https://doi.org/10.1002/ccd.27384.

49. Höllriegel R, Woitek F, Stativa R, Mangner N, Haußig S, Fuernau G, Holzhey D, Mohr FW, Schuler GC, Linke A. Hemodynamic assessment of aortic regurgitation after transcatheter aortic valve replacement:

the Diastolic Pressure-Time Index. JACC Cardiovasc Interv. 2016;9:1061–8.

50. Gilard M, Eltchaninoff H, Iung B, et al. Registry of transcatheter aortic-valve implantation in high-risk patients. N Engl J Med. 2012;366:1705–15.

51. Zoghbi WA, Chambers JB, Dumesnil JG, et al. Recommendations for evaluation of prosthetic valves with echocardiography and doppler ultrasound: a report from the American Society of Echocardiography's Guidelines and Standards Committee and the Task Force on Prosthetic Valves, Developed in Conjunction. J Am Soc Echocardiogr. 2009;22:975–1014.

52. Ruiz CE, Hahn RT, Berrebi A, et al. Clinical trial principles and endpoint definitions for paravalvular leaks in surgical prosthesis: an expert statement. J Am Coll Cardiol. 2017;69:2067–87.

53. Pibarot P, Hahn RT, Weissman NJ, Monaghan MJ. Assessment of paravalvular regurgitation following TAVR: a proposal of unifying grading scheme. JACC Cardiovasc Imaging. 2015;8: 340–60.

54. Ribeiro HB, Le Ven F, Larose É, et al. Cardiac magnetic resonance versus transthoracic echocardiography for the assessment and quantification of aortic regurgitation in patients undergoing transcatheter aortic valve implantation. Heart. 2014;100:1924 LP–1932.

55. Myerson SG, D'arcy J, Mohiaddin R, Greenwood JP, Karamitsos TD, Francis JM, Banning AP, Christiansen JP, Neubauer S. Aortic regurgitation quantification using cardiovascular magnetic resonance: association with clinical outcome. Circulation. 2012;126:1452–60.

56. Salaun E, Jacquier A, Theron A, et al. Value of CMR in quantification of paravalvular aortic regurgitation after TAVI. Eur Heart J Cardiovasc Imaging. 2016;17:41–50.

57. Ribeiro HB, Orwat S, Hayek SS, et al. Cardiovascular magnetic resonance to evaluate aortic regurgitation after transcatheter aortic valve replacement. J Am Coll Cardiol. 2016;68:577–85.

58. Cawley PJ, Hamilton-Craig C, Owens DS, et al. Prospective comparison of valve regurgitation quantitation by cardiac magnetic resonance imaging and transthoracic echocardiography. Circ Cardiovasc Imaging. 2013;6:48–57.

59. Sherif MA, Abdel-Wahab M, Beurich H-W, Stöcker B, Zachow D, Geist V, Tölg R, Richardt G. Haemodynamic evaluation of aortic regurgitation after transcatheter aortic valve implantation using cardiovascular magnetic resonance. EuroIntervention. 2011;7:57–63.

60. Hartlage GR, Babaliaros VC, Thourani VH, Hayek S, Chrysohoou C, Ghasemzadeh N, Stillman AE, Clements SD, Oshinski JN, Lerakis S. The role of cardiovascular magnetic resonance in stratifying paravalvular leak severity after transcatheter aortic valve replacement: an observational outcome study. J Cardiovasc Magn Reson. 2014;16:93.

61. Takagi H, Umemoto T. Impact of paravalvular aortic regurgitation after transcatheter aortic valve implantation on survival. Int J Cardiol. 2016;221:46–51.

62. Kodali SK, Williams MR, Smith CR, et al. Two-year outcomes after transcatheter or surgical aortic-valve replacement. N Engl J Med. 2012;366:1686–95.

63. Kodali S, Pibarot P, Douglas PS, et al. Paravalvular regurgitation after transcatheter aortic valve replacement with the Edwards sapien valve in the PARTNER trial: characterizing patients and impact on outcomes. Eur Heart J. 2015;36:449–56.

64. Popma JJ, Adams DH, Reardon MJ, et al. Transcatheter aortic valve replacement using a self-expanding bioprosthesis in patients with severe aortic stenosis at extreme risk for surgery. J Am Coll Cardiol. 2014;63:1972–81.

65. Outcomes C, Voskuil M, Shao C, Van BE, Wildbergh T, Politi L, Doevendans PA, Sangiorgi GM, Stella PR. First results of the DEB-AMI (drug eluting balloon in acute ST-segment elevation myocardial infarction) trial. J Am Coll Cardiol. 2012;59:2327–37.

66. Pibarot P, Hahn RT, Weissman NJ, et al. Association of paravalvular regurgitation with 1-year outcomes after transcatheter aortic valve replacement with the SAPIEN 3 valve. JAMA Cardiol. 2017;2:1208.

67. Baumgartner H, Falk V, Bax JJ, et al. 2017 ESC/EACTS guidelines for the management of valvular heart disease. Eur Heart J. 2017;38:2739–91.

68. Borz B, Durand E, Godin M, Tron C, Canville A, Hauville C, Bauer F, Cribier A, Eltchaninoff H. Does residual aortic regurgitation after transcatheter aortic valve implantation increase mortality in all patients? The importance of baseline natriuretic peptides. Int J Cardiol. 2014;173:436–40.

69. Jerez-Valero M, Urena M, Webb JG, et al. Clinical impact of aortic regurgitation after transcatheter aortic valve replacement: insights into the degree and acuteness of presentation. JACC Cardiovasc Interv. 2014;7:1022–32.

70. Colli A, Besola L, Salizzoni S, et al. Does pre-existing aortic regurgitation protect from death in patients who develop paravalvular leak after TAVI? Int J Cardiol. 2017;233:52–60.

71. Oh JK, Little SH, Abdelmoneim SS, et al. Regression of paravalvular aortic regurgitation and remodeling of self-expanding transcatheter aortic valve: an observation from the CoreValve U.S. Pivotal Trial. JACC Cardiovasc Imaging. 2015;8:1364–75.

72. Sinning JM, Vasa-Nicotera M, Chin D, Hammerstingl C, Ghanem A, Bence J, Kovac J, Grube E, Nickenig G, Werner N. Evaluation and management of paravalvular aortic regurgitation after transcatheter aortic valve replacement. J Am Coll Cardiol. 2013;62:11–20.

73. Nombela-franco L, Rodés-cabau J, Delarochellière R, et al. Predictive factors, efficacy, and safety of balloon post-dilation after transcatheter aortic valve implantation with a balloon-expandable valve. JACC Cardiovasc Interv. 2012;5:499–512.

74. Hahn RT, Pibarot P, Webb J, et al. Outcomes with post-dilation following transcatheter aortic valve

replacement: the PARTNER I trial (placement of aortic transcatheter valve). JACC Cardiovasc Interv. 2014;7:781–9.

75. Harrison JK, Hughes GC, Reardon MJ, Stoler R, Grayburn P, Hebeler R, Liu D, Chang Y, Popma JJ, Investigators CUC. Balloon post-dilation following implantation of a self-expanding transcatheter aortic valve bioprosthesis. JACC Cardiovasc Interv. 2017;10:168–75.

76. Ussia GP, Barbanti M, Ramondo A, et al. The valve-in-valve technique for treatment of aortic bioprosthesis malposition: an analysis of incidence and 1-year clinical outcomes from the Italian CoreValve Registry. J Am Coll Cardiol. 2011;57:1062–8.

77. Makkar RR, Jilaihawi H, Chakravarty T, et al. Determinants and outcomes of acute transcatheter valve-in-valve therapy or embolization: a study of multiple valve implants in the U.S. PARTNER trial (placement of aortic transcatheter valve trial Edwards SAPIEN transcatheter heart valve). J Am Coll Cardiol. 2013;62:418–30.

78. Sinning J-M, Vasa-Nicotera M, Werner N, Nickenig G, Hammerstingl C. Interventional closure of paravalvular leakage after transcatheter aortic valve implantation. Eur Heart J. 2012;33:2498.

79. Saia F, Martinez C, Gafoor S, et al. Long-term outcomes of percutaneous paravalvular regurgitation closure after transcatheter aortic valve replacement: a multicenter experience. JACC Cardiovasc Interv. 2015;8:681–8.

80. Leon MB, Smith CR, Mack M, et al. Transcatheter aortic-valve implantation for aortic stenosis in patients who cannot undergo surgery. N Engl J Med. 2010;363:1597–607.

81. Eltchaninoff H, Prat A, Gilard M, et al. Transcatheter aortic valve implantation: early results of the FRANCE (FRench Aortic National CoreValve and Edwards) registry. Eur Heart J. 2011;32:191–7.

82. Thomas M, Schymik G, Walther T, et al. Thirty-day results of the SAPIEN aortic bioprosthesis European outcome (SOURCE) registry. Circulation. 2010;122:62–9.

83. Smith C, Leon M, Mack M. Transcatheter versus surgical aortic-valve replacement in high-risk patients. N Engl J Med. 2011;364:2187–98.

84. Tamburino C, Capodanno D, Ramondo A, et al. Incidence and predictors of early and late mortality after transcatheter aortic valve implantation in 663 patients with severe aortic stenosis. Circulation. 2011;123:299–308.

85. Abdel-wahab M, Zahn R, Horack M, Gerckens U, Schuler G, Sievert H, Eggebrecht H, Senges J. Aortic regurgitation after transcatheter aortic valve implantation : incidence and early outcome. Results from the German transcatheter aortic valve interventions registry. Heart. 2011;97:899–907.

86. Moat NE, Ludman P, M a d B, et al. Long-term outcomes after transcatheter aortic valve implantation in high-risk patients with severe aortic stenosis: the U.K. TAVI (United Kingdom Transcatheter Aortic

Valve Implantation) Registry. J Am Coll Cardiol. 2011;58:2130–8.

87. Webb J, Gerosa G, Lefèvre T, Leipsic J, Spence M, Thomas M, Thielmann M, Treede H, Wendler O, Walther T. Multicenter evaluation of a next-generation balloon-expandable transcatheter aortic valve. J Am Coll Cardiol. 2014;64:2235–43.

88. Adams DH, Popma JJ, Reardon MJ, et al. Transcatheter aortic-valve replacement with a self-expanding prosthesis. N Engl J Med. 2014;370:1790–8.

89. Schofer J, Colombo A, Klugmann S, et al. Prospective multicenter evaluation of the direct flow medical transcatheter aortic valve. J Am Coll Cardiol. 2014;63:763–8.

90. Linke A, Wenaweser P, Gerckens U, et al. Treatment of aortic stenosis with a self-expanding transcatheter valve: the International Multi-centre ADVANCE Study Aortic stenosis Transcatheter aortic valve implantation CoreValve Valvuloplasty Mortality. Eur Heart J. 2014;35:2672–84.

91. Thyregod HGH, Steinbrüchel DA, Ihlemann N, et al. Transcatheter versus surgical aortic valve replacement in patients with severe aortic valve stenosis: 1-year results from the all-comers NOTION randomized clinical trial. J Am Coll Cardiol. 2015;65:2184–94.

92. Herrmann HC, Thourani VH, Kodali SK, et al. One-year clinical outcomes with SAPIEN 3 transcatheter aortic valve replacement in high-risk and inoperable patients with severe aortic stenosis. Circulation. 2016;134:130–40.

93. Vahanian A, Urena M, Walther T, et al. Thirty-day outcomes in patients at intermediate risk for surgery from the SAPIEN 3 European approval trial. EuroIntervention. 2016;12:e235–43.

94. Kodali S, Thourani VH, White J, et al. Early clinical and echocardiographic outcomes after SAPIEN 3 transcatheter aortic valve replacement in inoperable, high-risk and intermediate-risk patients with aortic stenosis. Eur Heart J. 2016;37:2252–62.

95. Popma JJ, Reardon MJ, Khabbaz K, et al. Early clinical outcomes after transcatheter aortic valve replacement using a novel self-expanding bioprosthesis in patients with severe aortic stenosis who are suboptimal for surgery. JACC Cardiovasc Interv. 2017;10:268–75.

96. Reardon MJ, Van Mieghem NM, Popma JJ, et al. Surgical or transcatheter aortic-valve replacement in intermediate-risk patients. N Engl J Med. 2017;376:1321–31.

97. Wendler O, Schymik G, Treede H, Baumgartner H, Dumonteil N, Ihlberg L, Neumann FJ, Tarantini G, Zamarano JL, Vahanian A. SOURCE 3 Registry: design and 30-day results of the European post-approval registry of the latest generation of the Sapien 3 transcatheter heart valve. Circulation. 2017;135:1123–32.

98. Hayashida K, Lefèvre T, Chevalier B, Hovasse T, Romano M, Garot P, Bouvier E. Impact of postprocedural aortic regurgitation on mortality after transcatheter aortic valve implantation. JACC Cardiovasc Interv. 2012;5:1247–56.

99. Zahn R, Gerckens U, Linke A, et al. Predictors of one-year mortality after transcatheter aortic valve implantation for severe symptomatic aortic stenosis. Am J Cardiol. 2013;112:272–9.

Leaflet Motion Abnormality Following Transcatheter Aortic Valve Implantation

Luca Testa, Matteo Casenghi,
Antonio Popolo Rubbio, Magdalena Cuman,
and Francesco Bedogni

Transcatheter aortic valve implantation (TAVI), also called transcatheter aortic valve replacement (TAVR), has become a well-established technique for treating severe aortic stenosis. Although to date reassuring data coming from PARTNER 1 trial shows no structural valve deterioration in TAVI group at 5 years, valve dysfunction may occur over time [1]. Causes of valve dysfunction can be classified in (1) structural valve deterioration (i.e., calcification, leaflet fibrosis, tear, or flail), (2) non-structural valve deterioration (i.e., intra- or para-prosthetic, regurgitation, prosthesis malposition, patient-prosthesis mismatch), (3) thrombosis, and (4) endocarditis.

Transcatheter aortic valve thrombosis (TAVT), albeit rare, is a known and potentially dramatic clinical manifestation. Part of the spectrum of valve thrombosis, subclinical leaflet motion abnormalities may result in "hypoattenuated leaflet thickening" (HALT) and/or "reduced leaflet motion" (RELM). HALT and RELM are relatively recent entities in the field of transcatheter aortic valves and are more frequent than symptomatic bioprosthetic aortic valve thrombosis.

L. Testa (✉) · M. Casenghi · F. Bedogni
Department of Cardiology, IRCCS Policlinico San
Donato, San Donato Milanese, Milan, Italy
e-mail: Francesco.Bedogni@grupposandonato.it

A. P. Rubbio
Department of Cardiology, University of Catania,
Catania, Italy

M. Cuman
Department of Cardiology, University of Verona,
Verona, Italy

Although valve thrombosis is a multifactorial phenomenon determined by the interplay of clinical, anatomic, procedural, and pharmacological factors, three main mechanisms according to Virchow's triad could be identified. These mechanisms involve valve surface, hemodynamic and homeostasis. Valve surface itself may promote thrombosis through adhesion of platelets, leukocytes, and red blood cells, thrombin generation, and complement activation. Incomplete prosthesis endothelialization, leaflet damage, and leaflet deterioration may further promote the activation of the coagulation cascade. Hemodynamic factors such as low cardiac output, valve malpositioning, and prosthetic hemodynamic profile may facilitate thrombus formation. Recently it has been hypothesized that TAV deployment may generate neo-sinus, the region between native and transcatheter aortic valve leaflets, in which complex flow patterns are implicated in valve thrombosis [2]. Lastly, homeostatic factors as primary or secondary hypercoagulable state or suboptimal anticoagulation therapy play a central role in pathogenesis of leaflet motion abnormalities.

15.1 Transcatheter Aortic Valve Thrombosis (TAVT)

Valve thrombosis has been defined, according to Valve Academic Research Consortium 2 criteria as "any thrombus attached to or near an implanted

© Springer Nature Switzerland AG 2019
A. Giordano et al. (eds.), *Transcatheter Aortic Valve Implantation*,
https://doi.org/10.1007/978-3-030-05912-5_15

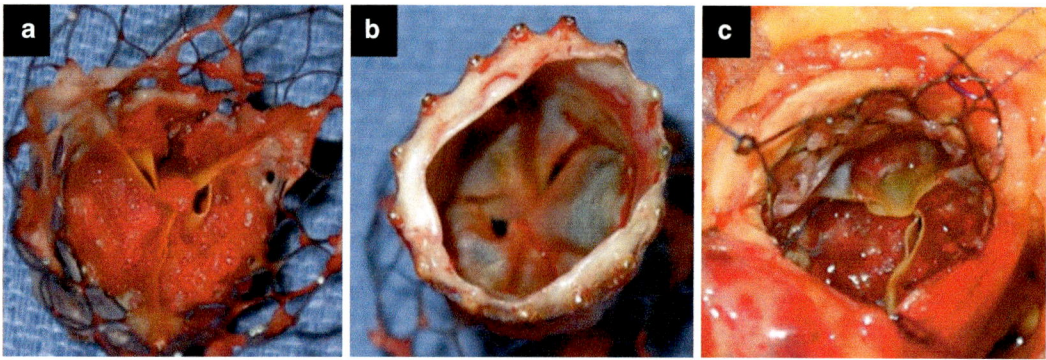

Fig. 15.1 (**a**) A normal seating of the CoreValve with a translucent neointimal sheath covering the upper portion of the nitinol frame; note the presence on the aortic side of the valve of a brown-colored thrombotic host tissue with-out calcification on the free edges of the valve leaflets; (**b**, **c**) white fibrous-like tissue covered the fabric skirt of the inflow portion of the device on outer and inner surfaces

valve that occludes part of the blood flow path, interferes with valve function, or is sufficiently large to warrant treatment" [3] (Fig. 15.1). Transcatheter aortic valve thrombosis has an incidence ranging from 0,61% to 2,8% [4, 5]. It can be classified, according to its timing, into acute (0–3 days after TAVI), subacute (3 days to 3 months after TAVI), late (3 months to 1 year after TAVI), and very late (>1 year after TAVI) [6]. In the study by Latib et al. on 4.266 patients undergoing TAVI, all cases of TAVT were detected within 2 years after valve implantation with a median time to thrombosis of 181 days [4].

Depending on diagnostic certainty, it can be classified also as (1) definite, when clinical, imaging, and pathological criteria are matched and there is a clinical response to initiation of anticoagulation therapy; (2) probable, on the basis of clinical and imaging (CT or echo) criteria; and (3) possible, based on uncertain clinical criteria [6].

The majority of patients with clinical TAVT presents at follow-up with new onset or worsening of dyspnea; seldom they may present non-ST-elevation myocardial infarction and embolic events such as stroke or cardiac arrest. Laboratory tests may be useful for diagnosis since serum NT-proBNP was found to be significantly elevated in patients with valve thrombosis [5]. Almost all patients (92.3%) present with significantly increased mean aortic valve pressure gradient, whereas 76.9% present with thickened leaflets or thrombotic apposition of leaflets, and only 23% had a thrombotic mass on leaflets [4].

Despite TAVT may occur without a specific underlying cause, several predisposing factors such as valve-in-valve procedures, obesity, use of a balloon-expandable valve, and a small prosthesis size (<23 mm) have been identified as independent predictor of TAVT [5, 7].

Several series showed higher postprocedural transprosthetic mean gradient after valve-in-valve TAVI [8]. Some authors suggest that valve-in-valve implantations may result in increased mechanical stress on leaflets and altered flow turbulence promoting thrombosis. Interestingly, in paper by Jose et al., all cases of valve-in-valve thrombosis involved Hancock II and Mosaic, valves that are also at high risk of thrombosis after surgical replacement [5].

Is it known that a higher BMI may contribute, through a lipid-mediated inflammatory mechanism, to aortic bioprosthesis degeneration. Moreover, diabetes and metabolic syndrome, two conditions strictly associated with obesity, may predispose to thrombosis [9]. The role of lipid-inflammatory pathway needs to be further elucidated in the future.

Mechanism involved in the increased risk of TAVT in balloon-expandable valve is still not known; however it seems that valve over- and under-expansion, poor stent endothelialization, and native leaflet fissuring during balloon expansion are implicated.

Although several studies demonstrated that patient-prosthesis mismatch is an independent predictor of bioprosthesis degeneration, whether a smaller prosthesis size is related to an augmented risk of valve thrombosis needs to be clarified [10, 11].

Treatment of choice in patients with TAVT is anticoagulation therapy which has been proven to be efficacious also in case of chronic and organized thrombi. Nowadays, preferred drugs for treatment of TAVT are vitamin K antagonist (VKA), but trial comparing novel oral anticoagulant versus dual antiplatelet therapy or VKA is currently on the way. In case of failure of anticoagulation therapy, the remaining option is transcatheter valve-in-valve procedure or surgical aortic valve replacement.

Since TAVT is a potential life-threatening condition and median time to diagnosis is 6 months, some authors suggest a closer surveillance with imaging at 1, 3, and 6 months and then annual follow-up. Further studies are needed to understand the optimal imaging technique among transthoracic echo, transesophageal echo, and CT.

15.2 Subclinical Leaflet Thrombosis

On 2015, during an ongoing clinical trial, reduced aortic valve leaflet motion was noted on computed tomography of patients undergoing TAVI. Makkar et al., referring to a "possible subclinical thrombosis," published data coming from Portico investigational device exemption (IDE) and two subsequent physician-initiated registries (SAVORY and RESOLVE), reporting an incidence of reduced leaflet motion of 40% in the Portico IDE study and of 13% in registries [12]. These findings lead the authors and the scientific community to raise question about safety and durability of TAVI, and the Food and Drug Administration was obligated to publish a perspective declaring: "We at the FDA believe that the available clinical evidence supports the conclusion that these valves remain safe and effective and that findings to date concerning reduced leaflet motion have not changed the overall favorable benefit–risk balance for these valves when they are used for their approved indications" [13]. The fact that leaflet motion abnormalities were not observed in anticoagulated patients and resolve with initiation of anticoagulation suggests that these findings were related to valve thrombosis.

Based on CT findings, subclinical leaflet thrombosis can be classified in "hypoattenuated leaflet thickening" (HALT) and/or "reduced leaflet motion" (RELM) (Fig. 15.2). Leaflet motion can be defined as normal, mildly reduced (<50%

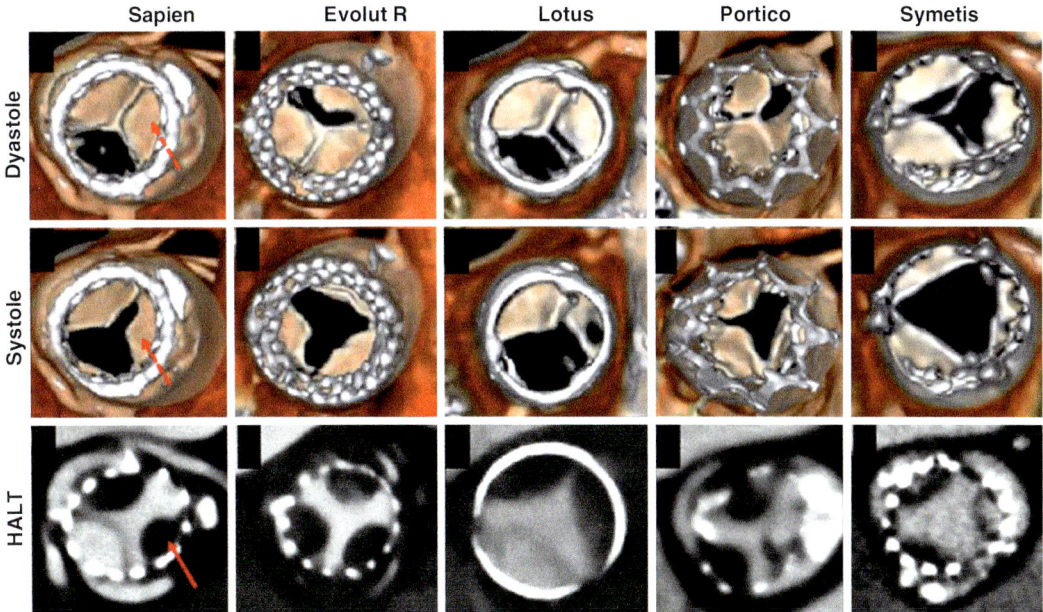

Fig. 15.2 Hypoattenuated leaflet thickening (HALT) on two-dimensional computed tomography (gray-scale images) and volume-rendered CT (color images) for multiple prosthesis types

reduction), moderately reduced (50–70% reduction), severely reduced (>70% reduction), or immobile. The prevalence of HALT/RELM has been reported in three studies. Makkar et al. reported their findings from 55 patients using 3D volume-rendered (VR) imaging. RELM was noted in 39 of 187 (20.9%) patients and in multiple transcatheter valve types, including the Portico valve, Edwards valves (Edwards SAPIEN, SAPIEN XT, and SAPIEN 3), Medtronic CoreValve, and the Lotus™ valve (Boston Scientific, Marlborough, MA, USA) [12]. Pache et al. performed contrast CT in 156 patients undergoing TAVR with the SAPIEN 3 valve at a median of 5 days post TAVR. HALT was noted in 16 (10.3%) patients [14]. Leetmaa et al. performed computed tomography (CT) in 140 patients with SAPIEN XT valves (Edwards Lifesciences) within 3 months postimplantation; TAVT (defined as HALT) was present in 5 patients (4%), 4 of these patients being asymptomatic with no echocardiographic evidence of significantly elevated gradients [15].

Recently, Chakravarty et al. published data on patients who had CT scans after surgical aortic valve replacement and TAVI, demonstrating a higher incidence of subclinical leaflet thrombosis in patients who underwent TAVI than in patients who underwent surgery (13% vs. 4%) [16].

Mylotte et al. hypothesized that several mechanisms may explain the higher incidence of leaflet thrombosis: (1) the elderly TAVI population is more likely to have coexisting prothrombotic conditions (e.g., cancer), (2) the metallic THV frame could potentially provide a nidus for thrombosis, (3) incomplete THV expansion can create leaflet folds and potential recesses for thrombus formation, (4) incomplete THV apposition to the aortic wall may delay endothelialization, and (5) the native leaflets may overhang balloon-expandable systems creating areas of diminished blood flow and stagnation [17].

Transthoracic echocardiography (TTE) plays a crucial role to exclude regurgitation and/or stenosis, but it provides inadequate details to assess the possible presence of HALT/RELM. Although a greater proportion of patients with subclinical leaflet thrombosis had aortic valve gradients of more than 20 mmHg, it is conceivable that, after calculating normal gradients (which are usually higher than the native valve), even an expert echocardiographer may not carefully search for HALT/RELM. The latter issue may imply that the real incidence of this phenomenon is far from being precisely depicted [16].

In some occasions, the transesophageal echocardiogram (TEE) may be helpful to detect the RELM, before or after the CT scan findings; however, it is impractical to advocate the use of TEE in all cases, especially when normal gradients and no suspicious findings come from the TTE.

Theoretically, the CT scan acquisition and reconstruction can be deemed as the gold standard imaging tool to visualize the leaflets; however, it gives no hemodynamic information; thus the CT scan is actually "complementary" to the TTE/TEE, although in all the published series the CT scan has been used to confirm the diagnosis.

All acquisition protocols enabling the formal assessment of leaflet motion and thickening employ contrast CT with retrospective gating. The acquisition is usually performed in the cranio-caudal direction from the aortic arch to the diaphragm and images reconstructed at 0.6 mm slices with 0.3 mm overlap with iterative reconstruction for evaluation at 10% intervals within the 0–90% RR range. To minimize radiation exposure, a dose-modulation approach can be used, thus reducing dose in the 55–100% RR range (diastole).

CT images are usually reconstructed in the systolic phase using 3mensio Valves Version 7.0 or Version 7.1 (3mensio Medical Imaging BV, Bilthoven, The Netherlands) and Vitrea® Software Version 6.7.2 (Vital Images, Inc., Minnetonka, MN, USA). The valve leaflets can be assessed using both 2D (axial cross-section assessment) and 3D-VR (volume rendered) imaging. The VR images can be generated using center line reconstructions and the hockey puck feature in 3mensio or using front-cut plane or five thick slab VR functions in Vitrea. In Vitrea, the medium denoising filter was employed.

Of note, while leaflets with normal motion are difficult to visualize on 4D VR-CT, leaflets with reduced motion can be clearly seen in 3D or 4D images. Hypo-attenuating lesions can be studied on maximum intensity projection (MIP) 2D CT and correlated to reduced leaflet motion on 3mensio software with the use of the marker feature and on Vitrea software using the VR auto-alignment with MIP feature.

A discrepancy must be acknowledged between CT and echocardiographic findings. Despite a 10–15% prevalence of subclinical thrombosis with CT, elevated gradients (a mean gradient of >20 mm Hg) with echocardiography are infrequent [12, 14, 15]. This observation implies that CT detects early subclinical thrombosis, whereas echocardiography detects the late consequences of thrombosis (i.e., valvular stenosis). This also indicates that not all thromboses result in valve degeneration, i.e., early thrombosis might resolve spontaneously.

Dynamic four-dimensional CT imaging was consistently used for detection of subclinical thrombosis although consensus definitions and quantification of leaflet thrombosis with CT are lacking, and it should be established before prospective study and clinical use are carried out.

Moreover, the CT timing after TAVI to detect meaningful leaflet thrombosis is actually unknown. It has been postulated that the timing of imaging might affect the proportions of leaflet thrombosis with different valve types; however there is no "evidence" supporting a specific risk linked to a specific type of bioprosthesis [13].

Most of the patients with HALT/RELM are asymptomatic, and subclinical leaflet thrombosis was incidentally found on CT. Laboratory tests may show higher level of D-dimer and NT-proBNP [5, 18].

Leetmaa et al. and Pache et al. provided limited clinical follow-up, with no strokes, transient ischemic attacks (TIAs), or thromboembolic complications in patients with HALT [14, 15]. Makkar et al. reported no difference in the incidence of stroke/TIA or thromboembolic complications in the Portico clinical trial; however, the presence of reduced leaflet motion was associated with a significant increase in the risk of TIA in the registries [19]. Chakravarty et al. demonstrated that subclinical leaflet thrombosis was associated with increased rates of transient ischemic attacks and all strokes or TIAs [16].

The appropriate management of HALT/RELM in asymptomatic patients with normal aortic valve pressure gradient remains unknown. Anticoagulation is associated with the resolution of the hypodense areas overlying the leaflets with restoration of normal leaflet motion, suggesting that thrombus formation is the primary event leading to reduced leaflet motion rather than contrary [12].

However, given the risks of chronic anticoagulation, questions remain:

- Should all patients be offered such therapy?
- Should patients be selected according to imaging findings?
- What is the optimal duration of treatment?
- With new oral anticoagulants being considered to be preferable over vitamin K antagonists, how and when should we reassess the efficacy of the treatment?

Before robust evidence that the imaging finding of HALT/RELM alone is clinically relevant, the management of patients with TAVR should not change (both ESC and ACC/AHA guidelines provide a Class IIb recommendation for DAPT but do not recommend routine anticoagulation). Two randomized clinical trials, GALILEO and ATLANTIS, are currently ongoing and may provide important additional information on whether NOACs prevent thrombosis and improve outcomes in patients undergoing TAVI.

References

1. Mack MJ, Leon MB, Smith CR, et al. 5-year outcomes of transcatheter aortic valve replacement or surgical aortic valve replacement for high surgical risk patients with aortic stenosis (PARTNER 1): a randomised controlled trial. Lancet. 2015;385(9986):2477–84.
2. Midha PA, Raghav V, Sharma R, et al. The fluid mechanics of transcatheter heart valve leaflet thrombosis in the neosinus. Circulation. 2017;136(17):1598–609.
3. Kappetein AP, Head SJ, Genereux P, et al. Updated standardized endpoint definitions for transcatheter aortic valve implantation: the Valve Academic Research Consortium-2 consensus document. J Am Coll Cardiol. 2012;60(15):1438–54.

4. Latib A, Naganuma T, Abdel-Wahab M, et al. Treatment and clinical outcomes of transcatheter heart valve thrombosis. Circ Cardiovasc Interv. 2015;8(4):e001779.

5. Jose J, Sulimov DS, El-Mawardy M, et al. Clinical bioprosthetic heart valve thrombosis after transcatheter aortic valve replacement: incidence, characteristics, and treatment outcomes. JACC Cardiovasc Interv. 2017;10(7):686–97.

6. Dangas GD, Weitz JI, Giustino G, Makkar R, Mehran R. Prosthetic heart valve thrombosis. J Am Coll Cardiol. 2016;68(24):2670–89.

7. Del Trigo M, Munoz-Garcia AJ, Wijeysundera HC, et al. Incidence, timing, and predictors of valve hemodynamic deterioration after transcatheter aortic valve replacement: multicenter registry. J Am Coll Cardiol. 2016;67(6):644–55.

8. Paradis JM, Del Trigo M, Puri R, Rodes-Cabau J. Transcatheter valve-in-valve and valve-in-ring for treating aortic and mitral surgical prosthetic dysfunction. J Am Coll Cardiol. 2015;66(18):2019–37.

9. Mahjoub H, Mathieu P, Senechal M, et al. ApoB/ApoA-I ratio is associated with increased risk of bioprosthetic valve degeneration. J Am Coll Cardiol. 2013;61(7):752–61.

10. Flameng W, Herregods MC, Vercalsteren M, Herijgers P, Bogaerts K, Meuris B. Prosthesis-patient mismatch predicts structural valve degeneration in bioprosthetic heart valves. Circulation. 2010;121(19):2123–9.

11. Mahjoub H, Mathieu P, Larose E, et al. Determinants of aortic bioprosthetic valve calcification assessed by multidetector CT. Heart. 2015;101(6):472–7.

12. Makkar RR, Fontana G, Jilaihawi H, et al. Possible subclinical leaflet thrombosis in bioprosthetic aortic valves. N Engl J Med. 2015;373(21):2015–24.

13. Laschinger JC, Wu C, Ibrahim NG, Shuren JE. Reduced leaflet motion in bioprosthetic aortic valves—the FDA perspective. N Engl J Med. 2015;373(21):1996–8.

14. Pache G, Schoechlin S, Blanke P, et al. Early hypo-attenuated leaflet thickening in balloon-expandable transcatheter aortic heart valves. Eur Heart J. 2016;37(28):2263–71.

15. Leetmaa T, Hansson NC, Leipsic J, et al. Early aortic transcatheter heart valve thrombosis: diagnostic value of contrast-enhanced multidetector computed tomography. Circ Cardiovasc Interv. 2015;8(4):e001596.

16. Chakravarty T, Sondergaard L, Friedman J, et al. Subclinical leaflet thrombosis in surgical and transcatheter bioprosthetic aortic valves: an observational study. Lancet. 2017;389(10087):2383–92.

17. Mylotte D, Andalib A, Theriault-Lauzier P, et al. Transcatheter heart valve failure: a systematic review. Eur Heart J. 2015;36(21):1306–27.

18. Yanagisawa R, Hayashida K, Yamada Y, et al. Incidence, predictors, and mid-term outcomes of possible leaflet thrombosis after TAVR. JACC Cardiovasc Imaging. 2016; https://doi.org/10.1016/j.jcmg.2016.11.005.

19. Chakravarty T, Abramowitz Y, Jilaihawi H, Makkar RR. Leaflet motion abnormality after TAVI: genuine threat or much ado about nothing? EuroIntervention. 2016;12(Y):Y28–32.

Gender-Related Differences in Transcatheter Aortic Valve Implantation

16

Brad Stair and John K. Forrest

16.1 Introduction

The natural history of aortic stenosis, as proposed by Ross and Braunwald in 1968 [1], has been confirmed in numerous studies over the last 50 years and is characterized by a relatively benign, asymptomatic beginning with a rapid mortality rate once symptoms develop. This onset of symptoms heralds an unfavorable outcome with more than half of patients succumbing to the disease over the next 2 years. Until recently, surgical aortic valve replacement (SAVR) was the mainstay of treatment. However, transcatheter aortic valve implantation (TAVI), also called transcatheter aortic valve replacement (TAVR), has emerged as a less invasive treatment option in inoperable, high, and intermediate surgical risk patients [2–7] with current, ongoing trials exploring low risk surgical patients [8, 9]. In contrast to most cardiovascular studies, females represent nearly half of patients undergoing TAVR. Through this, various distinctions in physiologic changes, clinical characteristics, and procedural outcomes have emerged between male and female patients. Here-in, these gender based differences in patients with AS are reviewed.

B. Stair · J. K. Forrest (✉)
Yale University School of Medicine, Yale New Haven Hospital, New Haven, CT, USA
e-mail: brad.stair@yale.edu; john.k.forrest@yale.edu

16.2 Physiologic Changes in Aortic Stenosis (Fig. 16.1)

16.2.1 Differences in Left Ventricular Response

Left ventricular hypertrophy as a response to pressure overload, such as that seen in aortic stenosis, is an interplay of the hemodynamic load exerted on the ventricle and the resultant cardiac remodeling and performance. Females more often exhibit a concentric remodeling or hypertrophy pattern [10–14]. This type of pattern is characterized by increased left ventricular wall thickness without associated left ventricular dilation, resulting in an increased relative left ventricular wall thickness. This type of remodeling is associated with lower end-systolic left ventricular wall stress and smaller ventricular size. This often results in a lower stroke volume and higher systolic ejection fraction [15]. Hachicha et al. showed that when stroke volume was indexed to body surface area, females with preserved left ventricular ejection fraction had a higher incidence of American Heart Association/American College of Cardiology (AHA/ACC) Guideline Stage D3 paradoxical low-flow (defined as a stroke volume index of <35 mL/m^2), low-gradient (PLFLG) aortic stenosis. Importantly, this hemodynamic profile, more common in women, conferred a lower 3-year survival compared with patients with normal left ventricular stroke

© Springer Nature Switzerland AG 2019
A. Giordano et al. (eds.), *Transcatheter Aortic Valve Implantation*,
https://doi.org/10.1007/978-3-030-05912-5_16

Fig. 16.1 Sex differences in aortic valve stenosis

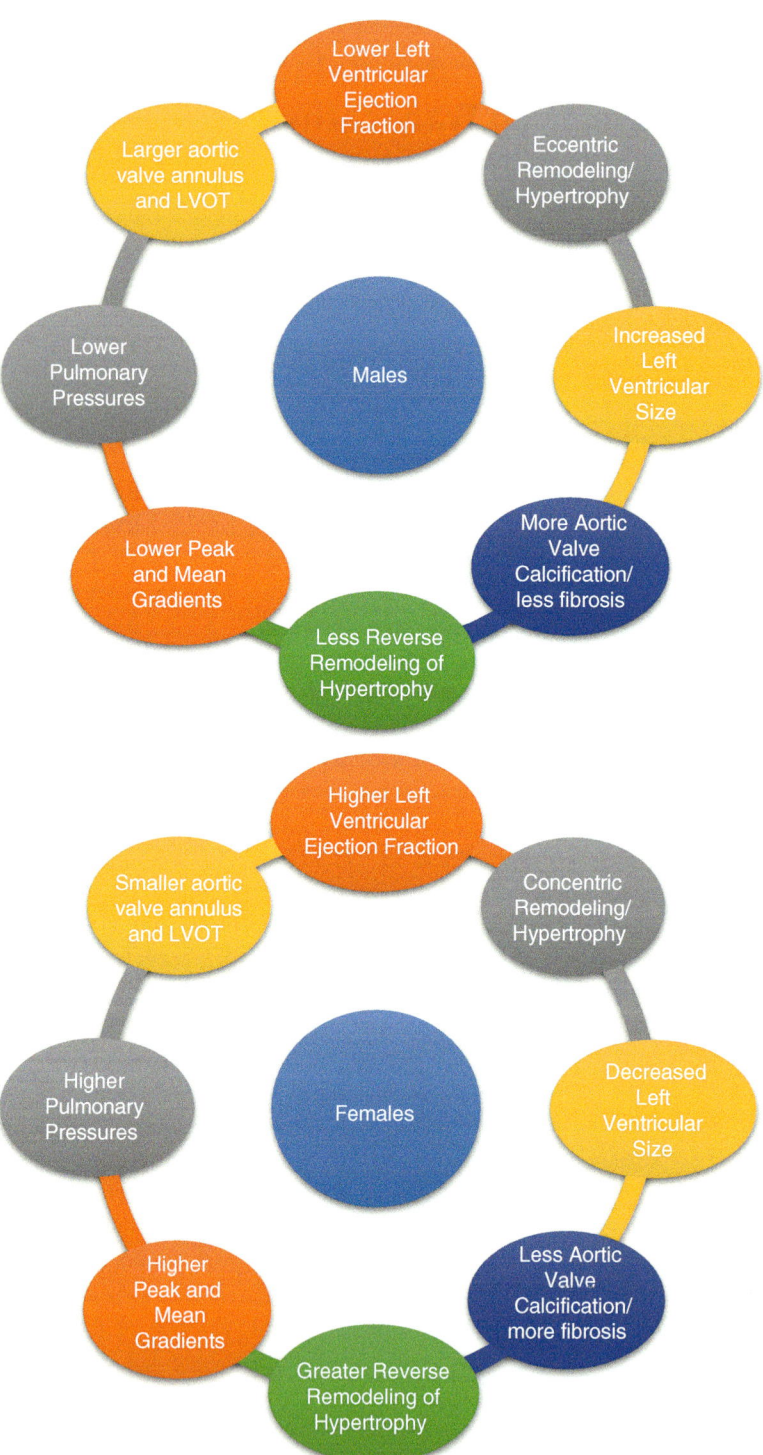

volume [16]. This is in contrast to their male counterparts who are more likely to exhibit an eccentric remodeling or hypertrophy pattern [10]. This type of pattern is characterized by a normal or a modest increase in left ventricular wall thickness with a more pronounced increase in ventricular cavity dimension and thus decreased relative wall thickness. This type of remodeling is associated with higher end-systolic left ventricular wall stress and a larger ventricular size. In turn, systolic ejection fraction is often low normal or mildly reduced with higher stroke volumes. Stangl et al. showed that following TAVR, both sexes showed regression of hypertrophy, but improvement of left ventricular ejection fraction (LVEF) was significant only in women, potentially reflecting a lower burden of irreversible myocardial damage before TAVR [14].

16.2.2 Differences in Aortic Valve Pathology

Valvular calcification is a unifying mechanism of AS in both men and women. Similar to data showing a lower overall volume of calcification in the coronary arteries in women as compared to men, the degree of aortic valve calcification (AVC) required to produce equivalent hemodynamic consequence appears to be less in women than in men [17]. This has been an area of interest recently with the advent of multidetector computed tomography (MDCT) and cardiac computed tomography (CCT). Multiple studies have shown that women tend to have less valvular calcification as compared to their male counterparts. Shivani et al. showed that women with similar AS severity as men, presented with lower AVC loads [18]. This held even after taking into account various parameters such has body size and normalization for body surface area, LVOT size, and cross-sectional annulus area. They also showed that, in women, AS severity increases at a greater magnitude with any given AVC load or density increase than it does in men. Current AHA/ACC guidelines list

moderate grade or greater AVC as one of the parameters to be considered in managing AS patients. This is due, in part, to the fact severe AVC and calcium density are independent predictors of mortality in AS patients. As a result, recommendations for sex-specific cutoffs for AVC have been established with score cutoffs for the identification of severe AS to be a total AVC of 2065 in men and 1275 in women. Use of these sex-specific measures of AVC has been shown to be predictive of survival in AS patients, independent of clinical and echocardiographic factors [19, 20].

16.2.3 Differences in Annulus, Left Ventricular Outflow Tract, and Sinus of Valsalva Dimensions

The aortic root has specific anatomic characteristics, and with the advent of TAVR, the ability to make precise measurements to allow proper valve sizing has been paramount. Multiple studies have shown that females have both smaller annular and left ventricular outflow tract (LVOT) dimensions but overall similar aortic dimensions as compared to their male counterparts. This similarity in ascending aortic dimensions between the sexes has been attributed to the more rapid growth of the ascending aorta experienced by women in the later years of life [21]. Buellesfeld et al. utilized computed tomography in consecutive patients undergoing TAVR and showed larger annular and LVOT dimensions in men than women (area annulus: 483.1 ± 75.6 mm^2 vs. 386.9 ± 58.5 mm^2, $p = 0.0002$; area LVOT: 478.2 ± 131.0 mm^2 vs. 374.0 ± 94.2 mm^2, $p = 0.0024$). Michelena et al. studied the impact that LVOT diameter has on AS severity grading in patients with normal left ventricular ejection fraction. The overwhelming majority (91%) of patients with small LVOT diameters were women [22]. LVOT diameter is a major determinant of AS severity as determined by echocardiography. Smaller LVOT diameters often result in AS assessment discordance, with valve areas consistent with severe AS and peak and mean gradients along with a dimensionless index suggestive of less severe AS. Sinus of Valsalva dimensions was significantly larger in men, whereas dimensions of the ascending aorta were comparable. They also showed that coronary heights were lower in women than in men [23]. Given these findings, to reduce the overdiagnosis of AS, the American Society of Echocardiography (ASE) has recommended indexing aortic valve area to body size in the setting of a height <135 cm, body surface area <1.5 m^2, or body mass index <22 kg/m^2. In these circumstances an indexed AVA <0.6 cm^2/m^2 can be used to define severe AS [24]. These findings are critically important when considering TAVR in both genders.

16.2.4 Differences in Bicuspid Aortic Valve Anatomy

The presence of a bicuspid aortic valve, the most common congenital cardiac defect, occurs more frequently in males than in females. Bicuspid aortic valve morphology is classified based on the Sievers classification according to the number of cusps and the presence of raphes, as well as spatial position and symmetry of raphes and cusps. Type 0 is characterized by the presence of two symmetric cusps and one commissure without evidence of a raphe, type 1 is characterized by the presence of one raphe, and type 2 when two raphes are present [25]. Aortic valve regurgitation, aortic aneurysm, and infective endocarditis are more commonly encountered in males, whereas aortic stenosis is more common in females. In patients with a bicuspid aortic valve undergoing SAVR, mortality is higher for both sexes as compared to the general population, and this difference is even more pronounced in females. Aortic regurgitation, though a more common finding in men, is a predictor of mortality only in females undergoing SAVR in bicuspid aortic valve morphology [26]. The experience of TAVR in bicuspid aortic valve stenosis is largely limited to small series [27–30] as TAVR trials excluded congenital bicuspid AS due to its unique morphological characteristics as compared to tri-

cuspid AS. Yoon et al., utilizing the Bicuspid AS TAVR registry, conducted the first large-scale study looking at clinical outcomes of TAVR in bicuspid AS compared to tricuspid AS. With the use of first-generation TAVR devices, more frequent adverse procedural events occurred when compared to those receiving these devices for tricuspid valve anatomy. When latest-generation devices were used, there was no significant difference in procedural complications, and the cumulative event rate for all-cause mortality at 2-year follow-up was similar between the bicuspid and tricuspid groups [31]. Ongoing research and trials are being conducted in this arena.

16.3 TAVR

16.3.1 Differences in Baseline Characteristics and Presentation

Gender differences in baseline characteristics and clinical presentation are quite pronounced in those patients undergoing TAVR. A secondary analysis of the PARTNER trial revealed women had lower rates of hyperlipidemia, diabetes, smoking, and renal disease but higher Society of Thoracic Surgeons Predicted Risk of Mortality scores (11.9% vs. 11.1%; $P < 0.001$) [15]. In addition, several meta-analyses have shown women had lower rates of prior myocardial infarction, higher left ventricular ejection fraction, lower rates of previous coronary revascularization including both percutaneous coronary intervention and coronary artery bypass surgery, and lower rates of both peripheral vascular disease and stroke despite older age at time of presentation [14, 15, 32]. Interestingly, women appear to have a higher incidence of pulmonary hypertension with pulmonary artery pressures often exceeding 60 mmHg which may be related to higher trans-aortic gradients though the exact mechanism has yet to be elucidated [32, 33].

Frailty is also an important determinant of mortality post-TAVR which is largely unaccounted for in the most commonly used risk assessment scores discussed below. At present, there are limited data regarding baseline gender differences with respect to frailty. Some studies showed no difference in baseline frailty [34–36], while others reported women to be more frail than men [36]. An analysis of the US CoreValve Trials demonstrated women tended to be more frail and had more physical limitations than men. Women had a higher incidence of being wheelchair.

bound, a greater number of deficits in Katz activities of daily living, a higher incidence of low body mass index, and a slower 5-min gait speed. There was no difference in baseline albumin between women and men [37]. This is an important subject that deserves further evaluation as frailty has been shown to be a predictor of mortality following TAVR independent of gender.

The most commonly used risk assessment scores to determine 30-day mortality and morbidity risks for patients undergoing cardiac surgery are the Society of Thoracic Surgeons (STS) risk score [38] and the European System for Cardiac Operative Risk Evaluation (EuroSCORE) risk score [39]. Female gender is an independent risk factor in both risk assessments. This holds true with both isolated coronary artery bypass graft surgery and isolated valvular surgery. Brown et al. conducted a STS database review over a 10-year period for patients who had undergone isolated aortic valve replacement in North America. This group found female patients had higher mortality, higher stroke rate, and longer postoperative stay relative to male patients. This was true for the overall population, the 1997 group, and the 2006 group [40]. A similar analysis using the EuroSCORE was conducted in patients undergoing any cardiac surgery in Europe with female gender being an independent predictor of increased mortality [41].

16.4 TAVR Approach and Valve Sizing

In the current era, transfemoral access is the most common and preferred implantation approach for patients undergoing TAVR. In patients without adequate iliofemoral anatomy, alternate access routes include, but are not limited to, trans-aortic, trans-apical, trans-subclavian, trans-axillary, trans-carotid, and trans-caval access. Given the sheath and delivery system diameters, the size of the femoral arteries, as measured most often by computed tomography angiography (CTA), is a deciding factor in determining route of access. On average, women presenting for TAVR have smaller vessel sizes than their male counterparts. Smaller vessel caliber contributes to increased complication rates including bleeding and blood vessel damage [42, 43] but also to the greater use of alternative access routes which have been associated with greater mortality [44].

CTA has now become the standard for annulus sizing as transthoracic and transesophageal 2-dimensional echocardiography, which was used as the primary sizing method in early TAVR studies, has been shown to underestimate annular size, thus increasing the risk of prosthesis-patient mismatch [2, 5]. Women have smaller aortic annuli then men, and, as a result, smaller transcatheter heart valve (THV) sizes are used in women. One meta-analysis showed greater than 90% of females received 26 mm or smaller THVs in contrast to greater than 30% of males who received 29 mm and greater THVs [32]. As new generations of THVs have come to market, the size ranges have expanded to include both smaller and larger valve sizes across both self- and balloon-expandable platforms. Despite this, annular size is still clinically important when it comes to TAVR especially with respect to complications and outcomes.

16.5 Procedural Complications

The Valve Academic Research Consortium (VARC) update defines vascular complications to include aortic or annular rupture, access-related injury, distal embolization, limb ischemia, and percutaneous closure device failure [45]. Data from the randomized control trial and continued access registry of the PARTNER I study have demonstrated higher vascular complications in females compared to males (17.3% vs. 10%; $p < 0.001$) [15]. Data from the US CoreValve Trials also demonstrated higher major vascular complication rates in females compared to males

(9.7% vs. 4.9%; $p < 0.01$ at 30 days and 9.9% vs. 5.3%; $p < 0.01$ at 1 year) [37]. These results are congruent with other meta-analyses. Hayashida et al. showed that although women have lower rates of baseline peripheral vascular disease, their minimal vascular diameter is smaller than their male counterparts, resulting in a reduced sheath-to-femoral artery ratio, and this difference may partly explain the higher rates of vascular complications [46]. The risk of aortic root and annular rupture also appears to be higher in women. In one series looking at 3067 patients undergoing TAVR, 37 developed annular rupture, of which 74% were women [47]. Several anatomical and procedurally related risk factors were identified including smaller annular size, subannular calcium, and oversizing with a balloon-expandable prosthesis >20% by area. As such, care should be taken when oversizing balloon-expandable prostheses in women with heavy subannular calcification. Women also have a higher incidence of bleeding, including major and life-threatening bleeds, than do men as confirmed by several meta-analyses [15, 32, 37, 48].

Several recent studies have suggested that women suffer from higher stroke rates than men. PARTNER trial data showed a trend toward higher stroke rates in females not reaching statistical significance [49]. CoreValve data showed an increased incidence of both all stroke and major stroke among women at both 30 days and 1 year [37] which was also seen in a meta-analysis by O'Connor [32]. Other meta-analyses have failed to demonstrate a significant gender difference in stroke rates [14, 48]. With growing experience and improved technology with newer-generation THV and the advent of cerebral protection devices, stroke rates continue to decline with TAVR. As these technologies continue to evolve, a better understanding of which patients are at increased risk of cerebrovascular complications will become increasingly important.

Another potential complication of TAVR is coronary artery obstruction. In general, coronary heights of 12 mm or less and sinus of Valsalva dimensions of 30 mm or less are identified as thresholds for increased risk [50, 51]. This has significant implications as women presenting for TAVR have lower coronary heights and smaller sinus of Valsalva dimensions as compared to men [23, 50]. This was shown by Ribeiro et al. where data collected from 81 centers worldwide revealed more than 80% of patients who developed coronary artery obstruction were women despite relatively equal gender representation in their registry data.

The presence of significant paravalvular leak (PVL), also referred to as paravalvular regurgitation, is a known predictor of mortality [52]. For both balloon and self-expanding valves, PVL is most commonly a result of undersizing of the THV, prosthesis mal-apposition to the native annulus due to extensive calcification, or malposition of the THV. Two specific studies evaluated the CoreValve and noted a lower depth of implantation, and a greater angle between the aorta and left ventricular outflow tract predicted PVL [53, 54]. Moderate or greater PVL is known to be associated with higher mortality rates, and 2-year results from the PARTNER trial showed that even mild PVL was associated with increased mortality [55]. Early studies have consistently shown decreased PVL in women as compared to men. This is likely multifactorial, due in part to women having smaller annular sizes and less annular calcification and also due to the fact that in the early years of TAVR, larger valve sizes were not available, thus resulting more frequently in the undersizing of valves in men as compared to women. As THV technology has advanced, the newest-generation valves have not only increased in maximum diameter but have also incorporated a skirt or wrap covering the inflow portion of the THV frame to help improve the better seal between the valve and native annulus. These advancements in THV design have led to a decrease in overall rates of PVL and may eventually help bridge the gap in the rates of PVL between the sexes.

Patient-prosthesis mismatch (PPM) results when the effective orifice area (EOA) of a prosthetic valve is too small for a given patient's body surface area. In the SAVR literature, studies have demonstrated that women experience PPM at significantly higher rates than men [56], and this has been associated with worse outcomes [57].

These higher rates have been attributed to the need for smaller valve sizes in women. In TAVR however, rates of PPM seem to be lower than that seen with SAVR. Both Pibarot et al. [58] and Popma et al. [59] demonstrated lower overall rates of PPM following TAVR compared with SAVR with a more pronounced difference in those patients with smaller aortic annular size. In patients with annular diameters <20 mm, severe PPM (defined as an indexed EOA <0.65 cm^2/m^2) occurred in 33.7% patients undergoing SAVR versus 19% undergoing TAVR ($p = 0.002$) [58]. These lower rates of PPM in TAVR may be explained in part by the presence of a sewing ring in surgical prostheses which is fixed in size and may result in a smaller annular diameter as compared to THVs lack sewing rings and have only a think stent structure between the valve and the native annulus. It appears that rates for PPM are similar between males and females across most studies in spite of the fact that women frequently need smaller THVs [60–62]. This highlights a critical point to the potential benefit of TAVR in women who are surgical candidates but have smaller annular dimensions, given the lower incidence of PPM as compared to SAVR where it is a known predictor of worse outcomes [63].

16.6   Outcomes

As previously discussed, women are generally at an increased risk for perioperative morbidity and mortality following SAVR as female gender is an independent risk factor in the STS risk stratification system. This increased mortality has not born out in the TAVR trials. Multiple studies have now demonstrated that the mortality benefit gained in having a TAVR vs. SAVR is greater for women than it is for men. Several reasons have been postulated including the fact women tend to have smaller chests and smaller aortic root and annular dimensions which may pose technical challenges during surgery and may increase post-procedural complications. Women also tend to have concentric remodeling and paradoxical low-flow low-gradient severe aortic stenosis, both of which are associated with increased risk of

hemodynamic instability, low output, and mortality following SAVR. In the PARTNER trial, mortality rates were lower for females who underwent TAVR, compared to SAVR, both at 6 months and 2 years, largely driven by the cohort who had undergone transfemoral TAVR [49]. In contrast, males did not demonstrate a survival advantage with TAVR, compared to SAVR. Similarly, 1-year survival for females who received self-expanding THVs was better than for females undergoing SAVR [5, 64]. Women also tend to have less incidence of moderate or greater PVL following TAVR which is a poor prognostic determinant. In addition, gender-related differences in left ventricular remodeling and fibrosis may lend to a more rapid and complete reversal of hypertrophy accounting for better outcomes following TAVR [36, 65].

Several studies and meta-analyses have evaluated gender differences in survival following TAVR. Despite higher rates of post-procedural complications including vascular complications, major bleeding, and stroke, female sex has been shown in a number of studies to be independently associated with improved survival at 1-year follow-up [32, 48, 66]. A recent risk-adjusted analysis of mortality using data from the Society of Thoracic Surgeons/American College of Cardiology TVT (Transcatheter Valve Therapies) registry concluded female sex was associated with improved survival [67]. O'Connor et al. showed women had improved survival at a median follow-up of 387 days regardless of valve type or access route [32]. Stangl et al. also showed a lower risk of death in women compared to men at both 30-day and >3 months follow-up even with the inclusion of two studies which demonstrated diminished or no benefit of TAVR in women [66]. Similarly, Conrotto et al. demonstrated a lower mortality rate in women versus men (24% vs. 34% at a median follow-up of 365 days) [48]. It is notable that the majority of these studies included patients treated early in the TAVR era using balloon-expandable valves, a time during which a complete range of valve sizes was not available (the first balloon-expandable valves were only available in 23 mm and 26 mm sizes, and the 29 mm size was not available until more recently). As such, undersizing was a frequent occurrence and likely contributed to some of the sex-related differences in outcomes. Data from the US CoreValve Trials showed that when larger valve sizes and dedicated CTA annular sizing were included, no significant mortality differences between the sexes existed out to 1 year [37].

The Women's International Transcatheter Aortic Valve Implantation (WIN-TAVI) real-world registry is a prospective, observational registry of women undergoing TAVR for AS. A recent report from this registry [68] evaluated VARC-2 [45] early safety endpoints at 30 days for 1019 women. In this study, the mean STS score was 8.3, and EuroSCORE was 17.8 with 90.6% having a transfemoral approach TAVR with newer-generation devices used in just under half (42.1%). The 30-day VARC-2 composite endpoint occurred in 14.0% with 3.4% all-cause mortality, 1.3% stroke, 7.7% major vascular complications, and 4.4% VARC life-threatening bleeding. The primary endpoint was driven largely by vascular or bleeding events, consistent with previous studies, though the observed rate of these events was lower than previously reported. Several independent predictors of the 30-day VARC-2 composite safety endpoint were increasing age, history of prior stroke, LVEF <30%, and TAVR device generation with remote history of pregnancy found to be associated with lower rate of the 30-day VARC-2 composite endpoint. Interestingly, both history of pregnancy and number of prior pregnancies were incremental predictors of the 30-day primary safety endpoint. Women who had never been pregnant were more frequently smokers with significant left main disease or more severely calcified aortic valves, and more often considered frail. Pregnancy did not appear to influence 30-day mortality and vascular or bleeding events but did impact death and stroke rates at 30 days. The all-cause mortality and stroke rates were lower than reported in the meta-analysis by O'Connor [32] which may largely be due to the use of newer-generation THVs, more experienced operators, smaller sheath sizes, as well as antithrombotic drug regimens at discharge.

16.7   Conclusion

TAVR trials are a unique setting with which to explore gender-related differences in aortic stenosis as women represent such a large proportion of the study population. Women present with various differences in morphologic and physiologic responses as compared to their male counterparts. Their symptomatology and baseline clinical profiles also differ greatly. While female sex is a risk factor for women undergoing SAVR, this has not played out in TAVR. As such, the mortality benefit of TAVR (as compared to SAVR) is greater for women than it is for men. In addition, despite higher rates of procedural complications as compared to men, early studies have shown improved survival in women as compared to men undergoing TAVR. While improvements in the latest generation of THVs, including expanded valve sizes and design elements to prevent PVL may result in a narrowing of the mortality differences between men and women, it remains clear that the benefits of TAVR for women are significant.

References

1. Ross J Jr, Braunwald E. Aortic stenosis. Circulation. 1968;38(1 suppl):61–7.
2. Leon MB, Smith CR, Mack M, Miller DC, Moses JW, Svensson LG, Tuzcu EM, Webb JG, Fontana GP, Makkar RR, Brown DL, Block PC, Guyton RA, Pichard AD, Bavaria JE, Herrmann HC, Douglas PS, Petersen JL, Akin JJ, Anderson WN, Wang D, Pocock S, for the PARTNER Trial Investigators. Transcatheter aortic-valve implantation for aortic stenosis in patients who cannot undergo surgery. N Engl J Med. 2010;363:1597–607.
3. Popma JJ, Adams DH, Reardon MJ, Yakubov SJ, Kleiman NS, Heimansohn D, James H Jr, Hughes GC, Harrison JK, Coselli J, Diez J, Kafi A, Schreiber T, Gleason TG, Conte J, Buchbinder M, Deeb GM, Carabello B, Serruys PW, Chenoweth S, Oh JK, for the CoreValve United States Clinical Investigators. CoreValve United States Clinical Investigators. Transcatheter aortic valve replacement using a self-expanding bioprosthesis in patients with severe aortic stenosis at extreme risk for surgery. J Am Coll Cardiol. 2014;63:1972–81.
4. Smith CR, Leon MB, Mack MJ, Miller DC, Moses JW, Svensson LG, Tuzcu EM, Webb JG, Fontana GP, Makkar RR, Williams M, Dewey T, Kapadia

S, Babaliaros V, Thourani VH, Corso P, Pichard AD, Bavaria JE, Herrmann HC, Akin JJ, Anderson WN, Wang D, Pocock SJ, for the PARTNER Trial Investigators. Transcatheter versus surgical aortic-valve replacement in high-risk patients. N Engl J Med. 2011;364:2187–98.

5. Adams DH, Popma JJ, Reardon MJ, Yakubov SJ, Coselli JS, Deeb GM, Gleason TG, Buchbinder M, Hermiller J Jr, Kleiman NS, Chetcuti S, Heiser J, Merhi W, Zorn G, Tadros P, Robinson N, Petrossian G, Hughes GC, Harrison JK, Conte J, Maini B, Mumtaz M, Chenoweth S, Oh JK, for the U.S. CoreValve Clinical Investigators. Transcatheter aortic-valve replacement with a self-expanding prosthesis. N Engl J Med. 2014;370:1790–8.

6. Leon MB, Smith CR, Mack MJ, Makkar RR, Svensson LG, Kodali SK, Thourani VH, Tuzcu EM, Miller DC, Herrmann HC, Doshi D, Cohen DJ, Pichard AD, Kapadia S, Dewey T, Babaliaros V, Szeto WY, Williams MR, Kereiakes D, Zajarias A, Greason KL, Whisenant BK, Hodson RW, Moses JW, Trento A, Brown DL, Fearon WF, Pibarot P, Hahn RT, Jaber WA, Anderson WN, Alu MC, Webb JG, for the PARTNER 2 Investigators. Transcatheter or surgical aortic-valve replacement in intermediate-risk patients. N Engl J Med. 2016;374:1609–20.

7. Reardon MJ, Van Mieghem NM, Popma JJ, Kleiman NS, Søndergaard L, Mumtaz M, Adams DH, Deeb GM, Maini B, Gada H, Chetcuti S, Gleason T, Heiser J, Lange R, Merhi W, Oh JK, Olsen PS, Piazza N, Williams M, Windecker S, Yakubov SJ, Grube E, Makkar R, Lee JS, Conte J, Vang E, Nguyen H, Chang Y, Mugglin AS, Serruys PWJC, Kappetein AP, for the SURTAVI Investigators. Surgical or transcatheter aortic-valve replacement in intermediate-risk patients. N Engl J Med. 2017;376:1321–31.

8. A prospective, randomized, controlled, multi-center study to establish the safety and effectiveness of the SAPIEN 3 transcatheter heart valve in low risk patients who have severe, calcific, aortic stenosis requiring aortic valve replacement. https://clinicaltrials.gov/ct2/show/NCT02675114

9. Transcatheter aortic valve replacement with the medtronic transcatheter aortic valve replacement system in patients at low risk for surgical aortic valve replacement. https://clinicaltrials.gov/ct2/show/NCT02701283

10. Carroll JD, Carroll EP, Feldman T, Ward DM, Lang RM, McGaughey D, Karp RB. Sex-associated differences in left ventricular function in aortic stenosis of the elderly. Circulation. 1992;86:1099–107.

11. Aurigemma GP, Silver KH, McLaughlin M, Mauser J, Gaasch WH. Impact of chamber geometry and gender on left ventricular systolic function in patients >60 years of age with aortic stenosis. Am J Cardiol. 1994;74:794–8.

12. Douglas PS, Otto CM, Mickel MC, Labovitz A, Reid CL, Davis KB. Gender differences in left ventricle geometry and function in patients undergoing balloon dilatation of the aortic valve for isolated aortic steno-

sis: NHLBI Balloon Valvuloplasty Registry. Br Heart J. 1995;73:548–54.

13. Kostkiewicz M, Tracz W, Olszowska M, Podolec P, Drop D. Left ventricular geometry and function in patients with aortic stenosis: gender differences. Int J Cardiol. 1999;71:57–61.

14. Stangl V, Baldenhofer G, Knebel F, Zhang K, Sanad W, Spethmann S, Grubitzsch H, Sander M, Ernecke K-DW, Baumann G, Stangl K, Laule M. Impact of gender on three-month outcome and left ventricular remodeling after transfemoral transcatheter aortic valve implantation. Am J Cardiol. 2012;110:884–90.

15. Kodali S, Williams MR, Doshi D, Hahn RT, Humphries KH, Nkomo VT, Cohen DJ, Douglas PS, Mack M, Xu K, Svensson L, Thourani VH, Tuzcu EM, Weissman NJ, Leon M, Kirtane AJ. Sex-specific differences at presentation and outcomes among patients undergoing transcatheter aortic valve replacement: a cohort study. Ann Intern Med. 2016;164(6):377–84.

16. Hachicha Z, Dumesnil JG, Bogaty P, Pibarot P. Paradoxical low-flow, low-gradient severe aortic stenosis despite preserved ejection fraction is associated with higher afterload and reduced survival. Circulation. 2007;115:2856–64.

17. Liyanange L, Lee NJ, Cook T, Herrmann HC, Jagasia D, Litt H, Han Y. The impact of gender on cardiovascular system calcification in very elderly patients with severe aortic stenosis. Int J Card Imaging. 2016;32:173–9.

18. Aggarwal SR, Clavel M-A, Messika-Zeitoun D, Cueff C, Malouf J, Araoz PA, Mankad R, Michelena H, Vahanian A, Enriquez-Sarano M. Sex differences in aortic valve calcification measured by multidetector computed tomography in aortic stenosis. Circ Cardiovasc Imaging. 2013;6:40–7.

19. Clavel M-A, Messika-Zeitoun D, Pibarot P, Aggarwal SR, Malouf J, Araoz PA, Michelena HI, Cueff C, Larose E, Capoulade R, Vahanian A, Enriquez-Sarano M. The complex nature of discordant severe calcified aortic valve disease grading: new insights from combined Doppler echocardiographic and computed tomographic study. J Am Coll Cardiol. 2013;62:2329–38.

20. Clavel M-A, Pibarot P, Messika-Zeitoun D, Capoulade R, Malouf J, Aggarval S, Araoz PA, Michelena HI, Cueff C, Larose E, Miller JD, Vahanian A, Enriquez-Sarano M. Impact of aortic valve calcification, as measured by MDCT, on survival in patients with aortic stenosis: results of an international registry study. J Am Coll Cardiol. 2014;64:1202–13.

21. Rylski B, Desjardins B, Moser W, Bavaria JE, Milewski RK. Gender-related changes in aortic geometry throughout life. Eur J Cardiothorac Surg. 2014;45:805–11.

22. Michelena HI, Margaryan FAM, Eleid M, Maalouf J, Suri R, Messika-Zeitoun D, Pellikka PA, Enriquez-Sarano M. Inconsistent echocardiographic grading of aortic stenosis: is the left ventricular outflow tract important? Heart. 2013;99:921–31.

23. Buellesfeld L, Stortecky S, Kalesan B, Gloekler S, Khattab AA, Nietlispach F, Delfine V, Huber C, Eberle B, Meier B, Wenaweser P, Windecker S. Aortic root dimensions among patients with severe aortic stenosis undergoing transcatheter aortic valve replacement. JACC Cardiovasc Interv. 2013;6:72–83.

24. Baumgartner H, Hung J, Bermejo J, Chambers JB, Evangelista A, Griffin BP, Iung B, Otto CM, Pellikka PA, Quiñones M. Echocardiographic assessment of valve stenosis: EAE/ASE recommendations for clinical practice. J Am Soc Echocardiogr. 2009;22:1–23; quiz 101–2

25. Sievers HH, Schmidtke C. A classification system for the bicuspid aortic valve from 304 surgical specimens. J Thorac Cardiovasc Surg. 2007;133:1226–33.

26. Michelena HI, Suri RM, Katan O, Eleid MF, Clavel M-A, Maurer MJ, Pellikka PA, Mahoney D, Enriquez-Sarano M. Sex differences and survival in adults with bicuspid aortic valves: verification in 3 contemporary echocardiographic cohorts. J Am Heart Assoc. 2016;5:e004211.

27. Mylotte D, Lefevre T, Søndergaard L, Watanabe Y, Modine T, Dvir D, Bosmans J, Tchetche D, Kornowski R, Sinning J-M, Thériault-Lauzier P, O'Sullivan CJ, Barbanti M, Debry N, Buithieu J, Codner P, Dorfmeister M, Martucci G, Nickenig G, Wenaweser P, Tamburino C, Grube E, Webb JG, Windecker S, Lange R, Piazza N. Transcatheter aortic valve replacement in bicuspid aortic valve disease. J Am Coll Cardiol. 2014;64:2330–9.

28. Perlman GY, Blanke P, Dvir D, Pache G, Modine T, Barbanti M, Holy EW, Treede H, Ruile P, Neumann F-J, Gandolfo C, Saia F, Tamburino C, Mak G, Thompson C, Wood D, Leipsic J, Webb JG. Bicuspid aortic valve stenosis: favorable early outcomes with a next-generation transcatheter heart valve in a multi-center study. J Am Coll Cardiol Intv. 2016;9:817–24.

29. Lee M, Yin W-H, Park D-W, Kang S-J, Lee S-W, Kim Y-H, Lee CW, Park S-W, Kim H-S, Butter C, Khalique OK, Schaefer U, Nietlispach F, Kodali SK, Leon MB, Ye J, Chevalier B, Leipsic J, Delgado V, Bax JJ, Tamburino C, Colombo A, Søndergaard L, Webb JG, Park S-J. Transcatheter aortic valve replacement with early- and new-generation devices in bicuspid aortic valve stenosis. J Am Coll Cardiol. 2016;68:1195–205.

30. Yousef A, Simard T, Webb J, Rodés-Cabau J, Costopoulos C, Kochman J, Hernández-Garcia JM, Chiam PTL, Welsh RC, Wijeysundera IIC, García E, Ribeiro HB, Latib A, Huczek Z, Shanks M, Testa L, Farkouh ME, Dvir D, Velianou JL, Lam B-K, Pourdjabbar A, Glover C, Hibbert B, Labinaz M. Transcatheter aortic valve implantation in patients with bicuspid aortic valve: a patient level multi-center analysis. Int J Cardiol. 2015;189:282–8.

31. Yoon S-H, Bleiziffer S, De Backer O, Delgado V, Arai T, Ziegelmueller J, Barbanti M, Sharma R, Perlman GY, Khalique OK, Holy EW, Saraf S, Deuschl F, Fujita B, Ruile P, Neumann F-J, Pache G, Takahashi M, Kaneko H, Schmidt T, Ohno Y, Schofer N, Kong WKF, Tay E, Sugiyama D, Kawamori H, Maeno Y, Abramowitz Y, Chakravarty T, Nakamura M, Kuwata

S, Yong G, Kao H-L, Lee M, Kim H-S, Modine T, Wong SC, Bedgoni F, Testa L, Teiger E, Butter C, Ensminger SM, Schaefer U, Dvir D, Blanke P, Leipsic J, Nietlispach F, Abdel-Wahab M, Chevalier B, Tamburino C, Hildick-Smith D, Whisenant BK, Park S-J, Colombo A, Latib A, Kodali SK, Bax JJ, Søndergaard L, Webb JG, Lefèvre T, Leon MB, Makkar R. Outcomes in transcatheter aortic valve replacement for bicuspid versus tricuspid aortic valve stenosis. J Am Coll Cardiol. 2017;69(21):2579–89.

32. O'Connor SA, Morice M-C, Gilard M, Leon MB, Webb JG, Dvir D, Rodés-Cabau J, Tamburino C, Capodanno D, D'Ascenzo F, Garot P, Chevalier B, Mikhail GW, Ludman PF. Revisiting sex equality with transcatheter aortic valve replacement outcomes: a collaborative, patient-level meta-analysis of 11,310 patients. J Am Coll Cardiol. 2015;66:221–8.

33. Buja P, Napodano M, Tamburino C, Petronio AS, Ettori F, Santoro G, Ussia GP, Klugmann S, Bedogni F, Ramondo A, Maisano F, Marzocchi A, Poli A, Gasparetto V, Antoniucci D, Colombo A, Tarantini G. Comparison of variables in men versus women undergoing transcatheter aortic valve implantation for severe aortic stenosis (from Italian Multicenter CoreValve registry). Am J Cardiol. 2013;111:88–93.

34. Green P, Arnold SV, Cohen DJ, Kirtane AJ, Kodali SK, Brown DL, Rihal CS, Xu K, Lei Y, Hawkey MC, Kim RJ, Alu MC, Leon MB, Mack MJ. Relation of frailty to outcomes after transcatheter aortic valve replacement (from the PARTNER trial). Am J Cardiol. 2015;116:264–9.

35. Green P, Woglom AE, Genereux P, Daneault B, Paradis J-M, Schnell S, Hawkey M, Maurer MS, Kirtane AJ, Kodali S, Moses JW, Leon MB, Smith CR, Williams M. The impact of frailty status on survival after transcatheter aortic valve replacement in older adults with severe aortic stenosis: a single-center experience. J Am Coll Cardiol Intv. 2012;5:974–81.

36. Humphries KH, Toggweiler S, Rodés-Cabau J, Nombela-Franco L, Dumont E, Wood DA, Willson AB, Binder RK, Freeman M, Lee MK, Gao M, Izadnegahdar M, Ye J, Cheung A, Webb JG. Sex differences in mortality after transcatheter aortic valve replacement for severe aortic stenosis. J Am Coll Cardiol. 2012;60:882–6.

37. Forrest JK, Adams DH, Popma JJ, Reardon MJ, Deeb GM, Yakubov SJ, Hermiller JB Jr, Huang J, Skelding Alexandra Lansky KA. Transcatheter aortic valve replacement in women versus men (from the US CoreValve Trials). Am J Cardiol. 2016;118(3):396–402.

38. Anderson RP. First publications from the Society of Thoracic Surgeons National Database. Ann Thorac Surg. 1994;57:6–7.

39. Nashef SA, Roques F, Michel P, Gauducheau E, Lemeshow S, Salamon R. European System or cardiac operative risk evaluation (EuroSCORE). Eur J Cardiothorac Surg. 1999;16:9–13.

40. Brown JM, O'Brien SM, Wu C, Sikora JAH, Griffith BP, Gammie JS. Isolated aortic valve replacement in North America comprising 108,687 patients in 10

years: changes in risks, valve types, and outcomes in the Society of Thoracic Surgeons National Database. J Thorac Cardiovasc Surg. 2009;137(1):82–90.

41. Roques F, Nashef SAM, Michel P, Gauducheau E, de Vincentiis C, Baudet E, Cortina J, David M, Faichney A, Gavrielle F, Gams E, Harjula A, Jones MT, Pinna Pintor P, Salamon R, Thulin L. Risk factors and outcome in European cardiac surgery: analysis of the EuroSCORE multinational database of 19030 patients. Eur J Cardiothorac Surg. 1999;15(6): 816–23.

42. Buchanan GL, Chieffo A, Montorfano M, Maisano F, Latib A, Godino C, Cioni M, Gullace MA, Franco A, Gerli C, Alfieri O, Colombo A. The role of sex on VARC outcomes following transcatheter aortic valve implantation with both Edwards SAPIEN and Medtronic CoreValve ReValving System devices: the Milan registry. EuroIntervention. 2011;7:556–63.

43. Humphries KH, Toggweiler S, Rodés-Cabau J, Nombela-Franco L, Dumont E, Wood DA, Wilson AB, Binder RK, Freeman M, Lee MK, Gao M, Izadnegahdar M, Ye J, Cheung A, Webb JG. Sex differences in mortality after transcatheter aortic valve replacement for severe aortic stenosis. J Am Coll Cardiol. 2012;60:882–6.

44. Mack MJ, Leon MB, Smith CR, Miller C, Moses JW, Tuzcu EM, Webb JG, Douglas PS, Anderson WN, Blackstone EH, Kodali SK, Makkar RR, Fontana GP, Kapadia S, Bavaria J, Hahn RT, Thourani VH, Babaliaros V, Pichard A, Herrmann HC, Brown DL, Williams M, Davidson MJ, Svensson LG, for the PARTNER 1 Trial Investigators. 5-year outcomes of transcatheter aortic valve replacement or surgical aortic valve replacement for high surgical risk patients with aortic stenosis (PARTNER 1): a randomised controlled trial. Lancet. 2015;385:2477–84.

45. Pieter Kappetein A, Head SJ, Genereux P, Piazza N, van Mieghem NM, Blackstone EH, Brott TG, Cohen DJ, Cutlip DE, van Es G-A, Hahn RT, Kirtane AJ, Krucoff MW, Kodali S, Mack MJ, Mehran R, Rodes-Cabau J, Vranckx P, Webb JG, Windecker S, Serruys PW, Leon MB. Valve Academic Research Consortium 2. Updated standardized endpoint definitions for transcatheter aortic valve implantation: the Valve Academic Research Consortium-2 consensus document. J Thorac Cardiovasc Surg. 2013;145:6–23.

46. Hayashida K, Morice M-C, Chevalier B, Hovasse T, Romano M, Garot P, Farge A, Donzeau-Gouge P, Bouvier E, Cormier B, Lefèvre T. Sex-related differences in clinical presentation and outcome of transcatheter aortic valve implantation for severe aortic stenosis. J Am Coll Cardiol. 2012;59:566–71.

47. Barbanti M, Yang T-H, Rodes-Cabau J, Tamburino C, Wood DA, Jilaihawi H, Blanke P, Makkar RR, Latib A, Colombo A, Tarantini G, Raju R, Binder RK, Nguyen G, Freeman M, Ribeiro HB, Kapadia S, Min J, Feuchtner G, Gurtvich R, Alqoofi F, Pelletier M, Ussia GP, Napodano M, de Brito FS Jr, Kodali S,

Norgaard BL, Hansson NC, Pache G, Canovas SJ, Zhang H, Leon MB, Webb JG, Leipsic J. Anatomical and procedural features associated with aortic root rupture during balloon expandable transcatheter aortic valve replacement. Circulation. 2013;128:244–53.

48. Conrotto F, D'Ascenzo F, Presbitero P, Humphries KH, Webb JG, O'Connor SA, Morice M-C, Lefèvre T, Grasso C, Sbarra P, Taha S, Omedè P, Marra WG, Salizzoni S, Moretti C, D'Amico M, Biondi-Zoccai G, Gaita F, Marra S. Effect of gender after transcatheter aortic valve implantation: a meta-analysis. Ann Thorac Surg. 2015;99:809–16.

49. Williams M, Kodali SK, Hahn RT, Humphries KH, Nkomo VT, Cohen DJ, Douglas PS, Mack M, Andrew TC, Svensson L, Thourani VH, Tuzcu EM, Weissman NJ, Kirtane AJ, Leon MB. Sex-related differences in outcomes after transcatheter or surgical aortic valve replacement in patients with severe aortic stenosis:insights from the PARTNER Trial (Placement of Aortic Transcatheter Valve). J Am Coll Cardiol. 2014;63:1522–8.

50. Ribeiro HB, Webb JG, Makkar RR, Cohen MG, Kapadia SR, Kodali S, Tamburino C, Barbanti M, Chakravarty T, Jilaihawi H, Paradis J-M, de Brito FS Jr, Cánovas SJ, Cheema AN, de Jaegere PP, del Valle R, Chiam PTL, Moreno R, Pradas G, Ruel M, Salgado-Fernández J, Sarmento-Leite R, Toeg HD, Velianou JL, Zajarias A, Babaliaros V, Cura F, Dager AE, Manoharan G, Lerakis S, Pichard AD, Radhakrishnan S, Perin MA, Dumont E, Larose E, Pasian SG, Nombela-Franco L, Urena M, Tuzcu EM, Leon MB, Amat-Santos IJ, Leipsic J, Rodés-Cabau J. Predictive factors, management, and clinical outcomes of coronary obstruction following transcatheter aortic valve implantation: insights from a large multicenter registry. J Am Coll Cardiol. 2013;62:1552–62.

51. Ribeiro HB, Sarmento-Leite R, Siqueira DA, Carvalho LA, Armando Mangione J, Rodés-Cabau J, Perin MA, de Brito FS Jr. Coronary obstruction following transcatheter aortic valve implantation. Arq Bras Cardiol. 2014;102:93–6.

52. Athappan G, Patvardhan E, Tuzcu EM, Svensson LG, Lemos PA, Fraccaro C, Tarantini G, Sinning J-M, Nickenig G, Capodanno D, Tamburino C, Latib A, Colombo A, Kapadia SR. Incidence, predictors, and outcomes of aortic regurgitation after transcatheter aortic valve replacement: meta-analysis and systematic review of literature. J Am Coll Cardiol. 2013;61:1585–95.

53. Sherif MA, Abdel-Wahab M, Stöcker B, Geist V, Richardt D, Tölg R, Richardt G. Anatomic and procedural predictors of paravalvular aortic regurgitation after implantation of the Medtronic CoreValve bioprosthesis. J Am Coll Cardiol. 2010;56:1623–9.

54. Takagi K, Latib A, Al-Lamee R, Mussardo M, Montorfano M, Maisano F, Godino C, Chieffo A, Alfieri O, Colombo A. Predictors of moderate-to-severe paravalvular aortic regurgitation immedi-

ately after CoreValve implantation and the impact of postdilatation. Catheter Cardiovasc Interv. 2011;78:432–43.

55. Kodali SK, Williams MR, Smith CR, Svensson LG, Webb JG, Makkar RR, Fontana GP, Dewey TM, Thourani VH, Pichard AD, Fischbein M, Szeto WY, Lim S, Greason KL, Teirstein PS, Malaisrie SC, Douglas PS, Hahn RT, Whisenant B, Zajarias A, Wang D, Akin JJ, Anderson WN, Leon MB, for the PARTNER Trial Investigators. Two-year outcomes after transcatheter or surgical aortic-valve replacement. N Engl J Med. 2012;366:1686–95.

56. Bonderman D, Graf A, Kammerlander AA, Kocher A, Laufer G, Lang IM, Mascherbaue J. Factors determining patient-prosthesis mismatch after aortic valve replacement—a prospective cohort study. PLoS One. 2013;8:e81940.

57. Head SJ, Mokhles MM, Osnabrugge RL, Pibarot P, Mack MJ, Takkenberg JJ, Bogers AJ, Kappetein AP. The impact of prosthesis–patient mismatch on long-term survival after aortic valve replacement: a systematic review and metaanalysis of 34 observational studies comprising 27 186 patients with 133 141 patient-years. Eur Heart J. 2012;33:1518–29.

58. Pibarot P, Weissman NJ, Stewart WJ, Hahn RT, Lindman BR, McAndrew T, Kodali SK, Mack MJ, Thourani VH, Miller DC, Svensson LG, Herrmann HC, Smith CR, Rodés-Cabau J, Webb J, Lim S, Xu K, Hueter I, Douglas PS, Leon MB. Incidence and sequelae of prosthesis-patient mismatch in transcatheter versus surgical valve replacement in high-risk patients with severe aortic stenosis: a PARTNER trial cohort—a analysis. J Am Coll Cardiol. 2014;64:1323–34.

59. Popma JJ, Khabbaz K. Prosthesis-patient mismatch after "high-risk" aortic valve replacement. J Am Coll Cardiol. 2014;64:1335–8.

60. Bleiziffer S, Hettich I, Hutter A, Wagner A, Deutsch MA, Piazz N, Lange R. Incidence and impact of prosthesis-patient mismatch after transcatheter aortic valve implantation. J Heart Valve Dis. 2013;22:309–16.

61. Jilaihawi H, Chin D, Spty T, Jeilan M, Vasa-Nicotera M, Bence J, Logtens E, Kovac J. Prosthesis patient mismatch after transcatheter aortic valve implantation with the Medtronic-CoreValve bioprosthesis. Eur Heart J. 2010;31:857–64.

62. Ewe SH, Muratori M, Delgado V, Pepi M, Tamborini G, Fusini L, Klautz RJM, Gripari P, Bax JJ, Fusari M, Schalij MJ, Marsan NA. Hemodynamic and clinical impact of prosthesis patient mismatch after transcatheter aortic valve implantation. J Am Coll Cardiol. 2011;58:1910–8.

63. Kalavrouziotis D, Rodés-Cabau J, Bagur R, Doyle D, De Larochellière R, Pibarot P, Dumont E. Transcatheter aortic valve implantation in patients with severe aortic stenosis and small aortic annulus. J Am Coll Cardiol. 2011;58:1016–24.

64. Skelding KA, Yakubov SJ, Kleiman NS, Reardon MJ, Adams DH, Huang J, Forrest JK, Popma JJ. Transcatheter aortic valve replacement versus surgery in women at high risk for surgical aortic valve replacement (from the CoreValve US High Risk Pivotal Trial). Am J Cardiol. 2016;118:560–6.

65. Petrov G, Regitz-Zagrosek V, Lehmkuhl E, Krabatsch T, Dunkel A, Dandel M, Dworatzek E, Mahmoodzadeh S, Schubert C, Becher E, Hampl H, Hetzer R. Regression of myocardial hypertrophy after aortic valve replacement: faster in women? Circulation. 2010;122:S23–8.

66. Stangl V, Baldenhofer G, Laule M, Baumann G, Stangl K. Influence of sex on outcome following transcatheter aortic valve implantation (TAVI): systematic review and meta-analysis. J Interv Cardiol. 2014;27:531–9.

67. Holmes DR Jr, Brennan JM, Rumsfeld JS, Dai D, O'Brien SM, Vemulapalli S, Edwards FH, Carroll J, Shahian D, Grover F, Tuzcu EM, Peterson ED, Brindis RG, Mack MJ, for the STS/ACC TVT Registry. Clinical outcomes at 1 year following transcatheter aortic valve replacement. JAMA. 2015;313:1019–28.

68. Chieffo A, Petronio AS, Mehilli J, Chandrasekhar J, Sartori S, Lefèvre T, Presbitero P, Capranzano P, Tchetche D, Iadanza A, Sardella G, Van Mieghem NM, Meliga E, Dumonteil N, Fraccaro C, Trabattoni D, Mikhail GW, Sharma S, Ferrer MC, Naber C, Kievit P, Faggioni M, Snyder C, Morice MC, Mehran R, on behalf of the WIN-TAVI Investigators. Acute and 30-day outcomes in women after TAVR results from the WIN-TAVI (Women's International Transcatheter Aortic Valve Implantation) Real-World Registry. JACC Cardiovasc Interv. 2016;9(15):1589–600.

Implementation Issues for Transcatheter Aortic Valve Implantation: Access, Value, Affordability, and Wait Times

17

Harindra C. Wijeysundera, Gabby Elbaz-Greener, Derrick Y. Tam, and Stephen E. Fremes

17.1 Introduction

Over the decade and a half since Cribier's description of the first human transcatheter aortic valve implantation (TAVI), also called transcatheter aortic valve replacement (TAVR), in 2002 [1], uptake has increased exponentially across the world [2, 3]. In 2004, high-surgical-risk TAVR feasibility studies were initiated, leading to the Conformité Européenne (CE) mark being granted in 2007 [2–4] followed by Food and Drug Administration (FDA) and Health Canada approval in 2011 [3, 5]. Over this period, over 350,000 procedures have been performed in more than 70 countries [3, 6]. Annually, there are over 17,000 new TAVR candidates in Europe and over 9000 in North America [7]. The indications for TAVR have evolved quickly from compassionate use as the last resort to being the first option for inoperable/high-risk patients [8, 9] and more recently as reasonable alternative for intermediate-risk populations [10–12]. TAVR has evolved from a challenging intervention to a standardized, simple, and streamlined procedure that has become standard of care [6, 13].

As TAVR has made this transition to standard of care, implementation issues are increasing importantly. Two conceptual models are helpful to frame a discussion around implementation. The first framework, known as the "life cycle" [14], describes the gradual penetration of a new product over time, from the development of the required threshold of robust clinical evidence to device iteration, physician training, and subsequent health system planning for dissemination [14, 15]. Superimposed on this is the cultural change within and across medical/surgical subspecialties required to embrace new therapies [15]. The shape of the life cycle curve can be affected by different economic factors such as initial capital costs, timeline of recovering these costs, and models of making the technology yield

H. C. Wijeysundera (✉)
Division of Cardiology, Department of Medicine, Schulich Heart Centre, Sunnybrook Health Sciences Centre, University of Toronto, Toronto, ON, Canada

Institute of Health Policy, Management and Evaluation, University of Toronto,
Toronto, ON, Canada

Institute for Clinical Evaluative Sciences (ICES),
Toronto, ON, Canada
e-mail: harindra.wijeysundera@sunnybrook.ca

G. Elbaz-Greener
Division of Cardiology, Department of Medicine, Schulich Heart Centre, Sunnybrook Health Sciences Centre, University of Toronto, Toronto, ON, Canada

D. Y. Tam · S. E. Fremes
Institute of Health Policy, Management and Evaluation, University of Toronto,
Toronto, ON, Canada

Division of Cardiac Surgery, Department of Surgery, Schulich Heart Centre, Sunnybrook Health Sciences Centre, University of Toronto, Toronto, ON, Canada
e-mail: stephen.Fremes@sunnybrook.ca

© Springer Nature Switzerland AG 2019
A. Giordano et al. (eds.), *Transcatheter Aortic Valve Implantation*,
https://doi.org/10.1007/978-3-030-05912-5_17

a profit proportionate to the costs and risks involved [14]. The second framework is termed the "disruptive technology or innovation" and describes a new technology that displaces an established one that shares the same market [14]; this would explain TAVR penetration as dependent on the sharing of the surgical aortic valve (SAVR) market and then displacing SAVR. This framework also has multiple economic and cultural aspects that influence the speed of dissemination. The focus of this chapter will be on these different concepts around TAVR implementation, specifically access, value, affordability, and the consequences of inadequate access, that of wait times and its adverse impacts. Finally, we will conclude a discussion on infrastructure needs, and how to balance access with quality of care, based on the relationship between procedural volume and outcomes.

17.2   TAVR Access

Despite the growth in TAVR demand, available data suggests that TAVR has remained relatively underutilized based on estimates of TAVR penetration in Europe and North America [5, 15]. The penetration rate of TAVR is a metric of the use of that therapy among eligible patients. Thus, TAVR penetration is a measure of actual TAVR use relative to potential use. Potential use is estimated by the prevalence of patients >75 years old, with symptomatic severe aortic stenosis at high or excessive surgical risk that could potentially be treated with TAVR [15]. Mylotte et al. reported a 17.9% TAVR penetration rate in 2011 in western Europe. The highest estimated nation-specific TAVR penetration rates were in Germany (36.2%) and Switzerland (34.5%). The lowest penetration rates were in Spain (8.4%) and Portugal (3.4%) [15]. TAVR penetration in Central and Eastern Europe have remained largely unreported; the exception is in Poland, where The Polish Interventional Cardiology TAVI Survey (PICTS) highlighted a lower rate of TAVR penetration in Poland in comparison to countries of Western Europe, 1.72% penetration rate in 2011 and 5.2% in 2015 [16]. Reported penetration rates in the United States and

Canada have been low compared to western Europe countries due to different regulatory requirements that delayed market access [5]; however, these have likely improved over time. Nonetheless, data from Canada suggests that even within the country across different regions, there is substantial inequity of access to TAVR [17].

Although the ideal penetration rate is not known, these statistics highlight the varied access to TAVR across jurisdictions [15]. The identification of inequitable access to medical technologies is important. It generates discussion and leads to initiatives to address inequalities and the corresponding impact on patient outcomes through payer- and physician-led programs [15]. Regional variation in the adoption of medical technology is not unique to TAVR. In Europe, disparate use of drug-eluting stents and implantable cardioverter-defibrillators (ICDs) has previously been described [18]. This inequity could partially be attributed to differences in health regulatory systems, limited economic resources, expanding technological capabilities, and demographically driven demands [14]. Differences in procedural reimbursement and healthcare funding are critical barriers in the implantation and access of new medical devices such as TAVR [19]. Indeed, TAVR-specific reimbursement systems were associated with a 3.3-fold higher number of TAVR implants per million population and 2.5 times more TAVR implants per center than constrained systems [15]. To understand and contrast reimbursement practices critically, one must first examine the value and subsequent affordability of TAVR.

17.3   Value and Affordability

Affordability and value are distinct concepts although both have an impact on reimbursement decisions and must be considered together. Affordability is the ability or inability to pay for an intervention from the perspective of the patient or the healthcare system. On the other hand, broadly speaking, value is measured as health outcomes achieved per dollar spent [20, 21]. Value is important as it defines the framework for measuring performance and efficiency in a healthcare system [21]. Thus, a discussion on affordability can only follow when value has been established via a cost-effectiveness analysis (CEA); assessing the affordability of an intervention of low value is a futile exercise. Here, we briefly describe important concepts in health economics in order to understand the cost-effectiveness of TAVR [22].

A new medical intervention, whether it is a drug or device, often displaces an existing standard; thus, the first step in a CEA is to determine the relevant comparators. In TAVR, the relevant comparator is either medical management or SAVR, depending on the population under study. After determining the relevant comparator(s), there are several means to compare the value of new interventions to the standard of care. A specific type of CEA, where costs and quality-adjusted life years (QALYs) are compared is termed a cost-utility analysis and is the criterion standard for most policy-makers and reimbursement agencies. These analyses output an incremental cost-effectiveness ratio (ICER), interpreted as the additional cost for each additional unit of health. When a new intervention offers clinical superiority at a lower cost compared to the standard of care, the intervention is deemed the "dominant" strategy and should be funded. Conversely, when a new intervention is clinically inferior and accompanied by higher costs, the new intervention is deemed economically "dominated" and should not be funded. However, most interventions provide incremental benefit at increased costs.

After the calculation of the ICER, in order to determine if the additional cost is reasonable, one must have a willingness-to-pay (WTP) threshold—the threshold at which the intervention is considered cost-effective and therefore should be adopted. The American College of Cardiology (ACC) and American Heart Association (AHA) consider WTP thresholds based on a country's gross domestic product (GDP) per capita: a WTP $\leq 1\times$ GDP per capita is high value, a WTP between 1 and 3$\times$ GDP per capita is of moderate value, and a WTP $\geq$ GDP per capita is of low value [23]. Thus, in the North American context, ICERs less than $50,000/QALY represent high value, while ICERs greater than $150,000/QALY are of low value [23]. The cost-effectiveness of TAVR must be discussed in the context of the specific population being treated with the intervention. As such, TAVR cost-effectiveness should be examined based on indications, which, at the present time, is related to estimated surgical risk as defined by the Society of Thoracic Surgeons (STS) Predicted Risk of Mortality (PROM) and restricted to patients with prohibitive, high, or intermediate surgical risk.

17.3.1 TAVR Versus Medical Therapy in Inoperable Patients

In patients at prohibitive surgical risk (STS-PROM 30 days >50%), balloon-expandable TAVR was compared against medical therapy in the Placement of Aortic Transcatheter Valves (PARTNER) 1B cohort [8]. A survival benefit was seen with TAVR along with marked improvement in quality of life at 1 month. Using prospective economic data collected alongside the PARTNER 1B trial, Reynolds et al. showed that TAVR was economically attractive compared to medical therapy with an ICER of USD $61,889/QALY over the lifetime time horizon from the US healthcare system perspective [24]. From the perspective of the Canadian healthcare system, Canadian cost data was combined with efficacy data from the PARTNER trial over a 3-year time horizon. An ICER of CAD $32,170/QALY was demonstrated [22]. Overall, these findings suggest that TAVR is cost-effective compared to medical management for patients at prohibitive surgical risk and of either good or moderate value based on ACC/AHA WTP thresholds [22]. Prohibitive surgical risk can be attributed to anatomical factors (i.e., porcelain aorta, previous CABG with patent grafts crossing midline) or irreversible medical comorbidities. One study found that TAVR was more economically attractive in prohibitive risk patients with anatomic factors compared to those with multiple comorbidities [25]. These findings suggest that careful patient selection plays an important role in containing costs and maximizing benefits.

17.3.2 TAVR Versus SAVR in High Surgical Risk

Patients at high surgical risk are defined as having a STS-PROM score greater than 15% at 30 days. An economic analysis performed using patient-level data from PARTNER 1A demonstrated that transfemoral (TF)-TAVR was a dominant strategy compared to SAVR, while non-TF TAVR was dominated by SAVR at 12 months [26]. A cost-effectiveness analysis of patients from the CoreValve Pivotal trial with a self-expandable valve system showed ICERs of USD $52,897/QALY and USD $62,767/QALY for TF and non-TF TAVR when compared to SAVR [22]. TAVR would be considered of moderate value with both ICERs. It is important to note that these results were obtained in an era where TAVR patients' average intensive care unit (ICU) length of stay (LOS) was 3 days in clinical trials. Total and ICU LOS may have decreased in the current era of a minimalist approach to TAVR. Overall, TAVR is likely to be cost-effective in the TF cohort compared to SAVR in the high-risk population, whereas non-TF TAVR may not be cost-effective compared to SAVR.

17.3.3 TAVR Versus SAVR in the Intermediate Surgical Risk

The efficacy for TAVR in the intermediate-risk population (STS-PROM 4–8%) has recently been examined in two large multicenter randomized clinical trials [10, 11]. A cost-effectiveness analysis using PARTNER 2 trial efficacy inputs and Canadian costing data showed that TAVR was likely to be cost-effective compared to SAVR although there was some uncertainty given the non-inferiority nature of the data [27]. This study demonstrated that important cost drivers in the intermediate-risk population included the cost of the TAVR system and ICU length of stay. A cost-effectiveness study by the study investigators for the PARTNER 2 trial was recently presented at TCT 2017 in Denver [28]. They used the as-treated population and compared the cost of 994 patients undergoing TAVR with Sapien XT with 944 patients undergoing SAVR from the perspective of the US healthcare system. They found that TAVR was the dominant strategy compared to SAVR.

In summary, TAVR has been shown to be cost-effective in the inoperable risk population, particularly for patients that were deemed inoperable due to anatomic factors. In the high-risk population, the literature suggests cost-effectiveness when the TF cohort was compared to SAVR. In the intermediate-risk population, a single cost-utility analysis from the perspective of the Canadian healthcare system has demonstrated that TAVR was likely to be cost-effective with moderate uncertainty. Given its value in several populations, affordability becomes an important criterion by which to inform TAVR reimbursement.

17.3.4 TAVR Affordability

The literature on healthcare affordability in TAVR is limited, as much of the research has focused on value rather than affordability. A budget impact analysis (BIA) allows for the analysis of the impact of a novel intervention on the payer's budget. Briefly, BIA forecasts the financial impact of implementing a new drug or intervention by considering future costs from the payer's perspective. Two scenarios are typically compared, the "reference case" and the "new intervention case" to evaluate the annual incremental cost over a period of interest. Guidelines recommend 3–5 years as the time horizon [29]. The incorporated treatment costs should reflect local practice patterns and include any relevant complication costs over the time period. The size of the market (i.e., number of patients eligible) for the new intervention must also be forecasted for both the new intervention and the reference case.

The size of the future TAVR market has been estimated by several investigators. Using decision analysis and Monte Carlo simulation, Osnabrugge estimated the number of patients with AS and number of TAVR candidates for several European and North American countries based on population demographic data [7]. In this analysis, there was an estimated 189,836 (95% CI: 80,281–347,372) TAVR candidates in Europe and 102,558 (95% CI 43,612–187,002) in North America, with an annual incidence of new TAVR candidates of 17,712 and 9189, respectively [7]. Importantly, this study only included patients at high or inoperable risk as the PARTNER 2 and SURTAVI trials were ongoing at the time of publication. They estimated in their sensitivity analyses an additional 145,000 intermediate-risk and 730,000 low-risk TAVR candidates across Europe and North America.

The enormous potential market of TAVR candidates, as well as the indication creep to lower-risk patients, is reflected by the temporal trends of TAVR adoption. In the TVT registry, there were 16,295 and 24,808 TAVR performed in 2014 and 2015 in the United States [30]. The median STS score for these patients declined from 6.8% in 2013 to 6.3% in 2015, suggesting that the majority of these patients were intermediate risk. Analysis of the Applied Quality Improvement and Research in Healthcare database, the mandatory quality control database for all SAVR and TAVR in Germany, showed that the number of TF-TAVR (10,299) exceeded the number of SAVR (9953) in 2014 [31]. Taken together, these findings suggest that the number of TAVRs will continue to rise substantially. These findings have tremendous implications for affordability, namely, what is the additional cost to treat all patients that are TAVR candidates. The authors estimated the budget impact of treating all eligible patients (inoperable and high risk) to be approximately $13.7 billion and $7.2 billion USD, respectively, based on an index hospitalization cost of $70,000 from two cost-effectiveness analyses [7, 24, 26]. However, the above figures did not consider the shift of patients out the SAVR arm and into the TAVR arm in their calculation of the cost impact of TAVR implementation.

The importance of shifting patient groups from SAVR to TAVR and the associated impact on affordability and budget impact cannot be overemphasized. Illustrating this point, a budget impact analysis performed in Canada's most populous province, Ontario (~13 million people), estimated the impact of shifting a proportion of high-risk patients from SAVR to TAVR over a 5-year time period in 2015 Canadian dollars from the perspective of the payer (Ontario's Ministry of Health) [32]. The target rate of TAVR in the BIA was 61.23 TAVR procedures per million population, translating to over 4351 high-risk patients shifted from SAVR to instead receive TAVR between 2016 and 2020. The total budget impact over 5 years was found to be only $8.2 million. This relatively modest amount recognizes that as TAVR extends into populations that are currently treated with SAVR, TAVR affordability is contingent on a shift of funds from SAVR—the required incremental new funds from outside the aortic valve envelop is modest. That said, a shift in funding has important implications on hospital capacity and infrastructure requirements, as well as physician and allied healthcare training and scope of practice. There will likely be substantial cultural barriers within and across specialties to such change that will require institutional leadership to overcome. As TAVR extends into lower-risk populations, this impact will be increasingly important.

17.3.5 Modifiable Costs

The costs of a TAVR procedure can be divided into the prosthesis and non-prosthesis costs, with the latter predominantly due to the index hospitalization. Cost drivers of care at index hospitalization for patients undergoing treatment with aortic valve replacement has been well studied using population databases housed in Ontario, Canada [33]. Using the Cardiac Care Network Registry to identify patients undergoing TAVR or SAVR with or without concomitant CABG, and micro-costing techniques, Wijeysundera et al. showed that the median index hospitalization costs were higher for TAVR ($42,742 CAD IQR: $37,295 to $56,196) compared to SAVR ($21,811, IQR $18,148 to $30,498) and SAVR with CABG (for $27,256, IQR $21,741 to $39,000). Patient-level cost drivers of care were identified: age >75 and renal impairment were significant predictors for both TAVR and SAVR, while lung disease was an important driver for TAVR only. Importantly, there were a number of potentially modifiable cost drivers, namely, that non-TF access TAVR was associated with a 30% increase in cost. Those with an ICU LOS less than 2 days had substantially lower costs, while those with overall hospital stays >3 days had substantially increased costs. Such modifiable cost drivers can be targets of quality improvement programs to improve overall efficiency of care delivery. Moreover, it is likely that there are areas for efficiency beyond the index hospitalization. It is an area of ongoing research as to the costs and their associated drivers in other relevant phases of TAVR care, specifically the pre-procedural period from referral and the post-procedural period beyond the index hospitalization.

McCarthy et al. compared Medicare payments for the cost of care of SAVR or TAVR in a propensity score (PS)-matched study of 3304 pairs [34]. This study found that in 2012, Medicare spent $215 million on 4083 patients undergoing TAVR. Hospital costs were higher for TAVR patients (median $50,200 USD 2012; IQR: 39,800–64,300) compared to PS-matched SAVR patients ($45,500; IQR: $34,500–$63,300; $p < 0.01$). This difference in cost was driven mainly by the higher TAVR prosthesis system. However, Medicare payments were lower for TAVR hospitalizations than for SAVR hospitalizations (median $49,500 vs. $50,400; $p < 0.01$). This meant that TAVRs contributed negatively to the margin of the hospital (i.e., on average, the hospital lost money per TAVR patient), while SAVR contributed positively to the margin of the hospital (−$3380 vs. +$2390). Importantly, this study found that there was a volume–outcome relationship; centers that performed more than 50 annual TAVR cases were able to achieve a net positive per patient contribution margin compared to those that performed less than 50 cases (median +$7761 vs. −$9037). These findings suggest that reimbursement for TAVR in 2012 was inadequate to cover the cost of performing the procedure. However, efficiencies in high-volume centers may have helped lower overall hospital costs to allow for a positive contribution margin for each case of TAVR. This study reinforces the importance of efficiencies from care pathways to reduce non-prosthesis-related costs to increase overall affordability. Moreover, it illustrates that funding models require updating to keep pace with the rapidly changing landscape of valve disease, such that hospitals are not penalized for pursuing appropriate percutaneous techniques such as TAVR.

17.3.6 TAVR Device Pricing and Procurement

Currently, the cost of TAVR prostheses ranges from $24,000 CAD to $36,000 USD, which is three- to fivefold greater than for surgical prostheses [26, 27, 35]. The cause for this price variability across TAVR devices remains unclear and has yet to be studied. However, cost variability for devices have been well studied in knee and hip arthroplasty surgery where the device implant accounts for the majority of the index episode of care hospitalization costs, similar to a TAVR procedure where the price of the device can account for almost half of the index hospitalization costs. A study examining the variability in knee or hip implant costs of 61 US hospitals found huge variation in the average implant cost (ranging from $1797 to $12,093 USD). Despite adjustment for patient and hospital characteristics, 37–60% of the total cost variance remain unexplained [36] and may be attributable to differences in hospital device procurement. Similarly, a wide variation in the cost of TAVR devices has been demonstrated across different countries. Currently, the vast majority of TAVRs in the United States are performed using either the Medtronic CoreValve or the Edward Life Sciences Sapien valve system. In Europe, other device manufacturers include JenaValve system. It is unclear whether the addition of new device manufacturers into the TAVR market will create sufficient competition to drive down the overall prices of the prosthesis. In orthopedics, there are five major joint implant manufacturers, and despite innovation and an increase in volume of patients requiring a prosthesis, device costs have not decreased with time but, in fact, have increased [37].

Importantly, for TAVR to be affordable, it requires that the procured prosthesis fits within a system of care where other cost drivers, such as LOS, and proportion of TF access are optimized. This sets the stage for innovative procurement practices such as value-based procurement, whereby a prosthesis is not selected purely based on lowest price, but instead there is industry support for process changes to achieve optimization on other non-prosthesis-related cost drivers, such as LOS. This can involve financial incentives for achieving these benchmarks, all of which is negotiated as part of the procurement process.

17.4 TAVR Wait Times

These issues regarding reimbursement and affordability have resulted in restricted capacity for TAVR. The imbalance between the demand and the TAVR capacity may result in long wait times. Wait-time management has been of increasing importance in many jurisdictions [38, 39]. Canada and the majority of the Organization for Economic Cooperation and Development (OECD) countries monitor national waiting time statistics and have procedural waiting time benchmarks, across multiple areas of medicine [40, 41]. However, the field of wait-time management has a number of inherent uncertainties, the first of which is how the wait-time metric is measured [42]. In the literature, there are different ways that are used to measure wait time for cardiovascular interventions [42]. Some studies define wait time as the interval between the referral to a cardiovascular surgeon and the date of surgery [43]. Others define the wait time as the period between the day of the clinical decision to perform an intervention to the actual intervention date [44]. It is important to consider the entire waiting interval measured from first contact with the medical care provider to procedure date, given the fact that the patient is at risk throughout this period and there are processes within this time period that can be potentially improved and streamlined [45, 46]. This may require fidelity in the wait-time monitoring system such that if a patient has comorbidities that require attention first or is not sufficiently symptomatic to warrant intervention, the wait time can be put on hold and not penalize the institution.

There is a limited literature on wait times in TAVR and its consequences. An evaluation of 378 patients from 3 hospitals during their early experience in TAVR showed a median wait time of 71 days [47]. An analysis of 4461 patients referred to TAVR in Ontario, Canada, from 2010 to 2016 showed a median wait time of approximately 80 days, which has stayed essentially unchanged since funding was initiated [48]. There are currently no guidelines for an appropriate TAVR wait time. The Canadian Wait-Time Alliance suggests a maximum wait time of 42 days for SAVR. Although TAVR wait times are markedly greater, the critical question is whether this is meaningful. A potential means to address this is to understand the magnitude of adverse consequences that occur during the waiting period for TAVR and if there is any relationship to the length of delay in treatment.

A previous paper estimated the hypothetical impact of increasing wait time on the effectiveness of TAVR [49], applying a mathematical simulation model with data from the seminal randomized clinical trials in this area. It was shown that TAVR wait time beyond 60 days would negate any potential benefit of TAVR over traditional surgical aortic valve replacement (SAVR) [49]. Data from the early period of use of TAVR showed mortality rates of 10–14% in patients waiting for TAVR [47, 50]. In Ontario, Canada, from 2010 to 2016, the cumulative probability of the TAVR wait-list mortality was 4.3% in a predominantly inoperable and high-risk population, with a relatively constant increase in mortality as wait time increased [48]. In other words, there did not appear to be a threshold wait time below which it was "safe" to delay the TAVR.

To place this mortality in context, previous contemporary registries and trials in TAVR show a 30-day all-cause mortality of 3.9% and 3.4% while that for SAVR is 4.1% and 6.5% for intermediate- and high-risk patients, respectively [9, 10, 51]. The latest randomized SURTAVI trial demonstrated even lower 30-day all-cause mortality 2.2% for TAVR and 1.7% for SAVR [51]. We would argue that it is rational to expect that mortality while waiting for a procedure should be less than the procedural mortality, suggesting that current wait-time mortality is unacceptably high. Although the wait-list mortality in intermediate-risk patients is not known, and we would hypothesize that it would be lower than that for higher-risk patients, this argument remains true, given the even lower post-procedural mortality in lower-risk patients.

In terms of other adverse events during the delay to TAVR treatment, approximately 14.7% of patients had a HF hospitalization while on the wait list [48]. HF hospitalization is also associated with substantial morbidity and healthcare costs. TAVR patients, whom require HF hospitalization prior to their TAVR, require a prolonged post-TAVR stay, which is associated with worse outcome and increased costs [52, 53].

Recently, it is increasingly recognized that a positive outcome for TAVR must include decrease in mortality and improvement in quality of life [54]. A critical determinant of post-TAVR improvement in quality of life is the pre-procedural status, and as such, any deterioration while waiting for TAVR is likely to have a substantial impact on post-TAVR recovery [55]. Indeed, patients awaiting TAVR have increasing symptoms with concomitant decreased quality of life [56], with a delay of greater than 6 weeks for TAVR associated with a significant higher decline in functional status and increase in frailty during the wait-time period [57].

Thus, if we accept that current TAVR wait times are excessive, the fundamental question is what should be considered the appropriate wait time for TAVR. As mentioned, to date, there is no consensus on the acceptable wait time for TAVR. As a conceptual framework, we would argue that a single wait-time benchmark is not logical, but instead benchmarks should reflect the risk profile of the patients and the potential for adverse clinical consequences. Methods for triaging patients on the wait list into low, medium, and high risk for wait-time deterioration should be informed by empiric evidence and remains an area of active research. The associated maximum

wait times for each of these groups remain undefined, with preliminary data suggest a wait time of between 42 and 60 days. To inform the required funding envelop and infrastructure needs, one must understand both the burden of disease and the maximum delay to treatment that is reasonable.

17.4.1 Infrastructure Complexities: Volume–Outcome Relationships

Optimizing TAVR capacity, and therefore wait times, requires both adequate funding and infrastructure. As more hospitals initiate TAVR programs, this can address the infrastructure needs; however, balanced against this is the expertise required for both safe and efficient care, which requires a sufficient volume of cases. To date, there are no volume-based guidelines for TAVR [58, 59].

Some have recommended centralization of TAVR procedures in high-volume tertiary referral centers to ensure adequate operator and center volume for these complex procedures [60–62]. Mylotte and colleagues observed substantial variation in hospital volume in Europe and highlighted that there were potentially an excessive number of TAVR centers in some countries [15]. Different factors such as national political and financial concerns, population density, and profile and different reimbursement strategies may have an important influence on the number of centers in each nation [15]. This topic has become of increasing importance after recent publications showing a clear inverse relationship between TAVR volume center and outcomes mortality [63–65], similar to that previously demonstrated for patients undergoing other surgical cardiac interventions [66, 67].

A volume–outcome association was assessed using data from the STS/ACC TVT registry including 42,988 TAVR procedures conducted at 395 hospitals from 2011 to 2015 [63–65]. Between the 1st case and the 400th case in the volume–outcome model, risk-adjusted adverse outcomes declined significantly in mortality

(3.57% to 2.15%), bleeding (9.56% to 5.08%), vascular complications (6.11% to 4.20%), and stroke (2.03% to 1.66%) [68]. Similar findings were also reported in the prospective German Quality Assurance Registry on TAVR comprising 9924 patients undergoing transfemoral (TR) TAVR in 2014. The average inhospital mortality in the highest-volume centers performing ≥ 200 TF-TAVR procedures annually was half of that of low-volume centers with <100 procedures [69]. Across the spectrum of hospital volumes ranging between 11 and 415 TF-TAVR patients per year, there was a statistically significant association between improved outcomes and increasing TF-TAVR volumes [69]. In a similar manner, Badheka and colleagues described an almost 50% reduction in mortality rates in high- versus low-volume centers. Above and beyond mortality, length of hospital LOS and hospitalization costs were significantly higher in lower-volume centers [65]. In addition, a recent meta-analysis that included seven European national TAVR registries (UK, Swiss, Belgium, Italy, Spain, France, Germany) reported that limiting the number of TAVR centers to selected ones with concentrated expertise led to reduction in 30-day mortality, reinforcing that notion that TAVR should be restricted to highly specialized centers [70]. This issue reflects the nuanced and difficult decision-making required of policy-makers, in order to balance access with quality of care.

17.5 Conclusions

We have highlighted some of the many issues regarding the implementation of a resource-intensive intervention such as TAVR that extends beyond acquisition of the prosthesis but rather adoption of a novel system of care. Despite its growth, TAVR has demonstrated marked variation of access across jurisdictions, with inadequate capacity manifested by prolonged wait times and adverse consequences due to delays in treatment. The underlying causes are multifactorial. Despite its high costs, there are modifiable drivers of cost, both prosthesis related and non-prosthesis related. Optimization of capacity, via

optimization of funding models and infrastructure, is paramount to address these implementation barriers.

References

1. Cribier A, Eltchaninoff H, Bash A, Borenstein N, Tron C, Bauer F, et al. Percutaneous transcatheter implantation of an aortic valve prosthesis for calcific aortic stenosis: first human case description. Circulation. 2002;106(24):3006–8.
2. Cribier A. Development of transcatheter aortic valve implantation (TAVI): a 20-year odyssey. Arch Cardiovasc Dis. 2012;105(3):146–52.
3. Cribier A. The development of transcatheter aortic valve replacement (TAVR). Glob Cardiol Sci Pract. 2016;2016(4):e201632.
4. Lawrie GM. Role of transcatheter aortic valve implantation (TAVI) versus conventional aortic valve replacement in the treatment of aortic valve disease. Methodist Debakey Cardiovasc J. 2012;8(2):4–8.
5. Dvir D, Barbash IM, Ben-Dor I, Okubagzi P, Satler LF, Waksman R, et al. The development of transcatheter aortic valve replacement in the USA. Arch Cardiovasc Dis. 2012;105(3):160–4.
6. Barbanti M, Webb JG, Gilard M, Capodanno D, Tamburino C. Transcatheter aortic valve implantation in 2017: state of the art. EuroIntervention. 2017;13(AA):AA11–21.
7. Osnabrugge RL, Mylotte D, Head SJ, Van Mieghem NM, Nkomo VT, LeReun CM, et al. Aortic stenosis in the elderly: disease prevalence and number of candidates for transcatheter aortic valve replacement: a meta-analysis and modeling study. J Am Coll Cardiol. 2013;62(11):1002–12.
8. Leon MB, Smith CR, Mack M, Miller DC, Moses JW, Svensson LG, et al. Transcatheter aortic-valve implantation for aortic stenosis in patients who cannot undergo surgery. N Engl J Med. 2010;363(17):1597–607.
9. Smith CR, Leon MB, Mack MJ, Miller DC, Moses JW, Svensson LG, et al. Transcatheter versus surgical aortic-valve replacement in high-risk patients. N Engl J Med. 2011;364(23):2187–98.
10. Leon MB, Smith CR, Mack MJ, Makkar RR, Svensson LG, Kodali SK, et al. Transcatheter or surgical aortic-valve replacement in intermediate-risk patients. N Engl J Med. 2016;374(17):1609–20.
11. Jones DA, Tchetche D, Forrest J, Hellig F, Lansky A, Moat N. The SURTAVI study: TAVI for patients with intermediate risk. EuroIntervention. 2017;13(5):e617–e20.
12. Hamm CW, Arsalan M, Mack MJ. The future of transcatheter aortic valve implantation. Eur Heart J. 2016;37(10):803–10.
13. Vahl TP, Kodali SK, Leon MB. Transcatheter aortic valve replacement 2016: a modern-day "through

the looking-glass" adventure. J Am Coll Cardiol. 2016;67(12):1472–87.

14. Brian D, Smith RT, Vella V. The role of product life cycle in medical technology innovation. J Med Market. 2013;13(1):37–43.

15. Mylotte D, Osnabrugge RLJ, Windecker S, Lefevre T, de Jaegere P, Jeger R, et al. Transcatheter aortic valve replacement in Europe: adoption trends and factors influencing device utilization. J Am Coll Cardiol. 2013;62(3):210–9.

16. Parma R, Dabrowski M, Ochala A, Witkowski A, Dudek D, Siudak Z, et al. The Polish Interventional Cardiology TAVI Survey (PICTS): adoption and practice of transcatheter aortic valve implantation in Poland. Postepy Kardiol Interwencyjnej. 2017;13(1):10–7.

17. Asgar AW, Lauck S, Ko D, Lambert LJ, Kass M, Adams C, et al. The transcatheter aortic valve implantation (TAVI) quality report: a call to arms for improving quality in Canada. Can J Cardiol. 2018;34(3):330–2.

18. Kearney P, Stokoe G, Breithardt G, Longson C, Marco J, Morgan J, et al. Improving patient access to novel medical technologies in Europe. Eur Heart J. 2006;27(7):882–5.

19. Ryden L, Stokoe G, Breithardt G, Lindemans F, Potgieter A. Task Force 2 of the Cardiovascular Round Table of the European Society of C. Patient access to medical technology across Europe. Eur Heart J. 2004;25(7):611–6.

20. Cerfolio RJ. What is value health care and who is the judge? Eur J Cardiothorac Surg. 2017;52(6):1015–7.

21. Porter ME. What is value in health care? N Engl J Med. 2010;363(26):2477–81.

22. Sud M, Tam DY, Wijeysundera HC. The economics of transcatheter valve interventions. Can J Cardiol. 2017;33(9):1091–8.

23. Anderson JL, Heidenreich PA, Barnett PG, Creager MA, Fonarow GC, Gibbons RJ, et al. ACC/AHA statement on cost/value methodology in clinical practice guidelines and performance measures: a report of the American College of Cardiology/American Heart Association Task Force on Performance Measures and Task Force on Practice Guidelines. Circulation. 2014;129(22):2329–45.

24. Reynolds MR, Magnuson EA, Wang K, Lei Y, Vilain K, Walczak J, et al. Cost-effectiveness of transcatheter aortic valve replacement compared with standard care among inoperable patients with severe aortic stenosis: results from the placement of aortic transcatheter valves (PARTNER) trial (Cohort B). Circulation. 2012;125(9):1102–9.

25. Neyt M, Van Brabandt H, Devriese S, Van De Sande S. A cost-utility analysis of transcatheter aortic valve implantation in Belgium: focusing on a well-defined and identifiable population. BMJ Open. 2012;2(3):e001032.

26. Reynolds MR, Magnuson EA, Lei Y, Wang K, Vilain K, Li H, et al. Cost-effectiveness of transcatheter aortic valve replacement compared with surgical aortic valve replacement in high-risk patients with severe aortic stenosis: results of the PARTNER (Placement of Aortic Transcatheter Valves) trial (Cohort A). J Am Coll Cardiol. 2012;60(25):2683–92.

27. Tam DY, Hughes A, Fremes SE, Youn S, Hancock-Howard RL, Coyte PC, et al. A cost-utility analysis of transcatheter versus surgical aortic valve replacement for the treatment of aortic stenosis in the population with intermediate surgical risk. J Thorac Cardiovasc Surg. 2018;155:1978–1988.e1.

28. Cohen D. Surgical aortic valve replacement in intermediate risk patients results from the PARTNER 2A and Sapien 3 Intermediate Risk Trials. https://www.acc.org/~/media/Clinical/PDF-Files/Approved-PDFs/2017/10/24/TCT17_Presentation_Slides/Tue_Oct31/PARTNER-2A-SAPIEN-3-Cost-Effectiveness-TCT-2017.pdf. TCT; October 31, 2017.

29. CADTH. Guidelines for the economic evaluation of health technologies. 4th ed. https://www.cadth.ca. Ottawa: Canadian Agency for Drugs and Technologies; 2017.

30. Grover FL, Vemulapalli S, Carroll JD, Edwards FH, Mack MJ, Thourani VH, et al. 2016 annual report of the Society of Thoracic Surgeons/American College of Cardiology Transcatheter Valve Therapy Registry. J Am Coll Cardiol. 2017;69(10):1215–30.

31. Gaede L, Kim WK, Blumenstein J, Liebetrau C, Dorr O, Nef H, et al. Temporal trends in transcatheter and surgical aortic valve replacement: an analysis of aortic valve replacements in Germany during 2012–2014. Herz. 2017;42(3):316–24.

32. Health Quality Ontario. Transcatheter aortic valve implantation for treatment of aortic stenosis: a health technology assessment. 2016;16:1–94.

33. Wijeysundera HC, Li L, Braga V, Pazhaniappan N, Pardhan AM, Lian D, et al. Drivers of healthcare costs associated with the episode of care for surgical aortic valve replacement versus transcatheter aortic valve implantation. Open Heart. 2016;3(2):e000468.

34. McCarthy FH, Savino DC, Brown CR, Bavaria JE, Kini V, Spragan DD, et al. Cost and contribution margin of transcatheter versus surgical aortic valve replacement. J Thorac Cardiovasc Surg. 2017;154(6):1872–80.e1.

35. Ribera A, Slof J, Andrea R, Falces C, Gutierrez E, Del Valle-Fernandez R, et al. Transfemoral transcatheter aortic valve replacement compared with surgical replacement in patients with severe aortic stenosis and comparable risk: cost-utility and its determinants. Int J Cardiol. 2015;182:321–8.

36. Robinson JC, Pozen A, Tseng S, Bozic KJ. Variability in costs associated with total hip and knee replacement implants. J Bone Joint Surg Am. 2012;94(18):1693–8.

37. http://www.nytimes.com/2013/08/04/health/for-medical-tourists-simple-math.html?pagewanted=all.

38. Siciliani L, Borowitz M, Moran V. Waiting time policies in the health sector: what works? OECD health policy studies. Paris: OECD Publishing; 2013.

39. Ansell D, Crispo JAG, Simard B, Bjerre LM. Interventions to reduce wait times for primary care

appointments: a systematic review. BMC Health Serv Res. 2017;17(1):295.

40. Viberg N, Forsberg BC, Borowitz M, Molin R. International comparisons of waiting times in health care—limitations and prospects. Health Policy. 2013;112(1–2):53–61.

41. http://www.waittimealliance.ca/about-us/.

42. Legare JF, Li D, Buth KJ. How established wait time benchmarks significantly underestimate total wait times for cardiac surgery. Can J Cardiol. 2010;26(1):e17–21.

43. Kent H. Waiting-list web site "inaccurate" and "misleading," BC doctors complain. CMAJ. 1999;161(2):181–2.

44. Lund O, Nielsen TT, Emmertsen K, Flo C, Rasmussen B, Jensen FT, et al. Mortality and worsening of prognostic profile during waiting time for valve replacement in aortic stenosis. Thorac Cardiovasc Surg. 1996;44(6):289–95.

45. Munt BI, Humphries KH, Gao M, Moss RR, Thompson CR. True versus reported waiting times for valvular aortic stenosis surgery. Can J Cardiol. 2006;22(6):497–502.

46. Lauck S, Stub D, Webb J. Monitoring wait times for transcatheter aortic valve implantation: a need for national benchmarks. Can J Cardiol. 2014;30(10):1150–2.

47. Nuis RJ, Dager AE, van der Boon RM, Jaimes MC, Caicedo B, Fonseca J, et al. Patients with aortic stenosis referred for TAVI: treatment decision, in-hospital outcome and determinants of survival. Neth Heart J. 2012;20(1):16–23.

48. Elbaz-Greener G, Masih S, Fang J, Ko DT, Lauck SB, Webb JG, et al. Temporal trends and clinical consequences of wait-times for trans-catheter aortic valve replacement: a population based study. Circulation. 2018;138:483–93.

49. Wijeysundera HC, Wong WW, Bennell MC, Fremes SE, Radhakrishnan S, Peterson M, et al. Impact of wait times on the effectiveness of transcatheter aortic valve replacement in severe aortic valve disease: a discrete event simulation model. Can J Cardiol. 2014;30(10):1162–9.

50. Bainey KR, Natarajan MK, Mercuri M, Lai T, Teoh K, Chu V, et al. Treatment assignment of high-risk symptomatic severe aortic stenosis patients referred for transcatheter AorticValve implantation. Am J Cardiol. 2013;112(1):100–3.

51. Reardon MJ, Van Mieghem NM, Popma JJ, Kleiman NS, Sondergaard L, Mumtaz M, et al. Surgical or transcatheter aortic-valve replacement in intermediate-risk patients. N Engl J Med. 2017;376(14):1321–31.

52. Arbel Y, Zivkovic N, Mehta D, Radhakrishnan S, Fremes SE, Rezaei E, et al. Factors associated with length of stay following trans-catheter aortic valve replacement—a multicenter study. BMC Cardiovasc Disord. 2017;17(1):137.

53. Sud M, Qui F, Austin PC, Ko DT, Wood D, Czarnecki A, et al. Short length of stay after elective transfemoral transcatheter aortic valve replacement is not associated with increased early or late readmission risk. J Am Heart Assoc. 2017;6(4):e005460.

54. Arnold SV, Reynolds MR, Lei Y, Magnuson EA, Kirtane AJ, Kodali SK, et al. Predictors of poor outcomes after transcatheter aortic valve replacement: results from the PARTNER (Placement of Aortic Transcatheter Valve) trial. Circulation. 2014;129(25):2682–90.

55. Arnold SV, Spertus JA, Lei Y, Green P, Kirtane AJ, Kapadia S, et al. How to define a poor outcome after transcatheter aortic valve replacement: conceptual framework and empirical observations from the placement of aortic transcatheter valve (PARTNER) trial. Circ Cardiovasc Qual Outcomes. 2013;6(5):591–7.

56. Olsson K, Naslund U, Nilsson J, Hornsten A. Experiences of and coping with severe aortic stenosis among patients waiting for transcatheter aortic valve implantation. J Cardiovasc Nurs. 2016;31(3):255–61.

57. Forman JM, Currie LM, Lauck SB, Baumbusch J. Exploring changes in functional status while waiting for transcatheter aortic valve implantation. Eur J Cardiovasc Nurs. 2015;14(6):560–9.

58. Levine GN, Bates ER, Blankenship JC, Bailey SR, Bittl JA, Cercek B, et al. 2011 ACCF/AHA/SCAI guideline for percutaneous coronary intervention. A report of the American College of Cardiology Foundation/American Heart Association Task Force on Practice Guidelines and the Society for Cardiovascular Angiography and Interventions. J Am Coll Cardiol. 2011;58(24):e44–122.

59. Bridgewater B, Hooper T, Munsch C, Hunter S, von Oppell U, Livesey S, et al. Mitral repair best practice: proposed standards. Heart. 2006;92(7):939–44.

60. Holmes DR Jr, Mack MJ. Transcatheter valve therapy a professional society overview from the american college of cardiology foundation and the society of thoracic surgeons. J Am Coll Cardiol. 2011;58(4):445–55.

61. Tommaso CL, Bolman RM 3rd, Feldman T, Bavaria J, Acker MA, Aldea G, et al. Multisociety (AATS, ACCF, SCAI, and STS) expert consensus statement: operator and institutional requirements for transcatheter valve repair and replacement, part 1: transcatheter aortic valve replacement. J Am Coll Cardiol. 2012;59(22):2028–42.

62. Vahanian A, Alfieri O, Al-Attar N, Antunes M, Bax J, Cormier B, et al. Transcatheter valve implantation for patients with aortic stenosis: a position statement from the European Association of Cardio-Thoracic Surgery (EACTS) and the European Society of Cardiology (ESC), in collaboration with the European Association of Percutaneous Cardiovascular Interventions (EAPCI). Eur Heart J. 2008;29(11):1463–70.

63. Kim LK, Minutello RM, Feldman DN, Swaminathan RV, Bergman G, Singh H, et al. Association between transcatheter aortic valve implantation volume and outcomes in the United States. Am J Cardiol. 2015;116(12):1910–5.

64. de Biasi AR, Paul S, Nasar A, Girardi LN, Salemi A. National analysis of short-term outcomes and volume-outcome relationships for transcatheter aortic valve replacement in the era of commercialization. Cardiology. 2016;133(1):58–68.

65. Badheka AO, Patel NJ, Panaich SS, Patel SV, Jhamnani S, Singh V, et al. Effect of hospital volume on outcomes of transcatheter aortic valve implantation. Am J Cardiol. 2015;116(4):587–94.

66. Patel HJ, Herbert MA, Drake DH, Hanson EC, Theurer PF, Bell GF, et al. Aortic valve replacement: using a statewide cardiac surgical database identifies a procedural volume hinge point. Ann Thorac Surg. 2013;96(5):1560–5; discussion 5–6

67. Gonzalez AA, Dimick JB, Birkmeyer JD, Ghaferi AA. Understanding the volume-outcome effect in cardiovascular surgery: the role of failure to rescue. JAMA Surg. 2014;149(2):119–23.

68. Carroll JD, Vemulapalli S, Dai D, Matsouaka R, Blackstone E, Edwards F, et al. Procedural experience for transcatheter aortic valve replacement and relation to outcomes: the STS/ACC TVT registry. J Am Coll Cardiol. 2017;70(1):29–41.

69. Bestehorn K, Eggebrecht H, Fleck E, Bestehorn M, Mehta RH, Kuck KH. Volume-outcome relationship with transfemoral transcatheter aortic valve implantation (TAVI): insights from the compulsory German Quality Assurance Registry on Aortic Valve Replacement (AQUA). EuroIntervention. 2017;13(8):914–20.

70. Krasopoulos G, Falconieri F, Benedetto U, Newton J, Sayeed R, Kharbanda R, et al. European real world trans-catheter aortic valve implantation: systematic review and meta-analysis of European national registries. J Cardiothorac Surg. 2016;11(1):159.

Part III

Interventional Perspectives

Access Management for Transfemoral Transcatheter Aortic Valve Implantation

18

Francesco Burzotta, Osama Shoeib,
and Carlo Trani

18.1 Introduction

Transcatheter aortic valve implantation (TAVI), also called transcatheter aortic valve replacement (TAVR), is a promising alternative to surgical aortic valve replacement. Even if TAVI may be successfully accomplished using various arterial accesses, the vast majority of scientific evidences on TAVI efficacy has been collected using the transfemoral approach. Both surgical and percutaneous insertion of the femoral sheath required for transfemoral access are contemporary practiced. Yet, as compared with surgical arteriotomy, percutaneous approach represents the less invasive technique for TAVI and is associated with the advantages of not requiring anesthesia and to facilitate patient recovery. The major drawback of transfemoral TAVI is represented by the fact that vascular complication after the procedure is a major source of TAVI-related complications [1] which have the potential to affect the patient's outcome after successful prosthesis implantation. We herein overview the main issues related with transfemoral access selection in TAVI procedures.

18.2 Femoral Access Anatomy

The common femoral artery (CFA) is a short, large artery defined as the continuation of the external iliac artery (EIA) staring behind the inguinal ligament after giving the inferior epigastric artery branch. The CFA, approximately 3–4 cm distal to the inguinal ligament, gives the profunda femoris artery and continues to be the superficial femoral artery (SFA). At the origin, it is accompanied by the anterior crural nerve laterally and the femoral vein medially all enclosed in inferior extension of the transversalis fascia.

The surface anatomy of the CFA is indicated by the upper two thirds of the line drawn between the anterior superior iliac spine and symphysis pubis to the prominent tuberosity of the inner condyle of the femur, while the patient's thigh is abducted and rotated outward. The relation of the femoral artery to the surface landmarks as the inguinal crease and the point of maximal pulsation is variable [2–4].

The size of the CFA artery is variable with an average diameter of 5–7 mm and average length of 3–5 cm; both diameter and length are larger in men and vary according to different demographic and clinical factors such as age, diabetes mellitus, body surface area, and race [2, 5–7].

F. Burzotta (✉) · C. Trani
Institute of Cardiology, Fondazione Policlinico Universitario A. Gemelli IRCCS,
Università Cattolica del Sacro Cuore, Rome, Italy
e-mail: francesco.burzotta@unicatt.it

O. Shoeib
Cardiology Department, Tanta University, Tanta, Egypt

© Springer Nature Switzerland AG 2019
A. Giordano et al. (eds.), *Transcatheter Aortic Valve Implantation*,
https://doi.org/10.1007/978-3-030-05912-5_18

From the percutaneous intervention point, the safest site for arterial puncture is the anterior wall of the CFA over the femoral bone's head [8, 9]. Too high puncture, above the level of the inguinal ligament, is associated with increased incidence of retroperitoneal hematoma which represents a dreadful complication [10]. Too low puncture, below the femoral bifurcation, implies higher risk of both ischemic complications (increased risk of arterial damage resulting in lumen compromise due to smaller artery size) and hemorrhagic complications (increased risk of hemostasis failure due to reduced compression efficacy in the absence of underlying femoral head) [11, 12].

18.3 Evaluation of the Femoral Artery Before Intervention

Preprocedural patient screening should include appropriate methods for full understanding of femoral artery features including the luminal size, vessel tortuosity, extension of atherosclerosis, and calcification. Only after this deep understanding, the patient's eligibility for transfemoral TAVI can be assessed [13].

Various techniques have the potential to provide information regarding the suitability of the femoral artery for TAVI. The most common methods for femoral artery evaluation include angiography, ultrasound, multidetector computed tomography (MDCT), and magnetic resonance angiography (MRA). Such techniques may provide different insights over various arterial features that might influence TAVI procedures. MDCT is actually regarded as the gold standard for effective workout in unselected TAVI patients since it allows both high-resolution three-dimensional bilateral aorto-iliofemoral arterial axis assessment and careful annulus size measurement. The main disadvantage of MDCT is the use of contrast media. Of note, in the presence of heavy calcifications, MDCT may underestimate the arterial luminal dimensions.

18.4 Access Management Hardware

The main hardware used during transfemoral access management are the sheath, stiff guidewire, and the closure devices.

18.4.1 Sheaths

The TAVI procedure usually requires a sheath that should be able to accommodate the insertion and removal of the aortic prosthesis delivery system. The sheath length is usually 30–35 cm in order to reach and cross the entire iliac artery course. Some TAVI manufactures offer sheaths which are specifically dedicated to the corresponding prosthesis to warrant the best compatibility between sheath and delivery systems. Recently, the delivery system of the last evolutions of CoreValve systems has been equipped with a dedicated and premounted 14 F sheath.

The aim of reducing the minimal arterial lumen necessary for prosthesis deployment produced the availability of "dynamic" sheaths. These are sheathes that can change their diameter after their insertion into the arteries. SoloPath (Terumo medical) is one of these examples which is a folded sheath with entry diameter of 11.5 Fr (3.8 mm) and, once inside the arterial access, has an inflatable balloon dilator allowing for radial dilatation allowing to reach 14 Fr (4.67 mm) internal diameter (ID) and 17 Fr (5.67) outer diameter [14]. This sheath has been safely applied in femoral arteries smaller than 5 mm [15].

The other main "dynamic" sheath is the eSheath (Edwards Lifesciences) which has a "sheet" technology that allows transient expansion during the prosthesis passage. The 14 Fr eSheath has an outer diameter of 5.8 mm that reaches 7.65 mm during the prosthesis passage and turns down to 7.14 mm in case of 23 mm Sapien prosthesis and 7.26 mm in case of 26 mm Sapien prosthesis.

The 16 Fr version has 6.5 mm outer diameter that reaches 8.18 mm during the prosthesis passage and turns down to 8.1 mm after the prosthesis passage [16].

An overview of the main characteristics of the sheaths required for the different TAVI systems is provided in Table 18.1.

18.4.2 Stiff Guidewires

The second important access management hardware is the stiff guidewire which should be used to support the insertion of TAVI sheath. They are essential in order to reduce the risk of vascular damages potentially associated with the advancement of stiff sheaths inside tortuous, frail, and atherosclerotic arteries. The stiff guidewires are

also used to track the valvuloplasty balloons and the TAVI prosthesis into the left ventricle outflow tract. Recently, a novel use of stiff guidewires has been proposed in the context of TAVI to reduce its invasiveness: stiff guidewires may conduct the electrical energy allowing for retrograde left ventricular pacing [17].

To date, vascular stiff guidewires which are not specific for TAVI are commonly used (Amplatz super stiff, Amplatz extra stiff, Backup Meier, Hi-Torque supra core, and Lunderquist extra stiff wire). It is important to keep in mind that adjectives associated with stiff guidewires named as "superstiff," "extra stiff," and "ultra-stiff" do not provide any accurate expression of the stiffness degree [18]. More recently, new guidewires dedicated to TAVI become available, and they share the characteristics of continuous tapered core and pre-shaped tips which should facilitate prosthesis delivery (Confida Brecker and Safari 2 wires).

Table 18.2 provides the main characteristics of the most popular stiff guidewires, while the degree of stiffness in relation to each other is graphically represented in Fig. 18.1.

All stiff guidewires can be used to support the sheath advancement, but not all of them can be used to support the prosthesis advancement. In particular, it is recommended to avoid the Lunderquist extra stiff wire for prosthesis advancement because its extraordinary stiff tip increases the risk of left ventricular damage.

Table 18.1 List of available transfemoral TAVI prosthesis and their compatible sheaths

Device name	Sheath size	Recommended min. artery size
Sapien 3	14 F (20, 23, 26 mm) 16 F (29 mm)	>5 mm (20, 23, 26) >5.5 mm (29 mm)
Evolut R	14 F outer diameter (23, 26, 29, 34 mm)	>5 mm (23, 26, 29) >5.5 mm (34)
Portico	18 F (23, 25 mm) 19 F (27, 29 mm)	>6 mm
Acurate Neo	18 F outer diameter	>6 mm
Allegra	18 F	>6 mm
LOTUS edge	14 F (23 mm) 15 F (25, 27 mm)	Not available

Table 18.2 Technical specification of main stiff guidewires used in TAVI

Name	Maximal length (cm)	Tip shape	Soft tip length	Key structural features
Amplatz extra stiff (Cook Medical Inc.)	260	Straight or small J-tip	Available in 1, 3, and 6 cm	PTFE-coated stainless steel
Amplatz super stiff (Boston Scientific)	260	Straight or small J-tip	Available in 1, 3, and 6 cm	PTFE-coated stainless steel
Backup Meier (Boston Scientific)	260	J-tip C-tip	15 cm 10 cm	PTFE-stainless steel, except distal 4 cm
Hi-Torque supra core (Abbott Vascular Inc.)	300	Straight tip	10 cm	PTFE-coated with atraumatic tip
Lunderquist extra stiff (Cook Medical Inc.)	260	J-tip	4 cm	PTFE-coated stainless steel
Confida Brecker guidewire (Medtronic Inc.)	260	Pre-shaped loop	Curve diameter 3 cm	Continuous tapered core
Safari 2 (Boston Scientific)	275	Pre-shaped loop	Available in 2.9 cm, 4.2 cm, and 4.9 cm curve diameter	Continuous tapered core

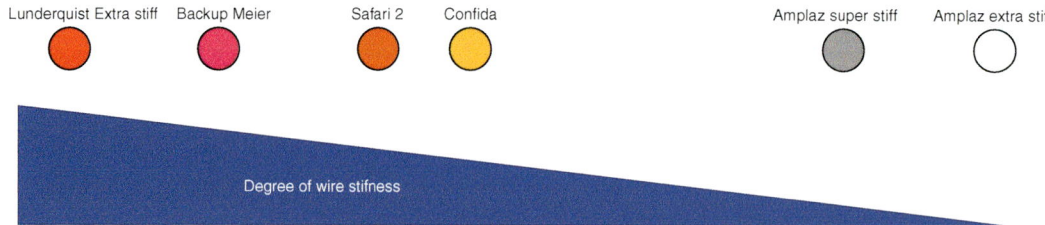

Fig. 18.1 Scale showing the degree of different stiff wire stiffness and their relation to each other

18.4.3 Vascular Closure Devices (VCD)

VCD represents a step through the management of transfemoral TAVI vascular access since their use has the recognized potential to render this procedure fully percutaneous.

To date, the most commonly used VCD for TAVI are two suture-based devices: the Prostar XL10F and Perclose ProGlide (Abbott Vascular Devices, Redwood City, CA, USA). These devices are designed to close 10 F and 8 F vascular access, respectively, but, in the case of large-bone sheath insertions, they may be deployed using the "preclosure" technique. This technique is based on the concept that the VCD suture is deployed before the sheath insertion (when the entry site has not been stretched beyond the size that is compatible with the specific device).

Prostar preclosure technique. The Prostar XL10F is a 0.035-in. guidewire-compatible 10 F device with a rotating barrel and four needles allowing to deploy two braided polyester sutures. When the device is in the correct position, indicated by pulsatile blood return from the dedicated marker lumen, the needles are unlocked and pulled through the arterial wall. After device deployment, the sutures are secured with mosquito clamps. At procedure end, the sheath and the guidewire are removed, while proximal pressure is maintained, and sutures are fastened individually with a sliding knot. A knot pusher is used to ensure the approximation of the knot to the surface of the vessel wall [19].

Double Proglide preclosure technique. The Perclose ProGlide device is based on two needles that can deploy a single monofilament polypropylene suture. To close the large sheath needed for TAVI, the preclosure technique is practiced by sequentially inserting two Proglide devices rotated in opposite sides 30–45°, to create an interrupted X-figure closure. After device deployment, the sutures are secured with mosquito clamps, and the TAVI sheath is inserted. At procedure end, arteriotomy closure is achieved by tying down the two knots using sequentially the two node pushers [20–22]. A newly proposed technique is the "parallel suture technique" which is based on the deployment of both Proglides with medial and lateral tension instead of applying any rotation. This results in a parallel suture deployment (instead of "X" configuration) which should resemble a standard surgical vascular suture [23].

Regarding the comparison between these devices, controversial results have been reported in different studies. A recent meta-analysis of TAVI and EVAR studies suggested higher safety for Double Proglide preclosure technique [24]. Yet, besides the technical differences between the two devices and the inherent limits of comparison study protocols, the individual operator's experience with each of these techniques is a main modulator of preclosure technique efficacy.

18.5 Obtaining the Access

18.5.1 Surgical Access

The surgical access is obtained by transverse incision at the groin followed by careful dissection of the subcutaneous tissue to expose the femoral artery. Then a U-shaped suture is deployed into the common femoral artery, and artery puncture and sheath insertion are performed. At procedure end, two sutures are tightened to achieve hemostasis [25].

The main advantages of the surgical access are the ability to perform a controlled puncture with the ability to select the puncture site, and in case of complications, it provides the ability to repair the femoral artery under direct vision.

18.5.2 Percutaneous Access

18.5.2.1   Arterial Stick

The percutaneous access is based on the Seldinger technique. Theoretically, the ideal percutaneous access in TAVI procedures is a single needle stick at the level of a healthy spot of the anterior wall of the common femoral artery during its course over the femoral head. Any deviation from these assumptions is associated with increased risk of complications which may have dreadful consequences in the specific setting of TAVI.

As a consequence, techniques for meticulous guidance of TAVI access femoral puncture are usually practiced in percutaneous TAVI. The more commonly adopted guidance for arterial stick is angiographic guidance using another (ancillary) arterial access that is previously been obtained. The "ancillary" arterial access may be either the contralateral femoral artery (routinely selected by most operators) or by the radial or brachial arteries and is used for both access guidance and TAVI implantation guidance. To achieve high-quality angiography, from the ancillary access, a diagnostic (or guiding) catheter should selectively advance to cannulate the common iliac artery of the side selected for TAVI. More rarely, some operators use to stick the distal superficial femoral artery (with micropuncture kit). This technique has the advantage of facilitating both angiographic guidance (no need of catheter manipulation for femoral artery angiography) and bailout interventions in the case of complications (direct access to the common femoral artery) but implies to have three simultaneous arterial accesses for a single TAVI procedure (since a further arterial access is needed for ascending aortography).

Independently, from the ancillary access selection, different angiography-based techniques may be practiced:

1. Simple angiography before (to recognize arterial track and anatomy) and after (to confirm appropriate entry site) arterial stick.
2. Road mapping-guided arterial stick: angiography is used to obtain (with the dedicated roadmap tool of the angiographic machine) persisting image of the artery during arterial stick.
3. Guidewire-guided arterial stick: under angiographic guidance, the J-tip of a regular 0.035 in. guidewire is placed in the common femoral artery, and arterial stick is performed under fluoroscopy aiming at reaching the guidewire tip.
4. *Angio-guidewire-ultrasound (AGU) guidance:* After J-tip placement in the common femoral artery, arterial stick is performed under ultrasound guidance (since the guidewire J is easily detected by ultrasound, the X-ray exposition for the operator's hand is spared).

18.5.2.2   Safety Wire

In case of vascular complication at the procedure, the possibility to achieve successful complication management by endovascular interventions is the guidewire advancement across the injured vessel segment. To warrant fast endovascular management of vascular complications, some operators use to early place and leave a guidewire across the TAVI access. This technique may be practiced with different guidewires (usually 0.014′ or 0.018′) according to the local attitudes and requires full knowledge and availability of the endovascular equipment. This technique was proven to have significant reduction in serious complication and mortality [26].

18.6   Access Site Complications and Their Classification

Serious vascular access complication can occur in association with TAVI procedures, ranging from minor hematomas and small non-flow-limiting dissection to a life-threatening condition as arterial rupture and avulsion; to obtain standardized definition for TAVI outcomes, the Valve Academic Research Consortium (VARC) has proposed a

Table 18.3 Valve Academic Research Consortium-2 classification of vascular access site and access-related complications

Major vascular complications

– Any aortic dissection, aortic rupture, annulus rupture, left ventricle perforation, or new apical aneurysm/ pseudoaneurysm

– Access site or access-related vascular injury (dissection, stenosis, perforation, rupture, arteriovenous fistula, pseudoaneurysm, hematoma, irreversible nerve injury, compartment syndrome, percutaneous closure device failure) leading to death, life-threatening or major bleeding, visceral ischemia, or neurological impairment

– Distal embolization (non-cerebral) from a vascular source requiring surgery or resulting in amputation or irreversible end-organ damage

  – The use of unplanned endovascular or surgical intervention associated with death, major bleeding, visceral ischemia, or neurological impairment

– Any new ipsilateral lower extremity ischemia documented by patient symptoms, physical exam, and/or decreased or absent blood flow on lower extremity angiogram

– Surgery for access site-related nerve injury

– Permanent access site-related nerve injury

Minor vascular complications

– Access site or access-related vascular injury (dissection, stenosis, perforation, rupture, arteriovenous fistula, pseudoaneurysm, hematomas, percutaneous closure device failure) not leading to death, life-threatening or major bleeding, visceral ischemia, or neurological impairment

– Distal embolization treated with embolectomy and/or thrombectomy and not resulting in amputation or irreversible end-organ damage

– Any unplanned endovascular stenting or unplanned surgical intervention not meeting the criteria for a major vascular complication

– Vascular repair or the need for vascular repair (via surgery, ultrasound-guided compression, transcatheter embolization, or stent graft)

Percutaneous closure device failure

– Failure of a closure device to achieve hemostasis at the arteriotomy site leading to alternative treatment (other than manual compression or adjunctive endovascular ballooning)

definition which then was updated (VARC-2) which include standardization for both vascular and bleeding complications following TAVI procedure (Table 18.3).

The occurrence of vascular complications has a high impact on both procedural and clinical outcomes, as it increases blood transfusion, renal impairment, and hospital stay. Furthermore, in the critical setting of fragile patient populations like TAVI candidates, vascular complications have been observed to predict late mortality. Table 18.4 summarizes the main studies assessing the clinical impact of vascular complications TAVI outcome.

18.7   Predictors of Vascular Complications

Several factors may predispose to the development of vascular complications. The non-modifiable risk factors include the female gender [27], advanced age, and history of peripheral artery dis-

ease [28]. Of note, peripheral artery disease (especially in the presence of critical limb ischemia) has been found to independently affect the in-hospital mortality after TAVI procedure [29] (see Table 18.5). For instance, beyond peripheral atherosclerosis, other adverse iliofemoral anatomic features like arterial tortuosities and vessel lumen size are known to influence vascular complication risk. Some authors suggested to stratify vascular complication risk by a simple scoring system which includes three simple points (minimal arterial diameter, extension of iliac artery calcification, and the degree of tortuosity) [30].

The modifiable factors include the sheath size [27] and sheath-to-femoral artery ratio. A careful evaluation of the perfect matching between sheath size and artery segment is actually routinely suggested in order to limit the risk of vascular complications. To facilitate this aim in the preoperative workout, dedicated softwares have been developed. As an example, Fig. 18.2 shows that, in a patient with complex arterial anatomy,

Table 18.4 Studies reporting on the frequency and clinical impact of vascular complication on TAVI outcome

Study	Year	Total number of patients	Vascular complications definition	Vascular complications frequency (%)	End points	Conclusion
Ducrocq et al. [53]	2010	54		16.7	Transfusion Reintervention 30-day mortality	Vascular complications are associated with a high need for transfusion and could lead to major events such as death or reintervention
Généreux et al. [54]	2012	419		27.2	Bleeding Transfusion Acute renal failure 30-day mortality 1-year mortality	Major VCs are associated with high mortality. However, the incidence and impact of major VC on 1-year mortality decreased in lower-risk populations
Czerwinska-Jelonkiewiez et al. [55]	2013	83		53.01	Early and late mortality (follow-up ranged 1–23 months, median 12 ± 15.5 months)	Vascular complications are predictors of late mortality after TAVI
Mwipatayi et al. [56]	2013	100 (81 transfemoral)		19.7	Blood transfusion Length of stay in hospital In-hospital mortality 30-day mortality	Vascular complications are associated with increased blood transfusion need, hospital stay, and costs
Steinvil et al. [57]	2015	403		19	In-hospital mortality 1- and 6-month mortality 1-year mortality	The implementation of the VARC-2 criteria results in a higher rate of reported major VC after TAVI
Perrin et al. [58]	2015	102		22	Bleeding Transfusion 30-day mortality	Major but not minor VCs are associated with increased mortality
Uguz et al. [59]	2016	211		16.1	Mortality	The major vascular complications are predictive of 30-day mortality
Okuyama et al. [60]	2016	376			1-year mortality	The VARC-2 definition of VC offers better predictive value of survival than the VARC-1 definition

Table 18.5 Studies assessing the prevalence and clinical impact of known peripheral arterial disease in TAVI

Study	Year	Total number of patients	PAD prevalence (%)	Main findings
Sinning et al. [61]	2012	1315	25.1	PAD was an independent predictor of mortality in patients with percutaneous and surgical TAVI
Kim et al. [62]	2018	115	31.3	Presence of PAD was significantly associated with increased rates of major vascular complication and immediate and late mortality
Malyar et al. [29]	2017	32,044	12.5	PAD is associated with an increased risk of periprocedural complications, while only CLI independently predicts increased in-hospital mortality
Fanaroff et al. [63]	2017	27,440 (19,660 transfemoral approach)	24.5	PAD is associated with a higher incidence of 1-year adverse outcomes compared with absence of PAD

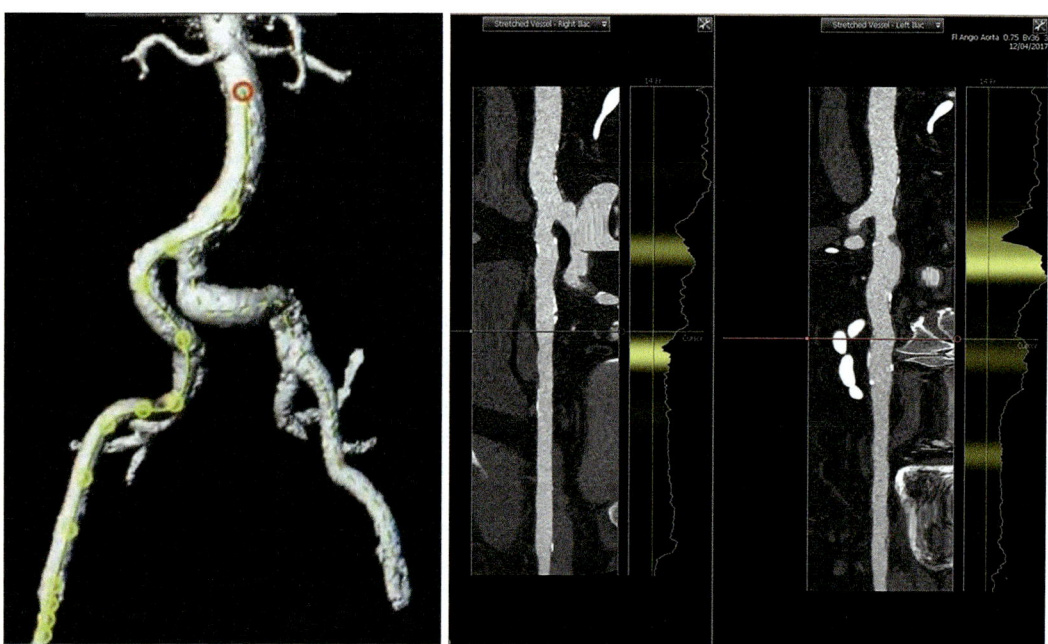

Fig. 18.2 A real-life example showing a "straightened" iliofemoral artery lumen reconstruction by a dedicated computed tomographic software

compatibility with 14 F sheath has been assessed using the "straightened" iliofemoral artery lumen reconstruction by a dedicated computed tomographic software.

18.8 Management of Vascular Complications

Surgical management for vascular complications is associated with prolonged hospitalizations and risk of wound infection that can delay patient mobilization [31]. With the advances in endovascular techniques, bailout vascular complication treatment may be effectively managed percutaneously with a high success rate and good short- and long-term outcomes [32]. To attempt endovascular management of vascular complications, operators should be familiar with different techniques and need to have basic peripheral intervention tools. Table 18.6 summarizes the endovascular equipment that should be available in the catheterization laboratory when percutaneous management of TAVI-related vascular complications is planned.

Table 18.6 Materials for bailout endovascular management of vascular complications

Device	Rationale
Sheaths or catheters	
Diagnostic 5 F catheters	Selective angiography to establish vascular complication type (when remote from access site sheath or when occurring after access site sheath removal)
Long (armored) sheaths	Selective access to the iliac artery for bailout intervention in the case of contralateral femoral artery access availability
125 cm, 6 F guiding catheter	Selective access to the iliac artery for bailout intervention in the case of contralateral radial/brachial artery access availability
Guidewires	
0.035′ hydrophilic wire	Easy access and support to cross with a diagnostic catheter the aortic bifurcation (crossover technique)
0.035′ stiff guidewire, 300 cm	Deployment of long armored sheaths by contralateral femoral artery ("crossover" technique)
0.014′ or 0.018′, 300 cm, hydrophilic guidewires	Injured vessel fast crossing in the case of absence for sentinel wire
Balloons	
Peripheral balloons (diameter: 6–9 mm)	– Restoration of antegrade flow to avoid acute limb ischemia in the case of occlusion/stenosis in the iliofemoral arteries – Immediate hemostasis in the case of hemorrhagic complications in the iliofemoral arteries
Large compliant aortic balloons	Immediate hemostasis by endovascular balloon occlusion of the aorta in the case of descending aorta rupture
Stents	
Peripheral self-expandable nitinol stents (diameter: 7–10 mm)	Iliofemoral arteries' flow-limiting dissection/stenosis
Peripheral self-expandable covered stent (diameter: 7–10 mm)	Vascular sealing in case of persistent blood extravasation after prolonged balloon inflation

18.8.1 Percutaneous Vascular Closure Device Failure

The failure of vascular closure devices (VCD) is now considered by the VARC-2 as a specific entity. Risk factors for these VCD failure include excessive femoral artery calcifications, female gender, obese patients [33], and operator's learning curve with such devices [34].

Prolonged manual compression may be sufficient to manage VCD failure. Yet, operators who are familiar with endovascular technique use to practice "balloon-assisted hemostasis." This technique consists in the inflation of an appropriately sized peripheral balloon (inserted through the ancillary access) in the arterial leak caused by VCD failure. To speedup balloon-assisted hemostasis, angiographic wire may be inserted before sheath removal.

18.8.2 Iliofemoral Dissection

Dissection of the iliofemoral arteries can occur with either surgical cut down or percutaneous sheath insertion. The key point to reduce arterial dissection risk is gentile sheath advancement. In case of resistance, the operator should avoid aggressive maneuvers and carefully check by fluoroscopy sheath progression (and eventual arterial calcification movement). Vaseline can be used to reduce the friction with the arterial wall.

Since most of these dissections are retrograde generated, the antegrade blood flow tends to keep the vessel open by favorably displacing the wall "flap" from the lumen. More extensive arterial dissection can lead to acute vessel occlusion which may have dreadful clinical consequences (extensive lower limb ischemia).

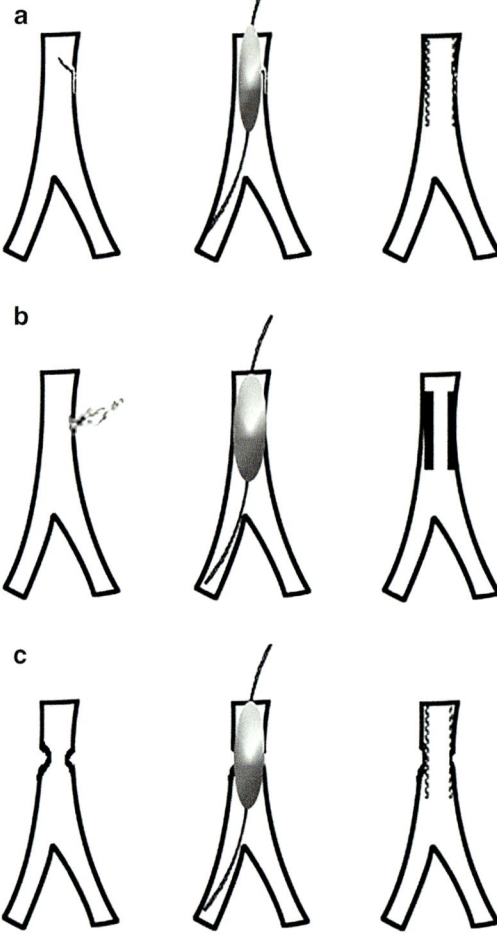

Fig. 18.3 Schematic representation of common vascular complication and their management. (**a**) Shows iliofemoral artery dissection which can be treated with appropriately sized balloon inflation, and in case of failure, a stent can be implanted to seal the dissection. (**b**) Shows iliofemoral artery perforation which can be treated with prolonged balloon inflation assisted with manual compression, and in case of failure, a covered stent can be implanted. (**c**) Shows iliofemoral artery stenosis/obstruction; the vessel can be dilated with a balloon; if the flow is still impaired, a stent can be implanted to maintain the flow

In such cases, prolonged peripheral balloon inflation may be attempted in order to restore flow (Fig. 18.3a). When balloon inflation fails to steadily restore arterial patency, peripheral self-expandable stent implantation of the appropriate size may safely seal the dissections (Fig. 18.3a).

18.8.3 Arterial Obstruction

The whole iliofemoral axis may be damaged during the TAVI-related catheters' manipulations. Arterial wall injury, especially when the artery wall is diseased, and the vessel has adverse features like tortuosity, may result in acute arterial lumen obstruction due to vessel dissections and thrombus development (these two mechanisms often being simultaneously present in the worse cases). Vessel wall obstruction, in the absence of extensive dissections, occurs more commonly where the vessel lumen is smaller like into the distal iliac artery and the common femoral artery. This latter artery, particularly prone to lumen obstruction also due to the direct damage induced by TAVI sheath insertion. A recent study demonstrated significant femoral artery lumen shrinkage may commonly be induced by percutaneous TAVI with the use of suture-based closure devices [28]. This is probably the result of a focal geometric deformation of the common femoral artery induced by the device's sutures. It is reasonable to speculate that this systematic subclinical entry site shrinkage may represent a predisposing factor for the occurrence of thrombotic phenomena or that this may exacerbate the hemodynamic consequences of eventually occurring dissections. For instance, femoral shrinkage has been reported to be associated with vascular complications [28]. Despite the underlying mechanism (dissection/thrombus), acute lumen obstructions may cause significant lower limb ischemia. Accordingly, anytime lower limb ischemia is suspected (antegrade flow perturbation at angiography or Doppler), peripheral angioplasty balloon may be used to treat and dilate the injured arterial site. Usually, prolonged dilations of appropriately sized balloons are able (Fig. 18.3c) to restore appropriate lumen size. Yet, in the cases of significant recoil, peripheral stent implantation may be considered (Fig. 18.3c).

18.8.4 Pseudoaneurysm

The failure of arterial access sealing (or its reopening after initial sealing) may lead to insidious, continuous blood leak into the surrounding soft tissue. In such condition, a fibrin shell may limit huge blood extravasation by determining pseudoaneurysm formation. Routine digital subtraction angiography of the access site at the procedure end will help arterial leak identification and prompt early management by balloon-assisted hemostasis with or without external compression.

If the angiographic diagnosis was not made immediately, it should be suspected in any patient with painful, pulsatile groin mass with possible murmur after the procedure.

Risk factors for pseudoaneurysm development include [35] advanced age, female gender, increased body mass index, low platelet count, and low puncture site (below the bifurcation), anticoagulation and antiplatelet administration, and continuation after the procedure [36].

The initial step of diagnosis remains the physical examination as it has a high sensitivity and accuracy approaching 100% especially the presence of a pulsatile mass [37, 38]. The physical examination should be followed by duplex scan where diagnosis is based on a triad of ultrasound findings: the hypoechoic sac near the femoral artery, a swirling high-resistance Doppler flow within the sac, and the "to and fro" or "yin-yang" waveform at the sac's neck [39]. Doppler wave allows ruling out the presence of concomitant arteriovenous fistula (which has a characteristic low resistance with continuous diastolic flow pattern). Once the pseudoaneurysm is diagnosed, prompt management is recommended since treatment delay adversely affects the probability of success for nonsurgical strategies. The main predictors of favorable pseudoaneurysm outcome include low-volume flow inside the sac [40] and the sac neck length [41]. Small (<3.5 cm) pseudoaneurysms with favorable anatomy may be initially managed conservatively by local compression. Anyway, an active nonsurgical management is actually considered as the first-line therapy in the vast majority of clinical conditions and includes ultrasound-guided compression [42] and ultrasound-guided thrombin injection [43–45]. Of note, thrombin injection is not recommended when the neck for the sac is not evident and when arteriovenous fistula has not been ruled out [46]. Most of centers actually use to consider vascular surgery only when large residual pseudoaneurysm is present after attempted ultrasound-guided compression and/or thrombin injection.

18.8.5 Iliofemoral Perforation and Rupture

The bulky and rigid TAVI sheaths and TAVI delivery systems have the potential for causing extreme damages into the arterial wall during their advancement. As previously discussed, stiff guidewires should reduce this risk by reducing the friction between devices and vessel wall. Nevertheless, vessel tortuosity, especially in calcific arteries, has the potential for hindering device advancement onto stiff guidewires. In such circumstances, the most dangerous condition is associated by the occurrence of guidewire kinking. This situation should carefully be avoided, and anytime it occurs, guidewire replacement (eventually with a stiffer guidewire) is recommended.

Once iliofemoral perforation/rupture occurred, adverse clinical consequences inexorably follow and may range from immediate hemorrhagic shock to insidious developing retroperitoneal hematoma. Accordingly, prompt diagnosis may be pivotal, and it may easily be obtained by subtraction angiography which usually allows immediate recognition of presence, site, and size of blood leakage. Intraprocedural angiography is highly recommended since (as compared with other diagnostic tests like CT scan) it allows immediate diagnosis on the operative table and may guide for appropriate endovascular management. If blood extravasation is recognized, the main rescue maneuver is a balloon inflation proximal to the vascular lesion and heparin reversal using protamine sulfate. This maneuver blocks blood loss thus preventing hemorrhagic shock. If the vascular injury is extensive, it is advisable to use an occlusion balloon which is a specified highly compliant balloon that can elongate easily and accommodate a wide range of vessel diameter without the application of radial force to the lacerated vessel [47]. Available 0.035′-compatible occlusion balloons include the Coda occlusion balloon catheter (Cook Medical Inc., Bloomington, IN) which is available in two sizes according to the balloon maximum diameter 32 mm and 40 mm and the Equalizer occlusion balloon catheter (Boston Scientific, Natick, MA) available in four different sizes 20, 27, 33, and 40 mm.

In the case of small perforations, prolonged balloon inflation may induce complete hemostasis. Yet, if bleeding persists, an appropriately sized covered stent can be used as definitive treatment [48] (Fig. 18.3b). Indeed, covered stents are now recommended as the first-line treatment of iatrogenic vascular injury [49].

18.8.6 Arterial Avulsion

A very rare subset of complication that can happen due to adherence of the large sheath to the arterial endothelium. The risk of avulsion can be reduced by early sheath removal and sheath rotation during withdrawal (of note, rotation is not recommended with expandable sheaths [50]).

If there is arterial avulsion suspicion due to resistance at sheath withdrawal, angiographic diagnosis and endovascular hemostasis should be prepared before the sheath is removed in order to prompt, recognize, and manage this dreadful complication. Surgical repair may be the only treatment in the worse cases, while covered stents may stabilize short arterial lesions.

18.8.7 Access Site Infection

Access site infection appears to be more prevalent among patients undergoing surgical as compared with percutaneous femoral artery approach. Superficial skin infection may response well to antibiotics and appropriate wound medications. Yet, since deep infections may lead to serious complication as septicemia and death [51, 52], prompt and careful diagnosis and management with eventual surgical curettage are recommended.

Disclosures Dr. Burzotta discloses to have been involved in advisory board meetings or having received speaker's fees from Medtronic, St Jude Medical, Abiomed, Biotronic. Dr. Trani discloses to have been involved in advisory board meetings or having received speaker's fees from St Jude Medical, Abiomed, Biotronic.

References

1. Dato I, Burzotta F, Trani C, Crea F, Ussia GP. Percutaneous management of vascular access in transfemoral transcatheter aortic valve implantation. World J Cardiol. 2014;6:836–46.
2. Irani F, Kumar S, Colyer WR Jr. Common femoral artery access techniques: a review. J Cardiovasc Med. 2009;10:517–22.
3. Lechner G, Jantsch H, Waneck R, Kretschmer G. The relationship between the common femoral artery, the inguinal crease, and the inguinal ligament: a guide to accurate angiographic puncture. Cardiovasc Intervent Radiol. 1988;11:165–9.
4. Grier D, Hartnell G. Percutaneous femoral artery puncture: practice and anatomy. Br J Radiol. 1990;63:602–4.
5. Johnson LW, Krone R. Cardiac catheterization 1991: a report of the Registry of the Society for Cardiac Angiography and Interventions (SCA&I). Catheter Cardiovasc Diagn. 1993;28:219–20.
6. Sandgren T, Sonesson B, Ahlgren R, Lanne T. The diameter of the common femoral artery in healthy human: influence of sex, age, and body size. J Vasc Surg. 1999;29:503–10.
7. Ahn HY, Lee HJ, Lee HJ, Yang JH, Yi JS, Lee IW. Assessment of the optimal site of femoral artery puncture and angiographic anatomical study of the common femoral artery. J Korean Neurosurg Soc. 2014;56:91–7.
8. Altin RS, Flicker S, Naidech HJ. Pseudoaneurysm and arteriovenous fistula after femoral artery catheterization: association with low femoral punctures. AJR Am J Roentgenol. 1989;152:629–31.
9. Cole PL, Krone RJ. Approach to reduction of vascular complications of percutaneous valvuloplasty. Catheter Cardiovasc Diagn. 1987;13:331–2.
10. Raphael M, Hartnell G. Femoral artery catheterization and retroperitoneal haematoma formation. Clin Radiol. 2001;56:933–4; author reply 934–5
11. Gabriel M, Pawlaczyk K, Waliszewski K, Krasinski Z, Majewski W. Location of femoral artery puncture site and the risk of postcatheterization pseudoaneurysm formation. Int J Cardiol. 2007;120:167–71.
12. Kim D, Orron DE, Skillman JJ, et al. Role of superficial femoral artery puncture in the development of pseudoaneurysm and arteriovenous fistula complicating percutaneous transfemoral cardiac catheterization. Catheter Cardiovasc Diagn. 1992;25:91–7.
13. Olasinska-Wisniewska A, Grygier M, Lesiak M, et al. Femoral artery anatomy-tailored approach in

transcatheter aortic valve implantation. Adv Interv Cardiol. 2017;13:150–6.

14. Krajcer Z, Parekh D. Dynamic sheaths, in the nick of time or past their prime? Catheter Cardiovasc Interv. 2016;88:1153–4.

15. Abu Saleh WK, Tang GH, Ahmad H, et al. Vascular complication can be minimized with a balloon-expandable, re-collapsible sheath in TAVR with a self-expanding bioprosthesis. Catheter Cardiovasc Interv. 2016;88:135–43.

16. Koehler T, Buege M, Schleiting H, Seyfarth M, Tiroch K, Vorpahl M. Changes of the eSheath outer dimensions used for transfemoral transcatheter aortic valve replacement. Biomed Res Int. 2015;2015:572681.

17. Hilling-Smith R, Cockburn J, Dooley M, et al. Rapid pacing using the 0.035-in. Retrograde left ventricular support wire in 208 cases of transcatheter aortic valve implantation and balloon aortic valvuloplasty. Catheter Cardiovasc Interv. 2017;89:783–6.

18. Harrison GJ, How TV, Vallabhaneni SR, et al. Guidewire stiffness: what's in a name? J Endovasc Ther. 2011;18:797–801.

19. Haas PC, Krajcer Z, Diethrich EB. Closure of large percutaneous access sites using the Prostar XL Percutaneous Vascular Surgery device. J Endovasc Surg. 1999;6:168–70.

20. Burzotta F, Paloscia L, Trani C, et al. Feasibility and long-term safety of elective Impella-assisted high-risk percutaneous coronary intervention: a pilot two-centre study. J Cardiovasc Med. 2008;9:1004–10.

21. Krajcer Z, Howell M. A novel technique using the percutaneous vascular surgery device to close the 22 French femoral artery entry site used for percutaneous abdominal aortic aneurysm exclusion. Catheter Cardiovasc Interv. 2000;50:356–60.

22. Lee WA, Brown MP, Nelson PR, Huber TS, Seeger JM. Midterm outcomes of femoral arteries after percutaneous endovascular aortic repair using the Preclose technique. J Vasc Surg. 2008;47:919–23.

23. Ott I, Shivaraju A, Schaffer NR, et al. Parallel suture technique with ProGlide: a novel method for management of vascular access during transcatheter aortic valve implantation (TAVI). EuroIntervention. 2017;13:928–34.

24. Maniotis C, Andreou C, Karalis I, Koutouzi G, Agelaki M, Koutouzis M. A systematic review on the safety of Prostar XL versus ProGlide after TAVR and EVAR. Cardiovasc Revasc Med. 2017;18:145–50.

25. Spitzer SG, Wilbring M, Alexiou K, Stumpf J, Kappert U, Matschke K. Surgical cut-down or percutaneous access-which is best for less vascular access complications in transfemoral TAVI? Catheter Cardiovasc Interv. 2016;88:E52–8.

26. Garcia E, Martin-Hernandez P, Unzue L, Hernandez-Antolin RA, Almeria C, Cuadrado A. Usefulness of placing a wire from the contralateral femoral artery to improve the percutaneous treatment of vascular complications in TAVI. Revista Esp Cardiol. 2014;67:410–2.

27. Van Mieghem NM, Tchetche D, Chieffo A, et al. Incidence, predictors, and implications of access site complications with transfemoral transcatheter aortic valve implantation. Am J Cardiol. 2012;110:1361–7.

28. Shoeib O, Burzotta F. Percutaneous transcatheter aortic valve replacement induces femoral artery shrinkage: angiographic evidence and predictors for a new side effect. Catheter Cardiovasc Interv. 2018;91:938–44.

29. Malyar NM, Kaier K, Freisinger E, et al. Prevalence and impact of critical limb ischaemia on in-hospital outcome in transcatheter aortic valve implantation in Germany. EuroIntervention. 2017;13:1281–7.

30. Blakeslee-Carter J, Dexter D, Mahoney P, et al. A novel iliac morphology score predicts procedural mortality and major vascular complications in transfemoral aortic valve replacement. Ann Vasc Surg. 2018;46:208–17.

31. Torsello GB, Kasprzak B, Klenk E, Tessarek J, Osada N, Torsello GF. Endovascular suture versus cutdown for endovascular aneurysm repair: a prospective randomized pilot study. J Vasc Surg. 2003;38:78–82.

32. Stortecky S, Wenaweser P, Diehm N, et al. Percutaneous management of vascular complications in patients undergoing transcatheter aortic valve implantation. JACC Cardiovasc Interv. 2012;5:515–24.

33. Vidi VD, Matheny ME, Govindarajulu US, et al. Vascular closure device failure in contemporary practice. JACC Cardiovasc Interv. 2012;5:837–44.

34. Hayashida K, Lefevre T, Chevalier B, et al. True percutaneous approach for transfemoral aortic valve implantation using the Prostar XL device: impact of learning curve on vascular complications. JACC Cardiovasc Interv. 2012;5:207–14.

35. Stone PA, Campbell JE, AbuRahma AF. Femoral pseudoaneurysms after percutaneous access. J Vasc Surg. 2014;60:1359–66.

36. Stone PA, Martinez M, Thompson SN, et al. Ten-year experience of vascular surgeon management of iatrogenic pseudoaneurysms: do anticoagulant and/or antiplatelet medications matter? Ann Vasc Surg. 2016;30:45–51.

37. Mlekusch W, Haumer M, Mlekusch I, et al. Prediction of iatrogenic pseudoaneurysm after percutaneous endovascular procedures. Radiology. 2006;240:597–602.

38. Kent KC, McArdle CR, Kennedy B, Baim DS, Anninos E, Skillman JJ. Accuracy of clinical examination in the evaluation of femoral false aneurysm and arteriovenous fistula. Cardiovasc Surg. 1993;1:504–7.

39. Hanson JM, Atri M, Power N. Ultrasound-guided thrombin injection of iatrogenic groin pseudoaneurysm: Doppler features and technical tips. Br J Radiol. 2008;81:154–63.

40. Paulson EK, Hertzberg BS, Paine SS, Carroll BA. Femoral artery pseudoaneurysms: value of color Doppler sonography in predicting which ones will thrombose without treatment. AJR Am J Roentgenol. 1992;159:1077–81.

41. Samuels D, Orron DE, Kessler A, et al. Femoral artery pseudoaneurysm: Doppler sonographic features predictive for spontaneous thrombosis. J Clin Ultrasound. 1997;25:497–500.

42. Fellmeth BD, Roberts AC, Bookstein JJ, et al. Postangiographic femoral artery injuries: nonsurgical repair with US-guided compression. Radiology. 1991;178:671–5.

43. Khoury M, Rebecca A, Greene K, et al. Duplex scanning-guided thrombin injection for the treatment of iatrogenic pseudoaneurysms. J Vasc Surg. 2002;35:517–21.

44. Stone P, Lohan JA, Copeland SE, Hamrick RE Jr, Tiley EH 3rd, Flaherty SK. Iatrogenic pseudoaneurysms: comparison of treatment modalities, including duplex-guided thrombin injection. W V Med J. 2003;99:230–2.

45. Lonn L, Olmarker A, Geterud K, Risberg B. Prospective randomized study comparing ultrasound-guided thrombin injection to compression in the treatment of femoral pseudoaneurysms. J Endovasc Ther. 2004;11:570–6.

46. Dzijan-Horn M, Langwieser N, Groha P, et al. Safety and efficacy of a potential treatment algorithm by using manual compression repair and ultrasound-guided thrombin injection for the management of iatrogenic femoral artery pseudoaneurysm in a large patient cohort. Circ Cardiovasc Interv. 2014;7:207–15.

47. Masson JB, Al Bugami S, Webb JG. Endovascular balloon occlusion for catheter-induced large artery perforation in the catheterization laboratory. Catheter Cardiovasc Interv. 2009;73:514–8.

48. Lagana D, Carrafiello G, Mangini M, et al. Emergency percutaneous treatment of arterial iliac axis ruptures. Emerg Radiol. 2007;14:173–9.

49. Goltz JP, Basturk P, Hoppe H, Triller J, Kickuth R. Emergency and elective implantation of covered stent systems in iatrogenic arterial injuries. RoFo. 2011;183:618–30.

50. Masson JB, Kovac J, Schuler G, et al. Transcatheter aortic valve implantation: review of the nature, management, and avoidance of procedural complications. JACC Cardiovasc Interv. 2009;2:811–20.

51. Hayashida K, Lefevre T, Chevalier B, et al. Transfemoral aortic valve implantation new criteria to predict vascular complications. JACC Cardiovasc Interv. 2011;4:851–8.

52. Van Mieghem NM, Nuis RJ, Piazza N, et al. Vascular complications with transcatheter aortic valve implantation using the 18 Fr Medtronic CoreValve System: the Rotterdam experience. EuroIntervention. 2010;5:673–9.

53. Ducrocq G, Francis F, Serfaty JM, et al. Vascular complications of transfemoral aortic valve implantation with the Edwards SAPIEN prosthesis: incidence and impact on outcome. EuroIntervention. 2010;5:666–72.

54. Généreux P, Webb JG, Svensson LG, et al. Vascular complications after transcatheter aortic valve replacement: insights from the PARTNER (Placement of AoRTic TraNscathetER Valve) trial. J Am Coll Cardiol. 2012;60:1043–52.

55. Czerwinska-Jelonkiewicz K, Michalowska I, Witkowski A, et al. Vascular complications after transcatheter aortic valve implantation (TAVI): risk and long-term results. J Thromb Thrombolysis. 2014;37:490–8.

56. Mwipatayi BP, Picardo A, Masilonyane-Jones TV, et al. Incidence and prognosis of vascular complications after transcatheter aortic valve implantation. J Vasc Surg. 2013;58:1028–36.e1.

57. Steinvil A, Leshem-Rubinow E, Halkin A, et al. Vascular complications after transcatheter aortic valve implantation and their association with mortality reevaluated by the valve academic research consortium definitions. Am J Cardiol. 2015;115:100–6.

58. Perrin N, Ellenberger C, Licker M, et al. Management of vascular complications following transcatheter aortic valve implantation. Arch Cardiovasc Dis. 2015;108:491–501.

59. Uguz E, Gokcimen M, Ali S, et al. Predictability and outcome of vascular complications after transfemoral transcatheter aortic valve implantation. J Heart Valve Dis. 2016;25:173–81.

60. Okuyama K, Jilaihawi H, Abramowitz Y, et al. The clinical impact of vascular complications as defined by VARC-1 vs. VARC-2 in patients following transcatheter aortic valve implantation. EuroIntervention. 2016;12:e636–42.

61. Sinning JM, Horack M, Grube E, et al. The impact of peripheral arterial disease on early outcome after transcatheter aortic valve implantation: results from the German Transcatheter Aortic Valve Interventions Registry. Am Heart J. 2012;164:102–10.e1.

62. Kim BG, Ko YG, Hong S-J, Ahn C-M, Kim JS, Kim B-K, Choi D, Jang Y, Hong MK, Lee SH, Lee S, Chang B-C. Impact of peripheral artery disease on early and late outcomes in patients who underwent transcatheter aortic valve implantation CCT. Int J Cardiol. 2018;255:206–11.

63. Fanaroff AC, Manandhar P, Holmes DR, et al. Peripheral artery disease and transcatheter aortic valve replacement outcomes: a report from the Society of Thoracic Surgeons/American College of Cardiology Transcatheter Therapy Registry. Circ Cardiovasc Interv. 2017;10:e005456.

Challenging Anatomy in Transcatheter Aortic Valve Implantation

19

Antonio Colombo and Nicola Buzzatti

19.1 Introduction

Transcatheter aortic valve implantation (TAVI), also called transcatheter aortic valve replacement (TAVR), emerged over the last decade as a valuable tool to treat patients affected by severe symptomatic aortic stenosis [1]. Thanks to the promising results achieved over the years, the population of patients who can be candidate to receive TAVI is continuously growing.

Careful preoperative anatomical assessment through computed tomography, procedural planning and technical execution are key to ensure the safety and the efficacy of the procedure. Indeed, some specific anatomies are associated with increased technical complexity, risk of complications and impaired results. Of note, multiple anatomical challenges can be present at the same time, possibly transforming what should have been a quick low-risk minimally invasive intervention in a true nightmare.

The purpose of this chapter is to discuss the most common of these unfavourable anatomical features for TAVI in the setting of native aortic stenosis. Unfortunately, for most of them, few data are still available. Several other even more rare anatomies can also be encountered, but reports are far too few to draw reliable evidence.

19.2 Bicuspid Aortic Valve

Bicuspid aortic valve (BAV) is a complex spectrum of disease, including several valvular anatomical variants ranging from true type 0 bicuspid valve (with no raphe) to forms in which three cusps can be identified, but they are unified by variably located raphes, Fig. 19.1a, b. Pure valve stenosis, pure regurgitation or both can be present.

The proportion of patients submitted to TAVI affected by BAV is about 2–6% [2, 3], but it is about 22% in octogenarians treated with SAVR [4]. BAV disease arise at younger age compared to tricuspid valves with calcifications progressing significantly after the forth decade of life. Vascular aortopathy due to aortic media abnormalities is present in up to 50% of affected persons, and it is an expression of the genetic basis of BAV [5].

Two are the major concerns regarding TAVI in BAV stenosis:

- BAV asymmetric shape and calcifications may impair adequate prosthesis expansion, function and durability, Fig. 19.2a.
- The associated aortopathy may increase the risk of aortic dissection and aortic annulus rupture, Fig. 19.2b.

A. Colombo
Interventional Cardiology Department, San Raffaele Scientific Institute, Milan, Italy
e-mail: colombo.antonio@hsr.it

N. Buzzatti (✉)
Cardiac Surgery Department, San Raffaele Scientific Institute, Milan, Italy
e-mail: buzzatti.nicola@hsr.it

© Springer Nature Switzerland AG 2019
A. Giordano et al. (eds.), *Transcatheter Aortic Valve Implantation*,
https://doi.org/10.1007/978-3-030-05912-5_19

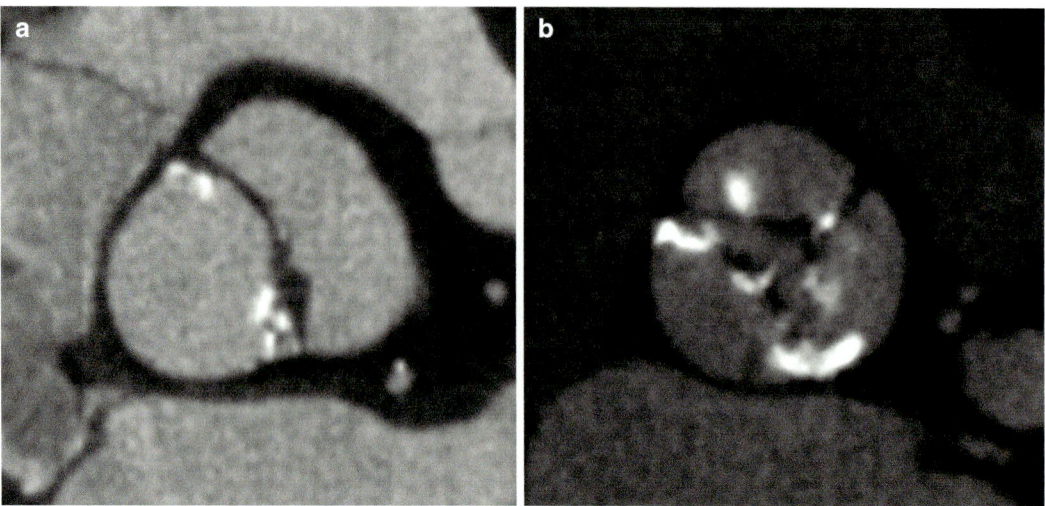

Fig. 19.1 Bicuspid aortic valve variants at preoperative computed tomography. (**a**) Type 0, "true" bicuspid valve. (**b**) Type 1, with raphe between the right and left coronary cusps

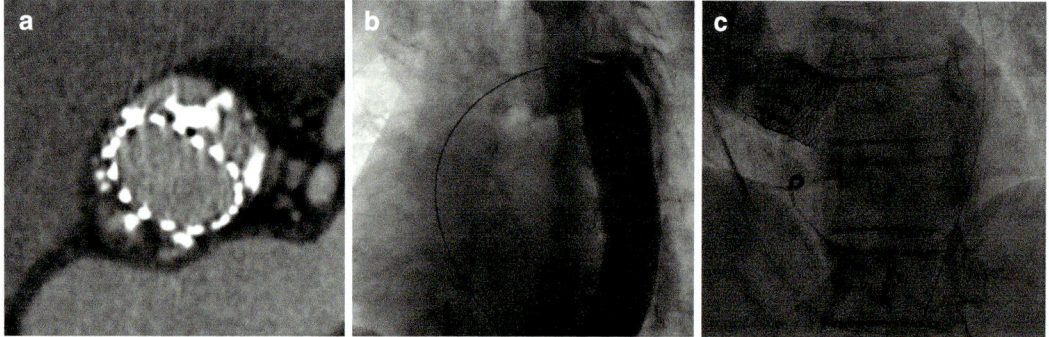

Fig. 19.2 TAVI in bicuspid aortic valve. (**a**) Incomplete asymmetrical CoreValve stent expansion after implantation. (**b**) Distal aortic arch dissection during attempt of valve shaft advancement. (**c**) Successful implantation of a new-generation device (Lotus valve) with no residual aortic regurgitation

Despite these concerns, a number of high-risk or inoperable patients affected by BAV have been actually treated with TAVI over the years.

In a recent large multicentre experience, the outcomes of 546 matched pairs of patients affected by BAV vs. tricuspid aortic stenosis have been compared [6]. Overall, BAV was associated with higher rate of conversion to surgery (2.0% vs. 0.2%, $P = 0.006$) mainly due to aortic root injury (9 out of 11 cases), need of second valve (4.8% vs. 1.5%, $P = 0.002$) and higher rate of paravalvular regurgitation ≥moderate (10.4% vs. 6.8%, $P = 0.04$). However, in spite of these pro-cedural pitfalls, no difference in survival was observed at 30-day nor at 2-year. Of note, the increased rate of procedural complications in BAV was only observed in patients who received old-generation devices. Specifically, aortic rupture was observed more frequently with the SAPIEN XT (Edwards Lifesciences Ltd., Irvine, CA, USA), whereas second valve need and paravalvular regurgitation were more frequent with the CoreValve (Medtronic Inc., MN, USA) prosthesis. On the other hand, in patients who received new-generation devices (in particular SAPIEN 3 and Lotus (Boston Scientific, Natick,

MA, USA), the results improved; nevertheless, there was a numerical trend highlighting the problems related to TAVI in BAV (conversion to surgery 1.3% vs. 0%, second valve need 1.3% vs. 0.4%, paravalvular leak 2.7% vs. 1.8%, all $P > 0.05$) Fig. 19.2c.

The number of treated cases is still limited, and more experience is needed to fully clarify the role of TAVI in the setting of BAV. Nevertheless, the results provided by new-generation devices show promising low rates of complications, similar to conventional tricuspid aortic stenosis. As a general rule, compared to tricuspid valves, a more cautious gentle approach to the procedure should still be adopted, trying to minimize the tissue trauma on the aorta and the aortic valve, for example, avoiding excessive prosthesis oversizing or even allowing some downsizing.

BAV in itself should not be considered an absolute contraindication to TAVI. Instead, the anatomy of each single case should be carefully assessed prior to the procedure to rule out possible issues (concomitant aortic dilatation, valve size, location of calcifications) and choose the best prosthesis type for the specific anatomy.

19.3 Severe Aortic Calcifications

Severe calcifications are frequently seen in the setting of aortic stenosis. In SAVR, the aortic annulus is carefully decalcified, and the prosthesis is sutured to the heart leaving no space between the two; on the contrary, in TAVI, a stent is expanded pushing/crushing/accommodating to the native calcific annular leaflets to provide adequate sealing. For this reason, the rocky irregular, sometimes bulky calcium of aortic valve may lead to several issues following TAVI, and therefore it may require special technical attentions during procedure planning and execution. Preprocedural computed tomography assessment of calcium location, shape, size, hardness and homogeneity is the first fundamental step for patient selection and procedure planning, Figs. 19.3 and 19.4. Unfortunately, precise shared criteria for calcium assessment are not yet available, and therefore personal experience currently still guides the decision-making.

When facing a patient who presents with severe calcifications of the aortic complex, the most important aspects to consider are:

- Increasing degrees of calcium, especially when located in the left ventricle outflow tract (LVOT), have been associated with increased paravalvular aortic regurgitation with all kinds of prostheses, and differences in incidence of aortic regurgitation have also been observed with regard to prostheses type [7–9]. Indeed, in moderate/severe calcifications, paravalvular leak appears to be higher with self-expandable compared to balloon-expandable valves, Fig. 19.5a. Of note, new-generation devices, thanks to the addition of a "skirt" outside the valve stent, have shown reduced paravalvular leak compared to previous-generation devices, independently from valve calcium severity [10], Fig. 19.5b. With these new prostheses, therefore the need of ample oversizing has been much reduced. Indeed, especially in the setting of severe calcifications, the use of a new-generation prosthesis allows to perform a minimal oversizing or even a small downsizing without increased risk of paravalvular leak.
- In case of severe calcifications, incomplete and asymmetric deployment can be observed with self-expandable prostheses [11], which in turn can cause not only paravalvular aortic regurgitation but possibly impaired leaflet long-term durability.
- Rupture of aortic root/annulus/LVOT/left ventricle has been repeatedly reported [9, 12, 13], Fig. 19.6. The estimated incidence of tissue rupture after TAVI is actually low, ranging 0.5–0.9%, but mortality after such complication is very high, up to ≈50%. The small incidence makes difficult to draw definitive information; nevertheless, aortic rupture has been more frequently observed in balloon-expandable compared to self-expandable prostheses, aortic annulus and LVOT being

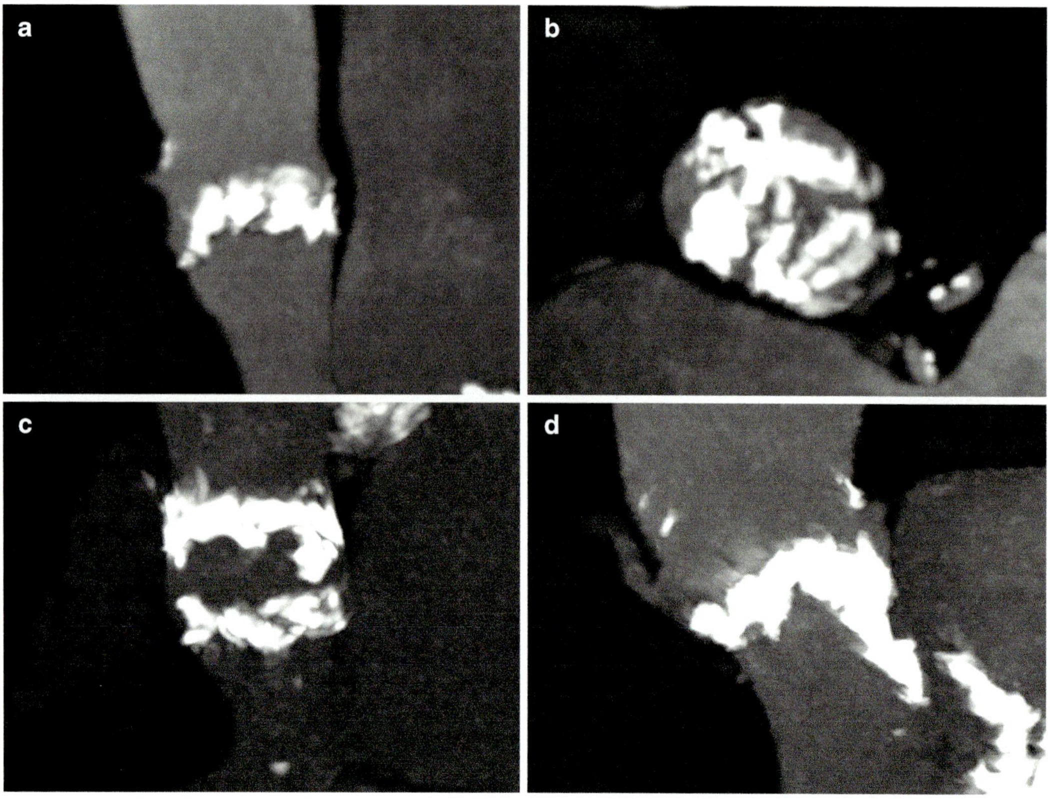

Fig. 19.3 Severe aortic complex calcifications at preoperative computed tomography. (**a**, **b**) Isolated, mostly leaflets, valve calcifications. (**c**) Severe circumferential sinotubular junction calcifications, care should be taken in this case not to stretch and rupture the sinotubular junction with a balloon (pre-dilatation, valve nor post-dilatation). (**d**) Severe left ventricle outflow tract calcification at the level of the mitro-aortic continuity

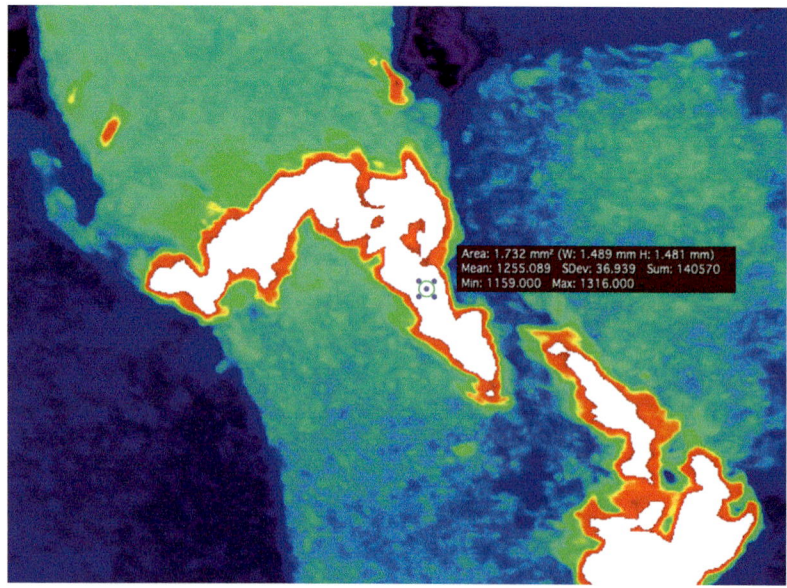

Fig. 19.4 Preoperative computed tomography assessment of calcium hardness and homogeneity

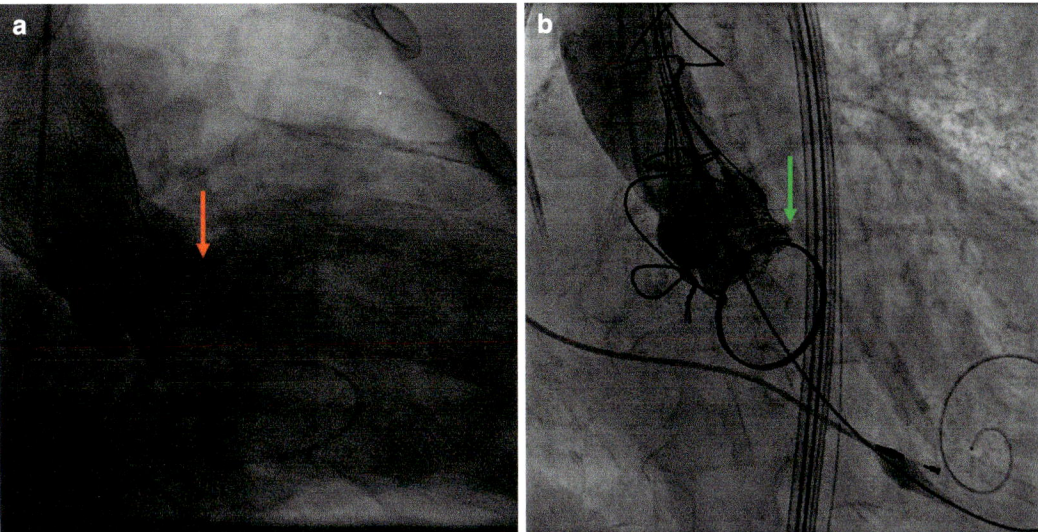

Fig. 19.5 Residual aortic regurgitation after TAVI. (**a**) Red arrow points the origin of aortic regurgitation from a calcific spot with an under-expanded CoreValve prosthe- sis. (**b**) Green arrow points the lack of any regurgitation despite visible calcium with a new-generation device (Lotus valve)

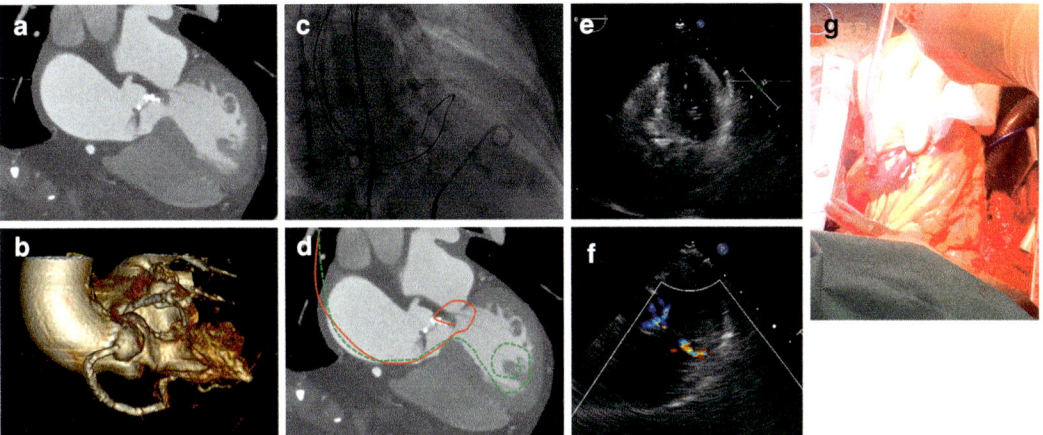

Fig. 19.6 A case of left ventricle perforation during TAVI in which multiple unfavourable anatomical features were present at the same time. (**a**) Preoperative computed tomography showed calcifications extending in the LVOT, increased aortic angulation and bulgy interventricular septum. (**b**) Preoperative computed tomography 3D reconstruction underlined the misalignment between the aorta and the left ventricle. (**c**) Abnormal position of the stiff wire inside the left ventricle prior to valve insertion during the procedure. (**d**) Expected correct wire position (green) compared to actual wrong observed wire position (red). (**e**) After the development of hypotension, pericardial effusion was documented. (**f**) Perforation of the lateral wall of the left ventricle was observed. (**g**) Emergent surgery was required, confirming and correcting the lateral wall perforation

the most common sites of lesion, Fig. 19.7. Indeed, moderate/severe LVOT calcifications and excessive prosthesis oversizing ($\geq 20\%$) have been associated with aortic rupture with balloon-expandable TAVI. Notably, calcium can express its effect through direct tissue compression/rupture at the site of calcium location itself but also, acting as a cornerstone, through prosthesis shift away from its location towards the opposite direction or

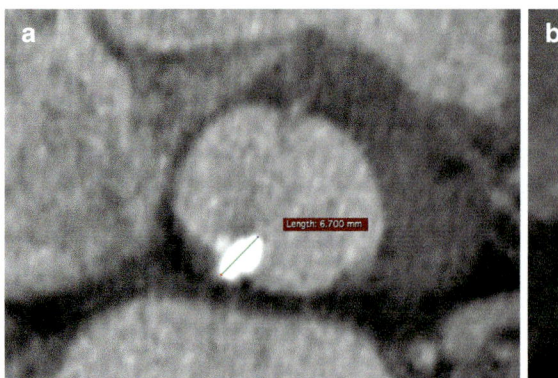
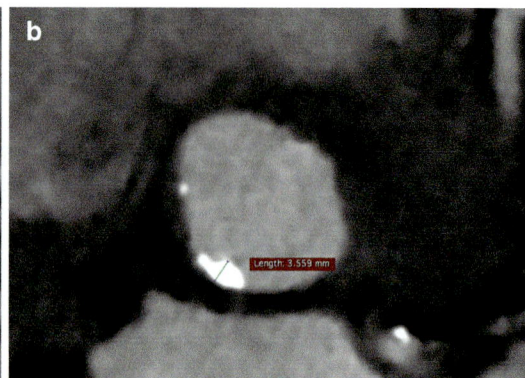

Fig. 19.7 Calcifications in the left ventricle outflow tract with different dimensions, shapes and risk of rupture. (**a**) Oblong high-risk calcium. (**b**) Flat low-risk calcium

through indirect transmitted tension on other weaker tissues. New-generation devices, thanks to their reduced need for oversizing, promise to limit the risk of tissue rupture, but no data to confirm this theory is available yet.

• The risk of definitive PM implantation is also increased [9, 14].

The role of predilatation is still debated in very calcified anatomies. On one side, it may facilitate valve crossing and positioning of the device as well as preparing the landing zone to minimize paravalvular leak and favour adequate valve expansion. Of course, this last aspect would be more important for self-expandable than for balloon-expandable valves. On the other side, the balloon itself can carry a risk of tissue rupture. A reasonable approach therefore could be to avoid predilatation with balloon-expandable devices and perform just a soft predilatation with other devices.

19.4 Increased Aortic Angulation

Since the early days of TAVI, increased angulation between the aortic root and the LVOT has been reported to be associated with increased residual aortic regurgitation after the implantation of CoreValve devices [15]. Over the years, the angle between the horizontal plane and the plane of the aortic annulus became more commonly used to describe aortic angulation, and the

term "horizontal aorta" defined extreme forms of angulation in which the aortic annulus is nearly vertical, causing technical difficulty in achieving optimal CoreValve prosthesis positioning [16]. Indeed, angulation >70° has been an exclusion criteria for randomized trials on CoreValve transfemoral TAVI [17].

A recent study compared the outcomes of patients with vs. without significant aortic angulation, separately in balloon Edwards and self-expandable CoreValve prostheses [18]. While in the balloon-expandable devices, no impact was observed; in the self-expandable group, increased aortic angulation adversely influenced procedural success. In this last group, the numerical cut-off for aortic angulation with the highest sum of sensitivity and specificity for device success was ≥48°. Patients whose angulation was ≥48° were associated with an increased need for a second valve and, post-dilation, had increased fluoroscopy time and increased valve embolization and had increased post-procedural paravalvular regurgitation. Follow-up mortality however up to 6 months was similar. Commonly advocated reasons for the difference between self- vs. balloon-expandable valves are the longer stent frame of self-expandable prostheses, which suffers from the dimensions and relative positions of ascending aorta-sinotubular junction-aortic annulus-LVOT, and the lack of flexibility and active steering of the delivery shaft, Fig. 19.8.

Several technical tips and tricks have been proposed to mitigate the effect of increased

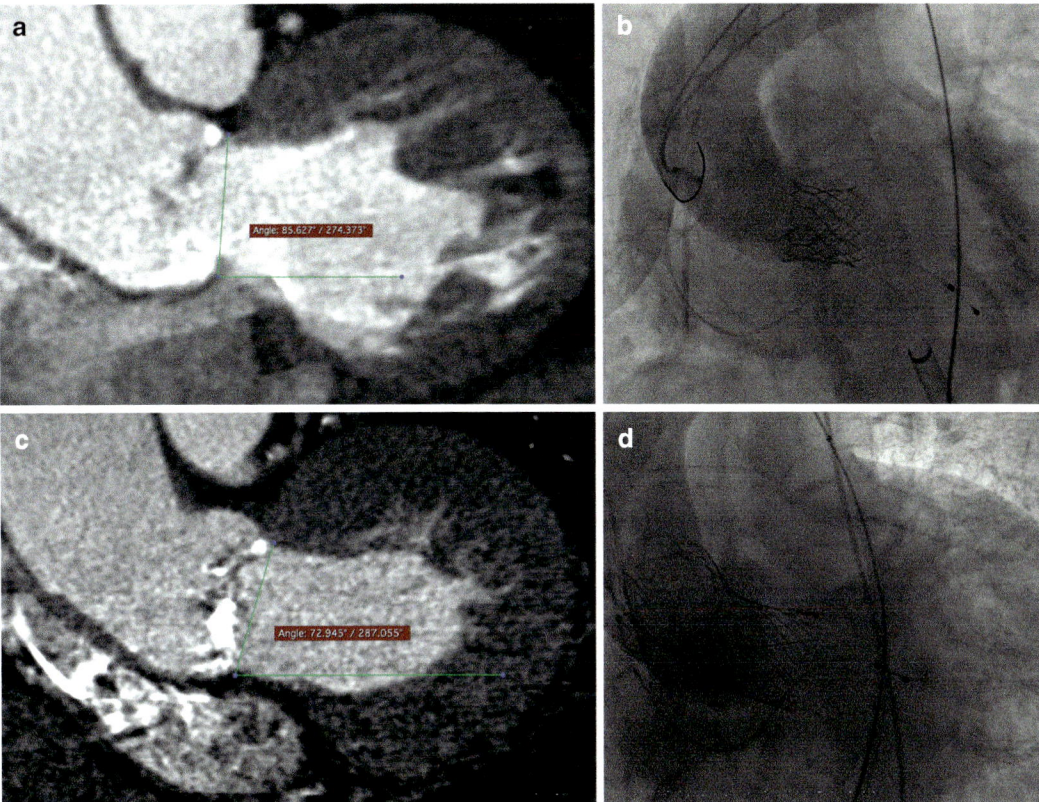

Fig. 19.8 Pre-procedure CT showes an almost vertical aortic annulus (**a**), successfully treated with a SAPIEN 3 prosthesis with no residual paravalvular leak (**b**). Pre-procedure CT showes a severely (>70%) horizontal aorta (**c**), treated with a CoreValve prosthesis. The device remained too low with residual moderate paravalvular leak (**d**).

aortic angulation during CoreValve implantation [19]. The most effective would be the use of a direct transaortic approach that would provide the best manoeuvrability and precision. In case of transfemoral route, best practice techniques include alignment of the delivery catheter along the greater curvature of the aorta using stiffer guidelines (e.g. Super Stiff Amplatz or Lunderquist 0.035-in. guidewires), stabilization of the delivery catheter using gentle forward force on the delivery catheter guidewire positioned in the left ventricular apex, alignment of the delivery catheter marker to allow visualization of the inflow of the prosthesis in a coaxial alignment, slow deployment and controlled annular contact to stabilized the valve frame, avoidance of deeper implantation by forward tension on the delivery guidewire and retraction on the catheter.

New-generation self-expandable valves as well as other devices may be useful in the setting of angulated aorta, but no evidence is currently available.

It should also be remembered that while the horizontal aorta is routinely easily used to find patients with challenging aortic angulation, it remains a raw approximation. The true problem lies in the misalignment between the ascending aorta—virtual basal ring—left ventricle and its consequences on bending of the device shaft, valve stent and LV guidewire. Indeed, recent evidences suggest that the angulation between ascending aorta—left ventricle inflow long axis would best predict residual aortic regurgitation after TAVI [20]. Finally the aortic angulation only takes into account a single two-dimensional angle between the aorta and the LV, whose real relationship on the other hand is three-dimensional, but no clear knowledge is currently established on three-dimensional aorta-LV alignment and its impact on TAVI.

19.5 Low Coronary Arteries

With old-generation devices, coronary obstruction after TAVI was a rare complication occurring in <1% of cases, but it could lead to a high 30-day mortality (≈40%) despite prompt intervention [21]. The left main was most frequently involved. Low-lying coronary ostium and shallow sinus of Valsalva were observed to be predictive anatomical factors. Also, coronary obstruction was found to be more frequent in patients receiving balloon-expandable valves.

In the common practice, the safety threshold for coronary ostium distance from the aortic valve virtual basal ring is usually considered 10 mm, but most cases below 10 mm can also easily be treated since the aortic root is usually wide enough, Fig. 19.9. Once again, preoperative careful assessment of the specific anatomy with computed tomography is key to identify patients who are at high risk for coronary obstruction, above all those with narrow aortic root.

In such risky anatomies, the choice, sizing and implantation technique of the device should be individualized for each single patient, the use of a repositionable device, avoidance of excessive oversizing and a slightly lower-than-usual implantation being reasonable decisions. When high risk is anticipated, similar to the valve-in-valve setting, coronary protection [22] with wiring and stent standby should be considered.

Together with the increasing experience of operators, the use of new-generation devices also seems to reduce the incidence of coronary obstruction [23], although few data are still available.

19.6 Challenging Femoral Access

The transfemoral route has by now become the preferred option for TAVI because of the advantages associated with its reduced invasiveness [24]. Over the years, the rapid evolution of devices and sheaths led to significant a reduction in the rate of transfemoral complications; nevertheless, vascular injuries remain still today observed in a not negligible ≈5% of patients [23]. Small vessel calibre (minimal artery diameter smaller than the external sheath diameter or sheath-to-femoral artery ratio >1.05), severe vessel calcification (especially when circumferential) and centre experience have been identified as major predictors of iliofemoral vascular complications [25].

Smaller introducers currently available in the clinical practice are down to 14Fr. Notably, in most cases and unless otherwise specified, the Fr size refers to *inner* sheath diameter, which means that the true *outer* diameter will be ≈2Fr larger. Indeed, vascular minimal lumen diameter ≥5.5 mm is currently considered safe for TAVI.

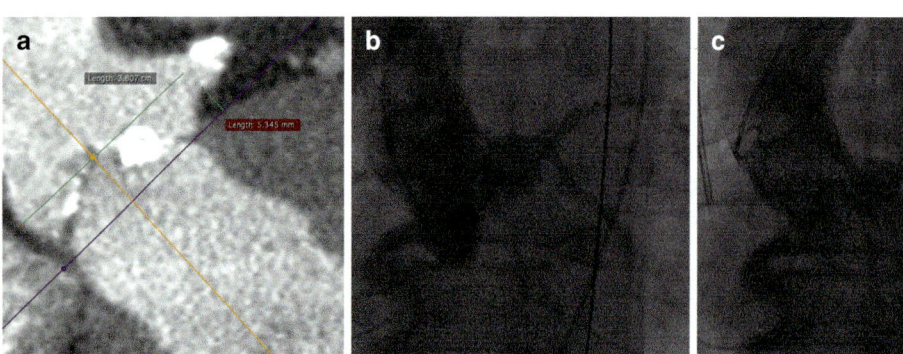

Fig. 19.9 A case of low left main treated with TAVI. (**a**) Preoperative computed tomography showed low ostium of the left main but wide sinus of Valsalva. (**b**) Angiography prior to TAVI procedure confirms wide aortic root. (**c**) Final angiography after TAVI confirms good left main perfusion

A limited number of cases of transfemoral TAVI in iliofemoral axes <5.5 mm have been reported [26]. In all these patients, pre-dilatation with semi-compliant balloons or dilatation with a Solopath sheath (Terumo, Somerset, NJ, USA) was used to allow the passage of the valve shaft, Fig. 19.10. Periprocedural vascular complications occurred in one fourth of patients. Recently, intra-vascular lithotripsy has provided initial promising results in selected TAVI patients affected by severely calcified ilio-femoral vessels.

Unlike vessel size and calcifications, tortuosity of the arterial route has not been clearly associated with increased vascular complications [25] because the arteries usually straighten out in the presence of a stiff wire. Nevertheless, severe tortuosity can make the procedure extremely difficult due to impossible advancement of the catheters or impaired manoeuvrability. Tortuosity remains difficult to define, measure and standardize. The most useful technical trick to overcome a difficult tortuosity in case a single stiff wire is not enough is to add a second stiff wire in the aortic root to be used as a "buddy-wire" [27]: this second wire will not only straighten the route but also provide direct support to the valve shaft to advance Fig. 19.11.

As a general safety rule, when a difficult access is anticipated, stiff wire should be used to insert even small introducers, and wiring of the superficial femoral artery from crossover or

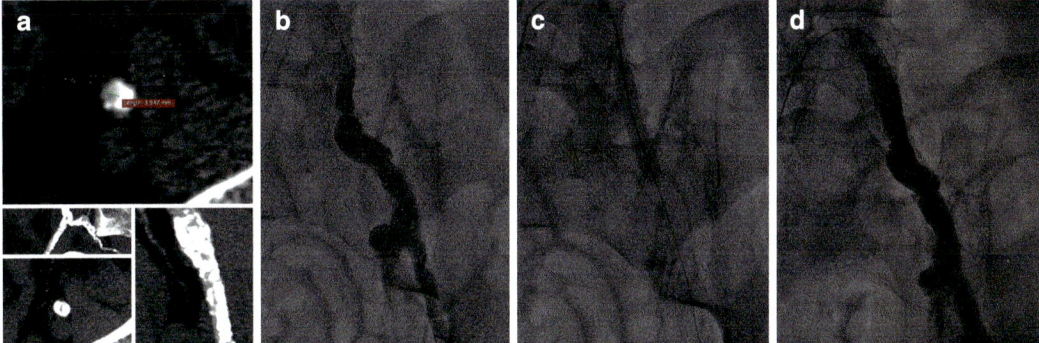

Fig. 19.10 Severely calcific iliofemoral axis successfully treated with TAVI. (**a**) Diffused calcium, minimal lumen diameter ≈4 mm. (**b**) Pre-procedure angiography, diffused atherosclerosis with severe stenosis impairing wires and catheter passage. (**c**) 8 mm semi-compliant balloon dilatation of the axis prior to TAVI sheath insertion. (**d**) Final angiography after TAVI sheath removal, adequate flow with no residual issue

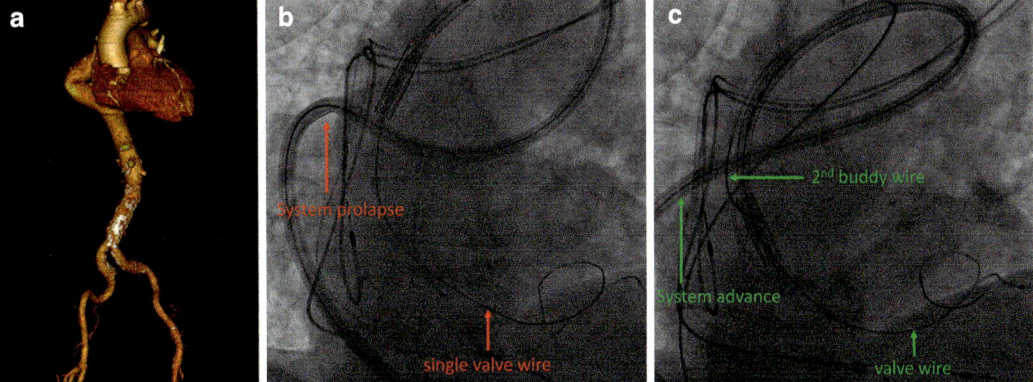

Fig. 19.11 Severely tortuous transfemoral route successfully treated with TAVI. (**a**) Preoperative 3D computed tomography reconstruction. (**b**) With conventional single stiff wire, the valve shaft prolapses with impossible advancement. (**c**) With two ("buddy technique") stiff wires, the valve shaft successfully advances to the aortic valve

radial access should be pre-performed to allow the positioning of a balloon or even a covered stent if required [28].

Although today the boundaries of transfemoral TAVI can be pushed to treat almost all patients that come at the cost of increased complication rate. Other approaches are available for TAVI and should be considered to offer the patients the lowest possible risk procedure. Specifically, trans-axillary access should be preferred as the top second option, provided that anatomy is suitable, because it is now feasible in a totally percutaneous fashion [29], and it is the only "alternative" route to have shown similar outcomes to those of the transfemoral approach (better than transapical and transaortic) [30].

19.7 Flipping the Therapy of Aortic Stenosis Upside Down?

Figure 19.12 depicts what has been in the past the evolution of other therapies for the correction of structural heart diseases (such as atrial septal defect and mitral stenosis).

Where does TAVI stand today in such process?

In the early days, patients submitted to TAVI have been inoperable or very high-risk patients for SAVR. In such extreme cases, despite the roughness of initial devices, TAVI provided a benefit compared to medical therapy [31],

yielding similar if not even a better clinical outcome compared to surgery [32, 33].

Over the following years, thanks to its promising results and rapid technological improvement, TAVI has become increasingly adopted in intermediate-risk elderly patients. In this healthier setting, TAVI confirmed to be a non-inferior alternative to surgery [34], and a survival benefit with the transfemoral approach compared to SAVR was actually observed [35, 36]. Indeed, TAVI has now become as a matter of fact the first-choice treatment for aortic stenosis in intermediate- and high-risk elderly patients.

Today the use of TAVI is currently under investigation in low-risk patients [37], and outside the clinical trials, low-risk patients have been treated already [38]. Moreover, besides the risk profile, a trend towards treating a "younger" age population has also recently emerged, and indeed according to the 2017 European Guidelines, the "younger" age threshold of 75 years now favours TAVI over SAVR [1].

The expansion of TAVI to younger, lower-risk patients (with a longer and more active life expectancy) makes more important than in the past the ability to provide optimal sustained long-term outcomes. In this scenario, it becomes crucial that, as discussed in this chapter, some specific patient's anatomies can increase the TAVI procedural risks (tissue perforation, coronary obstruction, vascular complications) and leave suboptimal acute results (residual aortic regurgitation, conduction disturbances, prosthesis under-expansion) which in turn can undermine

Fig. 19.12 Evolution of structural heart interventions, courtesy of Francesco Maisano

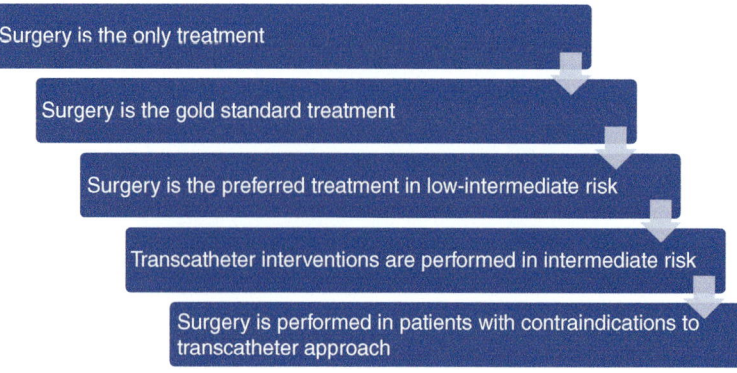

the long-term outcomes [25, 39]. Of note, although some of TAVI weak points may be reduced in the less diseased younger low-risk patients (e.g. less vascular complications in less calcific iliofemoral routes), others are likely to remain noteworthy or maybe become even more important (e.g. BAV, valve durability).

Today, we have reached the point where we start to face younger, low-risk, operable patients who have unfavourable anatomy for TAVI. In such cases, we should pause and carefully assess if TAVI can provide the patient the safest, good, durable result he deserves and critically recognize it that is not the case. If contraindications to TAVI are found and an optimal result cannot be anticipated, rediscussion within the Heart Team and with the patient should be done. After rebalancing the individual pros and cons, TAVI may be confirmed to be acceptable or SAVR may be reconsidered, to provide to each person the safest, more effective and more durable result.

Today, in the setting of younger, low-risk, operable patients, the quality bar for TAVI has been raised.

19.8   Conclusions

Some anatomical features may increase the TAVI procedure complexity and its risks, as well as impair the outcomes. Several technological improvement and technical expedients allow to overcome most challenges, but careful individual approach to each single patient is required. In the setting of younger, lower-risk, operable patients, an unfavourable anatomy should prompt towards a Heart Team patient-tailored rediscussion, and surgery may be reconsidered to provide each person the best possible result.

Conflict of Interest None.

References

1. Baumgartner H, Falk V, Bax JJ, De Bonis M, Hamm C, Holm PJ, Iung B, Lancellotti P, Lansac E, Munoz DR, Rosenhek R, Sjogren J, Tornos Mas P, Vahanian A, Walther T, Wendler O, Windecker S, Zamorano JL. 2017 ESC/EACTS Guidelines for the management of valvular heart disease: The Task Force for the Management of Valvular Heart Disease of the European Society of Cardiology (ESC) and the European Association for Cardio-Thoracic Surgery (EACTS). Eur Heart J. 2017;38:2739–279.
2. Mack MJ, Brennan JM, Brindis R, Carroll J, Edwards F, Grover F, Shahian D, Tuzcu EM, Peterson ED, Rumsfeld JS, Hewitt K, Shewan C, Michaels J, Christensen B, Christian A, O'Brien S, Holmes D, Registry SAT. Outcomes following transcatheter aortic valve replacement in the United States. JAMA. 2013;310:2069–77.
3. Yoon SH, Ahn JM, Hayashida K, Watanabe Y, Shirai S, Kao HL, Yin WH, Lee MK, Tay E, Araki M, Yamanaka F, Arai T, Lin MS, Park JB, Park DW, Kang SJ, Lee SW, Kim YH, Lee CW, Park SW, Muramatsu T, Hanyu M, Kozuma K, Kim HS, Saito S, Park SJ, Asian TI. Clinical outcomes following transcatheter aortic valve replacement in Asian population. JACC Cardiovasc Interv. 2016;9:926–33.
4. Roberts WC, Janning KG, Ko JM, Filardo G, Matter GJ. Frequency of congenitally bicuspid aortic valves in patients ≥80 years of age undergoing aortic valve replacement for aortic stenosis (with or without aortic regurgitation) and implications for transcatheter aortic valve implantation. Am J Cardiol. 2012;109:1632–6.
5. Siu SC, Silversides CK. Bicuspid aortic valve disease. J Am Coll Cardiol. 2010;55:2789–800.
6. Yoon SH, Bleiziffer S, De Backer O, Delgado V, Arai T, Ziegelmueller J, Barbanti M, Sharma R, Perlman GY, Khalique OK, Holy EW, Saraf S, Deuschl F, Fujita B, Ruile P, Neumann FJ, Pache G, Takahashi M, Kaneko H, Schmidt T, Ohno Y, Schofer N, Kong WKF, Tay E, Sugiyama D, Kawamori H, Maeno Y, Abramowitz Y, Chakravarty T, Nakamura M, Kuwata S, Yong G, Kao HL, Lee M, Kim HS, Modine T, Wong SC, Bedgoni F, Testa L, Teiger E, Butter C, Ensminger SM, Schaefer U, Dvir D, Blanke P, Leipsic J, Nietlispach F, Abdel-Wahab M, Chevalier B, Tamburino C, Hildick-Smith D, Whisenant BK, Park SJ, Colombo A, Latib A, Kodali SK, Bax JJ, Sondergaard L, Webb JG, Lefevre T, Leon MB, Makkar R. Outcomes in transcatheter aortic valve replacement for bicuspid versus tricuspid aortic valve stenosis. J Am Coll Cardiol. 2017;69:2579–89.
7. Seiffert M, Fujita B, Avanesov M, Lunau C, Schon G, Conradi L, Prashovikj E, Scholtz S, Borgermann J, Scholtz W, Schafer U, Lund G, Ensminger S, Treede H. Device landing zone calcification and its impact on residual regurgitation after transcatheter aortic valve implantation with different devices. Eur Heart J Cardiovasc Imaging. 2016;17:576–84.
8. Kim WK, Blumenstein J, Liebetrau C, Rolf A, Gaede L, Van Linden A, Arsalan M, Doss M, Tijssen JGP, Hamm CW, Walther T, Mollmann H. Comparison of outcomes using balloon-expandable versus self-expanding transcatheter prostheses according to the

extent of aortic valve calcification. Clin Res Cardiol. 2017;106:995–1004.

9. Maeno Y, Abramowitz Y, Jilaihawi H, Israr S, Yoon S, Sharma RP, Kazuno Y, Kawamori H, Miyasaka M, Rami T, Mangat G, Takahashi N, Okuyama K, Kashif M, Chakravarty T, Nakamura M, Cheng W, Makkar RR. Optimal sizing for SAPIEN 3 transcatheter aortic valve replacement in patients with or without left ventricular outflow tract calcification. EuroIntervention. 2017;12:e2177–85.

10. Kong WK, van Rosendael PJ, van der Kley F, de Weger A, Kamperidis V, Regeer MV, Marsan NA, Bax JJ, Delgado V. Impact of different iterations of devices and degree of aortic valve calcium on paravalvular regurgitation after transcatheter aortic valve implantation. Am J Cardiol. 2016;118:567–71.

11. Di Martino LFM, Soliman OII, van Gils L, Vletter WB, Van Mieghem NM, Ren B, Galema TW, Schultz C, de Jaegere PPT, Di Biase M, Geleijnse ML. Relation between calcium burden, echocardiographic stent frame eccentricity and paravalvular leakage after corevalve transcatheter aortic valve implantation. Eur Heart J Cardiovasc Imaging. 2017;18:648–53.

12. Barbanti M, Yang TH, Rodes Cabau J, Tamburino C, Wood DA, Jilaihawi H, Blanke P, Makkar RR, Latib A, Colombo A, Tarantini G, Raju R, Binder RK, Nguyen G, Freeman M, Ribeiro HB, Kapadia S, Min J, Feuchtner G, Gurtvich R, Alqoofi F, Pelletier M, Ussia GP, Napodano M, de Brito FS Jr, Kodali S, Norgaard BL, Hansson NC, Pache G, Canovas SJ, Zhang H, Leon MB, Webb JG, Leipsic J. Anatomical and procedural features associated with aortic root rupture during balloon-expandable transcatheter aortic valve replacement. Circulation. 2013;128:244–53.

13. Rojas P, Amat-Santos IJ, Cortes C, Castrodeza J, Tobar J, Puri R, Sevilla T, Vera S, Varela-Falcon LH, Zunzunegui JL, Gomez I, Rodes-Cabau J, San Roman JA. Acquired aseptic intracardiac shunts following transcatheter aortic valve replacement: a systematic review. JACC Cardiovasc Interv. 2016;9:2527–38.

14. Fujita B, Kutting M, Seiffert M, Scholtz S, Egron S, Prashovikj E, Borgermann J, Schafer T, Scholtz W, Preuss R, Gummert J, Steinseifer U, Ensminger SM. Calcium distribution patterns of the aortic valve as a risk factor for the need of permanent pacemaker implantation after transcatheter aortic valve implantation. Eur Heart J Cardiovasc Imaging. 2016;17:1385–93.

15. Sherif MA, Abdel-Wahab M, Stocker B, Geist V, Richardt D, Tolg R, Richardt G. Anatomic and procedural predictors of paravalvular aortic regurgitation after implantation of the Medtronic CoreValve bioprosthesis. J Am Coll Cardiol. 2010;56:1623–9.

16. Chan PH, Alegria-Barrero E, Di Mario C. Difficulties with horizontal aortic root in transcatheter aortic valve implantation. Catheter Cardiovasc Interv. 2013;81:630–5.

17. Adams DH, Popma JJ, Reardon MJ, Yakubov SJ, Coselli JS, Deeb GM, Gleason TG, Buchbinder M, Hermiller J Jr, Kleiman NS, Chetcuti S, Heiser J, Merhi W, Zorn G, Tadros P, Robinson N, Petrossian G, Hughes GC, Harrison JK, Conte J, Maini B, Mumtaz M, Chenoweth S, Oh JK, Investigators USCC. Transcatheter aortic-valve replacement with a self-expanding prosthesis. N Engl J Med. 2014;370:1790–8.

18. Abramowitz Y, Maeno Y, Chakravarty T, Kazuno Y, Takahashi N, Kawamori H, Mangat G, Cheng W, Jilaihawi H, Makkar RR. Aortic angulation attenuates procedural success following self-expandable but not balloon-expandable TAVR. JACC Cardiovasc Imaging. 2016;9:964–72.

19. Popma JJ, Reardon MJ, Yakubov SJ, Hermiller JB Jr, Harrison JK, Gleason TG, Conte JV, Deeb GM, Chetcuti S, Oh JK, Boulware MJ, Huang J, Adams DH, CoreValve USCI. Safety and efficacy of self-expanding TAVR in patients with aortoventricular angulation. JACC Cardiovasc Imaging. 2016;9:973–81.

20. Roule V, Placente A, Sabatier R, Bignon M, Saplacan V, Ivascau C, Milliez P, Beygui F. Angles between the aortic root and the left ventricle assessed by MDCT are associated with the risk of aortic regurgitation after transcatheter aortic valve replacement. Heart Vessel. 2018;33:58–65.

21. Ribeiro HB, Webb JG, Makkar RR, Cohen MG, Kapadia SR, Kodali S, Tamburino C, Barbanti M, Chakravarty T, Jilaihawi H, Paradis JM, de Brito FS Jr, Canovas SJ, Cheema AN, de Jaegere PP, del Valle R, Chiam PT, Moreno R, Pradas G, Ruel M, Salgado-Fernandez J, Sarmento-Leite R, Toeg HD, Velianou JL, Zajarias A, Babaliaros V, Cura F, Dager AE, Manoharan G, Lerakis S, Pichard AD, Radhakrishnan S, Perin MA, Dumont E, Larose E, Pasian SG, Nombela-Franco L, Urena M, Tuzcu EM, Leon MB, Amat-Santos IJ, Leipsic J, Rodes-Cabau J. Predictive factors, management, and clinical outcomes of coronary obstruction following transcatheter aortic valve implantation: insights from a large multicenter registry. J Am Coll Cardiol. 2013;62:1552–62.

22. Abramowitz Y, Chakravarty T, Jilaihawi H, Kashif M, Kazuno Y, Takahashi N, Maeno Y, Nakamura M, Cheng W, Makkar RR. Clinical impact of coronary protection during transcatheter aortic valve implantation: first reported series of patients. EuroIntervention. 2015;11:572–81.

23. Barbanti M, Buccheri S, Rodes-Cabau J, Gulino S, Genereux P, Pilato G, Dvir D, Picci A, Costa G, Tamburino C, Leon MB, Webb JG. Transcatheter aortic valve replacement with new-generation devices: a systematic review and meta-analysis. Int J Cardiol. 2017;245:83–9.

24. Siontis GC, Praz F, Pilgrim T, Mavridis D, Verma S, Salanti G, Sondergaard L, Juni P, Windecker S. Transcatheter aortic valve implantation vs. surgical aortic valve replacement for treatment of severe aortic stenosis: a meta-analysis of randomized trials. Eur Heart J. 2016;37:3503–12.

25. Toggweiler S, Leipsic J, Binder RK, Freeman M, Barbanti M, Heijmen RH, Wood DA, Webb JG. Management of vascular access in transcatheter aortic valve replacement: part 2: vascular complications. JACC Cardiovasc Interv. 2013;6:767–76.

26. Ruparelia N, Buzzatti N, Romano V, Longoni M, Figini F, Montorfano M, Kawamoto H, Miyazaki T, Spagnolo P, Alfieri O, Colombo A, Latib A. Transfemoral transcatheter aortic valve implantation in patients with small diseased peripheral vessels. Cardiovasc Revasc Med. 2015;16:326–30.

27. Buzzatti N, Mangieri A, Cota L, Ruparelia N, Romano V, Alfieri O, Colombo A, Montorfano M. Use of double stiff wire allows successful transfemoral transcatheter aortic valve implantation through extreme thoracic aorta tortuosity. Circ Cardiovasc Interv. 2015;8:e002331.

28. Curran H, Chieffo A, Buchanan GL, Bernelli C, Montorfano M, Maisano F, Latib A, Maccagni D, Carlino M, Figini F, Cioni M, La Canna G, Covello RD, Franco A, Gerli C, Alfieri O, Colombo A. A comparison of the femoral and radial crossover techniques for vascular access management in transcatheter aortic valve implantation: the Milan experience. Catheter Cardiovasc Interv. 2014;83:156–61.

29. Schafer U, Deuschl F, Schofer N, Frerker C, Schmidt T, Kuck KH, Kreidel F, Schirmer J, Mizote I, Reichenspurner H, Blankenberg S, Treede H, Conradi L. Safety and efficacy of the percutaneous transaxillary access for transcatheter aortic valve implantation using various transcatheter heart valves in 100 consecutive patients. Int J Cardiol. 2017;232:247–54.

30. Frohlich GM, Baxter PD, Malkin CJ, Scott DJ, Moat NE, Hildick-Smith D, Cunningham D, MacCarthy PA, Trivedi U, de Belder MA, Ludman PF, Blackman DJ, National Institute for Cardiovascular Outcomes R. Comparative survival after transapical, direct aortic, and subclavian transcatheter aortic valve implantation (data from the UK TAVI registry). Am J Cardiol. 2015;116:1555–9.

31. Kapadia SR, Leon MB, Makkar RR, Tuzcu EM, Svensson LG, Kodali S, Webb JG, Mack MJ, Douglas PS, Thourani VH, Babaliaros VC, Herrmann HC, Szeto WY, Pichard AD, Williams MR, Fontana GP, Miller DC, Anderson WN, Akin JJ, Davidson MJ, Smith CR, PARTNER Trial Investigators. 5-year outcomes of transcatheter aortic valve replacement compared with standard treatment for patients with inoperable aortic stenosis (PARTNER 1): a randomised controlled trial. Lancet. 2015;385:2485–91.

32. Mack MJ, Leon MB, Smith CR, Miller DC, Moses JW, Tuzcu EM, Webb JG, Douglas PS, Anderson WN, Blackstone EH, Kodali SK, Makkar RR, Fontana GP, Kapadia S, Bavaria J, Hahn RT, Thourani VH, Babaliaros V, Pichard A, Herrmann HC, Brown DL, Williams M, Akin J, Davidson MJ, Svensson LG, PARTNER 1 Trial Investigators. 5-year outcomes of transcatheter aortic valve replacement or surgical aortic valve replacement for high surgical risk patients with aortic stenosis (PARTNER 1): a randomised controlled trial. Lancet. 2015;385:2477–84.

33. Deeb GM, Reardon MJ, Chetcuti S, Patel HJ, Grossman PM, Yakubov SJ, Kleiman NS, Coselli JS, Gleason TG, Lee JS, Hermiller JB Jr, Heiser J, Merhi W, Zorn GL 3rd, Tadros P, Robinson N, Petrossian G, Hughes GC, Harrison JK, Maini B, Mumtaz M, Conte J, Resar J, Aharonian V, Pfeffer T, Oh JK, Qiao H, Adams DH, Popma JJ, CoreValve USCI. 3-year outcomes in high-risk patients who underwent surgical or transcatheter aortic valve replacement. J Am Coll Cardiol. 2016;67:2565–74.

34. Reardon MJ, Van Mieghem NM, Popma JJ, Kleiman NS, Sondergaard L, Mumtaz M, Adams DH, Deeb GM, Maini B, Gada H, Chetcuti S, Gleason T, Heiser J, Lange R, Merhi W, Oh JK, Olsen PS, Piazza N, Williams M, Windecker S, Yakubov SJ, Grube E, Makkar R, Lee JS, Conte J, Vang E, Nguyen H, Chang Y, Mugglin AS, Serruys PW, Kappetein AP, Investigators S. Surgical or transcatheter aortic-valve replacement in intermediate-risk patients. N Engl J Med. 2017;376:1321–31.

35. Leon MB, Smith CR, Mack MJ, Makkar RR, Svensson LG, Kodali SK, Thourani VH, Tuzcu EM, Miller DC, Herrmann HC, Doshi D, Cohen DJ, Pichard AD, Kapadia S, Dewey T, Babaliaros V, Szeto WY, Williams MR, Kereiakes D, Zajarias A, Greason KL, Whisenant BK, Hodson RW, Moses JW, Trento A, Brown DL, Fearon WF, Pibarot P, Hahn RT, Jaber WA, Anderson WN, Alu MC, Webb JG, PARTNER 2 Investigators. Transcatheter or surgical aortic-valve replacement in intermediate-risk patients. N Engl J Med. 2016;374:1609–20.

36. Thourani VH, Kodali S, Makkar RR, Herrmann HC, Williams M, Babaliaros V, Smalling R, Lim S, Malaisrie SC, Kapadia S, Szeto WY, Greason KL, Kereiakes D, Ailawadi G, Whisenant BK, Devireddy C, Leipsic J, Hahn RT, Pibarot P, Weissman NJ, Jaber WA, Cohen DJ, Suri R, Tuzcu EM, Svensson LG, Webb JG, Moses JW, Mack MJ, Miller DC, Smith CR, Alu MC, Parvataneni R, D'Agostino RB Jr, Leon MB. Transcatheter aortic valve replacement versus surgical valve replacement in intermediate-risk patients: a propensity score analysis. Lancet. 2016;387:2218–25.

37. Tarantini G, Nai Fovino L, Gersh BJ. Transcatheter aortic valve implantation in lower-risk patients: what is the perspective? Eur Heart J. 2018;39:658–66.

38. Thyregod HG, Steinbruchel DA, Ihlemann N, Nissen H, Kjeldsen BJ, Petursson P, Chang Y, Franzen OW, Engstrom T, Clemmensen P, Hansen PB, Andersen LW, Olsen PS, Sondergaard L. Transcatheter versus surgical aortic valve replacement in patients with severe aortic valve stenosis: 1-year results from the all-comers NOTION randomized clinical trial. J Am Coll Cardiol. 2015;65:2184–94.

39. Athappan G, Patvardhan E, Tuzcu EM, Svensson LG, Lemos PA, Fraccaro C, Tarantini G, Sinning JM, Nickenig G, Capodanno D, Tamburino C, Latib A, Colombo A, Kapadia SR. Incidence, predictors, and outcomes of aortic regurgitation after transcatheter aortic valve replacement: meta-analysis and systematic review of literature. J Am Coll Cardiol. 2013;61:1585–95.

Abbott Structural Heart Program for Transcatheter Aortic Valve Implantation

20

Vincent J. Nijenhuis, Jorn Brouwer, Pierfrancesco Agostoni, and Jurrien M. ten Berg

20.1 Introduction

Transcatheter aortic valve implantation (TAVI), also called transcatheter aortic valve replacement (TAVR), plays a key role in the treatment of severe aortic stenosis. Pivotal TAVI studies that form the base for this treatment were carried out using the balloon-expandable Edwards SAPIEN and SAPIEN XT valves (Edwards Lifesciences, Irvine, CA) and the self-expanding CoreValve system (Medtronic Inc., Minneapolis, MN). These TAVI devices have achieved favorable results in terms of clinical outcomes and valve performance. However, complications such as valve malpositioning, paravalvular leak (PVL), and conduction disturbances requiring permanent pacemaker implantation have emerged as important limitations of this procedure.

The Portico™ TAVI valve (Abbott Vascular, Abbott Park, IL) is a bovine pericardial tri-leaflet valve mounted inside a self-expanding nitinol stent. A porcine pericardial tissue skirt is sutured to the inside of the lower stent section and acts as

V. J. Nijenhuis (✉) · J. Brouwer · J. M. ten Berg
Department of Cardiology, St. Antonius Hospital, Nieuwegein, The Netherlands
e-mail: v.nijenhuis@antoniusziekenhuis.nl;
j.brouwer1@antoniusziekenhuis.nl;
j.ten.berg@antoniusziekenhuis.nl

P. Agostoni
Hartcentrum ZNA Middelheim, Antwerp, Belgium

a sealing cuff intended to reduce PVL. The device is designed for intra-annular placement and is fully re-sheathable, repositionable, and retrievable until deployed. The Abbott Structural Heart Portico™ TAVI system has been available commercially in Europe and other geographies since 2012. At the time of this publication, the Portico™ valve and accessory components are investigational devices in the United States and Canada. In the current chapter, we describe the properties of the valve system and the implantation techniques, summarize the experience and available data, and provide an outlook to future developments.

20.2 Abbott Portico™ TAVI System

20.2.1 Portico™ Transcatheter Aortic Valve

The Abbott Portico™ TAVI valve (Fig. 20.1) is a bovine pericardial tri-leaflet valve treated with Linx™ anti-calcification technology, mounted inside a self-expanding nitinol stent. A porcine pericardial tissue skirt is sutured to the inside of the lower stent section and acts as a sealing cuff intended to reduce PVL and to minimize leaflet contact with the stent. The device is designed for intra-annular placement and is fully re-sheathable, repositionable, and retrievable until deployed.

The Portico™ valve is available in four sizes (23 mm, 25 mm, 27 mm, and 29 mm) that are intended to treat patients with a native annulus

© Springer Nature Switzerland AG 2019
A. Giordano et al. (eds.), *Transcatheter Aortic Valve Implantation*,
https://doi.org/10.1007/978-3-030-05912-5_20

Fig. 20.1 Portico™ transcatheter aortic valve. Courtesy of Abbott Vascular, Abbott Park, IL

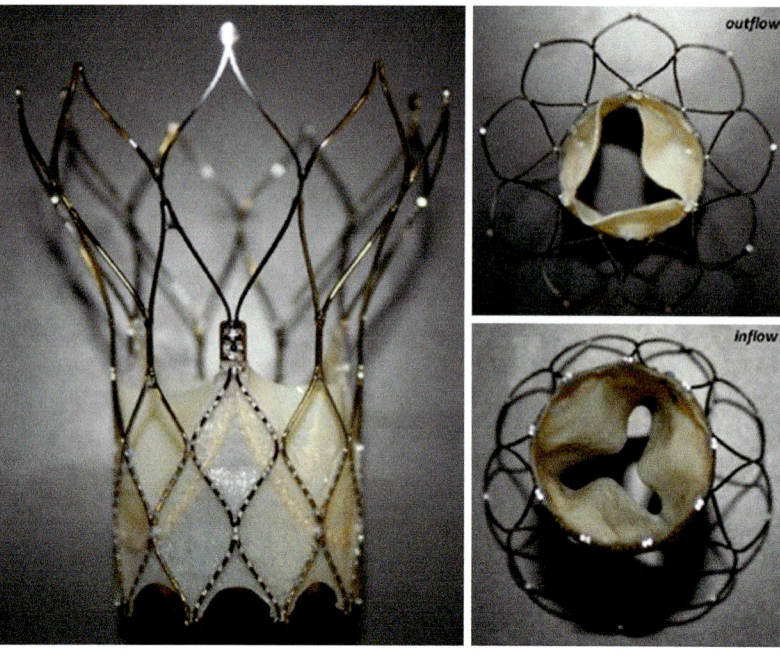

Table 20.1 Patient anatomical measurements

Portico™ valve size (mm)	Model number	Annulus size treated (mm)	Ascending aorta diameter (mm)	Vascular access diameter (mm)
23	PRT-23	19–21	26–36	≥6.0
25	PRT-25	21–23	28–38	≥6.0
27	PRT-27	23–25	30–40	≥6.5
29	PRT-29	25–27	32–42	≥6.5

size ranging from 19 to 27 mm, respectively (see Table 20.1).

20.2.2 Abbott Portico™ Delivery Systems

Dedicated delivery systems for the Portico™ valve (Figs. 20.2 and 20.3) are available for transfemoral access with a working length of 110 cm and alternative access (axillary/subclavian and transaortic) with a working length of 65 cm. Both configurations share the same basic design for the distal deployment end, the sheath body, and the proximal handle.

Portico™ delivery systems are over-the-wire, 0.035″ compatible systems and are 14 French (F) expandable sheath compatible. Both delivery systems use the same loading system according to the selected valve size.

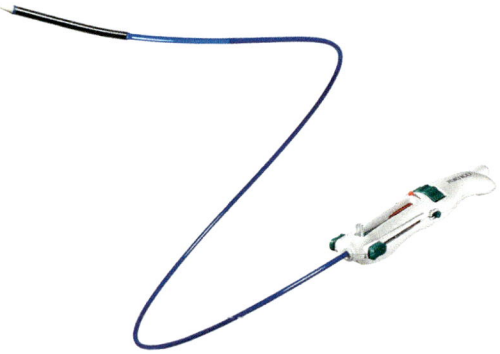

Fig. 20.2 Portico™ transfemoral delivery system. Courtesy of Abbott Vascular, Abbott Park, IL

The distal deployment end of the delivery system features an atraumatic radiopaque tip along with a radiopaque inner member marker band. The radiopaque marker band provides a reference point for alignment of the Portico™ valve with the native annulus during initial valve deploy-

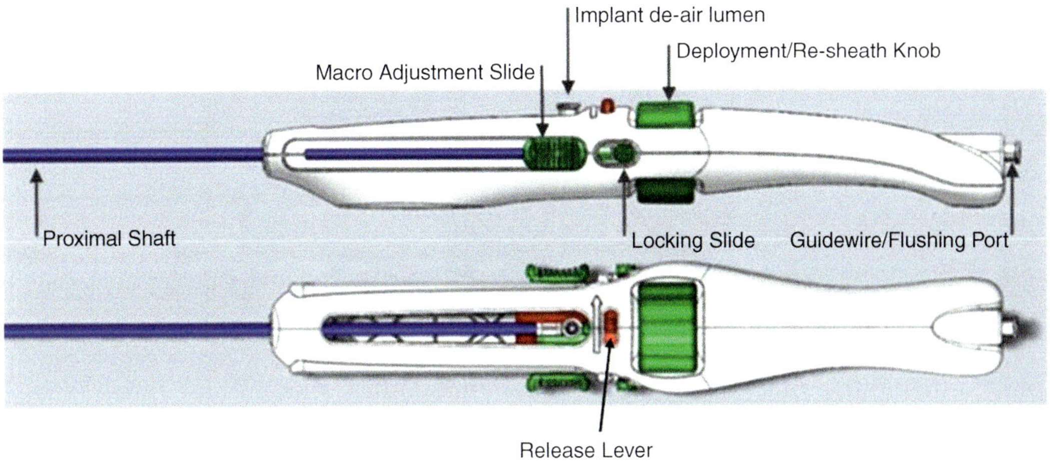

Fig. 20.3 Portico™ delivery system handle. Courtesy of Abbott Vascular, Abbott Park, IL

ment. A protective outer sheath covers and contains the valve in a collapsed profile, while the valve is held by the retainer receptacle. The outer sheath features a radiopaque distal marker band that serves as a reference point to determine the extent of valve deployment.

The macro adjustment slide on the proximal handle is used to open the distal sheath during valve loading and close the sheath after valve deployment.

When the deployment/re-sheath knob is turned, the outer sheath is retracted into the delivery system, allowing gradual deployment of the valve. The delivery system deploys the annulus end of the valve first. The position of a partially deployed valve can be evaluated, and if needed, the valve can be re-sheathed and redeployed for optimal placement in the native anatomy. Valve re-sheathing and redeployment can be performed provided that the valve has not been fully released from the delivery system. The valve is re-sheathed by reversing the deployment/re-sheath knob.

The Portico™ TAVI system has been available commercially in Europe and other geographies since 2012. At the time of this publication, the Portico™ valve and accessory components are investigational devices in the United States and Canada.

20.2.3 Implantation of the Portico™ Valve

Important recommendations for optimal implantation of the Portico™ valve include the use of balloon pre-dilation and slow, gradual deployment of the valve.

Balloon pre-dilation provides more room for the self-expanding TAVI implant to move freely during deployment, allowing a more precise, well-controlled deployment, and allows for stable hemodynamics. Usually, a 20 mm balloon is appropriate to achieve these benefits while minimizing the chance of aortic regurgitation or annular damage.

Following pre-dilation, a very slow and gradual deployment technique provides maximum positioning control and predictable deployment behavior, allowing the valve to be implanted at the position chosen by the operators.

The main steps of the optimal positioning and deployment of the Portico™ valve are discussed below.

20.2.3.1   Valve Positioning

The target implant depth is 3–5 mm below the annulus, i.e., relative to the bottom of the pigtail catheter in the non-coronary cusp (Fig. 20.4). The Portico™ valve provides stable

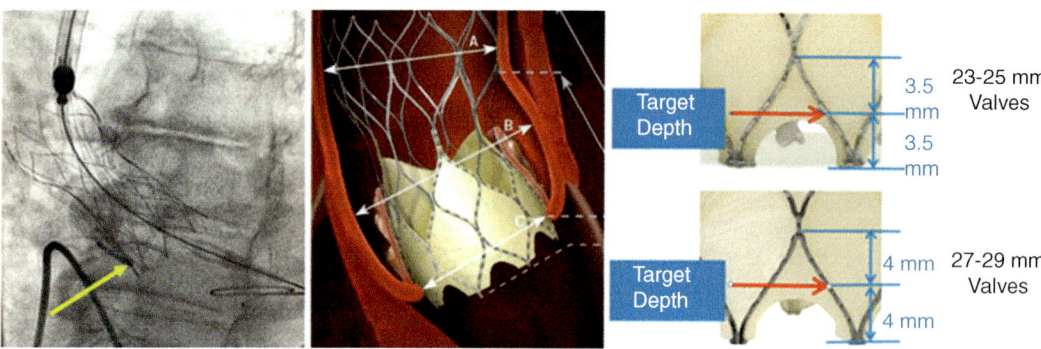

Fig. 20.4 Positioning of the Portico™ valve. Target depth can be related to the height of the stent cells. Courtesy of Abbott Vascular, Abbott Park, IL

hemodynamics throughout the deployment phase, and rapid pacing is usually not required. Once the target implant depth is reached, the dial knob on the proximal handle is turned relatively quickly until the delivery sheath reaches the struts. At this point, the operator should wait for 45 s to release any retained energy in delivery system cable.

20.2.3.2 Deployment

During deployment, one operator should keep the struts at 3–5 mm below the annulus, while a second operator slowly deploys the valve. Deployment should be done in small, sequential steps, each involving a single turn of the deployment knob followed by waiting approximately 10 s to allow the nitinol stent to expand uniformly and settle into the annulus. Once the frame has started to "flower," the struts need to be aligned to be able to evaluate the true depth below the annulus. These steps are repeated until 80–90% deployment is achieved.

20.2.3.3 PVL Assessment

PVL is usually assessed after full release. The presence and degree of PVL is best assessed by a combination of aortogram, echocardiography, and hemodynamics. If more than trace PVL is observed, balloon post-dilation should be considered, using a balloon size that is not greater than the mean diameter of the native annulus, as measured by CT.

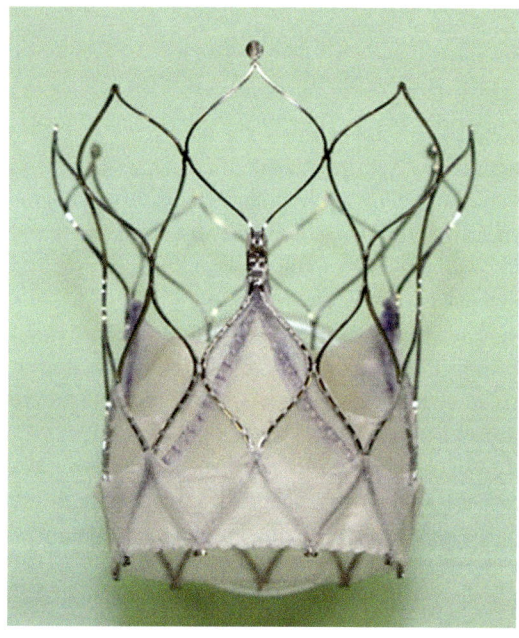

Fig. 20.5 Abbott SH Next-Generation TAVI Implant. Courtesy of Abbott Vascular, Abbott Park, IL

20.2.4 Future Outlook

20.2.4.1 Abbott Structural Heart Next-Generation TAVI Implant

The Abbott Structural Heart Next-Generation TAVI Implant (Fig. 20.5) will incorporate further design enhancements to minimize/eliminate PVL. Furthermore, design adaptations are aimed at further improvement of implant stability while

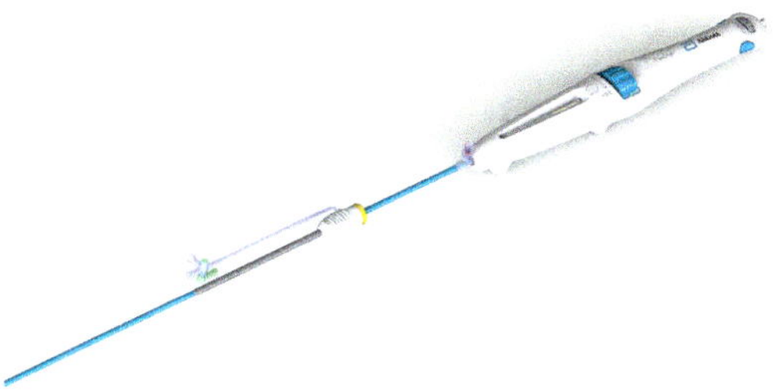

Fig. 20.6 Abbott's Next-Generation TAVR FlexNav™ Delivery System. Courtesy of Abbott Vascular, Abbott Park, IL

maintaining excellent valve hemodynamics and durability, without any increase to the delivery profile.

20.2.4.2 Next-Generation FlexNav™ Transcatheter Valve Delivery System

Abbott's Next-Generation FlexNav™ Transcatheter Valve Delivery System (Fig. 20.6) is being designed to facilitate low-profile access with an integrated sheath (14F and 15F equivalent inner diameter for the two smaller and two larger valve sizes, respectively). In addition, design enhancements are intended to achieve advanced trackability and placement accuracy to reduce manipulation at the access site. A hydrophilic coating is being added to enhance insertion and deliverability. The handle is being redesigned with additional ergonomic and ease of use elements.

20.3 Summary of Clinical Experience with the Portico™ TAVI System

20.3.1 Overview

Following an extensive preclinical test program, clinical investigations on the Portico™ TAVI valve and its delivery systems were started in 2011. Meanwhile, prospective clinical studies have been completed in six cohorts, and four additional clinical trials are currently ongoing (Table 20.2). The series of evaluations were designed to establish a robust portfolio of safety and performance data on the Portico™ transcatheter heart valve and transfemoral delivery system in patients with severe symptomatic aortic stenosis, who are at high and extreme risk for conventional surgical aortic valve replacement.

All clinical evaluations were completed under the following key considerations for consistency and to facilitate interpretation of results:

- Comparable patient cohort and outcome definitions, eligibility criteria, safety and effectiveness endpoints, sample size, and overall methods across studies.
- Criteria and assessment methods follow Valve Academic Research Consortium (VARC I or II) definitions and standards.
- Neurological assessment methods follow US FDA guidance.
- Global expert advisory committee utilized for oversight, including a subject selection committee to confirm all subjects were appropriate candidates for transcatheter aortic valve placement and met the high-risk designation.

Results from the two first-in-human (FIH) studies were published in 2012 [1, 2]. These studies were the foundation for the Portico™ TAVI System Conformité Européenne (CE) Mark study which included three separate cohorts and supported CE Mark approval for all four valve sizes in Europe. At completion, this study enrolled a total of 222 patients. Initial 30-day results of patients implanted with the 23 mm and 25 mm valves ($n = 100$) were published in 2016 [3]. Thirty-day and 1-year outcome data for all four Portico™ valve sizes were published shortly thereafter [4, 5].

20.3.2 First-in-Human (FIH) Studies

Two FIH clinical investigations were conducted in Canada [2] and Europe [1] in 2011 to assess the technical feasibility and procedural safety of transfemoral implantation of the first available size (23 mm) Portico™ valve.

Table 20.2 Clinical investigations for the Portico™ TAVI system

Study series	Sample size	Geography	Status	Published results
Portico™ EU First-in-Human TF-23 mm	10	UK (1 site)	12-month follow-up completed	30-day results published (n = 10) [1]
Portico™ Canadian Special Access First-in-Human TF-23 mm	10	Canada (2 sites)	Follow-up completed	30-day results published (n = 10) [2]
Portico™ Canadian Special Access Long Term Follow-up	10	Canada (2 sites)	12-month follow-up completed	–
Portico™ TAVI system CE Mark study: 23 mm	50	EU (5 sites)	12-month follow-up completed	30-day results published (23/25 mm; n = 100) [3]
Portico™ TAVI system CE Mark study: 25 mm	50	EU (7 sites)	12-month follow-up completed	30-day results published (23/25 mm; n = 100) [3]
Portico™ TAVI system CE Mark study: 27/29 mm	120	EU/AUS (12 sites)	12-month follow-up complete	30-day and 1-year results published (23/25/27/29 mm; n = 222) [4, 5]
Portico™ I PMCF study	1046	Worldwide (65 sites)	Enrollment and 30-day follow-up completed 1032 total (973 cohort A; 59 cohort B)	30-day results on cohort A to be presented at EuroPCR 2018
Portico™ US Pivotal IDE Trial	758 (randomized vs. commercially available valve)	USA and Australia (70 sites)	Enrollment completed in randomized arm. Enrollment in registries and follow-up ongoing	–
Portico™ Alternative Access CE Mark Trial	90	EU (12 sites)	Enrollment and follow-up ongoing	–
Portico™ Japan PMA study	50	Japan (8 sites)	Enrollment and follow-up ongoing	–

The Canadian FIH study enrolled ten patients from June to September 2011 from St. Paul's Vancouver Hospital and Quebec Heart and Lung Institute, Quebec City, Canada. Shortly thereafter, the European FIH study was initiated, and ten additional high-risk patients were enrolled from August to September 2011 from the Royal Victoria Hospital, Belfast, Northern Ireland, UK. All patients enrolled in the FIH studies were followed up to 1 year.

Key inclusion criteria for patients enrolled in the FIH studies are listed in Table 20.3.

Baseline characteristics of the 20 subjects enrolled across the two FIH studies are presented in Table 20.4. All enrolled patients were female due to the annulus size range suitable for implantation of the Portico™ 23 mm valve.

Procedural and 30-day safety outcomes in the FIH studies are summarized in Table 20.5 [1, 2]. Prosthetic valve delivery, deployment, removal of the delivery system, and percutaneous vascular closure were successful in all patients. Initial positioning of the Portico™ valve was suboptimal in 6 of the 20 patients. In all six cases, resheathing and repositioning of the valve was easily accomplished without withdrawing the system out of the aortic root. One patient had a moderate PVL because the valve was positioned too low; this resolved after snaring and pulling the valve a little higher. However, this patient required a second Portico™ 23 mm valve (TAVI-in-TAVI) to be implanted at 7 days post procedure to resolve intermittent prosthetic leaflet dysfunction.

Table 20.3 Portico™ 23 mm valve FIH studies—key inclusion criteria

Symptomatic severe aortic stenosis, confirmed by echocardiography

Native annulus diameter 19–21 mm

No atrial or ventricular thrombus

Mitral regurgitation < Grade 3

Normal–mild left ventricular hypertrophy (0.6–1.8 cm)

No subaortic stenosis

Annulus to aorta angle <70%

Sinus of Valsalva width ≥27 mm

Sinus of Valsalva height ≥15 mm

Ascending aortic diameter 28–36 mm

Aortic arch angulation: large radius turn. Patients with high angulation or sharp bend were excluded

Vascular access diameter >6 mm

Annulus eccentricity: maximum/minimum annulus diameter ratio ≥0.7

Table 20.4 Portico™ 23 mm valve FIH studies—baseline characteristics

Characteristic	Canadian FIH ($n = 10$)	European FIH ($n = 10$)
Age at consent date (years)	82.4 ± 5.7	85.8 ± 2.7
Sex (female)	10 (100%)	10 (100%)
STS risk score (%)	8.1 ± 3.2	6.5 ± 2.4
Logistic EuroSCORE (%)	NA	18.9 (9.6)
NYHA II	2/10 (20.0%)	3/10 (30.0%)
NYHA III/IV	8/10 (80.0%)	7/10 (70.0%)
Mean AVA (cm²)	0.62 ± 0.15	0.7 ± 0.2[a]
Mean transaortic gradient (mmHg)	44.5 ± 17.5	40.7 ± 12.6
LVEF (%)	57.3 ± 13.8	64.4 ± 6.8
Prior CABG	1 (10%)	2 (20.0%)
Prior pacemaker	1 (10%)	1 (10.0%)
Frailty	7 (70%)	NA
Porcelain aorta	1 (10%)	2 (20.0%)
Diabetes	5 (50%)	1 (10.0%)
Renal failure	3 (30%)	1 (10%)

Data presented as mean ± SD or n (%)
NA not available, STS Society of Thoracic Surgeons, NYHA New York Heart Association
[a]Based on data from six patients

Table 20.5 Portico™ 23 mm valve FIH studies—procedural and 30-day outcomes

Characteristic	Canadian FIH ($N = 10$)	European FIH ($N = 10$)
Procedural outcomes		
Local anesthesia	0	10 (100%)
Procedural time (min)	NA	54 (10.4)
Valve-in-valve	1 (10%)	0
Re-sheathing (%)	4 (40%)	2 (20%)
30-day outcomes		
Mortality	0	0
Major (disabling) stroke	0	0
Minor (non-disabling) stroke	1 (10%)	0
Myocardial infarction	0	0
Acute kidney disease, stage III	0	0
Major vascular complications	0	0
Minor vascular complications	1 (10%)	0
Life-threatening or disabling bleeding	0	0
Permanent pacemaker	0	0
New left bundle branch block	2 (20%)	3 (30%)
Readmission to hospital	0	0
Paravalvular aortic regurgitation		
None/trivial	5 (50%)	7 (70%)
Mild	4 (40%)	3 (30%)
Moderate	1 (10%)	0
Severe	0	0
Aortic valve area (cm²)	1.3 ± 0.2	1.5 ± 0.3[a]
Mean transaortic gradient (mmHg)	10.9 ± 3.8	7.8 ± 3.2

Data presented as mean ± SD or n (%). NA not available
[a]Based on data from four patients

At 30 days post-TAVI, there were no reported deaths, myocardial infarctions, life-threatening or disabling bleeding events, or major vascular complications. One patient reported a minor stroke (modified Rankin score 1), and one patient experienced a minor vascular complication (hematoma). New left bundle branch block developed in five patients. None of the 18 patients without a pre-existing pacemaker required insertion of a permanent pacemaker. Echocardiography at 30 days showed significant improvements in aortic valve area and mean transaortic gradient compared with baseline and none/trivial paravalvular aortic regurgitation in 14 patients (70%). Moderate paravalvular regurgitation was reported in only one case at 30 days. Compared to baseline, all patients improved in functional status, with 16 patients (80%) classified as New York

Heart Association (NYHA) functional class I and 4 patients (25%) as NYHA functional class II at 30 days.

Results from the two FIH studies showed that implantation of the Portico™ 23 mm device using the transfemoral delivery system in a population of elderly patients with symptomatic severe aortic stenosis who are at high surgical risk was feasible and safe. Acceptable safety and performance were confirmed by low adverse event rates and appropriate valve performance at 30 days and improvements in NYHA classification compared to baseline. These results justified further investigation of the Portico™ valve in larger, multicenter clinical trials (Courtesy of Abbott Vascular, Abbott Park, IL).

Early clinical results were further reported by Perlman et al. [6] from 57 patients, including the Canadian FIH cohort and additional early clinical experience in Canada, using all four valve sizes of the Portico™ TAVI system. Implantations were performed by transfemoral approach ($n = 41$) and non-transfemoral approach ($n = 16$). All-cause mortality rates at 30 days and 1 year were 3.5% and 15.8%, respectively. Compared with non-transfemoral cases, transfemoral cases were associated with numerically lower rates of 30-day mortality (0% vs. 12.5%), stroke (4.9% vs. 12.5%), and life-threatening bleeding (2.4% vs. 12.5%), although none of the differences reached statistical significance. More-than-moderate PVL was observed in two cases (3.5%) at 30 days and in four cases (10.3% of 39 patients) at 1-year post-TAVI. Implantation of a new pacemaker was required in five patients (10.4% of patients without previous pacemaker).

20.3.3 Portico™ TAVI System CE Mark Study

The Portico™ TAVI system CE Mark study was a prospective, non-randomized, multicenter clinical study designed to assess the safety and performance of the full family of Portico™ valve sizes at 30 days through to 1 year [3–5]. Between December 2011 and September 2015, the study enrolled 222 patients with symptomatic, severe aortic stenosis at high surgical risk across 12 centers in Europe ($n = 11$) and Australia ($n = 1$). Due to the sequential release of valve sizes into the study in Europe, subjects were enrolled in three separate cohorts commencing with the Portico™ 23 mm valve cohort on December 6, 2011, the 25 mm valve cohort on January 14, 2013, and the 27/29 mm valve cohort on February 13, 2014.

All patients had senile degenerative aortic valve stenosis confirmed by echocardiography. Valve selection was based on CT-derived annulus sizing, and an independent Subject Selection Committee confirmed the eligibility of all patients.

A total of 220 patients had a Portico™ valve implanted; 50 patients were each implanted with the 23 mm and 25 mm valve, and 60 patients were each implanted with the 27 mm and 29 mm valve. Two subjects had an unsuccessful implantation attempt of a Portico™ 25 mm valve. These two subjects were followed through to 30 days. Table 20.6 summarizes demographics and baseline data of the 222 enrolled patients.

The procedural outcomes are presented in Table 20.7. The re-sheathing feature was used in 73 procedures (33.0%) and was successful with-

Table 20.6 Portico™ TAVI system CE Mark study—demographics and baseline characteristics [4, 5]

Characteristic	$N = 222$
Age at consent date (years)	83.0 ± 4.6
Sex (female)	165 (74.3%)
STS risk score (%)	5.8 ± 3.3
Logistic EuroSCORE (%) (23/25 mm only)	16.7 ± 7.5
EuroSCORE II (27/29 mm only)	6.0 ± 5.6
NYHA II	47 (21.2%)
NYHA III/IV	175 (78.8%)
Prior CABG	22 (9.9%)
Permanent pacemaker	24 (10.8%)
Porcelain aorta	8 (3.6%)
Diabetes	69 (31.1%)
Renal failure	73 (32.9%)
Pulmonary disease (any type)	74 (33.3%)
Renal failure/insufficiency	73 (32.9%)

Data presented as mean ± SD or n (%)
STS Society of Thoracic Surgeons, NYHA New York Heart Association

Table 20.7 Portico™ TAVI system CE Mark study—procedural outcomes for enrolled patients [4]

Characteristic	N = 222
Local anesthesia	162 (73.0%)
Procedural time (min)	37.7 ± 18.8
Valve-in-valve	4 (1.8%)
Balloon dilation pre-implant	220 (99.5%)
Balloon dilation post implant	72 (32.7%)
Number of inflations if post-dilation	1.1 ± 0.3
Valve re-sheathed	73 (33.0%)
Successful re-sheathing	73 (100%)
Stent protrusion into LVOT (mm)	6.1 ± 2.2
Use of cardiopulmonary bypass	3 (1.4%)

Data presented as mean ± SD (n) or n (%)

Table 20.8 Portico™ TAVI system CE Mark study—Kaplan-Meier adverse events rates at 30 days and 1 year [5]

Characteristic	30 days	12 months
All-cause mortality	3.6% (8)	13.8% (29)
Cardiovascular mortality	3.6% (8)	9.4% (20)
Major (disabling) stroke	3.2% (7)	15.8% (12)
Myocardial infarction	3.2% (7)	3.2% (7)
Acute kidney disease, stage III	1.4% (3)	3.0% (6)
Major vascular complications	7.3% (16)	8.8% (19)
Life-threatening or disabling bleeding	3.6% (8)	5.2% (11)
Permanent pacemaker	13.6% (30)	14.7% (33)

Data presented as Kaplan-Meier event rates % (n)
Adverse events were adjudicated by an independent Clinical Event Committee using standardized VARC I criteria

Table 20.9 Portico™ TAVI system CE Mark study—echocardiographic valve hemodynamics [5]

Variable	Baseline	30 days	1 year
Effective orifice area (cm²)	0.7 ± 0.2	1.9 ± 0.5	1.7 ± 0.5
Mean aortic valve gradient (mmHg)	43.3 ± 14.6	8.3 ± 3.8	8.5 ± 3.6
Peak velocity (m/s)	411.2 ± 68.0	192.1 ± 42.3	194.3 ± 38.9
More-than-mild PVL		5.7	7.5

Data presented as mean ± standard error of the mean or %. Data adjudicated by an independent echocardiographic core laboratory

Compared with baseline, effective orifice area, mean aortic valve gradient, and peak velocity significantly improved at 30 days and at 1 year (all comparisons $p < 0.0001$; Table 20.9).

Of the 198 patients with analyzable PVL data at discharge, more-than-mild PVL was seen in 5%, with no cases of severe PVL reported. More-than-mild PVL was present in 5.7% and 7.5% at 30 days and 1 year, respectively.

Significant improvements in functional status were observed at 1 year compared to baseline. An improvement of at least 1 NYHA functional class was reported in 74.8% of the patients ($p < 0.0001$) at 1 year, while mean 6-min walk distance increased from 206 ± 117 m to 243 ± 108 m ($p = 0.0001$).

Overall, results through 1 year demonstrate that the full family of Portico™ valves is safe and has good clinical, functional, and hemodynamic outcomes.

out complications in all cases. Post-dilation was performed in approximately one-third of the procedures (32.7%) to ensure full device expansion and annular sealing.

Kaplan-Meier estimates of key safety event rates at 30 days and 1-year post-TAVI are presented in Table 20.8. The study achieved a primary safety endpoint of 3.6% for all-cause mortality at 30 days across all four valve sizes. Overall permanent pacemaker implantation rate at 30 days was 13.5% and increased marginally to 14.9% at 1 year. Intraoperative factors, such as implant depth, valve re-sheathing, and post-dilation, which are generally known to be predictive for the need for a new pacemaker, were not shown to be significant predictors in this study.

20.3.4 Ongoing Portico™ Clinical Studies

Currently, several studies with the Portico™ TAVI system are enrolling patients and/or are in active follow-up (see Table 20.2). These studies are aimed at gaining access to additional geographies and expanding indications for the Portico™ TAVI system in existing markets.

20.3.4.1 Portico™ I Post-Market Clinical Follow-Up Study

The Portico™ I Post-Market Clinical Follow-Up (PMCF) study is expected to report on 30-day results for the full cohort of prospectively enrolled patients at EuroPCR 2018. This study is a prospective, multicenter, non-randomized, single-arm post-market clinical follow-up investigation. The study will provide long-term (5 years) safety and performance data on the Portico™ TAVI system from a large population of high surgical risk patients with symptomatic severe aortic stenosis. Performance and safety data of the Portico™ TAVI system are evaluated at 30 days and 1 year and annually thereafter for 5 years, with 1-year all-cause mortality as the primary endpoint.

Study enrollment was completed in June 2017, and 1-year follow-up data collection is expected to be complete for publication by late 2018.

20.3.4.2 Portico™ US Pivotal IDE Trial

The Portico™ US Pivotal IDE Trial is a prospective, randomized, controlled, multicenter pivotal trial intended to demonstrate the safety and effectiveness of the Portico™ System compared to commercially available devices in patients with symptomatic, severe, native aortic stenosis, who are considered high or extreme surgical risk. The Portico™ US Pivotal IDE Trial was paused for new enrollments, along with implants outside the United States on September 12, 2014, pending the results of a detailed investigation to gain better insight into a leaflet motion observation exhibited on four-dimensional computed tomography (4D-CT) videos of several patients in the Portico™ US Pivotal IDE Trial. Following a comprehensive investigation, it was determined that the leaflet motion observation was due to subclinical thrombus formation. All available data were meticulously reviewed, and it was determined that the presence of subclinical thrombus was not limited to the Portico™ valve and did not pose an increased safety risk. The FDA approved to reinitiate enrollment in the trial in 2015.

20.3.4.3 Portico™ Alternative Access CE Mark Trial

The Portico™ Alternative Access CE Mark Trial is a prospective, multicenter, non-randomized CE Mark study to assess the safety and early performance of the Portico™ valve, implanted via subclavian and transaortic access, using the Portico™ transfemoral or alternative access delivery system. Data from the study will be used to support an expanded indication of the Portico™ TAVI system and to obtain CE Mark approval of the Portico™ alternative access delivery system for valve implantation via a subclavian/axillary or transaortic access site.

20.4 Discussion

The Abbott Structural Heart Portico™ TAVI system provides a safe and effective treatment for patients with severe, symptomatic aortic stenosis who are considered to be at high or extreme risk for surgical aortic valve replacement. Early clinical results with outcome up to 1-year post-TAVI have been reported in the literature from approximately 300 patients [1–6]. Accounting for the inevitable learning curve effect associated with the use of a new device, relatively low rates of mortality, stroke, and other major adverse events were reported, compared with other self-expanding and balloon-expandable TAVI systems [7]. The observed rates of early mortality as well as of disabling stroke are comparable with those reported from first- and second-generation TAVI systems [8–11], and 30-day mortality approaches the low procedural mortality rates reported for third-generation aortic valves implanted via transfemoral access [12, 13].

Results demonstrate the utility of the re-sheathing feature, facilitating optimal positioning of the valve [4, 6]. As an optimal valve position is a key prerequisite for valve performance and hemodynamic efficacy, the re-sheathing and repositioning capabilities of this self-expanding valve are highly appreciated among clinical users. Optimal valve positioning with minimal protrusion of the stent into the left ventricular outflow tract, facilitated by the re-sheathing capability, may reduce the risk of permanent injury to the cardiac conduction system. In addition, the low frame height and non-flared annular skirt with the porcine pericardial sealing cuff provide a uniform distribution of radial forces to the native annular tissue, minimizing trauma to the conduction system. Indeed, permanent pacemaker implantation rates reported from studies with the Portico™ valve are relatively low (approximately 10–15% [1, 2, 4, 6]), compared with those from other TAVI devices [14].

Other favorable implant-related characteristics of the Portico™ TAVI system, reported in the literature, include the low insertion profile and the flexible delivery system. These properties were suggested to contribute to acceptably low rates of major vascular complications (7.3%) and life-threatening or disabling bleeding (3.6%) at 30 days after implantation [5], comparable with other low-profile TAVI systems [13].

Reported results and experiences of early clinical users of the Portico™ valve suggest that pre-dilation and gradual, slow valve deployment are crucial elements with regard to achieving appropriate, uniform stent deployment and minimal PVL. Pre-dilation is recommended by the manufacturer and was performed in approximately 80–95% of the reported cases [4, 6]. Slow valve deployment allows the stent to accommodate within the native annulus and around calcific nodules. Throughout the deployment phase, the Portico™ valve is hemodynamically functional, eliminating the need for rapid pacing, which allows the operator to apply a slow, stepwise valve deployment. While slow valve deployment may be contra-intuitive to new users of this self-expanding aortic valve, a learning curve effect may be anticipated among operators introducing the Portico™ valve into their clinical routine. Publications of clinical data illustrating the learning curve effect with regard to the beneficial effect of slow deployment and pre-dilation on PVL reduction are expected shortly.

Implantation of the Portico™ valve was associated with good hemodynamic function, characterized by low (usually single-digit) transaortic valve gradients, improved aortic valve areas, and

a low incidence of more-than-mild PVL [1–6]. The Portico™ TAVI CE Mark study [5] reported more-than-mild PVL at rates of 5.7% and 7.5% at 30 days and 1 year, respectively. Severe PVL was rarely seen in any study with the Portico™ device. Overall, the totality of available clinical data indicates that the safety and performance profile associated with Portico™ use is comparable to other self-expanding valves [8, 10, 15]. Moreover, the early occurrence of PVL did not significantly differ between the four available sizes of the Portico™ valve [4]. Other hemodynamic outcomes were comparable with those reported from other balloon-expandable or self-expanding aortic valves [8, 10, 16].

20.5 Summarizing Conclusions

– The Abbott Structural Heart Portico™ TAVI system comprises a self-expanding, bioprosthetic aortic valve to be implanted intra-annularly using dedicated delivery systems. Additional design optimization is ongoing to further reduce the delivery profile and the degree of PVL.
– Recommendations for valve implantation include the use of balloon pre-dilation and slow, gradual stent deployment.
– Clinical studies at 1-year follow-up have shown acceptable safety and performance profile of the Portico™ valve, including appropriate hemodynamic function, low gradients, improved valve area, and a low degree of PVL.
– While the Portico™ TAVI system for trans-femoral delivery is CE marked in Europe, clinical studies are ongoing to obtain approval for other geographies including the United States and Japan and to expand the approved indications.

References

1. Manoharan G, Spence M, Rodés-Cabau J, Webb J. St Jude Medical Portico™ valve. EuroIntervention. 2012;8(Suppl Q):Q97–Q101.
2. Willson A, Rodès-Cabau J, Wood D, et al. Transcatheter aortic valve replacement with the St.

Jude Medical Portico™ valve: first-in-human experience. J Am Coll Cardiol. 2012;60:581–6.

3. Manoharan G, Linke A, Moellmann H, et al. Multicentre clinical study evaluating a novel resheathable annular functioning self-expanding transcatheter aortic valve system: safety and performance results at 30 days with the Portico™ system. EuroIntervention. 2016;12:768–74.

4. Möllmann H, Linke A, Holzhey D, et al. Implantation and 30-day follow-up on all 4 valve sizes within the portico™ transcatheter aortic bioprosthetic family. JACC Cardiovasc Interv. 2017;10:1538–47.

5. Linke A, Holzhey D, Möllmann H, et al. Treatment of aortic stenosis with a self-expanding, resheathable transcatheter valve: one-year results of the international multicenter portico™ transcatheter aortic valve implantation system study. Circ Cardiovasc Interv. 2018;11:e005206.

6. Perlman G, Cheung A, Dumont E, et al. Transcatheter aortic valve replacement with the Portico™ valve: one-year results of the early Canadian experience. EuroIntervention. 2017;12:1653–9.

7. Barbanti M, Buccheri S, Rodes-Cabau J, et al. Transcatheter aortic valve replacement with new-generation devices: a systematic review and meta-analysis. Int J Cardiol. 2017;245:83–9.

8. Leon M, Smith C, Mack M. Transcatheter aortic-valve implantation for aortic stenosis in patients who cannot undergo surgery. N Engl J Med. 2010;363:1597–607.

9. Smith C, Leon M, Mack M, et al. Transcatheter versus surgical aortic-valve replacement in high-risk patients. N Engl J Med. 2011;364:2187–98.

10. Popma J, Adams D, MJ R, et al. Transcatheter aortic valve replacement using a self-expanding bioprosthesis in patients with severe aortic stenosis at extreme risk for surgery. J Am Coll Cardiol. 2014;63:1972–81.

11. Meredith I, Walters D, Dumonteil N, et al. Transcatheter aortic valve replacement for severe symptomatic aortic stenosis using a repositionable valve system—30-day primary endpoint results from the REPRISE II study. J Am Coll Cardiol. 2014;64:1339–48.

12. Webb J, Gerosa G, Lefevre T, et al. Multicenter evaluation of a next-generation balloon-expandable transcatheter aortic valve. J Am Coll Cardiol. 2014;64:2235–43.

13. Manoharan G, Walton A, Brecker S, et al. Treatment of symptomatic severe aortic stenosis with a novel resheathable supra-annular self-expanding transcatheter aortic valve system. J Am Coll Cardiol Intv. 2015;8:1359–67.

14. Marzahn C, Koban C, Seifert M, et al. Conduction recovery and avoidance of permanent pacing after transcatheter aortic valve implantation. J Cardiol. 2018;71:101–8.

15. Adams D, Popma J, Reardon M, et al. Transcatheter aortic-valve replacement with a self-expanding prosthesis. N Engl J Med. 2014;370:1790–8.

16. Webb J, Doshi D, Mack MMR, et al. A randomized evaluation of the SAPIEN XT transcatheter heart valve system in patients with aortic stenosis who are not candidates for surgery. J Am Coll Cardiol. 2015;8:1797–806.

Boston Scientific Program for Transcatheter Aortic Valve Implantation

21

Mohammad Abdelghani
and Mohamed Abdel-Wahab

21.1 The Lotus Valve System

21.1.1 System Description

21.1.1.1 Frame and Leaflet Composition and Design

The Lotus valve (Boston Scientific, Marlborough, MA, USA) consists of a glutaraldehyde-fixed (or cross-linked) bovine trileaflet bioprosthesis and a frame made of continuous braided nitinol with an outer polycarbonate-based urethane seal at its ventricular end. The device is magnetic resonance conditional (i.e., poses no known hazards under specified conditions). The braided structure of the transcatheter heart valve (THV) frame is designed to shorten axially and expand radially during delivery and is then locked in this position using the "post and buckle" locking mechanism (Fig. 21.1 and Video 21.1).

Electronic Supplementary Material The online version of this chapter (https://doi.org/10.1007/978-3-030-05912-5_21) contains supplementary material, which is available to authorized users.

M. Abdelghani (✉)
Heart Center, Segeberger Kliniken,
Bad Segeberg, Germany
e-mail: mohammad.abdelghani@segebergerkliniken.de

Cardiology Department, The Academic Medical Center, University of Amsterdam,
Amsterdam, The Netherlands

M. Abdel-Wahab
Heart Center, Segeberger Kliniken, Bad Segeberg,
Germany

It is available in three sizes (23, 25, 27 mm), corresponding to native annulus diameters ranging from 20 to 27 mm (Table 21.1).

21.1.1.2 Delivery and Deployment

The Lotus valve is a 100% recapturable, repositionable, and retrievable THV that is partly self-expanding and mainly mechanically expanding [1]. During deployment, the frame shortens axially and expands radially, and the THV starts functioning early during deployment (Video 21.1). This latter property ensures stable hemodynamics during deployment which, together with repositionability, facilitates a comfortable and controlled THV release that does not require rapid pacing [1].

The Lotus valve is provided pre-attached to the delivery system through a post- and buckle-locking mechanism. Transfemoral and transaortic approaches are possible, and the minimal vascular lumen diameter required is 6 mm for the 18-Fr Lotus introducer sheath (for the 23 mm valve) and 6.5 mm for the 20-Fr introducer sheath (for the 25 and 27 mm valves).

The proximal end of the delivery system carries the Lotus Controller which comprises two mechanisms (Fig. 21.2 and Videos 21.1 and 21.2):

- A sheathing/locking control knob: Rotating this knob counterclockwise unsheathes and locks the THV, while clockwise rotation unlocks and progressively resheathes it back.

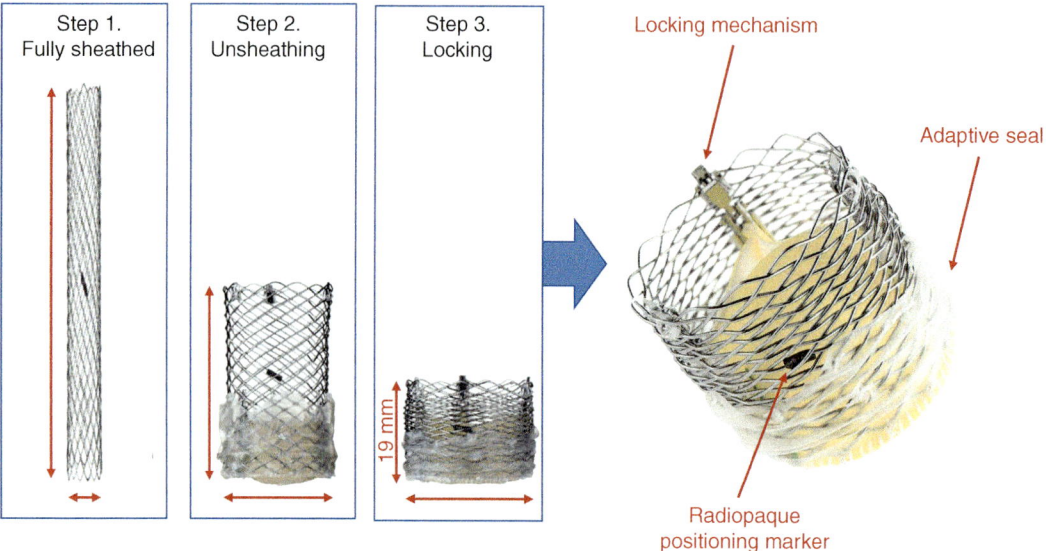

Fig. 21.1 The mechanical expansion and locking mechanisms of the Lotus Valve System. The sheathed device is 70 mm long, the intermediate (unsheathed) configuration is shorter and broader, and the final (locked) configuration has a height of 19 mm and a transverse diameter of 23–27 mm

Table 21.1 Dimensional data of the Lotus Valve System

Valve size		23 mm	25 mm	27 mm
Annulus	Diameter (mm)	20–23	23–25	25–27
	Area (mm²)	314–415.5	415.5–490.9	490.9–572.6
	Perimeter (mm)	62.8–72.3	72.3–78.5	78.5–84.8
Device/annulus perimeter oversizing (%)		0–13	0–8	0–7
Left ventricular outflow tract	Diameter (mm)	20–23	23–25	25–27
	Perimeter (mm)	314–415.5	415.5–490.9	490.9–572.6
	Area (mm²)	62.8–72.3	72.3–78.5	78.5–84.8
Sinus of Valsalva	Area too small (mm²)	<540	<595	<650
	Ideal area (mm²)	>600	>700	>800
	Area too large (mm²)	>1100	>1200	>1300
Delivery catheter outer diameter (mm)		6.9	7.2	7.2
Access artery minimal diameter (mm)		≥ 6	≥6.5	≥6.5

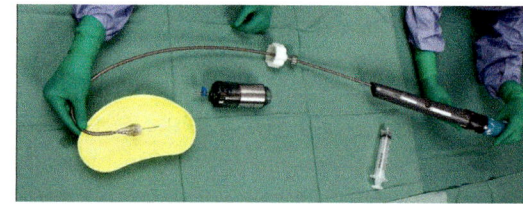

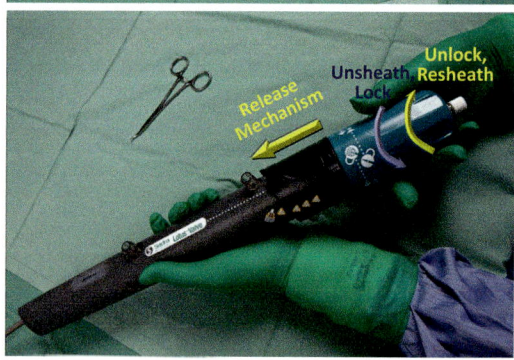

Fig. 21.2 Lotus Valve System deployment Controller (lower panel). The valve is provided pre-mounted to the delivery system (upper panel)

The locking mechanism should be checked before attempting implantation. Counter-clockwise rotation should lead to locking before a "click" is heard or felt, and further rotation should end up with a hard stop.

- A release ring: Turning the release mechanism detaches the THV from the delivery system. The release ring is protected from inadvertent manipulation by a safety cover, which should be pushed forward (toward the patient's head) to reach the release ring. The ring is rotated clockwise, leading to retraction of the release pin from inside the valve, until it is aligned with the first set of lines (pause sign) on the Lotus Controller. At this stage, the final check of valve position and function is performed, and, if satisfactory, the release ring rotation is resumed leading to detachment of the three fingers from the valve followed by a hard stop on further rotation.

21.1.2 Implantation Technique

The introducer sheath is placed in the descending aorta, and the aortic valve is crossed by a guidewire (a 0.035 in. super/extra stiff guidewire, at least 260 cm long for a 23 mm device or 275 cm long for a 25/27 mm device) which is then parked in the left ventricle. The delivery system is then advanced to the annular plane until the radiopaque mark (Fig. 21.1) is centered slightly above the annular plane. As mentioned above, valve deployment is initiated by rotating the delivery handle counterclockwise until the THV is fully expanded and locked and final valve release is accomplished by sliding the release ring and turning the release mechanism. The device can be completely resheathed during the procedure (Video 21.2), but should be replaced with a new device if a second full resheathing is performed.

21.1.3 Iterations

The manufacturer developed at least two improved generations of the Lotus Valve System, Lotus with Depth Guard™ and LOTUS Edge™ Valve Systems (Table 21.2). The latest version (LOTUS Edge™), while maintaining the advantages of an adaptive seal, a full repositionability, and an early function during deployment, has the advantages of a wider size range, a lower profile,

Table 21.2 Design features of the iterations of the Lotus valve[a]

Design feature	Lotus	Lotus with Depth Guard™	Lotus Edge™
Adaptive seal	+	+	+
Full repositionability	+	+	+
Early valve function	+	+	+
Sizes (mm)	23, 25, and 27	23, 25, and 27	21, 23, 25, 27, and 29
Sheath size	18/20 Fr	18/20 Fr	14/15 Fr
Delivery system	Pre-shaped	Pre-shaped	Flexible
Depth Guard[b]	−	+	+
One view locking[c]	−	−	+

[a]Lotus Mantra™ is a further upcoming generation of the Lotus valve planned to have a lower frame height and a lower delivery profile
[b]The Depth Guard™ mechanism aims at an early anchor during mechanical expansion of the valve frame leading to less initial axial elongation. The result is reduction of the depth that the frame reaches during deployment and the interaction with the left ventricular outflow tract and, eventually, a lower risk of conduction system injury
[c]Additional radio-opaque markers enable the operator to confirm locking in one view

and a more controlled deployment with less interaction with the left ventricular outflow tract (LVOT) and potentially the conduction system (Fig. 21.3).

21.1.4 Outcomes

Table 21.3 summarizes the concluded and the ongoing manufacturer-sponsored clinical trials of the Lotus Valve System and its subsequent iterations. The RESPOND study is a large all-comers registry that included a total of 1014 patients (age, 80.8 ± 6.5 years; 51% females; Society of Thoracic Surgeons (STS) predicted operative mortality risk, 6.0 ± 6.9%) [2]. The Lotus valve was successfully implanted in 98.2%. Repositioning of the valve was attempted in 29.2% of implantations and was successful in 99% of attempts. The 30-day rates of all-cause mortality and stroke were 2.6% and 3%, respectively. After transcatheter aortic valve implantation (TAVI), the mean aortic valve

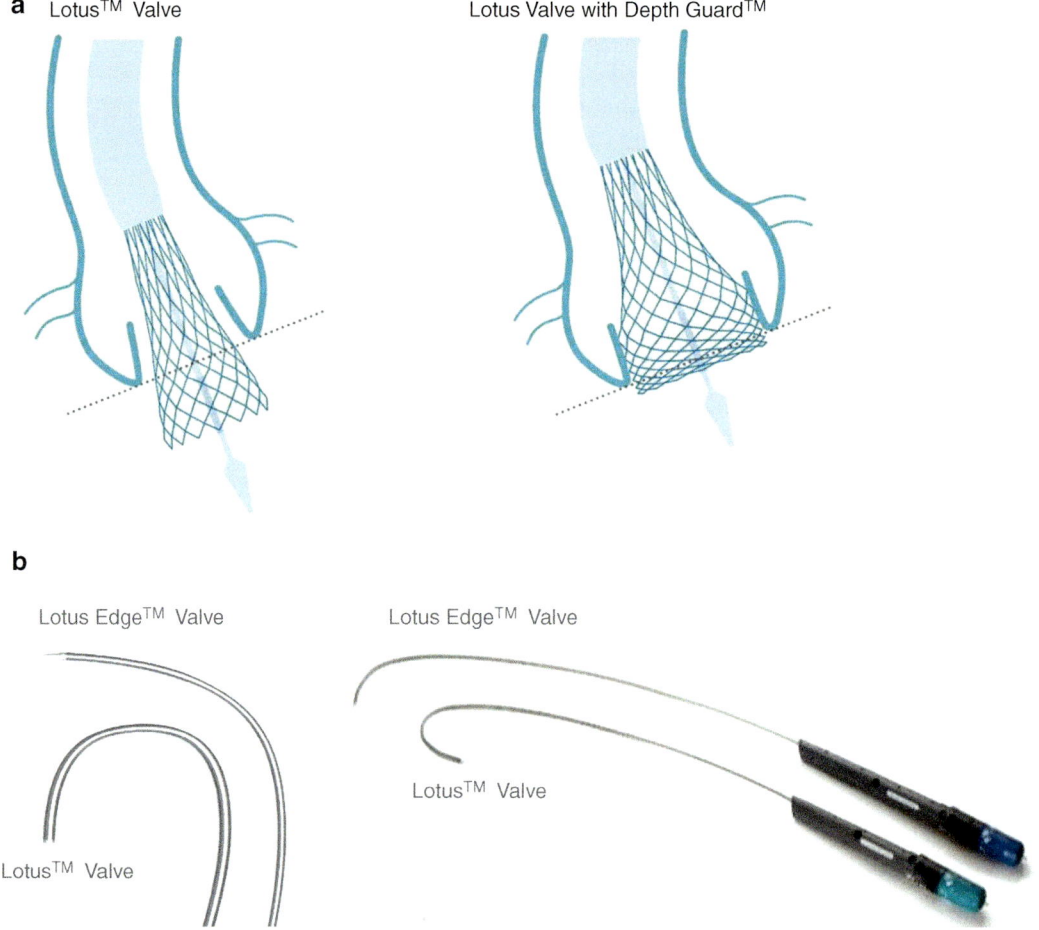

Fig. 21.3 Design features of the Lotus Edge™ Valve System. (**a**) The Lotus Edge™ Valve System is provided with the Depth Guard™ mechanism which minimizes the axial elongation of the valve frame during mechanical expansion and hence its interaction with the left ventricu-lar outflow tract and the risk of conduction system injury. (**b**) The delivery catheter of the Lotus Edge™ System is characterized by increased flexibility, a pre-shaped curve, and a reduced proximal catheter profile (3.0–4.0 Fr). *Image provided courtesy of Boston Scientific Corporation*

pressure gradient (PG) was 10.8 ± 4.6 mmHg, the effective orifice aortic valve area was 1.8 ± 0.4 cm², and paravalvular leakage (PVL) was absent or trace in 92% of patients, mild in 7.7%, and moderate in 0.3%. New permanent pacemaker was required in 34.6% of cases [3].

21.1.5 Relative Indications

The Lotus valve combines the advantages of a complete repositionability, an effective paravalvular sealing, and a low risk of annular injury. Therefore, it could be a practical option in cases with unfavorable landing zone anatomy (e.g., excessive/asymmetric calcification and/or borderline coronary ostial height) where the risks of annular injury, paravalvular leakage, and coronary obstruction are worrisome. Figure 21.4 represents two cases of "saber-toothed" LVOT calcification treated with either a balloon-expandable THV or the repositionable Lotus valve. The implantation of a balloon-expandable THV resulted in severe PVL (Videos 21.3a and 21.3b) that did not respond to balloon post-dilatation and required urgent

Table 21.3 Manufacturer-sponsored clinical trials involving the Lotus Valve System and its subsequent iterations

Study name (ClinicalTrials.gov Identifier)	Description	1ry endpoint	n	Device	Latest data
REPRISE I (NCT01383720)	Feasibility study Acute safety in high-risk patients Single arm	Device success (VARC) without MACCE	11	Lotus: 23 mm	5-year FUPTCT 2017
REPRISE II/II EXT (NCT01627691)	CE mark study and an extended cohort in high-risk patients Single arm	30 days mortality	250	Lotus: 23 and 27 mm	3-year FUPPCR London Valves 2017
REPRISE III (NCT02202434)	Pivotal study for FDA approval in high-risk and inoperable patients RCT; Lotus vs. CoreValve (52% CoreValve and 48% Evolut R)	30 days mortality, stroke, life-threatening/major bleed, AKI stage 2/3, or major vascular complications	912	Lotus: 23, 25, and 27 mm	1-year results PCR 2017
REPRISE III Continued Access (NCT02202434)	Continued access in high-risk and inoperable patients Single arm	30 days mortality, stroke, life-threatening/major bleed, AKI stage 2/3, or major vascular complications	250	Lotus Edge: 21, 23, 25, and 27 mm	Enrollment voluntarily suspended
REPRISE Japan (NCT02491255)	Safety for PMDA approval Safety and effectiveness in high-risk and inoperable patients	30 days mortality, stroke, life-threatening/major bleed, AKI stage 2/3, or major vascular complications + safety at 30 days, effectiveness at 6 months	50	Lotus: 23, 25, and 27 mm	6-month results CVIT 2017
RESPOND (NCT02031302)	Post-market study Safety and performance in all comers Single arm	Mortality at 30 days and 1 year	1014	Lotus: 23, 25, and 27 mm	1-year FUPPCR 2017
RESPOND Extension (NCT02031302)	Post-market study Safety and performance of Lotus with Depth Guard	Mortality at 30 days and 1 year	50	Lotus with Depth Guard: 23 and 25 mm	30-day results PCR 2017

Abbreviations: *AKI* acute kidney injury, *CE* Conformité Européenne, *FDA* food and drug administration, *FUP* follow-up, *MACCE* major adverse cardiovascular and cerebrovascular event, *PMDA* pharmaceuticals and medical devices agency, *RCT* randomized controlled trial, *VARC* valve academic research consortium

conversion to surgery. The second patient who received a Lotus valve developed a high-grade PVL on initial implantation attempt that was largely corrected upon repositioning (Videos 21.3c–21.3e).

21.1.6 Special Clinical Dilemmas

21.1.6.1 Pre-dilatation

Although the manufacturer recommends routine pre-dilatation before valve implantation, direct deployment without pre-dilatation seems to be safe and effective. In the RESPOND study, balloon pre-dilatation was not performed in 46% of implantations. The rate of any (≥trace) paravalvular leakage was 21.0% in patients who received pre-dilatation and 17.8% in those who did not receive pre-dilatation. Similar results were reported by Tarantini et al. in a small single-center experience [4]. In one study [5], balloon pre-dilatation before Lotus valve implantation was associated with increased risk of new left bundle branch block.

Fig. 21.4 Two patients with saber-toothed LVOT calcification. The short-axis cuts (upper panels) show two spots of LVOT calcification, and both are revealed in long-axis cuts (lower panels) as long pillars of calcium extending deep through the device landing zone. TAVI was performed with an Edwards Sapien XT valve in patient **a** and with a Lotus valve in patient **b**

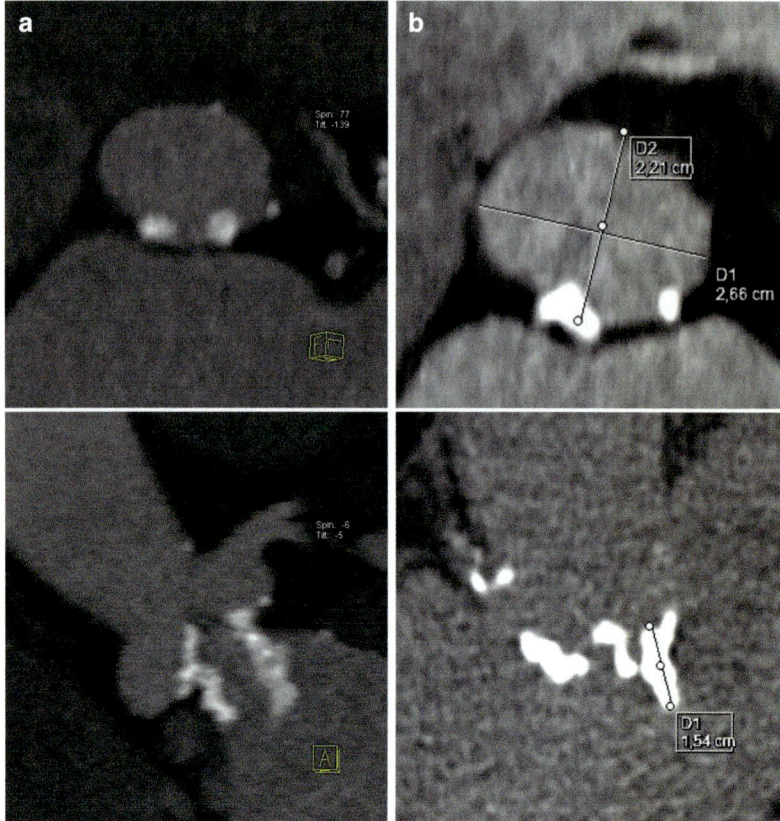

21.1.6.2 New Permanent Pacemaker

In the RESPOND trial, the rate of permanent pacemaker requirement in pacemaker-naïve patients was 34.6% at 30 days [2]. Predictors of new pacemaker implantation were the STS score, right bundle branch block at baseline, the implantation depth, and repositioning or retrieval attempt. In the REPRISE II Extension cohort, the rate of permanent pacemaker requirement in pacemaker-naïve patients was 32%. Multivariable predictors of pacemaker requirement were baseline right bundle branch block (odds ratio, 12.7), LVOT area oversizing $\geq 10\%$ (OR, 3.4), baseline first-degree atrioventricular block (OR, 2.5), and LVOT calcium volume (OR, $1.8/100$ mm^3 increment) [6]. In the UK Lotus valve registry [5, 7], the rates of new left bundle branch block and new pacemaker implantation were 55% and 31.8%, respectively. Pre-procedural conduction abnormality (atrioventricular block or bundle branch block) and

the absence of aortic valve calcification—but not implantation depth, valve oversizing, or balloon post-dilatation—were independently associated with the need for permanent pacemaker [5].

In the Nordic Lotus Registry [8], the overall pacemaker implantation rate was 27.9% but was as low as 12.8% in case of a combined implantation depth < 4 mm and a device/annulus ratio < 1.05. In another single-center experience, a systematic shallow implantation yielded a new pacemaker implantation rate of only 10% [9].

The modified Lotus valve iterations (with Depth Guard™ and Lotus Edge™) have a modified way of deployment, in which the inflow edge of the valve frame is anchored into the LVOT early during deployment (unlike the older version which allows deep protrusion into the LVOT before anchoring) minimizing the interaction with the LVOT and, potentially, the risk of conduction system injury (Fig. 21.3a).

21.1.6.3 Thrombosis and Hemodynamics

While TAVI with the Lotus Valve System is associated with exceedingly low rate of paravalvular leakage, it tends to yield a higher residual mean PG (12 ± 6 vs. 8 ± 4 mmHg, $p < 0.001$), a smaller effective orifice area (1.5 ± 0.5 vs. 1.7 ± 0.5 cm^2, $p < 0.001$), and a higher rate of leaflet thrombosis (1.5% vs. 0%, $p = 0.03$) at One year when compared with an approved self-expanding THV [10]. Other signals of a higher risk of bioprosthetic valve thrombosis after Lotus valve implantation come from rather small single-center series [11]. Further large-scale studies are required to assess the risks of thrombosis and unfavorable prosthetic valve hemodynamics after Lotus valve implantation.

21.1.6.4 Off-Label Use of the Lotus Valve

Lotus valve-in-valve implantation to treat degenerated surgical bioprosthesis has been shown to be safe and effective, with a residual gradient comparable to transcatheter valve-in-valve using other THV platforms [12–14]. There are also case reports of successful implantation of the Lotus valve in pure native aortic valve regurgitation [15, 16] and in bicuspid aortic valve stenosis [17, 18].

21.2 The ACURATE *neo*™ Transfemoral Valve System

21.2.1 System Description

21.2.1.1 Frame and Leaflet Composition and Design

The ACURATE *neo* valve (Symetis SA, a Boston Scientific company, Ecublens, Switzerland) consists of a self-expanding nitinol frame and BioFix™-treated non-coronary porcine leaflets that function at a supra-annular plane. The frame is made of a large cell stent (to which the leaflets are sewn) and three stabilizing arches for axial self-alignment (Fig. 21.5). At the lower and upper ends of the stent lie the lower and upper crowns. The former is 3 mm and the latter is

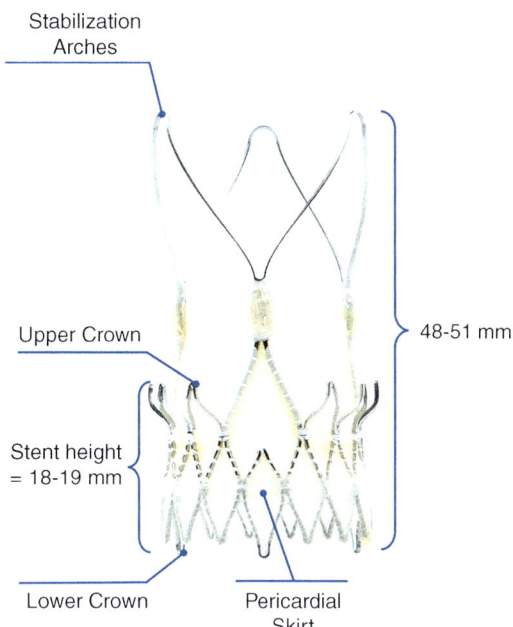

Fig. 21.5 The ACURATE *neo*™ transfemoral aortic valve. *Image provided courtesy of Boston Scientific Corporation*

5 mm larger than the waist of the valve frame. The upper crown contributes a supra-annular anchorage, holds the native leaflets away from coronary ostia, and allows for some tactile feedback during valve positioning. The frame has an outer and an inner porcine pericardial skirts covering and lining its landing portion (between the lower and upper crowns). The device is compatible with an 18 Fr sheath. The valve is available in three sizes (S, small; M, medium; and L, large) accommodating an annulus diameter of 21–27 mm (Table 21.4) and is CE marked since 2014 [19].

21.2.1.2 Delivery and Deployment

The ACURATE *neo* valve is deployed through rotation of a release knob in two steps, separated by an intermediate stop. Deployment is top-down (stabilizing arches and upper crown first). After the upper crown is released, it is gently pushed until it hooks onto the native annulus (Videos 21.4a and 21.4b). Routine balloon pre-dilatation is recommended by the manufacturer, and the valve is not repositionable after deployment.

Table 21.4 Dimensional data of the ACURATE *neo*™ transfemoral valve system

THV size	Aortic annulus diameter (mm)	Aortic annulus perimeter (mm)	Aortic annulus area (mm²)
S	≥21 to ≤23	66–72	346–415
M	≥23 to ≤25	72–79	415–491
L	≥ 25 to ≤27	79–85	491–573

21.2.2 Outcomes

The Symetis ACURATE *neo*™ Valve Implantation using TransFemoral access registry (SAVI-TF) is a European, multicenter, all-comers registry that included 1000 patients representing consecutive series at each of the participating centers (NCT02306226) [20]. One third of patients had severe aortic valve calcification, 96% received pre-dilatation, 49% were rapidly paced during valve deployment, 45% required post-dilatation, and 1% required valve-in-valve implantation. At discharge, effective orifice area was 1.77 ± 0.46 cm², mean PG was 8.4 ± 4.0 mmHg, and 4% of the patients had a significant PVL. The STS predicted risk of mortality was 6.0 ± 5.6, and the observed 30-day mortality rate was 1.4%. Disabling stroke occurred in 1.2%, a new permanent pacemaker implantation was required in 8.3%, and coronary obstruction was reported in one patient at 30 days. Although the registry was intended to be all-comers, the informed consent was prospectively collected in 58% of the study population and retrospectively collected in the rest (i.e., only patients who survived the procedure could be enrolled). The "all-comers" label can thus be disputed.

Although recommended by the manufacturer to be routinely performed, balloon pre-dilatation was shown in one study to be avoidable in a cohort of patients with mild-moderate aortic valve calcification, a relatively small annulus, and an adequate device oversizing (median [IQR], 8 [6–11]%). In this context, ACURATE neo valve could be implanted without pre-dilatation without increasing the risk of device failure [21].

Table 21.5 Relative advantages and disadvantages of the ACURATE *neo* valve

Advantages	Disadvantages
Easy controlled deployment	Requires 18 Fr delivery catheter
Anchorage is not completely dependent on radial force, enabling adequate anchor with little calcium (e.g., pure aortic regurgitation)	Difficult system assembly/loading
Supra-annular leaflet function; low residual pressure gradient and less prosthesis-patient mismatch than Sapien 3, especially in small annulus [22, 24]	No reliable radio-opaque implantation markers[a] Non-repositionable
Relatively low pacemaker rate [20, 25]; lower than Sapien 3 [24] and CoreValve [26]	More paravalvular leakage and balloon post-dilatation [20, 25] than Sapien 3 [22, 24]

[a]A new delivery system with radiopaque markers has been developed and is undergoing regulatory approval.

21.2.3 Relative Indications

The ACURATE *neo* valve with its supra-annular leaflets and generous oversizing is suitable in cases when prosthesis-patient mismatch is a concern (e.g., small annulus) [22]. As anchorage is secured by a combination of oversizing and the upper crown, the ACURATE *neo* valve can be an option in patients with pure native aortic valve regurgitation and little/no aortic valve calcification to help anchorage [23]. Although the upper crown can theoretically prevent coronary obstruction (by pushing the native leaflets) in patients with borderline coronary ostial height/relatively small sinus of Valsalva, this is so far not supported by clinical data [24]. Relative advantages and disadvantages of the ACURATE *neo* valve system are summarized in Table 21.5.

References

1. Gomes B, Katus HA, Bekeredjian R. Repositionable self-expanding aortic bioprosthesis. Expert Rev Med Devices. 2017;14(7):565–76.
2. Falk V, Wohrle J, Hildick-Smith D, Bleiziffer S, Blackman DJ, Abdel-Wahab M, et al. Safety and efficacy of a repositionable and fully retrievable aortic

valve used in routine clinical practice: the RESPOND study. Eur Heart J. 2017;38(45):3359–66.

3. Bagur R, Choudhury T, Mamas MA. Transcatheter aortic valve implantation with the repositionable and fully retrievable Lotus Valve System™. J Thorac Dis. 2017;9(9):2798–803.

4. Tarantini G, Nai Fovino L, Tellaroli P, Purita P, Masiero G, Napodano M, et al. TAVR with mechanically expandable prostheses: is balloon aortic valvuloplasty really necessary? Int J Cardiol. 2017;246:37–40.

5. Rampat R, Khawaja MZ, Hilling-Smith R, Byrne J, MacCarthy P, Blackman DJ, et al. Conduction abnormalities and permanent pacemaker implantation after transcatheter aortic valve replacement using the repositionable LOTUS device: the United Kingdom experience. JACC Cardiovasc Interv. 2017;10(12):1247–53.

6. Dumonteil N, Meredith IT, Blackman DJ, Tchetche D, Hildick-Smith D, Spence MS, et al. Insights into the need for permanent pacemaker following implantation of the repositionable LOTUS valve for transcatheter aortic valve replacement in 250 patients: results from the REPRISE II trial with extended cohort. EuroIntervention. 2017;13(7):796–803.

7. Rampat R, Khawaja MZ, Byrne J, MacCarthy P, Blackman DJ, Krishnamurthy A, et al. Transcatheter aortic valve replacement using the repositionable LOTUS valve: United Kingdom Experience. JACC Cardiovasc Interv. 2016;9(4):367–72.

8. De Backer O, Gotberg M, Ihlberg L, Packer E, Savontaus M, Nielsen NE, et al. Efficacy and safety of the Lotus Valve System for treatment of patients with severe aortic valve stenosis and intermediate surgical risk: results from the Nordic Lotus-TAVR registry. Int J Cardiol. 2016;219:92–7.

9. Krackhardt F, Kherad B, Krisper M, Pieske B, Laule M, Tschope C. Low permanent pacemaker rates following Lotus device implantation for transcatheter aortic valve replacement due to modified implantation protocol. Cardiol J. 2017;24(3):250–8.

10. Feldman TE, Reardon MJ, Rajagopal V, Makkar RR, Bajwa TK, Kleiman NS, et al. Effect of mechanically expanded vs. self-expanding transcatheter aortic valve replacement on mortality and major adverse clinical events in high-risk patients with aortic stenosis: the REPRISE III randomized clinical trial. JAMA. 2018;319(1):27–37.

11. Salido-Tahoces L, Hernandez-Antolin RA, Fernandez-Golfin C, Palomera-Rico A, Ayala-Carbonero A, Jimenez-Nacher JJ, et al. Three cases of early Lotus valve thrombosis. JACC Cardiovasc Interv. 2016;9(9):983–6.

12. Castriota F, Nerla R, Micari A, Cavazza C, Bedogni F, Testa L, et al. Transcatheter aortic valve-in-valve implantation using Lotus valve for failed surgical bioprostheses. Ann Thorac Surg. 2017;104(2):638–44.

13. Ruparelia N, Thomas K, Newton JD, Grebenik K, Keiralla A, Krasopoulos G, et al. Transfemoral transcatheter aortic valve-in-valve implantation for aortic valve bioprosthesis failure with the fully repositionable and retrievable Lotus valve: a single-center experience. J Invasive Cardiol. 2017;29(9):315–9.

14. Dvir D, Webb JG, Bleiziffer S, Pasic M, Waksman R, Kodali S, et al. Transcatheter aortic valve implantation in failed bioprosthetic surgical valves. JAMA. 2014;312(2):162–70.

15. Saraf S, Khawaja MZ, Hilling-Smith R, Dooley M, Cockburn J, Trivedi U, et al. Use of the Lotus transcatheter valve to treat severe native aortic regurgitation. Ann Thorac Surg. 2017;103(4):e305–e7.

16. Wohrle J, Rodewald C, Rottbauer W. Transfemoral aortic valve implantation in pure native aortic valve insufficiency using the repositionable and retrievable Lotus valve. Catheter Cardiovasc Interv. 2016;87(5):993–5.

17. Chan AW, Wong D, Charania J. Transcatheter aortic valve replacement in bicuspid aortic stenosis using Lotus Valve System. Catheter Cardiovasc Interv. 2017;90(1):157–63.

18. Seeger J, Gonska B, Rodewald C, Rottbauer W, Wohrle J. Bicuspid aortic stenosis treated with the repositionable and retrievable Lotus valve. Can J Cardiol. 2016;32(1):135 e17–9.

19. Kumar R, Latib A, Colombo A, Ruiz CE. Self-expanding prostheses for transcatheter aortic valve replacement. Prog Cardiovasc Dis. 2014;56(6):596–609.

20. Mollmann H, Hengstenberg C, Hilker M, Kerber S, Schafer U, Rudolph T, et al. Real-world experience using the ACURATE neo prosthesis: 30-day outcomes of 1,000 patients enrolled in the SAVI TF registry. EuroIntervention. 2018;13(15):e1764–e70.

21. Kim WK, Liebetrau C, Renker M, Rolf A, Van Linden A, Arsalan M, et al. Transfemoral aortic valve implantation using a self-expanding transcatheter heart valve without pre-dilation. Int J Cardiol. 2017;243:156–60.

22. Mauri V, Kim WK, Abumayyaleh M, Walther T, Moellmann H, Schaefer U, et al. Short-term outcome and hemodynamic performance of next-generation self-expanding versus balloon-expandable transcatheter aortic valves in patients with small aortic annulus: a multicenter propensity-matched comparison. Circ Cardiovasc Interv. 2017;10(10)

23. Toggweiler S, Biaggi P, Grunenfelder J, Reho I, Buhler I, Corti R. First-in-man transfemoral transcatheter aortic valve implantation with the ACURATE neo for the treatment of aortic regurgitation. EuroIntervention. 2016;12(1):78.

24. Husser O, Kim WK, Pellegrini C, Holzamer A, Walther T, Mayr PN, et al. Multicenter comparison of novel self-expanding versus balloon-expandable transcatheter heart valves. JACC Cardiovasc Interv. 2017;10(20):2078–87.

25. Toggweiler S, Nissen H, Mogensen B, Cuculi F, Fallesen C, Veien KT, et al. Very low pacemaker rate following ACURATE neo transcatheter heart valve implantation. EuroIntervention. 2017;13(11):1273–80.

26. Jatene T, Castro-Filho A, Meneguz-Moreno RA, Siqueira DA, Abizaid AAC, Ramos AIO, et al. Prospective comparison between three TAVR devices: ACURATE neo vs. CoreValve vs. SAPIEN XT. A single heart team experience in patients with severe aortic stenosis. Catheter Cardiovasc Interv. 2017;90(1):139–46.

Edwards Program for Transcatheter Aortic Valve Implantation

22

Grant W. Reed, Rachel Easterwood, and Samir R. Kapadia

22.1 Introduction

Implantation of a prosthetic aortic valve via the transcatheter approach was first performed in a living human in 2002 by Dr. Alain G. Cribier [1, 2]. This early clinical experience was the catalyst for continued innovation in transcatheter aortic valve technologies, culminating in several landmark clinical trials. This eventually led to approval of transcatheter aortic valve implantation (TAVI), also called transcatheter aortic valve replacement (TAVR), for patients with symptomatic severe aortic stenosis with prohibitive or high surgical risk profiles, and TAVR eventually met the international cardiovascular scene in 2010 [3, 4]. Continued success in major clinical trials led to the expeditious implementation of TAVR across an ever-expanding population of patients [5–12]. Concurrently, increasing operator experience and improvements in device design have extended the application of TAVR to lower risk and more technically challenging subsets of patients [13].

Many different transcatheter heart valve systems have been developed and refined since the initial introduction of the TAVR technique. Most of the various heart valve systems can be categorized into either balloon-expandable or self-expandable valve systems. Both the balloon-expandable and the self-expandable valve systems have revealed their own particular sets of benefits and challenges [2–13].

The only balloon-expandable TAVR systems available in the United States today are produced by Edwards Lifesciences (Irvine, CA). The efficacy and safety of the Edwards family of transcatheter aortic valves have been extensively evaluated in many of the major randomized controlled trials for TAVR, named the Placement of AoRtic TraNscathetER Valves (PARTNER) clinical trials. Many important lessons were learned from the PARTNER trials using the SAPIEN valves [14–16]. The very first conception of transcatheter aortic valve implantation was with balloon-expandable systems. Edwards built upon this concept, and over the years, there has been significant evolution of the Edwards family of balloon-expandable transcatheter heart valves, advancing across the SAPIEN, SAPIEN XT, and SAPIEN 3 systems (Fig. 22.1).

G. W. Reed · R. Easterwood · S. R. Kapadia (✉)
Department of Cardiovascular Medicine, Heart and Vascular Institute, Cleveland Clinic, Cleveland, OH, USA
e-mail: EASTERR@ccf.org; REEDG2@ccf.org; kapadis@ccf.org

© Springer Nature Switzerland AG 2019
A. Giordano et al. (eds.), *Transcatheter Aortic Valve Implantation*,
https://doi.org/10.1007/978-3-030-05912-5_22

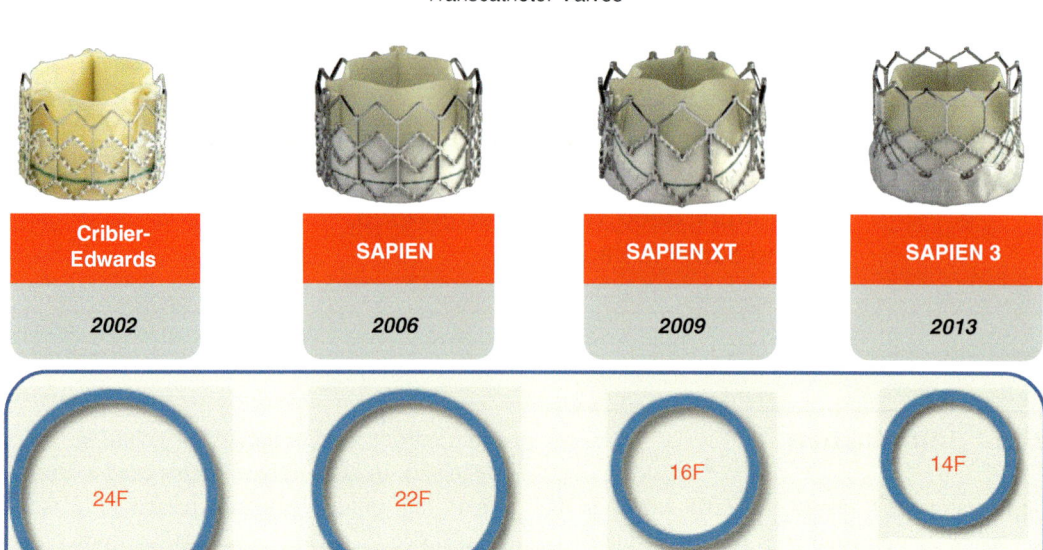

Evolution of the Edwards Balloon-Expandable Transcatheter Valves

Cribier-Edwards	SAPIEN	SAPIEN XT	SAPIEN 3
2002	2006	2009	2013
24F	22F	16F	14F

Kodali, S. Clinical and Echocardiographic Outcomes at 30 Days with the SAPIEN S3 Valve System in Inoperable, High-Risk, and Intermediate-Risk AS Patients, ACC 2015, San Diego.

Fig. 22.1 Evolution of Edwards transcatheter valves

22.2 SAPIEN Transcatheter Heart Valve System

22.2.1 History of Balloon-Expandable Transcatheter Aortic Valves

The first catheter-based balloon aortic valvuloplasty (BAV) was performed in a human by Cribier in 1985. It was observed that the main limitation of BAV was restenosis of the aortic valve within 6–12 months, an issue that remains prevalent after BAV today [17]. In 1989, Dr. Henning Rud Andersen sought to solve this issue and developed a bioprosthetic porcine valve sutured onto a stainless steel frame made from surgical wiring. The valve was subsequently compressed onto a balloon catheter. Using various deployments in pig cardiac models, the feasibility of TAVR using a balloon-expandable system was shown [18, 19].

In 1999, after several attempts to provoke commercial interest, Alain Cribier, Martin Leon, Stanley Rabinovich, and Stanton Rowe created a start-up company named Percutaneous Valve Technologies (PVT). The mission of PVT was to develop a balloon-expandable valve system to treat human stenotic aortic valves under the supposition that the bioprosthetic valve could be successfully expanded and stabilized inside of the stenotic valve. Similar to the initial versions, the PVT valve system consisted of a balloon-expandable stainless steel stent frame with equine pericardial leaflets fashioned onto a balloon catheter. In 2002, the first-in-human transcatheter aortic valve was deployed via a transseptal approach by Cribier in a 57-year-old male with inoperable, critical calcific aortic stenosis and was considered a major advance for the field of TAVR [1, 2].

In 2004, PVT was acquired by Edwards Lifesciences, leading to a rapid, continued acceleration in the evolution of transcatheter heart valve therapies. The initial PVT valve evolved into the Edwards SAPIEN transcatheter heart valve. The SAPIEN valve used the equine pericardial leaflet design of the Carpentier-Edwards PERIMOUNT surgical bioprosthetic valve but mounted the valve onto a balloon-expandable stainless steel stent frame. To prevent paravalvular leak, a polyethylene terephthalate (PET) fabric skirt was added at the inferior margin of the valve to improve seal around the aortic annulus. The SAPIEN transcatheter heart valve was available in 23- and 26-mm sizes for trans-femoral access and required 22- or 24-Fr sheaths for delivery, respectively (Fig. 22.1).

The SAPIEN transcatheter heart valve received CE Mark approval in 2007. Based on the PARTNER trials, the US Food and Drug Administration (FDA) approved SAPIEN transcatheter heart valve for use in patients that were deemed prohibitive-risk surgical aortic valve replacement candidates in 2011 and for patients that were considered high-risk surgical aortic valve replacement candidates in 2012. Tables 22.1 and 22.2 provide summaries of the design and pivotal results of each of the PARTNER trials.

22.2.2 PARTNER I (Cohort B)

The initial results of the PARTNER trial, Cohort B (PARTNER IB), were published in the *New England Journal of Medicine* (NEJM) in 2010. This randomized trial is unique in cardiovascular medicine, as it inverted the traditional paradigm of drug and device development, where traditional therapeutics are typically studied in healthier populations first. Instead, PARTNER B was a prospective, randomized trial designed to study patients with severe, symptomatic aortic stenosis considered poor (or "inoperable") surgical candidates (Fig. 22.2). Key inclusion criteria included a Society of Thoracic Surgeons [STS] Predicted Risk of Mortality within 30 days [PROM] ≥10%, co-existing conditions with ≥15% death, or a ≥50% risk of death or a serious irreversible complication within 30 days. Included patients were randomized 1:1 to either TAVR using the balloon-expandable SAPIEN valve system vs. medical therapy, which included BAV as a means of symptomatic relief. The study included 358 patients total, with 179 TAVR patients and 179 medical therapy patients. The trial had a superiority design with co-primary endpoints of all-cause mortality and the composite endpoint of all-cause mortality or repeat hospitalization for valve or procedure-related deterioration at 1 year [3].

PARTNER IB met its co-primary endpoint, as TAVR dramatically lowered all-cause mortality compared with medical therapy at 1 year (30.7% vs. 49.7%, hazard ratio [HR] 0.55, 95% confidence interval [CI] 0.40–0.74; $p < 0.001$; a 20% absolute survival advantage, NNT 5). Patients treated with TAVR also had lower rates of all-cause mortality or

Table 22.1 Major TAVR trial characteristics

Trial	Year	Design	Population	Groups	TAVR valve(s) used	Primary outcome(s)	Mean STS (%)[a]
PARTNER IB	2010	RCT	Inoperable	TAVR vs. OMT	SAPIEN	Death from any cause at 1 year	11.6
PARTNER IA	2011	RCT	High risk	TAVR vs. SAVR	SAPIEN	Death from any cause at 1 year	11.8 vs. 11.7
PARTNER IIA	2016	RCT	Intermediate risk	TAVR vs. SAVR	SAPIEN XT	Death from any cause or major stroke at 2 years	5.8 vs. 5.8
PARTNER II-S3i[b]	2016	Propensity score-adjusted analysis	Intermediate risk	TAVR vs. SAVR	SAPIEN 3	Death from any cause, stroke, or ≥ moderate PVL at 1 year	5.2 vs. 5.4

Abbreviations: *TAVR* transcatheter aortic valve replacement, *RCT* randomized controlled trial, *OMT* optimal medical therapy, *SAVR* surgical aortic valve replacement, *PVL* paravalvular leak
[a]TAVR vs. control
[b]PARTNER II-S3i was a non-randomized study that compared outcomes for the S3 valve to the surgical control group of PARTNER II in a propensity score-adjusted analysis

Table 22.2 Outcomes of randomized trials

Trial	Follow-up	All-cause mortality (%)	Cardiac mortality (%)	Major stroke (%)	Major bleeding (%)	Major vascular (%)	Atrial fibrillation (%)	PPM[a] (%)	PVL[b] (%)
PARTNER IB[c]	30 days	5.0 vs. 2.8 (p = 0.41)	4.5 vs. 1.7 (p = 0.22)	5.0 vs. 1.1 (p = 0.06)	16.8 vs. 3.9 (p < 0.001)	16.2 vs. 1.1 (p < 0.001)	0.6 vs. 1.1 (p = 1.00)	3.4 vs. 5.0 (p = 0.60)	12 vs. 0 (p < 0.001)
	1 year	30.7 vs. 49.7 (p < 0.001)	19.6 vs. 41.9 (p < 0.001)	7.8 vs. 3.9 (p = 0.18)	22.3 vs. 11.2 (p = 0.007)	16.8 vs. 2.2 (p < 0.001)	0.6 vs. 1.7 (p = 0.62)	4.5 vs. 7.8 (p = 0.27)	11 vs. 0 (p < 0.001)
PARTNER IA	30 days	3.4 vs. 6.5 (p = 0.07)	3.2 vs. 3.0 (p = 0.90)	3.8 vs. 2.1 (p = 0.20)	9.3 vs. 19.5 (p < 0.001)	17.0 vs. 3.8 (p < 0.001)	8.6 vs. 16.0 (p = 0.006)	3.8 vs. 3.6 (p = 0.89)	12.2 vs. 0.9 (p < 0.001)
	1 year	24.2 vs. 26.8 (p = 0.44)	14.3 vs. 13.0 (p = 0.63)	5.1 vs. 2.4 (p = 0.07)	14.7 vs. 25.7 (p < 0.001)	18.0 vs. 4.8 (p < 0.001)	12.1 vs. 17.1 (p = 0.07)	5.7 vs. 5.0 (p = 0.68)	6.8 vs. 1.9 (p < 0.001)
PARTNER IIA	30 days	3.9 vs. 4.1 (p = 0.78)	3.3 vs. 3.2 (p = 0.92)	3.2 vs. 4.3 (p = 0.20)	10.4 vs. 43.4 (p < 0.001)	7.9 vs. 5.0 (p = 0.008)	9.1 vs. 26.4 (p < 0.001)	8.5 vs. 6.9 (p = 0.17)	3.7 vs. 0.53 (p < 0.001)
	1 year	12.3 vs. 12.9 (p = 0.69)	7.1 vs. 8.1 (p = 0.40)	5.0 vs. 5.8 (p = 0.46)	15.2 vs. 45.5 (p < 0.001)	8.4 vs. 5.3 (p = 0.007)	10.1 vs. 27.2 (p < 0.001)	9.9 vs. 8.9 (p = 0.43)	3.4 vs. 0.33 (p < 0.001)
	2 years	16.7 vs. 18.0 (p = 0.45)	10.1 vs. 11.3 (p = 0.38)	6.2 vs. 6.4 (p = 0.83)	17.3 vs. 47.0 (p < 0.001)	8.6 vs. 5.5 (p = 0.006)	11.3 vs. 27.3 (p < 0.001)	11.8 vs. 10.3 (p = 0.29)	8.0 vs. 0.6 (p < 0.001)

[a]*PPM* permanent pacemaker (PPM) placement required

[b]At least moderate paravalvular leak

[c]All results reported as intention to treat outcomes for TAVR vs. SAVR except PARTNER IB, which was TAVR vs. medical therapy in patients at extreme surgical risk

PARTNER I: Study Design

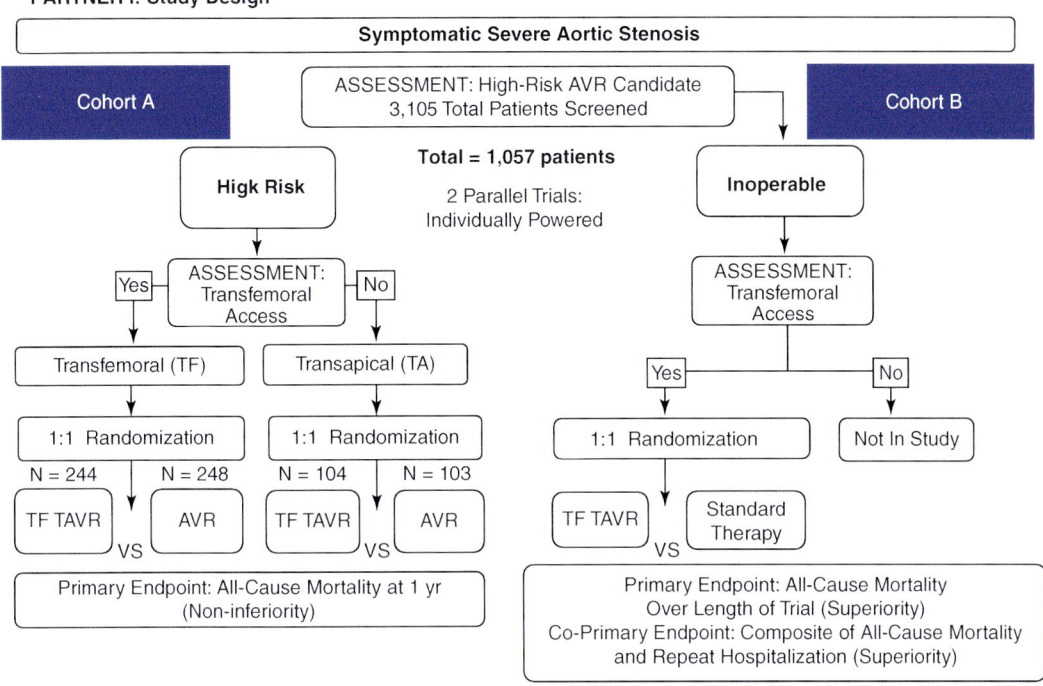

Fig. 22.2 PARTNER IA and PARTNER IB

repeat hospitalization at 1 year (42.5% vs. 70.4%, HR 0.46, 95% CI 0.35–0.59; $p < 0.001$, NNT 4) [3]. In addition, among patients surviving at 1 year, the rate of New York Heart Association (NYHA) class III or IV heart failure symptoms was less frequent in patients treated with TAVR compared to medical therapy (25.2% vs. 58.0%, $p < 0.001$). The results of PARTNER IB were the impetus for FDA approval of the SAPIEN valve system in inoperable patients in 2011.

The long-term 5-year results of PARTNER IB reflect that while there was a persistent reduction in death with TAVR, mortality rates among patients with inoperable AS are high (71.8% with TAVR vs. 93.6% with standard therapy; HR 0.50, 95% CI 0.39–0.65; $p < 0.0001$); only one patient in the medical management group was alive at 5 years. Echocardiography after TAVR showed durable hemodynamic results (aortic valve area [AVA] 1.52 cm^2 and mean gradient 10.6 mmHg at 5 years), with no evidence of structural valve deterioration [20].

Despite the mortality and symptom advantage of TAVR, the main results from PARTNER IB indicate that at 30 days TAVR associated with an increased rate of major stroke compared to medical therapy (5.0% vs. 1.1%, $p = 0.06$), a finding that reached statistical significance when including major stroke, minor stroke, and transient ischemic attack (TIA) (6.7% vs. 1.7%, $p = 0.03$). Major bleeding (16.8% vs. 3.9%, $p < 0.001$) and major vascular complications (16.2% vs. 1.1%) at 30 days were also increased with TAVR [3]. Similar results were seen for stroke, major bleeding, and major vascular complications at 1 year. It is important to note that the incidence of bleeding and vascular complications in PARTNER I reflect the SAPIEN transcatheter aortic valve devices that required 22- and 24-French sheaths and the earliest operator experiences with TAVR. Since PARTNER I, technology has improved, and sheath size has been reduced with iteration of the SAPIEN XT and S3 valves. Increased operator experience has further led to refinement in procedural techniques to mitigate vascular complications. As a result, access complications have fallen over the years, as described in the following sections.

A cost-effectiveness analysis of PARTNER IB demonstrated that among patients not candidates for surgery, TAVR increases life expectancy at an incremental cost per life year gained of $50,200, within well-accepted values for commonly used cardiovascular treatments and other non-cardiac therapies [21].

22.2.3 PARTNER I (Cohort A)

On the heels of the PARTNER IB, the results of the PARTNER I Cohort A (PARTNER IA) trial were published in the *New England Journal of Medicine* (NEJM) in 2011. PARTNER IA was a randomized controlled trial of patients with severe, symptomatic aortic stenosis classified as high-risk surgical candidates, with key inclusion criteria including a STS PROM score $\geq 10\%$ or co-existing conditions with a $\geq 15\%$ 30-day post-op risk of death (Fig. 22.2). Patients were randomized 1:1 to either TAVR using the SAPIEN valve vs. surgical AVR. Transcatheter aortic valve replacement patients were also stratified by access approach (transfemoral vs. transapical). The trial randomized 699 patients, with 348 assigned to TAVR and 351 to surgical AVR. The trial used a non-inferiority design, and the primary endpoint was all-cause mortality at 1 year [4].

The PARTNER IA trial demonstrated that TAVR was non-inferior to surgical AVR in high-risk surgical patients for mortality at 30 days (3.4% vs. 6.5%; $P = 0.07$) and 1 year (24.2% vs. 26.8%; $P = 0.44$ for superiority, $P = 0.001$ for non-inferiority). However, there was a trend toward increased major stroke with TAVR compared to surgical AVR at 30 days (3.8% vs. 2.1%; $p = 0.20$) and 1 year (5.1% vs. 2.4%; $p = 0.07$). Major vascular complications were higher with TAVR compared to surgical AVR (11.0% vs. 3.2%; $p < 0.001$), but major bleeding was lower with TAVR (9.3% vs. 19.5%; $p < 0.001$) due to blood loss during surgery. The need for permanent pacemaker implantation was equivalent between groups [4]. Of note, TAVR patients had a 2-day shorter intensive care unit stay and a 4-day shorter overall hospital length of stay. More patients in the TAVR group had improvement of their symptoms to NYHA class II or lower as compared to surgical AVR at 30 days;

but among subjects assessable at 1 year, this was equivalent [4].

Long-term follow-up from PARTNER IA demonstrates a durable mortality benefit for TAVR, similar to SAVR at 2 years (33.9% vs. 35.0%; $p = 0.78$) and 5 years (67.8% vs. 62.4%; $p = 0.76$). As in the 1-year results, there was a trend toward increased stroke or TIA with TAVR vs. surgical AVR at 2 years (11.2% vs. 6.5%; $p = 0.05$) [22], a hazard which peaked within 1 week of TAVR and declined to a constant late hazard out to 2 years related to patient comorbidities rather than randomization to TAVR or surgical AVR [23]. Consistent with this finding, there was no difference in stroke rates between TAVR and SAVR at 5 years [16].

Other valuable lessons were learned with long-term follow-up from PARTNER IA. Importantly, moderate or severe aortic paravalvular regurgitation was observed to be higher with TAVR vs. surgical AVR at 30 days (12.2% vs. 0.9%), 1 year (6.8% vs. 1.9%), 2 years (6.9% vs. 0.9%), and 5 years (14.0% vs. 1.0%) ($p < 0.001$ for all comparisons) [4, 16, 22]. The presence of moderate or severe aortic regurgitation was associated with an increased rate of late deaths at 2-year and 5-year follow-up; however there was an increased risk of late death seen with even mild aortic regurgitation, emphasizing the importance of optimizing procedural outcomes. In addition, while 1-year results from PARTNER suggested similar mortality rates between transfemoral and transapical approaches, it was underpowered for this assessment [4]. A larger analysis of both PARTNER IA and IB patients adjusted for patient differences using propensity score matching found that compared to the transfemoral approach, transapical access was associated with higher mortality at 6 months (19% vs. 12%; $p = 0.01$), more adverse procedural events, longer length of stay, and slower recovery. In addition, TAVR was found to have equivalent hemodynamic parameters (mean gradient, AVA) to surgical AVR at every point in follow-up out to 5 years with no signal of valve deterioration [4, 16, 22, 24, 25].

Similar to with PARTNER IB, a cost-effectiveness analysis of PARTNER IA revealed that among patients at high surgical risk, 12-month costs and quality-adjusted life years were similar for TAVR and surgical AVR. However, patients treated with transfemoral access had lower costs than surgery, making TAVR an economically attractive alternative to surgical AVR if transfemoral access is possible [26]. Avoidance of complications was demonstrated to be paramount for the cost-effectiveness of TAVR, as a pooled analysis of PARTNER IB and PARTNER IA demonstrated that approximately 25% of non-implant-related costs were attributed to complications from the procedure [27].

22.3 SAPIEN XT Transcatheter Heart Valve System

The Edwards SAPIEN XT transcatheter heart valve system was a modified and improved version of the SAPIEN valve. The SAPIEN XT was a balloon-expandable system with a cobalt chromium stent frame and trileaflet bovine valve tissue, with the addition of a fabric skirt

on the ventricular side to minimize paravalvular leak. The valve system's improved design and its ability to mount the valve on the deployment balloon inside the abdominal aorta allowed for a smaller delivery sheath. Additionally, a larger 29-mm valve was introduced so that in total three valve sizes were available (23, 26, and 29 mm), allowing for patients with annulus sizes ranging from 18 to 27 mm average diameter. The SAPIEN XT transcatheter heart valve system received CE Mark approval in Europe in 2010 and FDA approval in the United States in 2014 based on the results of the PARTNER II trials, discussed herein (Figs. 22.2, 22.3, and 22.4).

22.3.1 Partner IIA

The results of PARTNER IIA were published in the *New England Journal of Medicine* (NEJM) in 2016. PARTNER IIA was a randomized controlled trial of patients with severe, symptomatic aortic stenosis at intermediate surgical risk—not

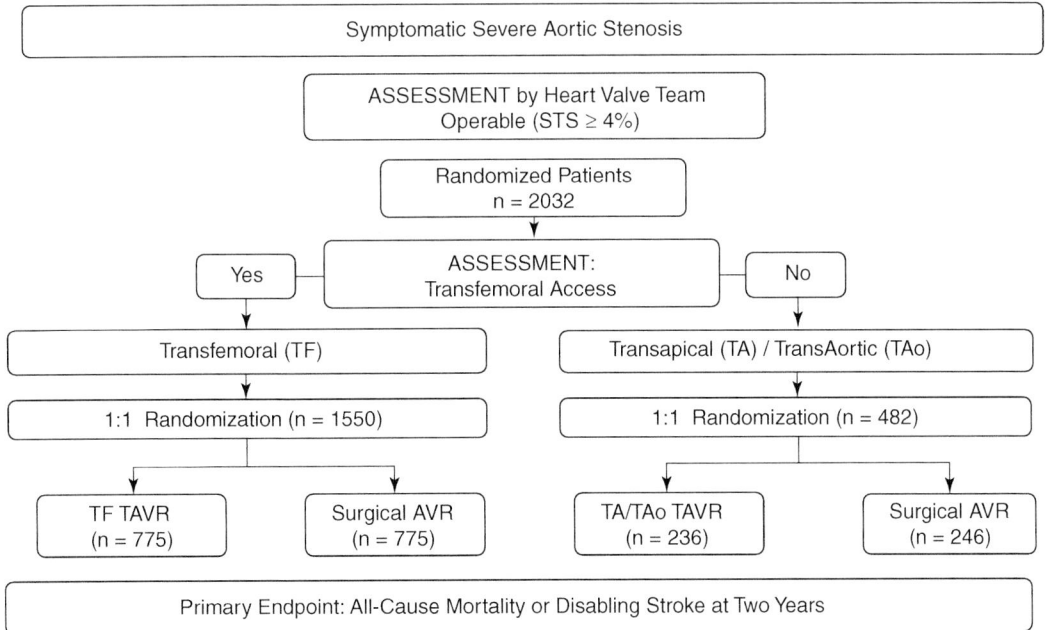

Smith, CR. Transcatheter or Surgical Aortic Valve Replacement in Intermediate Risk Patients with Aortic Stenosis: Final Results from the PARTNER 2A Trial. ACC 2016. Chicago.

Fig. 22.3 PARTNER IIA study design

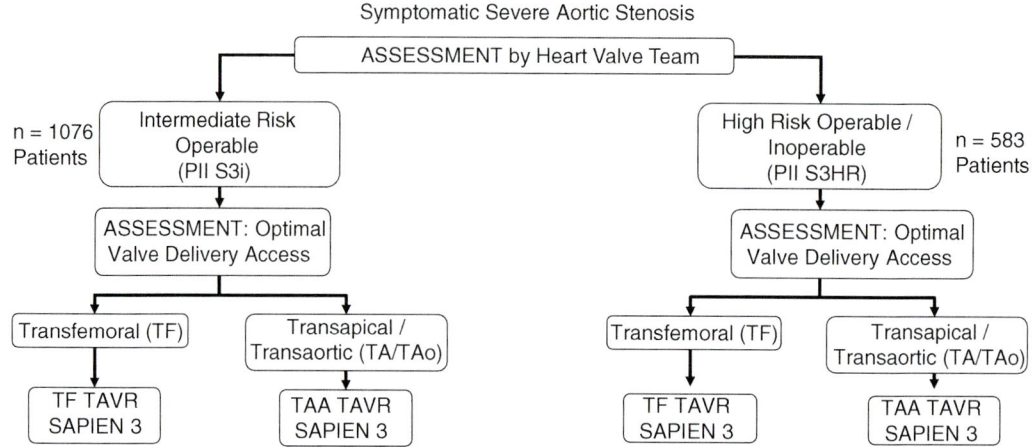

Kodali, S. Clinical and Echocardiographic Outcomes at 30 Days with the SAPIEN S3 Valve System in Inoperable, High-Risk and Intermediate -Risk AS Patients, ACC 2015, San Diego.

Fig. 22.4 PARTNER II S3 study design

inoperable or high-risk surgical candidates as included in PARTNER I (Fig. 22.3). Key inclusion criteria were an STS PROM score ≥4% or a <4% with a heart team determination of intermediate surgical risk based on characteristics not represented in the STS score. Patients were randomized 1:1 to TAVR using the SAPIEN XT valve system vs. surgical AVR. Transcatheter aortic valve replacement patients were further stratified into transfemoral access vs. transthoracic (transapical or transaortic) access based on pre-procedural evaluation. The trial included a total of 2032 patients, with 1011 patients randomized to TAVR and 1021 to surgical AVR. A non-inferiority design was used with a primary composite endpoint of all-cause mortality or disabling stroke at 2 years [7].

The PARTNER IIA trial succeeded in establishing TAVR with the SAPIEN XT valve as an alternative to surgical AVR in patients at intermediate surgical risk. At 2 years, the primary composite endpoint occurred in 19.3% with TAVR vs. 21.1% with surgical AVR ($p = 0.33$), meeting pre-specified non-inferiority criteria. That said, in a pre-specified analysis separating patients by access route, in patients in the transfemoral access cohort, TAVR resulted in a lower rate of death or disabling stroke than surgery (HR 0.79,

95% CI 0.62–1.00; $p = 0.05$), while in the transapical or transthoracic cohort, there was no difference. Reassuringly, there was no difference in disabling stroke or new pacemaker implantation between TAVR and surgical AVR at (6.2% vs. 6.4%; $p = 0.83$ and 11.8% vs. 10.3%; $p = 0.29$, respectively). Further, TAVR was associated with less major bleeding (17.3% vs. 47.0%; $p < 0.001$), less acute kidney injury (3.8% vs. 6.2%; $p = 0.02$), and less incident atrial fibrillation (11.3% vs. 27.3%; $p < 0.001$) at 2 years [7]. PARTNER 2A resulted in FDA approval of SAPIEN XT for use as an alternative to surgical aortic valve replacement in intermediate-risk patients.

22.4   SAPIEN 3 Transcatheter Heart Valve System

The SAPIEN 3 valve design was built upon the prior SAPIEN XT and was engineered to minimize aortic insufficiency and to further reduce the diameter of the delivery system. It is also constructed with a cobalt chromium frame, with the addition of a polyethylene terephthalate (PET) fabric cuff and an internal skirt on the ventricular side to reduce paravalvular leak. The crimped profile is smaller, and the stent frame is longer to prevent native leaflet prolapse and allow for better positioning during deployment. The SAPIEN 3 valve comes in four sizes (20-, 23-, 26-, and 29-mm); the 20-, 23-, and 26-mm valves are capable of delivery by a 14-French sheath, although the 29 mm requires a 16-French sheath (Fig. 22.1).

22.4.1 SAPIEN 3 Registry in Patients Inoperable and at High Surgical Risk

The initial experience with the SAPIEN 3 valve was in a large adjudicated registry of 583 patients to evaluate if there was an improvement in outcomes in high-risk or inoperable patients (average STS PROM 8.6%) compared to the results of the PARTNER I trial – known as the PII S3HR study (Fig. 22.4). In this registry, all-cause mortality and disabling stroke were 2.2% and 0.9% at 30 days, respectively. All-cause mortality was 17.7% for inoperable patients and 12.7% for high-risk patients. Among transfemoral patients, mortality was even lower at 12.3% for inoperable patients and 6.7% for high-risk patients. There was no severe aortic PVL, moderate aortic PVL was present in only 2.7% of patients, and there were significant improvements in NYHA classification and quality of life. Compared to the results of PARTNER IB and PARTNER IA, results of the SAPIEN 3 inoperable and high-risk registry demonstrate continued improvement in TAVR outcomes with experience and use of the third-generation SAPIEN 3 valve [28].

22.4.2 PARTNER II S3i

Building on the results of the inoperable and high-risk study, PARTNER II S3i was a prespecified, prospective study of 1077 patients with severe, symptomatic AS at intermediate surgical risk treated with the SAPIEN 3 valve (Fig. 22.4). Unlike the earlier PARTNER trials, the PARTNER II S3i study compared utilized the

controls from the PARTNER IIA trial, propensity score matched to eliminate differences in patient characteristics. At 30 days, all-cause mortality and disabling stroke were 1.1% and 1.0%, respectively. At 1-year follow-up, 7.4% of patients died (6.5% in the transfemoral group), disabling stroke occurred in 2% of patients, and moderate or severe aortic PVL in 2% of patients [8]. In the propensity score analysis, 963 patients treated with SAPIEN 3 were compared to 747 patients with surgical AVR. For the primary endpoint of composite all-cause mortality, disabling or minor stroke, and moderate or severe aortic PVL, TAVR was both non-inferior ($p < 0.0001$) and superior ($p < 0.0001$) to surgical AVR. In further superiority analysis, both all-cause mortality and stroke were lower with the SAPIEN 3 valve, although the incidence of paravalvular leak remained higher with TAVR compared to surgery. The results of this trial resulted in FDA approval of the SAPIEN 3 valve system as an alternative to surgical aortic valve replacement for intermediate-risk patients [8].

Data on the cost-effectiveness based on PARTNER 2A and S3i data have yet to be published but were presented at the Transcatheter Therapeutics (TCT) conference in 2017 and suggest that in intermediate-risk patients, TAVR with either the SAPIEN XT or SAPIEN 3 valve may lead to long-term cost-savings compared to surgical AVR. Results from PARTNER II indicate that among intermediate-risk patients, both TAVR and SAVR lead to significant improvements in health status and QOL. Patients treated with TAVR have greater gains in QOL at 1 month; however this was driven by patients treated with transfemoral access; patients with alternative access had no difference compared to surgery. In addition, QOL appeared to equalize between TAVR and surgery by 2 years [29].

The main results from the PARTNER randomized controlled trials are summarized in Table 22.2. A graphical depiction of the improvement in 30-day outcomes over the course of the PARTNER trials in as-treated patients is shown in Figs. 22.5, 22.6, 22.7, and 22.8. Figure 22.5 shows the improvements in all-cause

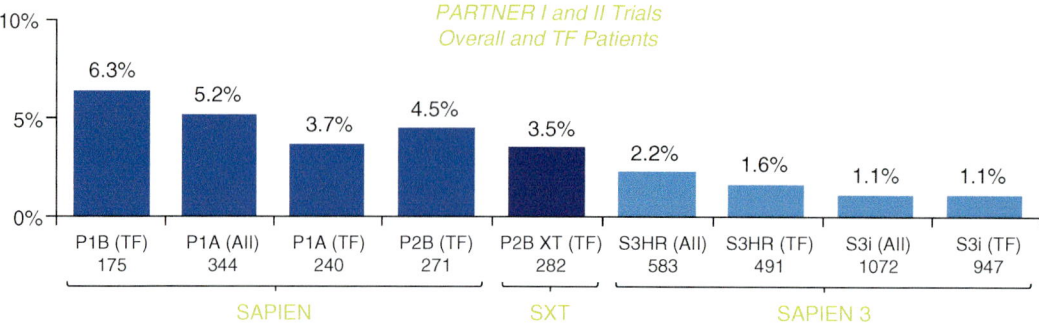

Fig. 22.5 Trend in all-cause mortality at 30 days in PARTNER trials (all patients and transfemoral patients)

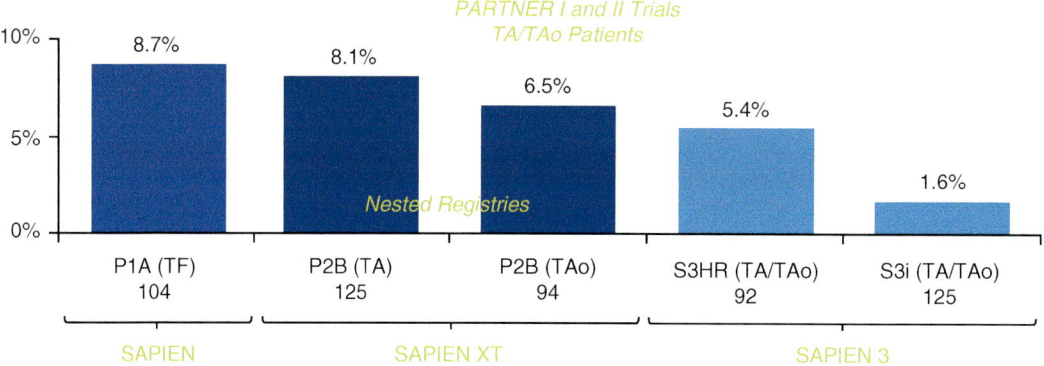

Fig. 22.6 Trend in all-cause mortality at 30 days in PARTNER trials (alternative access patients)

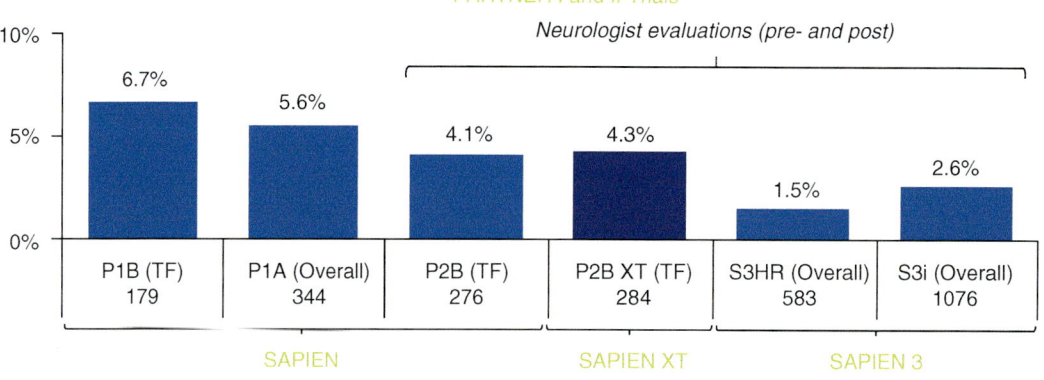

Fig. 22.7 Trend in strokes at 30 days in PARTNER trials

mortality among all access routes and transfemoral cases, while Fig. 22.6 depicts outcomes for alternative access cases via transapical and transaortic routes. Figure 22.7 shows trends for improvement in stroke, and Fig. 22.8 shows improvement in moderate or severe aortic paravalvular leak PVL over time.

22.5 CENTERA Transcatheter Heart Valve System

The Edwards CENTERA transcatheter heart valve system is a next-generation, self-expanding bioprosthesis to compliment the Edwards

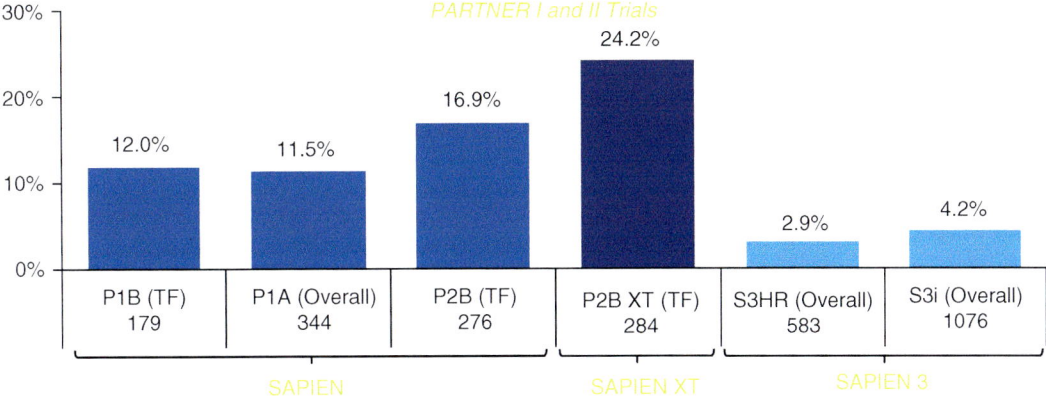

Fig. 22.8 Trend in moderate or severe PVL at 30 days in PARTNER trials

balloon-expandable portfolio. Unlike SAPIEN 3, CENTERA uses a motorized delivery system designed for delivery by a single operator. The CENTERA valve is made of a nitinol frame with a PET skirt that is available in 23-, 26-, and 29-mm sizes. CENTERA can be delivered by transfemoral or subclavian approach using 14-French sheaths, even up to the 29-mm size. The self-expanding frame allows for partial valve repositioning and retrieval, if necessary; the valve system can be re-sheathed and repositioned until 70% of the valve is deployed. The final valve deployment is performed with rapid ventricular pacing, and the valve is ultimately released by pressing a single button.

The feasibility study of the CENTERA valve was performed in 15 patients by Binder et al. The valve was successfully implanted in all cases, and no case required the placement of a second valve. Survival was 87% at 30 days and 80% at 1 year. Paravalvular leak at 30 days was none or trivial in 23% of patients, mild in 69%, and moderate in 8%. In this small feasibility study, four patients (27%) required pacemaker implantation, a challenge that has consistently arisen during the use of self-expanding valves [30].

The results of CENTERA-EU multicenter trial were published in the *Journal of American Cardiology* (JACC) in December 2017, showing the initial 30-day outcomes of CENTERA implantation in 203 patients with severe symptomatic aortic stenosis considered to be at high surgical risk. This was designed as a single-arm study. The primary endpoint was all-cause mortality at 30 days [14] and occurred in 1% of the as-treated population. Major stroke at 30 days occurred in 2.5%, life-threatening or disabling bleeding was in 4.9%, major vascular complications in 6.4%, and moderate or greater aortic PVL in only 0.6% of patients. Quite notably, the requirement for pacemaker implantation was relatively low at 4.5%—this is especially an accomplishment when compared to older versions of self-expandable valve systems [31]. CENTERA-EU ultimately resulted in CE Mark approval of the CENTERA valve in February 2018 but has yet to be approved in the United States.

22.6 Conclusions

There has been a great amount of innovation and evolution in the field of the TAVR over a relatively short amount of time, and the advancements in the field show no signs of slowing down. There are several ongoing studies in patients with symptomatic severe AS at low-surgical risk, patients with asymptomatic severe AS, and patients with moderate AS and reduced left ventricular ejection fraction and heart failure symptoms. In this chapter, the Edwards family of transcatheter aortic valve systems was reviewed. Through the lens of one transcatheter valve system family, the incredible progress in the field can be appreciated.

References

1. Cribier A, Eltchaninoff H, Borenstein N, et al. Transcatheter implantation of balloon-expandable prosthetic heart valves: early results in an animal model [abstract]. Circulation. 2001;104(Suppl II):II–552.
2. Cribier A, Eltchaninoff H, Bash A, et al. Percutaneous transcatheter implantation of an aortic valve prosthesis for calcific aortic stenosis: first human case description. Circulation. 2002;106(24):3006–8.
3. Leon MB, Smith CR, Mack M, et al. Transcatheter aortic-valve implantation for aortic stenosis in patients who cannot undergo surgery. N Engl J Med. 2010;363(17):1597–607.
4. Smith CR, Leon MB, Mack MJ, et al. Transcatheter versus surgical aortic-valve replacement in high-risk patients. N Engl J Med. 2011;364(23):2187–98.
5. Popma JJ, Adams DH, Reardon MJ. Transcatheter aortic valve replacement using a self-expanding bioprosthesis in patients with severe aortic stenosis at extreme risk for surgery. J Am Coll Cardiol. 2014;63(19):1972–81.
6. Adams DH, Popma JJ, Reardon MJ. Transcatheter aortic-valve replacement with a self-expanding prosthesis. N Engl J Med. 2014;370(19):1790–8.
7. Leon MB, Smith CR, Mack M, et al. Transcatheter or surgical aortic-valve replacement in intermediate-risk patients. N Engl J Med. 2016;374:1609–20.
8. Thourani VH, Kodali S, Makkar RR, et al. Transcatheter aortic valve replacement versus surgical valve replacement in intermediate-risk patients: a propensity score analysis. Lancet. 2016;387(10034):2218–25.
9. Reardon MJ, Van Mieghem NM, Popma JJ, et al. Surgical or transcatheter aortic-valve replacement in intermediate-risk patients. N Engl J Med. 2017;376:1321–31.
10. Yakubov SJ, Adams DH, Watson DR, et al. 2-year outcomes after iliofemoral self-expanding transcatheter aortic valve replacement in patients with severe Aortic stenosis deemed extreme risk for surgery. J Am Coll Cardiol. 2015;66(12):1327–34.
11. Reardon MJ, Adams DH, Kleiman NS, et al. 2-year outcomes in patients undergoing surgical or self-expanding transcatheter aortic valve replacement. J Am Coll Cardiol. 2015;66(2):113–21.
12. Kapadia SR, Leon MB, Makkar RR, et al. 5-year outcomes of transcatheter aortic valve replacement compared with standard treatment for patients with inoperable aortic stenosis (PARTNER 1): a randomised controlled trial. Lancet. 2015;385(9986):2485–91.
13. Harjai KJ, Grines CL, Paradis JM, Kodali S. Transcatheter aortic valve replacement: the year in review 2016. J Interv Cardiol. 2017;30(2):105–13.
14. Svensson LG, Tuzcu M, Kapadia S, Blackstone EH, Roselli EE, Gillinov AM, Sabik JF 3rd, Lytle BW. A comprehensive review of the PARTNER trial. J Thorac Cardiovasc Surg. 2013;145(3 Suppl):S11–6. https://doi.org/10.1016/j.jtcvs.2012.11.051.
15. Svensson LG, Blackstone EH, Rajeswaran J, Brozzi N, Leon MB, Smith CR, Mack M, Miller DC, Moses JW, Tuzcu EM, Webb JG, Kapadia S, Fontana GP, Makkar RR, Brown DL, Block PC, Guyton RA, Thourani VH, Pichard AD, Bavaria JE, Herrmann HC, Williams MR, Babaliaros V, Généreux P, Akin JJ. Comprehensive analysis of mortality among patients undergoing TAVR: results of the PARTNER trial. J Am Coll Cardiol. 2014;64(2):158–68. https://doi.org/10.1016/j.jacc.2013.08.1666.
16. Mack MJ, Leon MB, Smith CR, Miller DC, Moses JW, Tuzcu EM, Webb JG, Douglas PS, Anderson WN, Blackstone EH, Kodali SK, Makkar RR, Fontana GP, Kapadia S, Bavaria J, Hahn RT, Thourani VH, Babaliaros V, Pichard A, Herrmann HC, Brown DL, Williams M, Akin J, Davidson MJ, Svensson LG. 5-year outcomes of transcatheter aortic valve replacement or surgical aortic valve replacement for high surgical risk patients with aortic stenosis (PARTNER 1): a randomised controlled trial. Lancet. 2015;385(9986):2477–84.
17. Kumar A, Paniagua D, Hira RS, Alam M, Denktas AE, Jneid H. Balloon aortic valvuloplasty in the transcatheter aortic valve replacement era. J Invasive Cardiol. 2016;28(8):341–8.
18. Andersen HR, Knudsen LL, Hasenkam JM. Transluminal catheter implantation of a new expandable artificial cardiac valve (the stent–valve) in the aorta and the beating heart of closed chest pigs [abstract]. Eur Heart J. 1990;11(Suppl):224a.
19. Andersen HR, Knudsen LL, Hasenkam JM. Transluminal implantation of artificial heart valves. Description of a new expandable aortic valve and initial results with implantation by catheter technique in closed chest pigs. Eur Heart J. 1992;13(5):704–8.
20. Kapadia SR, Leon MB, Makkar RR, Tuzcu EM, Svensson LG, Kodali S, Webb JG, Mack MJ, Douglas PS, Thourani VH, Babaliaros VC, Herrmann HC, Szeto WY, Pichard AD, Williams MR, Fontana GP, Miller DC, Anderson WN, Akin JJ, Davidson MJ, Smith CR. 5-year outcomes of transcatheter aortic valve replacement compared with standard treatment for patients with inoperable aortic stenosis (PARTNER 1): a randomised controlled trial. Lancet. 2015;385(9986):2485–91.
21. Reynolds MR, Magnuson EA, Wang K, Lei Y, Vilain K, Walczak J, Kodali SK, Lasala JM, O'Neill WW, Davidson CJ, Smith CR, Leon MB, Cohen DJ. Cost-effectiveness of transcatheter aortic valve replacement compared with standard care among inoperable patients with severe aortic stenosis: results from the placement of aortic transcatheter valves (PARTNER) trial (Cohort B). Circulation. 2012;125(9):1102–9.
22. Kodali SK, Williams MR, Smith CR, Svensson LG, Webb JG, Makkar RR, Fontana GP, Dewey TM, Thourani VH, Pichard AD, Fischbein M, Szeto WY, Lim S, Greason KL, Teirstein PS, Malaisrie SC, Douglas PS, Hahn RT, Whisenant B, Zajarias A, Wang D, Akin JJ, Anderson WN, Leon MB. Two-year outcomes after transcatheter or surgical aortic-valve replacement. N Engl J Med. 2012;366(18):1686–95.

23. Miller DC, Blackstone EH, Mack MJ, Svensson LG, Kodali SK, Kapadia S, Rajeswaran J, Anderson WN, Moses JW, Tuzcu EM, Webb JG, Leon MB, Smith CR. Transcatheter (TAVR) versus surgical (AVR) aortic valve replacement: occurrence, hazard, risk factors, and consequences of neurologic events in the PARTNER trial. J Thorac Cardiovasc Surg. 2012;143(4):832–43.

24. Douglas PS, Leon MB, Mack MJ, Svensson LG, Webb JG, Hahn RT, Pibarot P, Weissman NJ, Miller DC, Kapadia S, Herrmann HC, Kodali SK, Makkar RR, Thourani VH, Lerakis S, Lowry AM, Rajeswaran J, Finn MT, Alu MC, Smith CR, Blackstone EH. Longitudinal hemodynamics of transcatheter and surgical aortic valves in the PARTNER trial. JAMA Cardiol. 2017;2(11):1197–206.

25. Blackstone EH, Suri RM, Rajeswaran J, Babaliaros V, Douglas PS, Fearon WF, Miller DC, Hahn RT, Kapadia S, Kirtane AJ, Kodali SK, Mack M, Szeto WY, Thourani VH, Tuzcu EM, Williams MR, Akin JJ, Leon MB, Svensson LG. Propensity-matched comparisons of clinical outcomes after transapical or transfemoral transcatheter aortic valve replacement: a placement of aortic transcatheter valves (PARTNER)-I trial substudy. Circulation. 2015;131(22):1989–2000.

26. Reynolds MR, Magnuson EA, Lei Y, Wang K, Vilain K, Li H, Walczak J, Pinto DS, Thourani VH, Svensson LG, Mack MJ, Miller DC, Satler LE, Bavaria J, Smith CR, Leon MB, Cohen DJ. Cost-effectiveness of transcatheter aortic valve replacement compared with surgical aortic valve replacement in high-risk patients with severe aortic stenosis: results of the PARTNER (Placement of Aortic Transcatheter Valves) trial (Cohort A). J Am Coll Cardiol. 2012;60(25):2683–92.

27. Arnold SV, Lei Y, Reynolds MR, Magnuson EA, Suri RM, Tuzcu EM, Petersen JL 2nd, Douglas PS, Svensson LG, Gada H, Thourani VH, Kodali SK, Mack MJ, Leon MB, Cohen DJ. Costs of periprocedural complications in patients treated with transcatheter aortic valve replacement: results from the placement of aortic transcatheter valve trial. Circ Cardiovasc Interv. 2014;7(6):829–36.

28. Herrmann HC, Thourani VH, Kodali SK, Makkar RR, Szeto WY, Anwaruddin S, Desai N, Lim S, Malaisrie SC, Kereiakes DJ, Ramee S, Greason KL, Kapadia S, Babaliaros V, Hahn RT, Pibarot P, Weissman NJ, Leipsic J, Whisenant BK, Webb JG, Mack MJ, Leon MB. One-year clinical outcomes with SAPIEN 3 transcatheter aortic valve replacement in high-risk and inoperable patients with severe aortic stenosis. Circulation. 2016;134(2):130–40.

29. Baron SJ, Arnold SV, Wang K, Magnuson EA, Chinnakondepali K, Makkar R, Herrmann HC, Kodali S, Thourani VH, Kapadia S, Svensson L, Brown DL, Mack MJ, Smith CR, Leon MB, Cohen DJ. Health status benefits of transcatheter vs. surgical aortic valve replacement in patients with severe aortic stenosis at intermediate surgical risk: results from the PARTNER 2 randomized clinical trial. JAMA Cardiol. 2017;2(8):837–45.

30. Binder RK, Schäfer U, Kuck KH, Wood DA, Moss R, Leipsic J, Toggweiler S, Freeman M, Ostry AJ, Frerker C, Willson AB, Webb JG. Transcatheter aortic valve replacement with a new self-expanding transcatheter heart valve and motorized delivery system. JACC Cardiovasc Interv. 2013;6(3):301–7.

31. Reichenspurner H, Schaefer A, Schäfer U, Tchétché D, Linke A, Spence MS, Søndergaard L, LeBreton H, Schymik G, Abdel-Wahab M, Leipsic J, Walters DL, Worthley S, Kasel M, Windecker S. Self-expanding transcatheter aortic valve system for symptomatic high-risk patients with severe aortic stenosis. J Am Coll Cardiol. 2017;70(25):3127–36.

The JenaValve Program for Transcatheter Aortic Valve Implantation

23

Hans R. Figulla, Markus Ferrari, Vicky Carr-Brendel, and Alexander Lauten

23.1 JenaValve Technology at Present

The JenaValve (JenaValve Technology Inc., Irvine, CA, USA) transfemoral system is regarded as the first **third-generation** transcatheter aortic valve implantation (TAVI), also called transcatheter aortic valve replacement (TAVR), device, because of its unique features, which aim to address:

- Aortic stenosis and aortic regurgitation patients,
- Easy positioning because of feelers,
- Very low pacemaker rate, because of high outflow tract implantation,
- Little paravalvular leak (PVL),
- Anatomic positioning, which means that the new leaflets of the prosthetic valve precisely overlap the native leaflets, so that the commissures remain in their native orientation,
- Easy coronary ostium access.

The JenaValve transfemoral system is presently in its Conformité Européenne (CE)-mark trial in Europe, and in the United States it is in the investigational device exemption (IDE) trial for TAVI and aortic regurgitation.

The market in Europe and the United States deserves a transfemoral device that can also treat aortic regurgitation (AR). The valve will address annulus sizes of 23, 25, and 27 mm, and a larger, 29-mm, valve is under development (Fig. 23.1).

For the future a very low pacemaker (PM) rate is a need, especially if TAVI will be performed in younger and low-risk patients. The JenaValve has the potential to especially address this low-risk and young patient group, owing to its low PM rate and anatomical positioning, which might be superior to all other valve types, because the pulsed outflow bloodstream will be anatomically directed and will not be impeded by randomly orientated leaflets and commissures within the bloodstream.

23.2 The Beginning of TAVI

As with many new disruptive technologies, the road to success is bumpy and frequently paved with setbacks and delays.

H. R. Figulla (✉)
Jena University Hospital, Jena, Germany
e-mail: figulla@figulla.org

M. Ferrari
Dr Horst Schmidt Kliniken Klinik Innere MED I:
Kardiologie und konservative Intensivmedizin,
Wiesbaden, Germany
e-mail: Markus.Ferrari@helios-gesundheit.de

V. Carr-Brendel
JenaValve Technology Inc., Irvine, CA, USA
e-mail: Carr-Brendel@jenavalve.com

A. Lauten
Klinik für Kardiologie, Charité Campus Benjamin
Franklin, Universitätsmedizin Berlin,
Berlin, Germany
e-mail: alexander.lauten@charite.de

© Springer Nature Switzerland AG 2019
A. Giordano et al. (eds.), *Transcatheter Aortic Valve Implantation*,
https://doi.org/10.1007/978-3-030-05912-5_23

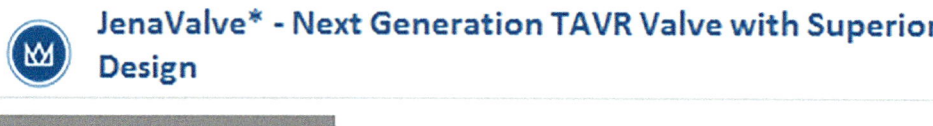

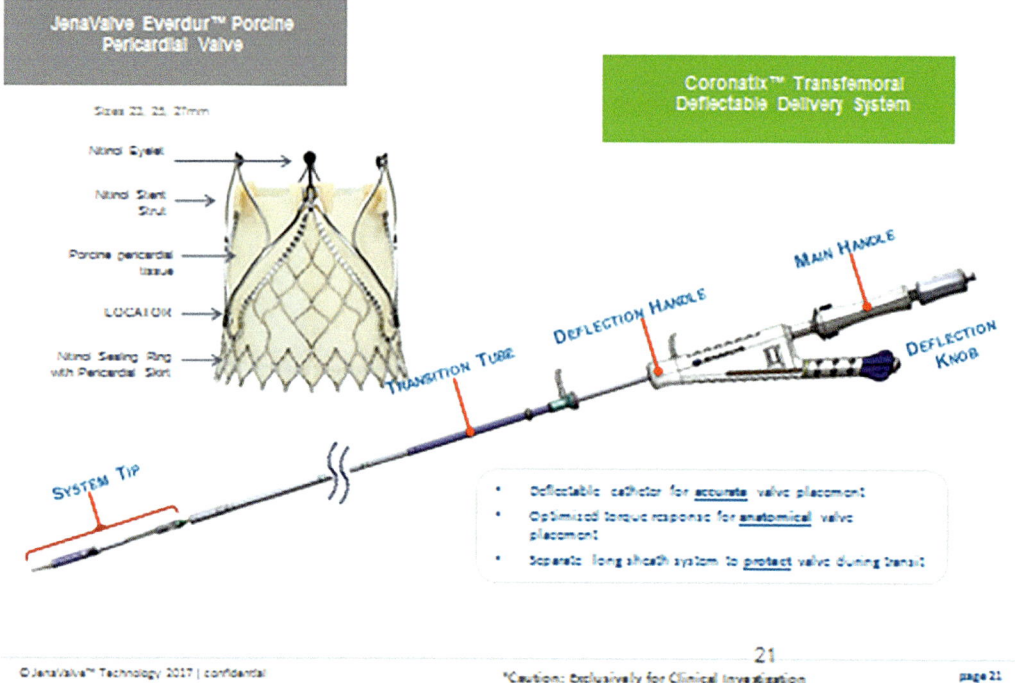

Fig. 23.1 The JenaValve (JV) transfemoral pericardial valve and introducing catheter, which is coming to the European market in 2018 (courtesy JenaValve)

After our personal experience in finding that aortic balloon valvuloplasty created no durable results, it was realized that stenting of the valvuloplasty, as in coronary vessels, should be an option for the prevention of restenosis. So a stent with a valve had to be constructed. Easy!!! (Fig. 23.2a). The first German patent application for a self-expanding stent valve to treat aortic stenosis was filed in 1995 (Fig. 23.2b).

Just a nitinol frame armed with a trileaflet valve would be sufficient.

However, two important issues remained:

- would it be possible to construct a device with a diameter that allowed for transfemoral access?
- would the device generate enough friction on the ascending aorta so that it would not cause embolization?

- would the coronary ostia stay open if the native leaflets stayed in place?
- would the valve tissue be resistant to the stretch stress during crimping?

Many questions to be solved, but a fascinating idea. Initially no one shared the idea; many in the field discouraged its development, and attempts to become supported by scientific grants failed. At this time surgeons dominated the field, as "valve specialists." The first publication of our valve design and the in vitro testing results, displayed at the annual meeting of the German Society of Cardiology as a poster, did not attract much attention [1].

Some attempts to approach the industry also failed. The concept was offered to large companies, who either showed no interest or who observed our animal trials in the late 1990s, and

Fig. 23.2 (**a, b**)
Percutaneous valve
technology in 1995, our
first prototypes, and the
first patent application
for a self-expanding
valve stent system to
treat aortic stenosis

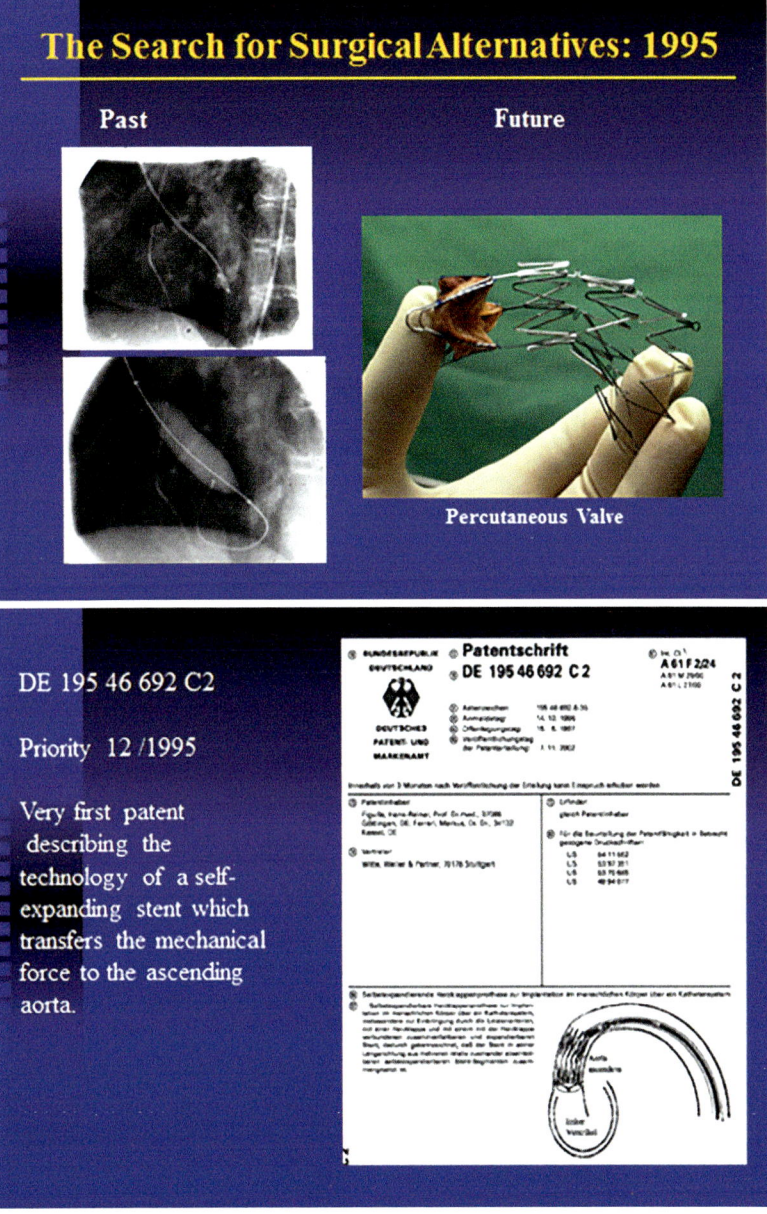

started their own developments thereafter. So lack of funding delayed the evolution of the idea, until 2001 some research grants could be collected. Animal experiments at that time showed that, although many of the above questions could be solved, it was difficult to cross the aortic arch with the rigid compressed long stented valve, because our device did not kink.

We needed to shorten the stent, but then the friction would be reduced, with the risk of dislodgement of the device. So the stent was shortened and barbs were added to prevent embolization. The hemodynamic profile was tested in vitro in a pig aorta and showed promising hemodynamic results. Also, the fixation, measured by retention forces within the aortic tissue, was satisfying (Fig. 23.3a).

The foundation of a company named JEN.cardiotec in 2001 allowed cooperation with the Fraunhofer Institute for Micromechanics and

Optics (Jena, Germany) and the first bulky catheter was built to allow transvascular implantation, and the first animal tests with this device
were performed (Fig. 23.3b). The valve showed a
good hemodynamic profile and stayed in place in
an adult sheep model even under dopamine stress
(Fig. 23.3c).

23.3 The JenaValve Clipping Idea

Fifteen years ago we had the feeling that a stent
with barbs in the ascending aorta incorporated
inherent unacceptable risks. To keep the stent
short, allowing it to cross the aortic arch, and to
eliminate the barbs, the revolutionary idea of a

a **Percutaneous Aortic Valve Replacement**
1995-97

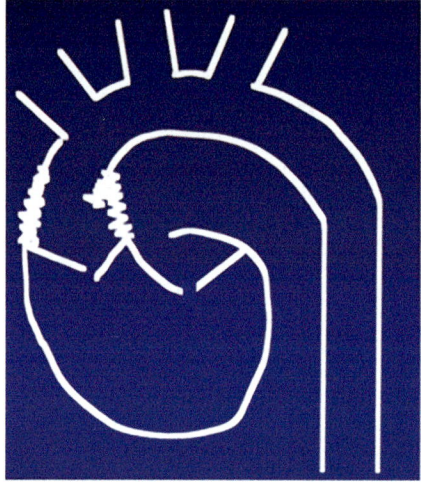

Expansion: 20-26 mm
Compression to: 8-9 mm
Dislocation force: >800 grams
Regurgitant flow: <150 ml/min
Flow gradient: 6mmHg/10l/min

b Concept of JEN.cardiotec
product description, production facilities (3)
2001

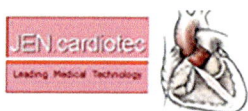

presentation of the current system

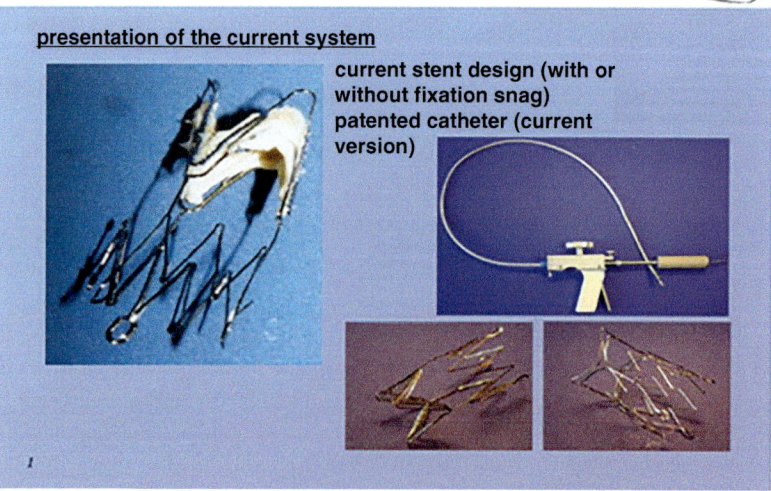

current stent design (with or
without fixation snag)
patented catheter (current
version)

Fig. 23.3 (**a**) In vitro testing of a self-expanding aortic
valve and its mechanical and hemodynamic profile (courtesy of H.R.F. and M.F.). (**b**) Stent valve design with barbs
for fixation in the ascending aorta and transvascular delivery catheter (courtesy of H.R.F. and M.F.). (**c**) The first
in vivo experiments with a percutaneously implanted aortic valve in an adult sheep model showed satisfying hemodynamic results even after dopamine stress (courtesy of
H.R.F. and M.F.)

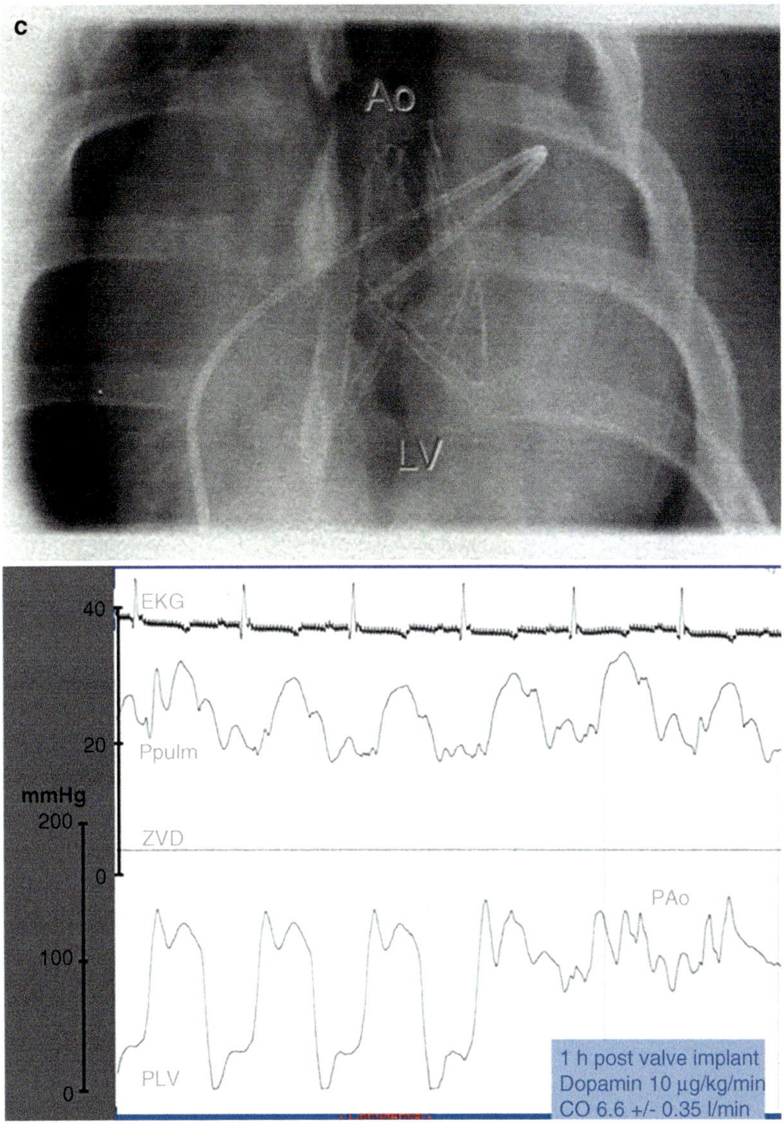

Fig. 23.3 (continued)

short stent with so-called clips came up. These clips could grip the native leaflets like a paper clip and would prevent any embolization toward the left ventricle.

This idea was patent protected in 2003/4 (Fig. 23.4). Besides clipping the native leaflets, this technology also allows:

- *the construction of a rather fragile stent,*
- *the positioning of the device during deployment with less traumatic effects on underlying*

tissues, making septum irritation with consequent atrioventricular (AV) block less likely,
- *leaflets that are always anatomically orientated.*

This idea allowed us to start with animal testing, because no calcification of the native leaflets was needed. The valve did fix itself by its clipping mechanism [1, 2].

However, the clipping mechanism required a catheter design that allowed, first, the exposure

Fig. 23.4 **Fig. 23.4** The
revolutionary idea of a
stent valve that clips
onto the native leaflets
(courtesy of H.R.F. and
M.F.)

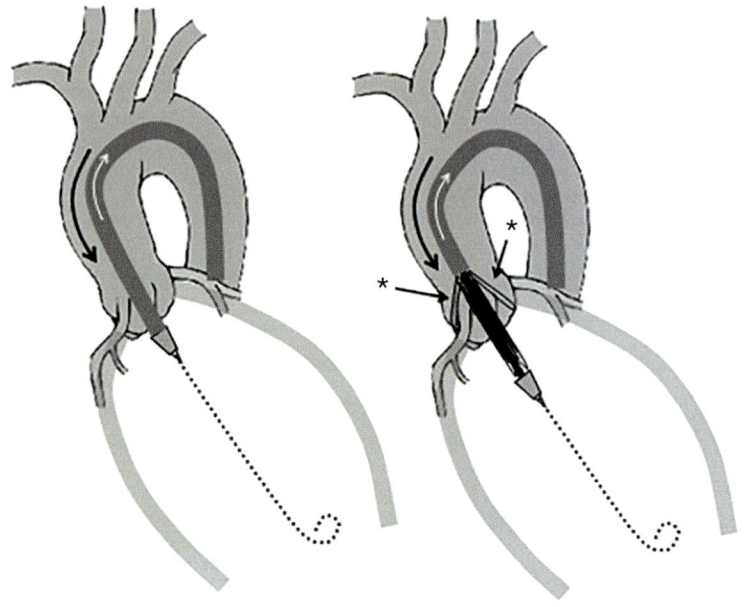

Clipping: shorter stent allows easy crossing of the aortic arch

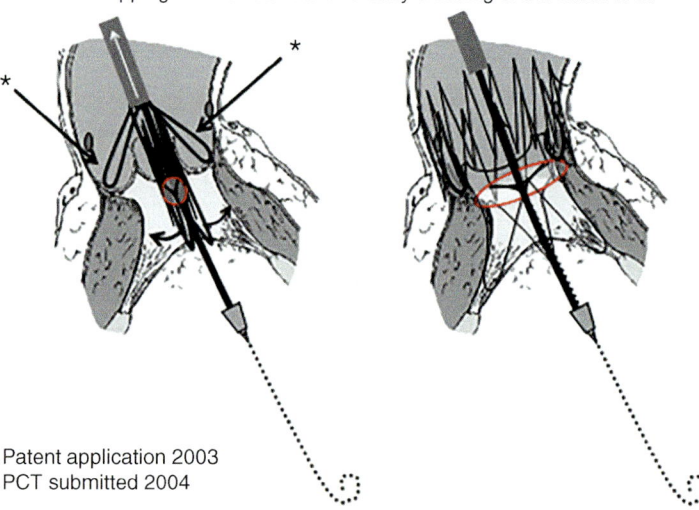

Patent application 2003
PCT submitted 2004

of the clippers (now called "feelers"), and in a second step, the deployment of the valve. This could be realized only with a very bulky catheter design, as shown in Fig. 23.3b.

Owing to the technical difficulties in realizing a small transvascular device, a company for the manufacture of such devices was founded in 2006 and named JenaValve. In 2011 the company marketed the first transapical device (32-French) with a full porcine valve (Fig. 23.5).

Market acceptance was good; however, the transapical market began to shrink at that time. In 2013 the JenaValve transapical system got the additional CE mark, owing to its technical finesse and good clinical results in also treating atrial regurgitation [3].

The same concept of clips on the valve was employed by Medtronic (Minneapolis, MN, USA) and a transapical valve named Engager came onto the market 2 years later. The clips were

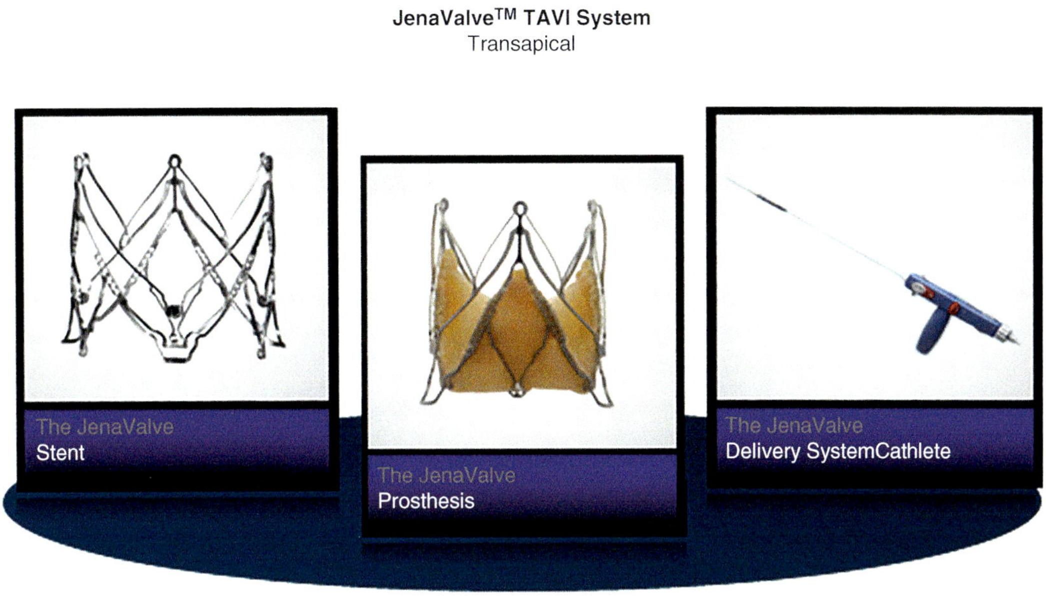

JenaValve™ TAVI System
Transapical

Fig. 23.5 The JenaValve (JV) transapical system with clips and full porcine root valve

connected to the stent as a second piece; however, that valve was withdrawn from the market later on, as the two-piece construction made the device very bulky, so that with this device a transfemoral system could probably never be realized.

In 2016 the JenaValve transapical system was also removed from the market, because recertification was necessary and the transapical market had become very small. In addition, a clinical trial for a transfemoral device with a new pericardial valve had begun.

However, owing to technical modifications the trial was interrupted and the clinical launch of the so-called third-generation TAVI device had to be postponed until the end of 2018 (Fig. 23.6).

Note that it took more than 15 years from its first concept until the first JenaValve device came onto the market. Disruptive technical medical solutions are highly regulated before market entry is possible. The safety and efficiency concerns of regulatory authorities have to be counterbalanced against the medical need to replace older and more invasive surgical procedures that are usually unregulated and applied according to individual surgeons' decisions and are not followed by clinical trials.

At present other new TAVI devices are still under development. The evolution of TAVI began in the early 1990s, but it is

"… not at its end,
Not even at the beginning of its end.
Maybe at the end of the beginning"
(Winston Churchill).

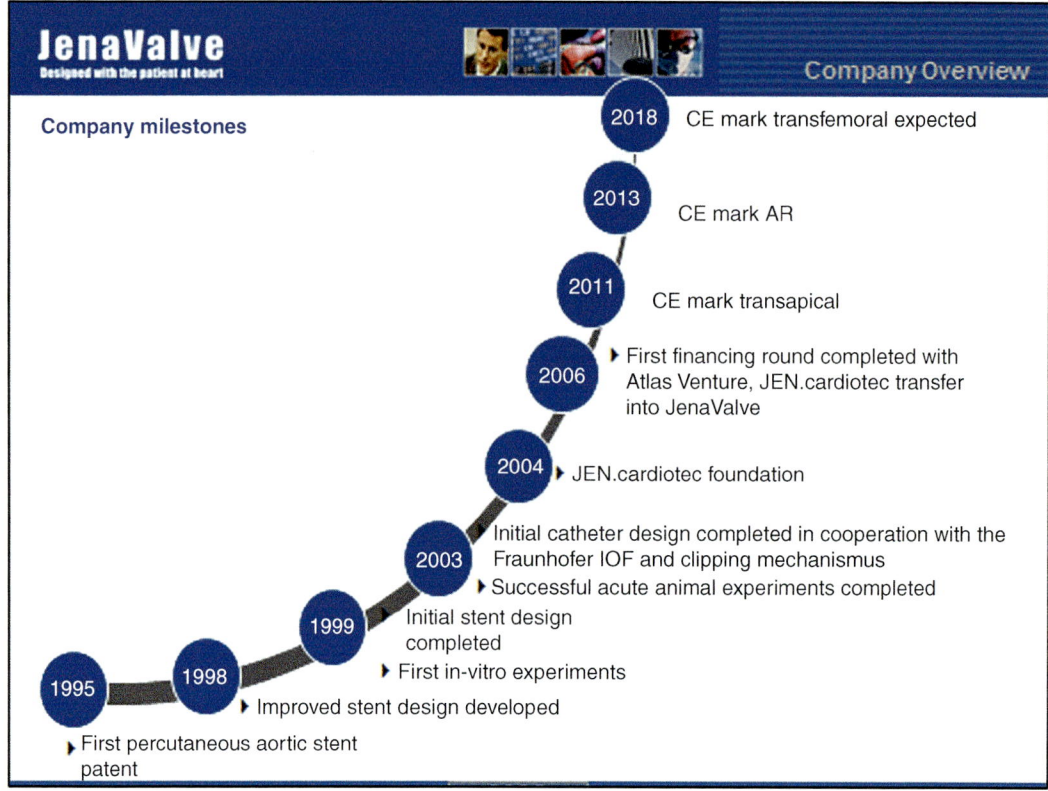

Fig. 23.6 JenaValve company milestones

References

1. Ferrari M, Figulla HR, Schlosser M, et al. Transarterial aortic valve replacement with a self-expanding stent in pigs. Heart. 2004;90:1326–31.
2. Lauten A, Ferrari M, Petri A, et al. Experimental evaluation of the JenaClip transcatheter aortic valve. Catheter Cardiovasc Interv. 2009;74:514–9.
3. Seiffert M, Diemert P, Koschyk D, et al. Transapical implantation of a second-generation transcatheter heart valve in patients with noncalcified aortic regurgitation. JACC Cardiovasc Interv. 2013;6:590–7.

Medtronic Program for Transcatheter Aortic Valve Implantation

Yasuhiro Ichibori, Sandeep M. Patel, Ankur Kalra, and Guilherme F. Attizzani

24.1 Introduction

Transcatheter aortic valve implantation (TAVI), also called transcatheter aortic valve replacement (TAVR), has been accepted as an alternative therapeutic option to surgical aortic valve replacement (SAVR) in severe aortic stenosis patients who have moderate or high perioperative risk for mortality [1, 2]. Ongoing improvements in devices and techniques have contributed to better TAVI outcomes with the decreased rate of 30-day mortality [3, 4]. Medtronic CoreValve (Medtronic, Inc., Minneapolis, Minnesota) is the first self-expandable transcatheter heart valve introduced in the market after obtaining Conformité Européenne (CE) Mark in 2007 and is characterized by supra-annular design to enhance valve function. The US Food and Drug Administration (FDA) approved CoreValve for commercial use in patients at high perioperative mortality risk for SAVR in January 2014. The next-generation CoreValve Evolut R device was approved in June 2015 for use in high or extreme surgical-risk patients. This second-generation device has four sizes (23 mm, 26 mm, 29 mm, and 34 mm) (Fig. 24.1), designed to obtain the following advantages compared with the previous CoreValve device:

1. Accurate positioning: EnVeo R delivery catheter system (Fig. 24.2) allows 1:1 torque response when the valve is released and allows recapturing and repositioning of the valve up to three times before reaching the point of no recapture.
2. Less trauma to the left ventricular outflow tract: valve inflow is redesigned to reduce the force applied by the inflow tip and subsequent incidence of pacemaker implantation.
3. Enhanced sealing: the improved inflow part of the valve, equipped with an extended skirt, produces consistent radial force and reduces paravalvular leak.
4. Smaller delivery profile: the built-in InLine sheath enables the insertion of the EnVeo R delivery catheter system without an additional sheath, allowing 14 Fr (for 23 mm, 26 mm, 29 mm) or 16 Fr (for 34 mm) equivalent delivery profiles of the device.

Y. Ichibori · A. Kalra · G. F. Attizzani (✉)
Division of Cardiovascular Medicine,
The Valve & Structural Heart Disease Intervention Center, Harrington Heart and Vascular Institute, University Hospitals Cleveland Medical Center, Cleveland, OH, USA
e-mail: Guilherme.Attizzani@uhhospitals.org

S. M. Patel
Division of Cardiovascular Medicine,
The Valve & Structural Heart Disease Intervention Center, Harrington Heart and Vascular Institute, University Hospitals Cleveland Medical Center, Cleveland, OH, USA

Structural Heart Center, St. Rita's Medical Center (Mercy), Lima, OH, USA
e-mail: SMPatel@mercy.com

© Springer Nature Switzerland AG 2019
A. Giordano et al. (eds.), *Transcatheter Aortic Valve Implantation*,
https://doi.org/10.1007/978-3-030-05912-5_24

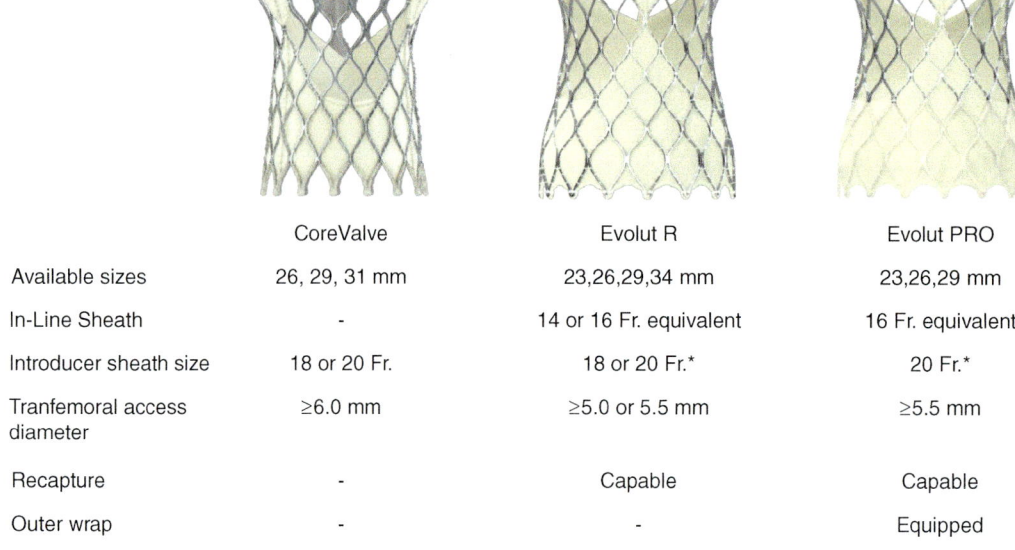

	CoreValve	Evolut R	Evolut PRO
Available sizes	26, 29, 31 mm	23,26,29,34 mm	23,26,29 mm
In-Line Sheath	-	14 or 16 Fr. equivalent	16 Fr. equivalent
Introducer sheath size	18 or 20 Fr.	18 or 20 Fr.*	20 Fr.*
Tranfemoral access diameter	≥6.0 mm	≥5.0 or 5.5 mm	≥5.5 mm
Recapture	-	Capable	Capable
Outer wrap	-	-	Equipped

*if necessary

Fig. 24.1 Device characteristics. Permission by © Medtronic 2018

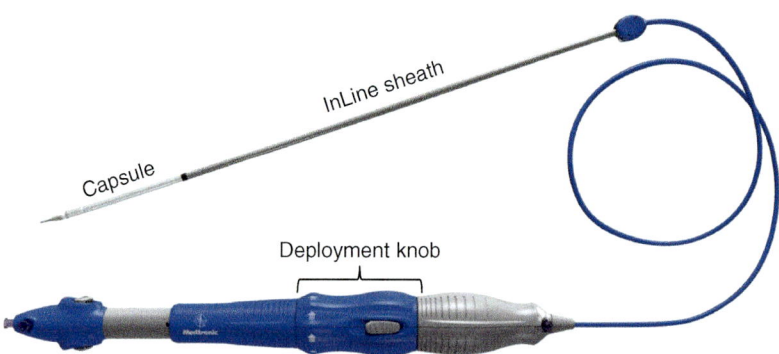

Fig. 24.2 EnVeo R delivery catheter system. Built-in InLine sheath enables to insert the EnVeo R delivery catheter system without additional sheath, which allows 14 Fr (for CoreValve Evolut R 23 mm, 26 m, 29 mm) or 16 Fr (for CoreValve Evolut R/PRO 34 mm) equivalent delivery profile of the device. Permission by © Medtronic 2018

When the additional sheath is required to deliver the catheter, 18 Fr sheath is used for the 23 mm, 26 mm, and 29 mm valves, and 20 Fr sheath is used for the 34 mm valve. Recently, the latest CoreValve Evolut PRO was approved in Europe and the United States. The CoreValve Evolut PRO has an outer wrap made from por-cine pericardial tissue that enhances contact between the valve and the aortic annulus, to further address the occurrence of paravalvular leak. This device is currently available in 23 mm, 26 mm, and 29 mm sizes (34 mm is not available) and has a 16 Fr equivalent delivery profile with the InLine sheath. Medtronic has a large global market share of TAVI devices, and until October 2017, Medtronic devices had been implanted in more than 160,000 patients worldwide.

24.2 Implantation Procedure

24.2.1 Valve and Access Selection

Computed tomography (CT) is the essential imaging modality for TAVI planning, including access and selection of valve type and size [5–7]. CoreValve size is decided by multi-detector CT-derived annulus perimeter in accordance with the sizing chart. Other information, such as the dimensions of sinus of Valsalva, coronary height, and severity of leaflet calcification, are also considered for sizing, especially when the annulus perimeter is at the borderline of two different valve sizes. Although an ideal cutoff value has not been established, oversizing of CoreValve is currently recommended to reduce the risk of paravalvular leak (PVL) [7–10]. Previous studies have shown a direct relationship between the rate of pacemaker implantation and the degree of oversizing [11, 12], and a recent study demonstrated that 9.6–16.2% perimeter oversizing is associated with better outcomes, including a lower rate of post-dilation and stroke [13].

Transfemoral route is considered to be less invasive and is the gold standard compared with other approaches. When the access vessel is small in size (<5.0 mm), or has severe calcification or tortuosity, an alternative route is optional, such as the subclavian artery or the direct aortic approach, as the vascular complications are still an issue in TAVI and are significantly associated with increased early and late mortality [14–16]. However, with the emergence of a lower-profile device and technique development, the need for alternative access is currently decreasing. In the International FORWARD Study, a multicenter, observational study of real-world clinical practice including 1083 patients with CoreValve Evolut R, only 1.9% of patients underwent TAVI via alternative access, 1.6% via the subclavian artery, and 0.3% with a direct aortic approach [17].

24.2.2 Implantation Technique

It is recommended that CoreValve Evolut R/PRO is implanted between 3 and 5 mm of depth from the annular line. Previous studies have shown that when the CoreValve is implanted deeper (lower), the patient is more likely to have PVL or permanent pacemaker implantation [8, 18–20]. An implantation depth less than 10 mm or 3 stent cells in relation to the aortic annulus is suggested to reduce PVL in previous reports [8, 20], while more precise implantation seems to be required to reduce the risk of pacemaker implantation. Although the rate of pacemaker implantation varies among reports, a depth of more than 6–10 mm has been reportedly associated with permanent pacemaker implantation [21, 22]. The option of recapture and new stent frame design of the CoreValve Evolut R has shown to allow precise implantation depth compared with CoreValve (4.0 mm vs. 5.3 mm, $p = 0.03$) [23]. On the other hand, shallow implanting position still has the possible risk of device migration to the aorta at the final release of the valve, which support importance of operator experience for better implantation position and clinical outcomes, including rates of pacemaker implantation or significant PVL [9, 24].

24.2.3 Transfemoral Approach

Femoral arterial access is achieved in the common femoral artery segment using open technique with surgical cutdown or percutaneous technique with suture-mediated vascular closure devices. Arterial puncture should be a bit more parallel to the vessel than conventional puncture to reduce the resistance when EnVeo R delivery catheter is inserted through the arterial wall. A 14 Fr (or 16 Fr) sheath is placed in femoral artery when EnVeo R delivery catheter is delivered directly using the InLine sheath. However, in cases with severe calcification and tortuosity, it is recommended to use an 18 Fr (or 20 Fr) sheath and deliver the EnVeo R delivery catheter through the sheath, because the EnVeo R delivery catheter has less pushability due to the gap between the nose cone and the capsule. A stiff wire, like Safari (Boston Scientific, Natick, Massachusetts), Confida (Medtronic), or Amplatz Super Stiff (Boston Scientific) wire, is placed at the left ventricular (LV) apex. A Lunderquist Extra Stiff wire (Cook Medical, Bloomington, Indiana) can also be used when greater support is required to deliver the catheter. Safari and Confida are dedicated pre-shaped wires that sit stable in the left ventricle, while manually shaped wires should be "created" carefully to minimize the risk of injury of left ventricle. The wire should be placed at the apex of the left ventricle to facilitate coaxial positioning and deployment of the valve as well as to avoid injuring the left ventricle or the mitral valve apparatus. Position of the wire is confirmed by echocardiography or fluoroscopy (right anterior oblique view).

Inspection of the loaded valve on the delivery catheter by fluoroscopy is imperative before balloon predilation of the native aortic valve, in case of ensuing acute severe aortic regurgitation or hemodynamic collapse after valvuloplasty that may require immediate implantation of the valve. Since the loaded valve is invisible from outside due to the nitinol capsule, the delivery catheter should be placed under fluoroscopy. Then, inspection can be performed in an anteroposterior view with a high frame rate ($\geq$30 frames per second) while rotating the entire valve. The two paddles of the CoreValve Evolut R/PRO are carefully inspected to ensure that they are perfectly inserted in the pocket and are completely symmetric, equidistant from the paddle attachment of the EnVeo R delivery catheter (Fig. 24.3). The outflow crowns should be parallel to the paddle attachment and straight. The capsule should be straight without any deformity, and the marker bands or nodes must be straight and aligned without a crease or bend of the loaded valve.

Balloon aortic valvuloplasty (BAV) before implantation can be performed to facilitate the delivery and expansion of the CoreValve Evolut R/PRO device across the native valve. BAV can also potentially stabilize hemodynamics during the implantation of the transcatheter valve and allow a slow deployment, as BAV can mitigate

LV outflow obstruction when the CoreValve Evolut R/PRO begins to expand. In contrast, BAV is reported to be associated with complications, such as stroke, conduction disturbances, severe aortic regurgitation, and hemodynamic collapse [25, 26], while safety of TAVI without predilation has been reported [27, 28]. In the absence of established recommendation, BAV before implantation should be determined by the experience of operator, as well as clinical and anatomical characteristics, including aortic valve calcification, aortic valve area, and left ventricular function.

The delivery system is advanced over the stiff wire positioned at the apex of the left ventricle while keeping an eye on the LV wire position under fluoroscopy. When the EnVeo R delivery catheter is directly inserted from the groin using an InLine sheath, confirm that the flush port of the delivery catheter is pointing upward and that the InLine sheath is in contact with the proximal end of the capsule. The delivery catheter is further advanced under fluoroscopy with no gap between the nose cone and the capsule, especially in tortuous vessels or heavily calcified vessels. When the gap is generated or the operator feels resistance during advancement, refrain from pushing too hard; instead pull back the delivery catheter and try to change the trajectory of the catheter by wire manipulation or, in some cases, rotating the catheter by a quarter turn. Replacement with a stiffer wire, e.g., Lunderquist Extra Stiff wire, or inserting an 18 Fr or 20 Fr standard sheath may also be helpful in advancing the delivery catheter.

The device is then advanced through the aortic valve, keeping it toward the outer curve of the ascending aorta. It is important to confirm that the pigtail catheter is in position at the bottom of the non-coronary cusp by an angiogram. Projection angle is adjusted to remove the parallax in the device, which is basically achieved by left anterior oblique and caudal rotation of the C-arm. Then, the inflow end of the mounted CoreValve Evolut R/PRO is positioned within a depth of 3–5 mm below the annulus, referring to the first node that indicates 6 mm proximal from the inflow end. After attaining optimal position of

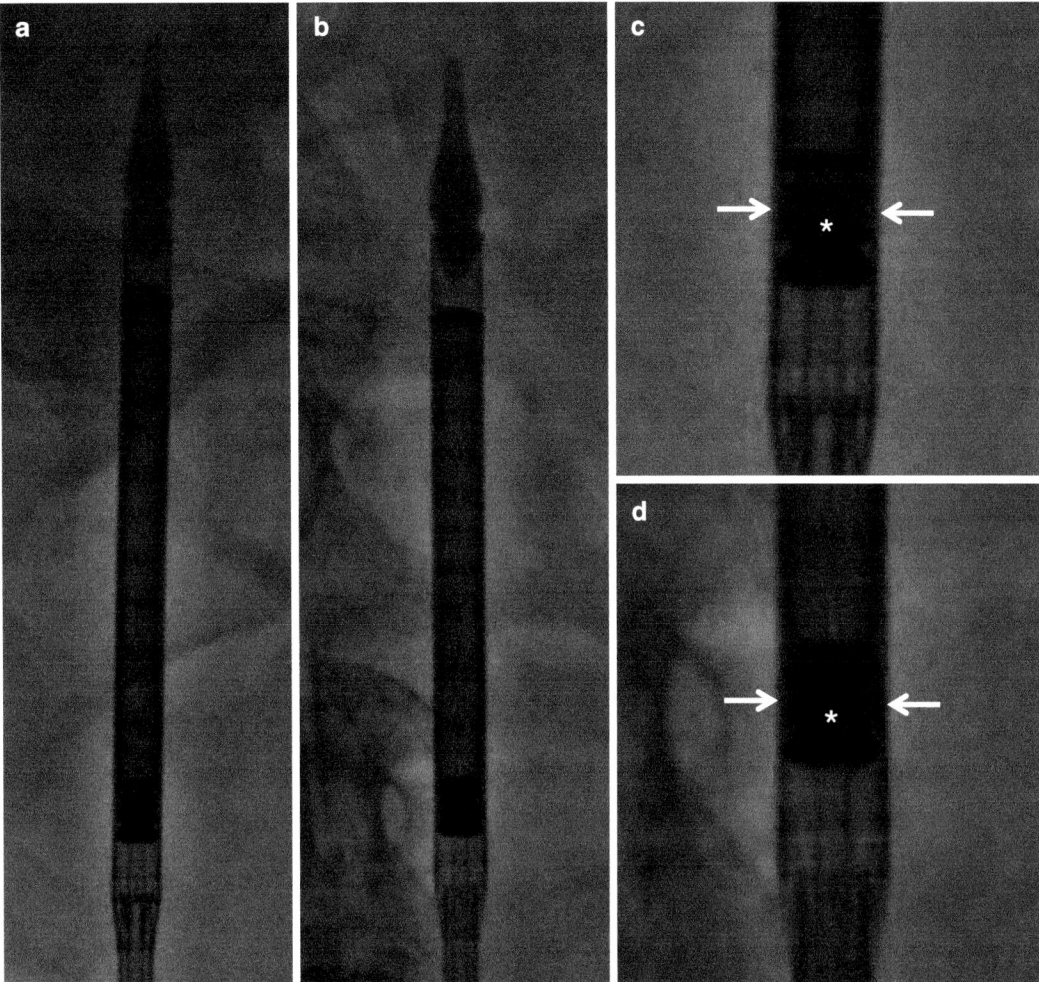

Fig. 24.3 Device inspection. (**a** and **c**) Proper loading: two paddles (arrows) of the CoreValve Evolut R/Pro are perfectly inserted in the pocket and completely symmetric equidistant from the paddle attachment (asterisk) of EnVeo R delivery catheter. (**b** and **d**) Improper loading: two paddles are not symmetric from the paddle attachment

the device, any tension in the delivery catheter is released, and the handle is turned slowly to flare the inflow portion of the bioprosthesis. The transcatheter valve is deployed slowly, and the position is monitored and adjusted using the pigtail catheter as a landmark for the nadir of the annulus with contrast injection (Fig. 24.4). Gentle pulling and pushing of the delivery system or LV wire is done to attain optimal adjustment with ventricular pacing at 90–120 beats per minute, if necessary, to stabilize device position. Once annular contact is made, there is a precipitous drop in the blood pressure, and, therefore, deployment should proceed quickly until the point of no

recapture—confirmed by the relationship between the radiopaque marker band and the radiopaque paddle attachment. During the rotation of the handle, the operator can also feel the tactile feedback that deployment is nearing the point of no return. It is important to confirm recovery of normal pressure. The position of CoreValve Evolut R/PRO is assessed by the injection of contrast after removing the parallax. When the position is not optimal, CoreValve Evolut R/PRO can be recaptured partially or fully at this point. After achievement of satisfactory position, the LV wire is retracted to centralize the nose cone to avoid interference with the valve

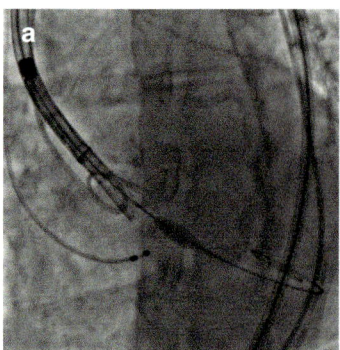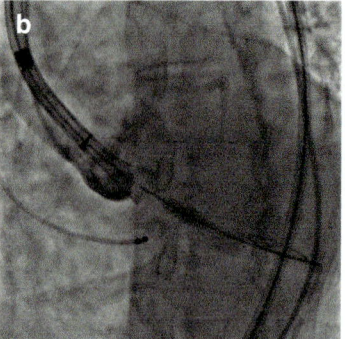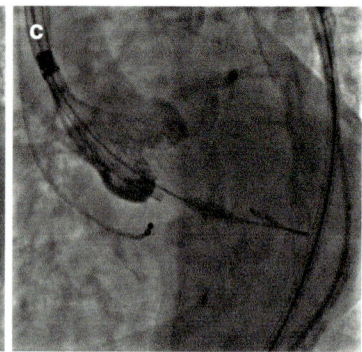

Fig. 24.4 Implantation procedure. (**a**) Device depth can be confirmed in relation to the pigtail placed on the bottom of the non-coronary cusp as a landmark for the aortic annulus. (**b**) Contrast injection further clarifies the depth of the device, including the left coronary cusp side. (**c**) At the point of no return, the device position is carefully assessed before final release

frame. The handle is turned very slowly until both paddles disengage, in some cases, with a gentle push of the delivery catheter. Complete detachment of the paddles should be carefully assessed. The capsule is recaptured in the descending aorta, and the delivery system is removed from the body. When balloon post-dilatation is considered, a 14 Fr (or 16 Fr) sheath is reinserted.

24.2.4 Alternative Access

In cases where transfemoral approach is unsuitable or at high risk for vascular complications, trans-subclavian/axillary or direct aortic approach can be alternative options. Both left and right subclavian arteries can be used, but the left is better due to delivery angulation relative to the aortic valve. Aortic root angulation (angle between the aortic valve annulus plane and the horizontal plane) of <30° is recommended for right subclavian access and <70° for left subclavian access. The subclavian artery is usually less calcified and tortuous, but can be relatively small in caliber and is subject to vascular injury, such as dissection and occlusion. Caution should be paid especially in patients with previous coronary artery bypass surgery and a patent left or right internal mammary artery graft; ≥6.5 mm of minimum vessel diameter for InLine sheath system and ≥7.5 mm for 18 Fr sheath are recom-

mended. In direct aortic approach, the operator can directly deliver the device at a short distance from the aortic valve through the ascending aorta. Surgical incision is required, either an upper partial sternotomy or a small right anterior thoracotomy. The access site of the ascending aorta should be ≥6 cm from the annular plane without calcification. The InLine sheath system is not recommended for the direct aortic approach.

Currently, the most common alternatives to transfemoral access are transapical (not available for CoreValve) or trans-subclavian approach. Until now, these two alternative procedures have been rarely compared in clinical study, and superiority of one approach to the other has yet to be established [29, 30]. Thus, the choice of alternative access can be made depending on the operators' experience and preference, as well as patient comorbidities and anatomical feasibility.

24.2.5 Valve-in-Valve Procedure

Valve-in-valve (VIV) TAVI is a less invasive approach for patients with failed surgical bioprosthesis, representing a useful alternative to reoperative surgical aortic valve replacement in patients with high-risk surgical profiles. Under-expansion of transcatheter valve can occur after VIV implantation because a rigid and nonelastic surgical valve hampers dilation of the valve, resulting in a tendency of higher post-procedural transvalvular gradients and a higher prevalence of patient-prosthesis mismatch [31]. Under-expansion may also have negative impact on the long-term durability of the valve, supporting the advantage of supra-annular transcatheter valve with higher positioning, because the device can function above the rigid frame of the surgical valve [32]. In an in vitro VIV model, CoreValve demonstrated better valve performance (i.e., transvalvular gradient and effective orifice area), when compared with the intra-annular valve [33]. Moreover, when the inflow of CoreValve is juxta-posed with inflow of the surgical valve, i.e., 0 mm of depth, the performance was highest among different depths of implantation. A clinical study also demonstrated that higher implantation, defined as an implantation depth ≤5 mm from ventricular border of the surgical valve, correlated with lower post-procedural transvalvular gradient using CoreValve Evolut R [32]. In higher implantations, the rate of elevated transvalvular gradient (mean gradient ≥ 20 mHg) was significantly lower than in lower implantations (depth > 5 mm). These results suggest repositionable supra-annular CoreValve Evolut R/PRO can be the first-line device for VIV, especially in patients with small surgical bioprosthesis [34].

For device sizing, the true inner diameter of the surgical valve at the level of the sewing ring is used and is commonly 1–4 mm smaller than the manufacturer's labeled size. This information can be obtained from manufacturer websites or publications. Multi-detector CT or transesophageal echocardiography is recommended to confirm smallest inner diameter of the surgical valve, given that valve design and size information will not always be correct after more than 10 years since replacement. The device size is based on the method used for native aortic valve selection with appropriate oversizing. The VinV app is also useful in obtaining important information for a successful VIV procedure, including TAVI valve sizing and image-based guidance for the ideal placement of the valve.

The sewing ring level is used as a reference plane of the surgical valve, similar to the annulus plane being used in TAVI for the native aortic valve. A perpendicular view of the surgical valve is achieved by adjusting the fluoroscopic projection using a radiopaque maker, such as the basal ring or stent frame. The sewing ring position must be confirmed using the radiopaque component of the surgical valve as a relative marker or using valvuloplasty to identify the neck and transesophageal echocardiography in cases without a radiopaque part [35]. CoreValve is implanted within the depth of 5 mm below the sewing ring for better hemodynamics as previously described (Fig. 24.5). The repositionable feature of CoreValve Evolut R/PRO is useful to obtain ideal depth and coaxiality to the surgical valve.

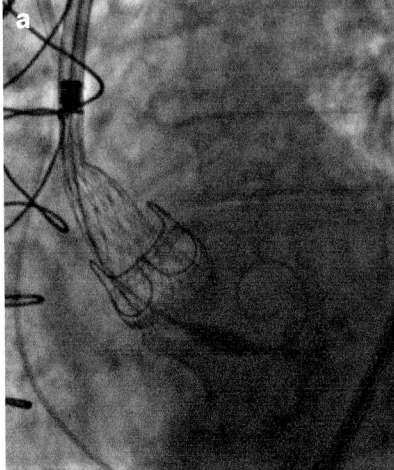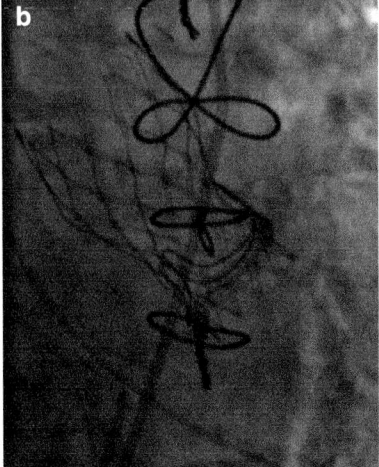

Fig. 24.5 Valve-in-valve procedure. (**a** and **b**) The deployment of CoreValve Evolut R 23 mm inside of Carpentier-Edwards Perimount 23 mm. Stent frame of the surgical valve can be used as a reference of the deployment

24.2.6 Post-procedure Monitoring

In recent trials of CoreValve Evolut R, 14.7–17.5% [4, 17, 36] of patients required PPM within 30 days following the procedure. Procedure-related high-degree atrioventricular block (HAVB) occurs mainly in the periprocedural period within 24 h following TAVI; however 2–7% of patients [37, 38] were shown to experience delayed HAVB ≥48 h after the procedure as self-expandable valve keeps expanding even after the implantation. Therefore, continuous rhythm monitoring is currently recommended up to 72 h [39]. On the other hand, a recent report [37] demonstrated that no patient with normal post-TAVI electrocardiogram experienced delayed HAVB up to 8 days after TAVI. Until now, an evidence-based strategy has not been established for monitoring duration, and the minimum required duration remains unclear. Therefore, operators should carefully assess the risk of HAVB in each patient according to the risk factors, such as the presence of intraoperative heart block and new-onset left bundle branch block.

24.3   The Results of Clinical Trials (Table 24.1)

24.3.1 CoreValve US Pivotal Trial

Extreme Risk Study of the CoreValve US Pivotal Trial [40] is the initial multicenter, nonrandomized study that investigated the safety and efficacy of CoreValve in patients at prohibitive risk for SAVR. A total of 486 patients from 41 clinical sites underwent TAVI with average age of 83.2 years old and predicted mortality at 30 days based on Society of Thoracic Surgeons (STS) scores of 10.3%. The primary endpoint of all-cause death or major stroke at 1 year was 26% and was significantly lower than a prespecified objective performance goal (43%; $P < 0.0001$). The rate of major stroke was 2.3% at 1 month and remained low throughout a year with 4.1%. The US CoreValve High-Risk Study [41] was a first multicenter, randomized, non-inferiority trial using CoreValve including 795 patients from 45 US centers. Patients who had symptomatic severe aortic stenosis and are at increased surgical risk were randomized in a 1:1 fashion to TAVI with CoreValve vs. SAVR. Average patient age was 83.2 years old, and the average STS score was 7.4%. All-cause death at 1 year was significantly lower in the TAVI group than in the SAVR group (14.2 vs. 19.1%, $P < 0.001$ for non-inferiority and $P = 0.04$ for superiority). Exploratory analyses of the secondary endpoint suggested that the rate of major adverse cardiovascular or cerebrovascular events at 1 year, including all-cause mortality, myocardial infarction, any stroke, and re-intervention, was significantly lower in the TAVI group than in the surgical group (20.4% vs. 27.3%, $P = 0.03$). Valve functions such as mean aortic valve gradient and effective orifice area were non-inferior in TAVI compared to SAVR shown by hierarchical testing. Rates of moderate or severe paravalvular regurgitation, new permanent pacemaker implantation, and major vascular complications were higher in TAVI, while bleeding, acute kidney injury, and new-onset or worsening atrial fibrillation were significantly more frequent in SAVR. These data supported the US FDA's decision to approve the device for patients at high risk for surgery. At the 3-year outcome presented at ACC 2016 Chicago, IL., the trend was still consistent; the rate of mortality or stroke was significantly lower in TAVI than SAVR (37.3% vs. 46.7%, $P = 0.006$).

24.3.2 NOTION Trial

NOTION (Nordic Aortic Valve Intervention) trial [42] was the first all-comers trial to randomize patients to TAVI with CoreValve or SAVR and enrolled 280 patients older than 70 years with severe aortic stenosis at 3 Nordic centers. Mean age was 79 years, and 81.8% were low-risk patients with predicted mortality at 30 days based on STS score of less than 4. One-year results showed no significant differences in the primary

Table 24.1 Clinical trials

Trial (Ref. #)	Location	Surgical risk	Device	Patients	Age	STS score
CoreValve US Pivotal (extreme risk) [40]	41 sites (United States)	Prohibitive risk	CoreValve	Single arm $N = 489$	83.2 years	10.3%
CoreValve US Pivotal (high risk) [41]	45 sites (United States)	High risk	CoreValve	Intention-to-treat/as treatedTAVR $N = 394/390$SAVR $N = 401/357$	TAVR 83.1 yearsSAVR 83.2 years	TAVR 7.3%SAVR 7.5%
Notion trial [42]	2 sites in Denmark and 1 in Sweden	All comer>70 years old	CoreValve	Intention-to-treat/as treatedTAVR $N = 145/139$SAVR $N = 135/135$	TAVR 79.2 yearsSAVR 79.0 years	TAVR 2.9%SAVR 3.1%
SURTAVI trial [2]	87 sites international	Intermediate risk	CoreValve 86%CoreValve Evolut R 14%	Intention-to-treat/modified intention-to-treatTAVR $N = 879/864$SAVR $N = 867/796$	TAVR 79.9 yearsSAVR 79.7 years	TAVR 4.4%SAVR 4.5%

Trial (Ref. #)	Access	30-day outcome	Long-term outcome
CoreValve US Pivotal (extreme risk) [40]	Iliofemoral 100%	All-cause mortality 8.3%Any stroke 4.0%	All-cause mortality or major stroke at 1 year (primary) 26.0%; $P < 0.001$ compared with prespecified objective performance goal (43.0%)All-cause mortality at 1 year 24.3%
CoreValve US Pivotal (high risk) [41]	Iliofemoral 82.8%Alternative 17.2%	All-cause mortality TAVR 3.3% vs. SAVR 4.5%; $P = 0.43$Any stroke TAVR 4.9% vs. SAVR 6.2%; $P = 0.46$	All-cause mortality at 1 year (primary) TAVR 14.2% vs. SAVR 19.1%; $P < 0.001$ for non-inferiority; $P = 0.04$ for superiorityStroke at 1 year TAVR 8.8% vs. SAVR 12.6%; $P = 0.10$
Notion trial [42]	Iliofemoral 96.5%Subclavian 3.5%	All-cause mortality TAVR 2.1% vs. SAVR 3.7%; $P = 0.43$Any stroke TAVR 1.4% vs. SAVR 3.0%; $P = 0.37$	All-cause mortality, stroke, or myocardial infarction at 1 year (primary) TAVR 13.1% vs. SAVR 16.3%; $P = 0.43$ for superiorityAll-cause mortality at 1 year TAVR 4.9% vs. SAVR 7.5%; $P = 0.38$
SURTAVI trial [2]	Iliofemoral 93.6%Direct aortic 4.1%Subclavian 2.3%	All-cause mortality TAVR 2.2% vs. SAVR 1.7%; 95% Credible interval −0.9 to 1.8Any stroke TAVR 3.4% vs. SAVR 5.6%; Credible interval −4.2 to −0.2	All-cause mortality or disabling stroke at 2 years (primary) TAVR 12.6% vs. SAVR 14.0%; $P = 0.43$ for non-inferiority, >0.999All-cause mortality at 1 year TAVR 6.7% vs. SAVR 6.8%; Credible interval −2.7 to 2.4All-cause mortality at 2 year TAVR 11.4% vs. SAVR 11.6%; Credible interval −3.8 to 3.3

endpoint, composite rate of death from any cause, stroke, or myocardial infarction, between those undergoing TAVI and those undergoing SAVR (13.1% vs. 16.3%; $p = 0.43$ for superiority). TAVI group had higher rate of pacemaker implantation, higher incidence of aortic valve regurgitation, and higher New York Heart Association (NYHA) functional class at 1 year. On the other hand, SAVR group showed smaller effective orifice area after surgery and more episodes of bleeding, cardiogenic shock, acute kidney injury, and new-onset or worsening atrial fibrillation. The higher incidence of post-procedural aortic valve regurgitation and conduction abnormality of TAVI may be associated with worse NYHA functional class at 1 year.

24.3.3 SURTAVI Trial

The SURTAVI (Surgical Replacement and Transcatheter Aortic Valve Implantation) trial [2] is a global, multicenter, randomized trial evaluating TAVI with CoreValve (86%) or CoreValve Evolut R (14%) vs. SAVR for 2 years in intermediate surgical-risk patients. Intermediate surgical risk was determined by the value of STS score or nontraditional factors like coexisting illnesses, frailty, and disability. In 1660 patients who underwent an attempted TAVI ($n = 864$) or SAVR ($n = 796$), the average patient age was 79.8 years old and STS score was 4.5%. The estimated incidence of the primary endpoint at 24 months, consisting of a composite of death from any cause or disabling stroke, was 12.6% in the TAVI group and 14.0% in the surgery group (95% credible interval for difference, −5.2 to 2.3%; posterior probability of non-inferiority, >0.999). Similar to previous trials, TAVI was associated with higher rate of post-procedural pacemaker implantation, while SAVR had higher rates of acute kidney injury and atrial fibrillation. Although TAVI resulted in more frequent moderate or severe paravalvular regurgitation, TAVI had greater aortic valve area and lower mean pressure gradient than SAVR. Structural valve deterioration was not detected in either group during 24 months of follow-up.

From these results, TAVI is currently increasingly being used in patients who have lower-risk profiles of SAVR and longer life expectancy. In August of 2016, Medtronic has received CE marking for CoreValve Evolut R system to include patients considered at intermediate risk for SAVR, and, thereafter, in July of 2017, the FDA cleared an additional indication to expand CoreValve Evolut R use for intermediate-risk patients. Recently, Medtronic started a new clinical trial comparing TAVI vs. SAVR in patients who have a low predicted risk of operative mortality for SAVR, i.e., predicted risk of mortality <3% at 30 days. This clinical trial will include 1200 patients with a randomization in a 1:1 fashion and aims to investigate non-inferiority of TAVI to SAVR in terms of all-cause mortality or disabling stroke at 2 years. The result of this study may support further shifting of TAVI toward lower surgical-risk patients. However, as demonstrated in clinical trials, TAVI is consistently associated with higher rates of PVL and permanent pacemaker implantation compared with SAVR. New-generation Medtronic devices are addressing these issues, and recent retrospective studies have demonstrated superiority of CoreValve Evolut R to Corevalve [43, 44]. The need for new permanent pacemaker implantation was shown to be significantly lower in CoreValve Evolut R than CoreValve (22.7% vs. 35.3%; $p = 0.008$) with the lower rate of moderate or severe PVL in CoreValve Evolut R (9.0% vs. 16.7%; $p = 0.044$). The recapture technology can optimize the valve position, which allows one to obtain better sealing of the native aortic annulus and less trauma to the conduction system of the left ventricular outflow tract. The newest CoreValve Evolut PRO with an outer wrap also showed favorable outcomes in the Medtronic Evolut PRO Clinical Study ($n = 60$) [45]. No incident of moderate or severe PVL was reported at 30 days, and 72.4% of patients experienced none or traces of paravalvular leak. In addition, incidence of new permanent pacemaker implantation is reported to be 10%. Until now, no study has directly compared CoreValve Evolut PRO with the previous devices, and results are currently being awaited.

24.4 Future Perspective

Medtronic transcatheter heart valve redesign, together with the operators' experience, has reduced TAVI-related complications such as vascular complications, paravalvular leak, and pacemaker implantation. Evolut R provides an option for valve recapture and repositioning that can assist the precise deployment of the valve, together with the reduced delivery profile using the InLine system, adding compatibility with small iliofemoral vessels and contributing to less vascular complications. The most recent commercially available Evolut PRO is equipped with an outer wrap designed to enhance contact between the valve and the aortic annulus.

Ongoing and future clinical studies, as well as experience in clinical practice, will prove its efficacy to reduce paravalvular leak. However, many challenges are still ahead for the evolution of the device, as the indication of TAVI has continuously been broadened to patients who have lower surgical-risk profiles and longer life expectancy. Future technologies will address the remaining issues associated with TAVI, such as coronary access and long-term durability of bioprosthesis including possibility of TAVI in TAVI, and continue to pursue reduction in delivery profile and the rate of pacemaker implantation as well as the delivery system that facilitates easy and precise positioning of the valve.

24.5 Conclusion

Since it emerged as the first self-expandable transcatheter heart valve, Medtronic devices have been widely used for the treatment of patients who have severe aortic stenosis with higher surgical risk. Clinical trials have shown their efficacy on various patients with different comorbidities and surgical risks, with the development of designs to reduce the complications associated with TAVI. Ongoing randomized trials on low surgical-risk patients are expected to demonstrate non-inferiority to SAVR and broaden indications for younger and lower surgical-risk patients. However, there still remain issues of TAVI to be solved for the better outcomes and to secure long-term safety especially for durability of device, which warrants further effort and challenge for the improvement of the device, together with the robust results from clinical trials with long-term follow-up.

Acknowledgments Armando Vergara-Martel: The Valve and Structural Heart Disease Intervention Center, Division of Cardiovascular Medicine, Harrington Heart and Vascular Institute, University Hospitals Cleveland Medical Center.

COI Disclosure Dr. Patel reports honoraria and personal fees from Abbott Vascular, Boston Scientific, and Medtronic. Dr. Kalra reports personal fees from Medtronic and Philips. Dr. Attizzani is a consultant and proctor for Edwards Lifesciences and Medtronic; consultant for Abbott Vascular. The remaining authors report no conflicts of interest.

References

1. Leon MB, Smith CR, Mack MJ, Makkar RR, Svensson LG, Kodali SK, Thourani VH, Tuzcu EM, Miller DC, Herrmann HC, Doshi D, Cohen DJ, Pichard AD, Kapadia S, Dewey T, Babaliaros V, Szeto WY, Williams MR, Kereiakes D, Zajarias A, Greason KL, Whisenant BK, Hodson RW, Moses JW, Trento A, Brown DL, Fearon WF, Pibarot P, Hahn RT, Jaber WA, Anderson WN, Alu MC, Webb JG, Investigators P. Transcatheter or surgical aortic-valve replacement in intermediate-risk patients. N Engl J Med. 2016;374:1609–20.

2. Reardon MJ, Van Mieghem NM, Popma JJ, Kleiman NS, Sondergaard L, Mumtaz M, Adams DH, Deeb GM, Maini B, Gada H, Chetcuti S, Gleason T, Heiser J, Lange R, Merhi W, Oh JK, Olsen PS, Piazza N, Williams M, Windecker S, Yakubov SJ, Grube E, Makkar R, Lee JS, Conte J, Vang E, Nguyen H, Chang Y, Mugglin AS, Serruys PW, Kappetein AP, Investigators S. Surgical or transcatheter aortic-valve replacement in intermediate-risk patients. N Engl J Med. 2017;376:1321–31.

3. Husser O, Pellegrini C, Kessler T, Burgdorf C, Thaller H, Mayr NP, Ott I, Kasel AM, Schunkert H, Kastrati A, Hengstenberg C. Outcomes after transcatheter aortic valve replacement using a novel balloon-expandable transcatheter heart valve: a single-center experience. JACC Cardiovasc Interv. 2015;8:1809–16.

4. Kalra SS, Firoozi S, Yeh J, Blackman DJ, Rashid S, Davies S, Moat N, Dalby M, Kabir T, Khogali SS, Anderson RA, Groves PH, Mylotte D, Hildick-Smith D, Rampat R, Kovac J, Gunarathne A, Laborde JC, Brecker SJ. Initial experience of a second-generation self-expanding transcatheter aortic valve: the UK & Ireland Evolut R Implanters' registry. JACC Cardiovasc Interv. 2017;10:276–82.

5. Binder RK, Webb JG, Willson AB, Urena M, Hansson NC, Norgaard BL, Pibarot P, Barbanti M, Larose E, Freeman M, Dumont E, Thompson C, Wheeler M, Moss RR, Yang TH, Pasian S, Hague CJ, Nguyen G, Raju R, Toggweiler S, Min JK, Wood DA, Rodes-Cabau J, Leipsic J. The impact of integration of a multidetector computed tomography annulus area sizing algorithm on outcomes of transcatheter aortic valve replacement: a prospective, multicenter, controlled trial. J Am Coll Cardiol. 2013;62:431–8.

6. Okuyama K, Jilaihawi H, Kashif M, Takahashi N, Chakravarty T, Pokhrel H, Patel J, Forrester JS, Nakamura M, Cheng W, Makkar RR. Transfemoral access assessment for transcatheter aortic valve replacement: evidence-based application of computed

tomography over invasive angiography. Circ Cardiovasc Imaging. 2015;8:e001995.

7. Willson AB, Webb JG, Labounty TM, Achenbach S, Moss R, Wheeler M, Thompson C, Min JK, Gurvitch R, Norgaard BL, Hague CJ, Toggweiler S, Binder R, Freeman M, Poulter R, Poulsen S, Wood DA, Leipsic J. 3-dimensional aortic annular assessment by multidetector computed tomography predicts moderate or severe paravalvular regurgitation after transcatheter aortic valve replacement: a multicenter retrospective analysis. J Am Coll Cardiol. 2012;59:1287–94.

8. Takagi K, Latib A, Al-Lamee R, Mussardo M, Montorfano M, Maisano F, Godino C, Chieffo A, Alfieri O, Colombo A. Predictors of moderate-to-severe paravalvular aortic regurgitation immediately after CoreValve implantation and the impact of postdilatation. Catheter Cardiovasc Interv. 2011;78:432–43.

9. Detaint D, Lepage L, Himbert D, Brochet E, Messika-Zeitoun D, Iung B, Vahanian A. Determinants of significant paravalvular regurgitation after transcatheter aortic valve: implantation impact of device and annulus discongruence. JACC Cardiovasc Interv. 2009;2:821–7.

10. Abdel-Wahab M, Mehilli J, Frerker C, Neumann FJ, Kurz T, Tolg R, Zachow D, Guerra E, Massberg S, Schafer U, El-Mawardy M, Richardt G, investigators C. Comparison of balloon-expandable vs self-expandable valves in patients undergoing transcatheter aortic valve replacement: the CHOICE randomized clinical trial. JAMA. 2014;311:1503–14.

11. Khawaja MZ, Rajani R, Cook A, Khavandi A, Moynagh A, Chowdhary S, Spence MS, Brown S, Khan SQ, Walker N, Trivedi U, Hutchinson N, De Belder AJ, Moat N, Blackman DJ, Levy RD, Manoharan G, Roberts D, Khogali SS, Crean P, Brecker SJ, Baumbach A, Mullen M, Laborde JC, Hildick-Smith D. Permanent pacemaker insertion after CoreValve transcatheter aortic valve implantation: incidence and contributing factors (the UK CoreValve Collaborative). Circulation. 2011;123:951–60.

12. Debry N, Sudre A, Elquodeimat I, Delhaye C, Schurtz G, Bical A, Koussa M, Fattouch K, Modine T. Prognostic value of the ratio between prosthesis area and indexed annulus area measured by MultiSlice-CT for transcatheter aortic valve implantation procedures. J Geriatr Cardiol. 2016;13:483–8.

13. Dvir D, Webb JG, Piazza N, Blanke P, Barbanti M, Bleiziffer S, Wood DA, Mylotte D, Wilson AB, Tan J, Stub D, Tamburino C, Lange R, Leipsic J. Multicenter evaluation of transcatheter aortic valve replacement using either SAPIEN XT or CoreValve: degree of device oversizing by computed-tomography and clinical outcomes. Catheter Cardiovasc Interv. 2015;86:508–15.

14. Genereux P, Webb JG, Svensson LG, Kodali SK, Satler LF, Fearon WF, Davidson CJ, Eisenhauer AC, Makkar RR, Bergman GW, Babaliaros V, Bavaria JE, Velazquez OC, Williams MR, Hueter I, Xu K, Leon MB, Investigators PT. Vascular complications after

transcatheter aortic valve replacement: insights from the PARTNER (Placement of AoRTic TraNscathetER Valve) trial. J Am Coll Cardiol. 2012;60:1043–52.

15. Ducrocq G, Francis F, Serfaty JM, Himbert D, Maury JM, Pasi N, Marouene S, Provenchere S, Iung B, Castier Y, Leseche G, Vahanian A. Vascular complications of transfemoral aortic valve implantation with the Edwards SAPIEN prosthesis: incidence and impact on outcome. EuroIntervention. 2010;5:666–72.

16. Toggweiler S, Gurvitch R, Leipsic J, Wood DA, Willson AB, Binder RK, Cheung A, Ye J, Webb JG. Percutaneous aortic valve replacement: vascular outcomes with a fully percutaneous procedure. J Am Coll Cardiol. 2012;59:113–8.

17. Grube E, Van Mieghem NM, Bleiziffer S, Modine T, Bosmans J, Manoharan G, Linke A, Scholtz W, Tchetche D, Finkelstein A, Trillo R, Fiorina C, Walton A, Malkin CJ, Oh JK, Qiao H, Windecker S, Investigators FS. Clinical outcomes with a repositionable self-expanding transcatheter aortic valve prosthesis: the International FORWARD Study. J Am Coll Cardiol. 2017;70:845–53.

18. Lenders GD, Collas V, Hernandez JM, Legrand V, Danenberg HD, den Heijer P, Rodrigus IE, Paelinck BP, Vrints CJ, Bosmans JM. Depth of valve implantation, conduction disturbances and pacemaker implantation with CoreValve and CoreValve Accutrak system for transcatheter aortic valve implantation, a multi-center study. Int J Cardiol. 2014;176:771–5.

19. Petronio AS, Sinning JM, Van Mieghem N, Zucchelli G, Nickenig G, Bekeredjian R, Bosmans J, Bedogni F, Branny M, Stangl K, Kovac J, Schiltgen M, Kraus S, de Jaegere P. Optimal implantation depth and adherence to guidelines on permanent pacing to improve the results of transcatheter aortic valve replacement with the medtronic corevalve system: the CoreValve Prospective, International, Post-Market ADVANCE-II Study. JACC Cardiovasc Interv. 2015;8:837–46.

20. Sherif MA, Abdel-Wahab M, Stocker B, Geist V, Richardt D, Tolg R, Richardt G. Anatomic and procedural predictors of paravalvular aortic regurgitation after implantation of the Medtronic CoreValve bioprosthesis. J Am Coll Cardiol. 2010;56:1623–9.

21. Guetta V, Goldenberg G, Segev A, Dvir D, Kornowski R, Finckelstein A, Hay I, Goldenberg I, Glikson M. Predictors and course of high-degree atrioventricular block after transcatheter aortic valve implantation using the CoreValve Revalving System. Am J Cardiol. 2011;108:1600–5.

22. Ferreira ND, Caeiro D, Adao L, Oliveira M, Goncalves H, Ribeiro J, Teixeira M, Albuquerque A, Primo J, Braga P, Simoes L, Ribeiro VG. Incidence and predictors of permanent pacemaker requirement after transcatheter aortic valve implantation with a self-expanding bioprosthesis. Pacing Clin Electrophysiol. 2010;33:1364–72.

23. Schulz E, Jabs A, Gori T, von Bardeleben S, Hink U, Kasper-Konig W, Vahl CF, Munzel T. Transcatheter aortic valve implantation with the new-generation

Evolut R: comparison with CoreValve(R) in a single center cohort. Int J Cardiol Heart Vasc. 2016;12:52–6.

24. Alli OO, Booker JD, Lennon RJ, Greason KL, Rihal CS, Holmes DR Jr. Transcatheter aortic valve implantation: assessing the learning curve. JACC Cardiovasc Interv. 2012;5:72–9.

25. Ben-Dor I, Pichard AD, Satler LF, Goldstein SA, Syed AI, Gaglia MA Jr, Weissman G, Maluenda G, Gonzalez MA, Wakabayashi K, Collins SD, Torguson R, Okubagzi P, Xue Z, Kent KM, Lindsay J, Waksman R. Complications and outcome of balloon aortic valvuloplasty in high-risk or inoperable patients. JACC Cardiovasc Interv. 2010;3:1150–6.

26. Percutaneous balloon aortic valvuloplasty. Acute and 30-day follow-up results in 674 patients from the NHLBI balloon valvuloplasty registry. Circulation. 1991;84:2383–97.

27. Liao YB, Meng Y, Zhao ZG, Zuo ZL, Li YJ, Xiong TY, Cao JY, Xu YN, Feng Y, Chen M. Meta-analysis of the effectiveness and safety of transcatheter aortic valve implantation without balloon predilation. Am J Cardiol. 2016;117:1629–35.

28. Auffret V, Regueiro A, Campelo-Parada F, Del Trigo M, Chiche O, Chamandi C, Puri R, Rodes-Cabau J. Feasibility, safety, and efficacy of transcatheter aortic valve replacement without balloon predilation: a systematic review and meta-analysis. Catheter Cardiovasc Interv. 2017;90:839–50.

29. Ciuca C, Tarantini G, Latib A, Gasparetto V, Savini C, Di Eusanio M, Napodano M, Maisano F, Gerosa G, Sticchi A, Marzocchi A, Alfieri O, Colombo A, Saia F. Trans-subclavian versus transapical access for transcatheter aortic valve implantation: a multicenter study. Catheter Cardiovasc Interv. 2016;87:332–8.

30. Petronio AS, De Carlo M, Bedogni F, Maisano F, Ettori F, Klugmann S, Poli A, Marzocchi A, Santoro G, Napodano M, Ussia GP, Giannini C, Brambilla N, Colombo A. 2-year results of CoreValve implantation through the subclavian access: a propensity-matched comparison with the femoral access. J Am Coll Cardiol. 2012;60:502–7.

31. Dvir D, Webb JG, Bleiziffer S, Pasic M, Waksman R, Kodali S, Barbanti M, Latib A, Schaefer U, Rodes-Cabau J, Treede H, Piazza N, Hildick-Smith D, Himbert D, Walther T, Hengstenberg C, Nissen H, Bekeredjian R, Presbitero P, Ferrari E, Segev A, de Weger A, Windecker S, Moat NE, Napodano M, Wilbring M, Cerillo AG, Brecker S, Tchetche D, Lefevre T, De Marco F, Fiorina C, Petronio AS, Teles RC, Testa L, Laborde JC, Leon MB, Kornowski R, Valve-in-Valve International Data Registry I. Transcatheter aortic valve implantation in failed bioprosthetic surgical valves. JAMA. 2014;312:162–70.

32. Simonato M, Webb J, Kornowski R, Vahanian A, Frerker C, Nissen H, Bleiziffer S, Duncan A, Rodes-Cabau J, Attizzani GF, Horlick E, Latib A, Bekeredjian R, Barbanti M, Lefevre T, Cerillo A, Hernandez JM, Bruschi G, Spargias K, Iadanza A, Brecker S, Palma JH, Finkelstein A, Abdel-Wahab M, Lemos P, Petronio AS, Champagnac D, Sinning JM,

Salizzoni S, Napodano M, Fiorina C, Marzocchi A, Leon M, Dvir D. Transcatheter replacement of failed bioprosthetic valves: large multicenter assessment of the effect of implantation depth on hemodynamics after aortic valve-in-valve. Circ Cardiovasc Interv. 2016;9:e003651.

33. Midha PA, Raghav V, Condado JF, Okafor IU, Lerakis S, Thourani VH, Babaliaros V, Yoganathan AP. Valve type, size, and deployment location affect hemodynamics in an in vitro valve-in-valve model. JACC Cardiovasc Interv. 2016;9:1618–28.

34. Diemert P, Seiffert M, Frerker C, Thielsen T, Kreidel F, Bader R, Schirmer J, Conradi L, Koschyk D, Schnabel R, Reichenspurner H, Blankenberg S, Kuck KH, Treede H, Schaefer U. Valve-in-valve implantation of a novel and small self-expandable transcatheter heart valve in degenerated small surgical bioprostheses: the Hamburg experience. Catheter Cardiovasc Interv. 2014;84:486–93.

35. Bapat V, Adams B, Attia R, Noorani A, Thomas M. Neo-annulus: a reference plane in a surgical heart valve to facilitate a valve-in-valve procedure. Catheter Cardiovasc Interv. 2015;85:685–91.

36. Popma JJ, Reardon MJ, Khabbaz K, Harrison JK, Hughes GC, Kodali S, George I, Deeb GM, Chetcuti S, Kipperman R, Brown J, Qiao H, Slater J, Williams MR. Early clinical outcomes after transcatheter aortic valve replacement using a novel self-expanding bioprosthesis in patients with severe aortic stenosis who are suboptimal for surgery: results of the Evolut R US study. JACC Cardiovasc Interv. 2017;10:268–75.

37. Toggweiler S, Stortecky S, Holy E, Zuk K, Cuculi F, Nietlispach F, Sabti Z, Suciu R, Maier W, Jamshidi P, Maisano F, Windecker S, Kobza R, Wenaweser P, Luscher TF, Binder RK. The electrocardiogram after transcatheter aortic valve replacement determines the risk for post-procedural high-degree AV block and the need for telemetry monitoring. JACC Cardiovasc Interv. 2016;9:1269–76.

38. Chorianopoulos E, Krumsdorf U, Pleger ST, Katus HA, Bekeredjian R. Incidence of late occurring bradyarrhythmias after TAVI with the self-expanding CoreValve((R)) aortic bioprosthesis. Clin Res Cardiol. 2012;101:349–55.

39. Kappetein AP, Head SJ, Genereux P, Piazza N, van Mieghem NM, Blackstone EH, Brott TG, Cohen DJ, Cutlip DE, van Es GA, Hahn RT, Kirtane AJ, Krucoff MW, Kodali S, Mack MJ, Mehran R, Rodes-Cabau J, Vranckx P, Webb JG, Windecker S, Serruys PW, Leon MB. Updated standardized endpoint definitions for transcatheter aortic valve implantation: the valve academic research consortium-2 consensus document. J Am Coll Cardiol. 2012;60:1438–54.

40. Popma JJ, Adams DH, Reardon MJ, Yakubov SJ, Kleiman NS, Heimansohn D, Hermiller J Jr, Hughes GC, Harrison JK, Coselli J, Diez J, Kafi A, Schreiber T, Gleason TG, Conte J, Buchbinder M, Deeb GM, Carabello B, Serruys PW, Chenoweth S, Oh JK, CoreValve United States Clinical I. Transcatheter aortic valve replacement using a self-expanding biopros-

thesis in patients with severe aortic stenosis at extreme risk for surgery. J Am Coll Cardiol. 2014;63:1972–81.

41. Adams DH, Popma JJ, Reardon MJ, Yakubov SJ, Coselli JS, Deeb GM, Gleason TG, Buchbinder M, Hermiller J Jr, Kleiman NS, Chetcuti S, Heiser J, Merhi W, Zorn G, Tadros P, Robinson N, Petrossian G, Hughes GC, Harrison JK, Conte J, Maini B, Mumtaz M, Chenoweth S, Oh JK, Investigators USCC. Transcatheter aortic-valve replacement with a self-expanding prosthesis. N Engl J Med. 2014;370:1790–8.

42. Thyregod HG, Steinbruchel DA, Ihlemann N, Nissen H, Kjeldsen BJ, Petursson P, Chang Y, Franzen OW, Engstrom T, Clemmensen P, Hansen PB, Andersen LW, Olsen PS, Sondergaard L. Transcatheter versus surgical aortic valve replacement in patients with severe aortic valve stenosis: 1-year results from the all-comers NOTION randomized clinical trial. J Am Coll Cardiol. 2015;65:2184–94.

43. Gomes B, Geis NA, Chorianopoulos E, Meder B, Leuschner F, Katus HA, Bekeredjian R. Improvements of procedural results with a new-generation self-expanding transfemoral aortic valve prosthesis in comparison to the old-generation device. J Interv Cardiol. 2017;30:72–8.

44. Giannini C, De Carlo M, Tamburino C, Ettori F, Latib AM, Bedogni F, Bruschi G, Presbitero P, Poli A, Fabbiocchi F, Violini R, Trani C, Giudice P, Barbanti M, Adamo M, Colombo P, Benincasa S, Agnifili M, Petronio AS. Transcathether aortic valve implantation with the new repositionable self-expandable Evolut R versus CoreValve system: a case-matched comparison. Int J Cardiol. 2017;243:126–31.

45. Forrest JK, Mangi AA, Popma JJ, Khabbaz K, Reardon MJ, Kleiman NS, Yakubov SJ, Watson D, Kodali S, George I, Tadros P, Zorn GL 3rd, Brown J, Kipperman R, Saul S, Qiao H, Oh JK, Williams MR. Early outcomes with the Evolut PRO repositionable self-expanding transcatheter aortic valve with pericardial wrap. JACC Cardiovasc Interv. 2018;11:160–8.

New Valve Technology Program for Transcatheter Aortic Valve Implantation

25

Nicola Corcione, Salvatore Giordano, Alberto Morello, and Arturo Giordano

25.1 Introduction

Since the pioneering efforts of Alain Cribier [1], there are now several different new-generation devices for transcatheter aortic valve implantation (TAVI), also called transcatheter aortic valve replacement (TAVR), in patients with severe aortic stenosis or degenerated bioprosthesis at intermediate or high surgical risk [2–4], which have clearly built their successes upon the foundations of first-generation devices, mainly SAPIEN XT (Edwards Lifesciences, Irvine, CA, USA) and CoreValve (Medtronic, Minneapolis, MN, USA) [5–9]. However, new developments continue, and indeed New Valve Technology (Hechingen, Germany) has recently obtained CE mark for a novel self-expandable device, the Allegra [10–12].

25.2 Technical Features

The Allegra TAVI system is a catheter-based, TAVI system (Fig. 25.1). It has received CE mark for the treatment of severe calcified aortic valve stenosis in high-risk patients with elevated surgical risk. Accordingly, this device is intended to replace a degenerative calcified aortic heart valve with the minimal invasive transcatheter implantation technique [10].

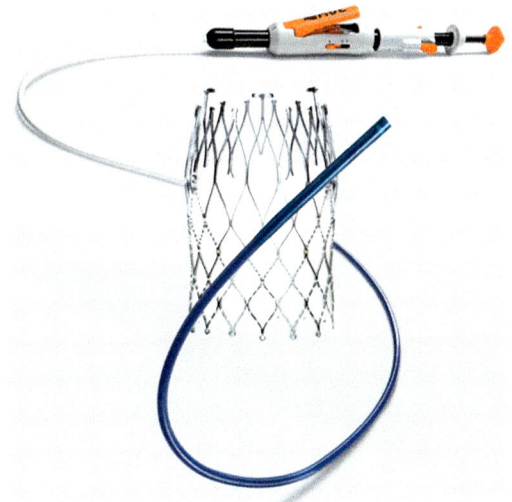

Fig. 25.1 The Allegra transcatheter aortic valve implantation system, consisting of the Allegra bioprosthesis, the delivery system, and the loading system. Courtesy of New Valve Technology

N. Corcione · S. Giordano · A. Giordano (✉)
Interventional Cardiology Unit, Pineta Grande Hospital, Castel Volturno, Italy
e-mail: arturogiordano@tin.it

A. Morello
Unità Operativa di Emodinamica, Casa di Salute Santa Lucia, San Giuseppe Vesuviano, Italy

© Springer Nature Switzerland AG 2019
A. Giordano et al. (eds.), *Transcatheter Aortic Valve Implantation*,
https://doi.org/10.1007/978-3-030-05912-5_25

The Allegra system consists of a bioprosthesis, a delivery system, and a loading system. Specifically, the bioprothesis is a trileaflet design supra-annular valve constructed with six individual parts of bovine pericardium. Three bovine pericardium segments constituting the skirt and three leaflets are sewed to the metallic frame in a semilunar fashion to form the valve coaptation plane. The stent is a nitinol laser-cut stent, with good radiopaque visibility and additional six gold radiopaque markers, where the valve is sutured in. The bioprosthesis is available in three different sizes, 23 mm, 27 mm, and 31 mm, for patients' native annulus size ranging from 19 mm up to 28 mm. The delivery system is based on the patented PermaFlow principle (Fig. 25.2), which ensures permanent blood flow condition during the bioprosthesis positioning and deployment sequences. The radiopaque marker rings provide a precise controlled release of the bioprosthesis in three steps. The catheter is characterized by an ideal balance of flexibility and stiffness. Finally, the loading system is a dedicated tool kit to load the bioprosthesis into the cartridge of the delivery system in a fast, easy, and intuitive loading. Notably, bioprostheses, delivery systems, and loading systems are developed, tested, and manufactured in Hechingen, Germany.

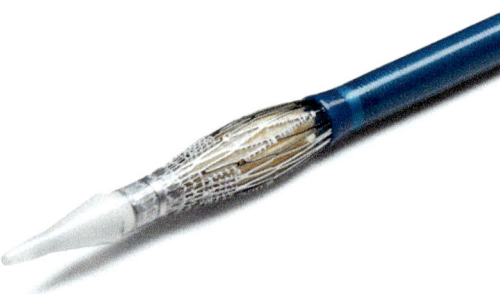

Fig. 25.2 The proprietary PermFlow deployment mechanism consists of the mechanically controlled delivery catheter unsheathing over the bioprosthesis coaptation plane, in order to expose the proximal free-cell stent frame. When the bioprothesis inflow is released, the valve is immediately competent in order to minimize any blood pressure drop. Courtesy of New Valve Technology

25.3   Peculiarities of Allegra

The benefits of the Allegra system are enabled by its design, which features a distinctive transcatheter aortic heart valve composed of a self-expandable stent frame with radiopaque gold markers and selected bovine pericardium [10–12]. The design of the stent frame allows a movement that can improve the bioprosthesis long-term durability. Tailored radial force distribution along the axis of the stent frame ensures safe anchoring in the annulus. In addition, movable points at the commissure reduce the mechanical stress on the leaflets by absorbing shocks. With the PermaFlow principle, the Allegra can be implanted in the correct position without compromising left ventricular outflow, allowing for implantation without rapid pacing. Finally, the supra-annular design leads to low gradients and high effective orifice areas.

25.4   Clinical Data

The Allegra system received CE mark in March 2017. Accordingly, and given the novelty of this device, only limited clinical evidence in support is available, but data to date appear promising. Specifically, Wenaweser et al. reported on the first-in-men study on the Allegra system in 2016 [10]. They included 21 patients with severe aortic stenosis, with device success in 86% of subjects and procedural success in 95% of patients, and a significant improvement in mean aortic gradient (from 48 mm to 9 mm) and aortic valve area (from 0.6 to 1.7 cm^2). Device success was not achieved because of aortic dissection shortly complicated by exitus (1 patient), valve embolization requiring bailout implantation of a different device (1 patient), and residual moderate aortic regurgitation (1 patient). Notably, permanent pacemaker implantation was required in 24% of cases. In addition, major vascular complications occurred in 14% of patients. Conversely, no case of stroke, transient ischemic attack, and life-threatening or major bleeding occurred. Clinical results were sustained from discharge up to 30 days of follow-up.

Similarly favorable results were reported in contemporary single-center series including 26 patients by Jagielak et al. [13]. Specifically, these authors highlighted that Allegra device success could be obtained in 96% of cases, despite one case of cardiac tamponade and another case of valve embolization requiring conversion to surgical aortic valve replacement. Intriguingly, in this series, no death occurred up to 1 month of follow-up, and in no patient was a permanent pacemaker implanted. Extended follow-up of these studies up to 12 months has shown favorable survival rates in such a high-risk cohort, without significant worsening post-procedural aortic regurgitation and consistently favorable valve hemodynamics.

Given its unique design, Allegra can be considered optimally suited for valve-in-valve procedures, as pioneered by Schäfer et al. [11]. Indeed, a dedicated in vitro study accompanied by a four-patient case series has been reported by Sedaghat et al. in 2018 [12], showing that this device can perform satisfactorily when implanted in Epic (St. Jude Medical, Saint Paul, MN, USA), Perimount (Edwards Lifesciences), Mosaic (Medtronic), Mitroflow (Sorin, Milan, Italy), Aspire (Vascutek, Inchinnan, UK), and Trifecta (St. Jude Medical) devices. Specifically, a dedicated hydronymic pulsatile model was used for in vitro testing, whereas all clinical procedures proved successful and uneventful.

These favorable pieces of evidence have provided support for ongoing trials on Allegra, which include the NVT ALLEGRA TAVI System TF in Failing Surgical Aortic Bioprosthesis (VIVALL) study [14] and the NVT ALLEGRA TAVI System TF in Failing Calcified Aortic Heart Valves in a Real-world Patient Population (FOLLOW) trial [15]. Specifically, the FOLLOW study will be a single-arm prospective study which will include 200 patients with severe aortic stenosis at high surgical risk, with a primary endpoint of cardiovascular death. The VIVALL trial is a single-arm prospective study aiming to enroll 30 patients requiring valve-in-valve transcatheter aortic valve implantation, with co-primary endpoints of post-procedural mean aortic gradient and 1 month survival.

25.5   Conclusions

The Allegra TAVI system appears as a useful adjunct to the interventionalist's armamentarium, given its favorable design features. Evidence to date support its expanded adoption for native valves as well as degenerated bioprostheses, with further insights coming from ongoing studies.

Conflicts of Interest Dr. Corcione has consulted for Abbott Vascular. Dr. A. Giordano has consulted for Abbott Vascular and Medtronic.

References

1. Cribier A, Eltchaninoff H, Bash A, Borenstein N, Tron C, Bauer F, Derumeaux G, Anselme F, Laborde F, Leon MB. Percutaneous transcatheter implantation of an aortic valve prosthesis for calcific aortic stenosis: first human case description. Circulation. 2002;106:3006–8.
2. Leon MB, Smith CR. Transcatheter aortic-valve replacement. N Engl J Med. 2016;375:700–1.
3. Giordano A, Corcione N, Biondi-Zoccai G, Berti S, Petronio AS, Pierli C, Presbitero P, Giudice P, Sardella G, Bartorelli AL, Bonmassari R, Indolfi C, Marchese A, Brscic E, Cremonesi A, Testa L, Brambilla N, Bedogni F. Patterns and trends of transcatheter aortic valve implantation in Italy: insights from RISPEVA. J Cardiovasc Med (Hagerstown). 2017;18:96–102.
4. Gatto L, Biondi-Zoccai G, Romagnoli E, Frati G, Prati F, Giordano A. New-generation devices for transcatheter aortic valve implantation. Minerva Cardioangiol. 2018;66(6):747–61. https://doi.org/10.23736/S0026-4725.18.04707-2.
5. Biondi-Zoccai G, Peruzzi M, Abbate A, Gertz ZM, Benedetto U, Tonelli E, D'Ascenzo F, Giordano A, Agostoni P, Frati G. Network meta-analysis on the comparative effectiveness and safety of transcatheter aortic valve implantation with CoreValve or Sapien devices versus surgical replacement. Heart Lung Vessel. 2014;6:232–43.
6. Makkar RR, Fontana GP, Jilaihawi H, Kapadia S, Pichard AD, Douglas PS, Thourani VH, Babaliaros VC, Webb JG, Herrmann HC, Bavaria JE, Kodali S, Brown DL, Bowers B, Dewey TM, Svensson LG, Tuzcu M, Moses JW, Williams MR, Siegel RJ, Akin JJ, Anderson WN, Pocock S, Smith CR, Leon MB, PARTNER Trial Investigators. Transcatheter aortic-valve replacement for inoperable severe aortic stenosis. N Engl J Med. 2012;366:1696–704.
7. Kodali SK, Williams MR, Smith CR, Svensson LG, Webb JG, Makkar RR, Fontana GP, Dewey TM, Thourani VH, Pichard AD, Fischbein M, Szeto WY, Lim S, Greason KL, Teirstein PS, Malaisrie SC,

Douglas PS, Hahn RT, Whisenant B, Zajarias A, Wang D, Akin JJ, Anderson WN, Leon MB, PARTNER Trial Investigators. Two-year outcomes after transcatheter or surgical aortic-valve replacement. N Engl J Med. 2012;366:1686–95.

8. Leon MB, Smith CR, Mack MJ, Makkar RR, Svensson LG, Kodali SK, Thourani VH, Tuzcu EM, Miller DC, Herrmann HC, Doshi D, Cohen DJ, Pichard AD, Kapadia S, Dewey T, Babaliaros V, Szeto WY, Williams MR, Kereiakes D, Zajarias A, Greason KL, Whisenant BK, Hodson RW, Moses JW, Trento A, Brown DL, Fearon WF, Pibarot P, Hahn RT, Jaber WA, Anderson WN, Alu MC, Webb JG, PARTNER 2 Investigators. Transcatheter or surgical aortic-valve replacement in intermediate-risk patients. N Engl J Med. 2016;374:1609–20.

9. Adams DH, Popma JJ, Reardon MJ, Yakubov SJ, Coselli JS, Deeb GM, Gleason TG, Buchbinder M, Hermiller J Jr, Kleiman NS, Chetcuti S, Heiser J, Merhi W, Zorn G, Tadros P, Robinson N, Petrossian G, Hughes GC, Harrison JK, Conte J, Maini B, Mumtaz M, Chenoweth S, Oh JK, U.S. CoreValve Clinical Investigators. Transcatheter aortic-valve replacement with a self-expanding prosthesis. N Engl J Med. 2014;370:1790–8.

10. Wenaweser P, Stortecky S, Schütz T, Praz F, Gloekler S, Windecker S, Elsässer A. Transcatheter aortic valve implantation with the NVT Allegra transcatheter heart valve system: first-in-human experience with a novel self-expanding transcatheter heart valve. EuroIntervention. 2016;12:71–7.

11. Schäfer U, Kalbacher D, Voigtländer L, Conradi L. First-in-human implantation of a novel self-expanding supra-annular transcatheter heart valve for transcatheter aortic valve implantation inside a small degenerated aortic surgical bioprosthesis. Catheter Cardiovasc Interv. 2018;92(7):1453–7. https://doi.org/10.1002/ccd.27466.

12. Sedaghat A, Sinning JM, Werner N, Nickenig G, Conradi L, Toggweiler S, Schäfer U. In vitro hydrodynamic and acute clinical performance of a novel self-expanding transcatheter heart valve in various surgical bioprostheses. EuroIntervention. 2018;13:2014–7.

13. Jagielak D, Kozaryn R, Ciecwierz D, Pawlaczyk R, Fijalkowski M, Rogowski J. Single-centre experience with the novel self-expanding NVT Allegra transcatheter aortic valve prosthesis. EuroPCR Book of Abstracts. 2016;1:427.

14. U.S. National Library of Medicine ClinicalTrials.gov—NVT ALLEGRA TAVI System TF in Failing Surgical Aortic Bioprosthesis (VIVALL). https://clinicaltrials.gov/ct2/show/NCT03287856. Accessed 8 Aug 2018.

15. U.S. National Library of Medicine ClinicalTrials.gov—NVT ALLEGRA TAVI System TF in Failing Calcified Aortic Heart Valves in a Real-world Patient Population (FOLLOW). https://clinicaltrials.gov/ct2/show/NCT03613246. Accessed 8 Aug 2018.

Self-Expanding vs. Balloon-Expandable Devices for Transcatheter Aortic Valve Implantation

26

Denise Todaro, Andrea Picci, Corrado Tamburino, and Marco Barbanti

26.1 Introduction

Since the first-in-human transcatheter aortic implantation (TAVI), also called transcatheter aortic valve replacement (TAVR), performed by Cribier in 2002 [1], the percutaneous treatment of aortic valve stenosis has had a widespread recognition, expanding his indications from the treatment of severe aortic stenosis in inoperable patients to high- and intermediate-risk patients [2–4].

The first prototype of transcatheter aortic valve (designed by Cribier and his start-up Percutaneous Valve Technologies) was a stainless steel stent (23 mm in diameter and 17 mm in height) that contained a trileaflet valve (at first made of polyurethane, but soon changed to bovine pericardium). The device was compatible with a 24-French introducer sheath and was initially implanted with an anterograde trans-septal approach. After a few years, this prototype evolved into the Cribier-Edwards valve (Edwards Lifesciences), and the original trans-septal route was abandoned in favor of the more reproducible transfemoral and transapical approaches [5]. At the same time, another device, the self-expanding CoreValve (Medtronic), made of a nitinol frame containing a porcine pericardial valve, had been developed. These two devices, which after a few

years obtained CE mark and US Food and Drug Administration (FDA) approval, can be considered the ancestors of all of the commercial devices now available.

In the last 15 years, TAVI technology has had an impressive advancement, transforming a challenging intervention into a very standardized and streamlined procedure [6]. The latest generation of TAVI devices have incorporated features to reduce the delivery catheter profile, facilitate deployment, and in some cases enable repositioning and retrieval capability [6]. According to the type of deployment, current TAVI devices can be divided into the categories of balloon-expandable, self-expanding, and mechanically expandable (Fig. 26.1).

Thus far, there are no clear indications for the use of transcatheter heart valve (THV) platform for different anatomical subsets. In this chapter we will provide a brief summary of the current TAVI technologies, and we will present several clinical scenarios in which a specific device could be more suitable than the others.

26.1.1 Balloon-Expandable Device

The Sapien 3 THV (Edwards Lifesciences) is the fourth-generation balloon-expandable by Edwards [7–12]. This is the only TAVI platform having a balloon-expandable deployment technique. Being available in four valve sizes (20, 23,

D. Todaro · A. Picci · C. Tamburino · M. Barbanti (✉)
Division of Cardiology, Ferrarotto Hospital,
University of Catania, Catania, Italy
e-mail: tambucor@uninct.it

© Springer Nature Switzerland AG 2019
A. Giordano et al. (eds.), *Transcatheter Aortic Valve Implantation*,
https://doi.org/10.1007/978-3-030-05912-5_26

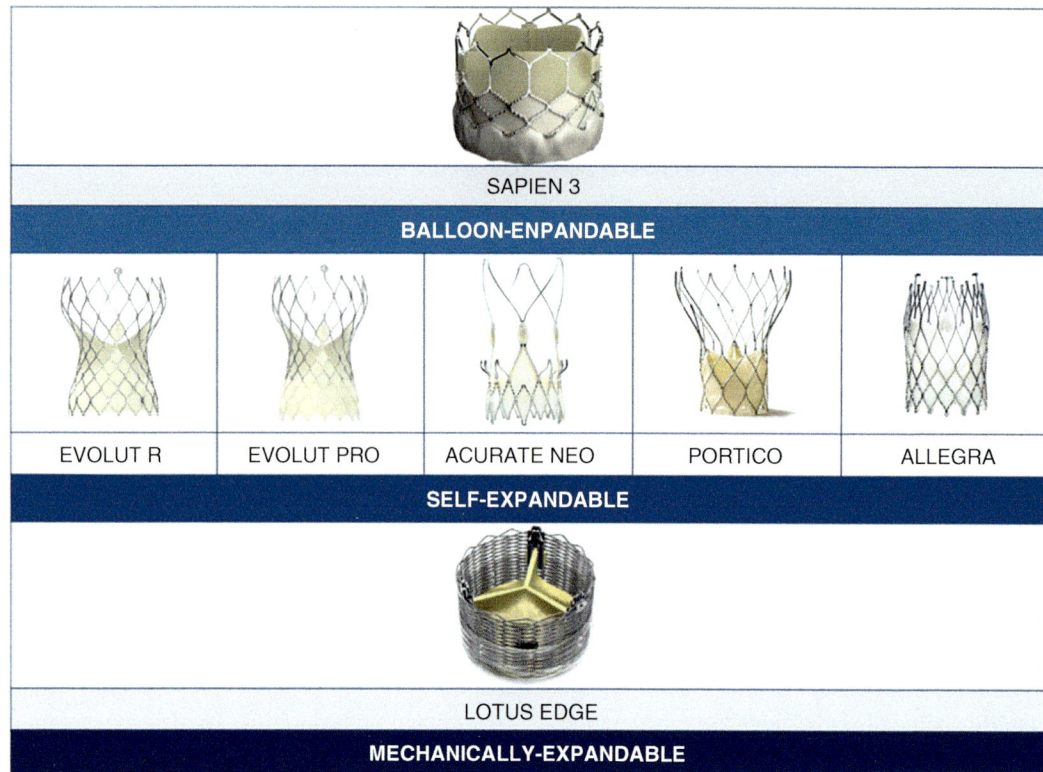

Fig. 26.1 Overview of the current TAVI devices used in clinical practice

26, and 29 mm), the Sapien 3 valve is designed with a cobalt-chromium frame, three bovine pericardial tissue leaflets, and a polyethylene terephthalate (PET) skirt at its inflow portion and outer PET skirt sealing skirt to reduce paravalvular leakage (Fig. 26.1 and Table 26.1).

The transfemoral Commander delivery system (Edwards Lifesciences) incorporates an inner balloon catheter, on which the prosthesis is crimped, and an outer deflectable flex catheter. The catheter offers dual articulation with partial and distal flew that enables crossing the aortic valve in challenging anatomies and controlled coaxial alignment. The handle incorporates a fine-adjustment wheel that allows advancing or retracting the balloon and that carries the valve several millimeters up or down within the annulus without pushing or pulling on the entire delivery system. The Commander delivery system is advanced through a 14-F (20-, 23-, 26-mm valves) and 16-F (29-mm valve) expandable eSheath (Edwards Lifesciences) (minimum

diameter, 5.5 mm). The Certitude delivery system (Edwards Lifesciences) is also commercially available for alternative access procedures in patients where transfemoral delivery may not be appropriate. The Certitude delivery system is compatible with an 18-F sheath for 20-, 23-, and 26-mm valves and a 21-F sheath for the 29-mm valve (Table 26.1).

26.1.2 Self-Expanding Devices

26.1.2.1 Evolut R and Evolut PRO

The CoreValve Evolut R device (Medtronic) (currently available in four device sizes of 23, 26, 29, and 34 mm, allowing the treatment of native valves with a perimeter of 56.5–94.2 mm) consists of a tricuspid valve obtained from porcine pericardial tissue, mounted and sutured inside a self-expanding nitinol frame (Fig. 26.1 and Table 26.1) [6]. The lower part of the device has a high radial force that allows for the

Table 26.1 Main characteristics of current transcatheter heart valves used in clinical practice

Device name	Valve structure	Access route, delivery system, and valve size	Reference access vessel diameter	Repositionable	Fully retrievable
Sapien 3 (Edwards Lifesciences)	Bovine pericardial tissue valve Balloon-expandable cobalt chromium frame	TF: Edwards eSheath 14 F (20, 23, 26 mm), 16 F (29 mm) TA, TAo: Certitude 18 F (20, 23, 26 mm), 21 F (29 mm)	≥5.0 mm (SAPIEN 3 20, 23, 26 mm) ≥5.5 mm (SAPIEN 3 29 mm)	No	No
Evolut R (Medtronic)	Porcine pericardial tissue valve Self-expanding nitinol frame	TF, TAo, TSc: EnVeo R 14Fr outer diameter (23, 26, 29 mm), EnVeo N 16Fr outer diameter (34 mm)	≥5.0 mm (Evolut R 23, 26, 29 mm) ≥5.5 mm (Evolut R 34 mm)	Yes	Yes
Evolut PRO (Medtronic)	Porcine pericardial tissue valve with outer porcine pericardial tissue wrap Self-expanding nitinol frame	TF, TAo, TSc: EnVeo N 16Fr outer diameter (23, 26, 29 mm)	≥5.5 mm	Yes	Yes
Portico (Abbott vascular)	Bovine pericardial tissue valve Self-expanding nitinol frame	TF, Tao, TSc: 18 F (23, 25 mm) 17 F (27, 29 mm)	≥6.0 mm	Yes	Yes
ACURATE neo (Boston Scientific)	Porcine pericardial tissue valve Self-expandable nitinol alloy stent	TF: 18 F outer diameter (S, M, L) TA: Sheathless 28 F (S, M, L)	≥6.0 mm	No	No
Lotus valve (Boston Scientific)	Bovine pericardial tissue valve Self-expanding, braided nitinol frame	TF: 18 F (23 mm) 20 F (25, 27 mm)	≥6.0 mm (lotus 23 mm) ≥6.5 mm (lotus 25, 27 mm)	Yes	Yes
Allegra (NVT AG)	Bovine pericardial tissue valve (annular skirt and leaflets) Self-expanding nitinol stent	TF: 18 F (23, 27, 31 mm)	≥6.0 mm	Yes	Yes

self-expansion and exclusion of native calcified valve leaflets. The central portion of the stent supports the valve.

As compared with the previous generation of CoreValve devices, the Evolut R provides several refinements to improve anatomical fit, annular sealing, and durability. In particular, the device is designed to enable recapturability and reposition-ability. The Evolut R frame is tailored to reduce the overall height while preserving the height of the pericardial skirt (13 mm) with an extended skirt of the inflow tract to provide a seal against paravalvular regurgitation (PVR). In addition, cell geometry has been redesigned to achieve optimized radial force.

The Evolut R has also been designed to be implanted through a 14-F compatible delivery system, the EnVeo R delivery system (Medtronic), which integrates an InLine sheath (Medtronic). This sheath slides against the capsule to allow vascular access that is the equivalent of a 14-F system (16 F for the Evolut R 34 mm). This means that the Evolut R system is now indicated to treat minimum access vessels of ≥5 mm (Evolut R 23, 26, 29 mm) and ≥5.5 mm (Evolut R 34 mm) (Table 26.1). Positioning accuracy is aided by the EnVeo R delivery system's 1:1 response. The EnVeo R provides the option to recapture and reposition up to three times before reaching the "point of no recapture."

The CoreValve Evolut PRO valve is the latest-generation Medtronic transcatheter aortic valve. The device obtained the FDA approval in March 2017 and the CE mark in July 2017. The Evolut PRO device follows the platform of the recapturable CoreValve Evolut R System, with the integration of an outer porcine pericardial tissue wrap that adds surface area contact between the valve and the native aortic annulus to further advance valve sealing performance. The device is currently available in the 23-mm, 26-mm, and 29-mm sizes (the 34-mm size will be also available in the next future). The Evolut PRO system is delivered through the 16-F equivalent EnVeo R Delivery Catheter System and is indicated for vessels down to 5.5 mm. The 14-F version of the delivery system of the Evolut PRO will be available soon.

26.1.3 Portico

The Portico valve (Abbott Vascular) is composed of a self-expanding stent, bovine leaflets, and a porcine pericardial sealing cuff. The large cell area and the annular positioning allow easy engagement of the coronary ostia after implantation (Fig. 26.1 and Table 26.1). The large cell area also minimizes the risk of PVR by allowing valve tissue to conform around calcific nodules at the annulus. The valve uses Linx anticalcification technology (as used on Trifecta and Epic surgical valves; St Jude Medical, Inc.). The 23- and 25-mm valves are loaded onto an 18-F delivery system, whereas the 27- and 29-mm valves are loaded onto a 19-F delivery system (Table 26.1). Clinical studies have been reported on alternative access sites including transaxillary, transaortic, and subclavian access, and case studies are currently underway to support this issue. The Portico valve is designed to be recaptured and repositioned at the implantation site, until it is fully deployed.

26.1.4 Acurate neo

The Acurate neo aortic bioprosthesis (Boston Scientific) is a second-generation valve with flaps composed of porcine pericardium sewn onto a stent made of self-expanding nitinol, covered both externally and internally by a porcine pericardium skirt (Fig. 26.1 and Table 26.1). The device includes three stabilization arches for the axial alignment to aortic annulus, a top crown for capping the aortic annulus, and a bottom that is open to the full distribution on the native valve. The prosthesis can be implanted through both the transapical (28 F) and the transfemoral (18 F) routes using a simple two-step deployment and stable positioning. The Acurate neo comes in three different sizes: small (21- to 23-mm aortic annulus), medium (23- to 25-mm aortic annulus), and large (25- to 27-mm aortic annulus).

26.1.5 Allegra

The Allegra THV (NVT AG) is a self-expanding valve consisting of a nitinol stent frame and bovine pericardium (annular skirt and leaflets). The annular portion of the frame is covered with a sealing skirt, above which the leaflets are sewn (i.e., the functional portion of the prosthesis is supra-annular). In addition, six radiopaque gold markers are incorporated to the stent frame indicating the level of the skirt/leaflet transition. The valve is available in three sizes (23, 27, and 31 mm) (Table 26.1), with a frame height of 37.3, 41.3, and 43 mm, respectively (Fig. 26.1 and Table 26.1). The stent frame uses a variable cell size design to allow for axially tailored radial force distribution with higher force in the annular sealing section of the valve for secure anchoring. The upper section of the stent frame has larger cells, created to allow for flexure of the stent frame and accommodation of conformational changes during the cardiac cycle, ultimately dissipating leaflet stresses. The transfemoral delivery system incorporates an 18-F cartridge and a 15-F catheter shaft. The Allegra device obtained CE mark approval in April 2017.

26.2 Clinical Trial Overview

A number of randomized clinical trials (RCTs) had been performed to evaluate the outcomes of TAVI vs. surgical aortic valve replacement (SAVR) in different clinical scenarios (high-risk, intermediate-risk, all-comers) [13–18]. Only two RCTs aimed at comparing two different TAVI devices: the Comparison of Transcatheter Heart Valves in High-Risk Patients With Severe Aortic Stenosis: Medtronic CoreValve vs. Edwards Sapien XT (CHOICE) trial and the Repositionable Percutaneous Replacement of Stenotic Aortic Valve Through Implantation of Lotus Valve System– Randomized Clinical Evaluation (REPRISE III) trial (Table 26.2).

The CHOICE trial was a multicenter trial enrolling 241 high-risk patients with symptomatic severe aortic stenosis undergoing TAVI and 1:1 randomly assigned to receive a balloon-expandable valve (Edwards Sapien XT, $n = 121$) or a self-expanding valve (Medtronic CoreValve,

Table 26.2 Randomized controlled trials comparing different THV types

	CHOICE	REPRISE III
First author name	M. Abdel-Wahab	T. Feldman
Objectives	To compare the clinical outcome of balloon-expandable vs. self-expandable valves in patients undergoing TAVI	To evaluate if a mechanically expanded valve (MEV) is non-inferior to an approved self-expanding valve (SEV) in high-risk patients with aortic stenosis undergoing TAVI
Study type	RCT	RCT
Randomization	1:1	2:1
Devices	BE (Edwards Sapien XT) SE (Medtronic)	ME (Lotus Valve) SE (Medtronic CoreValve Classic and Evolut R)
Patient population	High-risk patients with severe aortic stenosis and an anatomy suitable for the transfemoral TAVI procedure	High or extreme risk and severe, symptomatic aortic stenosis
No. of patients enrolled	241 (121 vs. 120)	912 (607 vs. 305)
No. of center involved	5	55
Countries	Germany	North America, Europe, and Australia
Enrolling time interval	March 2012–December 2013	September 2014–December 2015
Primary endpoints	Device success: • Successful vascular access and deployment of the device and retrieval of the delivery system • Correct position of the device • Intended performance of the heart valve without moderate or severe regurgitation • Only 1 valve implanted in the proper anatomical location	Composite endpoint: • All-cause mortality • Stroke • Life-threatening and major bleeding events • Stage 2/3 acute kidney injury • Major vascular complications at 30 days The primary effectiveness endpoint was the 1-year composite rate of all-cause mortality, disabling stroke, and moderate or greater PVL based on core laboratory assessment
Secondary endpoints	• Cardiovascular mortality • Bleeding and vascular complications • Postprocedural pacemaker placement • Combined safety endpoint at 30 days (including all-cause mortality, major stroke, and other serious complications)	• Moderate or greater PVL at 1 year
Timeframe (follow-up)	30-day and 1-year	30-day and 1-year
Conclusions	Balloon-expandable valve resulted in a greater rate of device success than use of a self-expandable valve 1-year follow-up, with limited statistical power, revealed not statistically significantly differences in clinical outcomes in both populations	The use of the MEV compared with the SEV did not result in inferior outcomes for the primary safety end point or the primary effectiveness end point

n = 120) between March 2012 and December 2013 at 5 centers in Germany [19, 20]. Device success occurred most frequently in the balloon-expandable valve group than in the self-expanding valve group (95.9% vs. 77.5%, $p < 0.001$). This was attributed to a significantly lower frequency of residual more-than-mild aortic regurgitation (4.1% vs. 18.3%; $p < 0.001$) and the less frequent need for implanting more than one valve (0.8% vs. 5.8%, $p = 0.03$) in the balloon-expandable valve group. Cardiovascular mortality at 30 days, bleeding, and vascular complications were not significantly different, and the combined safety endpoint occurred in 18.2% of those in the balloon-expandable valve group and 23.1% of the self-expanding valve (SEV) group ($p = 0.42$). Placement of a new permanent pacemaker was less frequent in the balloon-expandable valve group (17.3% vs. 37.6%, $p = 0.001$) [19]. At 1 year, the rates of death of any cause (17.4% vs. 12.8%; $p = 0.37$) and of cardiovascular causes (12.4% vs. 9.4%; $p = 0.54$) were not statistically significantly different in the balloon- and self-expanding groups, respectively. The frequencies of all strokes (9.1% vs. 3.4%; $p = 0.11$) and repeat hospitalization for heart failure (7.4% vs. 12.8%; $p = 0.19$) did not statistically significantly differ between the two groups. Elevated transvalvular gradients during follow-up were observed in four patients in the balloon-expandable group (3.4% vs. 0%; $p = 0.12$); all were resolved with anticoagulant therapy, suggesting a thrombotic etiology. More-than-mild PVR was more frequent in the self-expanding group (1.1% vs. 12.1%; $p = 0.005$) [20]. Despite the higher device success rate with the balloon-expandable valve, 1-year follow-up of patients in CHOICE, with limited statistical power, revealed clinical outcomes after transfemoral TAVI with both balloon- and self-expanding prostheses that were not statistically significantly different.

The more recent REPRISE III trial randomized 2:1 patients with high or extreme risk and severe, symptomatic aortic stenosis to receive the mechanically expanded Lotus Valve System (MEV; Boston Scientific) or the commercially available self-expanding CoreValve (either

CoreValve Classic or Evolut R; Medtronic). The trial was conducted at 55 sites and enrolled 912 patients in North America, Europe, and Australia between September 2014 and December 2015 [21]. The 30-day primary safety endpoint (all-cause mortality, stroke, life-threatening or major bleeding, stage 2/3 acute kidney injury, and major vascular complications) occurred in 20.3% of patients in the MEV group and in 17.2% of patients in the SEV group ($p = 0.003$ for noninferiority). The 1-year primary effectiveness endpoint (composite of all-cause mortality, disabling stroke, and moderate or greater paravalvular leak) occurred in 15.4% in the MEV group and in 25.5% in the SEV group ($p < 0.001$ for noninferiority). The 1-year rates of moderate or severe PVR were significantly reduced in MEV group (0.9% vs. 6.8%; $p < 0.001$), and the superiority analysis for primary effectiveness was statistically significant (difference, -10.2%; 95% CI, -16.3 to -4.0%; $p < 0.001$). Concurrently, the MEV had higher rates of new pacemaker implants (35.5% vs. 19.6%; $p < 0.001$) and valve thrombosis (1.5% vs. 0%) but lower rates of repeat procedures (0.2% vs. 2.0%), valve-in-valve deployments (0% vs. 3.7%), and valve malpositioning (0% vs. 2.7%). Concluding that among high-risk patients with aortic stenosis, the use of the MEV compared with the SEV did not result in inferior outcomes for the primary safety endpoint or the primary effectiveness endpoint [21]. A brief summary of two studies is reported in Table 26.2.

26.3   Clinical Scenarios

26.3.1 TAVI When the MDCT Is Not Available

The first consideration to do when selecting the type of device for a patient undergoing TAVI is whether a high-quality imaging screening (computed tomography, 3D transesophageal echocardiogram) is available. Between the different imaging techniques available for valve sizing, multidetector computed tomography (MDCT) has been recognized as the gold standard imaging technique in providing reproducible annular measurements [22, 23], but it is often denied in patients with very poor renal function, which it is frequent in TAVI populations, or not available in the setting of clinical urgency. Alternative strategies for aortic root measurements and anatomy assessment, including three-dimensional (3D) transesophageal [24] and 2D intracardiac echocardiography and magnetic resonance imaging (MRI) [25], have been studied. However, in daily practice, it usually happens to deal with patients requiring TAVI (particularly in an emergency setting) where operators should rely on angiography and 2D transthoracic echocardiography only for THV sizing.

On one hand, the balloon-expandable THV size selection requires an extremely accurate assessment of aortic root anatomy and dimensions, as excessive oversizing may increase the hazard of aortic annulus rupture [26, 27] and coronary occlusion [28], and undersizing increases the risk of PVR and valve migration [29, 30]. On the other hand, self-expanding devices may allow for even more aggressive oversizing providing better sealing without increasing the risk of annular rupture. Consequently, where aortic root measurements and calcium distribution are not known, the implantation of a self-expanding device might be safer [31].

Higher radial force of the balloon-expandable valve as compared with the self-expanding THVs has been well demonstrated by in vitro studies. Egron et al. [32] compared in the same bench test five THVs: CoreValve size 23 (CV-23) and size 26 (CV-26), the Acurate neo S (ACU-S), and the Sapien XT size 23 (XT-23) and size 26 (XT-26) to bring quantitative radial force profile information (Fig. 26.2). This study demonstrated that the radial force the balloon-expandable valves can exert are much higher (>100 Newton) than for the self-expanding valves (<50 Newton on recommended size ranges), which makes it unlikely for the surrounding anatomy to push back the Sapien XT valve frames [32]. This is in line with previous studies which showed balloon-expandable valves could keep a high degree of circularity after implantation in oval annuli [33].

26.3.2 Severe Calcific Native Aortic Valve

A severally calcified native aortic valve represents a big challenge because in this setting the operator has to find the better balance between the effectiveness of the procedure and safety of the patient. On one hand, the presence of severe calcified aortic complex increases the possibility of suboptimal deployment of the prosthesis and the presence of PVR [11, 12, 34, 35]. On the other hand, the presence of calcification involving the left ventricular outflow tract

Fig. 26.2 Comparison of the five valves: radial force (RF) profiles of self-expanding CV23, CV26, ACU-S inflow segments, and balloon-expandable XT23, XT26 valves, and respective recommended size windows (arrows). RF in Newton (N). Modified by Egron et al. [32]

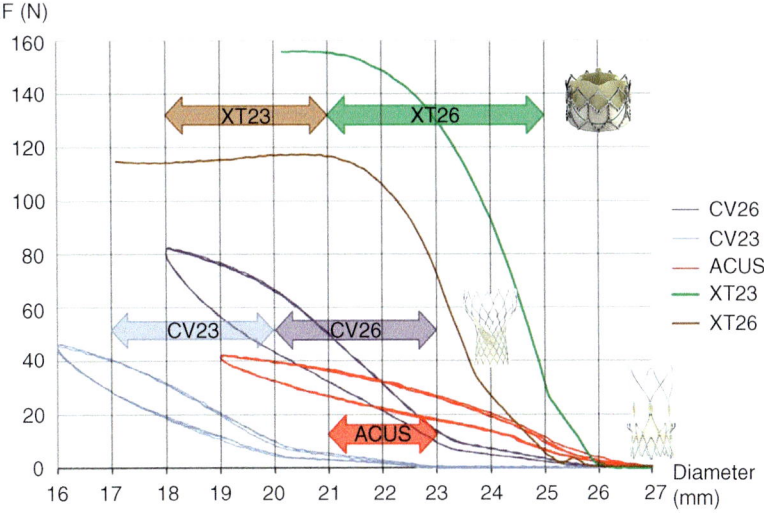

(LVOT) had been demonstrated to represent one of the major predictor of annular rupture during TAVI [20, 26].

Aortic valve calcification could be graded semiquantitatively as follows:

- Grade 1, no calcification.
- Grade 2, mildly calcified (small isolated spots).
- Grade 3, moderately calcified (multiple larger spots).
- Grade 4, heavily calcified (extensive calcifications of all cusps) [36].

When selecting a THV, the LVOT needs to be separately analyzed for the presence, amount, and location of calcification. If present, the distribution of calcification and extent can be assessed in a semiquantitative fashion as follows [26, 37]:

- Mild, 1 nodule of calcium extending <5 mm in any dimension and covering <10% of the perimeter of the LVOT.
- Moderate, 2 nodules of calcification or 1 extending >5 mm in any direction or covering >10% of the perimeter of the LVOT.
- Severe, multiple nodules of calcification of single focus extending >1 cm in length or covering >20% of the perimeter of the LVOT.

Formal LVOT calcification scoring was also performed by using a Hounsfield unit threshold of 800 to allow for determination of an Agatston score for the calcification in the LVOT on a contrast-enhanced computed tomography angiography as described by Ewe et al. [38].

Anatomically, THV device landing zone can be divided in three specific regions [39]:

- The overall LVOT (from the aortic annulus plane and 10 mm into the left ventricle).
- The upper LVOT (from the aortic annulus plane and 2 mm into the left ventricle).
- The aortic valve region (from the aortic annulus plane to the left coronary ostia).

Each region is further subdivided according to the aortic cups.

The first consideration to make when approaching a severe calcified valve regards safety; previous analyses of MDCT performed before TAVI suggested that there are at least two important features associated with annular rupture and periaortic hematoma: (1) moderate or severe LVOT/subannular calcification and (2) significantly oversized prostheses (≥20% area oversizing) [26, 27]. The severity of aortic valvular calcification instead did not appear to play a significant role in root rupture, perhaps because the calcified leaflets are generally accommodated within the capacious sinus of Valsalva. However, caution should still be exercised when performing TAVI on patients with heavily calcified aortic valve cusps in the setting of shallow sinuses of Valsalva, because this has been shown to result in perforation of a shallow sinus/narrow root and potentially increase the risk of coronary occlusion (Fig. 26.3) [26].

It is somewhat intuitive that upper LVOT calcium is more predictive of aortic root injury given its contact with the deployed THV and exposure to the force created during balloon expansion in this rigid, thin-walled structure. In particular, within the upper LVOT region, it is calcium located below the noncoronary cusp that was demonstrated to be most predictive of aortic root injury (Fig. 26.4), although previous case reports reported that the left aortic sinus may be the most vulnerable area with regard to aortic root injury possibly because of the lack of supporting cardiac structures in this area [26, 39]. Theoretically, trigonal calcification may impart greater rigidity to the annulus and make it prone to rupture, whereas more anterior calcification may not impart as great of a risk.

In light of these considerations, in terms of safety, THVs exerting low radial force (self-expanding) should be preferred over balloon-expandable THVs in a context of severe LVOT calcification. After implantation, eventual post-dilatation of self-expanding THVs should be performed with caution, preferably using undersized balloons (Fig. 26.5).

The second issue regards effectiveness of the procedure: heavy calcification of the device landing zone is commonly known to be an indepen-

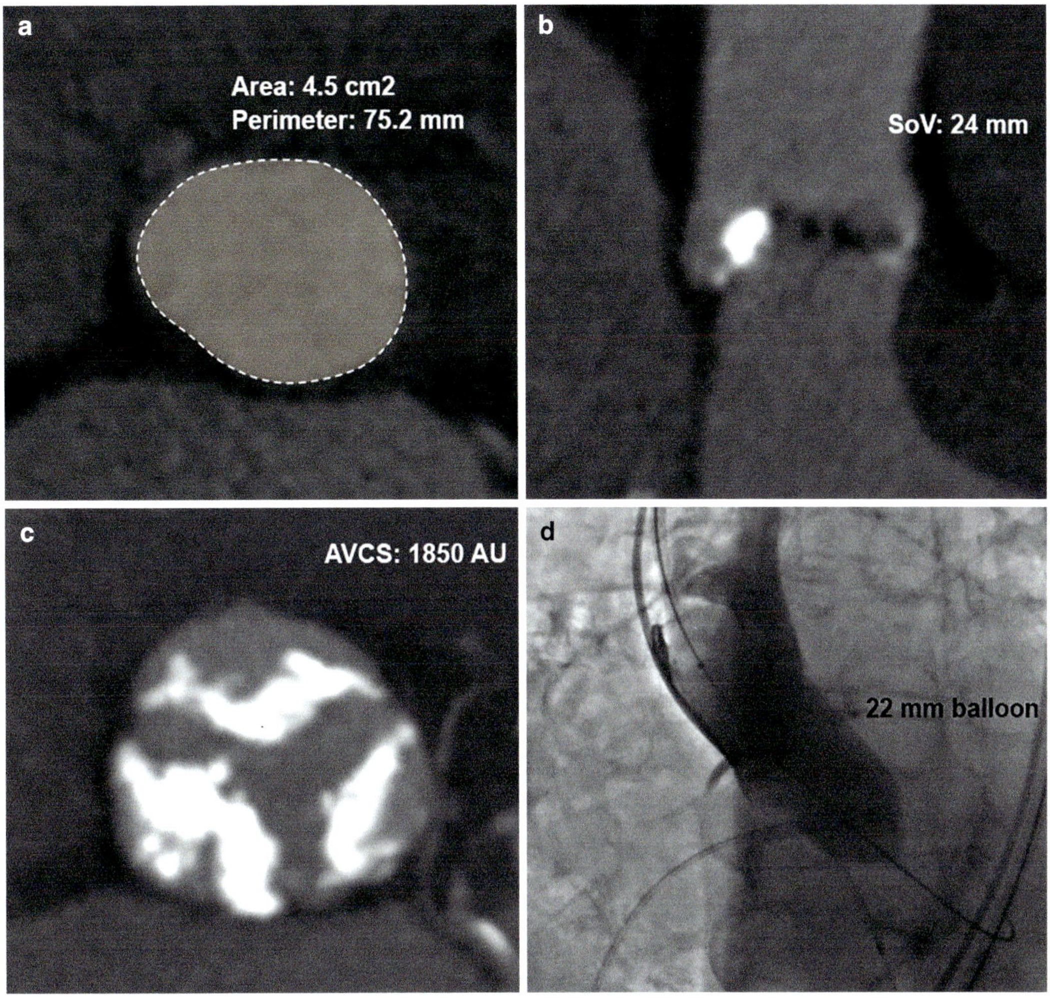

Fig. 26.3 Case example of one intermediate-risk patient candidate to TAVI. The MDCT (**a**) showed annular dimensions compatible with 29-mm Evolut, 26-mm Sapien 3, or 27-mm Portico (Acurate neo not feasible through either the transfemoral or transapical approaches due to not compatible iliofemoral accesses and poor left ventricular ejection fraction), but (**b**) shallow sinuses of Valsalva (SoV) and severely calcified aortic cusps (**c**). Balloon valvuloplasty performed with simultaneous aortography showed occlusion of the left main ostia by the aortic cusps (**d**). This patient underwent successful surgical aortic valve replacement due to the high-risk of TAVI-related complications

dent risk factor for residual PVR for all valve types, but especially for self-expanding THVs [35, 40].

As discussed previously, self-expanding prosthesis showed a more eccentric and underexpanded morphology, when compared to balloon-expandable valves. This needs to be counterbalanced with the risk of annular rupture in cases of severe calcification, in which prosthesis with less radial force might be beneficial [41, 42].

In patients undergoing self-expanding valve implantation, the volume of calcium appears to have more influence on the final geometry. Therefore, heavily calcified native valves might impose a higher resistance to valve deployment, and, in those cases, prosthesis with higher radial force, like balloon-expandable valves, may be more adequate [41]. It was demonstrated an independent association between calcium burden and eccentricity evaluated by MDCT and PVR in a

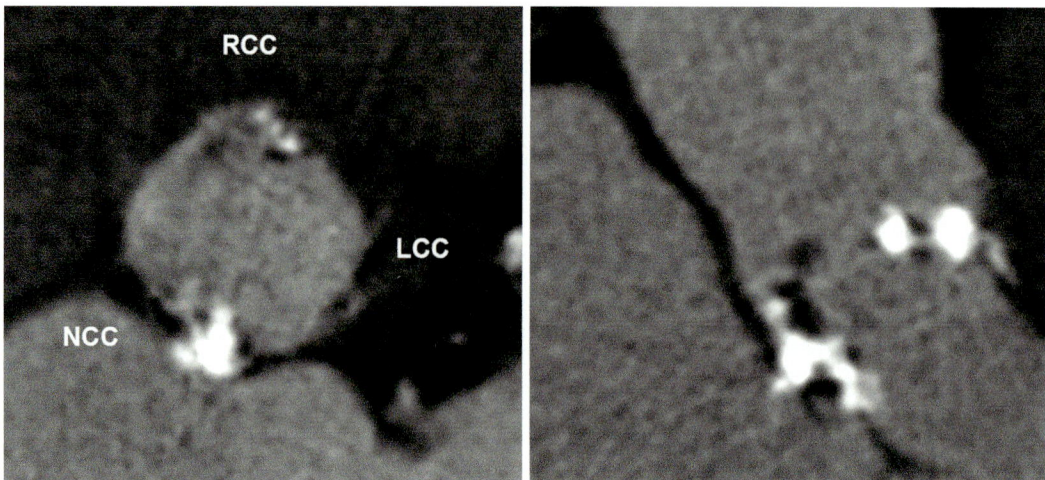

Fig. 26.4 Severe LVOT calcification located below the noncoronary cusp

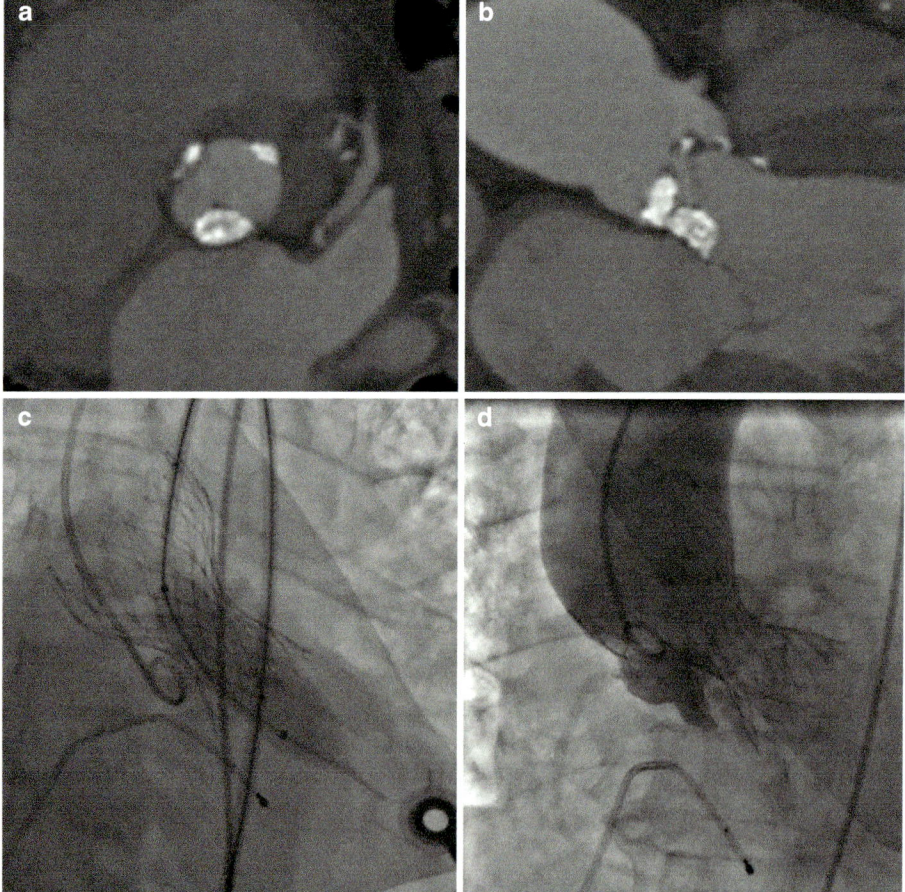

Fig. 26.5 Case example of a patient with candidate to TAVI and with severe LVOT calcification (**a** and **b**), This patient underwent 31-mm self-expanding CoreValve implantation. After release, the valve was significantly underexpanded. Post-dilatation with undersized balloon (24 mm) was performed. At the end of the procedure, PVR was mild and no signs of transvalvular gradient or aortic injury were reported (**c** and **d**)

cohort of patients undergoing TAVR with either self-expanding or balloon-expandable prosthesis [39]. Thus, the amount of radial force that is necessary to overcome the stenotic aortic valve directly correlates with the severity of calcification [43].

Walther et al. [44] suggested that diameter oversizing by ≈10% (based on transesophageal echocardiographic measurement) is desirable to avoid severe PVR, but, in the presence of a rigid aortic root, excessive oversizing should be avoided. Similarly, our and other groups have shown that annular area oversizing is essential to mitigate the risk of significant paravalvular regurgitation [22, 29].

Oversizing a patient with significant LVOT calcification should confer the greatest clinical concern: relative prosthesis area oversizing of ≥20% was found to be a strong predictor of contained or noncontained root rupture, but, importantly, it was suggested that that this risk may be amplified by other root modifiers such as significant LVOT/subannular calcification [26]. This might explain why significant annular area oversizing in historical cohorts does not necessarily result in annular rupture [45].

As recently demonstrated by Kim et al., in severe and moderate device landing zone (DLZ) calcification, BE devices may have advantages, whereas in mild DLZ calcification, low-radial force SE THV (Acurate neo) showed the most favorable profile [43].

The study confirmed the association of DLZ calcification and the use of BE devices with the onset of aortic root injury, but an association with a higher degree of oversizing was only found within the group treated with a BE device. The authors assumed that the underlying mechanism of aortic root injury in SE devices may not be spontaneous overexpansion due to oversizing, but rather aggressive post-dilatation [43]. Hence, in the presence of severe DLZ calcification, aortic root injury tended to be more frequent with BE devices, but this was without a significant difference to the incidence with SE devices, which might be explained by the high rate of post-dilation in the latter [46].

In this specific group with severe DLZ calcification, the lower rate of PVR ≥ moderate with BE devices was not at the cost of more clinically evident aortic root injuries, but due to the very low incidence of this complication and the limited sample size, it would not be appropriate to draw firm conclusions [43].

Moreover, it should be kept in mind that although rare, once aortic root injury occurs, this complication has a dismal prognosis, and contained ruptures of the aortic root may pose an additional risk of unknown extent. Thus, in patients with severe calcification, aggressive oversizing should be avoided, and it may be advisable to rather accept a certain degree of residual PVR. A strategy of less pronounced oversizing along with high implantation depth may also reduce the incidence of conduction disturbances [43].

A final consideration about this subset of patients regards the presence of higher transaortic mean gradients after TAVI, particularly in patients treated with BE THV, due to their intra-annular mounting of leaflets.

In conclusion, in a setting of severe aortic valve or LVOT calcifications, a more customized selection of THV that takes into account the severity of DLZ calcification is highly recommended. The use of BE prostheses may be favorable with respect to PVR, post-dilatation, and correct positioning, but this may be at the cost of higher mean gradients and an increased risk of aortic root injury.

A more patient-specific THV selection through integration of MDCT data is fundamental to allow the most appropriate valve choice with more modest oversizing (or even undersizing) of those patients with features that would predispose them to potential annular rupture through the selection of a smaller valve size or balloon underfilling [45] to control the degree of annular/LVOT stretch. It is important to recognize, however, that, although anatomic and procedural factors that are strongly predictive of annular rupture have been identified, this event remains rare, and the available models allow simply for the estimation of a probabilistic risk [26].

At the same time, we want to underline the fact that among currently available THVs, there is not one ideal device that fits all patients.

Therefore, it may be advantageous to store a certain number of different TAVI devices that allows a customized prosthesis selection, taking into consideration the learning curve with each new device and the minimum number of procedures necessary to become familiar with a system [47].

26.3.3 Extreme Sizing

The portfolio of THV currently available allows to cover a wide spectrum of annular dimensions (Fig. 26.6). Therefore while for the medium sizes the choice is various, the extreme sizes carry some additional issues. For a given valve size, self-expanding valves have a larger effective orifice area (EOA) compared with balloon-expandable valves, provided that these have a supra-annular location of the valve leaflets, which may be preferable in patients with small annulus.

26.3.4 Very Small Annuli

In surgical experience, aortic valve replacement in patients with small aortic annuli has been associated with a high incidence of prosthesis-patient mismatch (PPM) [48], which negatively impacts short- and long-term outcomes and predicts structural valve deterioration.

PPM has indeed been associated with diminished extent of regression of left ventricular hypertrophy, reduced coronary flow reserve,

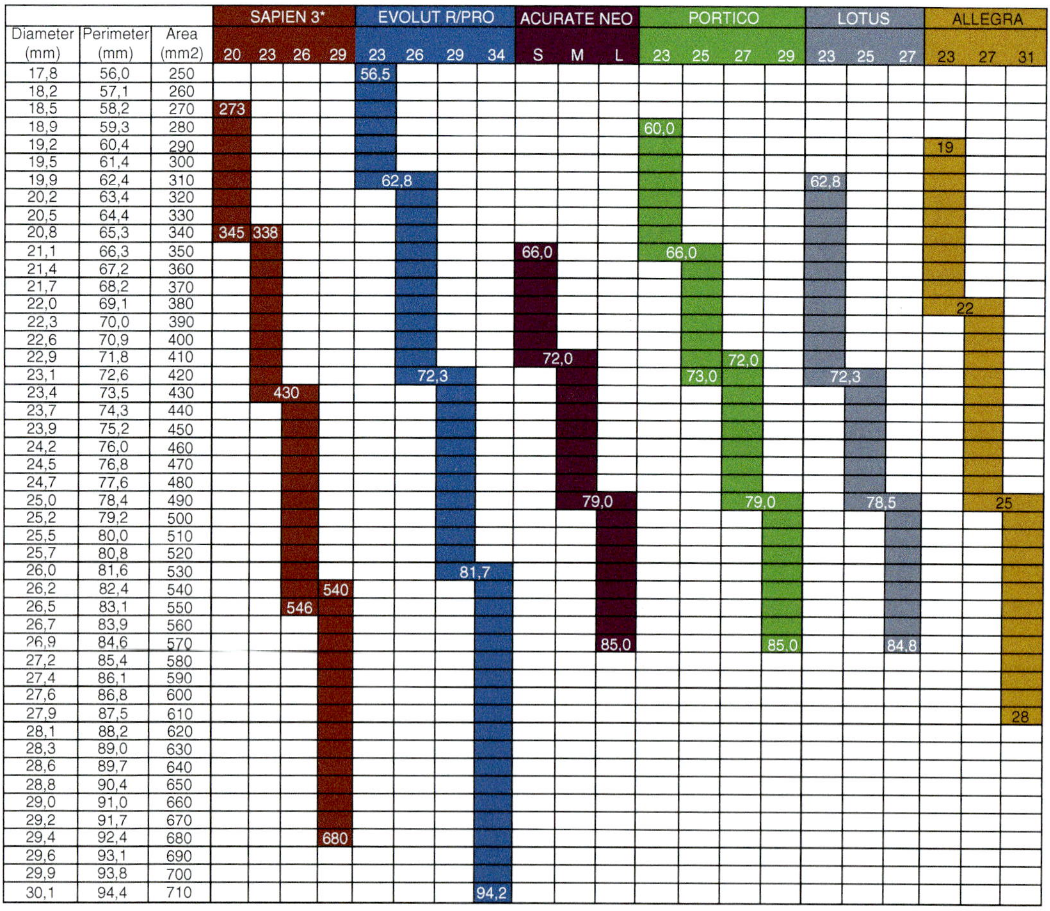

Diameter (mm)	Perimeter (mm)	Area (mm2)	SAPIEN 3*				EVOLUT R/PRO				ACURATE NEO			PORTICO				LOTUS			ALLEGRA		
			20	23	26	29	23	26	29	34	S	M	L	23	25	27	29	23	25	27	23	27	31
17,8	56,0	250					56,5																
18,2	57,1	260																					
18,5	58,2	270	273																				
18,9	59,3	280												60,0									
19,2	60,4	290																			19		
19,5	61,4	300																					
19,9	62,4	310						62,8										62,8					
20,2	63,4	320																					
20,5	64,4	330																					
20,8	65,3	340	345	338																			
21,1	66,3	350									66,0				66,0								
21,4	67,2	360																					
21,7	68,2	370																					
22,0	69,1	380																				22	
22,3	70,0	390																					
22,6	70,9	400																					
22,9	71,8	410										72,0				72,0							
23,1	72,6	420							72,3						73,0				72,3				
23,4	73,5	430			430																		
23,7	74,3	440																					
23,9	75,2	450																					
24,2	76,0	460																					
24,5	76,8	470																					
24,7	77,6	480																					
25,0	78,4	490											79,0			79,0			78,5			25	
25,2	79,2	500																					
25,5	80,0	510																					
25,7	80,8	520																					
26,0	81,6	530								81,7													
26,2	82,4	540				540																	
26,5	83,1	550			546																		
26,7	83,9	560																					
26,9	84,6	570											85,0				85,0			84,8			
27,2	85,4	580																					
27,4	86,1	590																					
27,6	86,8	600																					
27,9	87,5	610																					28
28,1	88,2	620																					
28,3	89,0	630																					
28,6	89,7	640																					
28,8	90,4	650																					
29,0	91,0	660																					
29,2	91,7	670																					
29,4	92,4	680				680																	
29,6	93,1	690																					
29,9	93,8	700																					
30,1	94,4	710								94,2													

Fig. 26.6 Sizing chart of current new-generation TAVI devices. *Cut-off expressed by area. †Cut-off expressed by perimeter

increased incidence of congestive heart failure, diminished functional capacity, and increased risk of early and late mortality [49–55].

Moreover, elevated transvalvular gradients have been identified as an important risk factor for decreased prostheses durability because of structural valve deterioration which occurs significantly more often in small bioprostheses [56].

Aortic root enlargement strategies or implantation of stentless bioprostheses has been proposed to reduce the risk of PPM after SAVR in this patient group. In this subset of patients, TAVI is associated with good inhospital and midterm outcomes, resulting in superior hemodynamics over surgery, with a significantly lower incidence of PPM and better post-procedural valve echocardiographic performance [57–59]. Although there is a paucity of comparative data available on this specific topic, the THV with a supra-annular design had demonstrated to achieve superior hemodynamic performances and EOA and thus a lower incidence of PPM [60].

A propensity score-based subanalysis of the OCEAN-TAVI registry (Optimized CathEter vAlvular iNtervention), which compared post-procedural hemodynamics and morphology between 20-mm and 23-mm Edwards Sapien XT-THVs in patients with extremely small annuli (<314 mm^2) [61], showed how the transvalvular gradient was higher and the EOA was lower in the 20-mm group than in the 23-mm group in both the overall cohort and matched cohort. However, the differences appeared to be subclinical, and the prevalence of severe PPM, which can influence the symptoms and prognoses after TAVI [62, 63], was very low in both the 20-mm and 23-mm groups. There was no increase of mean transvalvular gradient at 6-month follow-up in either group, and the THV expansion on post-procedural MDCT was lower in the 20-mm group than in the 23-mm group after matching, although the annular complex dimension on pre-procedural MDCT was similar between the two groups.

This finding indicates that larger Sapien XTs would be favorable for patients with an extremely small annulus. However, larger Sapien XTs have the potential risk of aortic root rupture or coronary obstruction [26, 64], and these data also suggest that a small 20-mm SXT would be useful for patients with a very small and heavily calcified aortic valve complex, because the incidence of severe PPM, which can influence prognosis after TAVI or SAVR, was quite low [61].

In a recent study, Theron et al. [65] used the regression adjustment for the propensity score to retrospectively compare the occurrence of moderate and severe PPM among patients with severe aortic stenosis implanted with new-generation Sapien 3-THV (S3; $n = 71$) and the older Sapien XT-THV (XT; $n = 50$). The main finding of the study was that S3-THV was associated with a higher risk of moderate and severe PPM than XT-THV implantation. The analysis shows that the iEOA was significantly lower (1.12 ± 0.34 vs. 0.96 ± 0.27 cm^2/m^2, $p = 0.009$) and the mean trans-prosthetic gradient was significantly higher (11.0 ± 5.5 and 13.5 ± 4.7 mmHg, $p = 0.002$) in S3-THV. Strikingly, S3-THV significantly decreased the iEOA by -0.21 cm^2/m^2 and increased the mean trans- prosthetic gradient by $+4.95$ mmHg compared with the XT-THV. Consequently, the risk of PPM increased nearly fivefold for S3-THV implantation. More specifically, the smallest aortic annulus patients who received a 23-mm S3-THV prosthesis demonstrated a 15-fold increased risk of PPM compared with 23-mm XT-THV, whereas aortic annuli were significantly lower with XT-THV (324 ± 38.8 vs. 376.8 ± 38 mm^2, $p < 0.001$). In concordance with previous studies, the reduction in rate and severity of PVR was confirmed (34 and 82%, $p < 0.001$) [7].

The increase in both the risk and severity of high trans-prosthetic gradients and PPM was explained by the authors by the outer sealing cuff, which is embedded in the new S3-THV. This new feature bulges into the annular space after deployment to fill up irregularities. However, although this novelty achieved a lower rate of PVR, the presence of a supplementary material occupying the annular space could have favored systolic blood obstruction and reduced hemodynamic performance, particularly in the case of a small aortic annulus. However, this observation needs to be better confirmed in larger analyses.

	SAPIEN 3 20	Evolut R 23	ACURATE neo S
	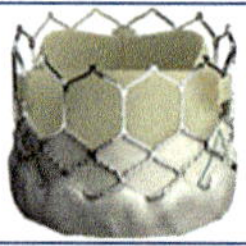	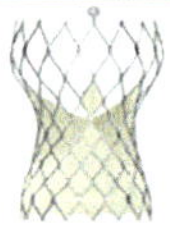	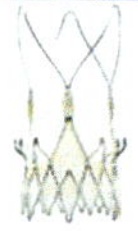
Annulus Diameter (mm)	18.6 – 21	18 – 20	21 – 23
Annulus Perimeter (mm)	58.4 – 65.9	56.5 – 62.8	66 – 72
Annulus Area (mm2)	273 – 345	254,4 – 314.1	346 – 415
Mean SOV (mm)	-	≧25	-
Mean SOV Height (mm)	-	≧15	-

Fig. 26.7 Characteristics of small-size THV. *SOV* sinus of Valsalva

In the comparison between different THV, two recent analyses compared hemodynamics and clinical outcomes of the balloon-expandable Edwards Sapien and a self-expanding device (Medtronic CoreValve/Evolut R and Acurate neo) in patients with small aortic annuli (Fig. 26.7).

Rogers et al. [60] compared valve hemodynamics and clinical outcomes according to aortic annulus size (small-medium-large) and type of valve (Sapien XT or S3 THV vs. CoreValve or Evolut R THV). In patients with small aortic annulus, SEV was associated with significantly higher dimensionless index (0.64 vs. 0.53, $p = 0.02$) and lower peak velocity (1.8 vs. 2.4 m/s, $p < 0.001$) and a trend toward lower mean gradient (7.5 vs. 10.0 mmHg, $p = 0.07$) compared with BEV. These differences in valve hemodynamics between valve types were diminished as aortic annulus size increased. In the study there was no significant association between aortic annulus size or valve type and PVR. No difference in

mortality at 1 year was observed between aortic annulus size tertiles [60].

Mauri et al. [66] performed a propensity score-matched analysis comparing hemodynamics and early to 1-year clinical outcomes after TAVI with a small-sized self-expanding Acurate neo valve ($n = 129$) or current-generation Sapien 3 23-mm balloon-expandable THV ($n = 117$) in five centers in Germany. PS matching resulted in 92 matched pairs.

TAVI with the self-expanding Acurate neo valve resulted in superior hemodynamics regarding mean transvalvular gradients (9.3 ± 3.9 mmHg vs.14.5 ± 5.5 mmHg; $p < 0.001$; Acurate neo vs. Sapien 3), indexed effective orifice area (iEOA) (0.96 ± 0.3 vs. 0.80 ± 0.2 cm^2/m^2; $p = 0.003$; Acurate neo vs. Sapien 3), and frequency of prosthesis-patient mismatch compared with TAVI with the balloon-expandable Sapien 3 (41% vs. 67%; $p = 0.002$; Acurate neo vs. Sapien 3). In particular, severe PPM was found in 3% of Acurate patients and 22% of Sapien 3 patients

($p = 0.004$). The observations were sustained at 1-year follow-up with mean transvalvular gradients of 6.6 ± 2.7 vs. 17.5 ± 6.5 mm Hg ($p < 0.008$) and iEOA of 1.01 ± 0.3 vs. 0.74 ± 0.2 cm^2/m^2 ($p = 0.031$) in Acurate neo and Sapien 3 patients, respectively.

Both prostheses provided efficient protection against PVR. Clinically relevant PVR $\geq$ moderate was low in both groups (discharge: 4.5% vs. 3.6%; $p = 0.208$; 1-year: 3.9% vs. 3.6%; $p = 0.527$; Acurate neo vs. Sapien 3, respectively).

In conclusion, these two latter analyses demonstrated that both THV systems (balloon-expandable and self-expanding) have similar safety profiles. However, SEV with supra-annular design had superior hemodynamics regarding transvalvular gradients, iEOA, and frequency of PPM (Fig. 26.8). This may be particularly beneficial in patients with small aortic annulus, who are at risk for PPM, which in turn might be a risk factor for structural valve deterioration and impaired outcome.

26.3.4.1   Oversized Annuli

Patients with large aortic root anatomy (annulus diameter > 29 mm), who otherwise would be suitable candidates, have until recently been excluded from TAVI due to the lack of an appropriately large prosthesis.

The largest prostheses actually available are the Sapien 3 29-mm valve (available for patients with a 3D area-derived annular diameter of up to 29.5 mm or a 3D annular area up to 683 mm^2) and the Evolut R 34-mm valve (available for patients with annulus diameter of up to 30 mm or a perimeter of up to 94.2 mm) (Fig. 26.9). However, some patients possess aortic anatomy that is still too large for TAVI and is out of range for manufacturer recommendations.

These two THVs have been recently tested in anatomies in which the dimension of the aortic annulus was greater than higher limit recommended by the companies.

Shivaraju et al. [67] first established the feasibility of using overexpanded 29-mm Sapien 3 valves to treat annular sizes >683 mm^2. They demonstrated that an additional 4 mL of contrast into the delivery balloon could treat annular areas as large as 740 mm^2 with good valve performance, acceptable rate of PVR, and no increased risk of annular rupture.

The success of this technique was further demonstrated by Mathur et al. [68] in a case series of three patients who received an overexpanded 29-mm Sapien 3 valve-in-valve areas >740 mm^2 (up to 793 mm^2), with no patients demonstrating greater than moderate PVR during short-term follow-up or valve migration or embolization (Table 26.3).

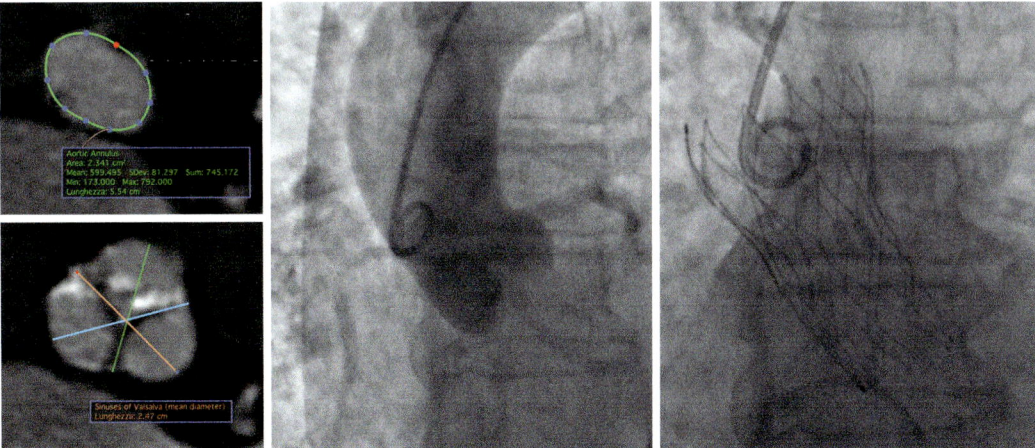

Fig. 26.8 Clinical case of a patient with very small aortic annulus treated with the 23-mm Portico THV. The leaflets of the Portico are sealed intrannularly. The patient was discharged with 23 mmHg of trans-prosthetic gradient post-TAVI

	SAPIEN 3 29	Evolut R 34
	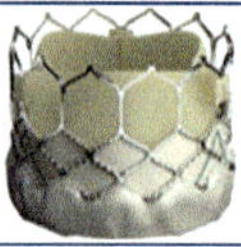	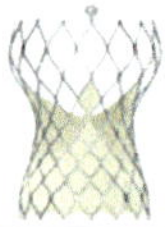
Annulus Diameter (mm)	26.2 – 29.5	26.2 – 29.5
Annulus Perimeter (mm)	82.3 – 92.6	82.3 – 92.6
Annulus Area (mm2)	540 – 683	540 – 683
Mean SOV (mm)	-	≧ 31
Mean SOV Height (mm)	-	≧ 16

Fig. 26.9 Characteristics of large-size THV. SOV sinus of Valsalva

Table 26.3 Overexpansion of the 29 mm SAPIEN 3 THV in patients with large aortic annuli: baseline and procedural features

	Patient #1	Patient #2	Patient #3
Annulus diameter (mm)	28.6/32.4	29.3/36.2	27/36
Eccentricity index	0.12	0.19	0.25
Annulus perimeter (mm)	97.7	101	101
Annulus area (mm^2)	748.1	793	787
Estimated % oversize by area with no overexpansion	−11.7	−16.71	−16.07
Overexpansion S3 29 (mL of contrast)	+4	+4	+4
Access site	Transfemoral	Transfemoral	Transfemoral
Pre-dilatation balloon (mm)	23	No	No
Post-dilatation balloon (mm)	No	+5 mL	No
Final TTE AR	Trace PVR and trace central AR	Mild PVR	Mild-moderate PVR

Abbreviations: *AR* aortic regurgitation, *TTE* transthoracic echocardiography, *PVR* paravalvular regurgitation [68]

In the study, the 29-mm S3 delivery balloon was bench-tested outside the body and was able to hold an additional 16 ml of contrast volume over nominal inflation. Balloon width measurements were made using digital calipers (Neiko 01407A 0–150 mm). Balloon rupture occurred at 17 mL of contrast and occurred along the longitudinal axis of the balloon (Table 26.4) [68].

Of course, overexpansion raises concerns over reduced leaflet coaptation, PVR, valve migration, and positioning challenges due to frame shortening [67]. For this reason a "low" positioning strategy, positioning the central marker of the 29 mm S3 at approximately 1.5 mm below the annular plane at the start of TAVI deployment, should be intentionally chosen to account for

Table 26.4 Edward Sapien 29 mm S3 delivery balloon (bench testing results) [68]

Volume (cc)	Diameter (mm)	Derived area (mm²)
33 mL (nominal)	29.0	660.48
+1 mL	29.5	683.45
+2 mL	29.9	702.11
+3 mL	30.1	711.53
+4 mL	30.2	716.27
+5 mL	30.5	730.57
+6 mL	31.1	759.6
+7 mL	Rupture	

Table 26.5 Baseline and procedural features

	Patient #1	Patient #2
Baseline AR	Moderate	Moderate
Annulus diameter (mm)	31.9	31.1
Annulus perimeter (mm)	100.2	97.7
Annulus area (mm²)	762	739.5
Annular calcium	Moderate	Moderate (with multiple protruding annular calcium nodules)
Oversizing (%)	5.7	9.3
Access site	Transfemoral	Transaortic
Pre-dilatation balloon (mm)	No	23
Pacing	Yes	No
Post-implantation PVR	Moderate	Moderate
Post-dilatation balloon (mm)	28	25
Final PVR	Mild	Mild

AR aortic regurgitation, *PVR* paravalvular regurgitation; oversizing is calculated as [(Valve perimeter—annulus perimeter)/annular perimeter] × 100 [69]

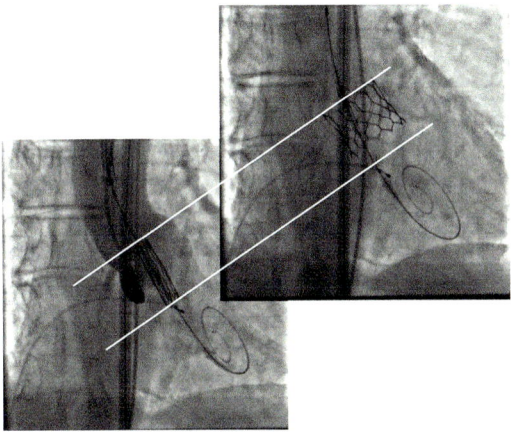

Fig. 26.10 Valve shortening during overexpansion of 29 mm SAPIEN S3. The top edge of the valve is noted to remain relatively stable, while the bottom edge translates in the aortic direction

valve shortening. In this way it could be anticipated valve shortening occurring from the "bottom" (ventricular) edge of the valve toward the "top" (aortic) edge (Fig. 26.10).

Recently Elmously et al. [69] described the clinical course of two high-risk patients with severe aortic stenosis (AS) and aortic annulus sizes well beyond range who underwent TAVI using the 34-mm Evolut R (Table 26.5). Both patients underwent postimplantation dilatation resulting in a significant decrease in PVR, with mild PVR at the end of the case in both patients.

When choosing a THV type in large annuli, a consideration must be done about the potential for physical restriction against overexpansion due to frame design and outer sealing skirt. The ability of the S3 to overexpand is contingent not only upon frame and cell geometry but also by a sealing skirt made of polyethylene terephthalate, whose elasticity limit may impose further restrictions to overexpansion. As such, there is an "upper limit" to overexpansion. On the other hand, the strategy of post-dilating a CoreValve Evolut is limited due to an inability to overexpand its nitinol frame beyond nominal diameter.

26.3.5 Bicuspid Aortic Valve

Bicuspid aortic valvulopathy (BAV) has a high prevalence in younger patients with AS. However, even in the elderly (>80 years of age), bicuspid valves comprise approximately 20% of surgical cases [70].

BAV is a spectrum of abnormal aortic valve morphology consisting of two functional cusps with less than three zones of parallel apposition between cusps [71]. BAV classification was assigned according to the number and spatial orientation of the raphe (Fig. 26.11).

Fig. 26.11
Classification of
Bicuspid Aortic Valve
according to the
description of Sievers
et al. [71]

Type 0 - No raphe

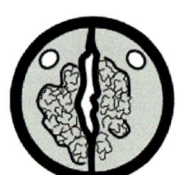

Type 2 - Two raphe

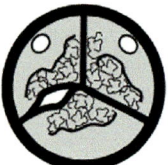

Type 1 - One raphe

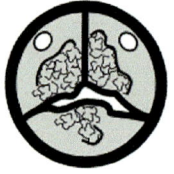

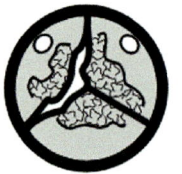

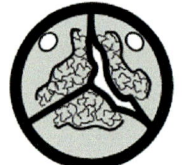

L-R

R-N

L-N

– Type 0, commonly referred to as "pure BAV," has two normally developed cusps, sinuses, and commissures and no raphe.
– Type 1 has three anlagen, two underdeveloped cusps, one fully developed cusp, one underdeveloped commissure, two fully developed commissures, and one raphe whose orientation in relation to the sinuses defined subcategorization (left-right, right-non, and left-non).
– Type 2 has three anlagen, two underdeveloped cusps, one fully developed cusp, two underdeveloped commissures, one fully developed commissure, and two raphe [71].

Early experience with TAVI in bicuspid valves demonstrated that this anatomical entity has several features that more often make the outcomes of TAVI suboptimal and less predictable [72]:

– An elliptically shaped annulus that may impair valve positioning and sealing.
– Asymmetrical and heavy calcification of leaflets may impede valve expansion and then compromise valve hemodynamics (e.g., higher transvalvular gradients and PVR).
– The presence of aortic disease may potentially increase the risk of dissection or rupture during valvuloplasty, post-dilatation, or implantation of balloon-expandable valves.

– Fused commissures are susceptible to disruption during balloon valvuloplasty, resulting in severe aortic regurgitation.
– Underexpansion and/or a noncircular shape of the THV may affect long-term durability.

BAV morphology presents potential advantages and disadvantages for balloon- and self-expanding TAV systems. The balloon-expandable valve exerts greater radial force and may circularize the native annulus, obliterating potential sites of PVR. Calcified nodules or raphe, however, may impair complete prosthesis expansion, thereby necessitating postimplantation balloon dilation or, potentially, resulting in residual PVR. The self-expanding THV could have greater propensity to such PVR given the reduced radial strength relative to balloon-expandable systems. The greater compliance of self-expanding prostheses and the supra-annular position of the leaflets could, however, mitigate the unequal circular stress at the level of the annulus and potentially improve long-term hemodynamic outcomes (Fig. 26.12) [70].

One multicenter study on early-generation TAVI devices evaluated clinical outcomes of a large cohort of patients undergoing TAV-in-BAV using either balloon- or self-expanding devices [70].

Incidence of type 0 BAV was 26.7%; type 1 BAV was 68.3%; and type 2 BAV was 5.0%.

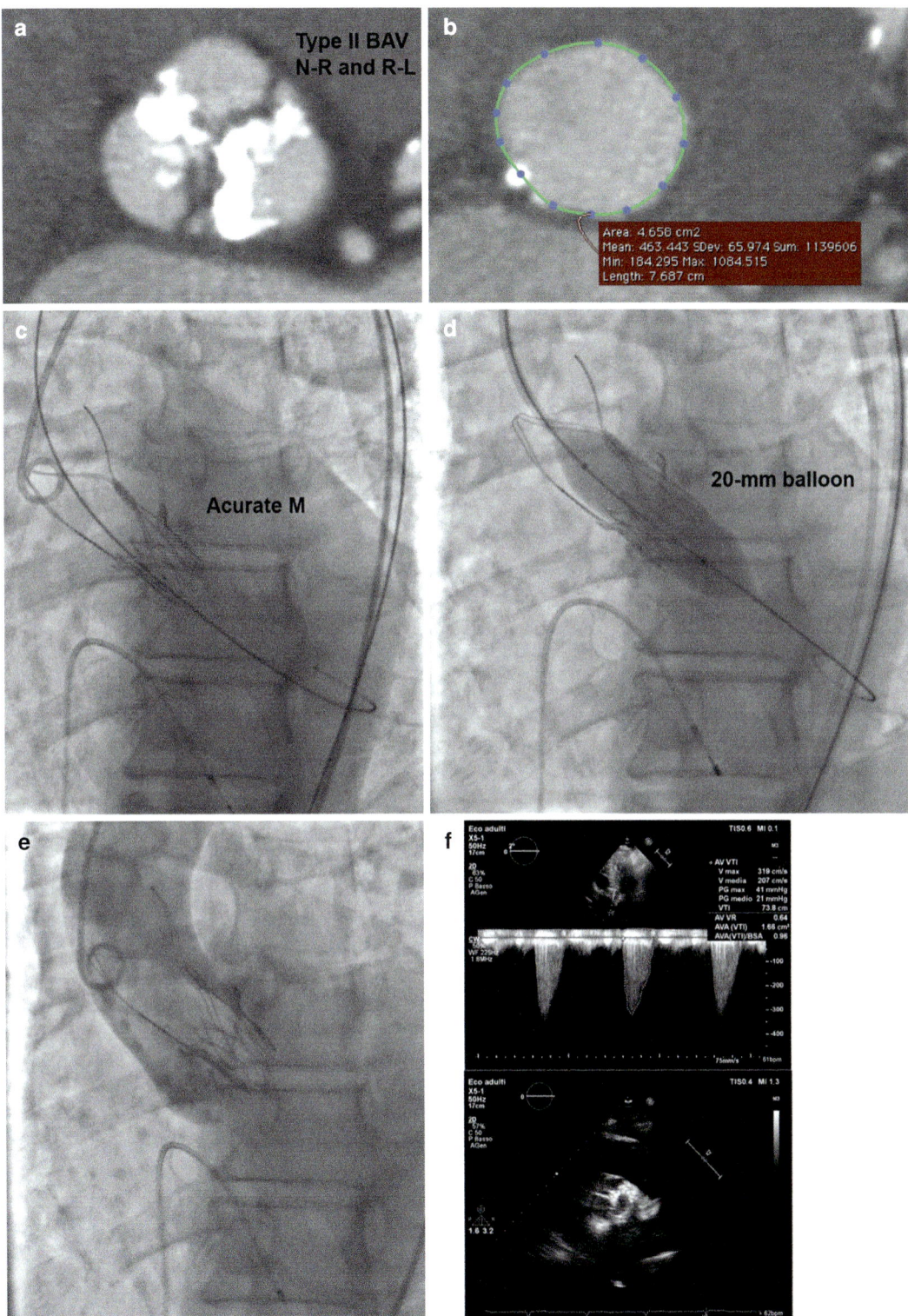

Fig. 26.12 Case example of a patient with a Type 2 BAV (**a** and **b**) who underwent TAVI using the self-expanding Acurate neo THV (**c**). After release the valve was highly underexpanded. Post-dilatation with an undersized balloon was then performed (**d**). The final aortography (**e**) showed the asymmetrical expansion of the THV with no PVR. The transthoracic echocardiogram (**f**) showed the oval shape of the THV with mild trans-prosthetic mismatch

MDCT-based TAV sizing was used in 63.5% of patients (77.1% balloon-expandable THV vs. 56.0% self-expanding THV, $p = 0.02$).

This study showed an overall higher incidence of THV malposition requiring a second valve implantation (3.6%) and moderate or severe PVR in 28.4% of patients.

Clinical outcomes among patients treated with balloon-expandable TAV were similar to those observed in patients treated with the self-expanding prostheses. In particular, there was a slightly major need for a second valve in patients treated with self-expanding devices (2.1% vs. 4.4%; $p = 0.66$; BE THV vs. SE THV). The procedural mortality was numerically higher for the self-expanding THV (4.9% vs. 2.1%, respectively; $p = 0.66$), whereas the 1-year mortality rate was lower for the self-expanding THV (12.5% vs. 20.8%, respectively; $p = 0.12$). The procedure was effective in most patients, with a 30-day combined efficacy endpoint achieved in 84.9% of the patients (87,5% vs. 84,5%; BE THV vs. SE THV; $p = 0,81$).

Significant aortic regurgitation was two times more frequent following implantation of the self-expandable THV than the balloon-expandable THV (32.2% vs. 19.6%, respectively; $p = 0.11$); however, the considerably lower use of MDCT-based TAV sizing in the self-expanding THV cohort might have accounted for this difference. Significant aortic regurgitation, indeed, decreased to 17.4% when pre-procedural annular assessment was performed by MDCT and subgroup analysis demonstrated no significant between-group differences in the rates of postimplantation AR (16.7% BE THV vs. 17.6% SE THV; $p = 0.99$).

Interestingly, significant aortic regurgitation was more frequent when the baseline BAV anatomy was type 0 (no raphe, classic bicuspid aortic valve).

The second-generation devices have demonstrated some advancement in overcoming the procedural limitations in tricuspid AS and now go beyond the challenges of treating bicuspid AS. The new-generation balloon-expandable Sapien 3, with an external sealing cuff allowing for effective sealing, eliminates the extreme over-sizing and mitigates the morphological challenges of bicuspid AS. Similarly, the mechanical-expanding Lotus valve, with an outer adaptive seal, as well as retrievability and repositioning capacity, may ameliorate the difficulties in optimal positioning and prevent paravalvular leak [73–78].

A recent large multicenter propensity-based analysis compared TAVI outcomes in 546 pairs of patients with bicuspid (BAV) and tricuspid (TrAV) aortic valves [79]. Compared with patients with tricuspid AS, patients with bicuspid AS had more frequent conversion to surgery (2.0% vs. 0.2%; $p = 0.006$) and a significantly lower device success rate (85.3% vs. 91.4%; $p = 0.002$). In the study early-generation devices (Sapien XT, CoreValve) were implanted in 320 patients with bicuspid and 321 patients with tricuspid AS, whereas new-generation devices (Sapien 3, Lotus, Evolut R) were implanted in 226 and 225 patients with bicuspid and tricuspid AS, respectively. When stratified according to whether they received early- vs. new-generation devices, patients with bicuspid AS had more frequent procedural complications than those with tricuspid AS when receiving the early- generation devices (conversion to surgery: 2.5% vs. 0.3%; $p = 0.02$; second valve implantation: 7.2% vs. 2.2%; $p = 0.003$; moderate or severe PVR: 15.9% vs. 10.3%; $p = 0.03$).

In particular, compared with patients with tricuspid AS, patients with bicuspid AS had more frequent aortic root injury (4.5% vs. 0.0%; $p = 0.015$) when receiving the Sapien XT and more frequent second valve implantation (11.6% vs. 2.9%; $p = 0.002$), moderate or severe paravalvular leak (19.4% vs. 10.5%; $p = 0.02$), and subsequent lower device success rate (72.1% vs. 86.0%; $p = 0.002$) than those with tricuspid AS when receiving the CoreValve. However, there were no significant differences in these adverse procedural events between groups when receiving the Sapien 3 and Lotus, that fact is probably related to the high radial force of both devices.

Similarly, a large multicenter analysis compared TAVI early and 1-year outcomes in bicuspid aortic valves in patient receiving early- and old-generation devices [80].

Of 301 patients, 199 patients (71.1%) were treated with early-generation devices (Sapien XT: $n = 87$; CoreValve: $n = 112$) and 102 with new-generation devices (Sapien 3: $n = 91$; Lotus: $n = 11$). The mean Society of Thoracic Surgeons score was 4.7 ± 5.2 without significant differences between groups (4.6 ± 5.1 vs. 4.9 ± 5.4; $p = 0.57$). Pre-procedural CT assessment was conducted for 157 patients with early-generation devices (78.9%) compared to all patients with new-generation devices. The more frequent anatomy was type 1 (86.2%).

Overall, all-cause mortality rates were 4.3% at 30 days and 14.4% at 1 year. Moderate or severe paravalvular leak was absent and significantly less frequent with new-generation compared to early-generation devices (0.0% vs. 8.5%; $p = 0.002$), which resulted in a higher device success rate (92.2% vs. 80.9%; $p = 0.01$). There were no differences between early- and new-generation devices in stroke (2.5% vs. 2.0%; $p > 0.99$), life-threatening bleeding (3.5% vs. 2.9%; $p > 0.99$), major vascular complication (4.5% vs. 2.9%; $p = 0.76$), stage 2 to 3 acute kidney injury (2.5% vs. 2.9%; $p > 0.99$), early safety endpoints (15.1% vs. 10.8%; $p = 0.30$), and 30-day all-cause mortality (4.5% vs. 3.9%; $p > 0.99$).

A multicenter study performed by Perlman et al. [81] collected baseline characteristics, procedural data, and 30-day clinical follow-up of 51 patients from 8 centers in Europe and Canada that had performed TAVI in bicuspid AS using the Sapien 3 valve. In the patient population, bicuspid valve types were type 0, 11.8%; type 1, 82.3%; and type 2, 1.9%. There were no cases of valve embolization or need for a second valve. There were no cases of moderate or severe post-implantation AR. At 30-day follow-up, there were 2 deaths (3.9%) and 2 major vascular complications, and 12 patients (23.5%) required pacemaker implantation.

In conclusions, it is undeniable that outcomes of TAVI in BAV are not as favorable as with tricuspid valves, and indications for TAVI must be carefully discussed based on patient-specific aortic root anatomy and calcium distribution. It is not clear whether one THV type is superior to another one. In this uncertainty, and waiting for stronger evidence, THV choice should be made by carefully assessing the morphology of the leaflets and the distribution of calcium, balancing the chances to obtain an optimal sealing with the risk of aortic root injury.

References

1. Cribier A, et al. Percutaneous transcatheter implantation of an aortic valve prosthesis for calcific aortic stenosis. Circulation. 2002;106(24):3006 LP–3008.
2. Baumgartner H, et al. 2017 ESC/EACTS guidelines for the management of valvular heart disease. Eur Heart J. 2017;38(36):2739–86.
3. Nishimura RA, et al. 2017 AHA/ACC focused update of the 2014 AHA/ACC guideline for the management of patients with valvular heart disease. J Am Coll Cardiol. 2017;17:735–1097.
4. Barbanti M, Webb JG, Gilard M, Capodanno D. Transcatheter aortic valve implantation in 2017: state of the art. EuroIntervention. 2017;13(AA):AA11–21.
5. Cribier AG. The odyssey of TAVR from concept to clinical reality. Texas Hear Inst J. 2014;41(2):125–30.
6. van Gils L, et al. TAVI with current CE-marked devices: strategies for optimal sizing and valve delivery. EuroIntervention. 2016;12(Y):Y22–7.
7. Binder RK, et al. Transcatheter aortic valve replacement with the SAPIEN 3. JACC Cardiovasc Interv. 2013;6(3):293–300.
8. Nijhoff F, Abawi M, Agostoni P, Ramjankhan FZ, Doevendans PA, Stella PR. Transcatheter aortic valve implantation with the new balloon-expandable sapien 3 versus sapien XT valve system. Circ Cardiovasc Interv. 2015;8(6)
9. Husser O, et al. Outcomes after transcatheter aortic valve replacement using a novel balloon-expandable transcatheter heart valve: a single-center experience. JACC Cardiovasc Interv. 2015;8(14):1809–16.
10. Wöhrle J, Gonska B, Rodewald C, Seeger J, Scharnbeck D, Rottbauer W. Transfemoral aortic valve implantation with the new Edwards Sapien 3 valve for treatment of severe aortic stenosis - impact of valve size in a single center experience. PLoS One. 2016;11(3):1–10.
11. De Torres-Alba F, et al. Changes in the pacemaker rate after transition from Edwards SAPIEN XT to SAPIEN 3 transcatheter aortic valve implantation the critical role of valve implantation height. JACC Cardiovasc Interv. 2016;9(8):805–13.
12. Reichenspurner H, et al. Self-expanding transcatheter aortic valve system for symptomatic high-risk patients with severe aortic stenosis. J Am Coll Cardiol. 2017;70(25):3127–36.
13. Mack MJ, et al. 5-year outcomes of transcatheter aortic valve replacement or surgical aortic valve

replacement for high surgical risk patients with aortic stenosis (PARTNER 1): a randomised controlled trial. Lancet. 2016;385(9986):2477–84.

14. Kapadia SR, et al. 5-year outcomes of transcatheter aortic valve replacement compared with standard treatment for patients with inoperable aortic stenosis (PARTNER 1): a randomised controlled trial. Lancet. 2015;385(9986):2485–91.

15. Leon MB, et al. PARTNER 2: Transcatheter or surgical aortic-valve replacement in intermediate-risk patients. N Engl J Med. 2016;374(17):1609–20.

16. Deeb GM, et al. 3-year outcomes in high-risk patients who underwent surgical or transcatheter aortic valve replacement. J Am Coll Cardiol. 2016;67(22):2565–74.

17. Søndergaard L, et al. Two-year outcomes in patients with severe aortic valve stenosis randomized to transcatheter versus surgical aortic valve replacement: the all-comers nordic aortic valve intervention randomized clinical trial. Circ Cardiovasc Interv. 2016;9(6):1–10.

18. Reardon MJ, et al. Surgical or transcatheter aortic-valve replacement in intermediate-risk patients. N Engl J Med. 2017;376(14):1321–31.

19. Abdel-Wahab M, et al. Comparison of balloon-expandable vs. self-expanding valves in patients undergoing transcatheter aortic valve replacement: the CHOICE randomized clinical trial. JAMA. 2014;311(15):1503–14.

20. Abdel-Wahab M, et al. 1-year outcomes after transcatheter aortic valve replacement with balloon-expandable versus self-expanding valves. J Am Coll Cardiol. 2015;46(2):791–800.

21. Feldman TE, et al. Effect of mechanically expanded vs. self-expanding transcatheter aortic valve replacement on mortality and major adverse clinical events in high-risk patients with aortic stenosis. JAMA. 2018;319(1):27.

22. Willson AB, et al. 3-dimensional aortic annular assessment by multidetector computed tomography predicts moderate or severe paravalvular regurgitation after transcatheter aortic valve replacement: a multicenter retrospective analysis. J Am Coll Cardiol. 2012;59(14):1287–94.

23. Zamorano JL, Gonçalves A, Lang R. Imaging to select and guide transcatheter aortic valve implantation. Eur Heart J. 2014;35(24):1578–87.

24. Hahn RT, et al. Recommendations for comprehensive intraprocedural echocardiographic imaging during TAVR. JACC Cardiovasc Imaging. 2015;8(3):261–87.

25. La Manna A, et al. Non-contrast three-dimensional magnetic resonance imaging for pre-procedural assessment of aortic annulus dimensions in patients undergoing transcatheter aortic valve implantation. Struct Hear. 2018;0(0):1–3.

26. Barbanti M, et al. Anatomical and procedural features associated with aortic root rupture during balloon-expandable transcatheter aortic valve replacement. Circulation. 2013;128(3):244–53.

27. Blanke P, et al. Prosthesis oversizing in balloon-expandable transcatheter aortic valve implantation is associated with contained rupture of the aortic root. Circ Cardiovasc Interv. 2012;5(4):540–8.

28. Gurvitch R, et al. Transcatheter aortic valve implantation: lessons from the learning curve of the first 270 high-risk patients. Catheter Cardiovasc Interv. 2011;78(7):977–84.

29. Jilaihawi H, et al. Cross-sectional computed tomographic assessment improves accuracy of aortic annular sizing for transcatheter aortic valve replacement and reduces the incidence of paravalvular aortic regurgitation. J Am Coll Cardiol. 2012;59(14):1275–86.

30. Détaint D, et al. Determinants of significant paravalvular regurgitation after transcatheter aortic valve implantation. JACC Cardiovasc Interv. 2009;2(9):821–7.

31. Barbanti M, et al. Prosthesis choice for transcatheter aortic valve replacement: improved outcomes with the adoption of a patient-specific transcatheter heart valve selection algorithm. Int J Cardiol. 2016;203:1009–10.

32. Egron S, et al. Radial force: an underestimated parameter in oversizing transcatheter aortic valve replacement prostheses: in vitro analysis with five commercialized valves. ASAIO J. 2018;64(4):536–43.

33. Schuhbaeck A, et al. Aortic annulus eccentricity before and after transcatheter aortic valve implantation: comparison of balloon-expandable and self-expanding prostheses. Eur Heart J. 2013;34(7):31–2.

34. Barbanti M, et al. Underexpansion and ad hoc post-dilation in selected patients undergoing balloon-expandable transcatheter aortic valve replacement. J Am Coll Cardiol. 2014;63(10):976–81.

35. John D, et al. Correlation of device landing zone calcification and acute procedural success in patients undergoing transcatheter aortic valve implantations with the self-expanding CoreValve prosthesis. JACC Cardiovasc Interv. 2010;3(2):233–43.

36. Tops LF, et al. Noninvasive evaluation of the aortic root with multislice computed tomography: implications for transcatheter aortic valve replacement. JACC Cardiovasc Imaging. 2008;1(3):321–30.

37. Maeno Y, et al. Relationship between left ventricular outflow tract calcium and mortality following transcatheter aortic valve implantation. Am J Cardiol. 2017;120(11):2017–24.

38. Ewe SH, et al. Location and severity of aortic valve calcium and implications for aortic regurgitation after transcatheter aortic valve implantation. Am J Cardiol. 2011;108(10):1470–7.

39. Hansson NC, et al. The impact of calcium volume and distribution in aortic root injury related to balloon-expandable transcatheter aortic valve replacement. J Cardiovasc Comput Tomogr. 2015;9(5):382–92.

40. Khalique OK, et al. Quantity and location of aortic valve complex calcification predicts severity and location of paravalvular regurgitation and frequency of post-dilation after balloon-expandable transcatheter aortic valve replacement. JACC Cardiovasc Interv. 2014;7(8):885–94.

41. Almeida JG, et al. Comparison of self-expanding and balloon-expandable transcatheter aortic valves

morphology and association with paravalvular regurgitation: evaluation using multidetector computed tomography. Catheter Cardiovasc Interv. 2018;92(3):533–41.

42. Delgado V, Kapadia S, Schalij MJ, Schuijf JD, Tuzcu EM, Bax JJ. Transcatheter aortic valve implantation: implications of multimodality imaging in patient selection, procedural guidance, and outcomes. Heart. 2012;98(9):743–54.

43. Kim WK, et al. Comparison of outcomes using balloon-expandable versus self-expanding transcatheter prostheses according to the extent of aortic valve calcification. Clin Res Cardiol. 2017;106(12):995–1004.

44. Walther T, et al. Transapical aortic valve implantation: step by step. Ann Thorac Surg. 2009;87(1):276–83.

45. Willson AB, et al. Computed tomography-based sizing recommendations for transcatheter aortic valve replacement with balloon-expandable valves: comparison with transesophageal echocardiography and rationale for implementation in a prospective trial. J Cardiovasc Comput Tomogr. 2012;6(6):406–14.

46. Barbanti M, et al. Impact of balloon post-dilation on clinical outcomes after transcatheter aortic valve replacement with the self-expanding CoreValve prosthesis. JACC Cardiovasc Interv. 2014;7(9):1014–21.

47. Kempfert J, et al. Transapical aortic valve implantation: analysis of risk factors and learning experience in 299 patients. Circulation. 2011;124(11 Suppl):S124–9.

48. Pibarot P, Dumesnil JG. Prosthetic heart valves: selection of the optimal prosthesis and long-term management. Circulation. 2009;119(7):1034–48.

49. Head SJ, et al. The impact of prosthesis patient mismatch on long-term survival after aortic valve replacement: a systematic review and meta-analysis of 34 observational studies comprising 27 186 patients with 133 141 patient-years. Eur Heart J. 2012;33(12):1518–29.

50. Dayan V, Vignolo G, Soca G, Paganini JJ, Brusich D, Pibarot P. Predictors and outcomes of prosthesis-patient mismatch after aortic valve replacement. JACC Cardiovasc Imaging. 2016;9(8):924–33.

51. Flameng W, Herregods MC, Vercalsteren M, Herijgers P, Bogaerts K, Meuris B. Prosthesis-patient mismatch predicts structural valve degeneration in bioprosthetic heart valves. Circulation. 2010;121(19):2123–9.

52. Walther T, et al. Patient prosthesis mismatch affects short- and long-term outcomes after aortic valve replacement. Eur J Cardiothorac Surg. 2006;30(1):15–9.

53. Bleiziffer S, et al. Impact of patient-prosthesis mismatch on exercise capacity in patients after bioprosthetic aortic valve replacement. Heart. 2008;94(5):637–41.

54. Bakhtiary F, et al. Impact of patient-prosthesis mismatch and aortic valve design on coronary flow reserve after aortic valve replacement. J Am Coll Cardiol. 2007;49(7):790–6.

55. Tasca G, et al. Impact of prosthesis-patient mismatch on cardiac events and midterm mortality after aortic valve replacement in patients with pure aortic stenosis. Circulation. 2006;113(4):570–6.

56. Johnston DR, et al. Long-term durability of bioprosthetic aortic valves: implications from 12,569 implants. Ann Thorac Surg. 2015;99(4):1239–47.

57. Pibarot P, et al. Incidence and sequelae of prosthesis-patient mismatch in transcatheter versus surgical valve replacement in high-risk patients with severe aortic stenosis: a PARTNER trial cohort-a analysis. J Am Coll Cardiol. 2014;64(13):1323–34.

58. Zorn GL, et al. Prosthesis-patient mismatch in high-risk patients with severe aortic stenosis: a randomized trial of a self-expanding prosthesis. J Thorac Cardiovasc Surg. 2016;151(4):1014–1023.e3.

59. Kalavrouziotis D, et al. Transcatheter aortic valve implantation in patients with severe aortic stenosis and small aortic annulus. J Am Coll Cardiol. 2011;58(10):1016–24.

60. Rogers T, et al. Choice of balloon-expandable versus self-expanding transcatheter aortic valve impacts hemodynamics differently according to aortic annular size. Am J Cardiol. 2017;119(6):900–4.

61. Yashima F, et al. Transcatheter aortic valve implantation in patients with an extremely small native aortic annulus: the OCEAN-TAVI registry. Int J Cardiol. 2017;240:126–31.

62. Ewe SH, et al. Hemodynamic and clinical impact of prosthesis patient mismatch after transcatheter aortic valve implantation. J Am Coll Cardiol. 2011;58(18):1910–8.

63. Kukucka M, et al. Patient-prosthesis mismatch after transapical aortic valve implantation: incidence and impact on survival. J Thorac Cardiovasc Surg. 2013;145(2):391–7.

64. Ribeiro HB, et al. Coronary obstruction following transcatheter aortic valve implantation: a systematic review. J Am Coll Cardiol Intv. 2013;6(5):452–61.

65. Theron A, et al. Patient-prosthesis mismatch in new generation trans-catheter heart valves: a propensity score analysis. Eur Heart J Cardiovasc Imaging. 2018;19(2):225–33.

66. Mauri V, et al. Short-term outcome and hemodynamic performance of next-generation self-expanding versus balloon-expandable transcatheter aortic valves in patients with small aortic annulus. Circ Cardiovasc Interv. 2017;10(10):e005013.

67. Shivaraju A, et al. Overexpansion of the SAPIEN 3 transcatheter heart valve: a feasibility study. JACC Cardiovasc Interv. 2015;8(15):2041–3.

68. Mathur M, Mccabe JM, Aldea G, Pal J, Don CW. Overexpansion of the 29 mm SAPIEN 3 transcatheter heart valve in patients with large aortic annuli (area > 683 mm^2): a case series. Catheter Cardiovasc Interv. 2018;91(6):1149–56.

69. Elmously A, Worku B, Wong SC, Salemi A. Pushing boundaries: implantation of the 34 mm Medtronic CoreValve in patients with a large aortic annulus. Catheter Cardiovasc Interv. 2018;92(7):1449–52.

70. Mylotte D, et al. Transcatheter aortic valve replacement in bicuspid aortic valve disease. J Am Coll Cardiol. 2014;64(22):2330–9.

71. Sievers HH, Schmidtke C. A classification system for the bicuspid aortic valve from 304 surgical specimens. J Thorac Cardiovasc Surg. 2007;133(5):1226–33.

72. Colombo A, Latib A. Bicuspid aortic valve: any room for TAVR? J Am Coll Cardiol. 2014;64(22):2340–2.

73. Barbanti M, et al. Transcatheter aortic valve replacement with new-generation devices: a systematic review and meta-analysis. Int J Cardiol. 2017;245:83–9.

74. Ando T, Briasoulis A, Holmes AA, Taub CC, Takagi H, Afonso L. Sapien 3 versus Sapien XT prosthetic valves in transcatheter aortic valve implantation: a meta-analysis. Int J Cardiol. 2016;220:472–8.

75. Grube E, et al. Clinical outcomes with a repositionable self-expanding transcatheter aortic valve prosthesis: the international FORWARD study. J Am Coll Cardiol. 2017;70(7):845–53.

76. Todaro D. et al. Early and mid-term outcomes of transcatheter aortic valve replacement using the new generation self-expanding Corevalve Evolut R device. 2018: 1–6

77. Forrest JK, et al. Early outcomes with the Evolut PRO repositionable self-expanding transcatheter aortic valve with pericardial wrap. JACC Cardiovasc Interv. 2018;11(2):181–91.

78. Möllmann H, et al. Real-world experience using the ACURATE neo prosthesis: 30-day outcomes of 1,000 patients enrolled in the SAVI TF registry. EuroIntervention. 2018;13(15):e1764–70.

79. Yoon S-H, et al. Outcomes in transcatheter aortic valve replacement for bicuspid versus tricuspid aortic valve stenosis. J Am Coll Cardiol. 2017;69(21):2579–89.

80. Yoon SH, et al. Transcatheter aortic valve replacement with early- and new-generation devices in bicuspid aortic valve stenosis. J Am Coll Cardiol. 2016;68(11):1195–205.

81. Perlman GY, et al. Bicuspid aortic valve stenosis: favorable early outcomes with a next-generation transcatheter heart valve in a multicenter study. JACC Cardiovasc Interv. 2016;9(8):817–24.

Individualized Device Choice for Transcatheter Aortic Valve Implantation

Nicola Corcione, Salvatore Giordano, Alberto Morello, and Arturo Giordano

The way a team plays as a whole determines its success. You may have the greatest bunch of individual stars in the world, but if they don't play together, the club won't be worth a dime

Babe Ruth

27.1 Introduction

In 2002, the treatment of aortic valve stenosis was revolutionized by Alain Cribier in Rouen, France [1]. Indeed, at that time, he performed the first transcatheter implant of a bioprosthesis in a compassionate case of severe valvular stenosis, and at this point, a new era began, the transcatheter aortic valve implantation (TAVI), also called transcatheter aortic valve replacement (TAVR), era. Thereafter, the treatment based on the first-generation balloon-expandable TAVI device obtained the CE mark of approval for patients deemed inoperable. Based on the results of trials such as Placement of AoRtic TraNscathetER Valves (PARTNER) study [2–4], the CoreValve

High-Risk US Pivotal trial [5], and the Surgical Replacement and Transcatheter Aortic Valve Implantation (SURTAVI) study [6], indications were extended to patients with high and intermediate surgical risk, with US Food and Drug Administration (FDA) approval following suite. Thus, this procedure immediately became commonplace in catheterization laboratories worldwide. This inevitably led to the comparison between the two leading technologies for TAVI: the CoreValve self-expandable prosthesis (Medtronic, Irvine, CA, USA) and the SAPIEN balloon-expandable prosthesis (Edwards Lifesciences, Irvine, CA, USA) [7]. Indeed, in a pioneering network meta-analysis comparing surgical valve replacement with transapical TAVI and transfemoral TAVI, distinguishing device type, Biondi-Zoccai et al. pooled data from four randomized trials (1805 patients) on TAVI.

Such comparisons did not only focus on delivery method and acute results but even more so on long-term effectiveness and safety. Specifically, the Comparison of Transcatheter Heart Valves in High-Risk Patients with Severe Aortic Stenosis: Medtronic CoreValve vs. Edwards SAPIEN XT (CHOICE) trial was the first trial to formally compare these two first-generation prostheses

N. Corcione · S. Giordano · A. Giordano (✉)
Interventional Cardiology Unit, Pineta Grande Hospital, Castel Volturno, Italy
e-mail: arturogiordano@tin.it

A. Morello
Unità Operativa di Emodinamica, Casa di Salute Santa Lucia, San Giuseppe Vesuviano, Italy

© Springer Nature Switzerland AG 2019
A. Giordano et al. (eds.), *Transcatheter Aortic Valve Implantation*,
https://doi.org/10.1007/978-3-030-05912-5_27

(CoreValve vs. SAPIEN), including a total of 241 high-risk patients with severe aortic stenosis [8]. Device success appeared higher with SAPIEN, with less residual aortic regurgitation, lower need for valve-in-valve procedures, and smaller risk of permanent pacemaker implantation. Yet, mortality and morbidity were not significantly different between the two devices.

Since then, huge scientific and economic resources have been invested on TAVI, bringing further developments and pieces of evidence, clearly changing the TAVI device landscape altogether. Specifically, second- and third-generation prostheses, which boast lower-profile delivery systems and controlled release, repositionability, and/or retrievability features, are now available for operators interested in TAVI [9]. Accordingly, one balloon-expandable and at least six different self-expandable devices are currently on the shelves, each yielding procedural success rate approaching 100%. Thus, in almost all cases, it is possible to perform the procedure with a reduced number of complications, irrespectively of the chosen device, as long as patient selection is carefully performed and operators are expert with their preferred device [10].

Yet, the choice of device continues to be a crucial strategic step, with important technical and procedural implications, which potentially also impact on acute device and procedural success, as well as short- and long-term outcomes. In particular, every device has several unique charac-teristics which must be known and weighed by the operator, in order to harmonize them with those of the patient during the pre-procedural screening phase as well as the very implant procedure (Table 27.1). However, much remains to be clarified regarding the durability of the prostheses over time and the mechanisms involved in TAVI prosthetic valve dysfunction, compared to the well-known alternatives which are surgically implanted.

In addition, the degeneration of TAVI prostheses, which is regarded as at least a moderate regurgitation or as a mean gradient ≥ 20 mmHg, has been observed in up to 50% of balloon-expandable prostheses at 8 years of follow-up [11]. The durability of the self-expandable CoreValve prosthesis has been reported recently by several groups, who were among the first users of the self-expandable prosthesis [12]. Notably, after almost 10 years of follow-up, few cases of valve dysfunction were recognized, albeit most with dire clinical consequences. These anecdotal data obviously call for continuous long-term follow-up of first- and second-generation TAVI devices, as well as for comparative effectiveness studies of third-generation devices.

In the following sections, we will review the leading TAVI devices, summarizing their key features, pros, cons, and clinical applications, highlighting which features make them ideal in different settings.

Table 27.1 Choice of transcatheter aortic valve implantation device based on patient features

	Acute aortic arch	Horizontal aorta	Bicuspid valve	Elliptical annulus	Extensive valve calcification	Small peripheral vessels	Depressed systolic function
Acurate neo	++	++	+/−	+/−	+	+/−	++
Allegra	+?	+?	+?	+?	−?	+/−	+
Evolut	--	−	++	++	+/−	++	+/−
Portico	++	++	+	++	++	+/−	++
Lotus edge	--	--	−	+/−	++	--	+/−
SAPIEN 3	++	++	--	--	--	++	++

++, favorable results can most likely be expected when using this device in this setting; +, favorable results can be expected when using this device in this setting; +/−, favorable results could possibly be expected when using this device in this setting; −, favorable results are not very likely to be expected when using this device in this setting; --, favorable results are most likely not to be expected when using this device in this setting; +?, favorable results might be expected when using this device in this setting, but additional data are required; -?, favorable results are unlikely using this devices in this setting, but additional data are required

27.2 Acurate Neo

The Acurate neo device (Boston Scientific, Natick, MA, USA) is a new-generation self-expandable TAVI device, which cannot be recaptured nor repositioned, although being particularly stable during the various release phases [13, 14]. It is comprised of a porcine pericardial supra-annular valve, which is built on a structure unique for its opening modality: the so-called top-down implantation. It is the indeed the only prosthesis which expands first in aorta and then in the aortic root. Regarding its implant, the first step involves the opening of three very large stabilization arches for possible subsequent access to the coronary ostia, and then the expansion of the upper crown determines the anchorage of the supra-annular prosthesis. Then the opening of the lower crown allows the adhesion of the prosthesis in LVOT with minimal protrusion. Therefore the Acurate neo easily reaches the implant position and keeps it steadily during the various phases of release, reducing turbulence and the risk of jumping. In addition, the Acurate neo is equipped with a pericardial skirt lining, the internal and external part of the landing zone, in order to reduce the paravalvular leak. The prosthesis is mounted on an 18 French compatible delivery system (Acurate TF), with a flexible shaft that allows the navigation of angular arches. The prosthesis demonstrated good performance, with particularly favorable results for all-cause mortality, periprosthetic residual regurgitation, and permanent pacemaker implantation rates [13–15]. Most importantly, recent data provided by Kim and colleagues highlight the importance of appropriate oversizing and taking into account patient anatomy and calcium distribution to minimize paravalvular leak and permanent implantation [16].

27.3 Allegra

The Allegra (New Valve Technology, Hechingen, Germany) is a self-expanding valve, constituted by a trileaflet bovine pericardial valve, attached to a nitinol stent frame [17]. Its nitinol stent frame presents cells of variable dimensions that lead to different levels of radial force and ease the access to coronary ostia. Six radiopaque gold markers are placed at the level of the valve plan to assist correct valve positioning, whereas the inflow section of the prosthesis is covered by a bovine pericardial sealing skirt to reduce paravalvular regurgitation. Notably, the outflow of the valve, which has smaller dimensions than the inflow, allows a leaflet stress reduction, that could be related to a reduction of the degeneration and calcification of the leaflets, which may increase the durability. Allegra is available in three sizes (23, 27, and 31 mm) to match aortic annulus dimensions ranging from 19 to 29 mm. Its delivery system consists of an 18 French sheath that is used for all sizes of prosthesis and includes a three-step releasing mechanism (PermaFlow) for the controlled positioning without interfering with the left ventricular outflow tract. Thanks to such features, it can be recaptured and fully retrieved. Currently little data are available regarding this prosthetic valve, but the characteristics of the valve such as the short height and those related to the delivery system seem to be interesting from a flexibility point of view. Hence, selective use of this device could be envisioned for complex aortic arches and horizontal aortas.

27.4 Evolut

Evolut R and Evolut PRO are, respectively, second- and third-generation devices succeeding the CoreValve device (Medtronic, Minneapolis, MN, USA) [18–21]. Evolut is a self-expanding valve, with a gradual release system which can then enable valve recapturing and repositioning. Although being characterized by a low profile structure of nitinol mesh, it exerts great radial force that allows an excellent ability to adapt to an elliptical or irregularly shaped annulus, such as one resulting from abundant calcification. Specifically, Evolut PRO also has a porcine pericardium skirt that wraps the outside of the prosthesis to a height of one cell and a half of the inflow (13 mm). This coating allows an increase of the contact surface between the prosthesis and the native annulus, reducing the gap, favoring endothelization, and reducing the risk of a possible periprosthetic regurgitation. Three cusps of porcine pericardium are mounted inside the metal structure in order to obtain supra-annular valve functioning that optimizes the coaptation in an elliptical annulus or in cases of bicuspid valve disease.

The prosthesis is mounted on a low-profile (14 French equivalent) releasing system (16 French for the Evolut PRO) which allows its use via femoral access in patients with a iliofemoral vessel caliber ≥5 mm. Prosthesis size ranges from 23 to 34 mm, such that Evolut covers the broadest range of annulus sizes. Moreover, currently the Evolut is the only TAVI system approved for annulus diameters up to 30 mm. The wide sizing range, the gradual release, and the possibility of recapture make the Evolut suitable for its implantation in failed surgical bioprostheses (valve-in-valve), as long as the original model and size are known. The two metal cores inside the delivery system contribute to maintain the coaxiality and give stability during the release. However on the other hand, they make the prosthesis unsuitable in anatomically complex cases such as horizontal aorta or particular tortuosities of the aortic arch. Whenever the angulation of the aortic arch is reduced, the bending of the nose cone may cause the loss of continuity with the capsule that, due to its rigidity, may cause fissures and tears in the vessel or may ease the displacement of atero-thrombotic material.

Several institutions and collaborative groups have provided clinical data in support of the strengths of Evolut while highlighting some of its limitations [20, 22–24]. Notably, in the Evolut R US study, 241 patients received this second-generation device. Short-term follow-up showed good mortality (2.5%) and morbidity results, with permanent pacemaker implantation in 16.4% and moderate paravalvular leak in 5.3% [22]. Forrest et al. have also provided preliminary data on Evolut PRO in 60 US patients, providing favorable 30-day outcome data, including 1.7% death, 11.8% permanent pacemaker

implantation, and 0% moderate or severe para-valvular leak rates [20].

27.5   Lotus Edge

Lotus Edge (Boston Scientific) is a self-expandable prosthesis, currently not available on international markets due to a safety recall, characterized by three bovine pericardial cusps mounted on a nitinol structure, boasting a polyurethane sealing membrane for the reduction of periprosthetic regurgitation [25–27]. There are two sizes of this prosthesis, 23 and 27 mm, which are, respectively, mounted on a pre-curved delivery system of 18 or 20 French, which therefore requires a specific proprietary introducer from 20.1 French (6.7 mm) to 22.5 French (7.5 mm), hence wider than the standard introducers. This system unfortunately has reduced flexibility that does not make it suitable for complex aortic arches [28]. The valve has an initial elongated conformation which, as it is released, is shortened to its final configuration that has a height of 19 mm. Although this device has shown excellent results in terms of reducing paravalvular leak, it pays duty for the high percentage of final post-procedural pacemaker implantation compared to the other prostheses [25–27]. Despite limited details on the reasons for the recall, it appears that excess tension in the pin mechanism inadvertently introduced during manufacturing caused issues in valve locking [29].

27.6   Portico

Portico (Abbott Vascular, Santa Clara, CA, USA) is a self-expandable prosthesis composed of a nitinol structure very similar to the Medtronic device, although presenting a different geometry characterized by large cells which facilitate the access to coronary ostia and increase the contact between the stent and the tissue, with excellent conformability and sealing capacity [30–32]. Three bovine pericardial cusps and a porcine pericardial skirt complete the prosthetic structure. Both components of the device are treated with anti-calcification substances (Linux anti-calcification treatment). The prosthesis can be mounted, in a relative short time, and its release system is characterized by an 18 French distal portion and 13 French proximal shaft. Most importantly, the delivery system is extremely flexible allowing its use also in cases of complex anatomy such as severe tortuosity, angulated aortic arch, and horizontal aorta.

The controlled and gradual release allows complete recapture and repositioning. A very important characteristic is correct functioning from the early phases of the opening. This allows hemodynamic stability during the whole procedure, avoiding the necessity of rapid-pacing during its release. This prosthesis has also an excellent capacity of adaptation and conformability, even to elliptical annuli, maintaining suitable performance over time, with a durability equal to the surgically implanted St. Jude biological prostheses [33].

27.7 SAPIEN 3

The SAPIEN 3 device (Edwards Lifesciences, Irvine, CA, USA) is a balloon-expandable prosthesis currently in the third-generation stage [34, 35]. It is composed of a cobalt-chromium structure, which is shorter than the anatomy of the aortic root, in which three cusps of bovine pericardium are mounted (exactly the same used in surgical prostheses). An inner and an outer layer of polyethylene, designed for paravalvular leak reduction, coats the prosthesis, which is pre-mounted on a balloon which, after being dilated, determines the expansion and the adhesion of the prosthetic valve to the aortic annulus, with a non-gradual mechanism. The releasing mechanism allows a simple and fast implantation, but on the other hand, it is not possible to recapture it nor reposition it. In addition, this device is suitable for circular and slightly calcified annuli. However, whenever there is abundant calcium, prosthetic oversize of >20% exposes the patient to a high-

risk, even if rare, complication: the rupture of the annulus [36].

The proprietary eSheath is a low-profile introducer, and it is expandable when the prosthesis passes through it. It is available in two sizes: 14 French, compatible with valves of 23 and 26 mm, and 16 French, compatible with valves of 29 mm, allowing the procedure to be performed by a femoral route even in patients with small femoral vessels. The proprietary Commander releasing system is equipped with a double joint to achieve perfect coaxiality, making the device suitable for excellent performance even in difficult anatomical conditions, such as the tortuosity of the aortic arch and the horizontal aorta [37, 38].

27.8 Comparative Effectiveness

Several studies have compared TAVI vs. competing treatments such as medical therapy including balloon aortic valvuloplasty or surgical aortic valve replacement or have focused on different devices for TAVI (Table 27.2) [39, 40]. Despite the accrual of data, substantial uncertainty persists, with data suggesting that balloon-expandable devices are associated with a lower risk of permanent pacemaker implantation and lower risk of significant paravalvular leak, albeit at the expense of a potential increase in periprocedural complications. Self-expandable devices have each specific feature which may make them more or less suitable for individual patients but in general are associated with a higher rate of permanenst pacemaker implantation and significant paravalvular leak. Yet, ongoing evolution of current devices (including balloon-expandable ones) suggests that eventually short- and long-term clinical outcomes will tend to become uniform across devices. Nonetheless, further insights will be provided by several trials currently ongoing and aiming at comparing last-generation devices [41]. Their results will help to establish each specific device characteristic, thus hopefully proving useful for choosing the right prosthesis for each individual patient.

Table 27.2 Completed or ongoing randomized clinical trials on the comparative effectiveness of transcatheter aortic valve implantation (TAVI)

Name	Experimental Rx	Comparator Rx	Sample	Status	Reference
CHOICE	CoreValve	SAPIEN XT	121	CoreValve and SAPIEN XT have similar outcomes	PMID 24682026
DEDICATE	Any CE marked TAVI device	SAVR	1600	Recruiting	NCT 03112980
EARLY TAVR	SAPIEN 3	Medical Rx	1109	Recruiting	NCT 03042104
ELECT	SAPIEN XT	CoreValve	108	Results pending	NCT 01982032
Evolut R Low Risk	CoreValve or Evolut	SAVR	1200	Recruiting	NCT 02701283
NOTION	CoreValve	SAVR	280	TAVI and SAVR have similar outcomes	PMID 27296202
NOTION 2	Any CE marked TAVI device	SAVR	992	Recruiting	NCT 02825134
PARTNER 1A	SAPIEN XT	SAVR	699	TAVI and SAVR have similar outcomes	PMID 22443479
PARTNER 1B	SAPIEN XT	Medical Rx (including valvuloplasty)	358	TAVI is superior to medical therapy	PMID 22443478
PARTNER 2	SAPIEN XT	SAVR	2032	TAVI and SAVR have similar outcomes	PMID 27040324
PARTNER 3	SAPIEN 3	SAVR	1328	Recruiting	NCT 02675114
PORTICO IDE	Portico	Evolut or SAPIEN 3	758	Recruiting	NCT 02000115
REBOOT	Lotus edge	SAPIEN 3	116	Suspended	NCT 02668484
REPRISE 3	Lotus edge	Evolut	2092	Suspended	NCT 02202434
SCOPE 1	Acurate neo	SAPIEN 3	730	Recruiting	NCT 03011346
SCOPE 2	Acurate neo	Evolut	764	Recruiting	NCT 03192813
STACCATO	SAPIEN XT	SAVR	70	TA TAVI is worse than SAVR	PMID 22581299
SURTAVI	CoreValve	SAVR	1746	TAVI and SAVR have similar outcomes	PMID 28304219
TAVR UNLOAD	SAPIEN 3	Medical Rx	600	Recruiting	NCT 02661451
US CoreValve High Risk	CoreValve	SAVR	795	TAVI is superior to SAVR	PMID 24678937

NCT US National Library of Medicine ClinicalTrials.gov ID; *PMID* PubMed ID; *SAVR* surgical

27.9 Conclusion

Transcatheter aortic valve implantation has already reached maturity in the field of structural heart disease therapies. Notably, several TAVI devices are available, each with its unique features. Most likely, no device is superior to the others for all technical and clinical dimensions, and some patients may benefit from a specific device and others from others. Awaiting additional comparative effectiveness studies, clinicians, interventional cardiologists, and surgeons need to become acquainted with the subtleties of each device, in order to maximize effectiveness and minimize risk, while remaining conscious of costs and resource use.

Conflicts of Interest Dr. Corcione has consulted for Abbott Vascular. Dr. A. Giordano has consulted for Abbott Vascular and Medtronic.

References

1. Cribier A, Eltchaninoff H, Bash A, Borenstein N, Tron C, Bauer F, Derumeaux G, Anselme F, Laborde F, Leon MB. Percutaneous transcatheter implantation of an aortic valve prosthesis for calcific aortic stenosis: first human case description. Circulation. 2002;106:3006–8.
2. Makkar RR, Fontana GP, Jilaihawi H, Kapadia S, Pichard AD, Douglas PS, Thourani VH, Babaliaros VC, Webb JG, Herrmann HC, Bavaria JE, Kodali S, Brown DL, Bowers B, Dewey TM, Svensson LG, Tuzcu M, Moses JW, Williams MR, Siegel RJ, Akin JJ, Anderson WN, Pocock S, Smith CR, Leon MB, PARTNER Trial Investigators. Transcatheter aortic-

valve replacement for inoperable severe aortic stenosis. N Engl J Med. 2012;366:1696–704.

3. Kodali SK, Williams MR, Smith CR, Svensson LG, Webb JG, Makkar RR, Fontana GP, Dewey TM, Thourani VH, Pichard AD, Fischbein M, Szeto WY, Lim S, Greason KL, Teirstein PS, Malaisrie SC, Douglas PS, Hahn RT, Whisenant B, Zajarias A, Wang D, Akin JJ, Anderson WN, Leon MB, PARTNER Trial Investigators. Two-year outcomes after transcatheter or surgical aortic-valve replacement. N Engl J Med. 2012;366:1686–95.

4. Leon MB, Smith CR, Mack MJ, Makkar RR, Svensson LG, Kodali SK, Thourani VH, Tuzcu EM, Miller DC, Herrmann HC, Doshi D, Cohen DJ, Pichard AD, Kapadia S, Dewey T, Babaliaros V, Szeto WY, Williams MR, Kereiakes D, Zajarias A, Greason KL, Whisenant BK, Hodson RW, Moses JW, Trento A, Brown DL, Fearon WF, Pibarot P, Hahn RT, Jaber WA, Anderson WN, Alu MC, Webb JG, PARTNER 2 Investigators. Transcatheter or surgical aortic-valve replacement in intermediate-risk patients. N Engl J Med. 2016;374:1609–20.

5. Adams DH, Popma JJ, Reardon MJ, Yakubov SJ, Coselli JS, Deeb GM, Gleason TG, Buchbinder M, Hermiller J Jr, Kleiman NS, Chetcuti S, Heiser J, Merhi W, Zorn G, Tadros P, Robinson N, Petrossian G, Hughes GC, Harrison JK, Conte J, Maini B, Mumtaz M, Chenoweth S, Oh JK, U.S. CoreValve Clinical Investigators. Transcatheter aortic-valve replacement with a self-expanding prosthesis. N Engl J Med. 2014;370:1790–8.

6. Reardon MJ, Van Mieghem NM, Popma JJ, Kleiman NS, Søndergaard L, Mumtaz M, Adams DH, Deeb GM, Maini B, Gada H, Chetcuti S, Gleason T, Heiser J, Lange R, Merhi W, Oh JK, Olsen PS, Piazza N, Williams M, Windecker S, Yakubov SJ, Grube E, Makkar R, Lee JS, Conte J, Vang E, Nguyen H, Chang Y, Mugglin AS, Serruys PW, Kappetein AP, SURTAVI Investigators. Surgical or transcatheter aortic-valve replacement in intermediate-risk patients. N Engl J Med. 2017;376:1321–31.

7. Biondi-Zoccai G, Peruzzi M, Abbate A, Gertz ZM, Benedetto U, Tonelli E, D'Ascenzo F, Giordano A, Agostoni P, Frati G. Network meta-analysis on the comparative effectiveness and safety of transcatheter aortic valve implantation with CoreValve or Sapien devices versus surgical replacement. Heart Lung Vessel. 2014;6:232–43.

8. Abdel-Wahab M, Mehilli J, Frerker C, Neumann FJ, Kurz T, Tölg R, Zachow D, Guerra E, Massberg S, Schäfer U, El-Mawardy M, Richardt G, CHOICE Investigators. Comparison of balloon-expandable vs self-expandable valves in patients undergoing transcatheter aortic valve replacement: the CHOICE randomized clinical trial. JAMA. 2014;311:1503–14.

9. Giordano A, Corcione N, Biondi-Zoccai G, Berti S, Petronio AS, Pierli C, Presbitero P, Giudice P, Sardella G, Bartorelli AL, Bonmassari R, Indolfi C, Marchese A, Brscic E, Cremonesi A, Testa L, Brambilla N, Bedogni F. Patterns and trends of transcatheter aortic

valve implantation in Italy: insights from RISPEVA. J Cardiovasc Med (Hagerstown). 2017;18:96–102.

10. Gatto L, Biondi-Zoccai G, Romagnoli E, Frati G, Prati F, Giordano A. New-generation devices for transcatheter aortic valve implantation. Minerva Cardioangiol. 2018;66:747–61. https://doi.org/10.23736/S0026-4725.18.04707-2.

11. Kappetein AP, Head SJ, Généreux P, Piazza N, van Mieghem NM, Blackstone EH, Brott TG, Cohen DJ, Cutlip DE, van Es GA, Hahn RT, Kirtane AJ, Krucoff MW, Kodali S, Mack MJ, Mehran R, Rodés-Cabau J, Vranckx P, Webb JG, Windecker S, Serruys PW, Leon MB. Updated standardized endpoint definitions for transcatheter aortic valve implantation: the valve academic research consortium-2 consensus document. Eur Heart J. 2012;33:2403–18.

12. Arora S, Vavalle JP. Transcatheter aortic valve replacement in intermediate and low risk patients-clinical evidence. Ann Cardiothorac Surg. 2017;6:493–7.

13. Möllmann H, Diemert P, Grube E, Baldus S, Kempfert J, Abizaid A. Symetis ACURATE TF™ aortic bioprosthesis. EuroIntervention. 2013;9:S107–10.

14. Möllmann H, Walther T, Siqueira D, Diemert P, Treede H, Grube E, Nickenig G, Baldus S, Rudolph T, Kuratani T, Sawa Y, Kempfert J, Kim WK, Abizaid A. Transfemoral TAVI using the self-expanding ACURATE neo prosthesis: one-year outcomes of the multicentre "CE-approval cohort". EuroIntervention. 2017;13:e1040–6.

15. Möllmann H, Hengstenberg C, Hilker M, Kerber S, Schäfer U, Rudolph T, Linke A, Franz N, Kuntze T, Nef H, Kappert U, Walther T, Zembala MO, Toggweiler S, Kim WK. Real-world experience using the ACURATE neo prosthesis: 30-day outcomes of 1,000 patients enrolled in the SAVI TF registry. EuroIntervention. 2018;13:e1764–70.

16. Kim WK, Möllmann H, Liebetrau C, Renker M, Rolf A, Simon P, Van Linden A, Arsalan M, Doss M, Hamm CW, Walther T. The ACURATE neo transcatheter heart valve: a comprehensive analysis of predictors of procedural outcome. JACC Cardiovasc Interv. 2018;11:1721–9. https://doi.org/10.1016/j.jcin.2018.04.039.

17. Wenaweser P, Stortecky S, Schütz T, Praz F, Gloekler S, Windecker S, Elsässer A. Transcatheter aortic valve implantation with the NVT Allegra transcatheter heart valve system: first-in-human experience with a novel self-expanding transcatheter heart valve. EuroIntervention. 2016;12:71–7.

18. Piazza N, Martucci G, Lachapelle K, de Varennes B, Bilodeau L, Buithieu J, Mylotte D. First-in-human experience with the Medtronic CoreValve Evolut R. EuroIntervention. 2014;9:1260–3.

19. Noble S, Stortecky S, Heg D, Tueller D, Jeger R, Toggweiler S, Ferrari E, Nietlispach F, Taramasso M, Maisano F, Grünenfelder J, Jüni P, Huber C, Carrel T, Windecker S, Wenaweser P, Roffi M. Comparison of procedural and clinical outcomes with Evolut R versus Medtronic CoreValve: a Swiss TAVI registry analysis. EuroIntervention. 2017;12:e2170–6.

20. Forrest JK, Mangi AA, Popma JJ, Khabbaz K, Reardon MJ, Kleiman NS, Yakubov SJ, Watson D, Kodali S, George I, Tadros P, Zorn GL 3rd, Brown J, Kipperman R, Saul S, Qiao H, Oh JK, Williams MR. Early outcomes with the Evolut PRO repositionable self-expanding transcatheter aortic valve with pericardial wrap. JACC Cardiovasc Interv. 2018;11:160–8.

21. Mahtta D, Elgendy IY, Bavry AA. From CoreValve to Evolut PRO: reviewing the journey of self-expanding transcatheter aortic valves. Cardiol Ther. 2017;6:183–92.

22. Popma JJ, Reardon MJ, Khabbaz K, Harrison JK, Hughes GC, Kodali S, George I, Deeb GM, Chetcuti S, Kipperman R, Brown J, Qiao H, Slater J, Williams MR. Early clinical outcomes after transcatheter aortic valve replacement using a novel self-expanding bioprosthesis in patients with severe aortic stenosis who are suboptimal for surgery: results of the Evolut R US study. JACC Cardiovasc Interv. 2017;10:268–75.

23. Kuhn C, Frerker C, Meyer AK, Kurz T, Schäfer U, Deuschl F, Abdel-Wahab M, Schewel D, Elghalban A, Kuck KH, Frey N, Frank D. Transcatheter aortic valve implantation with the 34 mm self-expanding CoreValve Evolut R: initial experience in 101 patients from a multicentre registry. EuroIntervention. 2018;14:e301–5.

24. Schwerg M, Stangl K, Laule M, Stangl V, Dreger H. Valve in valve implantation of the CoreValve Evolut R in degenerated surgical aortic valves. Cardiol J. 2018;25:301–7.

25. Gooley R, Lockwood S, Antonis P, Meredith IT. The SADRA lotus valve system: a fully repositionable, retrievable prosthesis. Minerva Cardioangiol. 2013;61:45–52.

26. Meredith IT, Worthley SG, Whitbourn RJ, Antonis P, Montarello JK, Newcomb AE, Lockwood S, Haratani N, Allocco DJ, Dawkins KD. Transfemoral aortic valve replacement with the repositionable lotus valve system in high surgical risk patients: the REPRISE I study. EuroIntervention. 2014;9:1264–70.

27. Meredith IT, Walters DL, Dumonteil N, Worthley SG, Tchétché D, Manoharan G, Blackman DJ, Rioufol G, Hildick-Smith D, Whitbourn RJ, Lefèvre T, Lange R, Müller R, Redwood S, Allocco DJ, Dawkins KD. Transcatheter aortic valve replacement for severe symptomatic aortic stenosis using a repositionable valve system: 30-day primary endpoint results from the REPRISE II study. J Am Coll Cardiol. 2014;64:1339–48.

28. Ruparelia N, Latib A, Kawamoto H, Buzzatti N, Giannini F, Figini F, Mangieri A, Regazzoli D, Stella S, Sticchi A, Tanaka A, Ancona M, Agricola E, Monaco F, Spagnolo P, Chieffo A, Montorfano M, Alfieri O, Colombo A. A comparison between first-generation and second-generation transcatheter aortic valve implantation (TAVI) devices: a propensity-matched single-center experience. J Invasive Cardiol. 2016;28:210–6.

29. Grover N. Boston Scientific recalls lotus valve heart devices. Reuters Health News. 2017. https://www.reuters.com/article/us-boston-scientific-recall/boston-scientific-recalls-lotus-valve-heart-devices-idUSKBN1621NA. Accessed 7 Aug 2018.

30. Manoharan G, Spence MS, Rodés-Cabau J, Webb JG. St Jude medical portico valve. EuroIntervention. 2012;8:Q97–101.

31. Manoharan G, Linke A, Moellmann H, Redwood S, Frerker C, Kovac J, Walther T. Multicentre clinical study evaluating a novel resheathable annular functioning self-expanding transcatheter aortic valve system: safety and performance results at 30 days with the portico system. EuroIntervention. 2016;12:768–74.

32. Linke A, Holzhey D, Möllmann H, Manoharan G, Schäfer U, Frerker C, Worthley SG, van Boven AJ, Redwood S, Kovac J, Butter C, Søndergaard L, Lauten A, Schymik G, Walther T. Treatment of aortic stenosis with a self-expanding, resheathable transcatheter valve: one-year results of the international multicenter portico transcatheter aortic valve implantation system study. Circ Cardiovasc Interv. 2018;11:e005206.

33. Tzikas A, Amrane H, Bedogni F, Brambilla N, Kefer J, Manoharan G, Makkar R, Möllman H, Rodés-Cabau J, Schäfer U, Settergren M, Spargias K, van Boven A, Walther T, Worthley SG, Sondergaard L. Transcatheter aortic valve replacement using the portico system: 10 things to remember. J Interv Cardiol. 2016;29:523–9.

34. Wendler O, Schymik G, Treede H, Baumgartner H, Dumonteil N, Ihlberg L, Neumann FJ, Tarantini G, Zamarano JL, Vahanian A. SOURCE 3 registry: design and 30-day results of the European Postapproval registry of the latest generation of the SAPIEN 3 transcatheter heart valve. Circulation. 2017;135:1123–32.

35. Mauri V, Reimann A, Stern D, Scherner M, Kuhn E, Rudolph V, Rosenkranz S, Eghbalzadeh K, Friedrichs K, Wahlers T, Baldus S, Madershahian N, Rudolph TK. Predictors of permanent pacemaker implantation after transcatheter aortic valve replacement with the SAPIEN 3. JACC Cardiovasc Interv. 2016;9:2200–9.

36. Miyasaka M, Tada N, Taguri M, Kato S, Enta Y, Otomo T, Hata M, Watanabe Y, Naganuma T, Araki M, Yamanaka F, Shirai S, Ueno H, Mizutani K, Tabata M, Higashimori A, Takagi K, Yamamoto M, Hayashida K, OCEAN-TAVI Investigators. Incidence, predictors, and clinical impact of prosthesis-patient mismatch following transcatheter aortic valve replacement in Asian patients: the OCEAN-TAVI lregistry. JACC Cardiovasc Interv. 2018;11(8):771–80.

37. Ohno Y, Tamburino C, Barbanti M. Transcatheter aortic valve implantation experience with SAPIEN 3. Minerva Cardioangiol. 2015;63:205–16.

38. Facchin M, Mojoli M, Covolo E, Tarantini G. The SAPIEN 3 valve: lights and shadows. Minerva Med. 2014;105:497–500.

39. Baumgartner H, Falk V, Bax JJ, De Bonis M, Hamm C, Holm PJ, Iung B, Lancellotti P, Lansac E, Rodriguez Muñoz D, Rosenhek R, Sjögren J, Tornos Mas P, Vahanian A, Walther T, Wendler O, Windecker

S, Zamorano JL, ESC Scientific Document Group. 2017 ESC/EACTS guidelines for the management of valvular heart disease. Eur Heart J. 2017;38:2739–91.

40. Nishimura RA, Otto CM, Bonow RO, Carabello BA, Erwin JP 3rd, Fleisher LA, Jneid H, Mack MJ, McLeod CJ, O'Gara PT, Rigolin VH, Sundt TM 3rd, Thompson A. 2017 AHA/ACC focused update of the 2014 AHA/ACC guideline for the management of patients with valvular heart disease: a report of the American College of Cardiology/American Heart Association Task Force on clinical practice guidelines. J Am Coll Cardiol. 2017;70:252–89.

41. Abawi M, Agostoni P, Kooistra NHM, Samim M, Nijhoff F, Voskuil M, Nathoe H, Doevendans PA, Chamuleau SA, Urgel K, Hendrikse J, Leiner T, Abrahams AC, van der Worp B, Stella PR. Rationale and design of the Edwards SAPIEN-3 periprosthetic leakage evaluation versus Medtronic CoreValve in transfemoral aortic valve implantation (ELECT) trial: a randomised comparison of balloon-expandable versus self-expanding transcatheter aortic valve prostheses. Neth Hear J. 2017;25:318–29.

Predilation in Transcatheter Aortic Valve Implantation

28

Alexander Sedaghat, Eberhard Grube, and Jan-Malte Sinning

The only thing I know, is that I know nothing

Socrates

28.1 Introduction

The notion that predilation calcific aortic stenosis in transcatheter aortic valve implantation (TAVI), also called transcatheter aortic valve replacement (TAVR), is required for procedural success derives from the concept of (coronary) angioplasty and stent (graft) implantation. Especially in severely calcified stenotic lesions, predilation and lesion preparation are necessary to facilitate crossing of the lesion with the stent (graft) and to ensure complete expansion of the subsequently implanted stent (graft) [1]. In TAVI, predilation has three aims: (1) increasing the aortic valve area to allow passage of the delivery catheter, (2) improving periprocedural hemodynamics, and (3) preventing recoil and thereby underexpansion of the transcatheter prosthesis by modifying the valvular calcium pattern [2]. Furthermore, predilation can be useful in other aspects of TAVI including prosthesis sizing or the anticipation of coronary obstruction [3, 4].

Although the scientific evidence supporting the necessity of predilation is limited, it has been con-

sidered mandatory in the early years of TAVI and is still part of the manufacturers' instructions for use. In contrast, more recently, several (mainly retrospective) studies and meta-analyses studies have been published, suggesting safety and feasibility of "direct TAVI" (i.e., TAVI without predilation), challenging the general need for predilation [5–9].

This chapter will give an overview of predilation in the context of TAVI including potential benefits and pitfalls of this technique as well as the current scientific evidence on this topic.

28.2 Predilation: Technical Aspects

In its essence, predilation of calcific aortic stenosis in TAVI follows the procedural characteristics of aortic valvuloplasty [10]. In transvascular procedures, after establishing arterial access, a guidewire is advanced toward the aortic valve in a retrograde fashion. The aortic valve is then crossed with the use of an Amplatz Left (e.g. AL 1) diagnostic catheter and a soft straight-tip 0.035″ wire in an RAO 30° projection. In severely calcified aortic stenosis, the use of a hydrophilic Terumo guidewire with a straight tip (e.g., Terumo, Kanagawa, Japan) may be useful. After successful crossing, the catheter is advanced into left ventricular (LV) cavity, and the soft wire is

A. Sedaghat · E. Grube (✉) · J.-M. Sinning
Heart Center Bonn, University Hospital Bonn, Bonn, Germany
e-mail: alexander.sedaghat@ukbonn.de; jan-malte.sinning@ukbonn.de

© Springer Nature Switzerland AG 2019
A. Giordano et al. (eds.), *Transcatheter Aortic Valve Implantation*, https://doi.org/10.1007/978-3-030-05912-5_28

exchanged for a regular J-tip steel wire which is then that a stiffer wire over a pigtail catheter. Several different types of stiff wires are available for use, e.g., Amplatz Super Stiff™ (Boston Scientific, Marlborough, MA, USA) or the Lunderquist Extra Stiff® wire (Cook Medical, Bloomington, IN, USA), providing different degrees of support during the procedure. Currently, the use of pre-shaped TAVI guidewires can be considered a therapeutic "gold-standard" owing to their less traumatic design to prevent ventricular injury (e.g., the Safari™ guidewire; Boston Scientific Inc., Marlborough, MA, USA; or the Confida™ guidewire, Medtronic Inc., Minneapolis, MN, USA).

Classically, prior to predilation, a temporary pacing wire (TPW) is inserted into the right ventricle via a transfemoral or transjugular venous access. Predilation is then performed during rapid ventricular overdrive pacing at 180–220/min to minimize cardiac output and to stabilize balloon position. In patients with implanted permanent pacemakers, overdrive pacing may be performed using the implanted system. Recently, single-wire techniques using the 0.035″ guidewire and left ventricular overdrive pacing have been found feasible and safe, suggesting a role of this approach for selected patients [11].

Predilation is usually performed with the use of either semi-compliant (e.g., Tyshak II, Braun International Systems) or non-compliant balloons (e.g., Z-Med™, Braun Interventional Systems Inc., Bethlehem, PA, USA). As an alternative, balloons with hourglass shapes have been implemented into clinical practice. These balloons, such as the V8™ (InterValve Inc., Minnetonka, MN, USA) or the NuCLEUS X™ (NuMed Inc., Hopkinton, NY, USA) can theoretically improve stability and reduce the risk of annular rupture [10]. More recently, a valvuloplasty balloon allowing continuous cardiac blood flow during predilation has been introduced and is currently under clinical investigation (ClinicalTrials.gov identifier: NCT02847546). Owing to a central open lumen, the True™ Flow balloon (BARD PV Inc., Tempe, AZ, USA) allows a cardiac output of ~1 L/min during inflation, thereby potentially obviating the need for rapid overdrive pacing and reducing predilation-associated systemic hypoperfusion.

Whereas the type of balloon used for predilation remains mostly at the discretion of the physician, balloon size is chosen based on preprocedural sizing of the aortic annulus determined either by (transesophageal) echocardiography or computed tomography (CT) imaging. Hereby, the size of the balloon is usually chosen slightly smaller than the mean diameter of the native aortic annulus (≤1:1 ratio) to avoid annular rupture and/or aortic root dissection. Recently, even more pronounced balloon undersizing has been advocated. In this context, aortic valve morphology (bicuspid/tricuspid) and amount and distribution of aortic valve calcium, as well as left ventricular outflow tract (LVOT) calcification, should be taken into account, to avoid aortic injury and annulus rupture.

During predilation, the balloon is usually inflated with 25–50 mL of saline/contrast (10:90 ratio) for ~3 s [10]. Complete expansion and stable positioning of the balloon should be documented by either periprocedural fluoroscopy or transesophageal echocardiography. The authors of this chapter prefer fluoroscopy due to the less invasive nature of this approach and due to the fact that complete deflation of the balloon can be appreciated.

Although its procedural success is not clearly defined, predilation should translate to a significant reduction of the transvalvular peak-to-peak gradient and an increase of the aortic valve area. Changes in peak aortic gradient can hereby be assessed periprocedurally by pressure tracings of two pigtail catheters (in left ventricle and aorta), a pigtail catheter (in the left ventricle) and the side port of the femoral access sheath or a dual-lumen pigtail catheter. Whereas a reduction of peak aortic gradients of 50 mmHg or 40–50% is warranted in balloon aortic valvuloplasty as bridging or definite therapy [10], smaller reductions can be expected after predilation with an undersized balloon to facilitate a TAVI procedure owing to the less aggressive approach. Hereby, increases in aortic valve area are best assessed with the use of (transesophageal) echocardiography. However, this information is usually not required in clinical practice, given the fact that predilation is usually followed by TAVI as final therapy. During predilation, outward movement of the bulky, calcified aortic cusps toward the coronary sinus is noted and can be helpful— combined with an aortic root angiography—to determine the risk of coronary obstruction.

28.3 Complications of Predilation

The potential complications inflicted by predilation reflect those of traditional balloon aortic valvuloplasty (BAV). Whereas most complications can be managed by the means of acute interventional strategies, major complications such as rupture of the aortic annulus or LV perforation may require emergency surgical intervention. It is therefore current consensus of the European Society of Cardiology (ESC) and the European Association of Cardio-Thoracic Surgeons (EACTS) that percutaneous aortic interventions such as TAVI should only be performed in centers with both departments of cardiology and cardiac surgery on-site [12].

28.3.1 Cardiac Perforation

Cardiac perforation with subsequent cardiac tamponade represents one of the most dreaded forms of periprocedural complications and usually requires emergency (surgical) therapy. During predilation cardiac perforation can be caused by annular rupture or perforation of the left ventricular wall by the stiff guidewire and should always be excluded immediately by echocardiography in case of sudden hemodynamic instability. Cardiac perforation and tamponade are hereby not restricted to the process of predilation but can occur during all procedural steps of TAVI including placement of the temporary pacing wire, crossing of the aortic valve, THV placement, and postdilation [13]. With increasing operator experience and the development of less traumatic pre-shaped wires, the incidence of LV perforation has been successfully reduced. In a recently published multicenter registry of >27,000 patients

treated between 2013–2016, guidewire-induced LV perforation necessitating emergent cardiac surgery was seen in 0,23% of patients [14].

28.3.2 Vascular Injury

Vascular complications represent a rather common entity in TAVI and may already occur during the process of balloon insertion and predilation. Generally, vascular injury is divided into minor and major complications by prespecified, standardized criteria of the Valve Academic Research Consortium [15]. In current randomized TAVI collectives, major vascular complications are observed in 6–7,9% [16, 17]. Furthermore, vascular complications may be distinguished according to their primary location. Hereby, access site and access-related vascular injury (ASARVI) such as bleeding, dissection, or vessel occlusion are usually caused by either the transfemoral sheath, the THV delivery system, or incomplete access site closure and can be managed by percutaneous techniques (e.g., manual compression, crossover balloon occlusion, or stent graft placement) in the majority of cases [18–21].

On the other hand, non-ASARVI complications, such as rupture/perforation of the aortic annulus/root and aortic (root) dissection, can result as the immediate consequence of BAV/predilation and are associated with increased morbidity.

Rupture of the aorta or the aortic annulus is described in the literature with an incidence of 0–2% and is associated with poor prognosis [22]. In the EuRECS-TAVI registry, the incidence of annular rupture requiring emergency cardiac surgery was 0.25%, with an inhospital mortality of 62,2% [14]. Generally, management strategies range from conservative therapy to emergent cardiac surgery and are dependent on location and clinical manifestation [23]. From clinical experience, it is known that the etiology of annular rupture is multifactorial and not linked merely to the mismatch of balloon/aortic annulus (i.e., oversizing). Predisposing factors for its occurrence include small annuli (<20 mm) combined with narrow aortic roots, circular aortic valve calcification, LVOT calcification, and LV hypertrophy [23]. Given the potentially fatal consequences of this complication, meticulous preprocedural imaging with computed tomography and 3D transesophageal echocardiography is warranted to evaluate landing zone dimensions, the extent of valvular/LVOT calcification, and its patterns in order to assess the potential risk of rupture.

Another dreaded complication of predilation (and TAVI) is aortic dissection. Aortic dissection is observed in approximately 0,2% [24] of patients and can occur either acutely or with delay [25]. Acute dissection should be suspected with unexplained hemodynamic instability, pericardial effusion, or signs of (cerebral) malperfusion.

Management of iatrogenic aortic dissection varies from conservative strategies ("watchful waiting") over endograft placement to emergent cardiac surgery [26]. Although robust evidence on this issue is lacking, the underlying pathophysiology is likely similar to that of annular rupture meaning that a combination of aortic (root) calcification and vessel wall stress exerted by the balloon and/or THV might lead to dissection.

28.3.3 Severe Aortic Regurgitation

Severe aortic regurgitation (AR) may result as the immediate consequence of predilation. Whereas paravalvular leakage after TAVI has been successfully reduced with newer-generation transcatheter heart valves and increasing operator experience [27], acute AR following predilation remains a potential pitfall. Severe AR can be detected by means of invasive hemodynamics (e.g., the AR-index) [28] or imaging techniques (i.e., aortography or echocardiography) [29] and should be expected when clinical signs of heart failure/congestion are paired with a sudden decrease in aortic diastolic pressure and/or an increase of LVEDP after predilation.

Due to reduced LV compliance as the consequence of the compensatory changes and LV remodeling processes in severe aortic stenosis, acute AR is usually not well tolerated in patients undergoing TAVI [30]. Thus, acute severe AR after predilation necessitates immediate therapy including pacing to induce tachycardia with decreased diastolic period and urgent implantation of the THV prosthesis itself.

28.3.4 Stroke/Embolism

Similar to aortic balloon valvuloplasty, predilation in TAVI can potentially result in the mobilization of aortic valve calcium/debris with subsequent embolization. Reported stroke rates in BAV either as destination or bridging to TAVI are low, ranging between 0,5 and 0,8% suggesting an acceptable safety profile of predilation with regard to embolization [31, 32]. In recent TAVI cohorts, the 30-day incidence of stroke ranges between 3,4 and 5,5% in intermediate-risk patients, indicating a difference in procedural risk between BAV and TAVI [16, 17].

Of interest, transcranial Doppler studies have suggested that the predominant embolic load in TAVI is not detected during predilation but rather during device positioning and implantation [33, 34]. Another retrospective analysis of patients undergoing TAVI with and without predilation has even suggested an increased volume of cerebral ischemic lesions detected by magnetic resonance imaging (MRI) in patients undergoing TAVI without predilation [35]. Provided this information, the role of predilation in the context of cerebral emboli during TAVI remains uncertain, overall indicating no overt risk of stroke/embolism associated with its use. Clinical management of stroke/emboli should incorporate a multidisciplinary approach including radiologists, neurologist, and interventional neuroradiologists and should adhere current therapeutic guidelines.

28.3.5 Conduction Disorders

Disorders of conduction, mainly new high-degree atrioventricular block (HAVB) and left bundle branch block (LBB), are commonly encountered in TAVI and may develop already during predilation. Hereby, new LBBB as well as (HAVB) may be transient or permanent [36]. The acute clinical relevance of new-onset conduction disorders during predilation is usually small, provided that a temporary pacing wire is placed. The details of conduction disorders in the context of TAVI are outlined in Chap. 33 of this book.

Mechanistically, a two-hit model has been suggested consisting of a first hit inflicted by the valvuloplasty balloon and a second hit applied by the subsequently implanted THV. In their retrospective analysis, Lange et al. found lower rates of permanent pacemaker implantation in patients undergoing TAVI with the use of a self-expanding THV when smaller valvuloplasty balloons ($\leq$23 mm) were used [37]. Another propensity-matched analysis has described lower rates of new-onset LBB in patients in whom direct TAVI without predilation was performed, however without influence on pacemaker rates [38]. Overall, data on the influence of predilation on new-onset conduction disturbances are limited, and the role of predilation conduction disorders will likely be elucidated in ongoing randomized studies.

28.3.6 Coronary Obstruction

Coronary obstruction is a rare (<1%) but potentially fatal complication of TAVI which usually inflicts occlusion of the left coronary artery (LCA) [39, 40]. Coronary obstruction is hereby seen mainly in patients with low takeoff of the LCA and/or narrow sinuses of Valsalva—especially when balloon-expandable THVs are used. Although there is no clinical data indicating a specific role of predilation in its pathophysiology, predilation can be useful to evaluate the potential risk of coronary obstruction [4]. Especially when CT angiographic data are inconclusive or unavailable, predilation can be helpful to assess displacement of the aortic valve calcium/leaflets towards the coronary ostia. Severe hypotension or ST-segment changes during predilation can be indicative of transient coronary obstruction during predilation. Hereby, predilation-induced coronary obstruction is likely reversible, due to the recoil of the native aortic valve. When coronary obstruction occurs after THV placement, interventional strategies including percutaneous coronary intervention and stent placement are usually warranted [39].

28.4 Routine Predilation or "Direct TAVI?"

With the beginning of TAVI as a treatment for patients with severe symptomatic aortic stenosis at high or prohibitive risk for surgery, predilation was considered a mandatory part of the procedure. In fact, pre-implant predilation was required as a part of the study protocol in the pivotal PARTNER trials using the first generation of the Edwards SAPIEN transcatheter heart valve (THV) and is still part of most instructions for use (IFUs) [41, 42]. With growing clinical expertise and operator experience, this notion has been challenged by clinicians headed by Eberhard Grube performing the TAVI procedure in a direct fashion without predilation, leading to a decreasing trend in the systematic use of predilation [2, 43]. In theory, the omission of routine predilation is associated with shorter procedure times and may reduce complications potentially associated with predilation. Accordingly, it has been speculated that omitting predilation can lead to a reduction in the incidence of stroke, acute kidney injury, or systemic inflammation which are associated with hypoperfusion [44, 45]. On the other hand, direct TAVI might theoretically result in an increased need for postdilation [5] or in THV underexpansion/noncircular valve deployment and thus unfavorable hemodynamics and increased paravalvular leakage [30, 46]. In this context, patient-specific variables are likely to influence the necessity for predilation including anatomical and morphological characteristics [47, 48]. However, relevant THV underexpansion may even occur despite the use of predilation [49], highlighting the need for systematic studies on this issue. To this point in time, the scientific evidence regarding predilation in TAVI remains limited mostly to retrospective non-randomized studies and meta-analyses. Although larger randomized comparative studies are currently being conducted, only one randomized study has been published so far [50].

28.4.1 Retrospective Analyses

There are ample retrospective analyses comparing outcome in patients undergoing TAVI with and without predilation. Whereas smaller studies have evaluated the performance of specific THV models, the largest studies available are multicenter analyses derived from national registries or single-center analyses including different types of THVs.

Safety and feasibility of TAVI without predilation was suggested by results from the UK TAVI registry. Including 5.888 patients treated with the Medtronic CoreValve and Edwards SAPIEN prosthesis, the study by Martin et al. demonstrated comparable clinical outcome as defined by the VARC-2 criteria in a propensity-matched analysis of TAVI treated with and without predilation [43].

A single-center analysis published by Pagnesi et al. studied the safety of predilation and direct TAVI in 837 patients undergoing TAVI with several different balloon- and self-expanding THVs (Medtronic CoreValve and Evolut R, Edwards SAPIEN and SAPIEN XT). As a result, the authors concluded a similar safety profile of direct TAVI compared to the routine use of predilation; however, after propensity score matching for baseline differences, direct TAVI appeared to be associated with a higher need for postdilation [5].

Results from the Brazilian TAVR registry including a total of 761 patients have been published recently. In this study of patients treated with the CoreValve (Medtronic Inc., Minneapolis, Minnesota, USA) and Edwards SAPIEN (Edwards LifeSciences, Irvine, Ca, USA), Bernardi et al. demonstrated similar clinical and echocardiographic outcome parameters

in patients treated by "direct TAVI" or TAVI with predilation after propensity score matching for baseline differences. However, patients treated with predilation experienced a higher incidence of new-onset left bundle branch blocks (LBB), which was confirmed in multivariate analysis [38].

28.4.2 Predilation in Self-Expanding THVs

Full expansion of self-expanding THVs relies on the radial force exerted by the nitinol frame on surrounding tissues. Therefore, it is conceivable that predilation may be required in self-expanding THVs to adequately displace valvular calcium to allow circular expansion of the THV frame.

Safety and feasibility of TAVI without predilation in 60 patients using the self-expanding CoreValve prosthesis was demonstrated by Eberhard Grube and colleagues already in 2011 [51]. In a single-center study evaluation of high-risk patients undergoing TAVI with the CoreValve prosthesis, Kochman et al. found similar rates of procedural success, survival, and hemodynamic results (i.e., transvalvular gradients and paravalvular leakage) in patients treated with and without predilation [52]. Similar findings regarding procedural success and survival were reported by Toutouzas et al., who published an analysis of 210 patients treated with the CoreValve prosthesis. In this retrospective study, lower rates of more than moderate paravalvular leakage were observed with "direct TAVI" [53]. Of interest, Lange et al. observed lower rates of pacemaker implantation in patients undergoing TAVI with the CoreValve prosthesis when smaller valvuloplasty balloons ($\leq$23 mm) for predilation were used [37].

The effect of predilation on the performance of the ACURATE neo transfemoral prosthesis (Boston Scientific Inc., Marlborough, MA, USA) was assessed by Kim and colleagues. In their study of patients with severe aortic stenosis and mild to moderate aortic valve calcification, propensity score matching revealed similar clinical outcome parameters but significantly shorter procedure and fluoroscopy times compared to patients undergoing TAVI with predilation [54].

28.4.3   Predilation in Balloon-Expandable THVs

In contrast to self-expanding THVs, balloon-expandable THVs are delivered and deployed with the use of a premounted valvuloplasty balloon. Predilation was considered mandatory in the pivotal trials using balloon-expandable THVs and is commonly performed in patients undergoing TAVI with balloon-expandable valves [43]. As certain TAVI-associated complications, such as rupture of the aortic annulus or coronary obstruction, appear to be predominantly associated with the use of balloon-expandable THVs, the role of predilation as a potential risk factor has been the topic of several retrospective analyses.

In patients with moderate aortic valve calcification, direct TAVI produces comparable clinical results with regard to early and mid-mortality as well as procedural safety [55]. In a case-matched analysis of patients undergoing both transfemoral and transapical TAVI with newer-generation Edwards SAPIEN prostheses, Conradi et al. were able to show comparable clinical and hemodynamic outcome when predilation was omitted. Hereby, procedural duration and contrast use were lower in "direct TAVI." Hamm et al. demonstrated shorter procedural duration in patients undergoing transfemoral implantation of the Edwards SAPIEN XT and SAPIEN 3 prostheses treated without predilation, whereas procedural safety and success were found to be similar [56]. Moderate predilation with smaller sized balloons (≤22 mm) was found to produce similar clinical outcome as direct TAVI in a study by Abramowitz and colleagues. Also in this study, direct TAVI was associated with less fluoroscopy time [6]. Of interest, direct TAVI without predilation was found to be linked to increased total volume of new cerebral ischemic lesions as assessed by magnetic resonance imaging, but this could not be reproduced in other studies [35].

28.4.4   Meta-analyses

Three meta-analyses on the safety and feasibility of TAVI with and without predilation have been published. Incorporating 18 studies and >2.000 patients, Liao et al. concluded that direct TAVI without predilation was not only safe but also associated with preferable short-term mortality and fewer complications (i.e., stroke, paravalvular leakage, and pacemaker implantation) [8]. In contrast, as a result of an analysis of 1395 patients enrolled in 16 studies, Bagur and colleagues found similar outcomes with regard to paravalvular leakage, stroke, and pacemaker implantation rates in direct TAVI vs. routine predilation [57]. The largest meta-analysis on this matter published by Auffret et al. indicated similar safety profiles of the two approaches but emphasized the need for randomized studies on this topic [9].

28.4.4.1   Randomized Studies
To this point only one randomized study on the topic of predilation has been published. This study included 60 patients undergoing both transfemoral and transapical TAVI with the use of the balloon-expandable Edwards SAPIEN XT THV. As a result, the authors found no significant differences with regard to early mortality as well as hemodynamic outcomes [50]. However, the small size and heterogeneity of this study make it difficult to draw significant conclusions. Several large-scale randomized studies on this topic are currently being conducted. Adequately powered, dedicated trials such as the SIMPLIFy TAVI study (NCT01539746), the DIRECT study (NCT02448927), or the EASE-IT trials (NCT02760771, NCT02127580) will hopefully elucidate the potential benefits and risks of systematic predilation in TAVI and its omission.

28.5   Conclusion

Technically, predilation in TAVI mimics classic balloon valvuloplasty in aortic valve stenosis and is thus associated with a similar risk profile and

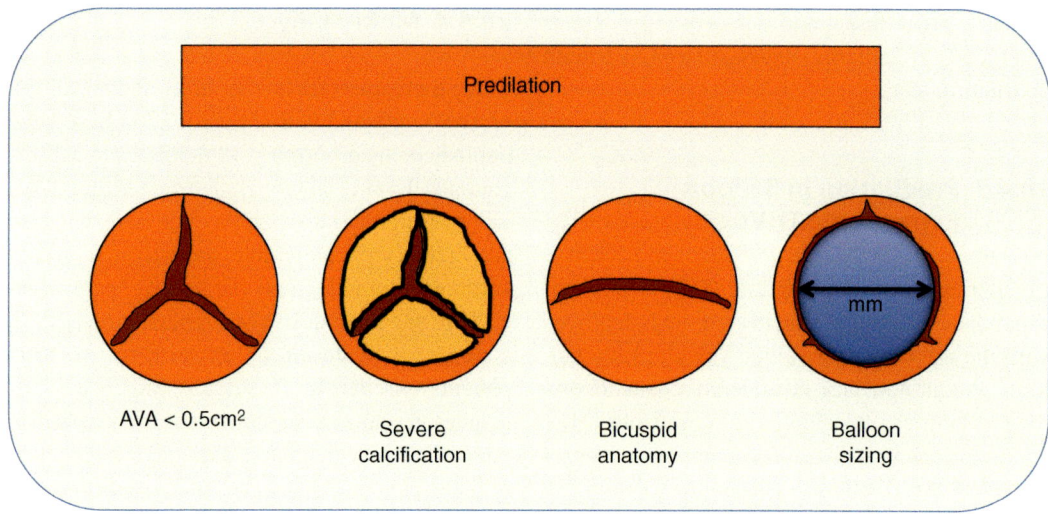

Fig. 28.1 Clinical factors indicating the need for predilation in TAVI

set of complications. A trend toward declining use of predilation in TAVI has been observed within the last years, mostly owing to increasing operator experience. Retrospective studies and meta-analyses have indicated safety and efficacy of the omission of predilation; however large-scale studies are lacking. In selected patients, "direct TAVI" without predilation appears to be associated with shorter procedural duration, less fluoroscopy time, and contrast use. However, clinical safety endpoints seem less effected when routine predilation is performed. Especially with regard to potentially fatal complications such as stroke, aortic rupture, or coronary obstruction, current evidence does not suggest an increased risk with predilation. With the lack of randomized clinical trials, the indication for predilation in TAVI remains at the discretion of the physician. However, patient-specific characteristics and individual risk profiles should be incorporated in the decision for or against predilation; especially in patients with heavily calcified aortic stenosis or bicuspid aortic disease, predilation may be beneficial and facilitate the procedure (Fig. 28.1). Ongoing clinical trials such as the SIMPLIFy TAVI, DIRECT, or EASE-IT study will further elucidate the potential risks and benefits of predilation in TAVI.

References

1. Levine GN, Bates ER, Blankenship JC, Bailey SR, Bittl JA, Cercek B, et al. 2011 ACCF/AHA/SCAI guideline for percutaneous coronary intervention. J Am Coll Cardiol. 2011;58(24):e44–e122.
2. Pagnesi M, Baldetti L, Sole PD, et al. Predilatation prior to transcatheter aortic valve implantation: is it still a prerequisite? Interv Cardiol. 2017;12(2):116–0.
3. Patsalis PC, Al-Rashid F, Neumann T, Plicht B, Hildebrandt HA, Wendt D, et al. Preparatory balloon aortic valvuloplasty during transcatheter aortic valve implantation for improved valve sizing. J Am Coll Cardiol Intv. 2013;6(9):965–71.
4. Furini FR, de Lima VC, de Brito FS Jr, de Oliveira AT, da Cunha Sales M, Lucchese FA. Coronary occlusion after TAVI: safety strategy report. Revista Brasileira de Cardiologia Invasiva (English Edition). Sociedade Brasileira de Hemodinâmica e Cardiologia Intervencionista. 2016;23(2):152–5.
5. Pagnesi M, Jabbour RJ, Latib A, Kawamoto H, Tanaka A, Regazzoli D, et al. Usefulness of predilation before transcatheter aortic valve implantation. Am J Cardiol. 2016;118(1):107–12.
6. Abramowitz Y, Jilaihawi H, Chakravarty T, Kashif M, Matar G, Hariri B, et al. Feasibility and safety of balloon-expandable transcatheter aortic valve implantation with moderate or without predilatation. EuroIntervention. 2016;11(10):1132–9.
7. Conradi L, Schaefer A, Seiffert M, Schirmer J, Schaefer U, Schön G, et al. Transfemoral TAVI without pre-dilatation using balloon-expandable devices: a case-matched analysis. Clin Res Cardiol. 2015;104(9):735–42.

8. Liao Y-B, Meng Y, Zhao Z-G, Zuo Z-L, Li Y-J, Xiong T-Y, et al. Meta-analysis of the effectiveness and safety of transcatheter aortic valve implantation without balloon predilation. Am J Cardiol. 2016;117(10):1629–35.

9. Auffret V, Regueiro A, Campelo-Parada F, Del Trigo M, Chiche O, Chamandi C, et al. Feasibility, safety, and efficacy of transcatheter aortic valve replacement without balloon predilation: a systematic review and meta-analysis. Catheter Cardiovasc Interv. 2017;90(5):839–50.

10. Keeble TR, Khokhar A, Akhtar MM, Mathur A, Weerackody R, Kennon S. Percutaneous balloon aortic valvuloplasty in the era of transcatheter aortic valve implantation: a narrative review. Open Heart. 2016;3(2):e000421–12.

11. Hilling-Smith R, Cockburn J, Dooley M, Parker J, Newton A, Hill A, et al. Rapid pacing using the 0.035-in. Retrograde left ventricular support wire in 208 cases of transcatheter aortic valve implantation and balloon aortic valvuloplasty. Cathet Cardiovasc Intervent. 2016;89(4):783–6.

12. Baumgartner H, Falk V, Bax JJ, De Bonis M, Hamm C, Holm PJ, et al. ESC/EACTS Guidelines for the management of valvular heart disease. Eur Heart J. 2017;38(36):2739–91.

13. Rezq A, Basavarajaiah S, Latib A, Takagi K, Hasegawa T, Figini F, et al. Incidence, management, and outcomes of cardiac tamponade during transcatheter aortic valve implantation: a single-center study. J Am Coll Cardiol Intv. 2012;5(12):1264–72.

14. Eggebrecht H, Vaquerizo B, Moris C, Bossone E, Lämmer J, Czerny M, et al. Incidence and outcomes of emergent cardiac surgery during transfemoral transcatheter aortic valve implantation (TAVI): insights from the European Registry on Emergent Cardiac Surgery during TAVI (EuRECS-TAVI). Eur Heart J. 2017;39(8):676–84.

15. Kappetein AP, Head SJ, Généreux P, Piazza N, van Mieghem NM, Blackstone EH, et al. Updated standardized endpoint definitions for transcatheter aortic valve implantation: the valve academic research consortium-2 consensus document. J Am Coll Cardiol. 2012;60(15):1438–54.

16. Reardon MJ, van Mieghem NM, Popma JJ, Kleiman NS, Søndergaard L, Mumtaz M, et al. Surgical or transcatheter aortic-valve replacement in intermediate-risk patients. N Engl J Med. 2017;376(14):1321–31.

17. Leon MB, Smith CR, Mack MJ, Makkar RR, Svensson LG, Kodali SK, et al. Transcatheter or surgical aortic-valve replacement in intermediate-risk patients. N Engl J Med. 2016;374(17):1609–20.

18. Sedaghat A, Neumann N, Schahab N, Sinning J-M, Hammerstingl C, Pingel S, et al. Routine endovascular treatment with a stent graft for access-site and access-related vascular injury in transfemoral transcatheter aortic valve implantation. Circ Cardiovasc Interv. 2016;9(8):e003834.

19. Généreux P, Kodali S, Leon MB, Smith CR, Ben-Gal Y, Kirtane AJ, et al. Clinical outcomes using a new crossover balloon occlusion technique for percutaneous closure after transfemoral aortic valve implantation. J Am Coll Cardiol Intv. 2011;4(8):861–7.

20. De Backer O, Arnous S, Sandholt B, Brooks M, BIASCO L, Franzen O, et al. Safety and efficacy of using the viabahn endoprothesis for percutaneous treatment of vascular access complications after transfemoral aortic valve implantation. Am J Cardiol. 2015;115(8):1123–9.

21. Stortecky S, Wenaweser P, Diehm N, Pilgrim T, Huber C, Rosskopf AB, et al. Percutaneous management of vascular complications in patients undergoing transcatheter aortic valve implantation. J Am Coll Cardiol Intv. 2012;5(5):515–24.

22. Toggweiler S, Leipsic J, Binder RK, Freeman M, Barbanti M, Heijmen RH, et al. Management of vascular access in transcatheter aortic valve replacement: part 2: vascular complications. J Am Coll Cardiol Intv. 2013;6(8):767–76.

23. Pasic M, Unbehaun A, Buz S, Drews T, Hetzer R. Annular rupture during transcatheter aortic valve replacement classification, pathophysiology, diagnostics, treatment approaches, and prevention. J Am Coll Cardiol Intv. 2015;8(1):1–9.

24. Möllmann H, Kim W-K, Kempfert J, Walther T, Hamm C. Complications of transcatheter aortic valve implantation (TAVI): how to avoid and treat them. Heart. 2015;101(11):900–8.

25. Al-Attar N, Himbert D, Barbier F, Vahanian A, Nataf P. Delayed aortic dissection after transcatheter aortic valve implantation. J Heart Valve Dis. 2013;22(5):701–3.

26. Conzelmann LO, Yousef M, Schnelle N, Grawe A, Ferrari M, Vahl CF, et al. How should I treat a DeBakey type I acute aortic dissection four weeks after transcatheter aortic valve implantation in an old, fragile patient? EuroIntervention. 2015;10(12):e1–6.

27. Jochheim D, Zadrozny M, Theiss H, Baquet M, Maimer-Rodrigues F, Bauer A, et al. Aortic regurgitation with second versus third-generation balloon-expandable prostheses in patients undergoing transcatheter aortic valve implantation. EuroIntervention. 2015;11(2):214–20.

28. Sinning J-M, Hammerstingl C, Vasa-Nicotera M, Adenauer V, Lema Cachiguango SJ, Scheer A-C, et al. Aortic regurgitation index defines severity of peri-prosthetic regurgitation and predicts outcome in patients after transcatheter aortic valve implantation. J Am Coll Cardiol. 2012;59(13):1134–41.

29. Abdelghani M, Tateishi H, Spitzer E, Tijssen JG, de Winter RJ, Soliman OII, et al. Echocardiographic and angiographic assessment of paravalvular regurgitation after TAVI: optimizing inter-technique reproducibility. Eur Heart J Cardiovasc Imaging. 2016;17(8):852–60.

30. Sinning J-M, Vasa-Nicotera M, Chin D, Hammerstingl C, Ghanem A, Bence J, et al. Evaluation and management of paravalvular aortic regurgitation after transcatheter aortic valve replacement. J Am Coll Cardiol. 2013;62(1):11–20.

31. Moretti C, Chandran S, Vervueren P-L, D'Ascenzo F, Barbanti M, Weerackody R, et al. Outcomes of patients undergoing balloon aortic valvuloplasty in the TAVI Era: a multicenter registry. J Invasive Cardiol. 2015;27(12):547–53.

32. Ben-Dor I, Maluenda G, Dvir D, Barbash IM, Okubagzi P, Torguson R, et al. Balloon aortic valvuloplasty for severe aortic stenosis as a bridge to transcatheter/surgical aortic valve replacement. Catheter Cardiovasc Interv. 2013;82(4):632–7.

33. Erdoes G, Basciani R, Huber C, Stortecky S, Wenaweser P, Windecker S, et al. Transcranial Doppler-detected cerebral embolic load during transcatheter aortic valve implantation. Eur J Cardiothorac Surg. 2012;41(4):778–83; discussion783–4

34. Kahlert P, Al-Rashid F, Döttger P, Mori K, Plicht B, Wendt D, et al. Cerebral embolization during transcatheter aortic valve implantation: a transcranial Doppler study. Circulation. 2012;126(10):1245–55.

35. Bijuklic K, Haselbach T, Witt J, Krause K, Hansen L, Gehrckens R, et al. Increased risk of cerebral embolization after implantation of a balloon-expandable aortic valve without prior balloon valvuloplasty. J Am Coll Cardiol Intv. 2015;8(12):1608–13.

36. Auffret V, Puri R, Urena M, Chamandi C, Rodriguez-Gabella T, Philippon F, et al. Conduction disturbances after transcatheter aortic valve replacement. Circulation. 2017;136(11):1049–69.

37. Lange P, Greif M, Vogel A, Thaumann A, Helbig S, Schwarz F, et al. Reduction of pacemaker implantation rates after CoreValve (R) implantation by moderate predilatation. EuroIntervention. 2014;9(10):1151–7.

38. Bernardi FLM, Ribeiro HB, Carvalho LA, Sarmento-Leite R, Mangione JA, Lemos PA, et al. Direct transcatheter heart valve implantation versus implantation with balloon predilatation insights from the Brazilian transcatheter aortic valve replacement registry. Circulation Cardiovasc Interv. 2016;9(8):e003605.

39. Ribeiro HB, Nombela-Franco L, Urena M, Mok M, Pasian S, Doyle D, et al. Coronary obstruction following transcatheter aortic valve implantation a systematic review. J Am Coll Cardiol Intv. 2013;6(5):452–61.

40. Ribeiro HB, Webb JG, Makkar RR, Cohen MG, Kapadia SR, Kodali S, et al. Predictive factors, management, and clinical outcomes of coronary obstruction following transcatheter aortic valve implantation insights from a large multicenter registry. J Am Coll Cardiol. 2013;62(17):1552 62.

41. Smith CR, Leon MB, Mack MJ, Miller DC, Moses JW, Svensson LG, et al. Transcatheter versus surgical aortic-valve replacement in high-risk patients. N Engl J Med. 2011;364(23):2187–98.

42. Leon MB, Smith CR, Mack M, Miller DC, Moses JW, Svensson LG, et al. Transcatheter aortic-valve implantation for aortic stenosis in patients who cannot undergo surgery. N Engl J Med. 2010;363(17):1597–607. https://doi.org/10.1056/NEJMoa1008232.

43. Martin GP, Sperrin M, Bagur R, de Belder MA, Buchan I, Gunning M, et al. Pre-implantation balloon aortic valvuloplasty and clinical outcomes following transcatheter aortic valve implantation: a propensity score analysis of the UK registry. J Am Heart Assoc. 2017;6(2):e004695–12.

44. Sinning J-M, Scheer A-C, Adenauer V, Ghanem A, Hammerstingl C, Schueler R, et al. Systemic inflammatory response syndrome predicts increased mortality in patients after transcatheter aortic valve implantation. Eur Heart J. 2012;33(12):1459–68. https://doi.org/10.1093/eurheartj/ehs002.

45. Sinning J-M, Ghanem A, Steinhäuser H, Adenauer V, Hammerstingl C, Nickenig G, et al. Renal function as predictor of mortality in patients after percutaneous transcatheter aortic valve implantation. J Am Coll Cardiol Intv. 2010;3(11):1141–9.

46. Kuetting M, Sedaghat A, Utzenrath M, Sinning J-M, Schmitz C, Roggenkamp J, et al. In vitro assessment of the influence of aortic annulus ovality on the hydrodynamic performance of self-expanding transcatheter heart valve prostheses. J Biomech. 2014;47(5):957–65.

47. Islas F, Almería C, García-Fernández E, Jiménez P, Nombela-Franco L, Olmos C, et al. Usefulness of echocardiographic criteria for transcatheter aortic valve implantation without balloon predilation: a single-center experience. J Am Soc Echocardiogr. 2015;28(4):423–9.

48. Pagnesi M, Baldetti L, Sole PD, Mangieri A, Ancona MB, Regazzoli D, et al. Predilatation prior to transcatheter aortic valve implantation: is it still a prerequisite? Interv Cardiol. 2017;12(02):116–0.

49. Sinning J-M, Vasa-Nicotera M, Ghanem A, Grube E, Nickenig G, Werner N. An exceptional case of frame underexpansion with a self-expandable transcatheter heart valve despite predilation. J Am Coll Cardiol Intv. 2012;5(12):1288–9.

50. Ahn HC, Nielsen N-E, Baranowski J. Can predilatation in transcatheter aortic valve implantation be omitted? - a prospective randomized study. J Cardiothorac Surg. 2016;11(1):124. https://doi.org/10.1186/s13019-016-0516-x.

51. Grube E, Naber C, Abizaid A, Sousa E, Mendiz O, Lemos P, et al. Feasibility of transcatheter aortic valve implantation without balloon pre-dilation a pilot study. J Am Coll Cardiol Intv. 2011;4(7):751–7.

52. Kochman J, Kołtowski L, Huczek Z, Scisło P, Bakoń L, Wilimski R, et al. Direct transcatheter aortic valve implantation - one-year outcome of a case control study. Postepy Kardiol Interwencyjnej. 2014;10(4):250–7.

53. Toutouzas K, Latsios G, Stathogiannis K, Drakopoulou M, Synetos A, Sanidas E, et al. One-year outcomes after direct transcatheter aortic valve implantation with a self-expanding bioprosthesis. A two-center international experience. Int J Cardiol. 2016;202:631–5.

54. Kim W-K, Liebetrau C, Renker M, Rolf A, Van Linden A, Arsalan M, et al. Transfemoral aortic valve implantation using a self-expanding transcatheter heart valve without pre-dilation. Int J Cardiol. 2017;243:156–60.

55. Spaziano M, Sawaya F, Chevalier B, Roy A, Neylon A, Garot P, et al. Comparison of systematic predilation, selective predilation, and direct transcatheter aortic valve implantation with the SAPIEN S3 valve. Can J Cardiol. 2017;33(2):260–8.

56. Hamm K, Reents W, Zacher M, Halbfass P, Kerber S, Diegeler A, et al. Omission of predilation in balloon-expandable transcatheter aortic valve implantation: retrospective analysis in a large-volume centre. EuroIntervention. 2017;13(2):e161–7.

57. Bagur R, Kwok CS, Nombela-Franco L, Ludman PF, de Belder MA, Sponga S, et al. Transcatheter aortic valve implantation with or without preimplantation balloon aortic valvuloplasty: a systematic review and meta-analysis. J Am Heart Assoc. 2016;5(6):e003191–20.

Balloon Post-dilation During Transcatheter Aortic Valve Implantation

29

Amit N. Vora, G. Chad Hughes IV, and J. Kevin Harrison

29.1 Introduction

Transcatheter aortic valve, also called transcatheter aortic valve replacement (TAVR), has emerged as a revolutionary alternative for the treatment of severe, symptomatic aortic valve stenosis, initially among patients at prohibitive risk for open surgical aortic valve replacement (SAVR) [1, 2] but more recently in patients at high [3, 4] and intermediate risk [5] for surgery, with current trials ongoing for the role of this therapy among low-risk patients. Because the valve is not implanted under direct visualization as in open surgery where the aortic valve leaflets and annulus can be removed and debrided, there is a risk of paravalvular aortic valve regurgitation (AR) with TAVR. The presence of more than mild AR has been associated with deleterious late clinical outcomes. Less frequently, TAVR fails to sufficiently relieve aortic stenosis, a situation most commonly encountered when treating bioprosthetic valve dysfunction.

As such, balloon post-dilation (BPD) has been recommended to optimize valve performance during TAVR. Although BPD may further expand the valve frame and reduce the severity of post-implantation AR and improve the systolic pressure gradient, risks include aortic annular rupture, migration and malposition of the newly implanted valve, damage to the newly implanted valve leaflets, and/or stroke. In this chapter, we review the impact of post-TAVR AR on outcomes, evaluate the benefits and risks associated with BPD, and describe best practices to optimize valve expansion with BPD. We also describe the early procedural data regarding bioprosthetic surgical valve fracture to optimize the hemodynamic performance of a valve-in-valve (ViV) TAVR. We will limit our discussion to the two FDA-approved THV systems in the United States.

29.2 Post-TAVR Aortic Valve Regurgitation

Rates of post-procedural paravalvular leak (PVL) following AVR have been reported to be higher in patients undergoing TAVR compared with SAVR. The incidence of PVL following TAVR is variable, and heterogeneity of published rates is due to a number of factors, including the imaging modality (cineangiography, hemodynamics, transthoracic echocardiography, transesophageal echocardiography), the time point of assessment (immediately after the procedure, prior to discharge, or at 30 days), and the grading system [6]. The grading system by cineangiography used most commonly is that which was initially described by sellers [7]: (1) grade 1 (mild AR) is a small amount of contrast entering the LV during diastole and clearing with each cardiac cycle, (2)

A. N. Vora · G. Chad Hughes IV · J. K. Harrison (✉)
Duke University Medical Center, Durham, NC, USA
e-mail: harri015@mc.duke.edu

© Springer Nature Switzerland AG 2019
A. Giordano et al. (eds.), *Transcatheter Aortic Valve Implantation*,
https://doi.org/10.1007/978-3-030-05912-5_29

grade 2 (moderate AR) is contrast filling the entire LV during diastole but with less density than the aorta, (3) grade 3 (moderate-severe AR) is contrast filling the entire LV during diastole with the same density as the aorta, and (4) grade 4 (severe AR) is contrast filling the entire LV in diastole on the first beat with greater density than in the aorta. With echocardiography, the Valve Academic Research Consortium (VARC II) has identified semiquantitative (diastolic flow reversal in descending aorta, circumferential extent of PVL) and quantitative parameters (regurgitant volume, regurgitant fraction, effective regurgitant orifice area) to classify mild, moderate, and severe AR following TAVR [8, 9]. The time point for assessment is also important, as immediate post-deployment assessment may overestimate the degree of overall AR. Prior data has demonstrated continued frame expansion with reduction in PVL from 30 days to 1 year [10].

Historically, the strongest predictors of PVL included undersizing of the device, incomplete apposition of the stent struts to the native annulus due to calcification [11], and/or valve malposition [6]. Undersizing of the device was more common with the use of TEE to determine aortic annular dimensions, but the current routine use of multidetector computed tomography (MDCR) imaging has led to the reduction of mis-sizing and lower rates of PVL [12–15]. Additionally, newer iterations of THV systems have specifically addressed the concern of PVL. The Edwards SAPIEN 3 is designed with a polyethylene terephthalate outer skirt along the stent frame inflow in an attempt to reduce PVL. The CoreValve Evolut Pro valve system allows the operator to recapture and reposition the stent valve, reducing the incidence of improper valve position. The stent valve itself is designed with an external porcine pericardial layer at the stent valve inflow in an attempt to minimize PVL.

The deleterious effects of post-TAVR aortic valve regurgitation have been well-documented. An analysis by Hayashida and colleagues evaluated clinical outcomes among 400 consecutive patients undergoing TAVR, stratified by post-AR grade 0/1 (75% of overall population), grade 2 (22% of cohort), or grade 3/4 (3.0%), and dem-

onstrated no significant differences in 30-day mortality but a stepwise increase in long-term mortality with increasing AR. Post-procedure AR ≥2 was identified as an independent predictor of long-term mortality (HR 1.68, 95% CI 1.21–1.44) after multivariable analysis [16] (Fig. 29.1). The PARTNER trials and registry reported similar short-term outcomes (<30 days) among patients with none/trace, mild, and moderate/severe PVL but higher rates of increased 1 year all-cause mortality (15.9 vs. 22.2 vs. 35.1%, $p < 0.0001$), cardiac mortality (6.1 vs. 7.4% vs. 16.3%, $p < 0.0001$), and rehospitalization (14.4 vs. 23.0 vs. 31.3%, $p < 0.0001$) with worsening PVL. In the multivariable analysis, even mild PVL was associated with higher 1-year mortality (HR 1.37, 95% CI 1.14–1.90, $p = 0.012$), though the risk of mortality was substantially higher among patients with moderate/severe PVL (HR 2.18, 95% CI 1.57–3.02, $p < 0.0001$) [17]. A meta-analysis of 45 studies with almost 13,000 patients reported the incidence of moderate or severe AR post-TAVR was 11.7% (95% CI 9.6–14.1%) and was associated with higher mortality at 30 days (OR 2.95, 95% CI 1.73–5.02) and 1 year (OR 2.27, 95% CI 1.84–2.81, $p = 0.001$) [18].

29.3 Indications and Outcomes for Balloon Post-dilation Following TAVR

Given the association between greater than mild paravalvular AR and adverse short- and long-term outcomes, BPD can be a safe and effective method to allow for appropriate expansion of the THV stent frame and therefore reduce overall PVL [19]. Experience with BPD has been described with both commercially available THV systems in the United States. Although BPD reduced post-procedure AR among patients receiving either CoreValve or SAPIEN valves, there were important differences in 1-year outcomes. Among patients enrolled in the CoreValve trials (Extreme Risk Pivotal Trial, High Risk Pivotal Trial, and the Continued Access Registries for both, $n = 3532$ patients),

Fig. 29.1 Cumulative survival of patients following TAVR with aortic valve regurgitation classified as: grade 0/1 (blue), grade 2 (green), grade 3/4 (red). From Hayashida et al., JACC Intv 2012

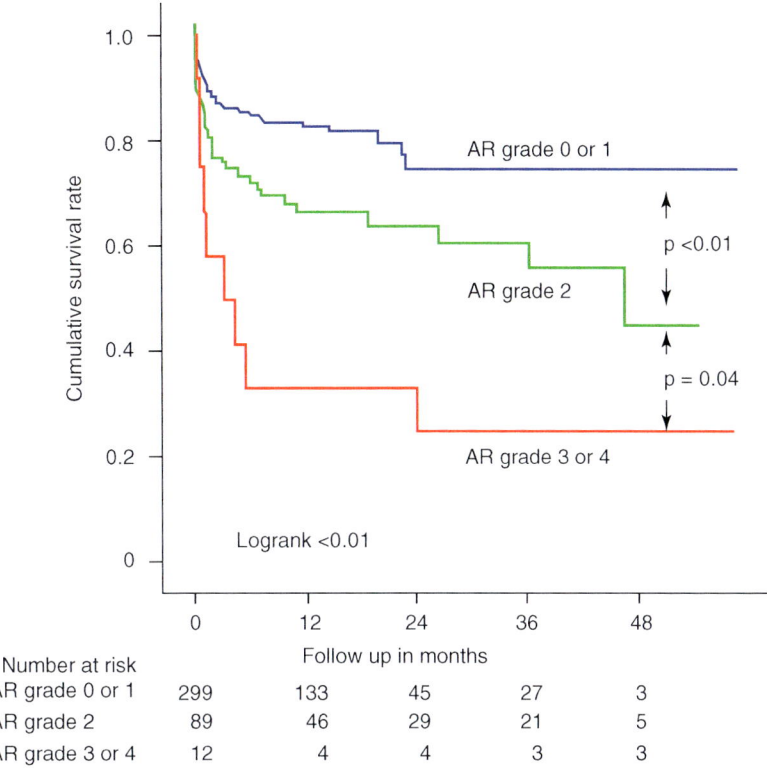

Number at risk				
AR grade 0 or 1	299	133	45	27	3
AR grade 2	89	46	29	21	5
AR grade 3 or 4	12	4	4	3	3

782 (22%) patients underwent BPD following initial valve deployment [20]. The most common indication for BPD was moderate or greater AR (58.1%). There was no difference among rates of BPD when stratified by whether predilation was not or was performed (25.2% vs. 21.6%, p = NS). There were no significant differences in rates of inhospital major adverse cardiovascular and cerebrovascular events (MACCE), all-cause mortality, stroke, or permanent pacemaker placement following TAVR between patients undergoing BPD and those not. However, rates of acute kidney injury (12.7% vs. 9.9%) and life-threatening/disabling bleeding (15.9% vs. 10.5%) were higher among patients undergoing BPD.

Overall, 12.4% of patients that were enrolled in the PARTNER I Trial (both cohorts A and B and the nonrandomized continue access registry, n = 2135 patients) underwent BPD following TAVR [21]. There was a higher incidence of procedural stroke among BPD patients (4.9% vs. 2.6%, p = 0.04). There was no statistically sig-

nificant difference at 7–30 days or >30 days postprocedure. Importantly, there was a trend toward higher all-cause mortality at 1 year (25.4% vs. 20.3%, HR 1.30 95% CI 0.99–1.70, p = 0.054) and a higher rate of all-cause mortality and stroke at 1 year (28.2% vs. 23.0%, HR 1.29 95% CI 1.01–1.66, p = 0.04), which persisted after multivariable adjustment.

29.4 Risks of Balloon Post-dilation Following TAVR

The most significant risk of BPD that can lead to imminent hemodynamic instability following TAVR is aortic injury and annular rupture. An analysis by Barbanti and colleagues described anatomic and procedural factors associated with aortic root rupture during balloon-expandable SAPIEN TAVR. Although greater amounts of subannular/LVOT calcium and more aggressive oversizing were associated with annular rupture among the 31 cases compared with matched patients without rupture, aortic rupture was also associated with BPD (22.6% vs. 0.0%, $p = 0.005$) [22].

However, it may be also possible to mitigate this risk by being conservative with the BPD balloon size. In the CoreValve experience across the initial Extreme Risk and High Risk Pivotal Trial and Continued Access studies, there were three cases of annular rupture leading to death, and all occurred with large diameter (28 mm) balloons. The authors speculated that these deaths were likely due to annular and left ventricular outflow tract calcification and due to oversizing of the BPD balloon relative to the native annulus dimension [20].

When performing BPD it is critical to ensure appropriate guidewire position across the aortic valve prosthesis. Noble and colleagues describe a case in which BPD was performed 6 days after initial implantation of a 26 mm SAPIEN XT valve via a transapical approach with resultant 2–3+ AR [23]. During the BPD the guidewire was inadvertently placed in the paravalvular space and was not recognized, resulting in a crushed SAPIEN XT valve and massive AR with hemodynamic instability, resolving after emergent placement of a CoreValve prosthesis.

29.5 Best Practices to Minimize PVL in TAVR

29.5.1 Before the Procedure

Prior to the TAVR procedure, the most important step in minimizing PVL and the potential need to perform BPD is meticulous pre-procedural planning. MDCT has emerged as the standard of care (over TTE or TEE) for the accurate assessment of annular dimensions, geometry, and degree of annular/leaflet and LVOT calcification that may influence valve platform selection as well as valve sizing [24]. For annular dimensions that are between sizes, using the larger of the two valve sizes may provide a better seal and lead to lower rates of PVL [25], providing that there is adequate coronary clearance for the larger of the two sizes being considered. Thus a detailed root

assessment by MDCT study must be performed to ensure adequate sinus of Valsalva dimensions and coronary ostial heights for the valve size selected.

29.5.2 After Valve Deployment

After the THV is fully deployed, the first step is to undertake a careful assessment of residual AR, and this includes a combination of transthoracic or transesophageal echocardiography, hemodynamic assessment, and cineangiography. This includes visual assessment of the valve to ensure appropriate, circumferential frame expansion as well as an assessment of valve implantation depth. There are conflicting reports regarding depth of CoreValve implantation and rates of PVL. Although earlier studies demonstrated increased rates of PVL with deeper implantation [26–28], a more recent analysis did not demonstrate higher rates of BPD in lower implant depths [20]. For the CoreValve, this assessment is typically performed about 10 min after valve implantation to allow time for the nitinol frame to warm and expand. If AR is visualized, the operator must try to determine if the AR is paravalvular.

If PVL is detected, BPD is generally recommended if feasible to obtain an optimal result. However, integrating this interim result with paravalvular regurgitation severity, pre-procedural anatomy, and the overall patient characteristics is important. For example, BPD may be tempered in the setting of heavy annular and LVOT calcium, where aggressive BPD carries a higher risk of catastrophic annular rupture. If the implant depth is high (i.e., stent valve inflow at the native annular plane), aggressive BPD carries a higher risk of dislodging the THV above the valve plane.

29.5.3 Steps to Ensure Successful BPD

Once the operator has decided to proceed with BPD, the most critical step in successful BPD is balloon type and sizing. For balloon-expandable systems such as the SAPIEN, typically 1–2 cc of diluted contrast can be added to the delivery balloon used to implant the THV prosthesis, obviating the need to remove the delivery system and position another aortic valvuloplasty balloon (Fig. 29.2). For other balloons, it is important to note that many semi-compliant balloons often achieve their nominal diameter at 5 atmospheres, which is not attainable with hand inflation of the balloon. Our experience has been that these balloons, like the Z-Med II, generally achieve a diameter 1 mm less than the indicated balloon diameter at pressures of ~2 atm, which is the internal balloon pressure generally achieved with

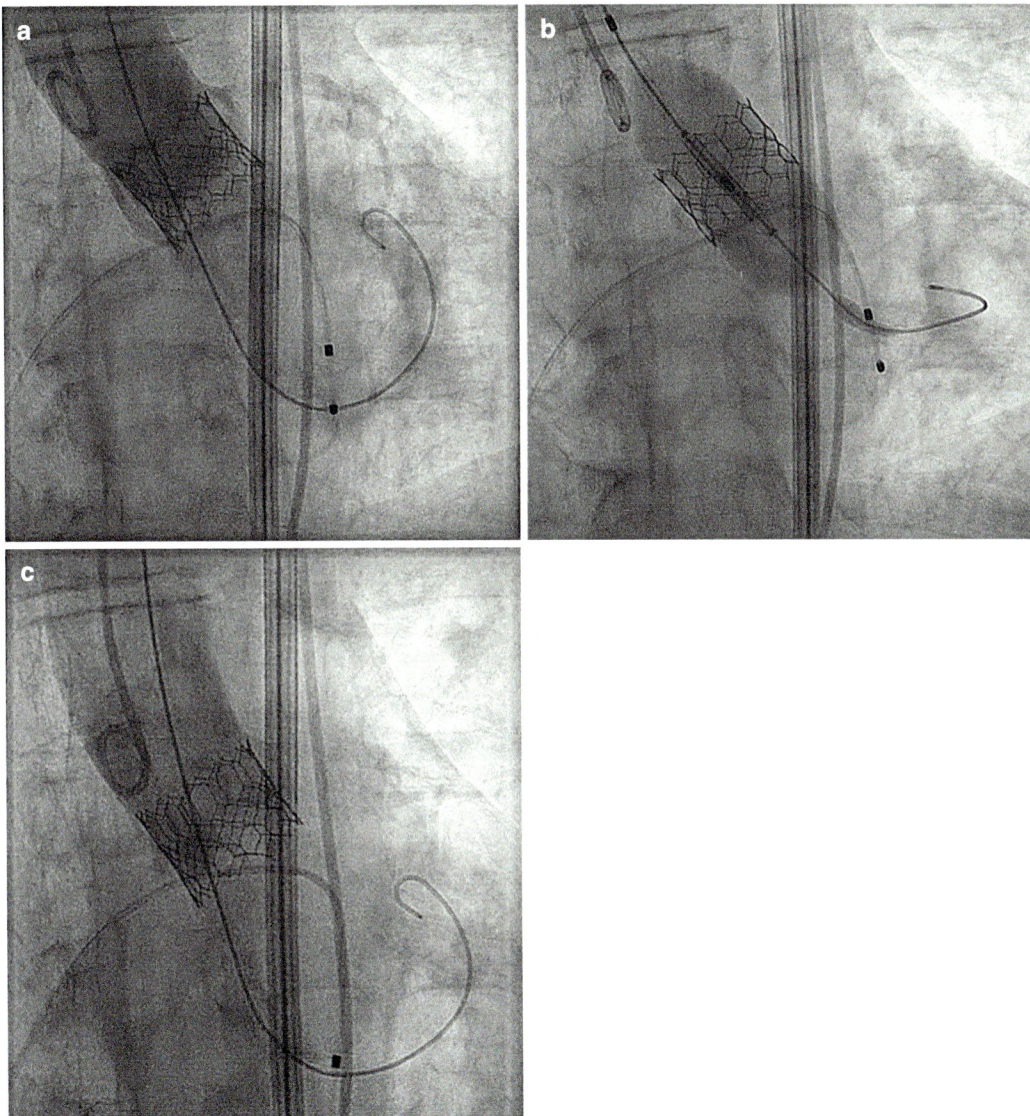

Fig. 29.2 A 74-year-old man with severe symptomatic AS underwent treatment a 23 mm SAPIEN S3. The CTA mean annular diameter was 22.1 mm, and there was no annular calcification. After initial deployment, there was mild aortic valve insufficiency with a <1 mm gap visible between the stent frame and the left coronary side of annulus (**a**). An additional 1 cc of volume was added to the deployment balloon, and the valve frame was post-dilated using the delivery system (**b**). There was no aortic regurgitation following post-dilation (**c**). The final transvalvular gradient was 5 mmHg

hand inflation. In contrast, noncompliant balloons (such as the Bard True Balloon) achieve their target diameter with hand inflation but exert minimal radial force until that particular diameter is achieved.

For most BPD, we generally prefer to use semi-compliant balloons (such as the Z-Med II) and use hand inflation. The selected balloon is sized to achieve an inflation diameter of ~1–2 mm smaller than the area-derived diameter on the MDCT study. For example, if the mean diameter of the annulus is 24.5 mm, the maximum diameter balloon we would select would be a 25 mm Z-Med II balloon, knowing that the maximal inflated diameter will be 24 mm when fully hand inflated. This balloon also allows the operator to stop prior to full hand inflation, should the desired expansion of the stent frame be observed by cineradiography prior to full hand inflation. It should be noted that a prior analysis of three deaths from annular rupture BPD involved balloon oversizing and/or presence of extensive annular/LVOT calcium. Therefore, we recommend an initial conservative balloon size selection (Fig. 29.3).

Less commonly BPD is needed for residual aortic stenosis. For example, this may be seen when self-expanding valves are implanted without balloon pre-dilation of the native valve. In extreme cases there may be an infold in stent valve frame that resolves with BPD.

The exception to the aforementioned BPD technique is for valve-in-valve (ViV) TAVR. In that instance, the precise annular dimension is known a priori, and the goal of the BPD is to allow for complete expansion of the THV frame at its inflow directly within the bioprosthetic valve ring. As a result, a noncompliant balloon that matches the internal diameter of the bioprosthetic valve ring is selected (Fig. 29.4).

Once the appropriate balloon is selected, it is positioned so that the distal marker of the balloon, marking the distal balloon shoulder, is at the inflow of the THV. During BPD, rapid ventricular pacing is critical (rates of 170–200 bpm are typical) to ensure that the precise balloon position is maintained during the inflation and deflation sequence. Balloon inflation should not begin until LV stroke volume produces <10 mmHg pulse pressure. If the balloon "watermelon seeds" into

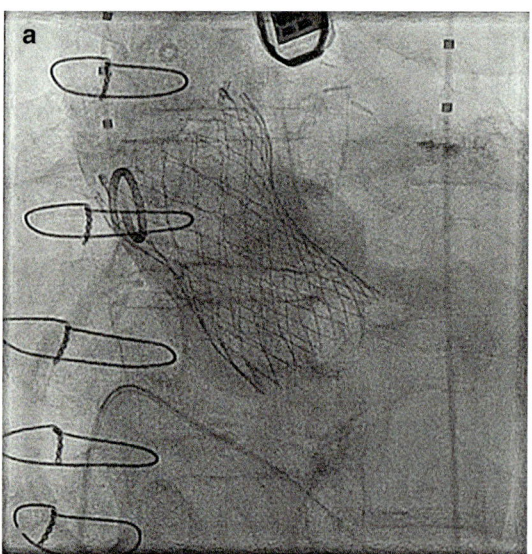
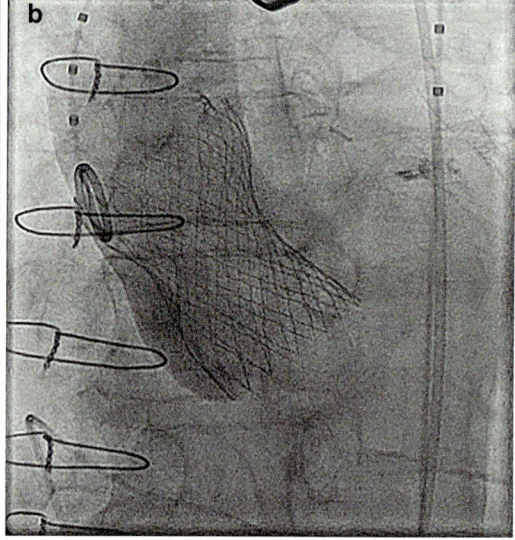

Fig. 29.3 The patient was a 62-year-old man with severe AS (mean gradient 40 mmHg with AVA 0.4 cm²). His aortic annular mean diameter was 27.9 mm (perimeter 90.3). A 34 mm CoreValve Evolut was implanted. After stent valve deployment, there was a 4 mm gap on the left coronary side of the valve with moderate paravalvular leak (**a**). Balloon post-dilation was performed with a 28 mm Z-Med II balloon resulting in trivial aortic insufficiency post-procedure (**b**)

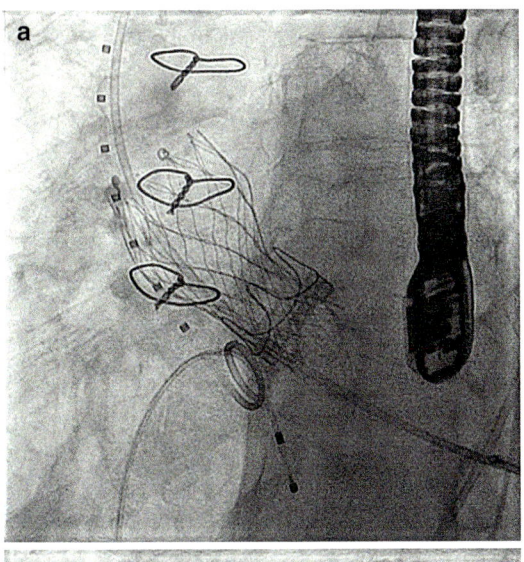
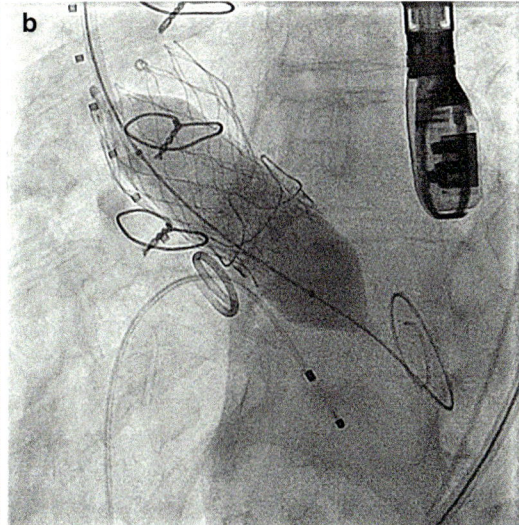
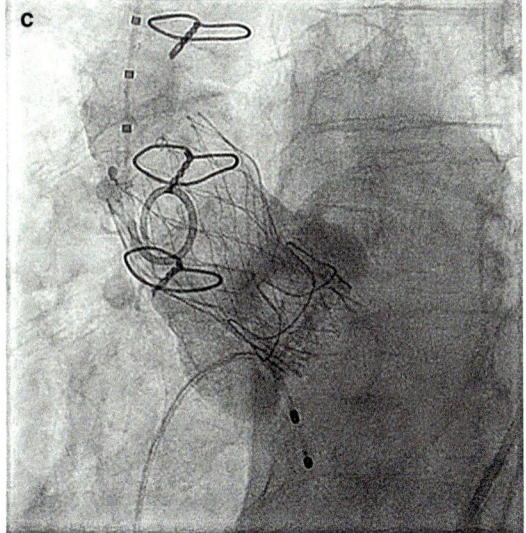

Fig. 29.4 A 68-year-old man was treated with a 23 mm CoreValve Evolut R valve for heart failure resulting from bioprosthetic valve dysfunction and severe AS (mean gradient 51 mmHg). The surgical valve was a 21 mm Carpentier-Edwards Magna valve surgically implanted 15 years previously (**a**). After placement of the 23 mm Evolut R, there was a mean transvalvular gradient of 18 mmHg. Post-dilation was performed with a 20 mm True Balloon (**b**). The final image (**c**) demonstrates appropriate frame expansion with no aortic insufficiency. The transvalvular gradient after post-dilation was 6 mmHg

the LV, direct trauma to the LV apex or mitral valve apparatus may result or the new THV may be dislodged from its annular position. We recommend continuing rapid pacing for 1 s after the balloon deflation begins to minimize the risk of trauma or stent valve movement from a partially deflated balloon. All necessary steps to ensure successful BPD are listed in Table 29.1.

29.6   Special Case: Bioprosthetic Valve Fracture in Valve-in-Valve TAVR

Recently, valve-in-valve (ViV) TAVR has emerged as a potentially less invasive treatment option for patients with bioprosthetic aortic valve dysfunction, and both self-expanding and

Table 29.1 Checklist for successful balloon post-dilation

Pre-procedure planning
- Appropriate pre-procedure imaging, including multidetector CT imaging to measure annular and root dimensions

After valve deployment
- Accurate assessment of residual AR
  - Transesophageal/transthoracic echocardiography
  - Invasive hemodynamic assessment
  - Cineangiography

Balloon post-dilation for balloon expandable systems
- Keep delivery system in place
- Add 1–2 cc of diluted contrast to delivery balloon
- Inflate balloon after rapid ventricular pacing while visually assessing stent frame expansion
- Reassess residual AR and aortic valve gradient

Balloon post-dilation for self-expanding systems
- Remove valve delivery system
- Select semi-compliant balloon to achieve inflation diameter of 1–2 mm smaller than area-derived mean diameter on MDCT
- Inflate balloon after rapid ventricular pacing while visually assessing stent frame expansion
- Reassess residual AR and aortic valve gradient

Balloon post-dilation valve-in-valve
- Remove valve delivery system
- Select non-compliant balloon (i.e., bard true balloon) to achieve inflation diameter equal to that of the internal dimension of existing stent frame
  - Inflate balloon after rapid ventricular pacing while visually assessing stent frame expansion
- Reassess residual AR and aortic valve gradient

balloon-expandable platforms approved by the US Food and Drug Administration for patients at increased risk for open surgical redo valve replacement. However, patient-prosthesis mismatch (PPM), generally defined as an indexed effective orifice area (EOA) of <0.65 cm^2/m^2 in patients with a BMI <30 kg/m^2 or < 0.6 cm^2/m^2 in patients with a BMI $\geq$ 30 kg/m, is a significant concern in these patients and may occur in >30% of patients undergoing ViV TAVR [29]. Recent data from the VIVID (Valve-in-Valve International Data) registry demonstrated that severe PPM was associated with higher mortality at 1 year, even after multivariable adjustment [30]. Additionally, patients treated with ViV TAVR with small bioprosthetic valves ($\leq$21 mm) may also be at increased risk of mortality at 1 year compared with patients with intermediate-

sized (21–25 mm) or large ($\geq$25 mm) surgical bioprosthetic valves.

There have been a few proposed strategies to reduce the risk of severe PPM in ViV TAVR and to increase the EOA, such as the use of a supra-annular CoreValve Evolut system and implanting the transcatheter inflow higher in the stent frame to improve the hemodynamic result. Both the CoreValve Evolut R and the SAPIEN XT valve are preferred over the Evolut Pro and SAPIEN 3 valves, as the former two lack outer sealing material in the prosthetic valve and yield less systolic obstruction for ViV TAVR. Because the TAVR valve frame sits inside the bioprosthetic valve stent frame, it is constrained by the bioprosthesis and is unable to expand fully, raising concern for potential underexpansion and suboptimal hemodynamic performance with residual prosthetic stenosis. BPD is used frequently, and is almost the rule, in ViV TAVR. Many patients meet criteria for PPM even when the original surgical valve was placed and was functioning normally. Recently, there have been case reports of successful balloon overexpansion and fracture of the existing bioprosthetic valve [31–35]. In the largest case series of bioprosthetic valve fracture, BVF resulted in a reduction in the mean gradient (from 20.5 ± 7.4 to 6.7 ± 3.7 mmHg, $p < 0.001$) and an increase in EOA (from 1.0 ± 0.4 to 1.8 ± 0.6 cm^2, $p < 0.001$) [33].

Fractured bioprosthetic stent frames have included the St. Jude Biocor Epic, Medtronic Mosaic, Sorin Mitroflow, Carpentier-Edwards Perimount, Edwards Magna Ease, and Edwards Magna. Importantly, the St. Jude Medical Trifecta and the Medtronic Hancock II are unable to be fractured. Generally, the noncompliant Bard True Balloon (occasionally the Bard Atlas Gold) is selected at a size 1 mm diameter larger than the labelled bioprosthetic valve size (i.e., 22 mm balloon for a 21 mm bioprosthetic valve). The noncompliant balloon is inflated from 10–24 atm using an indeflator until the bioprosthetic valve frame is fractured, typically visualized on fluoroscopy by the release of the balloon waist on expansion (Fig. 29.5). The timing of balloon valve fracture is controversial, and there are

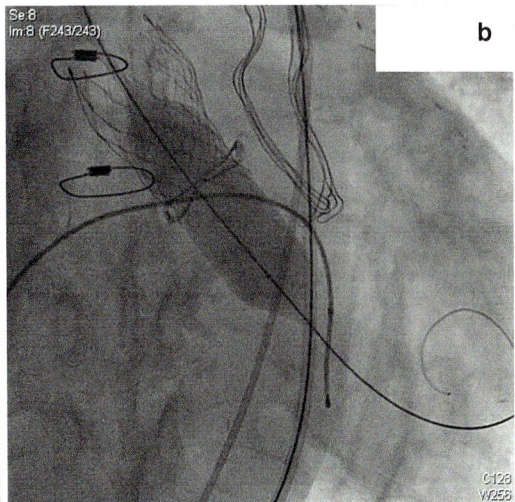

Fig. 29.5 Bioprosthetic valve frame fracture: An 82-year-old man with a dysfunctional 21 mm Sorin Mitroflow bioprosthetic valve underwent placement of a #23 CoreValve Evolut transcatheter heart valve (**a**). Due to a post-procedure gradient of 16 mmHg, the valve frame was post-dilated and fractured with a 22 mm True Balloon to 13 atm (**b**). Notice the "waist" expand in the two images. The gradient after BPD was 6 mmHg. Courtesy of Matthew Sherwood, MD

potential advantages in performing it either prior to transcatheter valve deployment or after. Fracturing the frame prior to transcatheter valve delivery may allow for potentially larger transcatheter valve; additionally, the new valve leaflets are not subjected to high pressure and the potential subclinical damage that may affect valve durability. Fracture prior to TAVR placement, however, runs the risk of hemodynamic instability if severe aortic regurgitation occurs. Fracturing the valve as part of a post-dilation process allows for assessment of hemodynamics after a traditional ViV procedure, potentially avoiding the need for valve fracturing. Saxon and colleagues offer recommendations on balloon selection and inflation pressures in Fig. 29.6 [36].

Importantly, there are potentially life-threatening risks to balloon overexpansion leading to bioprosthetic valve fracture. Although the largest case series did not report adverse outcomes, there is potential for the release of debris from the bioprosthetic valve, resulting in stroke and peripheral emboli or late neurologic sequelae; periprocedural stroke was observed in two patients ($n = 30$). There is also a potential risk of severe AR from leaflet damage, annular rupture, heart block requiring permanent pacemaker

placement, and coronary occlusion. Aortic annular rupture has not been reported in the case series. Additional study is needed to fully elucidate the safety, efficacy, and role for bioprosthetic valve fracture as part of ViV TAVR.

29.7   Conclusion

Although catheter-based valve therapies have revolutionized the treatment of severe, symptomatic aortic valve stenosis, paravalvular AR remains a potential liability of TAVR with greater than mild AR associated with adverse long-term outcomes. Residual stenosis, particularly in the case of valve-in-valve TAVR to treat bioprosthetic valve dysfunction, is also associated with adverse late clinical outcomes. Balloon post-dilation is an effective tool to minimize residual AR and to optimize valve performance during TAVR. Employing the best practices described in this chapter will minimize the risk of complications during BPD. Future directions in this field include the use of high pressure balloon dilation resulting in bioprosthetic valve fracture when treating patients with residual stenosis during valve-in-valve TAVR.

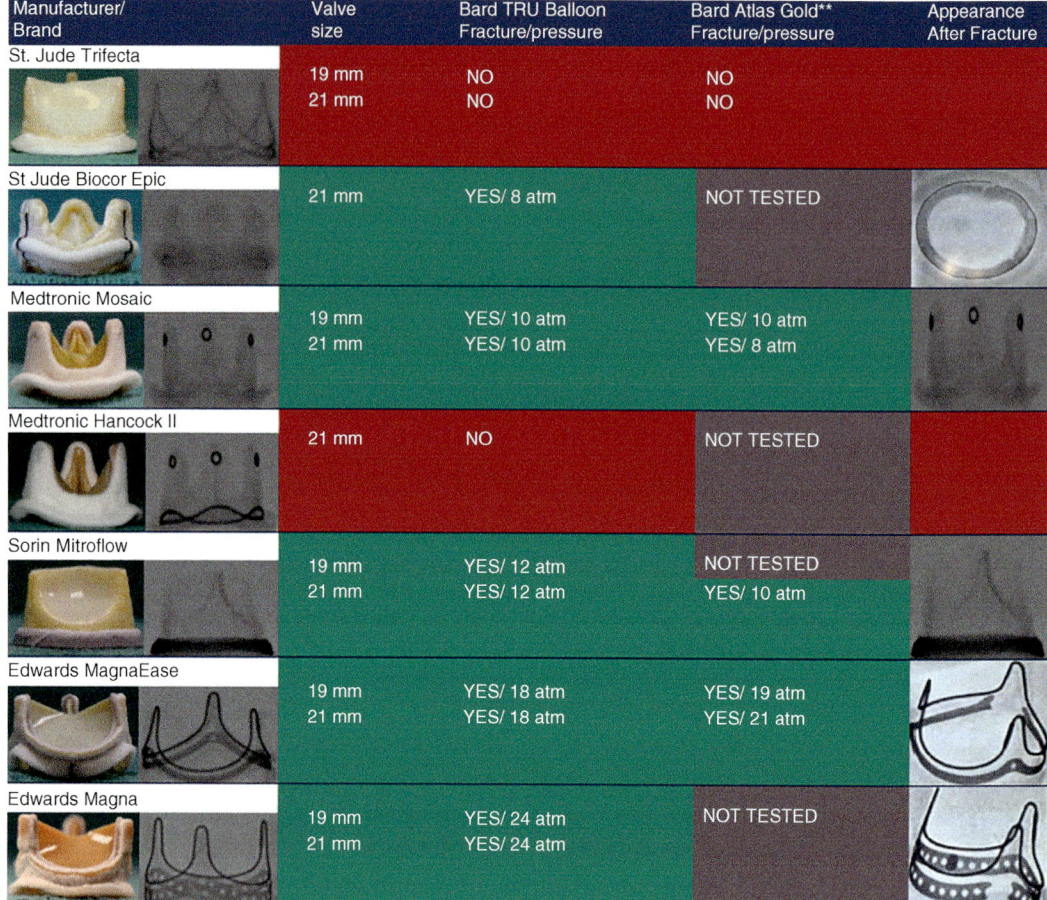

Manufacturer/ Brand	Valve size	Bard TRU Balloon Fracture/pressure	Bard Atlas Gold** Fracture/pressure	Appearance After Fracture
St. Jude Trifecta	19 mm	NO	NO	
	21 mm	NO	NO	
St Jude Biocor Epic	21 mm	YES/ 8 atm	NOT TESTED	
Medtronic Mosaic	19 mm	YES/ 10 atm	YES/ 10 atm	
	21 mm	YES/ 10 atm	YES/ 8 atm	
Medtronic Hancock II	21 mm	NO	NOT TESTED	
Sorin Mitroflow	19 mm	YES/ 12 atm	NOT TESTED	
	21 mm	YES/ 12 atm	YES/ 10 atm	
Edwards MagnaEase	19 mm	YES/ 18 atm	YES/ 19 atm	
	21 mm	YES/ 18 atm	YES/ 21 atm	
Edwards Magna	19 mm	YES/ 24 atm	NOT TESTED	
	21 mm	YES/ 24 atm		

Fig. 29.6 Considerations for balloon selection and pressure for fracture of bioprosthetic valve frame. From Saxon, Interventional Cardiology, 2018

References

1. Leon MB, Smith CR, Mack M, Miller DC, Moses JW, Svensson LG, et al. Transcatheter aortic-valve implantation for aortic stenosis in patients who cannot undergo surgery. N Engl J Med. 2010;363(17):1597–607.
2. Popma JJ, Adams DH, Reardon MJ, Yakubov SJ, Kleiman NS, Heimansohn D, et al. Transcatheter aortic valve replacement using a self-expanding bioprosthesis in patients with severe aortic stenosis at extreme risk for surgery. J Am Coll Cardiol. 2014;63(19):1972–81.
3. Adams DH, Popma JJ, Reardon MJ, Yakubov SJ, Coselli JS, Deeb GM, et al. Transcatheter aortic-valve replacement with a self-expanding prosthesis. N Engl J Med. 2014;370(19):1790–8.
4. Smith CR, Leon MB, Mack MJ, Miller DC, Moses JW, Svensson LG, et al. Transcatheter versus surgical aortic-valve replacement in high-risk patients. N Engl J Med. 2011;364(23):2187–98.
5. Reardon MJ, Van Mieghem NM, Popma JJ, Kleiman NS, Sondergaard L, Mumtaz M, et al. Surgical or transcatheter aortic-valve replacement in intermediate-risk patients. N Engl J Med. 2017;376(14):1321–31.
6. Généreux P, Head SJ, Hahn R, Daneault B, Kodali S, Williams MR, et al. Paravalvular leak after transcatheter aortic valve replacement: the new Achilles' heel? A comprehensive review of the literature. J Am Coll Cardiol. 2013;61(11):1125–36.
7. Sellers RD, Levy MJ, Amplatz K, Lillehei CW. Left retrograde cardioangiography in acquired cardiac disease: technic, indications and interpretations in 700 cases. Am J Cardiol. 1964;14:437–47.
8. Kappetein AP, Head SJ, Genereux P, Piazza N, van Mieghem NM, Blackstone EH, et al. Updated standardized endpoint definitions for transcatheter aortic valve implantation: the valve academic research Consortium-2 consensus document. J Am Coll Cardiol. 2012;60(15):1438–54.
9. Kappetein AP, Head SJ, Genereux P, Piazza N, van Mieghem NM, Blackstone EH, et al. Updated stan-

dardized endpoint definitions for transcatheter aortic valve implantation: the valve academic research Consortium-2 consensus document. J Thorac Cardiovasc Surg. 2013;145(1):6–23.

10. Oh JK, Little SH, Abdelmoneim SS, Reardon MJ, Kleiman NS, Lin G, et al. Regression of paravalvular aortic regurgitation and remodeling of self-expanding transcatheter aortic valve: an observation from the CoreValve US Pivotal Trial. JACC Cardiovasc Imaging. 2015;8(12):1364–75.

11. Haensig M, Rastan AJ, Kempfert J, Mukherjee C, Gutberlet M, Holzhey DM, et al. Aortic valve calcium scoring is a predictor of significant paravalvular aortic insufficiency in transapical-aortic valve implantation. Eur J Cardiothorac Surg. 2012;41(6):1234–41.

12. Jilaihawi H, Kashif M, Fontana G, Furugen A, Shiota T, Friede G, et al. Cross-sectional computed tomographic assessment improves accuracy of aortic annular sizing for transcatheter aortic valve replacement and reduces the incidence of paravalvular aortic regurgitation. J Am Coll Cardiol. 2012;59(14):1275–86.

13. Jabbour A, Ismail TF, Moat N, Gulati A, Roussin I, Alpendurada F, et al. Multimodality imaging in transcatheter aortic valve implantation and post-procedural aortic regurgitation: comparison among cardiovascular magnetic resonance, cardiac computed tomography, and echocardiography. J Am Coll Cardiol. 2011;58(21):2165–73.

14. Willson AB, Webb JG, Labounty TM, Achenbach S, Moss R, Wheeler M, et al. 3-dimensional aortic annular assessment by multidetector computed tomography predicts moderate or severe paravalvular regurgitation after transcatheter aortic valve replacement: a multicenter retrospective analysis. J Am Coll Cardiol. 2012;59(14):1287–94.

15. Hayashida K, Bouvier E, Lefevre T, Hovasse T, Morice MC, Chevalier B, et al. Impact of CT-guided valve sizing on post-procedural aortic regurgitation in transcatheter aortic valve implantation. EuroIntervention. 2012;8(5):546–55.

16. Hayashida K, Lefèvre T, Chevalier B, Hovasse T, Romano M, Garot P, et al. Impact of post-procedural aortic regurgitation on mortality after transcatheter aortic valve implantation. J Am Coll Cardiol Intv. 2012;5(12):1247–56.

17. Kodali S, Pibarot P, Douglas PS, Williams M, Xu K, Thourani V, et al. Paravalvular regurgitation after transcatheter aortic valve replacement with the Edwards sapien valve in the PARTNER trial: characterizing patients and impact on outcomes. Eur Heart J. 2015;36(7):449–56.

18. Athappan G, Patvardhan E, Tuzcu EM, Svensson LG, Lemos PA, Fraccaro C, et al. Incidence, predictors, and outcomes of aortic regurgitation after transcatheter aortic valve replacement: meta-analysis and systematic review of literature. J Am Coll Cardiol. 2013;61(15):1585–95.

19. Daneault B, Koss E, Hahn RT, Kodali S, Williams MR, Genereux P, et al. Efficacy and safety of postdilatation to reduce paravalvular regurgitation during

20. Harrison JK, Hughes GC, Reardon MJ, Stoler R, Grayburn P, Hebeler R, et al. Balloon post-dilation following implantation of a self-expanding transcatheter aortic valve bioprosthesis. JACC Cardiovasc Interv. 2017;10(2):168–75.

21. Hahn RT, Pibarot P, Webb J, Rodes-Cabau J, Herrmann HC, Williams M, et al. Outcomes with post-dilation following transcatheter aortic valve replacement: the PARTNER I trial (placement of aortic transcatheter valve). JACC Cardiovasc Interv. 2014;7(7):781–9.

22. Barbanti M, Yang TH, Rodes Cabau J, Tamburino C, Wood DA, Jilaihawi H, et al. Anatomical and procedural features associated with aortic root rupture during balloon-expandable transcatheter aortic valve replacement. Circulation. 2013;128(3):244–53.

23. Noble S, Cikirikcioglu M, Roffi M. Massive aortic regurgitation following paravalvular balloon valvuloplasty of an Edwards SAPIEN valve treated by emergent CoreValve implantation: never cross a transcatheter aortic valve without a pigtail. Catheter Cardiovasc Interv. 2013;82(4):E609–12.

24. Binder RK, Webb JG, Willson AB, Urena M, Hansson NC, Norgaard BL, et al. The impact of integration of a multidetector computed tomography annulus area sizing algorithm on outcomes of transcatheter aortic valve replacement: a prospective, multicenter, controlled trial. J Am Coll Cardiol. 2013;62(5):431–8.

25. Popma JJ, Gleason TG, Yakubov SJ, Harrison JK, Forrest JK, Maini B, et al. Relationship of annular sizing using multidetector computed tomographic imaging and clinical outcomes after self-expanding CoreValve transcatheter aortic valve replacement. Circ Cardiovasc Interv. 2016;9(7)

26. Sinning JM, Hammerstingl C, Vasa-Nicotera M, Adenauer V, Lema Cachiguango SJ, Scheer AC, et al. Aortic regurgitation index defines severity of peri-prosthetic regurgitation and predicts outcome in patients after transcatheter aortic valve implantation. J Am Coll Cardiol. 2012;59(13):1134–41.

27. Sherif MA, Abdel-Wahab M, Stocker B, Geist V, Richardt D, Tolg R, et al. Anatomic and procedural predictors of paravalvular aortic regurgitation after implantation of the Medtronic CoreValve bioprosthesis. J Am Coll Cardiol. 2010;56(20):1623–9.

28. Takagi K, Latib A, Al-Lamee R, Mussardo M, Montorfano M, Maisano F, et al. Predictors of moderate-to-severe paravalvular aortic regurgitation immediately after CoreValve implantation and the impact of postdilatation. Catheter Cardiovasc Interv. 2011;78(3):432–43.

29. Dvir D, Webb JG, Bleiziffer S, Pasic M, Waksman R, Kodali S, et al. Transcatheter aortic valve implantation in failed bioprosthetic surgical valves. JAMA. 2014;312(2):162–70.

30. Pibarot P, Simonato M, Barbanti M, Linke A, Kornowski R, Rudolph T, et al. Impact of pre-existing prosthesis-patient mismatch on survival following

aortic valve-in-valve procedures. JACC Cardiovasc Interv. 2018;11(2):133–41.

31. Allen KB, Chhatriwalla AK, Cohen DJ, Saxon JT, Aggarwal S, Hart A, et al. Bioprosthetic valve fracture to facilitate transcatheter valve-in-valve implantation. Ann Thorac Surg. 2017;104(5):1501–8.

32. Brown SC, Cools B, Gewillig M. Cracking a tricuspid perimount bioprosthesis to optimize a second transcatheter sapien valve-in-valve placement. Catheter Cardiovasc Interv. 2016;88(3):456–9.

33. Chhatriwalla AK, Allen KB, Saxon JT, Cohen DJ, Aggarwal S, Hart AJ, et al. Bioprosthetic valve fracture improves the hemodynamic results of valve-in-valve transcatheter aortic valve replacement. Circ Cardiovasc Interv. 2017;10(7)

34. Nielsen-Kudsk JE, Christiansen EH, Terkelsen CJ, Norgaard BL, Jensen KT, Krusell LR, et al. Fracturing the ring of small mitroflow bioprostheses by high-pressure balloon predilatation in transcatheter aortic valve-in-valve implantation. Circ Cardiovasc Interv. 2015;8(8):e002667.

35. Tanase D, Grohmann J, Schubert S, Uhlemann F, Eicken A, Ewert P. Cracking the ring of Edwards perimount bioprosthesis with ultrahigh pressure balloons prior to transcatheter valve in valve implantation. Int J Cardiol. 2014;176(3):1048–9.

36. Saxon JT, Allen KB, Cohen DJ, Chhatriwalla AK. Bioprosthetic valve fracture during valve-in-valve TAVR: bench to bedside. Interv Cardiol. 2018;13(1):20–6.

Embolic Protection Devices for Transcatheter Aortic Valve Implantation

30

Anna Franzone and Stefan Stortecky

Abbreviations and Acronyms

CI	Confidence intervals
CLEAN-TAVI	Claret Embolic Protection and TAVI
CVE	Cerebrovascular events
DW-MRI	Diffusion-weighted magnetic resonance imaging
EPDs	Embolic protection devices
FLAIR	Fluid-attenuated inversion recovery
HITS	High intensity transient signals
HR	Hazard ratio
MACCE	Major adverse cardiac and cerebrovascular events
MISTRAL-C	MRI Investigation in TAVI with Claret
MoCA	Montreal Cognitive Assessment
NOTION	Nordic Aortic Valve Intervention Trial
OR	Odds ratio
PARTNER	Placement of Aortic Transcatheter Valves
RR	Risk ratio
SAVR	Surgical aortic valve replacement
SENTINEL	Cerebral Protection in Transcatheter Aortic Valve Replacement
SMD	Standardized mean difference
SURTAVI	*Surgical Replacement and Transcatheter Aortic Valve Implantation*
TAVI	Transcatheter aortic valve implantation
TCD	Transcranial Doppler
TIA	Transient ischemic attack
VARC	Valve Academic Research Consortium

A. Franzone
Department of Advanced Biomedical Sciences,
Federico II University of Naples, Naples, Italy

S. Stortecky (✉)
Department of Cardiology,
Inselspital, Bern University Hospital,
University of Bern, Bern, Switzerland
e-mail: Stefan.Stortecky@insel.ch

30.1 Introduction

The occurrence of cerebrovascular events (CVE) represents a dramatic complication of interventional procedures and is associated with significant morbidity and mortality [1, 2]. Early studies showed an increased risk of CVE after transcatheter aortic valve implantation (TAVI), also called transcatheter aortic valve replacement (TAVR), with first-generation devices when compared with surgical aortic valve replacement (SAVR) [3]. Nevertheless, technological innovation, procedure simplification, and better patient selection have been paralleled by a progressive decline of

© Springer Nature Switzerland AG 2019
A. Giordano et al. (eds.), *Transcatheter Aortic Valve Implantation*,
https://doi.org/10.1007/978-3-030-05912-5_30

rates of CVE after TAVI [4]. Furthermore, a wide scientific investigation spreads light on mechanisms, timing, and clinical significance of CVE in patients undergoing TAVI. Embolization has been recognized as the leading mechanism of neurological complications that occur early after TAVI, supporting the rationale for the use of embolic protection devices (EPDs) during the procedure [5].

This chapter summarizes current knowledge about the incidence, timing, mechanisms, and clinical spectrum of CVE in the setting of TAVI; in addition, it describes features of EPDs and provides an overview of their safety and efficacy profile based on currently available evidence.

30.2 Timing and Frequency of Thromboembolic CVE in the Setting of TAVI

Assessing the burden of embolic CVE after TAVI poses unique challenges related to the variability of definitions adopted across the studies as well as differences in methodology used for the diagnosis of neurological complications. Figure 30.1 shows the typical temporal pattern of CVE among TAVI patients with relative potential preventive strategies [6].

Embolic CVE may occur in the early periprocedural period and at any time during follow-up as a consequence of different mechanisms and

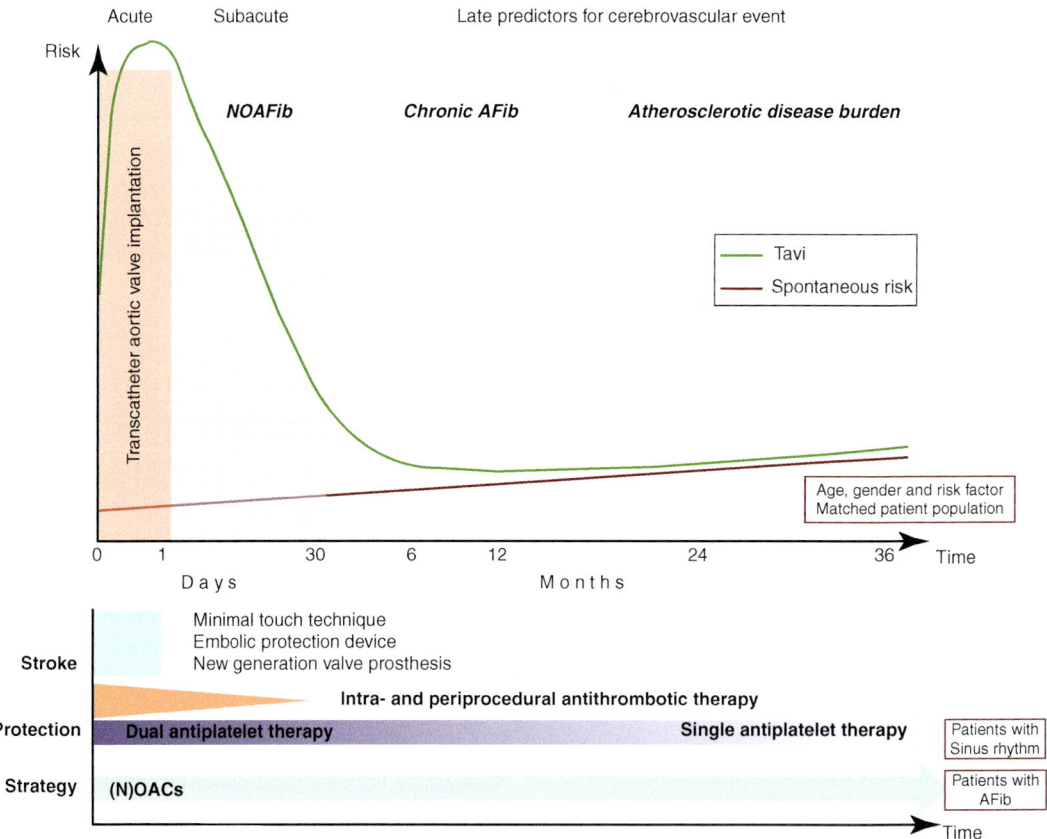

Fig. 30.1 Timing, risk, and potential strategies for prevention of cerebrovascular events in the setting of transcatheter aortic valve implantation. Green line indicates patients undergoing transcatheter aortic valve implantation (TAVI); red line displays the risk of an age-, sex-, and risk factor-matched population. AFib indicates atrial fibrillation; NOAFib, new onset atrial fibrillation; and (N) OAC, (novel) oral anticoagulants
Reproduced with permission from Stortecky S, Windecker S, Circulation. 2012;126:2921–2924

predisposing factors, as reported below. However, there is evidence that CVE occurring within 10 days from the procedure account for roughly 75% of all neurological events occurring during the first 2 years following TAVI. In a study of 1061 consecutive patients who underwent TAVI with either balloon-expandable or self-expanding valves, a total of 54 patients (5.1%) had a CVE within 30 days: 54% of these events occurred in the first 24 h after TAVI, while 25 CVE were sub-acute (occurred between 1 and 30 days after the procedure) [7]. An analysis of 2621 patients from the Placement of Aortic Transcatheter Valves (PARTNER) trial showed that 85% of CVE occurred within 1 week from the procedure; in addition, the instantaneous risk of stroke peaked on day 2 and then fell to a low prolonged risk of 0.8% by 1–2 weeks [8]. This biphasic shape of the hazard function was also observed among patients enrolled in the CoreValve US Extreme Risk and High Risk Pivotal Trials or Continued Access Study: there was an early phase during the first 10 days after the procedure during which 147 (4.1%) strokes occurred; this period was fol-lowed by a later phase that remained constant for the duration of follow-up [9].

Overall, clinically apparent stroke has ranged from 1.2% to 6.7% in studies assessing the perfor-mance of TAVI, whereas patients undergoing iso-lated SAVR have an estimated risk of stroke of 1.5% according to a report of the Society of Thoracic Surgeons [10]. Early randomized stud-ies showed a higher incidence of stroke after TAVI than standard therapy during the first 30 days. In the PARTNER-1B trial, stroke rates were 13.8% and 5.5% after TAVI and medical therapy, respec-tively, ($p = 0.01$); within 30 days after interven-tion, more ischemic events occurred in the TAVI group (6.7% vs. 1.7%, $p = 0.02$), while, beyond 30 days, a numerical difference of more hemor-rhagic strokes was observed in the TAVI patient population (2.2% vs. 0.6%, $p = 0.16$) [11]. Nevertheless, at the longest available follow-up (5 years), stroke risk was 16.0% in the TAVI group versus 18.2% in the standard treatment group (hazard ratio, HR, 1.39; 95% confidence intervals, CI, 0.62–3.11; $p = 0.555$) [12]. Among patients included in the PARTNER-1A trial, there was a twofold increased risk of all new neurological events after TAVI compared with SAVR, both at 30 days (5.5% vs. 2.4%, $p = 0.04$) and at 1 year (8.3% vs. 4.3%, $p = 0.04$). Specifically, rates of major stroke were 3.8% in the transcatheter group and 2.1% in the surgical group at 30 days ($p = 0.20$) and 5.1% and 2.4% at 1 year, respec-tively, ($p = 0.07$) [3]. However, the risk of stroke or transient ischemic attack (TIA) was compa-rable in each treatment group at 5 years (14.7% in the TAVI group vs. 15.9% in the SAVR group) [13]. Patient- and procedure-related factors may have contributed to these findings: multiple comorbidities predisposing to increased throm-boembolic risk featured inoperable and high-risk patients included in the PARTNER-1A and B, respectively; in addition, first-generation balloon-expandable transcatheter valves (Edwards SAPIEN—Edwards Lifesciences, Inc., Irvine, California) were used. The lower incidence (2.3%) of major stroke at 30 days among patients included in the CoreValve Extreme Risk Pivotal has been attributed to the lower profile of the first-generation self-expand-ing Medtronic CoreValve (Medtronic, Minneapolis, Minnesota) compared with the SAPIEN valves [14]. In the CoreValve High Risk trial, rates of any stroke were 4.9% in the TAVI group and 6.2% in the surgical group at 30 days ($p = 0.46$) and 8.8% and 12.6% at 1 year, respectively ($p = 0.10$) [15].

Studies involving intermediate risk patients found no significant difference between TAVI and SAVR in terms of any CVE. In the PARTNER-2A, rates of any neurological events were 6.4% and 6.5% ($p = 0.94$) and 12.7% and 11% ($p = 0.25$), at 30 days and 2 years after trans-catheter or surgical intervention, respectively [16]. Along the same line, rates of disabling stroke were similar between patients randomized to TAVI or SAVR in the Surgical Replacement and Transcatheter Aortic Valve Implantation (SURTAVI) trial [17]. The Nordic Aortic Valve Intervention Trial (NOTION)-I included 81.8% of patients with STS score <4%; at 30 days, neu-rological events were reported in 2.8% and 3% of patients in the TAVI and SAVR group, respec-tively ($p = 0.94$), and in 5% and 6.2% at 1 year, respectively ($p = 0.68$) [18]. Meta-analysis of randomized trials found no difference between TAVI and SAVR in terms of CVE rates (including stroke or TIA) [19, 20].

Rates of CVE from large national registries are in line with the results of more recent randomized trials. Furthermore, in real-world patients, a progressive decline of neurological complications has been observed over the time, probably as consequence of changing patients' characteristics and technical advances. Among patients included in the UK TAVI Registry, the frequency of stroke decreased from 3.6% in 2007 and 2008 to 2.4% in 2012 ($p = 0.022$) [21]. The 2016 Annual Report of The Society of Thoracic Surgeons/American College of Cardiology Transcatheter Valve Therapy (TVT) Registry showed a 30-day stroke rate of 2.1% that decreased from 2.3% in 2012 to 1.9% in 2015 ($p = 0.03$) [22]. Interestingly, another analysis from the same registry found a linear association between TAVI volume and inhospital stroke; although this association was lost after adjustment for patient and procedural characteristics, it supports the notion that operators' experience may play a role in the occurrence of periprocedural CVE [23].

30.3 Mechanisms of Cerebrovascular Events in Patients Undergoing TAVI

While the majority of neurological complications occurring in the periprocedural period is thought to be caused by athero- or thromboembolic events, also periprocedural hypotension and cerebral hypoperfusion may contribute to neurological injury. During the short period of rapid ventricular pacing to reduce cardiac motion and ventricular ejection for balloon valvuloplasty and valve deployment, cerebral hypoperfusion may be responsible for cerebral injury. Studies using transcranial cerebral oximetry were able to detect a reduction of regional oxygen saturation in cerebral areas during these procedural steps [5]. However, these abnormalities are usually well tolerated and rapidly recovering and may only be of clinical relevance in the setting of prolonged cerebral hypoperfusion.

Aortic plaque disruption with cerebral embolism has been found to be as frequent as 0.2–0.4% in patients undergoing percutaneous coronary intervention. The use of larger caliber and stiffer catheters and the presence of a significant calcium burden in the aortic wall of TAVI patients, however, significantly increase the risk of disruption of embolic debris. In particular, manipulation of catheters, wires, and devices through the calcified aortic arch and the native aortic valve has been considered the main mechanism of embolization to the brain. Van Mieghem and colleagues studied the histopathological characteristics of debris captured by the dual filter-based embolic protection device (Montage Dual Filter System, Claret Medical, Inc., Santa Rosa, California) in 81 patients undergoing TAVI: overall, thrombotic material was found in 74% of patients and tissue-derived debris in 63%; the embolized tissue originated from the native aortic valve leaflets, aortic wall, or left ventricular myocardium. In addition, in 33% of samples, amorphous calcified debris as well as collagenous and proteoglycan matrix were found [24]. Thrombus is the most common type of debris that has been found across published reports [25]. Studies on native valves from patients undergoing SAVR for severe aortic stenosis demonstrated that 83% had evidence of dystrophic calcium, supporting the notion that most debris originate from the bulky calcific atheroma in the peri-annular area or valve [26]. Air emboli originating from contrast injection or exchange of large catheters may also be cause of neurological complications. Among other procedural factors, post-dilation of the transcatheter heart valve has been hypothesized to promote debris disruption: a nearly sixfold increase in the rates of stroke after balloon post-dilation has been reported in a study of 221 patients treated with balloon-expandable transcatheter valves [27]. Along the same line, in a systematic review of 64 studies involving 72,318 patients, the use of balloon post-dilation tended to be associated with a higher risk of CVE (risk ratio (RR), 1.43; $p = 0.07$) [28]. For similar reasons, the role of balloon pre-dilation for facilitating crossing of the aortic valve and the deployment of the device has been questioned. However, a systematic review of 20 studies, including 3586 patients, showed no differences between TAVI with or without balloon pre-dilation in terms of early CVE (RR, 0.92; 95% CI, 0.58–1.46) [29].

Further evidence supporting the theory of particulate debris and embolization is provided by studies with intraprocedural transcranial Doppler (TCD). This test looks for high intensity transient signals (HITS) in the Doppler signal of an intracranial artery (usually the middle cerebral artery) representing microembolic events. These signs have been observed during all steps of TAVI procedure with peak rates detected during balloon aortic valvuloplasty and valve positioning [30]. Furthermore, the number of HITS detected with TCD during TAVI has been associated with postprocedural release of S100B, a marker of cerebral injury [31]. Consistently, initial diffusion-weighted magnetic resonance imaging (DW-MRI) reports have demonstrated the near ubiquitous presence of subclinical or silent cerebral lesions after TAVI, with a pattern typical of embolic processes [32–36]. This technique consists of mapping diffusion of molecules (mainly water) in biological tissues; specifically, territories of acute cerebral ischemia, where the water diffusion rate is low, appear brighter than surrounding tissues. The embolic origin of such lesions is supported by their typical distribution: they are usually disseminated and multiple. In addition, a greater vulnerability of the anterior than posterior circulation has been described. Moreover, the number and the size of lesions detected at baseline have been shown to correlate with the occurrence of new lesions after the procedure.

On the other side, the etiology of CVE presenting later after the procedure is less clear and likely involving patient- rather than procedure-related factors. Among these, new onset of atrial fibrillation can occur in up to 35% of patients after TAVI and is an independent predictor of stroke or other systemic embolic events (HR 5.0, 95% CI 1.29 to 19.35; $p = 0.020$) [37]. Additionally, a pro-thrombotic status that is typical of elderly patients with severe aortic stenosis

and delayed endothelialization of the stent frame of the prosthesis may further be associated with thromboembolic events.

30.4 Clinical Spectrum of Thromboembolic Events in TAVI Patients

Valve Academic Research Consortium (VARC)-2 criteria for assessing CVE in patients undergoing TAVI are reported in Table 30.1 [38]. More recently, the NeuroARC (Neurologic Academic Research Consortium Consensus) document proposed updated definitions and classification of neurological complications in the setting of interventional studies [39]. The upcoming Valve Academic Research Consortium-3 is planned to incorporate imaging for the diagnosis of stroke. Nevertheless, standardized criteria are less adopted in clinical investigations, especially in the context of observational studies. CVE after TAVI have been usually reported as stroke (disabling or non-disabling) and TIA. However, the spectrum of neurological events associated with TAVI is more complex and includes subclinical events whose impact on clinical outcomes is still to be defined. DW-MRI studies allowed for the identification of new ischemic lesion in a range of 66–90% of TAVI patients [33, 40, 41]. However, a correlation of such lesions with neurological symptoms, changes in neurocognitive behavior, or impaired survival has never been demonstrated. The main challenges of DW-MRI interpretation include preexisting cerebral pathologies that might be common in elderly patients and the difficulty to identify all new lesions. While 1.5-T imaging may fail to detect smaller emboli, 3-T imaging offers improved sensitivity with higher resolution that may lead to an overestimation of the lesions. In this context, although an analysis of the SENTINEL (Cerebral Protection in Transcatheter Aortic Valve Replacement) trial (that compared distal protection vs. no protection for brain embolization during TAVI, as detailed below) showed a significant relationship between baseline cognitive function and pre-procedural brain pathology as measured

Table 30.1 Valve Academic Research Consortium (VARC)-2 criteria for diagnosis of stroke or transient ischemic attack

Diagnostic criteria

Acute episode of a focal or global neurological deficit with at least one of the following: Change in the level of consciousness, hemiplegia, hemiparesis, numbness, or sensory loss affecting one side of the body, dysphasia or aphasia, hemianopia, amaurosis fugax, or other neurological signs or symptoms consistent with stroke

Stroke: Duration of a focal or global neurological deficit >24 h; OR <24 h if available neuroimaging documents a new hemorrhage or infarct; OR the neurological deficit results in death

TIA: Duration of a focal or global neurological deficit <24 h, any variable neuroimaging does not demonstrate a new hemorrhage or infarct

No other readily identifiable non-stroke cause for the clinical presentation (e.g., brain tumor, trauma, infection, hypoglycemia, peripheral lesion, pharmacological influences), to be determined by or in conjunction with the designated neurologist

Confirmation of the diagnosis by at least one of the following:

Neurologist or neurosurgical specialist; neuroimaging procedure (CT scan or brain MRI), but stroke may be diagnosed on clinical grounds alone

Stroke classification

Ischemic: An acute episode of focal cerebral, spinal, or retinal dysfunction caused by infarction of the central nervous system tissue

Hemorrhagic: An acute episode of focal or global cerebral or spinal dysfunction caused by intraparenchymal, intraventricular, or subarachnoid hemorrhage

A stroke may be classified as **undetermined** if there is insufficient information to allow categorization as ischemic or hemorrhagic

Stroke definitions

Disabling stroke: a modified Rankin scale score of 2 or more at 90 days and an increase in at least one category from an individual's pre-stroke baseline

Non-disabling stroke: a modified Rankin scale score of <2 at 90 days or one that does not result in an increase in at least one category from an individual's pre-stroke baseline

by 3-T T2 fluid-attenuated inversion recovery (FLAIR) imaging, the clinical significance of new lesions remains uncertain [42].

30.5 Rationale for Use and General Principles of EPDs

The evidence of embolic phenomena as main cause of periprocedural CVE supports the rationale for performing TAVI with the use of EPDs. They are intended to provide a mechanical protection from embolization of debris to the brain, by deflecting their route or by capturing them. The main fields of application of these devices other than TAVI include carotid stenting; in addition, they have also been used in SAVR cohorts [43, 44]. Initial human experience of EPDs in four TAVI patients (mean age 90 years) was reported in 2010: correct device placement was uncomplicated in all patients, there were no procedural complications, and the additional time

due to the use of the device was 13 min (interquartile range, 12–16 min) [45]. The ideal device should be able to protect the ostia of all three large branches of the aortic arch, remains in a stable position during the procedure, is easy to use, and does not cause any injury to the aortic arch. Currently available EPDs can be broadly divided in two families on the basis of the design: filter devices such as the Sentinel (Claret Medical Inc., Santa Rosa, CA) and the EMBOL-X (Edwards Lifesciences, Irvine, CA) and deflectors that include the Embrella (Edwards Lifesciences, Irvine, CA) and TriGuard (Keystone Heart Ltd., Caesarea, Israel) devices (Fig. 30.2).

30.6 Sentinel Cerebral Protection System

The Sentinel Cerebral Protection System (Fig. 30.2a) is made of two interconnected filters: the proximal filter is deployed in the brachiocephalic trunk and covers all areas of the brain sup-

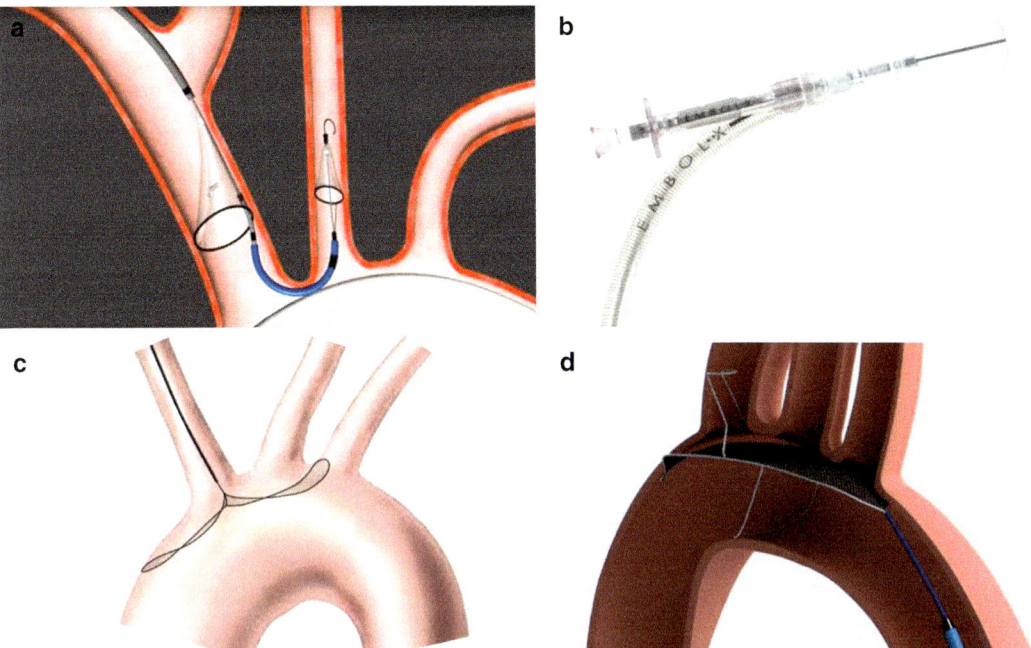

Fig. 30.2 Device studies for cerebral embolic protection in patients undergoing transcatheter aortic valve implantation. (**a**) Sentinel cerebral protection system (Claret Medical Inc., Santa Rosa, CA); (**b**) EMBOL-X (Edwards Lifesciences, Irvine, CA); (**c**) Embrella (Edwards Lifesciences, Irvine, CA); (**d**) TriGuard (Keystone Heart Ltd., Caesarea, Israel). *Reproduced with permission from Samim et al., J Thorac Cardiovasc Surg. 2015 Mar;149(3):799–805*

plied by the right vertebral and carotid arteries; the distal (SpiderFX™, Covidien, Mansfield, MA, USA, or FilterWire™, Boston Scientific, Natick, MA, USA) is released into the left common carotid artery. The left vertebral artery, which usually originates from the left subclavian artery, remains unprotected: as consequence, the current device provides protection only to 9 out of 28 brain regions. The proximal filter is made of a radiopaque nitinol frame containing a polyurethane filter with 140-μm-diameter pores that can be accommodated within vessels of 9–15 mm in diameter. The system can be delivered through a 6 Fr sheath introduced through either the brachial or radial artery of the right arm shortly prior to the passage of the prosthesis delivery catheter through the aortic arch. The safety of device implantation was explored in a first-in-man study including 40 TAVI patients: technical success rate (primary study endpoint) with the first-generation device (Claret CE Pro) was 60% and 87% for the second-generation device. Debris

was found in 54.3% of patients; however, no neurological events occurred during the procedure, and three strokes were reported at 30 days [46]. The second-generation device includes a central 0.014 guide wire lumen along with a modified curve on the distal, telescoping catheter to facilitate easier engagement of the left common carotid artery. It was employed in the randomized MISTRAL-C (MRI Investigation in TAVI with Claret) trial that included 65 patients. New brain lesions were found in 78% of patients at follow-up MRI; patients with the Sentinel had numerically fewer new lesions and a smaller total lesion volume (95 mm³, IQR 10–257 vs. 197 mm³). Neurocognitive deterioration was present in 4% of patients with Sentinel vs. 27% of patients without ($p = 0.017$). However, follow-up DW-MRI and neurocognitive testing were completed in 57% and 80%, respectively [47].

The Claret Embolic Protection and TAVI (CLEAN-TAVI) trial was a single-center, blinded trial that randomized 100 TAVI patients, in a 1:1

ratio, to receive cerebral embolic protection during the procedure or not. The use of the Sentinel EPD was associated with a significant reduction of the number of new lesions (4.00, interquartile range, IQR, 3.00–7.25 vs. 10.00, IQR, 6.75–7.00 in the control group; difference, 5.00, IQR, 2.00–8.00; $p < 0.001$) and total lesion volume on DW-MRI (242 mm³, 95% CI, 159–353 vs. 527 mm³, 95% CI, 364–830; difference, 234 mm³, 95% CI, 91–406; $p = 0.001$). Nevertheless, stroke rates and neurocognitive outcomes were not different between randomized arms [48].

Hitherto, the largest randomized trial that assessed the potential advantage associated with the use of EPDs was the Cerebral Protection in Transcatheter Aortic Valve Replacement (SENTINEL): 363 patients were randomized to the safety ($n = 123$), device imaging ($n = 121$), and control imaging ($n = 119$) arms. The two imaging arms included a serial assessment of new and preexisting brain lesions using DW-MRI and fluid-attenuated inversion recovery MRI (FLAIR). Furthermore, patients in the imaging arms underwent a comprehensive, neurocognitive function assessment. Debris was found in 99% of patients and included thrombus, calcification, valve tissue, artery wall, and foreign material. The primary safety endpoint consisting of major adverse cardiac and cerebrovascular events (MACCE) at 30 days was 7.3% (meeting the non-inferiority margin to the pre-specified performance goal of 18.3%) and was not statistically different from that of the control group (9.9%; $p = 0.41$). The primary efficacy endpoint was not met because new lesion volume in protected brain territories at 2–7 days after the procedure was 178.0 mm³ in control subjects and 102.8 mm³ in the device arm ($p = 0.33$). However, after adjusting for valve type and baseline T2/FLAIR lesion volume in a post hoc analysis, there were significant differences in new lesion volumes favoring embolic protection. Although there was a correlation between lesion volume and neurocognitive decline, no differences in stroke rates were reported. Several factors may have contributed to these results: among these, the lack of standardized criteria to characterize new ischemic lesions with DW-MRI and to take into account the burden of preexisting disease. Furthermore, several different transcatheter valves were employed with a significant interaction effect between the device and treatment (the effect of the EPD was statistically significant only with valves other than the Edwards SAPIEN 3) without clear explanation. Another important limitation, which is common in similar and comparable studies, was the lost-of-imaging-follow-up in 25% of patients [49].

A pooled analysis of study-level data from the three randomized trials investigating the Sentinel device (314 patients) showed a significant reduction of total new lesion volume in protected regions [50].

Nevertheless, earlier studies showed that at least one-fifth of all silent cerebral lesions were present in the posterior regions (brainstem and cerebellum), which are unprotected by the current Sentinel device [34, 51]. To address the issue of uncovered brain areas, the addition of the WIRION single filter in the left vertebral artery was studied in nine patients: no periprocedural strokes occurred, and debris, consisting of thrombus, tissue-derived debris, and foreign body material, was found in equal amount in the extra filter and the Sentinel device [52].

In contrast with the results of randomized studies, a propensity score matching analysis including 280 and 522 patients undergoing TAVI with and without the Sentinel device, respectively, showed a significant reduction of the composite of all-cause mortality or all-stroke according to VARC-2 criteria within 7 days in the protected group (OR 0.30; 95% CI 0.12–0.77, $p = 0.001$). Moreover, there was a significant reduction in disabling and non-disabling stroke from 4.6% without protection to 1.4% with the Sentinel embolic protection device ($p = 0.03$) [53]. It should be noted, however, that TAVI without cerebral protection were performed in 2014–2015, whereas EPDs were used in the context of procedures performed in 2016–2017: better operator experience, different transcatheter valves, and patients' features may have contributed to lower stroke rate in protected group.

The research program with the Sentinel device is going on with the PROTECT-TAVI trial

(NCT02895737), a four-arm study comparing the device in self-expanding vs. balloon-expandable valves, and trial results are expected in 2019.

30.7 EMBOL-X Device

The EMBOL-X device (Fig. 30.2b) is made of a self-expanding and self-fitting nitinol-based frame, covered by a semipermeable polyester mesh (120 mm pore diameter) that is placed inside the aorta. The TAo-EmbolX (Intraprocedural Intraaortic Embolic Protection With the EMBOL-X device in Patients Undergoing Transaortic Transcatheter Aortic Valve Implantation) included 30 high-risk patients randomly assigned to undergo transaortic TAVI with the SAPIEN XT prosthesis (Edwards Lifesciences) combined with either the EMBOL-X device (group-1, $n = 14$) or without (group-2, $n = 16$). New areas of ischemia on cerebral DW-MRI were found in 69% in group-2 and 50% in group-1. Lesion size was smaller in patients treated with the EMBOL-X device than in those without (88 ± 60 vs. 168 ± 217 mm^3, $p = 0.27$). There were no neurologic events in both groups [54].

30.8 Embrella Embolic Deflector Device

The Embrella device (Fig. 30.2c) is an umbrella-like device with 2 heparin-coated polyurethane membranes (whose pores are the smallest of any of the currently available EPDs) mounted on an oval-shaped nitinol frame. It can be loaded into a 6 Fr sheath and is delivered through the right arm using the radial or the brachial artery and has three markers for guiding the deployment under fluoroscopy. The petals protect the brachiocephalic trunk and the left carotid artery. In some patients, it further covers (sometimes partially) the left subclavian artery. The Embrella received CE mark approval in 2010. The feasibility of device use was explored in the PROTAVI-C trial that included an experimental group of 41 patients and a control group of 11 patients. The

system was successfully deployed at the level of the aortic arch in all patients without complications. TCD showed a higher total number of HITS in the EPD group ($p < 0.001$ vs. control group). DW-MRI performed within 7 days after TAVR showed the presence of new ischemic lesions in all patients in both groups, whereas the use of EPD was associated with a lower lesion volume compared with the control group ($p = 0.003$). All new cerebral lesions were not present on the DW-MRI performed at 30 days after TAVI [55]. No additional trials are ongoing, and the device has been withdrawn from the market by the manufacturer.

30.9 TriGuard Cerebral Protection Device

The TriGuard (Fig. 30.2d) is a biocompatible filter made of nickel titanium alloy wires and coated with an antithrombotic coating, which is delivered via a 9 Fr introducer sheath, positioned in the aortic arch, and anchored in position by an atraumatic stabilizer in the ostium of the innominate artery. It covers all three major cerebral arteries in the aortic arch (innominate, left common carotid, and subclavian) while preserving blood flow to the cerebral vessels through 250 μm pores.

The safety and the performance of the device was first assessed in the DEFLECT I trial, a prospective, multicenter, single-arm study including 37 patients. Successful cerebral coverage was achieved in 80% of cases. The primary safety endpoint (inhospital device- or procedure-related cardiovascular mortality, major stroke disability, life-threatening bleeding, distal embolization, major vascular complications, or need for acute cardiac surgery) occurred in 8.1% of subjects. Post-procedure DW-MRI was performed in 28 subjects and showed a total number of new cerebral ischemic lesions similar to historical controls. However, per-patient total lesion volume was 34% lower than reported historical data and 89% lower in patients with complete ($n = 17$) versus incomplete ($n = 10$) cerebral vessel coverage [56]. On this basis, the device obtained CE mark approval in October 2013.

The DEFLECT III trial was the first multi-center randomized controlled trial that assessed the performance of the TriGuard device in 85 subjects. Technical success was achieved in 88.9% of cases. The primary inhospital procedural safety endpoint (death, stroke, life-threatening or disabling bleeding, stage 2 or 3 acute kidney injury, or major vascular complications) occurred in 21.7% of TriGuard and 30.8% of control subjects ($p = 0.34$). The per-treatment population analysis (subjects with complete three-vessel cerebral coverage) showed a greater freedom from new ischemic brain lesions (26.9 vs. 11.5%), fewer new neurologic deficits detected by the National Institutes of Health Stroke Scale (3.1% vs. 15.4%), improved Montreal Cognitive Assessment (MoCA) scores, better performance on a delayed memory task ($p = 0.028$) at discharge, and a twofold increase in recovery of normal cognitive function at 30 days in protected patients [41].

The REFLECT trial (NCT02536196), powered for neurocognitive scores and cerebral ischemic lesions, has been halted after the introduction of the new-generation device TriGuard 3, featuring a threefold larger filter area in combination with smaller pores.

30.10 Combined Evidence

Data from four randomized trials ($n = 252$ patients) assessing the performance of EPDs in TAVI patients (CLEAN-TAVI, DEFLECT III, EMBOL-X, MISTRAL-C) were combined in a systematic review and meta-analysis with the aim to assess total lesion volume and number of new ischemic lesions (primary imaging efficacy endpoints) and any deterioration in National Institutes of Health Stroke Scale and Montreal Cognitive Assessment scores at hospital discharge (primary clinical efficacy endpoints). The use of EPDs was associated with lower total lesion volume (Montreal Cognitive Assessment (MoCA) SMD, 0.65; 95% CI 1.06 to 0.25; $p = 0.002$) and smaller number of new ischemic lesions (SMD 1.27; 95% CI 2.45 to 0.09; $p = 0.03$). In addition, a trend toward lower risk

for neurocognitive deterioration in National Institutes of Health Stroke Scale score at discharge (RR 0.55; 95% CI 0.27–1.09; $p = 0.09$) and higher Montreal Cognitive Assessment score (SMD 0.40; 95% CI 0.04–0.76; $p = 0.03$) was reported among patients with cerebral protection. Nevertheless, risk for overt stroke and all-cause mortality were not significantly lower in the EPD group [57]. An updated analysis, including data from the SENTINEL trial, showed an association between EPDs and lower risk of death or stroke on relative and absolute terms. Furthermore, results were consistent following stratification by type of EPD device used [58]. A larger meta-analysis, including also not randomized trials for a total of 16 studies and 1170 patients, found no difference in terms of clinically evident stroke (RR 0.70; 95% CI 0.38–1.29; $p = 0.26$) or 30-day mortality (RR 0.58; 95% CI 0.20–1.64; $p = 0.30$), whereas the use of EPD was associated with a significantly smaller ischemic volume per lesion and smaller total volume of lesion [59].

30.11 Conclusions

Current evidence on the performance of EPDs in the setting of TAVI can be summarized as follows:

- Particulate debris reaches cerebral circulation in almost all patients undergoing TAVI.
- The mere presence of debris is not associated with clinically relevant brain injury or cognitive dysfunction.
- Available studies were based on surrogate endpoints and were not powered for assessing major clinical outcomes.
- Some of the EPDs proved ability to reduce the number and the volume of new ischemic lesions; however their impact on clinically apparent adverse events remains unclear.
- Although technically feasible and safe, the use of EPDs in the context of TAVI requires further investigation and may only be recommended in routine clinical practice in case of strong evidence of cerebral protection from stroke emerging from randomized trials adequately powered for clinical endpoints.

References

1. Sabate M, Canovas S, Garcia E, Hernandez Antolin R, Maroto L, Hernandez JM, Alonso Briales JH, Munoz Garcia AJ, Gutierrez-Ibanes E, Rodriguez-Roda J, et al. In-hospital and mid-term predictors of mortality after transcatheter aortic valve implantation: data from the TAVI National Registry 2010–2011. Rev Esp Cardiol (Engl Ed). 2013;66(12):949–58.

2. Eggebrecht H, Schmermund A, Voigtlander T, Kahlert P, Erbel R, Mehta RH. Risk of stroke after transcatheter aortic valve implantation (TAVI): a meta-analysis of 10,037 published patients. EuroIntervention. 2012;8(1):129–38.

3. Smith CR, Leon MB, Mack MJ, Miller DC, Moses JW, Svensson LG, Tuzcu EM, Webb JG, Fontana GP, Makkar RR, et al. Transcatheter versus surgical aortic-valve replacement in high-risk patients. N Engl J Med. 2011;364(23):2187–98.

4. Bonow RO, Leon MB, Doshi D, Moat N. Management strategies and future challenges for aortic valve disease. Lancet. 2016;387(10025):1312–23.

5. Fanning JP, Walters DL, Platts DG, Eeles E, Bellapart J, Fraser JF. Characterization of neurological injury in transcatheter aortic valve implantation: how clear is the picture? Circulation. 2014;129(4):504–15.

6. Stortecky S, Windecker S. Stroke: an infrequent but devastating complication in cardiovascular interventions. Circulation. 2012;126(25):2921–4.

7. Nombela-Franco L, Webb JG, de Jaegere PP, Toggweiler S, Nuis RJ, Dager AE, Amat-Santos IJ, Cheung A, Ye J, Binder RK, et al. Timing, predictive factors, and prognostic value of cerebrovascular events in a large cohort of patients undergoing transcatheter aortic valve implantation. Circulation. 2012;126(25):3041–53.

8. Kapadia S, Agarwal S, Miller DC, Webb JG, Mack M, Ellis S, Herrmann HC, Pichard AD, Tuzcu EM, Svensson LG, et al. Insights into timing, risk factors, and outcomes of stroke and transient ischemic attack after Transcatheter aortic valve replacement in the PARTNER trial (placement of aortic Transcatheter valves). Circ Cardiovasc Interv. 2016;9(9)

9. Kleiman NS, Maini BJ, Reardon MJ, Conte J, Katz S, Rajagopal V, Kauten J, Hartman A, McKay R, Hagberg R, et al. Neurological events following transcatheter aortic valve replacement and their predictors: A report from the CoreValve trials. Circ Cardiovasc Interv. 2016;9(9).

10. Gallo M, Putzu A, Conti M, Pedrazzini G, Demertzis S, Ferrari E. Embolic protection devices for transcatheter aortic valve replacement. Eur J Cardiothorac Surg. 2017;

11. Makkar RR, Fontana GP, Jilaihawi H, Kapadia S, Pichard AD, Douglas PS, Thourani VH, Babaliaros VC, Webb JG, Herrmann HC, et al. Transcatheter aortic-valve replacement for inoperable severe aortic stenosis. N Engl J Med. 2012;366(18):1696–704.

12. Kapadia SR, Leon MB, Makkar RR, Tuzcu EM, Svensson LG, Kodali S, Webb JG, Mack MJ, Douglas PS, Thourani VH, et al. 5-year outcomes of transcatheter aortic valve replacement compared with standard treatment for patients with inoperable aortic stenosis (PARTNER 1): a randomised controlled trial. Lancet. 2015;385(9986):2485–91.

13. Mack MJ, Leon MB, Smith CR, Miller DC, Moses JW, Tuzcu EM, Webb JG, Douglas PS, Anderson WN, Blackstone EH, et al. 5-year outcomes of transcatheter aortic valve replacement or surgical aortic valve replacement for high surgical risk patients with aortic stenosis (PARTNER 1): a randomised controlled trial. Lancet. 2015;385(9986):2477–84.

14. Popma JJ, Adams DH, Reardon MJ, Yakubov SJ, Kleiman NS, Heimansohn D, Hermiller J, Jr., Hughes GC, Harrison JK, Coselli J et al: Transcatheter aortic valve replacement using a self-expanding bioprosthesis in patients with severe aortic stenosis at extreme risk for surgery. J Am Coll Cardiol 2014, 63(19):1972–1981.

15. Adams DH, Popma JJ, Reardon MJ, Yakubov SJ, Coselli JS, Deeb GM, Gleason TG, Buchbinder M, Hermiller J Jr, Kleiman NS, et al. Transcatheter aortic-valve replacement with a self-expanding prosthesis. N Engl J Med. 2014;370(19):1790–8.

16. Leon MB, Smith CR, Mack MJ, Makkar RR, Svensson LG, Kodali SK, Thourani VH, Tuzcu EM, Miller DC, Herrmann HC, et al. Transcatheter or surgical aortic-valve replacement in intermediate-risk patients. N Engl J Med. 2016;374(17):1609–20.

17. Reardon MJ, Van Mieghem NM, Popma JJ, Kleiman NS, Sondergaard L, Mumtaz M, Adams DH, Deeb GM, Maini B, Gada H, et al. Surgical or transcatheter aortic-valve replacement in intermediate-risk patients. N Engl J Med. 2017;376(14):1321–31.

18. Thyregod HG, Steinbruchel DA, Ihlemann N, Nissen H, Kjeldsen BJ, Petursson P, Chang Y, Franzen OW, Engstrom T, Clemmensen P, et al. Transcatheter versus surgical aortic valve replacement in patients with severe aortic valve stenosis: 1-year results from the all-comers NOTION randomized clinical trial. J Am Coll Cardiol. 2015;65(20):2184–94.

19. Siemieniuk RA, Agoritsas T, Manja V, Devji T, Chang Y, Bala MM, Thabane L, Guyatt GH. Transcatheter versus surgical aortic valve replacement in patients with severe aortic stenosis at low and intermediate risk: systematic review and meta-analysis. BMJ. 2016;354:i5130.

20. Siontis GC, Praz F, Pilgrim T, Mavridis D, Verma S, Salanti G, Sondergaard L, Juni P, Windecker S. Transcatheter aortic valve implantation vs. surgical aortic valve replacement for treatment of severe aortic stenosis: a meta-analysis of randomized trials. Eur Heart J. 2016;37(47):3503–12.

21. Duncan A, Ludman P, Banya W, Cunningham D, Marlee D, Davies S, Mullen M, Kovac J, Spyt T, Moat N. Long-term outcomes after transcatheter aortic valve replacement in high-risk patients with severe aortic stenosis: the UK Transcatheter Aortic

Valve Implantation Registry. JACC Cardiovasc Interv. 2015;8(5):645–53.

22. Grover FL, Vemulapalli S, Carroll JD, Edwards FH, Mack MJ, Thourani VH, Brindis RG, Shahian DM, Ruiz CE, Jacobs JP, et al. 2016 annual report of the Society of Thoracic Surgeons/American College of Cardiology transcatheter valve therapy registry. J Am Coll Cardiol. 2017;69(10):1215–30.

23. Carroll JD, Vemulapalli S, Dai D, Matsouaka R, Blackstone E, Edwards F, Masoudi FA, Mack M, Peterson ED, Holmes D, et al. Procedural experience for Transcatheter aortic valve replacement and relation to outcomes: The STS/ACC TVT Registry. J Am Coll Cardiol. 2017;70(1):29–41.

24. Van Mieghem NM, El Faquir N, Rahhab Z, Rodriguez-Olivares R, Wilschut J, Ouhlous M, Galema TW, Geleijnse ML, Kappetein AP, Schipper ME, et al. Incidence and predictors of debris embolizing to the brain during transcatheter aortic valve implantation. JACC Cardiovasc Interv. 2015;8(5):718–24.

25. Schmidt T, Akdag O, Wohlmuth P, Thielsen T, Schewel D, Schewel J, Alessandrini H, Kreidel F, Bader R, Romero M, et al. Histological findings and predictors of cerebral debris from transcatheter aortic valve replacement: the ALSTER experience. J Am Heart Assoc. 2016;5(11)

26. Mohler ER, 3rd, Gannon F, Reynolds C, Zimmerman R, Keane MG, Kaplan FS: Bone formation and inflammation in cardiac valves. Circulation 2001, 103(11):1522–1528.

27. Nombela-Franco L, Rodes-Cabau J, DeLarochelliere R, Larose E, Doyle D, Villeneuve J, Bergeron S, Bernier M, Amat-Santos IJ, Mok M, et al. Predictive factors, efficacy, and safety of balloon post-dilation after transcatheter aortic valve implantation with a balloon-expandable valve. JACC Cardiovasc Interv. 2012;5(5):499–512.

28. Auffret V, Regueiro A, Del Trigo M, Abdul-Jawad Altisent O, Campelo-Parada F, Chiche O, Puri R, Rodes-Cabau J. Predictors of early cerebrovascular events in patients with aortic stenosis undergoing Transcatheter aortic valve replacement. J Am Coll Cardiol. 2016;68(7):673–84.

29. Auffret V, Regueiro A, Campelo-Parada F, Del Trigo M, Chiche O, Chamandi C, Puri R, Rodes-Cabau J. Feasibility, safety, and efficacy of transcatheter aortic valve replacement without balloon predilation: a systematic review and meta-analysis. Catheter Cardiovasc Interv. 2017;90(5):839–50.

30. Erdoes G, Basciani R, Huber C, Stortecky S, Wenaweser P, Windecker S, Carrel T, Eberle B. Transcranial Doppler-detected cerebral embolic load during transcatheter aortic valve implantation. Eur J Cardiothorac Surg. 2012;41(4):778–83; discussion 783-774

31. Reinsfelt B, Westerlind A, Ioanes D, Zetterberg H, Freden-Lindqvist J, Ricksten SE. Transcranial Doppler microembolic signals and serum marker evidence of brain injury during transcatheter aortic valve implantation. Acta Anaesthesiol Scand. 2012;56(2):240–7.

32. Rodes-Cabau J, Dumont E, Boone RH, Larose E, Bagur R, Gurvitch R, Bedard F, Doyle D, De Larochelliere R, Jayasuria C, et al. Cerebral embolism following transcatheter aortic valve implantation: comparison of transfemoral and transapical approaches. J Am Coll Cardiol. 2011;57(1):18–28.

33. Ghanem A, Muller A, Nahle CP, Kocurek J, Werner N, Hammerstingl C, Schild HH, Schwab JO, Mellert F, Fimmers R, et al. Risk and fate of cerebral embolism after transfemoral aortic valve implantation: a prospective pilot study with diffusion-weighted magnetic resonance imaging. J Am Coll Cardiol. 2010;55(14):1427–32.

34. Arnold M, Schulz-Heise S, Achenbach S, Ott S, Dorfler A, Ropers D, Feyrer R, Einhaus F, Loders S, Mahmoud F, et al. Embolic cerebral insults after transapical aortic valve implantation detected by magnetic resonance imaging. JACC Cardiovasc Interv. 2010;3(11):1126–32.

35. Fairbairn TA, Mather AN, Bijsterveld P, Worthy G, Currie S, Goddard AJ, Blackman DJ, Plein S, Greenwood JP. Diffusion-weighted MRI determined cerebral embolic infarction following transcatheter aortic valve implantation: assessment of predictive risk factors and the relationship to subsequent health status. Heart. 2012;98(1):18–23.

36. Abdul-Jawad Altisent O, Ferreira-Gonzalez I, Marsal JR, Ribera A, Auger C, Ortega G, Cascant P, Urena M, Del Blanco BG, Serra V, et al. Neurological damage after transcatheter aortic valve implantation compared with surgical aortic valve replacement in intermediate risk patients. Clin Res Cardiol. 2016;105(6):508–17.

37. Amat-Santos IJ, Rodes-Cabau J, Urena M, DeLarochelliere R, Doyle D, Bagur R, Villeneuve J, Cote M, Nombela-Franco L, Philippon F, et al. Incidence, predictive factors, and prognostic value of new-onset atrial fibrillation following transcatheter aortic valve implantation. J Am Coll Cardiol. 2012;59(2):178–88.

38. Kappetein AP, Head SJ, Genereux P, Piazza N, van Mieghem NM, Blackstone EH, Brott TG, Cohen DJ, Cutlip DE, van Es GA, et al. Updated standardized endpoint definitions for transcatheter aortic valve implantation: the valve academic research Consortium-2 consensus document. J Am Coll Cardiol. 2012;60(15):1438–54.

39. Lansky AJ, Messe SR, Brickman AM, Dwyer M, van der Worp HB, Lazar RM, Pietras CG, Abrams KJ, McFadden E, Petersen NH, et al. Proposed standardized neurological endpoints for cardiovascular clinical trials: an academic research consortium initiative. J Am Coll Cardiol. 2017;69(6):679–91.

40. Kahlert P, Knipp SC, Schlamann M, Thielmann M, Al-Rashid F, Weber M, Johansson U, Wendt D, Jakob HG, Forsting M, et al. Silent and apparent cerebral ischemia after percutaneous transfemoral aortic valve implantation: a diffusion-weighted magnetic resonance imaging study. Circulation. 2010;121(7):870–8.

41. Lansky AJ, Schofer J, Tchetche D, Stella P, Pietras CG, Parise H, Abrams K, Forrest JK, Cleman M,

Reinohl J, et al. A prospective randomized evaluation of the TriGuard HDH embolic DEFLECTion device during transcatheter aortic valve implantation: results from the DEFLECT III trial. Eur Heart J. 2015;36(31):2070–8.

42. Lazar RM, Pavol MA, Bormann T, Dwyer MG, Kraemer C, White R, Zivadinov R, Wertheimer JC, Thone-Otto A, Ravdin LD, et al. Neurocognition and cerebral lesion burden in high-risk patients before undergoing transcatheter aortic valve replacement: insights from the SENTINEL trial. JACC Cardiovasc Interv. 2018;

43. Banbury MK, Kouchoukos NT, Allen KB, Slaughter MS, Weissman NJ, Berry GJ, Horvath KA. Investigators I: emboli capture using the Embol-X intraaortic filter in cardiac surgery: a multicentered randomized trial of 1,289 patients. Ann Thorac Surg. 2003;76(2):508–15; discussion 515.

44. Bolotin G, Huber CH, Shani L, Mohr FW, Carrel TP, Borger MA, Falk V, Taggart D, Nir RR, Englberger L, et al. Novel emboli protection system during cardiac surgery: a multi-center, randomized, clinical trial. Ann Thorac Surg. 2014;98(5):1627–33; discussion 1633-1624

45. Nietlispach F, Wijesinghe N, Gurvitch R, Tay E, Carpenter JP, Burns C, Wood DA, Webb JG. An embolic deflection device for aortic valve interventions. JACC Cardiovasc Interv. 2010;3(11):1133–8.

46. Naber CK, Ghanem A, Abizaid AA, Wolf A, Sinning JM, Werner N, Nickenig G, Schmitz T, Grube E. First-in-man use of a novel embolic protection device for patients undergoing transcatheter aortic valve implantation. EuroIntervention. 2012;8(1):43–50.

47. Van Mieghem NM, van Gils L, Ahmad H, van Kesteren F, van der Werf HW, Brueren G, Storm M, Lenzen M, Daemen J, van den Heuvel AF, et al. Filter-based cerebral embolic protection with transcatheter aortic valve implantation: the randomised MISTRAL-C trial. EuroIntervention. 2016;12(4):499–507.

48. Haussig S, Mangner N, Dwyer MG, Lehmkuhl L, Lucke C, Woitek F, Holzhey DM, Mohr FW, Gutberlet M, Zivadinov R, et al. Effect of a cerebral protection device on brain lesions following Transcatheter aortic valve implantation in patients with severe aortic stenosis: the CLEAN-TAVI randomized clinical trial. JAMA. 2016;316(6):592–601.

49. Kapadia SR, Kodali S, Makkar R, Mehran R, Lazar RM, Zivadinov R, Dwyer MG, Jilaihawi H, Virmani R, Anwaruddin S, et al. Protection against cerebral embolism during Transcatheter aortic valve replacement. J Am Coll Cardiol. 2017;69(4):367–77.

50. Latib A, Pagnesi M. Cerebral embolic protection during transcatheter aortic valve replacement: a disconnect between logic and data? J Am Coll Cardiol. 2017;69(4):378–80.

51. Samim M, Hendrikse J, van der Worp HB, Agostoni P, Nijhoff F, Doevendans PA, Stella PR. Silent ischemic brain lesions after transcatheter aortic valve replacement: lesion distribution and predictors. Clin Res Cardiol. 2015;104(5):430–8.

52. Van Gils L, Kroon H, Daemen J, Ren C, Maugenest AM, Schipper M, De Jaegere PP, Van Mieghem NM. Complete filter-based cerebral embolic protection with transcatheter aortic valve replacement. Catheter Cardiovasc Interv. 2017;

53. Seeger J, Gonska B, Otto M, Rottbauer W, Wohrle J. Cerebral embolic protection during transcatheter aortic valve replacement significantly reduces death and stroke compared with unprotected procedures. JACC Cardiovasc Interv. 2017;10(22):2297–303.

54. Wendt D, Kleinbongard P, Knipp S, Al-Rashid F, Gedik N, El Chilali K, Schweter S, Schlamann M, Kahlert P, Neuhauser M, et al. Intraaortic protection from embolization in patients undergoing transaortic transcatheter aortic valve implantation. Ann Thorac Surg. 2015;100(2):686–91.

55. Rodes-Cabau J, Kahlert P, Neumann FJ, Schymik G, Webb JG, Amarenco P, Brott T, Garami Z, Gerosa G, Lefevre T, et al. Feasibility and exploratory efficacy evaluation of the embrella embolic deflector system for the prevention of cerebral emboli in patients undergoing transcatheter aortic valve replacement: the PROTAVI-C pilot study. JACC Cardiovasc Interv. 2014;7(10):1146–55.

56. Baumbach A, Mullen M, Brickman AM, Aggarwal SK, Pietras CG, Forrest JK, Hildick-Smith D, Meller SM, Gambone L, den Heijer P, et al. Safety and performance of a novel embolic deflection device in patients undergoing transcatheter aortic valve replacement: results from the DEFLECT I study. EuroIntervention. 2015;11(1):75–84.

57. Giustino G, Mehran R, Veltkamp R, Faggioni M, Baber U, Dangas GD. Neurological outcomes with embolic protection devices in patients undergoing Transcatheter aortic valve replacement: a systematic review and meta-analysis of randomized controlled trials. JACC Cardiovasc Interv. 2016;9(20):2124–33.

58. Giustino G, Sorrentino S, Mehran R, Faggioni M, Dangas G. Cerebral embolic protection during TAVR: a clinical event meta-analysis. J Am Coll Cardiol. 2017;69(4):465–6.

59. Bagur R, Solo K, Alghofaili S, Nombela-Franco L, Kwok CS, Hayman S, Siemieniuk RA, Foroutan F, Spencer FA, Vandvik PO, et al. Cerebral embolic protection devices during Transcatheter aortic valve implantation: systematic review and meta-analysis. Stroke. 2017;48(5):1306–15.

Antithrombotic Therapy During and After Transcatheter Aortic Valve Implantation

31

Gennaro Sardella, Simone Calcagno, Nicolò Salvi, and Massimo Mancone

31.1 Introduction

Transcatheter aortic valve implantation (TAVI), also called transcatheter aortic valve replacement (TAVR), has become the therapy of choice for patients with severe aortic stenosis (AS) who are deemed to be inoperable or at high/intermediate risk for conventional surgical aortic valve replacement (SAVR). The number of TAVI procedures is increasing exponentially as it has been demonstrated to be a live-saving procedure. The TAVI population is frail and bears a high risk of both ischaemic stroke and major bleeds that is much higher than in conventional bioprosthetic aortic valve replacement. Importantly, the thrombotic risk also extends during follow-up, particularly in the presence of atrial fibrillation (AF). The 30-day rate of major bleeding and stroke exceeds 15% in this population, increasing the risk of mortality. Guidelines on antithrombotic therapy after TAVI are scarce, and no randomised evaluation has been performed to demonstrate what is the best strategy.

G. Sardella (✉) · S. Calcagno · N. Salvi
M. Mancone
Department of Cardiovascular, Respiratory, Nephrology, Anesthesiology and Geriatric Sciences, Umberto I Hospital, Sapienza University of Rome, Rome, Italy
e-mail: rino.sardella@uniroma1.it

31.2 Pathophysiology

The risk of stroke is highest in the periprocedural period owing to the mechanics of valve positioning and implantation [1]. Indeed, stenotic aortic valves, unlike normal aortic valve leaflets, are characterised by large amounts of tissue factor and thrombin that increase inflammation and thrombogenicity. Unlike SAVR, the diseased native valve remains in situ during (and after) TAVI and may be mechanically damaged, leading to the exposure and/or embolism of valvular components into the arterial circulation. Additionally, insertion of a prosthesis without removal of the diseased aortic valve creates an irregular zone around the valve frame with modified flow patterns that may predispose to thrombus formation, particularly in the case of small valve sizes with associated patient-prosthesis mismatch. It has been demonstrated that cerebral embolism associated with TAVI can be composed of thrombotic or calcific atherosclerotic material. It remains unclear whether the stroke potential of these two subtypes of embolic material is alike. Importantly, TAVI patients remain at risk of stroke throughout the first months after the procedure. In these patients, mechanisms other than valve manipulation seem to be involved, such as aortic wall injury, post-traumatic surface exposure with consequent activation of the haemostatic system, turbulence, or local blood stasis. In addition to the prothrombotic environment

© Springer Nature Switzerland AG 2019
A. Giordano et al. (eds.), *Transcatheter Aortic Valve Implantation*,
https://doi.org/10.1007/978-3-030-05912-5_31

related to valve implantation and procedure-related aortic damage, roughly one third of TAVI patients have pre-existing AF, and a further variable percentage (ranging from 1% to 30%) experience new-onset post-procedural AF, which is known to increase the risk of thrombotic complications further [2].

31.3 The Choice of Antithrombotic Therapy

Establishing the optimal antithrombotic therapy for TAVI patients remains a challenge, largely due to the lack of properly powered studies to inform practice. Unfractionated heparin (UFH) is the most common method of anticoagulation during the procedure. In the PARTNER [3] study, UFH was administered as a parenteral bolus of 5000 IU followed by additional doses to achieve an activated clotting time (ACT) ≥250 s. A subsequent American consensus document recommended a target ACT ≥300 s with reversal of UFH following the procedure with protamine sulphate at a milligram-to-milligram neutralisation dose [4]. Although the purpose of giving protamine at the end of the procedure is to reduce bleeding related to access closure, a prothrombotic effect of the protamine leading to an increase in cerebrovascular events (CVEs) cannot be excluded [5]. Therefore, the safety of reversing heparin effects after TAVI warrants further investigation.

The procedural bleeding may be decreased by using alternative parenteral anticoagulants, such as bivalirudin, an intravenous direct thrombin inhibitor, which has already shown to reduce the rate of bleeding during PCI [6]. Although bivalirudin might prove to be useful in the high bleeding risk population referred to TAVI, its role instead of UFH remains unclear. The multicentre open-label study BRAVO 3 [7] randomised 802 patients with AS to undergo TAVI with bivalirudin vs. UFH during the procedure. The results did not show a superiority role of bivalirudin to reduce rates of major bleeding at 48 h or net adverse cardiovascular events (all-cause mortality, myocardial infarction, stroke, and major bleeding) within 30 days compared with heparin. Although superiority was not shown, the noninferiority hypothesis was met with respect to the latter factor. Given the lower cost, heparin should remain the standard of care, and bivalirudin can be an alternative anticoagulant option in patients unable to receive heparin in TAVR. Moreover life-threatening vascular and bleeding complications occurring during the procedure, such as cardiac tamponade, aortic annulus rupture, or peripheral vascular rupture, often require immediate reversal of anticoagulation, which is not possible with bivalirudin, despite the rapid half-life of the drug.

Even more uncertain are the data about the optimal antithrombotic therapy after TAVI. Adequately studies addressing this topic are not designed. It may be reasonable to consider that TAVI patients may benefit from similar antithrombotic treatment as currently used after SAVR with a biological prosthesis. However, it is relevant to underline that percutaneous valves have leaflets composed of biological material and a metallic frame similar to vascular/coronary stents. Moreover, there are not strong evidences to identify the ideal antithrombotic therapy after SAVR with biological prostheses, and the international guidelines do not give the same indications. Indeed the European guidelines support use of aspirin (IIa recommendation) or vitamin K antagonists (VKA, IIb recommendation) for 3 months after SAVR [8]; AHA/ACC guidelines recommend long-term low-dose aspirin (IIa recommendation; level of evidence [LOE] B), while VKA are considered only for the first 3 months (IIb recommendation, LOE C) [9]; and ACCP guidelines support low-dose aspirin over VKA (Grade 2C) [10]. Therefore, some but not all guidelines recommend VKA in the first 3–6 months after SAVR, whereas aspirin may be a preferred long-term treatment.

31.4 The Choice of Antiplatelet Therapy

In TAVI patients, secondary prevention regimes based on antiplatelet therapy have been the most widely studied. Considering the increased thrombotic risks related to the valve structure, dual antiplatelet therapy (DAPT) with aspirin and clopidogrel, in the absence of an indication for anticoagulation treatment, is a commonly accepted strategy which has been incorporated into practice guidelines (Table 31.1).

However, the use of a loading dose of clopidogrel (300–600 mg) before TAVI is usually not specified, and the duration of clopidogrel therapy has varied widely across studies (usually 1–6 months). The ACCF/AATS/SCAI/STS panel recommends DAPT with aspirin and clopidogrel after TAVI to reduce the risk of thrombotic or thromboembolic events, but its duration and the use of a loading dose of clopidogrel are not specified [4]. A Canadian Cardiovascular Society statement on TAVI recommends the use of aspirin indefinitely and clopidogrel for 1–3 months [11]. The principal recommendations for antithrombotic treatment in the setting of TAVI are summarised in Table 31.1.

DAPT play a key role also for the many TAVI patients undergoing coronary stenting. The recommendation to add clopidogrel (75 mg/day) to low-dose aspirin for 1–6 months following TAVI is empirical, and no studies to date have clearly demonstrated the efficacy of this strategy. Moreover, the benefits of DAPT have been questioned, and recent observations showed that DAPT does not seem to improve the safety and this may trigger a paradigm shift in the choice of optimal antithrombotic therapy after TAVI. Pooled analysis of individual patient data from 672 participants comparing aspirin alone vs. DAPT after TAVI showed no difference in the rate of 30-day net adverse clinical and cerebral events, but a trend towards less life-threatening and major bleeding was observed in favour of aspirin alone [12].

It should be considered that only four studies based on small numbers of patients and events are available and in only two of them was treatment randomly allocated. In the first randomised trial comparing DAPT vs. aspirin alone following TAVI by Ussia et al., aspirin was recommended indefinitely (100 mg) in all patients and clopidogrel for 3 months (75 mg daily) in the clopidogrel arm [13]. In the Single Antiplatelet Therapy for TAVI (SAT-TAVI) trial, aspirin was recommended indefinitely (75–160 mg) in all patients and clopidogrel for 6 months (75 mg daily) in the clopidogrel arm [14]. Bleeding at 30 days was

Table 31.1 Recommendations for antithrombotic therapy in TAVI patients

	Aspirin	Additional Antiplatelet therapy	Oral anticoagulation
European guideline and consensus	Low-dose lifelong	Thienopyridine early after TAVI	VKA alone in patients with AF but no CAD (VKA + antiplatelet therapy if AF and recent stent implantation, as per CAD guidelines)
AHA/ACC guidelines	Low-dose (75–100 mg/day) indefinitely	Clopidogrel 75 mg/day for 6 months	
ACCF/AATS/SCAI/STS consensus	Low-dose indefinitely	Clopidogrel 75 mg/day for 3–6 months	VKA if indicated (no clopidogrel)
Canadian society position statement	Low-dose indefinitely	Clopidogrel 75 mg/day for 1–3 months	VKA if indicated (avoid triple therapy unless definite indication)

AF atrial fibrillation, *CAD* coronary artery disease, *TAVI* transcatheter aortic valve implantation, *VKA* vitamin K antagonist

not different for aspirin vs. DAPT in the trial by Ussia et al. (18% vs. 18%) and in the SAT-TAVI trial (10% vs. 15%). Also, in both trials were not found any differences in 30-day mortality, MI, and stroke. Aspirin monotherapy was superior on DAPT in the SAT-TAVI trial, showing a lower rate of vascular access site-related complications (VASC) (5% vs. 13%, $p < 0.05$) [14].

Poliacikova et al. retrospectively compared in a single centre, aspirin monotherapy ($N = 91$) with DAPT ($N = 58$) with clopidogrel administration for 6 months after TAVI [15]. The bleeding rate at 30 days trended higher for DAPT vs. aspirin (19.0% vs. 8.8%, $P = 0.069$) and was not found differences in mortality and thrombotic events. The composite of all-cause mortality, acute coronary event, stroke, and major bleeding was higher for DAPT than in aspirin (27.6% vs. 12.1%). Durand et al. prospectively compared DAPT ($N = 128$) and monotherapy ($N = 164$) after TAVI in patients enrolled in the FRANCE 2 registry in three centres [16]. Mortality rates and thromboembolic events were not different between groups. Aspirin alone had a lower rate of major and minor vascular complications (10% vs. 6% and 9% vs. 2%, respectively) and major and life-threatening bleeds (13% vs. 2% and 13% vs. 4%, respectively). Also the number of patients receiving blood transfusions was higher in the DAPT vs. aspirin group (25% vs. 7%).

Overall, these data are informative but not conclusive on the best antiplatelet strategy after TAVI. A prospective randomised controlled study, the ARTE trial [17], was prematurely stopped after the inclusion of 74% of the planned study population and was recently published. This compared DAPT (aspirin 80–100 mg/day plus clopidogrel 75 mg/day) vs. aspirin alone (single-antiplatelet therapy [SAPT]) in patients undergoing TAVR with a balloon-expandable valve. The primary endpoint was the occurrence of death, myocardial infarction (MI), stroke or transient ischaemic attack, or major or life-threatening bleeding within the 3 months following the procedure. A total of 222 patients were included, 111 allocated to DAPT and 111 to SAPT. The composite endpoint tended to occur more frequently in the DAPT group (15.3% vs.

7.2%, $p = 0.065$), while there were no differences between groups in the occurrence of death, MI, or stroke or transient ischaemic attack at 3 months. DAPT was associated with a higher rate of major or life-threatening bleeding events (10.8% vs. 3.6% in the SAPT group, $p = 0.038$). Also these data are not decisive to address the best antiplatelet strategies after TAVI procedure but showed that monotherapy tended to reduce the occurrence of major adverse events in particular reducing the risk for major or life-threatening events.

Additionally it should be considered [1] the high on-treatment platelet reactivity phenomenon, associated with clopidogrel or aspirin that can also occur in TAVI patients [18, 19], although its clinical correlations remain unclear, and [2] the impact of old vs. newer percutaneous valve technologies that remains elusive, introducing new characteristics and material could reduce the frequency of paravalvular leak and the potentially consequent thrombogenicity.

31.5 Anticoagulation Therapy After TAVI

Whether thrombi produced during and after TAVI have a platelet- or thrombin-based origin remains uncertain. Hence, antiplatelet-based strategies alone may still be suboptimal. Moreover, the need for oral anticoagulant (OAC) is also supported by the high burden of pre-existing and new-onset atrial fibrillation (AF) in TAVI patients, particularly since the large majority of these patients have a high CHA2DS2-VASc score. OAC in this context has great relevance in thrombosis prevention because new-onset and recurrent paroxysmal AF may be silent, clinically unrecognised and high risk unless specifically investigated [10].

Risk stratification is very relevant to guide the choice of antithrombotic therapy following a TAVI procedure. The CHA2DS2-VASc score has a key step in this elderly population. This approach to risk stratification of patients with non-valvular AF defines "major (definitive)" risk factors (e.g. previous stroke/transient ischaemic attack and age ≥75 years) and "clinically relevant nonmajor" risk factors (e.g. heart failure, hypertension, diabetes, female gender, age 65–74 years, and atherosclerotic vascular disease) [20]. It has the ability to identify AF patients with no net clinical benefit or even some disadvantage from anticoagulant treatment [21] but also to identify non-AF patients with a prior history of stroke and at very high risk of further cardiovascular events [22]. Of importance, this score was found to be associated with 1-year mortality in TAVI patients. Although the vast majority of TAVI patients with AF are eligible for chronic OAC given an average CHA2DS2-VASc score ≥4, whether non-AF patients with a CHA2DS2-VASc score ≥2 would benefit from chronic OAC is challenging.

Transcatheter valve thrombosis is rare but dangerous and may result in elevated transvalvular gradients requiring OAC. A finding of reduced leaflet motion on CT in a patient who had had a stroke after TAVR and similar findings in an asymptomatic patient at one clinical site led to closer scrutiny of this observation. Additional CT review by the core laboratory revealed that this finding was not isolated, which prompted a more extensive investigation that involved analysis of all available CT and echocardiographic data. A recent study reviewed a total of 18 published cases (SAPIEN = 17, CoreValve = 1) and reported 4 new cases (SAPIEN = 1, CoreValve = 3) [23], while a larger multicentre retrospective study analysed 4266 patients, reporting 26 cases of transcatheter valve thrombosis (mean follow-up 6 months; SAPIEN = 20, CoreValve = 6) [24]. Clinical presentation was principally with dyspnoea and increased gradients, and anticoagulation therapy was effective in reducing gradients in the majority of patients within 2 months of treatment. The frequency of transcatheter valve thrombosis may be underestimated, however, since clinical signs and symptoms can be masked by comorbidities, and early follow-up echocardiography is not uniformly performed. Nonetheless, pannus formation or thrombosis should be suspected in patients with sudden elevation in valve gradient, prompting further investigation and therapy with OAC plus single-antiplatelet therapy (SAPT) or DAPT. In case of failure, valve-in-valve TAVI or SAVR could be considered.

These events also led to the establishment of three ongoing studies to evaluate bioprosthetic leaflet function after TAVI or surgical aortic valve replacement: PORTICO IDE trial, the RESOLVE registry, and the SAVORY registry. Makkar et al. reported the findings of these investigations [25] evaluating the prevalence of reduced leaflet motion in bioprosthetic aortic valves, as assessed on four-dimensional, volume-rendered CT, the association between reduced leaflet motion and clinical event (strokes and transient ischaemic attacks), and the influence of anticoagulation on reduced leaflet motion. The data indicated that reduced leaflet motion was noted on CT in 22 of 55 patients (40%) in the clinical trial and in 17 of 132 patients (13%) in the two registries. Therapeutic anticoagulation with warfarin, as compared with DAPT, was associated with a significant decreased incidence of reduced leaflet motion. In patients who were reevaluated with follow-up CT, restoration of leaflet motion was noted in all 11 patients who were receiving anticoagulation and in 1 of 10 patients who were not receiving anticoagulation ($P < 0.001$). There was no significant difference in the incidence of stroke or TIA between patients with reduced leaflet motion and those with normal leaflet motion in the clinical trial, although in the pooled registries, a significant difference was detected. Even if a reduced aortic valve leaflet motion was shown in patients with bioprosthetic aortic valves and this condition resolved with therapeutic anticoagulation, the effect of this finding on clinical outcomes including stroke needs further investigation.

Neumann et al. published the results of systematic computed tomography (CT) 5 days after TAVI (SAPIEN 3 prosthesis), demonstrating valve leaflet thickening in 16/156 patients [26] without clinical events. At the CT follow-up (approximately after 2 months), 11 patients with OAC therapy (INR 2.5–3.5) showed a regression of these findings. Sondergaard et al. presented data concerning valve leaflet motion assessed with CT about 3 months after TAVI ($n = 47$) or SAVR ($n = 15$), demonstrating that the incidence of reduced leaflet motion was similar with different types of valve and that the phenomenon did not worsen the outcomes [27]. The data shown above suggest that therapeutic anticoagulation with warfarin, but not therapy with antiplatelet drugs, prevented and effectively treated the reduced aortic valve leaflet motion and the possible leaflet thrombosis in bioprosthetic aortic valves. Considering that these preliminary data need to confirm with dedicated trials, they may open new perspectives on the management of TAVI patients with the use of OAC after TAVI, even in the absence of specific indications (AF, mechanic valves). Conversely, the necessity of this approach remains the subject of discussion since all patients were asymptomatic and no clinical events were reported or prevented.

31.6 Patients with Atrial Fibrillation

In patients with atrial fibrillation (AF) undergoing TAVI to date, only few data have been published about the best antithrombotic treatment and its long prescription. The American and Canadian guidelines dissuade the administration of triple therapy with OAC plus aspirin and clopidogrel. In patient with AF and concomitant coronary atherosclerosis treated with stent implantation, the combination of OAC plus a single-antiplatelet agent, comparing with triple therapy, demonstrated the best safety profile in terms of lower rate of bleeding events without an increase of ischaemic ones [28, 29]. However, a recent European consensus about patient with FA and undergoing TAVI recommends to prefer the single therapy with warfarin instead of adding an antiplatelet agent, if there is not a concomitant coronary disease. Indeed this double therapy could be adding a higher haemorrhage risk with a doubt ischaemic benefit. On the contrary in patient with AF who received a coronary stent and undergoing TAVI was recommended the same strategy of care for patients treated for coronary stenosis, because actually no specific data were available in this setting of patients [30].

31.7 Upcoming Studies

In the field of TAVI, the POPular-TAVI trial [31] test in a total of 1000 patients, the hypothesis that monotherapy with aspirin or OAC after TAVI is safer than the addition of clopidogrel for 3 months, without compromising clinical benefit. This trial encompasses two cohorts: cohort A, patients are randomised to aspirin vs. aspirin + clopidogrel, and cohort B, patients on OAC therapy are randomised to OAC vs. OAC + clopidogrel. Primary outcome is freedom from non-procedure-related bleeding at 1 year. Secondary net clinical benefit outcome is freedom from the composite of cardiovascular death, non-procedural-related bleeding, myocardial infarction, or stroke at 1 year. Conversely, more insights into the appropriate use of non-vitamin K antagonist oral anticoagulants (NOACs) will come from the ongoing ATLANTIS trial and GALILEO trial. In the first one, the authors compare standard of care (SOC Group) vs. an apixaban-based strategy (anti-Xa group) after successful TAVI [32]. Randomization is stratified according to the need for chronic anticoagulation therapy for a reason other than the TAVI procedure. In the experimental arm, patients receive 5 mg bid of apixaban or a reduced dose of 2.5 mg bid according to the drug label or when apixaban is combined with antiplatelet therapy. In the control arm, patients receive VKA therapy if there is an indication for oral anticoagulation or antiplatelet therapy alone (single or dual) or the combination of both if needed. In GALILEO trial [33] conduct in more than 1520 patients without an indication for oral anticoagulation who underwent a successful TAVI. Patients are randomised, to either a rivaroxaban-based strategy or an antiplatelet-based strategy. In the experimental arm, subjects receive rivaroxaban (10 mg once daily) plus acetylsalicylic acid (ASA, 75–100 mg once daily) for 90 days followed by rivaroxaban

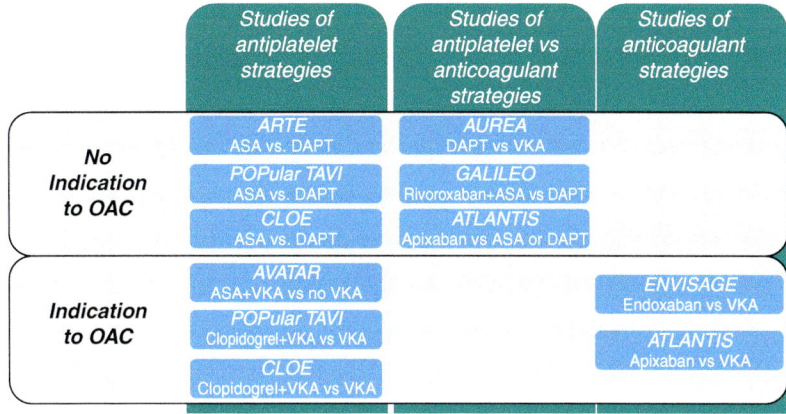

Fig. 31.1 Ongoing randomised trials on direct oral anticoagulant in TAVI patients

alone. In the control arm, subjects receive clopidogrel (75 mg once daily) plus ASA (as above) for 90 days followed by ASA alone.

Another study is ENVISAGE trial that uses edoxaban in patients with AF and indication to chronic OAC after transcatheter aortic valve implantation. The authors investigate the effect of edoxaban vs. vitamin K antagonist on net adverse clinical events (the composite of all-cause death, myocardial infarction, ischaemic stroke, systemic thromboembolism, valve thrombosis, and major bleeding). The above ongoing studies are reported in Fig. 31.1.

31.8 Conclusions

Despite improving practice and techniques, ischaemic and bleeding complications after TAVI remain prevalent and impair survival. Due to changing aetiology of complications over time, antithrombotic therapy after TAVI remains unclear. The justification for currently recommended regimes of DAPT after TAVI has recently been questioned, while arguments supporting the potential benefits of OAC therapy have now emerged. New anticoagulant therapies are promising and should be compared to the standard of care, including vitamin K antagonists. To support these recommendations, well-designed and appropriately powered trials are strongly warranted. Currently, randomised controlled trials are recruiting to gather more knowledge about the effects of clopidogrel after TAVI.

References

1. Rodés-Cabau J, Dauerman HL, Cohen MG, Mehran R, Small EM, Smyth SS, Costa MA, Mega JL, O'Donoghue ML, Ohman EM, Becker RC. Antithrombotic treatment in transcatheter aortic valve implantation: insights for cerebrovascular and bleeding events. J Am Coll Cardiol. 2013;62:2349–59.
2. Amat-Santos IJ, Rodés-Cabau J, Urena M, DeLarochellière R, Doyle D, Bagur R, et al. Incidence, predictive factors, and prognostic value of new-onset atrial fibrillation following transcatheter aortic valve implantation. J Am Coll Cardiol. 2012;59(2):178–88.
3. Leon MB, Smith CR, Mack M, Miller DC, Moses JW, Svensson LG, et al. Transcatheter aortic-valve implantation for aortic stenosis in patients who cannot undergo surgery. N Engl J Med. 2010;363(17):1597–607.
4. Holmes DR, Mack MJ, Kaul S, Agnihotri A, Alexander KP, Bailey SR, et al. ACCF/AATS/SCAI/STS expert consensus document on transcatheter aortic valve replacement. J Am Coll Cardiol. 2012;59(13):1200–54.
5. Levison JA, Faust GR, Halpern VJ, Theodoris A, Nathan I, Kline RG, et al. Relationship of protamine dosing with postoperative complications of carotid endarterectomy. Ann Vasc Surg. 1999;13(1):67–72.
6. Thompson KA, Philip KJ, Schwarz ER. Clinical applications of bivalirudin in the cardiac catheterization laboratory. J Cardiovasc Pharmacol Ther. 2011;16(2):140–9.

7. Dangas GD, Lefèvre T, Kupatt C, Tchetche D, Schäfer U, Dumonteil N, et al. Bivalirudin versus heparin anticoagulation in transcatheter aortic valve replacement: the randomized BRAVO-3 trial. J Am Coll Cardiol. 2015;66(25):2860–8.

8. Baumgartner H, Falk V, Bax JJ, De Bonis M, Hamm C, Holm PJ, et al. ESC/EACTS guidelines for the management of valvular heart disease. Eur Heart J. 2017;38(36):2739–91.

9. Nishimura RA, Otto CM, Bonow RO, Carabello BA, Erwin JP, Fleisher LA, et al. 2017 AHA/ACC focused update of the 2014 AHA/ACC guideline for the management of patients with valvular heart disease. J Am Coll Cardiol. 2017;70(2):252–89.

10. Whitlock RP, Sun JC, Fremes SE, Rubens FD, Teoh KH. Antithrombotic and thrombolytic therapy for valvular disease. Chest. 2012;141(2):e576S–600S.

11. Webb J, Rodés-Cabau J, Fremes S, Pibarot P, Ruel M, Ibrahim R, et al. Transcatheter aortic valve implantation: a Canadian cardiovascular society position statement. Can J Cardiol. 2012;28(5):520–8.

12. Hassell MECJ, Hildick-Smith D, Durand E, Kikkert WJ, Wiegerinck EMA, Stabile E, et al. Antiplatelet therapy following transcatheter aortic valve implantation. Heart. 2015;101(14):1118–25.

13. Ussia GP, Scarabelli M, Mulè M, Barbanti M, Sarkar K, Cammalleri V, et al. Dual antiplatelet therapy versus aspirin alone in patients undergoing transcatheter aortic valve implantation. Am J Cardiol. 2011;108(12):1772–6.

14. Stabile E, Pucciarelli A, Cota L, Sorropago G, Tesorio T, Salemme L, et al. SAT-TAVI (single antiplatelet therapy for TAVI) study: a pilot randomized study comparing double to single antiplatelet therapy for transcatheter aortic valve implantation. Int J Cardiol. 2014;174(3):624–7.

15. Poliacikova P, Cockburn J, de Belder A, Trivedi U, Hildick-Smith D. Antiplatelet and antithrombotic treatment after transcatheter aortic valve implantation—comparison of regimes. J Invasive Cardiol. 2013;25(10):544–8.

16. Durand E, Blanchard D, Chassaing S, Gilard M, Laskar M, Borz B, et al. Comparison of two antiplatelet therapy strategies in patients undergoing transcatheter aortic valve implantation. Am J Cardiol. 2014;113(2):355–60.

17. Rodés-Cabau J, Masson J-B, Welsh RC, Garcia Del Blanco B, Pelletier M, Webb JG, et al. Aspirin versus aspirin plus clopidogrel as antithrombotic treatment following transcatheter aortic valve replacement with a balloon-expandable valve: the ARTE (aspirin versus aspirin + clopidogrel following transcatheter aortic valve implantation) randomized clinical trial. JACC Cardiovasc Interv. 2017;10(13):1357–65.

18. Sardella G, Calcagno S, Mancone M, Lucisano L, Pennacchi M, Stio RE, et al. Comparison of therapy with Ticagrelor, Prasugrel or high Clopidogrel dose in PCI patients with high on treatment platelet reactivity and genotype variation. TRIPLETE RESET trial. Int J Cardiol. 2015;194:60–2.

19. Sardella G, Calcagno S, Mancone M, Palmirotta R, Lucisano L, Canali E, et al. Pharmacodynamic effect of switching therapy in patients with high on-treatment platelet reactivity and genotype variation with high clopidogrel dose versus prasugrel: the RESET GENE trial. Circ Cardiovasc Interv. 2012;5(5):698–704.

20. Lip GYH, Halperin JL. Improving stroke risk stratification in atrial fibrillation. Am J Med. 2010;123(6):484–8.

21. Friberg L, Rosenqvist M, Lip GYH. Net clinical benefit of warfarin in patients with atrial fibrillation: a report from the Swedish atrial fibrillation cohort study. Circulation. 2012;125(19):2298–307.

22. Ntaios G, Lip GYH, Makaritsis K, Papavasileiou V, Vemmou A, Koroboki E, et al. CHADS$_2$, CHA$_2$S$_2$DS$_2$-VASc, and long-term stroke outcome in patients without atrial fibrillation. Neurology. 2013;80(11):1009–17.

23. De Marchena E, Mesa J, Pomenti S, Marin Y, Kall C, Marincic X, Yahagi K, et al. Thrombus formation following transcatheter aortic valve replacement. JACC Cardiovasc Interv. 2015;8(5):728–39.

24. Latib A, Naganuma T, Abdel-Wahab M, Danenberg H, Cota L, Barbanti M, et al. Treatment and clinical outcomes of transcatheter heart valve thrombosis. Circ Cardiovasc Interv. 2015;8(4):e001779.

25. Makkar RR, Fontana G, Jilaihawi H, Chakravarty T, Kofoed KF, De Backer O, et al. Possible subclinical leaflet thrombosis in bioprosthetic aortic valves. N Engl J Med. 2015;373(21):2015–24.

26. Ruile P, Neumann F-J. Valve thrombosis after TAVI. Eur Heart J. 2017;38(36):2700–1.

27. Sondergaard L, Sigitas C, Chopra M, Bieliauskas G, De Backer O. Leaflet thrombosis after TAVI. Eur Heart J. 2017;38(36):2702–3.

28. Camm AJ, Lip GYH, De Caterina R, Savelieva I, Atar D, Hohnloser SH, et al. 2012 focused update of the ESC guidelines for the management of atrial fibrillation: an update of the 2010 ESC guidelines for the management of atrial fibrillation. Developed with the special contribution of the European heart rhythm association. Eur Heart J. 2012;33(21):2719–47.

29. Lip GYH, Windecker S, Huber K, Kirchhof P, Marin F, Ten Berg JM, et al. Management of antithrombotic therapy in atrial fibrillation patients presenting with acute coronary syndrome and/or undergoing percutaneous coronary or valve interventions: a joint consensus document of the European Society of Cardiology Working Group on thrombosis, European heart rhythm association (EHRA), European Association of Percutaneous Cardiovascular Interventions (EAPCI) and European Association of Acute Cardiac Care (ACCA) endorsed by the Heart Rhythm Society (HRS) and Asia-Pacific Heart Rhythm Society (APHRS). Eur Heart J. 2014;35(45):3155–79.

30. Capodanno D, Lip GYH, Windecker S, Huber K, Kirchhof P, Boriani G, et al. Triple antithrombotic therapy in atrial fibrillation patients with acute coronary syndromes or undergoing percutaneous coronary intervention or transcatheter aortic valve replacement. EuroIntervention. 2015;10(9):1015–21.

31. Nijenhuis VJ, Bennaghmouch N, Hassell M, Baan J, van Kuijk JP, Agostoni P, et al. Rationale and design of popular-TAVI: antiPlatelet therapy for patients undergoing transcatheter aortic valve implantation. Am Heart J. 2016;173:77–85.

32. Collet J-P, Berti S, Cequier A, Van Belle E, Lefevre T, Leprince P, et al. Oral anti-Xa anticoagulation after trans-aortic valve implantation for aortic stenosis: the randomized ATLANTIS trial. Am Heart J. 2018;200:44–50.

33. Windecker S, Tijssen J, Giustino G, Guimarães AHC, Mehran R, Valgimigli M, et al. Trial design: rivaroxaban for the prevention of major cardiovascular events after transcatheter aortic valve replacement: rationale and design of the GALILEO study. Am Heart J. 2017;184:81–7.

Contrast-Induced Acute Kidney Injury in Transcatheter Aortic Valve Implantation: Risk, Outcomes, Treatment, and Prevention

32

Andrew M. Goldsweig and J. Dawn Abbott

32.1 Introduction

Contrast-induced acute kidney injury (CIAKI) is a frequent and serious complication of transcatheter aortic valve implantation, also called transcatheter aortic valve replacement (TAVR). Acute kidney injury (AKI) has been variably defined in the literature, but in the field of structural heart disease, the most widely accepted contemporary definition comes from the Valve Academic Research Consortium-2 (VARC-2) and Acute Kidney Injury Network (AKIN) [1, 2] (Table 32.1), which defines three stages of AKI based upon serum creatinine and urine output. An important 2015 meta-analysis reported that CIAKI complicates on the order of 20% of TAVR procedures with hemodialysis required in up to 10% of CIAKI cases [3].

Table 32.1 Valve Academic Research Consortium-2 (VARC-2) Criteria [1] for CIAKI from Acute Kidney Injury Network (AKIN) [2]

Stage 1
Increase in serum creatinine to 150–199% (1.5–1.99 × increase compared with baseline) *or* increase of >0.3 mg/dL (>26.4 mmol/L) within 48 h of contrast *or*
Urine output <0.5 mL/kg/h for >6 but <12 h
Stage 2
Increase in serum creatinine to 200–299% (2.0–2.99 × increase compared with baseline) within 48 h of contrast *or*
Urine output <0.5 mL/kg/h for >12 but <24 h
Stage 3
Increase in serum creatinine to >300% (>3 × increase compared with baseline) *or* serum creatinine of >4.0 mg/dL (>354 mmol/L) with an acute increase of at least 0.5 mg/dL (44 mmol/L) *or*
Urine output <0.3 mL/kg/h for >24 h *or*
Initiation of renal replacement therapy

32.2 Risk of CIAKI

Iodinated contrast media directly cause apoptosis of renal tubule cells. Also, contrast decreases nitric oxide and prostaglandin secretion as well as free radical clearance in the renal medulla, contributing to vasoconstriction, ischemia, and delayed contrast clearance [4]. Several patient-specific factors contribute to the risk of AKI associated with TAVR (Table 32.2). While these factors may not be specific to CIAKI, kidney injury is additive, and non-contrast renal insults worsen CIAKI.

A. M. Goldsweig
University of Nebraska Medical Center,
Omaha, NE, USA
e-mail: andrew.goldsweig@unmc.edu

J. D. Abbott (✉)
Warren Alpert Medical School of Brown University
and Lifespan Cardiovascular Institute,
Providence, RI, USA
e-mail: jabbott@lifespan.org

© Springer Nature Switzerland AG 2019
A. Giordano et al. (eds.), *Transcatheter Aortic Valve Implantation*,
https://doi.org/10.1007/978-3-030-05912-5_32

Table 32.2 Risk factors for CIAKI in TAVR

Patient-specific factors

Age

Female gender (likely due to lower baseline GFR)

Hypertension

Diabetes

Baseline renal impairment

Anemia

Congestive heart failure (CHF)

Decreased left ventricular systolic function

Peripheral arterial disease (PAD)

Atrial fibrillation

Malignant arrhythmias

Hemodynamic instability

Procedure-related factors

Contrast volume

Blood transfusion

Concomitant nephrotoxins

Emergent TAVR

IABP

Hypotension from rapid pacing

Renal atheroemboli

Multiple primary studies and meta-analyses have shown that baseline renal impairment is the factor most predictive of post-procedural AKI [5, 6]. In patients with chronic kidney disease (CKD) identified by billing codes, the incidence of post-TAVR AKI was 34.1% vs. 10.6% in patients without CKD (adjusted odds ratio [OR] 4.70, 95% confidence interval [CI] 4.42–5.00). In the same population, the incidence of post-TAVR AKI requiring hemodialysis was 2.4% vs. 0.6% in patients without CKD (adjusted OR 3.55, 95% CI 2.88–4.38) [7]. Table 32.3 summarizes the major recent studies examining AKI associated with TAVR using the VARC-2 definition of AKI.

Other patient-specific factors related to baseline renal function also impact the risk of CIAKI. Increasing age and female gender, both components of the Cockcroft-Gault equation, are associated with lower numbers of glomeruli and hence lower baseline glomerular filtration rate (GFR) [8]. Similarly, hypertension [9, 10], diabetes [6, 11], congestive heart failure [12], and decreased left ventricular systolic function [13] may potentiate CIAKI, presumably through the mechanism of underlying renal impairment.

Peripheral arterial disease, a marker for renal vascular disease, predisposes patients to AKI post-TAVR [11], as does atrial fibrillation, which may be associated with renal emboli [14]. Hemodynamic instability [15], whether from pump failure, aortic regurgitation, or malignant arrhythmia, is also associated with renal impairment following TAVR.

In addition, procedure-related factors may increase the risk of CIAKI. Contrast volume has been well-documented to be the most important procedural risk factor in the setting of coronary intervention [16]. One study to date has confirmed this finding in TAVR and also cited blood transfusion as another significant CIAKI risk factor [13]. Other concomitant renal insults may synergistically worsen CIAKI. Among these insults is exposure to other nephrotoxins, including proximate contrast exposure. Because hemodynamic instability has been associated with AKI, emergent procedures [17] and periprocedural intra-aortic balloon pump (IABP) use have been associated with AKI. Similarly, hypotension from rapid ventricular pacing may decrease renal perfusion, thereby potentiating CIAKI [3]. The association of transapical access with AKI likely reflects the population of patients undoing transapical access, with more peripheral arterial and potentially renal vascular disease [18, 19]. Additionally, atheroemboli from catheter manipulation in the aorta may cause renal infarction.

32.3 Effect of CIAKI on TAVR Outcomes

AKI, including CIAKI, has significant ramifications for TAVR outcomes including development of CKD, new hemodialysis, length of hospital stay, and mortality. One study showed that in patients who developed AKI, the mean serum creatinine was increased by 0.17 mg/dL at 6 months post-TAVR [20]. In the general AKI literature, a multivariable model of patients with stage 1, 2, or 3a CKD who developed AKI during

Table 32.3 Major recent studies of AKI associated with TAVR using VARC-2 Criteria

Study	Year	Patients (n)	AKI rate (%)	Dialysis rate (%)	Factors predicting AKI
Gupta et al. [7]	2017	41,025	18.8	1.2	
Crowhurst et al. [25]	2015	209	39.2	2.4	CKD, respiratory failure, previous stroke, blood transfusion, valve repositioning
Schnabel et al. [47]	2014	458	16	2.4	Body-mass index (BMI), pre-TAVR GFR
Frerker et al. [48]	2013	323	10.3		
Généreux et al. [49]	2013	218	8.3	4.1	Bleeding
Yamamoto et al. [13]	2013	415	15.2	1.0	Diabetes, LVEF <40%, blood transfusion, post-TAVR aortic insufficiency
Khawaja et al. [11]	2012	248	35.9	10.0	PAD, diabetes, CKD
Nuis et al. [12]	2012	995	30.1	3.1	Blood transfusion, PAD, CHF, leukocytosis, EuroSCORE
Tchetche et al. [50]	2012	943	23.2		Blood transfusion
Ussia et al. [51]	2012	178	18.5	2.2	

hospitalization predicted a 2.7% risk of the development of sustained stage 4 or 5 CKD with six independent predictors: older age, female sex, higher baseline serum creatinine, albuminuria, greater severity of AKI, and higher serum creatinine at discharge [21].

The rate of new initiation of hemodialysis post-TAVR has decreased significantly from 6.1% in 2007–2008 to 2.3% in 2013–2014. An analysis from the STS/ACC TVT Registry found minimal effect with stages 1 and 2 CKD; however stages 3, 4, and 5 were associated with new hemodialysis with adjusted hazard ratios (HRs) of 3.22, 12.62, and 60.29, respectively [22]. In addition to baseline CKD, new initiation of hemodialysis has been associated with baseline reduced left ventricular systolic function, diabetes, use of Edwards SAPIEN valve (which requires rapid pacing, unlike the other FDA-approved TAVR valve, the Medtronic CoreValve), non-transfemoral access, and greater than mild post-TAVR aortic insufficiency [23, 24]. Because of the additional care necessary for patients with AKI, time in intensive care units may increase by 75% and total hospital length of stay by 56% [25].

AKI is an independent predictor of post-TAVR mortality [9, 26]. A meta-analysis reported a fourfold higher mortality rate with AKI, regardless of baseline or procedural characteristics [5]. This effect is most prominent in patients without

CKD who develop AKI, especially if dialysis is required. A study from the National Inpatient Sample registry reported that, in the absence of CKD, AKI was associated with a sevenfold increase in in-hospital mortality (17.3% vs. 2.2%, $p < 0.001$), and AKI requiring dialysis was associated with a 15-fold increase in in-hospital mortality (56.3% vs. 3.5%, $p < 0.001$) [7]. However, post-TAVR AKI patients whose renal function recovers completely or partially have lower mortality than those without renal recovery [27].

32.4 Treatment of CIAKI

Treatment of CIAKI revolves around maximizing renal perfusion. To maximize renal perfusion, hemodynamics should be optimized with hydration for volume depletion and inotropes as needed for hypotension not responsive to volume expansion. Vasopressors that reduce renal perfusion should be avoided. Afterload reduction with hydralazine, nitroprusside, or dihydropyridine calcium channel blockers may be employed, but angiotensin-converting enzyme (ACE) inhibitors should be avoided because they inhibit efferent arteriolar vasoconstriction, thereby reducing GFR. Invasive hemodynamic monitoring with a peripheral arterial line and central venous line or

Swan-Ganz catheter may facilitate management of vasoactive medications.

Adequate urine output is important, both as a sign of adequate renal blood flow and for clearing contrast from the body. Therefore, if hydration and hemodynamic support fail to correct oliguria (<0.5 mL/kg/h), administration of a loop diuretic may become necessary. As a last resort, renal replacement therapy (intermittent hemodialysis or, if not tolerated hemodynamically, continuous veno-venous hemofiltration) may be necessary in cases of electrolyte abnormalities or volume overload.

32.5   Prevention of CIAKI

The risk and severity of CIAKI may be reduced by minimizing contrast dose, maximizing renal perfusion with hydration and prevention of hypotension, and avoidance of concomitant nephrotoxins.

Many of the data on CIAKI prevention come from the percutaneous coronary intervention (PCI) literature. In a landmark 2007 study, Laskey et al. proposed the concept of the contrast volume to creatinine clearance ratio. Developing receiver-operator characteristic models, they reported that a ratio of less than 3.7 was a significant and independent predictor of AKI within 48 h after PCI [28]. In 2012, Gurm et al. used insurance registry data to devise a similar model, demonstrating that the risk for CIAKI became statistically significant when the ratio of the contrast volume to the creatinine clearance exceeded 2.0 [29]. In TAVR, Yamamoto et al. conducted a similar study in TAVR patients analyzing the product of the contrast media volume (mL) × [serum creatinine (mg/dL)/body weight (kg)]; they found that 2.7 was a threshold value above which this statistic predicted an increased risk of AKI [13].

Low-osmolar, nonionic contrast agents carry the lowest risk of CIAKI. In a meta-analysis of 25 studies, 4 studies suggested iodixanol to be minimally safer than iohexol, iopamidol, iopromide, and ioxaglate [30]. In addition, contrast may be diluted with saline to provide a similar volume of injection with fewer nephrotoxic contrast molecules. Multiple contrast exposures should be spaced at least 48 h apart to minimize cumulative toxicity and CIAKI. This includes pre-TAVR coronary angiography and PCI as well as computed tomographic angiography (CTA), which is usually performed to assess the annular dimensions and ensure sufficient diameter of peripheral vasculature through which the TAVR will be performed. Regarding this CTA, instead of using the traditional 80–100 mL of contrast injected intravenously, a low-contrast-dose imaging protocol may be used without compromising image and interpretability and without increased procedural complications [31]. Select patients with an extremely elevated risk of CIAKI may benefit from annular sizing by non-contrast MRI and peripheral CTA imaging using a 10–15 mL direct aortic injection through a multi-sidehole catheter [32].

Maximizing renal perfusion has been demonstrated to reduce the risk of CIAKI. In the definitive POSEIDON study of patients with CKD stage 3 or higher, the hydration strategy was guided by the left ventricular end-diastolic pressure resulting in a relative risk (RR) of AKI of 0.41 (95% CI 0.22–0.79, $p = 0.005$) [33]. A device called RenalGuard, which balances volume expansion with furosemide-induced diuresis, was developed to prevent AKI in PCI [34] and also been specifically trialed in the PROTECT-TAVI study. In 112 consecutive TAVR patients randomized to RenalGuard or standard normal saline treatment, the rate of AKI was significantly lower with RenalGuard (5.4% vs. 25.0% respectively, $p = 0.014$) [35].

Normal saline is appropriate for hydration; no benefit has been shown from treatment with sodium bicarbonate [36] or N-acetyl cysteine (NAC) [37, 38]. Limited evidence points to a utility in AKI of fenoldopam, a D1 dopamine receptor agonist and vasodilator [39], or atrial natriuretic peptide, a diuretic hormone [40]; however data are scarce, CIAKI and TAVR experience is absent, and no guidelines currently recommend use of these agents. Similarly, while embolic protection devices have been developed and approved for the cerebral vessels [41], there are no such devices designed for prevention of renal emboli during TAVR. In the surgical literature, prophylactic hemodialysis in patients with CKD has reduced AKI as well as mortality following coronary artery bypass grafting [42], but no such studies have been conducted in TAVR, and the cost of such an intervention is prohibitive.

In addition, because concomitant renal insults have a synergistic effect in potentiating CIAKI, additional insults such as hypotension and nephrotoxins must be assiduously avoided. Hypotension decreases renal perfusion and has been shown to cause AKI [43]; inotropes are indicated if hydration alone cannot maintain a mean arterial pressure less than 65 mmHg. Nephrotoxic drugs, including nonsteroidal anti-inflammatory drugs, must be withheld to prevent an increased risk of renal injury.

Lastly, case reports and small studies present strategies to minimize contrast usage using transesophageal and intracardiac echocardiography (TEE and ICE, respectively) to provide procedural imaging guidance. At least two groups have reported entirely contrast-free TAVR procedures, guided by TEE and fluoroscopy [44, 45]. In a study of 60 TAVR patients randomized to primary ICE guidance or primary angiography guidance, ICE yielded a mean of 51.9 mL less of contrast used and a 17% reduction in freedom AKI (freedom from AKI 80% vs. 63%, respectively) [46].

32.6 Conclusion

CIAKI is a common adverse clinical event associated with TAVR. Patient-specific factors and procedure-related factors determine the risk of CIAKI, which in turn significantly increases the risk of periprocedural mortality. Treatment of CIAKI by maximizing renal perfusion ex post facto is imperfect; the optimal strategy is prevention by minimizing contrast volume and maximizing renal perfusion a priori.

Disclosures The authors report that they have no relevant conflicts of interest to disclose.

References

1. Kappetein AP, Head SJ, Généreux P, Piazza N, van Mieghem NM, Blackstone EH, Brott TG, Cohen DJ, Cutlip DE, van Es GA, Hahn RT, Kirtane AJ, Krucoff MW, Kodali S, Mack MJ, Mehran R, Rodés-Cabau J, Vranckx P, Webb JG, Windecker S, Serruys PW, Leon MB. Updated standardized endpoint definitions for transcatheter aortic valve implantation: the valve academic research consortium-2 consensus document. J Am Coll Cardiol. 2012;60:1438–54.
2. Mehta RL, Kellum JA, Shah SV, Molitoris BA, Ronco C, Warnock DG, Levin A, Acute Kidney Injury Network. Acute kidney injury network: report of an initiative to improve outcomes in acute kidney injury. Crit Care. 2007;11:R31.
3. Najjar M, Salna M, George I. Acute kidney injury after aortic valve replacement: incidence, risk factors and outcomes. Expert Rev Cardiovasc Ther. 2015;13:301–16.
4. Persson PB, Hansell P, Liss P. Pathophysiology of contrast medium-induced nephropathy. Kidney Int. 2005;68:14–22.
5. Elhmidi Y, Bleiziffer S, Deutsch MA, Krane M, Mazzitelli D, Lange R, Piazza N. Acute kidney injury after transcatheter aortic valve implantation: incidence, predictors and impact on mortality. Arch Cardiovasc Dis. 2014;107:133–9.
6. Alassar A, Roy D, Abdulkareem N, Valencia O, Brecker S, Jahangiri M. Acute kidney injury after transcatheter aortic valve implantation: incidence, risk factors, and prognostic effects. Innovations (Phila). 2012;7:389–93.
7. Gupta T, Goel K, Kolte D, Khera S, Villablanca PA, Aronow WS, Bortnick AE, Slovut DP, Taub CC, Kizer JR, Pyo RT, Abbott JD, Fonarow GC, Rihal CS, Garcia MJ, Bhatt DL. Association of chronic kidney disease with in-hospital outcomes of transcatheter aortic valve replacement. JACC Cardiovasc Interv. 2017;10:2050–60.
8. Scherner M, Wahlers T. Acute kidney injury after transcatheter aortic valve implantation. J Thorac Dis. 2015;7:1527–35.
9. Bagur R, Webb JG, Nietlispach F, Dumont E, De Larochelliere R, Doyle D, Masson JB, Gutierrez MJ, Clavel MA, Bertrand OF, Pibarot P, Rodes-Cabau J. Acute kidney injury following transcatheter aortic valve implantation: predictive factors, prognostic value, and comparison with surgical aortic valve replacement. Eur Heart J. 2010;31:865–74.
10. Kong WY, Yong G, Irish A. Incidence, risk factors and prognosis of acute kidney injury after transcatheter aortic valve implantation. Nephrology (Carlton). 2012;17:445–51.
11. Khawaja MZ, Thomas M, Joshi A, Asrress KN, Wilson K, Bolter K, Young CP, Hancock J, Bapat V, Redwood S. The effects of VARC-defined acute kidney injury after transcatheter aortic valve implantation (TAVI) using the Edwards bioprosthesis. EuroIntervention. 2012;8:563–70.

12. Nuis RJ, Rodes-Cabau J, Sinning JM, van Garsse L, Kefer J, Bosmans J, Dager AE, van Mieghem N, Urena M, Nickenig G, Werner N, Maessen J, Astarci P, Perez S, Benitez LM, Dumont E, van Domburg RT, de Jaegere PP. Blood transfusion and the risk of acute kidney injury after transcatheter aortic valve implantation. Circ Cardiovasc Interv. 2012;5:680–8.

13. Yamamoto M, Hayashida K, Mouillet G, Chevalier B, Meguro K, Watanabe Y, Dubois-Rande JL, Morice MC, Lefevre T, Teiger E. Renal function-based contrast dosing predicts acute kidney injury following transcatheter aortic valve implantation. JACC Cardiovasc Interv. 2013;6:479–86.

14. Wang J, Yu W, Zhou Y, Yang Y, Li C, Liu N, Hou X, Wang L. Independent risk factors contributing to acute kidney injury according to updated valve academic research consortium-2 criteria after transcatheter aortic valve implantation: a meta-analysis and meta-regression of 13 studies. J Cardiothorac Vasc Anesth. 2017;31:816–26.

15. Villablanca PA, Ramakrishna H. The renal frontier in TAVR. J Cardiothorac Vasc Anesth. 2017;31:800–3.

16. Rihal CS, Textor SC, Grill DE, Berger PB, Ting HH, Best PJ, Singh M, Bell MR, Barsness GW, Mathew V, Garratt KN, Holmes DR Jr. Incidence and prognostic importance of acute renal failure after percutaneous coronary intervention. Circulation. 2002;105:2259–64.

17. Mihelis EA, Vidi VD, Sraow D, Scheinerman SJ, Palazzo RS, Kaplan B, Jauhar R, Meraj P. Acute kidney injury following transcatheter aortic valve replacement: utilizing STS/ACC-TVT registry to aid in improved capture of adverse outcomes and to perform internal audit as a quality improvement initiative. Washington, DC: National Cardiovascular Data Registry Annual Meeting; 2014.

18. Barbash IM, Ben-Dor I, Dvir D, Maluenda G, Xue Z, Torguson R, Satler LF, Pichard AD, Waksman R. Incidence and predictors of acute kidney injury after transcatheter aortic valve replacement. Am Heart J. 2012;163:1031–6.

19. Saia F, Ciuca C, Taglieri N, Marrozzini C, Savini C, Bordoni B, Dall'Ara G, Moretti C, Pilato E, Martin-Suarez S, Petridis FD, Di Bartolomeo R, Branzi A, Marzocchi A. Acute kidney injury following transcatheter aortic valve implantation: incidence, predictors and clinical outcome. Int J Cardiol. 2013;168:1034–40.

20. Thongprayoon C, Wisit C, Kittanamongkolchai W, Srivali N, Greason KL, Kashani K. Changes in kidney function among patients undergoing transcatheter aortic valve replacement. J Renal Inj Prev. 2017;6:216–21.

21. James MT, Pannu N, Hemmelgarn BR, Austin PC, Tan Z, McArthur E, Manns BJ, Tonelli M, Wald R, Quinn RR, Ravani P, Garg AX. Derivation and external validation of prediction models for advanced chronic kidney disease following acute kidney injury. JAMA. 2017;318:1787–97.

22. Hansen JW, Foy A, Yadav P, Gilchrist IC, Kozak M, Stebbins A, Matsouaka R, Vemulapalli S, Wang A, Wang DD, Eng MH, Greenbaum AB, O'Neill WO. Death and dialysis after transcatheter aortic valve replacement: an analysis of the STS/ACC TVT registry. JACC Cardiovasc Interv. 2017;10:2064–75.

23. Ferro CJ, Law JP, Doshi SN, de Belder M, Moat N, Mamas M, Hildick-Smith D, Ludman P, Townend JN: Dialysis following transcatheter aortic valve implantation, risk factors and outcomes: an analysis from the UK TAVI registry (transcatheter aortic valve implantation) registry. JACC Cardiovasc Interv 2017; 10(20):2040-2047.

24. Ladia V, Panchal HB, TJ ON, Sitwala P, Bhatheja S, Patel R, Ramu V, Mukherjee D, Mahmud E, Paul TK. Incidence of renal failure requiring hemodialysis following transcatheter aortic valve replacement. Am J Med Sci. 2016;352:306–13.

25. Crowhurst JA, Savage M, Subban V, Incani A, Raffel OC, Poon K, Murdoch D, Saireddy R, Clarke A, Aroney C, Bett N, Walters DL. Factors contributing to acute kidney injury and the impact on mortality in patients undergoing transcatheter aortic valve replacement. Heart Lung Circ. 2016;25:282–9.

26. Sinning JM, Ghanem A, Steinhauser H, Adenauer V, Hammerstingl C, Nickenig G, Werner N. Renal function as predictor of mortality in patients after percutaneous transcatheter aortic valve implantation. JACC Cardiovasc Interv. 2010;3:1141–9.

27. Thongprayoon C, Cheungpasitporn W, Srivali N, Kittanamongkolchai W, Sakhuja A, Greason KL, Kashani KB. The association between renal recovery after acute kidney injury and long-term mortality after transcatheter aortic valve replacement. PLoS One. 2017;12:e0183350.

28. Laskey WK, Jenkins C, Selzer F, Marroquin OC, Wilensky RL, Glaser R, Cohen HA, Holmes DR. Investigators NDR: volume-to-creatinine clearance ratio: a pharmacokinetically based risk factor for prediction of early creatinine increase after percutaneous coronary intervention. J Am Coll Cardiol. 2007;50:584–90.

29. Gurm HS, Dixon SR, Smith DE, Share D, Lalonde T, Greenbaum A, Moscucci M. Registry BBCBSoMCC: renal function-based contrast dosing to define safe limits of radiographic contrast media in patients undergoing percutaneous coronary interventions. J Am Coll Cardiol. 2011;58:907–14.

30. Eng J, Wilson RF, Subramaniam RM, Zhang A, Suarez-Cuervo C, Turban S, Choi MJ, Sherrod C, Hutfless S, Iyoha EE, Bass EB. Comparative effect of contrast media type on the incidence of contrast-induced nephropathy: a systematic review and meta-analysis. Ann Intern Med. 2016;164:417–24.

31. Zemedkun M, LaBounty TM, Bergman G, Wong SC, Lin FY, Reynolds D, Gomez M, Dunning AM, Leipsic J, Min JK. Effectiveness of a low contrast load CT angiography protocol in octogenarians and nonagenarians being evaluated for transcatheter aortic valve replacement. Clin Imaging. 2015;39:815–9.

32. Krishnaswamy A, Tuzcu EM. Minimizing acute kidney injury during TAVR: the importance of seeing the trees and the forest. Catheter Cardiovasc Interv. 2015;85:1254–5.

33. Brar SS, Aharonian V, Mansukhani P, Moore N, Shen AY, Jorgensen M, Dua A, Short L, Kane K. Haemodynamic-guided fluid administration for the prevention of contrast-induced acute kidney injury: the POSEIDON randomised controlled trial. Lancet. 2014;383:1814–23.

34. Putzu A, Boscolo Berto M, Belletti A, Pasotti E, Cassina T, Moccetti T, Pedrazzini G. Prevention of contrast-induced acute kidney injury by furosemide with matched hydration in patients undergoing interventional procedures: a systematic review and meta-analysis of randomized trials. JACC Cardiovasc Interv. 2017;10:355–63.

35. Barbanti M, Gulino S, Capranzano P, Imme S, Sgroi C, Tamburino C, Ohno Y, Attizzani GF, Patane M, Sicuso R, Pilato G, Di Landro A, Todaro D, Di Simone E, Picci A, Giannetto G, Costa G, Deste W, Giannazzo D, Grasso C, Capodanno D. Acute kidney injury with the RenalGuard system in patients undergoing transcatheter aortic valve replacement: the PROTECT-TAVI trial (PROphylactic effecT of furosEmide-induCed diuresis with matched isotonic intravenous hydraTion in Transcatheter aortic valve implantation). JACC Cardiovasc Interv. 2015;8:1595–604.

36. Maioli M, Toso A, Leoncini M, Gallopin M, Tedeschi D, Micheletti C, Bellandi F. Sodium bicarbonate versus saline for the prevention of contrast-induced nephropathy in patients with renal dysfunction undergoing coronary angiography or intervention. J Am Coll Cardiol. 2008;52:599–604.

37. Xu R, Tao A, Bai Y, Deng Y, Chen G. Effectiveness of N-acetylcysteine for the prevention of contrast-induced nephropathy: a systematic review and meta-analysis of randomized controlled trials. J Am Heart Assoc. 2016;5

38. Weisbord SD, Gallagher M, Jneid H, Garcia S, Cass A, Thwin SS, Conner TA, Chertow GM, Bhatt DL, Shunk K, Parikh CR, McFalls EO, Brophy M, Ferguson R, Wu H, Androsenko M, Myles J, Kaufman J, Palevsky PM. Outcomes after angiography with sodium bicarbonate and acetylcysteine. N Engl J Med:2017.

39. Landoni G, Biondi-Zoccai GG, Marino G, Bove T, Fochi O, Maj G, Calabro MG, Sheiban I, Tumlin JA, Ranucci M, Zangrillo A. Fenoldopam reduces the need for renal replacement therapy and in-hospital death in cardiovascular surgery: a meta-analysis. J Cardiothorac Vasc Anesth. 2008;22:27–33.

40. Nigwekar SU, Navaneethan SD, Parikh CR, Hix JK. Atrial natriuretic peptide for management of acute kidney injury: a systematic review and meta-analysis. Clin J Am Soc Nephrol. 2009;4:261–72.

41. Giustino G, Sorrentino S, Mehran R, Faggioni M, Dangas G. Cerebral embolic protection during TAVR: a clinical event meta-analysis. J Am Coll Cardiol. 2017;69:465–6.

42. Durmaz I, Yagdi T, Calkavur T, Mahmudov R, Apaydin AZ, Posacioglu H, Atay Y, Engin C. Prophylactic dialysis in patients with renal dysfunction undergoing on-pump coronary artery bypass surgery. Ann Thorac Surg. 2003;75:859–64.

43. Vincent JL, Zapatero DC. The role of hypotension in the development of acute renal failure. Nephrol Dial Transplant England. 2009;24:337–8.

44. Pershad A, Fraij G, Girotra SV, Fang HK, Gellert G. TEE-guided transcatheter aortic valve implantation with "zero contrast"—a viable alternative for patients with chronic kidney disease. J Invasive Cardiol. 2015;27:E25–6.

45. Latib A, Maisano F, Colombo A, Klugmann S, Low R, Smith T, Davidson C, Harreld JH, Bruschi G, DeMarco F. Transcatheter aortic valve implantation of the direct flow medical aortic valve with minimal or no contrast. Cardiovasc Revasc Med. 2014;15:252–7.

46. Bartel T, Bonaros N, Edlinger M, Velik-Salchner C, Feuchtner G, Rudnicki M, Muller S. Intracardiac echo and reduced radiocontrast requirements during TAVR. JACC Cardiovasc Imaging. 2014;7:319–20.

47. Schnabel RB, Seiffert M, Wilde S, Schirmer J, Koschyk DH, Conradi L, Ojeda F, Baldus S, Reichenspurner H, Blankenberg S, Treede H, Diemert P. Kidney injury and mortality after transcatheter aortic valve implantation in a routine clinical cohort. Catheter Cardiovasc Interv. 2015;85:440–7.

48. Frerker C, Schewel D, Kuck KH, Schafer U. Ipsilateral arterial access for management of vascular complication in transcatheter aortic valve implantation. Catheter Cardiovasc Interv. 2013;81:592–602.

49. Genereux P, Kodali SK, Green P, Paradis JM, Daneault B, Rene G, Hueter I, Georges I, Kirtane A, Hahn RT, Smith C, Leon MB, Williams MR. Incidence and effect of acute kidney injury after transcatheter aortic valve replacement using the new valve academic research consortium criteria. Am J Cardiol. 2013;111:100–5.

50. Tchetche D, Van der Boon RM, Dumonteil N, Chieffo A, Van Mieghem NM, Farah B, Buchanan GL, Saady R, Marcheix B, Serruys PW, Colombo A, Carrie D, De Jaegere PP, Fajadet J. Adverse impact of bleeding and transfusion on the outcome post-transcatheter aortic valve implantation: insights from the Pooled-RotterdAm-Milano-Toulouse in Collaboration Plus (PRAGMATIC Plus) initiative. Am Heart J. 2012;164:402–9.

51. Ussia GP, Barbanti M, Petronio AS, Tarantini G, Ettori F, Colombo A, Violini R, Ramondo A, Santoro G, Klugmann S, Bedogni F, Maisano F, Marzocchi A, Poli A, De Carlo M, Napodano M, Fiorina C, De Marco F, Antoniucci D, de Cillis E, Capodanno D, Tamburino C. Transcatheter aortic valve implantation: 3-year outcomes of self-expanding CoreValve prosthesis. Eur Heart J. 2012;33:969–76.

Conduction Disorders and Permanent Pacemaker Implantation After Transcatheter Aortic Valve Implantation

33

Jorn Brouwer, Vincent J. Nijenhuis, Uday Sonker, and Jurrien M. ten Berg

33.1 Introduction

Aortic valve stenosis is the most common valvular heart disease with increasing incidence due to ageing population [1]. Transcatheter aortic valve implantation (TAVI), also called transcatheter aortic valve replacement (TAVR), has been rapidly adopted as minimal invasive therapeutic alternative to surgical aortic valve replacement (SAVR) for patients with severe aortic stenosis, who are considered inoperable or at intermediate to high surgical risk [2–5]. As a result, the number of patients undergoing TAVI is increasing.

The development of conduction disorders is the most prevalent complication associated with TAVI and is of clinical importance [6]. Most TAVI-related complications decreased due to improved technology, minimalistic invasive approach (i.e. transfemoral approach over transapical approach) as well as rising experience of surgeons. However, the incidence of conduction disorders has not decreased over time [7]. The most prevalent TAVI-induced conduction disorders are new-onset left bundle branch block (LBBB) and high-degree atrioventricular block (HAVB) requiring permanent pacemaker implantation (PPI).

Compared to surgical aortic valve replacement, the rate of severe conduction disorders requiring PPI following TAVI is higher (around 17% for TAVI vs. 3–6.9% for SAVR) [1, 3–5]. Lower rates of PPI after SAVR can be explained by different techniques of valve replacement and differences in patient populations. Compared to patients suitable for SAVR, TAVI patients are older and often have more pre-existent conduction disorders and other comorbidities (e.g. renal impairment, respiratory disease, previous myocardial infarction, poor mobility) [8].

Due to close anatomical relation between cardiac conduction system and aortic valvular complex, any surgical or percutaneous intervention can result in conduction disorders [9]. Despite the negative influences of ageing on the conduction system, there is also evidence for an association between severity of aortic stenosis and conduction disorders. This is suspected to be due to similar calcium deposition on the conduction system and aortic valve, which makes the conduction system more vulnerable for external influences [10].

This chapter provides a brief overview of the different aspects of conduction disorders following TAVI: the anatomy of the conduction system and its relation to the aortic valvular complex;

J. Brouwer (✉) · V. J. Nijenhuis · J. M. ten Berg
Department of Cardiology, St. Antonius Hospital Nieuwegein, Nieuwegein, The Netherlands
e-mail: j.brouwer1@antoniusziekenhuis.nl;
v.nijenhuis@antoniusziekenhuis.nl;
j.ten.berg@antoniusziekenhuis.nl

U. Sonker
Department of Cardiothoracic Surgery, St. Antonius Hospital Nieuwegein, Nieuwegein, The Netherlands
e-mail: u.sonker@antoniusziekenhuis.nl

© Springer Nature Switzerland AG 2019
A. Giordano et al. (eds.), *Transcatheter Aortic Valve Implantation*,
https://doi.org/10.1007/978-3-030-05912-5_33

the pathophysiology; the incidence, development, risk factors, outcome and prognosis of LBBB and HAVB requiring pacemaker; and the management.

33.2 Anatomical Relationship Between Aortic Valvular Complex and the Conduction System

Conduction disorders after TAVI can be explained by the conduction system being positioned close to the aortic valvular complex (see Fig. 33.1).

The atrioventricular node lies within the triangle of Koch, which is located in the right atrium. This triangle is delineated by the tendon of Todaro, the orifice of the coronary sinus and the septal leaflet attachment of the tricuspid valve. The ostium of the coronary sinus forms the base of this triangle, while the apex is formed by the convergence of the tendon of Todaro and the insertion of the septal leaflet of the tricuspid valve. Just inferior to the apex lies the atrioventricular node, which continues as the bundle of His once it penetrates the central fibrous body. The bundle of His passes the membranous septum and emerges on the left side directly within the aortic root and left ventricular outflow tract, positioned superficially on the crest of the ventricular septum. From this point the fascicles of the left bundle branch originate, which is directly related to the base of the interleaflet triangle which separates the right coronary and noncoronary leaflets of the aortic valve [6, 7, 11, 12].

33.3 Mechanism of Conduction Disorders After Tavi

Conduction disorders result mainly from mechanical compression of the prosthetic valve or calcified native aortic valve to the atrioventricular conduction system, in TAVI. Based on the close position of the bundle of His, conduction disorders can easily arise if the expansion of the prosthetic valve or calcified native aortic valve exerts pressure to the relating tissues. Autopsied tissues from patients with HAVB after TAVI showed local oedema, hematoma and infarction with compression of the His bundle causing the conduction disorder [13]. On the other hand, several other factors, such as anatomical variations, can determine the susceptibility of the conduction system to injury during TAVI procedures.

First of all, there is a great anatomical variability of atrioventricular node position inside the triangle of Koch and the non-penetrating part of the His bundle. Three major variants are described based on autopsy series. In approximately 50%, the non-penetrating His bundle crosses the right side of the ventricular septum, in approximately 30% of the left side, whereas in 20% the bundle crosses under the membranous septum, just below the endocardium. Especially the last two variants are prone to a higher risk of TAVI procedure-related conduction disorders, due to its superficial course within the aortic valvular complex [14].

A short membranous septum measured by computer tomography is related to a higher rate of conduction disorders after TAVI. The distal end of the membranous septum is considered as anatomical landmark for the left ventricular exit point of the His bundle, with the total length of the membranous septum equalling the aortic annulus-to-His bundle distance. In patients with a short membranous septum and therefore a shorter aortic annulus-to-His bundle distance, it is more difficult to avoid pressure on the His bundle during expansion of the prosthetic valve [15]. There is also evidence for an association between aortic stenosis and conduction disorders. The hypothesis is that there is a calcium deposition on the conduction system as well as on the aortic valve as a result of its proximity to the aortic valve, which makes the conduction system more vulnerable for external influences [10]. Therefore, the close anatomical proximity of the atrioventricular conduction axis within the aortic valvular complex in combination with increased age and senile conduction system explains the origin and induction of conduction abnormalities after TAVI.

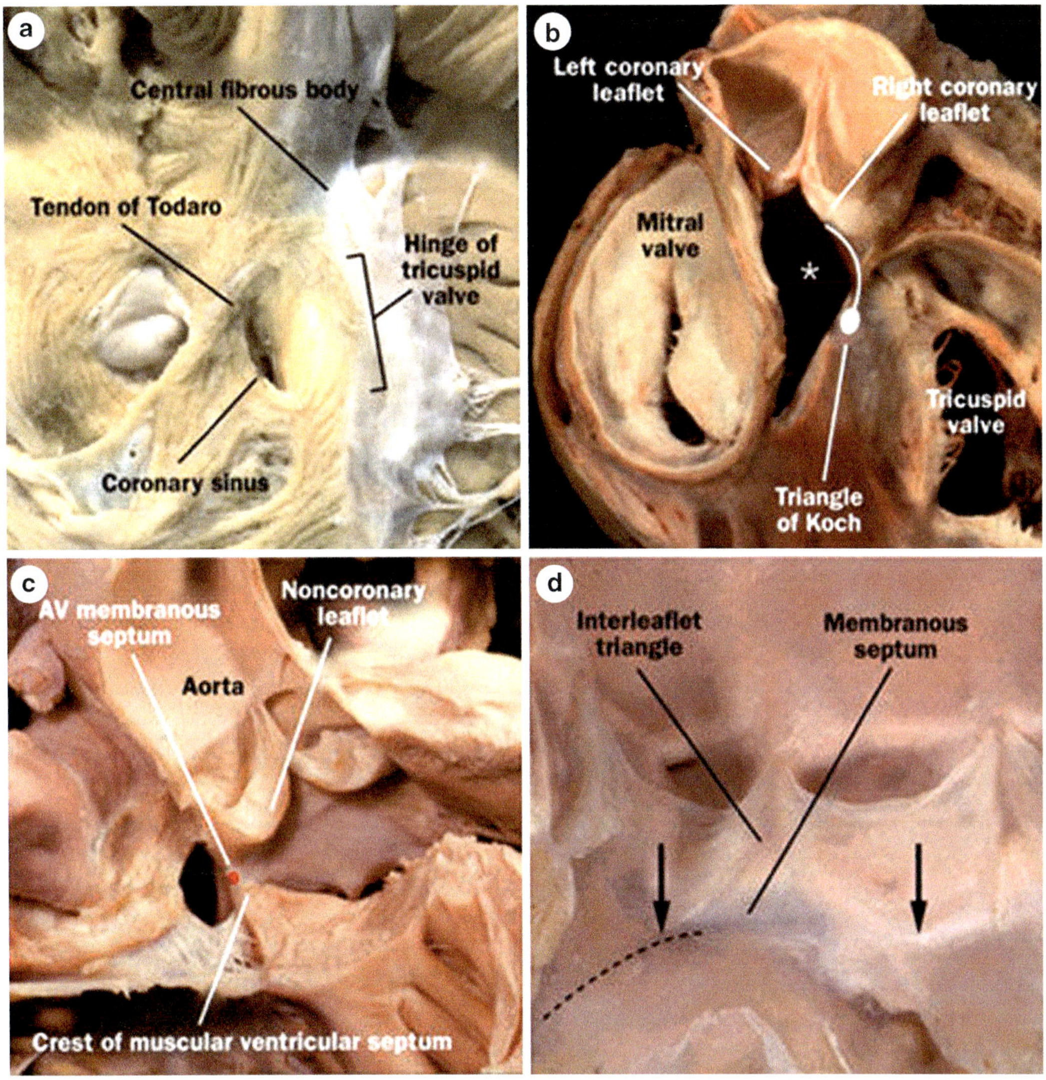

Fig. 33.1 Anatomy and relationship between the aortic valvular complex and the atrioventricular conduction system. (**a**) A view of the right side of the atrial and ventricular septa, illustrating the landmarks of the triangle of Koch. The atrioventricular node is located at the apex of the triangle, and the bundle of His penetrates the central fibrous body. (**b**) The course of the axis as it penetrates, created by removing the noncoronary sinus of the aortic root, which reveals the deep diverticulum (star) that interposes between the mitral valve and the ventricular septum. The location of the atrioventricular node (oval) and the course of the conduction axis (line emanating from the oval) are marked. (**c**) The position of the bundle of His as it is sandwiched between the membranous and muscular parts of the ventricular septum (red circle), created by dissecting away the right ventricular outflow tract to reveal the posterior components of the aortic root. (**d**) The opened aortic root viewed from the left ventricle. The basal attachments of the right and noncoronary leaflets of the aortic valve (arrows), with the location of the most superior part of the left bundle branch as it originates from the branching component of the conduction axis (broken black line). Reproduced from Van der Boon RM et al. Nat Rev. Cardiol. 2012;9:454–463 with permission from the publisher

33.4 Left Bundle Branch Block

33.4.1 Incidence

New-onset LBBB is the most common conduction disorder after TAVI with variable incidence reported in currently available literature, explained by several methodological discrepancies between studies. Incidence depends on the TAVI prosthesis used during the procedure and whether transient LBBB is included.

The reported incidence of new-onset left bundle branch block after TAVI ranges from 4% to 65% using first generations TAVI prostheses of Medtronic and Edwards Lifesciences [1, 7, 12, 16]. New-onset LBBB occurred in 4–30% using the balloon-expandable Edwards SAPIEN and SAPIEN XT valve and 18–65% using the self-expandable Medtronic CoreValve device [12]. Data on newer generation TAVI system are limited. New-onset LBBB after TAVI using the Edwards SAPIEN 3 varies from 12% to 22% [7, 17]. A study using self-expandable Portico TAVI device (St. Jude) reported similar incidence, whereas two studies using the mechanical expendable Lotus system (Boston Scientific) reported higher rates of LBBB (55 and 77%) [18–20].

33.4.2 Timing of Left Bundle Branch Block

Most conduction disturbances develop during the periprocedural period; 85–94% of TAVI-induced LBBB arises during that period [21]. New-onset LBBB occurs mainly during different stages of the procedure before implantation and not only during actual valve implantation. One study continuously monitored all patients with electrocardiography during TAVI procedure and observed that new-onset LBBB occurred in 62% before the actual valve implantation (i.e. stiff wire insertion and balloon predilation of aortic valve) [22]. New-onset LBBB developing after the procedure occurs less frequently and is rare after discharge. Resolution of new-onset LBBB after discharge is uncommon. Moreover reported incidence of LBBB after 1-year follow-up is 60% [23].

33.4.3 Risk Factors

Risk factors for TAVI-induced LBBB can be divided in patient-related, procedural and anatomical factors. The risk factors are displayed in Table 33.1.

The main predictive risk factors of new-onset LBBB are procedure related. First of all, the implantation depth of the TAVI prosthesis into the LVOT is recognised as the main predictor: deeper implantation is correlated with higher risk of LBBB [7, 24]. In line with this observation, Medtronic TAVI devices are associated with higher occurrence of LBBB compared to Edwards SAPIEN valves [25, 26]. The self-expandable Medtronic device expands from the ventricular side of the aortic valve and therefore exerts higher radial forces on the LVOT and the membranous septum [27]. Valve oversizing, small aortic annulus and small LVOT diameter also predict a higher risk of new-onset LBBB after TAVI procedures [28]. Standard TAVI procedure aortic valvuloplasty, such as crossing the valve with a stiff wire, and catheter removal may induce conduction disturbances as well [22].

Multiple patient-related factors are associated with new-onset LBBB after TAVI and include female gender, diabetes mellitus, preprocedural

Table 33.1 Risk factor for new-onset LBBB after TAVI

Anatomical	Patient related	Procedure related
Severe calcification aortic annulus and LVOT	Female sex	Implantation depth
Short membranous septum	Diabetes mellitus	Use of Medtronic CoreValve
Small LVOT diameter	Pre-existent conduction disorder (prolonged QRS duration)	Overexpansion aortic annulus
		Larger valve sizes
		Insertion guiding wire
		Balloon valvuloplasty

conduction disorders (mainly prolonged QRS duration), severe calcification of aortic annulus and LVOT [26, 28].

33.4.4 Outcome and Prognosis

One large meta-analysis, including 8 studies observing new-onset LBBB post-TAVI with a total of 4756 patients, investigated 3 different 1-year outcomes: risk of permanent pacemaker implantation, all-cause mortality and cardiac mortality [16]. 17–24% of the patients with new-onset LBBB required PPI [24, 29]. There was no increased risk of all-cause mortality 1-year post implantation and no difference in all-cause mortality amongst different TAVI prostheses. There was, however, a higher 1-year cardiac mortality risk related to new-onset LBBB [30].

33.5 High-Degree Atrioventricular Block Requiring Permanent Pacemaker Implantation

33.5.1 Incidence

HAVB requiring PPI is a common and clinically relevant complication after TAVI. The use of PPI after TAVI as an outcome variable has some limitations. It is highly dependable on the timing of the pacemaker implantation and different indications used. The latest European Cardiology Society Guidelines recommend cardiac pacing in the occurrence of a HAVB (third- or second-degree type II) irrespective of symptoms [31]. In literature PPI is the most used outcome variable for severe conduction disorders after TAVI and therefore used in this chapter.

Around 17% (ranging incidence of 2–51% between studies) of patients developed severe conduction disorders requiring PPI after implantation of first-generation TAVI device [7, 9, 32]. The first randomised trials with TAVI, the PARTNER I-II and the US CoreValve Clinical trial, reported PPI rates from 3.6% to 19.8% [2–5].

Data on newer generation TAVI valves observed lower periprocedural complications, such as paravalvular leakage, but no evident reduction of PPI rates after the procedure. PPI rates of the latest commonly used TAVI devices are Edwards SAPIEN 3 11–14%, Medtronic Evolut R 15–22%, Boston Scientific Lotus 28–37%, Symetis Acurate Neo 5–11%, JenaValve 12–15% and St. Jude Portico 4.5–10% [7, 18, 19, 33–47].

PPI rates mentioned above could be an underestimation as most studies included patients with PPI prior to the TAVI procedure into the control non-PPI group [48]. On the other hand, many practitioners may undertake PPI earlier to reduce post-procedure hospital stay and for prophylactic reasons (thus not following the current guidelines).

33.5.2 Timing of HAVB

As previously mentioned, most conduction disturbances develop during the periprocedural period. TAVI-induced HAVB develops in 60–96% during periprocedural period. Occurrence of HAVB more than 24–48 h after TAVI is considered as delayed HAVB and occurs less frequently (2–7%) [7, 16]. Late development of HAVB after discharge is unlikely to occur, if no conduction disorders are present at discharge. New-onset LBBB will regress to HAVB in 17% [16, 49]. Moreover, PPI within the first year after TAVI is very rare when no conduction orders were present during hospitalisation for TAVI procedure [32, 49].

Interesting is pacemaker dependency after TAVI procedure. Up to 86% of patients with PPI after TAVI exhibited ventricular pacing >1% of the time during median follow-up of 4 years [50]. Almost all patients with TAVI-induced HAVB underwent PPI procedure within 5 days after TAVI procedure with a median of 3 days [31, 32]. Resolution of HAVB without pacemaker dependency and a low ventricular pacing rate (<1%) can occur over time. Observed recovery rates after 30 days are 59% for acute-onset HAVB (within 24 h) and 25% for delayed HAVB. Acute-onset HAVB showed faster recovery compared to delayed HAVB (longer than 6 days) [7].

Table 33.2 Risk factor for PPI following TAVI

Anatomical	Patient related	Procedure related
Severe calcification aortic annulus and LVOT	Female sex	Implantation depth
Short membranous septum	Pre-existent RBBB	Use of Medtronic CoreValve
	Pre-existent first-degree AV block	Oversizing aortic valve
	Pre-existent left anterior hemiblock	Overextension aortic valve
		Periprocedural HAVB

33.5.3 Risk Factors

Similar to risk factors of new-onset LBBB, a distinction is made between patient-related and procedural-related factors, beside the earlier mentioned anatomical factors. See Table 33.2 for an overview of predictors of PPI after TAVI.

Patient-related risk factors for PPI after TAVI include male gender and pre-existent conduction disorders such as right bundle branch block (RBBB), first-degree atrioventricular block or left anterior hemiblock. Calcifications of the aortic annulus, LVOT and mitral annulus are also associated with PPI after TAVI [7, 9, 21, 32].

Two to three times higher risk of severe conduction disorder after TAVI requiring PPI is reported in self-expandable CoreValve prosthesis compared to balloon-expandable Edwards's device. Other procedural factors are intraoperative HAVB, more than 10% oversizing and a lower implantation depth. Left ventricular function and access route (transfemoral vs. transapical) seem not to be related with increased PPI risk after TAVI [7, 9, 21, 32].

Focussing on delayed HAVB (>24 h after TAVI), male gender, pre-existent RBBB, new-onset LBBB or RBBB after TAVI and a specific prolonged QRS duration are independent risk factors.

33.5.4 Outcome and Prognosis

A large meta-analysis investigated the all-cause and cardiac mortality rates after 1-year follow-up

[16]. No increased risk of all-cause mortally and cardiac mortality was observed for patients with PPI after TAVI. Even more, there was a trend towards a lower cardiac mortality in favour of PPI [51]. However, a more recent large American registry showed a higher mortality rate after 1 year in the PPI group [32]. Left ventricular dysfunction and heart failure may develop more often due to long-term right ventricle pacing [50, 51]. The average TAVI population are usually elderly with other noncardiac comorbidities and reduced life expectancy though.

33.6 Management of Tavi-Induced LBBB and HAVB

Currently, no hard evidence on best management strategies is available for conduction disorders after TAVI. Based on current literature, a recommended strategy consists of electrocardiographic analysis preprocedural and periprocedural rhythm observation (24–48 h after TAVI) till discharge [7]. The presence of one or multiple pre-existent conduction disorders such as RBBB, first-degree atrioventricular block, anterior hemiblock and prolonged QRS duration makes patients more vulnerable to severe conduction disorder. This may influence the choice of TAVI device used, in favour of TAVI prostheses with a lower rate of HAVB such as the balloon-expandable SAPIEN valves, in combination with higher positioning of the prosthetic valve [52]. In the periprocedural period, rhythm monitoring at a cardiac care unit is advised, since most conduction disorders develop periprocedural. Continuous rhythm monitoring till discharge is a simple solution for observing possible conduction disorders and to diagnose new-onset rhythm disorders such as atrial fibrillation [53].

A proposal of management of new-onset LBBB is shown in Fig. 33.2. A temporary pacemaker is always inserted during TAVI procedures. When new-onset LBBB occurs during procedure, observation is advised for 24 h due to possible evolution towards HAVB. In case of TAVI-induced LBBB resolution, the temporary pacemaker can be removed, and observation with continuous rhythm monitoring will be sufficient

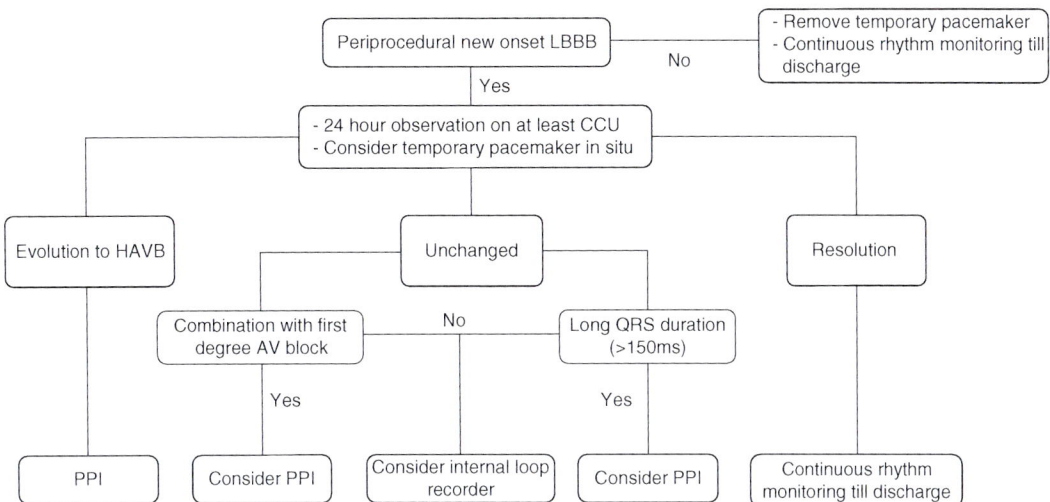

Fig. 33.2 Suggested management of new-onset left bundle branch block (LBBB). *AV* atrioventricular, *CCU* cardiac care unit, *HAVB* high-degree atrioventricular block, *PPI* permanent pacemaker implantation

till discharge. When new-onset LBBB persists, further investigations (e.g. internal loop recorder) should be considered. Consider PPI when combined with prolonged QRS duration (>150 ms) or first-degree AV block. Unchanged pre-existent LBBB or other minor conduction disorders after TAVI will not require further observation [7]. During follow-up, electrocardiographic examination after 30 days and 1 year is advised in order to monitor possible evolution towards more severe conduction disorders.

Suggested management of new-onset HAVB is shown in Fig. 33.3. When a HAVB occurs during the procedure, an observational period with temporary pacemaker for 24–48 h is advised, while it is uncommon for periprocedural emerged HAVB to recover after 24–48 h. In case of HAVB resolution, the temporary pacemaker can be removed, and observation with rhythm monitoring will be sufficient till discharge. When HAVB is persistent (after observation) or recurrent, PPI is indicated before discharge [7]. In case of evolution of HAVB towards LBBB, we refer to the management of LBBB as mentioned above.

The latest European Cardiology Society Guidelines recommend a clinical observation up to 7 days in patients with HAVB or complete heart block after TAVI, in order to assess whether the conduction disorder is transient and resolves over time (class I, level of evidence C indication) [31]. However, this observation period can be shortened in the case of complete heart block with slow ventricular response rate and when HAVB occurred in the periprocedural period and persists >48 h [31]. As mentioned in this guideline, most PPI were performed within 3–5 days after procedure, which differs from the guideline recommendations [31]. PPI shortly after TAVI does not result in increased risk of hospitalisation and cardiac mortality [54, 55]. A longer observational period may avoid inappropriate PPI in patients with transient HAVB and therefore prevent these patients from PPI complications and long-term ventricular pacing-induced complications, such as left ventricular impairment, heart failure and hospitalisation [32, 51]. On the other hand, longer observational period for TAVI-induced HAVB results in longer hospitalisation and longer temporary external pacing period with its own inherent complications such as longer immobilisation, infection, thromboembolism and perforation [7]. During follow-up, electrocardiographic analysis in combination with pacemaker function control at 30 days and regularly afterwards is advised in order to monitor the conduction disorder and functionality of the pacemaker.

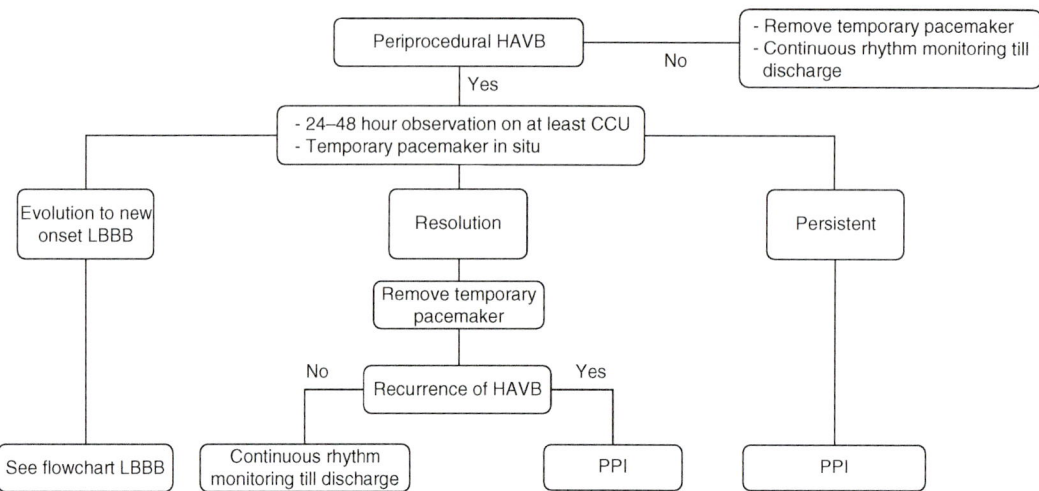

Fig. 33.3 Suggested management of new-onset high-degree atrioventricular block (HAVB). *AV* atrioventricular, *CCU* cardiac care unit, *LBBB* left bundle branch block, *PPI* permanent pacemaker implantation

33.7 Conclusion

This chapter provides an overview of the general aspects of TAVI-induced conduction disorders. Patients undergoing TAVI are prone to develop conduction disorders due to the close relationship between the aortic valvular complex and the conduction system. In the setting of TAVI, conduction disorders mainly result from mechanical trauma of the prosthetic valve or native calcified aortic valve to the atrioventricular conduction system. New-onset LBBB and HAVB are observed frequently following TAVI despite several improvements and have implications in the post-implantation period and on prognosis. Furthermore, the latest generation TAVI valves reduced other procedural complications, but PPI rate remains similar. Electrocardiographic observation during the entire admission is recommended in order to determine the severity of potential conduction disorders. Also, several anatomical, patient- and procedure-related factors may predict which patients are vulnerable to onset of conduction disorders. The best predictive risk factors are pre-existent RBBB, implantation of self-expandable TAVI devices, implantation deep into the LVOT and oversizing or overstretching aortic annulus and LVOT. TAVI-induced LBBB is associated with higher cardiac mortality and PPI (due to HAVB with long-term

ventricle pacing complication) and possible higher mortality rate. More studies are necessary to investigate the occurrence and outcome in the latest generation TAVI devices and specially to determine optimal timing of treatment for conduction disorders following TAVI.

Conflict of Interest None.

References

1. Martinez-Selles M, Bramlage P, Thoenes M, Schymik G. Clinical significance of conduction disturbances after aortic valve intervention: current evidence. Clin Res Cardiol. 2015;104(1):1–12.
2. Leon MB, Smith CR, Mack M, Miller DC, Moses JW, Svensson LG, et al. Transcatheter aortic-valve implantation for aortic stenosis in patients who cannot undergo surgery. N Engl J Med. 2010;363(17):1597–607.
3. Smith CR, Leon MB, Mack MJ, Miller DC, Moses JW, Svensson LG, et al. Transcatheter versus surgical aortic-valve replacement in high-risk patients. N Engl J Med. 2011;364(23):2187–98.
4. Leon MB, Smith CR, Mack MJ, Makkar RR, Svensson LG, Kodali SK, et al. Transcatheter or surgical aortic-valve replacement in intermediate-risk patients. N Engl J Med. 2016;374(17):1609–20.
5. Adams DH, Popma JJ, Reardon MJ, Yakubov SJ, Coselli JS, Deeb GM, et al. Transcatheter aortic-valve replacement with a self-expanding prosthesis. N Engl J Med. 2014;370(19):1790–8.

6. Young Lee M, Chilakamarri Yeshwant S, Chava S, Lawrence Lustgarten D. Mechanisms of heart block after transcatheter aortic valve replacement: cardiac anatomy, clinical predictors and mechanical factors that contribute to permanent pacemaker implantation. Arrhythmia Electrophysiol Rev. 2015;4:81–5.

7. Auffret V, Puri R, Urena M, Chamandi C, Rodriguez-Gabella T, Philippon F, et al. Conduction disturbances after transcatheter aortic valve replacement: current status and future perspectives. Circulation. 2017;136(11):1049–69.

8. Jilaihawi H, Chakravarty T, Weiss RE, Fontana GP, Forrester J, Makkar RR. Meta-analysis of complications in aortic valve replacement: comparison of Medtronic-Corevalve, Edwards-Sapien and surgical aortic valve replacement in 8,536 patients. Catheter Cardiovasc Interv. 2012;80(1):128–38.

9. Siontis GC, Juni P, Pilgrim T, Stortecky S, Bullesfeld L, Meier B, et al. Predictors of permanent pacemaker implantation in patients with severe aortic stenosis undergoing TAVR: a meta-analysis. J Am Coll Cardiol. 2014;64(2):129–40.

10. Yater WM, Cornell VH. Heart block due to calcareous lesions of the bundle of his: review and report of a case with detailed histopathologic study. Ann Intern Med. 1935;8:777–89.

11. Piazza N, de Jaegere P, Schultz C, Becker AE, Serruys PW, Anderson RH. Anatomy of the aortic valvar complex and its implications for transcatheter implantation of the aortic valve. Circ Cardiovasc Interv. 2008;1:74–81.

12. van der Boon RM, Nuis RJ, Van Mieghem NM, Jordaens L, Rodes-Cabau J, van Domburg RT, et al. New conduction abnormalities after TAVI—frequency and causes. Nat Rev Cardiol. 2012;9(8):454–63.

13. Moreno R, Dobarro D, Lopez de Sa E, Prieto M, Morales C, Calvo Orbe L, et al. Cause of complete atrioventricular block after percutaneous aortic valve implantation: insights from a necropsy study. Circulation. 2009;120(5):e29–30.

14. Kawashima T, Sato F. Visualizing anatomical evidences on atrioventricular conduction system for TAVI. Int J Cardiol. 2014;174(1):1–6.

15. Hamdan A, Guetta V, Klempfner R, Konen E, Raanani E, Glikson M, et al. Inverse relationship between membranous septal length and the risk of atrioventricular block in patients undergoing transcatheter aortic valve implantation. JACC Cardiovasc Interv. 2015;8(9):1218–28.

16. Regueiro A, Abdul-Jawad Altisent O, Del Trigo M, Campelo-Parada F, Puri R, Urena M, et al. Impact of new-onset left bundle branch block and periprocedural permanent pacemaker implantation on clinical outcomes in patients undergoing transcatheter aortic valve replacement: a systematic review and meta-analysis. Circ Cardiovasc Interv. 2016;9(5):e003635.

17. Husser O, Pellegrini C, Kessler T, Burgdorf C, Thaller H, Mayr NP, et al. Predictors of permanent pacemaker implantations and new-onset conduction abnormalities with the SAPIEN 3 balloon-expandable transcatheter heart valve. JACC Cardiovasc Interv. 2016;9(3):244–54.

18. Rampat R, Khawaja MZ, Byrne J, MacCarthy P, Blackman DJ, Krishnamurthy A, et al. Transcatheter aortic valve replacement using the repositionable LOTUS valve: United Kingdom experience. JACC Cardiovasc Interv. 2016;9(4):367–72.

19. Zaman S, McCormick L, Gooley R, Rashid H, Ramkumar S, Jackson D, et al. Incidence and predictors of permanent pacemaker implantation following treatment with the repositionable Lotus transcatheter aortic valve. Catheter Cardiovasc Interv. 2017;90(1):147–54.

20. Manoharan G, Linke A, Moellmann H, Redwood S, Frerker C, Kovac J, et al. Multicentre clinical study evaluating a novel resheathable annular functioning self-expanding transcatheter aortic valve system: safety and performance results at 30 days with the portico system. EuroIntervention. 2016;12(6):768–74.

21. Erkapic D, De Rosa S, Kelava A, Lehmann R, Fichtlscherer S, Hohnloser SH. Risk for permanent pacemaker after transcatheter aortic valve implantation: a comprehensive analysis of the literature. J Cardiovasc Electrophysiol. 2012;23(4):391–7.

22. Nuis RJ, Van Mieghem NM, Schultz CJ, Tzikas A, Van der Boon RM, Maugenest AM, Cheng J, Piazza N, van Domburg RT, Serruys PW, de Jaegere PP. Timing and potential mechanisms of new conduction abnormalities during the implantation of the Medtronic CoreValve system in patients with aortic stenosis. Eur Heart J. 2011;32:2067–74.

23. Nazif TM, Williams MR, Hahn RT, Kapadia S, Babaliaros V, Rodes-Cabau J, et al. Clinical implications of new-onset left bundle branch block after transcatheter aortic valve replacement: analysis of the PARTNER experience. Eur Heart J. 2014;35(24):1599–607.

24. Aktug O, Dohmen G, Brehmer K, Koos R, Altiok E, Deserno V, et al. Incidence and predictors of left bundle branch block after transcatheter aortic valve implantation. Int J Cardiol. 2012;160(1):26–30.

25. Franzoni I, Latib A, Maisano F, Costopoulos C, Testa L, Figini F, et al. Comparison of incidence and predictors of left bundle branch block after transcatheter aortic valve implantation using the CoreValve versus the Edwards valve. Am J Cardiol. 2013;112(4):554–9.

26. Schymik G, Tzamalis P, Bramlage P, Heimeshoff M, Würth A, Wondraschek R, Gonska BD, Posival H, Schmitt C, Schröfel H, Luik A. Clinical impact of a new left bundle branch block following TAVI implantation: 1-year results of the TAVIK cohort. Clin Res Cardiol. 2015;104:351–62.

27. Tzamtzis S, Viquerat J, Yap J, Mullen MJ, Burriesci G. Numerical analysis of the radial force produced by the Medtronic-CoreValve and Edwards-SAPIEN after transcatheter aortic valve implantation (TAVI). Med Eng Phys. 2013;35(1):125–30.

28. Hein-Rothweiler R, Jochheim D, Rizas K, Egger A, Theiss H, Bauer A, et al. Aortic annulus to left coronary distance as a predictor for persistent left bundle

branch block after TAVI. Catheter Cardiovasc Interv. 2017;89(4):E162–8.

29. Nijenhuis VJ, Van Dijk VF, Chaldoupi SM, Balt JC, Ten Berg JM. Severe conduction defects requiring permanent pacemaker implantation in patients with a new-onset left bundle branch block after transcatheter aortic valve implantation. Europace. 2017;19(6):1015–21.

30. Zannad F, Huvelle E, Dickstein K, van Veldhuisen DJ, Stellbrink C, Kober L, et al. Left bundle branch block as a risk factor for progression to heart failure. Eur J Heart Fail. 2007;9(1):7–14.

31. Brignole M, Auricchio A, Baron-Esquivias G, Bordachar P, Boriani G, Breithardt OA, et al. 2013 ESC guidelines on cardiac pacing and cardiac resynchronization therapy: the task force on cardiac pacing and resynchronization therapy of the European Society of Cardiology (ESC). Developed in collaboration with the European Heart Rhythm Association (EHRA). Eur Heart J. 2013;34(29):2281–329.

32. Fadahunsi OO, Olowoyeye A, Ukaigwe A, Li Z, Vora AN, Vemulapalli S, et al. Incidence, predictors, and outcomes of permanent pacemaker implantation following transcatheter aortic valve replacement: analysis from the US Society of Thoracic Surgeons/ American College of Cardiology TVT Registry. JACC Cardiovasc Interv. 2016;9(21):2189–99.

33. Kodali S, Thourani VH, White J, Malaisrie SC, Lim S, Greason KL, et al. Early clinical and echocardiographic outcomes after SAPIEN 3 transcatheter aortic valve replacement in inoperable, high-risk and intermediate-risk patients with aortic stenosis. Eur Heart J. 2016;37(28):2252–62.

34. Wendler O, Schymik G, Treede H, Baumgartner H, Dumonteil N, Ihlberg L, et al. SOURCE 3 registry: design and 30-day results of the European postapproval registry of the latest generation of the SAPIEN 3 transcatheter heart valve. Circulation. 2017;135(12):1123–32.

35. Seeger J, Gonska B, Rottbauer W, Wohrle J. Outcome with the repositionable and retrievable Boston Scientific Lotus valve compared with the balloon-expandable Edwards Sapien 3 valve in patients undergoing transfemoral aortic valve replacement. Circ Cardiovasc Interv. 2017;10(6):e004670. https://doi.org/10.1161/CIRCINTERVENTIONS.116.004670.

36. Pilgrim T, Stortecky S, Nietlispach F, Heg D, Tueller D, Toggweiler S, et al. Repositionable versus balloon-expandable devices for transcatheter aortic valve implantation in patients with aortic stenosis. J Am Heart Assoc. 2016;5(11) https://doi.org/10.1161/JAHA.116.004088.

37. Kalra SS, Firoozi S, Yeh J, Blackman DJ, Rashid S, Davies S, et al. Initial experience of a second-generation self-expanding transcatheter aortic valve: the UK & Ireland Evolut R Implanters' Registry. JACC Cardiovasc Interv. 2017;10(3):276–82.

38. Popma JJ, Reardon MJ, Khabbaz K, Harrison JK, Hughes GC, Kodali S, et al. Early clinical outcomes after transcatheter aortic valve replacement using a novel self-expanding bioprosthesis in patients with severe aortic stenosis who are suboptimal for surgery: results of the Evolut R US study. JACC Cardiovasc Interv. 2017;10(3):268–75.

39. Noble S, Stortecky S, Heg D, Tueller D, Jeger R, Toggweiler S, et al. Comparison of procedural and clinical outcomes with Evolut R versus Medtronic CoreValve: a Swiss TAVI registry analysis. EuroIntervention. 2017;12(18):e2170–6.

40. Meredith Am IT, Walters DL, Dumonteil N, Worthley SG, Tchetche D, Manoharan G, et al. Transcatheter aortic valve replacement for severe symptomatic aortic stenosis using a repositionable valve system: 30-day primary endpoint results from the REPRISE II study. J Am Coll Cardiol. 2014;64(13):1339–48.

41. Del Trigo M, Dahou A, Webb JG, Dvir D, Puri R, Abdul-Jawad Altisent O, et al. Self-expanding portico valve versus balloon-expandable SAPIEN XT valve in patients with small aortic annuli: comparison of hemodynamic performance. Rev Esp Cardiol (Engl Ed). 2016;69(5):501–8.

42. Perlman GY, Cheung A, Dumont E, Stub D, Dvir D, Del Trigo M, et al. Transcatheter aortic valve replacement with the portico valve: one-year results of the early Canadian experience. EuroIntervention. 2017;12(13):1653–9.

43. Bagur R, Teefy PJ, Kiaii B, Diamantouros P, Chu MWA. First North American experience with the transfemoral ACURATE-neo(TM) self-expanding transcatheter aortic bioprosthesis. Catheter Cardiovasc Interv. 2017;90(1):130–8.

44. Jatene T, Castro-Filho A, Meneguz-Moreno RA, Siqueira DA, Abizaid AAC, Ramos AIO, et al. Prospective comparison between three TAVR devices: ACURATE neo vs. CoreValve vs. SAPIEN XT. A single heart team experience in patients with severe aortic stenosis. Catheter Cardiovasc Interv. 2017;90(1):139–46.

45. Treede H, Mohr FW, Baldus S, Rastan A, Ensminger S, Arnold M, et al. Transapical transcatheter aortic valve implantation using the JenaValve system: acute and 30-day results of the multicentre CE-mark study. Eur J Cardiothorac Surg. 2012;41(6):e131–8.

46. Kempfert J, Meyer A, Kim WK, Van Linden A, Arsalan M, Blumenstein J, et al. Comparison of two valve systems for transapical aortic valve implantation: a propensity score-matched analysis. Eur J Cardiothorac Surg. 2016;49(2):486–92.

47. Kempfert J, Holzhey D, Hofmann S, Girdauskas E, Treede H, Schrofel H, et al. First registry results from the newly approved ACURATE TA TAVI systemdagger. Eur J Cardiothorac Surg. 2015;48(1):137–41.

48. Chamandi C, Regueiro A, Auffret V, Rodriguez-Gabella T, Chiche O, Barria A, et al. Reported versus "real" incidence of new pacemaker implantation post-transcatheter aortic valve replacement. J Am Coll Cardiol. 2016;68(21):2387–9.

49. Toggweiler S, Stortecky S, Holy E, Zuk K, Cuculi F, Nietlispach F, et al. The electrocardiogram after transcatheter aortic valve replacement determines the

risk for post-procedural high-degree AV block and the need for telemetry monitoring. JACC Cardiovasc Interv. 2016;9(12):1269–76.

50. Chamandi C, Barbanti M, Munoz-Garcia A, Latib A, Nombela-Franco L, Gutierrez-Ibanez E, et al. Long-term outcomes in patients with new permanent pacemaker implantation following transcatheter aortic valve replacement. JACC Cardiovasc Interv. 2018;11(3):301–10.

51. Urena M, Webb JG, Tamburino C, Muñoz-García AJ, Cheema A, Dager AE, Serra V, Amat-Santos IJ, Barbanti M, Immè S, Briales JH, Benitez LM, Al Lawati H, Cucalon AM, García Del Blanco B, López J, Dumont E, Delarochellière R, Ribeiro HB, Nombela-Franco L, Philippon F, Rodés-Cabau J. Permanent pacemaker implantation after transcatheter aortic valve implantation: impact on late clinical outcomes and left ventricular function. Circulation. 2014;129:1233–43.

52. van Gils L, Tchetche D, Lhermusier T, Abawi M, Dumonteil N, Rodriguez Olivares R, et al. Transcatheter heart valve selection and permanent pacemaker implantation in patients with pre-existent right bundle branch block. J Am Heart Assoc. 2017;6(3) https://doi.org/10.1161/JAHA.116.005028.

53. Amat-Santos IJ, Rodes-Cabau J, Urena M, DeLarochelliere R, Doyle D, Bagur R, et al. Incidence, predictive factors, and prognostic value of new-onset atrial fibrillation following transcatheter aortic valve implantation. J Am Coll Cardiol. 2012;59(2):178–88.

54. Durand E, Eltchaninoff H, Canville A, Bouhzam N, Godin M, Tron C, et al. Feasibility and safety of early discharge after transfemoral transcatheter aortic valve implantation with the Edwards SAPIEN-XT prosthesis. Am J Cardiol. 2015;115(8):1116–22.

55. Leclercq F, Iemmi A, Lattuca B, Macia JC, Gervasoni R, Roubille F, et al. Feasibility and safety of transcatheter aortic valve implantation performed without intensive care unit admission. Am J Cardiol. 2016;118(1):99–106.

Radiation Exposure in Transcatheter Aortic Valve Implantation Procedure

34

Florian Stierlin, Nick Ryck, Stéphane Cook, and Jean-Jacques Goy

Abbreviations

ACC	American College of Cardiology
ALARA	As low as reasonably achievable
CA	Coronary angiogram
Gy	Gray
ICRP	International Commission on Radiological Protection
IRP	Interventional reference point
$K_{a,r}$	Cumulative air kerma at the interventional reference point (IRP)
LRA	Left radial access
mSv	Millisievert
NC	Cine angiogram
PCI	Percutaneous intervention
RFA	Right femoral access
RRA	Right radial access
TAVI	Transcatheter aortic valve implantation

34.1 Introduction

Utilization of ionizing radiation in the form of X-rays is mandatory during cardiac interventions such as coronary angiogram (CA) or transcatheter aortic valve implantation (TAVI), also called transcatheter aortic valve replacement (TAVR), procedures and inevitably leads to patient and medical personnel radiation exposure. CA with or without percutaneous intervention (PCI) is more frequently performed than TAVI, but advancements in TAVI are increasing the utilization of this relatively new technique. Initial concerns about patient safety regarding radiation have facilitated equipment improvements and lessened X-ray exposure. Despite these improvements, cardiologists are responsible for 45% of the entire cumulative radiation dose per person per year to the United States population induced by medical sources excluding radiotherapy [1]. Therefore, a major concern for interventional cardiologists must be the avoidance of unjustified or non-optimized radiation use among their patients. More recently, increased incidence of long-term malignancies in interventional cardiologists has raised awareness of medical personnel safety. Despite years of experience in procedures requiring radiation use, improvements in medical staff safety during cardiac procedures such as TAVI are still needed. Our objective is to summarize what is known about radiation exposure for patients and operators, its risks and consequences and the means of protection.

34.2 Measures of Radiation

Radiation exposure leads to potential adverse effects in both patients and medical staff. These risks are usually described as deterministic and

F. Stierlin · N. Ryck · S. Cook · J.-J. Goy (✉)
Hôpital Universitaire Fribourg Switzerland and Clinique Cecil Lausanne, Lausanne, Switzerland
e-mail: jjgoy@goyman.com

© Springer Nature Switzerland AG 2019
A. Giordano et al. (eds.), *Transcatheter Aortic Valve Implantation*,
https://doi.org/10.1007/978-3-030-05912-5_34

stochastic effects [2–4]. The deterministic effect (or tissue reaction) is a direct health dose-dependent effect of radiation exposure and is characterized by a threshold. A threshold is defined as the absorbed dose at which 1% of the population will begin expressing symptoms, and after which this proportion grows dramatically. Examples of deterministic effects are the development of a patient skin burn due to prolonged procedure time (threshold of about 2 Gy of absorbed dose) or cataract formation in doctors (threshold of about 0.5 Gy). Stochastic effects are defined as the biologic effect of radiation that occurs by chance to a specific population. The probability of the effect is linearly proportional to the dose, with a slope of 5% per Sievert (Sv) effective dose, but the severity is independent of the dose [3]. Malignancy development after radiation exposure is an example of stochastic effect, and its severity is independent of the radiation dose, as a cancer induced by a high radiation dose will not be worse than one induced by a smaller dose.

Quantification of the radiation dose is needed to study these adverse effects. During interventions, measurements are usually registered with dosimetry instrumentation such as individual electronic dosimeters which can be placed on almost any body part (e.g., chest, hands, or feet) to quantify localized dose. In order to study and compare patient exposure, standard dose indicators are used. These parameters usually include fluoroscopic time (FT), cumulative air kerma at the interventional reference point IRP ($K_{a,r}$), and cumulated kerma-area product (P_{KA})$K_{a,r}$. FT represents the utilization of fluoroscopy in minutes. Different X-ray imaging modes exist during fluoroscopy in TAVI procedures including cine (or digital) acquisition. Cine mode permits high-contrast/low-noise images but needs a high radiation dose and is usually not included in the FT [5]. Therefore, FT may underestimate the total beam-on time and is often used as an indicator for procedural complexity but not as a patient radiation dose parameter [6]. Kerma, an acronym for "Kinetic Energy Released per unit Mass," quantifies the amount of energy transferred from the impinging ionizing radiation (e.g., X-rays) to

electrons at a given location[1] and is expressed in Joules (J) of energy released in a given mass (kg). A unit of Joules/kg is called a Gray (Gy). The cumulative air kerma measures the quantity of X-ray energy delivered to the air at a predefined reference point, called the "interventional reference point" (IRP). This virtual location, 15 cm from the angiography unit isocenter in the direction of the X-ray focal point, is designed to be located at the entrance of the patient's skin for isocentric procedures, as is the case in interventional cardiology, and is therefore a convenient measure of the risks of deterministic effects. The P_{KA}, expressed in gray-square centimeters ($Gy*cm^2$), is the integral of air kerma over the exposed area. The P_{KA} permits assessment of radiation risks from ionizing procedures (namely, stochastic effect) and is therefore often used to evaluate patient radiation dose. For example, some detailed conversion factors between patient P_{KA} and effective dose have been established [7] such as a generic conversion of approximately 0.2 mSv/($Gy*cm^2$) for the chest region.

CA and PCI are older procedures compared to TAVI and have been more studied regarding radiation dose, thus permitting the development of different protection means. Several studies on patient exposure during TAVI describe a comparable range of radiation between TAVI and PCI or CA [8, 9]. Occupational radiation doses are certainly less investigated, and differences in the number and/or position of physicians and assistants during TAVI procedures in comparison to PCI or CA vary sufficiently to considerably modify radiation exposure. Nonetheless, occupational radiation doses during PCI or CA are more studied and thus provide interesting and applicable information for the operating staff.

---

[1]In the energy range of diagnostic imaging (~10–100 keV), the location at which the electrons are ejected from their atoms and the location where these electrons deposit their energy as absorbed dose are sufficiently close to allow for a gross approximation, i.e., kerma and absorbed dose are numerically considered identical. This is not the case in radiation therapy, where photon energy is in the order of several MeV.

34.3   Radiation Doses

34.3.1   Recommendations

Ionizing radiation and its adverse effects arise from human and natural sources, but the largest man-made source in Western countries is currently due to medical X-ray imaging and nuclear medicine [10]. Coinciding with the rise in therapeutic and diagnostic cardiologic procedures [11], ionizing radiation exposure has doubled during the past two decades [12]. As a protective goal, maximum radiation doses are set for the general population and medical staff by the International Commission on Radiological Protection (ICRP). Those limits are thought to sufficiently protect against deterministic and stochastic effects of radiation. For the general population, a dose of 1 mSv per year (or exceptionally higher for 1 year if the average over 5 years is not more than 1 mSv per year) is tolerated. As a comparison, 1 mSv corresponds to the same amount of radiation as approximately 50 chests X-rays. Recommendations for workers are 20 mSv per year, and specific equivalent doses per year are set for different organs, e.g., 20 mSv per year for eye lens, 500 mSv per year for skin, and 500 mSv per year for extremities (hands, feet) [13]. These limitations are created for planned exposure situations. In regard to patients, no threshold is set for medical interventions or imaging, as radiation exposure is always counterbalanced by the expected benefit of the investigation.

34.4   Exposure During TAVI Procedures

34.4.1   Patients

A prospective study in 2012 involving 105 TAVI patients among whom 79 underwent a transfemoral approach and 26 a transapical approach compares patient exposure during this procedure [8]. Radiation doses were measured by dosimetry instrumentation attached to the fluoroscope and analyzed using P_{KA}. Results showed a median radiation dose for all patients of 188 Gy*cm^2

which is within a reasonable range in comparison to other cardiologic percutaneous interventions. The authors concluded that deterministic side effects for patients were unlikely within this range of radiation. They suggest that clinical cancers due to radiation exposure are probably lower in patients undergoing TAVI than PCI. In fact, even though the amount of radiation used in TAVI and PCI procedures is similar, TAVI is performed in a patient population approximately two decades older than PCI patients thus reducing the time to develop symptomatic radiogenic cancer. They also found that patients with higher body mass index and therefore higher body weight received higher radiation doses [14]. This observation is explained by the larger amount of radiation needed in obese patients to obtain proper imaging. Interestingly, lower radiation doses and FT with a transapical approach in comparison to a transfemoral approach were also reported. This observation was probably due to extra FT needed to access and close the right femoral artery compared to the surgical access of a transapical approach and to the included occurrence of two vascular complications during transfemoral approaches which prolonged FT time.

More recently, data on patient exposure was collected in eight Swiss centers during numerous cardiac procedures such as CA (with or without PCI), defibrillator implantation, and TAVI. For TAVI only, a total of 221 patients were analyzed and compared to PCI procedures. The following parameters were recorded: $K_{a,r}$ in mGy, number of images, P_{KA} in Gy*cm^2, and fluoroscopy time (FT) [15]. The P_{KA} during TAVI was 55 ± 33 Gy*cm^2 and is approximately similar to the dose delivered during PCI. However, as shown in Fig. 34.1, a particularity during TAVI is the presence of a second peak of radiation at 130 Gy*cm^2 that is not found in PCI procedures. This higher radiation exposure is likely due to the greater complexity of the TAVI intervention. Of course, PCI procedures may also have elevated complexity but typically never reach the same level of difficulty as TAVI.

The cumulative air kerma, in this case the total dose of radiation received by the patient during TAVI or PCI time, is shown in Fig. 34.2. It is

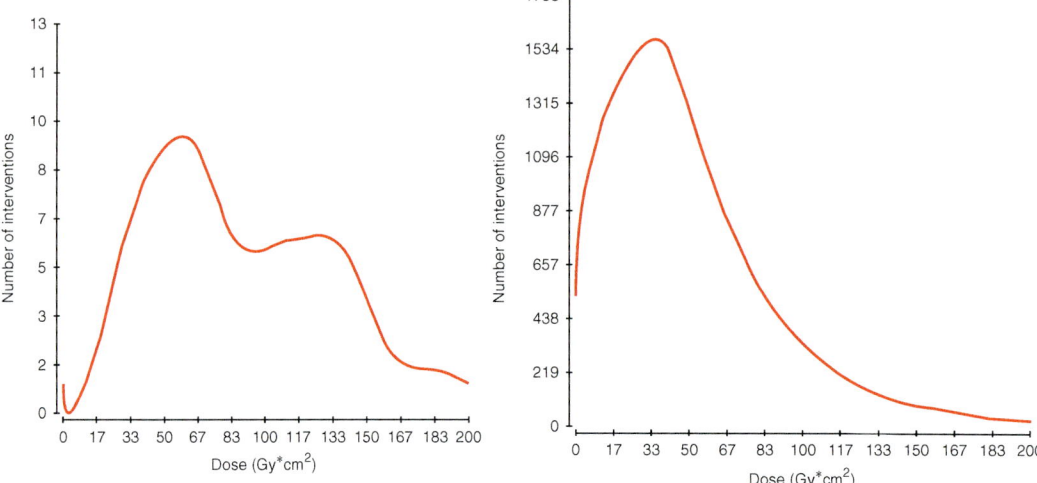

Fig. 34.1 Dose area product in Gy*cm². This graph shows two curves: on the left the curve of TAVI procedures and on the right the curve of PCI procedures in Switzerland. There are two peaks for the TAVI proce-

dures. The first peak around 55 Gy*cm² is very similar to the one obtained during PCI. The second peak is around 130 Gy*cm² and reflects higher radiation exposition during more complex procedures

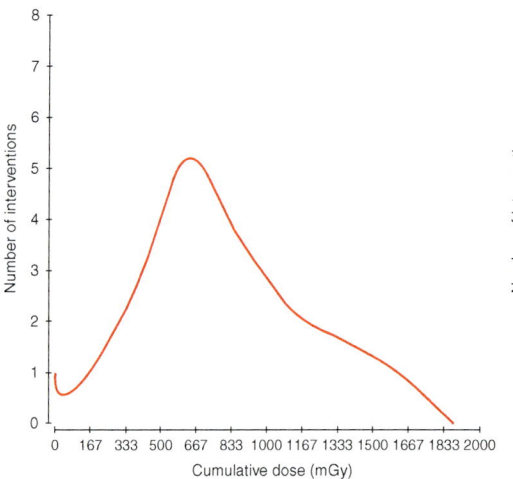

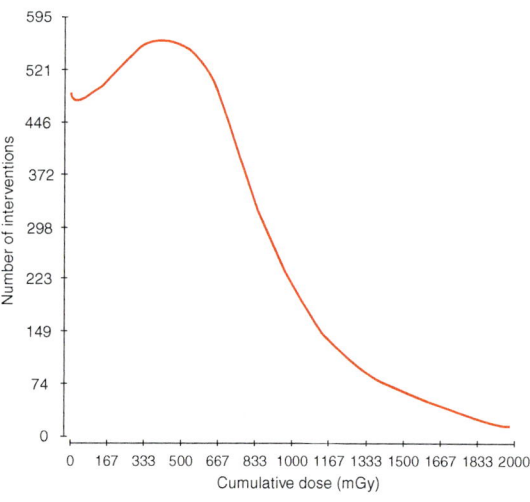

Fig. 34.2 Cumulative air kerma ($K_{a,r}$) in milligray. This graph shows two curves: on the left, the curve of the TAVI procedures and on the right the curve of PCI procedures in Switzerland. The mean cumulative dose is very similar for

the 2 procedures with a slightly lower, but not significant, dose for PCI. Complex procedures induced higher cumulative dose

similar during the two procedures, with slightly but not significantly lower dose for PCI than TAVI ($p = 0.3$).

Fluoroscopy time measured in minutes, as represented in Fig. 34.3, was higher during TAVI procedures. As previously explained, FT is often used to compare procedural complexity. This

observation is compatible with the higher complexity of TAVI, already seen in Fig. 34.1.

Figure 34.4 shows the number of images done during the two procedures. For TAVI, the mean number of images is 620 ± 350 and is significantly lower than for PCI with 980 ± 380 images ($p < 0.05$). The number of images does not reflect

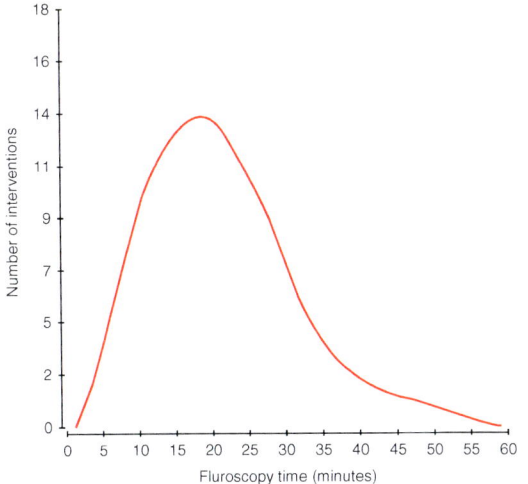

Fig. 34.3 Fluoroscopy time (FT) in minutes. This graph shows two curves: on the left, the curve of FT during TAVI procedures and, on the right, the curve of FT during PCI procedures in Switzerland. The FT during TAVI procedures is longer reflecting the greater complexity of the latter

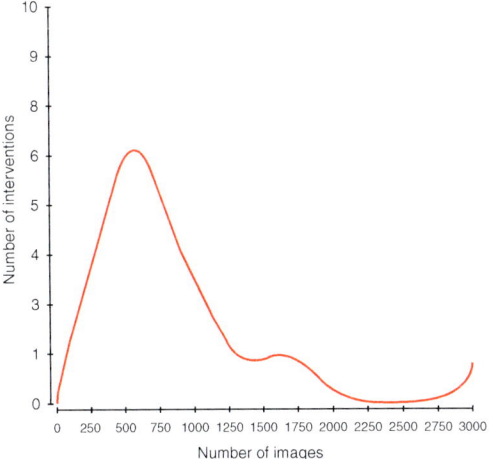

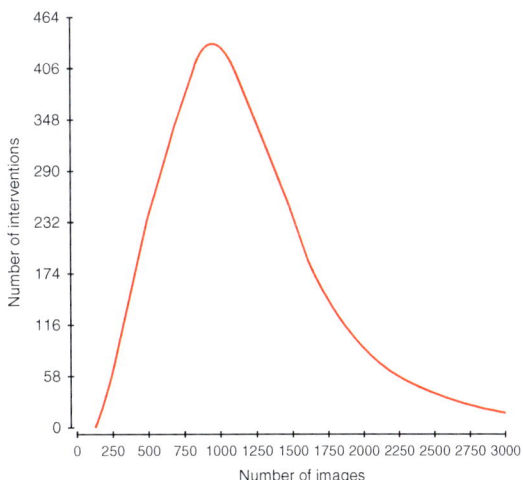

Fig. 34.4 Number of images. This graph shows two curves: on the left, the curve of the TAVI procedure and on the right the curve of PCI procedures in Switzerland. The mean number of images is significantly lower for TAVI (620 images) than for PCI (980 images) ($p < 0.001$)

the radiation dose. In fact, this is influenced principally by the differing utilization of fluoroscopy time and cineradiography time. During TAVI, the use of cineradiography is preferred, which requires more contrast medium and therefore more radiation. During PCI, fluoroscopic X-ray imaging without contrast agent is more typical.

Overall occupational radiation exposure during cardiac interventions and TAVI.

In 2008, an analysis of several PubMed studies reviewing different cardiac interventions (diagnostic catheterizations, PCI, ablations, or pacemaker/defibrillator implantations) was conducted and reported effective radiation doses between 0.02 and 31.2 μSv/procedure. Equivalent extremity doses ranged between 50 and 4160 μSv/procedure [16] raising concerns about extremity radiation exposure. Due to proximity with the primary beam, a left-sided predominance of radiation to the operator was noted. Also, the authors mentioned considerable difficulty in comparing results as dosimetry methods were not standardized in the different studies and multiple cofactors influenced radiation doses.

A previous study in 2011 aimed to compare occupational radiation doses during two different methods of TAVI, namely, transfemoral and transapical approaches [17]. Dosimeters were used on the chest of all staff, on the hands and feet of the cardiothoracic surgeons and cardiologists, and on the eyes of the cardiothoracic surgeon. Significantly higher total body radiation doses were observed for the cardiothoracic surgeon, including measured doses at the hands, eyes, and feet during the transapical approach (reported doses of 0.03 mSv) as opposed to the transfemoral approach (reported doses of 0.003 mSv). Their explanation for this higher dose was proximity with the X-ray beam and a lack of protection above the table in order to facilitate the surgeon's access to the apex of the heart. The most prominent observation was the elevated radiation dose endured by the left hand of the cardiothoracic surgeon during transapical approach (almost 2 mSv per procedure). With 500 mSv/year tolerated on the extremities, 250 transapical TAVI procedures per year would be the maximal limit. On the contrary, no significant total body radiation difference in the transapical vs. transfemoral approach was noted for the cardiologists; however both hands were significantly more irradiated during the transapical (0.08 mSv for the left and 0.09 mSv for the right) than the transfemoral approach (0.03 mSv for the left and 0.01 mSv for the right). Of note, the occupational radiation doses in this study are similar to the doses reported by Kim et al. during other cardiac interventions.

A publication from our group sought to compare occupational radiation doses during CA and CA followed by PCI, regarding different access locations, right femoral access (RFA), right radial access (RRA), and left radial access (LRA). The study included 830 consecutives procedures with 457 CA and 373 CA followed by ad hoc PCI [18]. Radiation exposure was measured using individual chest dosimeters with several parameters recorded such as operator cumulative dose ($K_{a,r}$), FT, number of cine angiogram (NC), and the P_{KA}-normalized $K_{a,r}$, defined as the dose (mSv) received by the operator with each Gy*cm^2 applied to the patient. Most procedures (55%) were performed using RFA, 33% used RRA, and 12% used LRA. Access choice was operator dependent. The conclusions of this non-randomized single center study were as follows: a lower degree of radiation is achieved for the cardiologist when performing CA or CA and PCI using RFA rather than RRA and similarly using LRA rather than RRA. These results are consistent with the literature as transradial access is known to increase operator radiation exposure [19]. Explanations for this observation are proximity to the X-ray beam and the patient (a source of scattered radiation to the operator) and in this particular study, the presence of an increased radioprotection gap between the leaded glass mobile and the patient table to facilitate RRA. Finally, despite less operator radiation exposure, RFA seems to display a higher complexity as shown by increased NC in comparison to RRA and LRA (but with no significant difference in FT). With TAVI being performed mostly via right femoral access, these results are somewhat reassuring.

The abovementioned publication also sought to analyze occupational exposure specifically from one center. These results showed an air kerma dose of 249 Gy for medical staff with a FT time of 9 min 35 s and a P_{KA} of 36.55 Gy*cm^2. These FT and P_{KA} are lower than usual and are positively influenced by the experience of the operators. Cardiologists working in this center are all well trained on TAVI intervention, thus promoting shorter procedure times and, therefore, reduced radiation exposure.

34.5   Discussion

Contemporary literature shows a comparable radiation exposure for patients during TAVI vs. other cardiac interventions such as CA. Most importantly, this exposure is shown to be in a safe range. However, deterministic and stochastic effects exist. For patients, deterministic effects range from erythema to more severe permanent skin damage [20] as well as hair loss [2]. These reactions occur when a threshold is exceeded and causes a change in tissue, predominately cell death [21]. For erythema, a dose of about 2Gy is thought to be sufficient, whereas a higher dose of 5Gy is needed before long-term skin damage occurs [22].

Stochastic effect, namely, cancer development, is more difficult to study as the latency period can be years and complicates the analysis. Ionizing radiation is known to directly alter DNA or to induce radical hydroxyl formation through water molecule ionization which then leads to DNA damage. If unrepaired, this damage can favor cancer development [23]. Studies on radiation exposure conducted in several exposed groups such as Japanese atomic bomb survivors or other medically or environmentally exposed populations have established a clear causative link between radiation exposure and cancer induction at doses above 50 mSv [24]. For lower doses, the cancer risk remains difficult to estimate. The limit of >50 mSv can be reached with some cardiologic procedures such as myocardial perfusion imaging [25] and also during TAVI, where a median P_{KA} of 188 Gy*cm² has been reported [8]. Furthermore, repetitive cardiac procedures and/or combinations with other medical imaging can accumulate to finally reach this threshold and must therefore be considered.

Occupational radiation is a more recent but equally significant concern. With lifelong radiation exposure, the risk of deterministic and stochastic adverse effects for cardiologists is among the highest in medical practice. Here again, estimation of the development of adverse effects due to occupational radiation is not simple, but impact on the health of interventional cardiologists has been reported regarding several organs, mainly the brain and eyes. The effect of radiation on other organs obviously exists but is not specific to interventional cardiology.

Concern about occupational radiation was first raised in 1998 with a case report of two Canadian cardiologists displaying brain tumors [26]. The possible causative link was reinforced in 2012 by another case report of brain tumors in four interventional cardiologists [27] with more described cases following afterward [28]. Interestingly, the majority of these brain tumors were left-sided coinciding with the known sidedness of radiation exposure [29]. Along with brain tumors, a higher incidence of cataracts has been shown by a French multicenter observational study in 2013 [30]. This study compared interventional cardiologists to an unexposed control group of nonmedical workers and showed a significant increased risk of posterior subcapsular cataracts among cardiologists. Despite being the least common of age-related cataracts, posterior subcapsular cataracts are proven to be the most frequent type associated with ionizing radiation exposure [1]. Due to the increase in interventional cardiology, an exposure per person per year two to three times higher than in radiologists has been reported among cardiologists [31].

The majority of actual literature concentrates on occupational radiation exposure during CA with or without PCI and is less focused on TAVI procedures. However, it is generally seen that operator as well as patient exposure is similar during TAVI and PCI and both stay in an acceptable range. Ever-increasing cardiac procedures and medical imaging may lead to severe adverse effects, mainly stochastic. Unfortunately, difficulties in standardizing dose measurement and estimating long-term cancer risk, as well as high intra-operator variability, hamper literature clarity. Nonetheless, radiation protection for both patients and operators include several means and techniques which are proven effective and must definitely be used.

34.5.1 Recommendations for TAVI Procedures Regarding Radiation Protection

Diverse methods and techniques have been proposed to lessen X-ray exposure. In order to protect the population against ionizing radiation due to medical exposure, the Council of Ministers approved the European directive which is simply referred as the ALARA principle [32]. This acronym stands for "As Low As Reasonably Achievable" and is based on the principle that no absolutely safe radiation dose exists. As suggested by the name, the ALARA principle aims for the optimum diagnostic efficacy coinciding with the lowest radiation exposure possible and the reduction of unnecessary use of ionizing radiation. No fixed radiation threshold exists, but a plan counterbalancing the risks and benefits must be considered before any intervention requiring ionizing radiation.

In conjunction with the ALARA principle, several methods and techniques have been developed to specifically reduce patient and operator exposure during interventional cardiology. These were studied during various cardiac interventions, not specifically for TAVI procedures, but can logically be translated to all cardiac procedures. While some of these methods permit reductions for both patient and operator, others are more specific to either patient or operator protection alone.

For patients, minimizing fluoroscopic and acquisition time is, of course, the first step. However, additional proven techniques include variation of the beam angle to avoid prolonged exposure to the same skin area [33], increasing table height to maximize the distance between the patient and the X-ray source [34] and keeping the patient's arms out of the beam as this can deliver high radiation doses. In order to minimize the patient's skin area exposed and to limit scattered radiation, the patient should always be kept close to the detector [34]. The utilization of steep angles of the radiation beam is also known to favor scattered radiation and needs to be avoided or minimized [35]. As previously mentioned, different acquisition modes exist during cardiologic interventions with various degrees of radiation exposure. In order to minimize radiation exposure, a comparison between two modes, namely, digital acquisition or "cine" angiography and fluoroscopy with last fluoroscopic hold (LFH), has been studied during coronary angiogram [5]. LFH is a mode where the last image is automatically stored and shown on the monitor, therefore decreasing the need of continuous fluoroscopy. LFH in comparison to cine mode permits a decrease in radiation exposure. A remaining problem is the lower diagnostic quality of the fluoroscopic LFH images when compared to cine coronary angiography, a problem that could be solved with improvement in the

new angiographic systems. Some newer devices store the last fluoroscopy run in a buffer memory that could potentially be stored instead of performing a cineradiography sequence, thus sparing substantial skin dose, as the dose rates between fluoroscopy and cineradiography differ by a factor of approximately 10. Other simple radiological techniques such as decreasing the frame rate of fluoroscopy or cine [36, 37] or replacing the use of magnification modes by using software magnification algorithms that allow zoom without necessitating more radiation [36] also permit reduced radiation exposure. Finally, both the American College of Cardiology (ACC) and the ICRP recommend monitoring of radiation dose with dosimeters to avoid exceeding the safe range and to incorporate feedback on radiation exposure [38].

For medical staff, utilization of appropriate personal protection garments, including a full suit, a thyroid collar [39], and head protection [29], is of paramount importance. Although adverse orthopedic effects caused by the weight of these devices have been reported [40], lighter aprons are being studied. Development of cataracts may be prevented by wearing lead-lined glasses during interventions [41]. Depending on the use of radial or femoral access, a protective shield and/or drape between the operator and the patient will further help reduce operator radiation exposure [42]. Similar to patient recommendations, it is essential for operators to keep extremities free of the ionizing beam and to maximize the distance between themselves, the ionizing ray source, and the patient in order to protect against scattered radiation. Scattered radiation is a known source of incidental procedural radiation and affects both the operating staff and patient areas not directly inside the primary X-ray beam [33].

34.6 Conclusion

Medical use of ionizing radiation is of paramount importance in the modern practice of medicine and will likely continue to increase in the near future. While the benefit of procedures requiring radiation often exceeds the potentially harmful effects, attention must be given to the consequences of repetitive radiation exposure to patients as well as to healthcare professionals. While the TAVI procedure is a relatively new technique, the side effects and quantification of radiation exposure in this intervention is less studied and is hampered by a lack of standardization and intra-operator variability. However, a review of current literature indicates that the radiation exposure for both patient and operator is similar to a coronary angiogram and is therefore in a safe range. As concern over radiation exposure has grown, simple methods to protect both patient and medical staff have been developed and must be followed imperatively. Well-trained cardiologists benefit from higher procedural speed thus realizing a reduction of radiation exposure. Accordingly, recent increases in interventional cardiology and a growing number of TAVI procedures should foster improvement in cardiologist's technical skills. Moreover, in the near future TAVI procedures will surely be widened to a younger and healthier population, thus facilitating improvements in the procedure itself leading to reduced procedural times. Finally, technical progress with radiological materials can also contribute to diminishing radiation exposure for both patient and medical staff.

In conclusion, TAVI procedures expose patient and medical staff to radiation and its subsequent risks. Operators seem to be more at risk through repetitive exposures as opposed to patients, but use of several simple protections means and following recommendations regarding X-ray material utilization will help keep radiation exposure in a safe range. Progress with radiology materials in addition to improvements in cardiologist's technical skills will further help decrease the radiation exposure inherent in TAVI procedures.

Conflict of Interest None.

References

1. Picano E, Vano E. The radiation issue in cardiology: the time for action is now. Cardiovasc Ultrasound. 2011;9:35.
2. Balter S, Hopewell JW, Miller DL, Wagner LK, Zelefsky MJ. Fluoroscopically guided interventional procedures: a review of radiation effects on patients' skin and hair. Radiology. 2010;254(2):326–41.
3. Chambers CE, Fetterly KA, Holzer R, Lin PJ, Blankenship JC, Balter S, et al. Radiation safety program for the cardiac catheterization laboratory. Catheter Cardiovasc Interv. 2011;77(4):546–56.
4. Little MP. Risks associated with ionizing radiation. Br Med Bull. 2003;68:259–75.
5. Olcay A, Guler E, Karaca IO, Omaygenc MO, Kizilirmak F, Olgun E, et al. Comparison of fluoro and cine coronary angiography: balancing acceptable outcomes with a reduction in radiation dose. J Invasive Cardiol. 2015;27(4):199–202.
6. Padovani R, Bernardi G, Malisan MR, Vano E, Morocutti G, Fioretti PM. Patient dose related to the complexity of interventional cardiology procedures. Radiat Prot Dosimetry. 2001;94(1–2):189–92.
7. Struelens L, Vanhavere F, Bacher K, Thierens H. DAP to effective dose conversion in cardiology and vascular/interventional radiology: FANC/SCK/UGent; 2009.
8. Daneault B, Balter S, Kodali SK, Williams MR, Genereux P, Reiss GR, et al. Patient radiation exposure during transcatheter aortic valve replacement procedures. EuroIntervention. 2012;8(6):679–84.
9. Sharma D, Ramsewak A, O'Conaire S, Manoharan G, Spence MS. Reducing radiation exposure during transcatheter aortic valve implantation (TAVI). Catheter Cardiovasc Interv. 2015;85(7):1256–61.
10. Mettler FA Jr, Bhargavan M, Faulkner K, Gilley DB, Gray JE, Ibbott GS, et al. Radiologic and nuclear medicine studies in the United States and worldwide: frequency, radiation dose, and comparison with other radiation sources—1950–2007. Radiology. 2009;253(2):520–31.
11. Picano E, Vano E, Rehani MM, Cuocolo A, Mont L, Bodi V, et al. The appropriate and justified use of medical radiation in cardiovascular imaging: a position document of the ESC associations of cardiovascular imaging, percutaneous cardiovascular interventions and electrophysiology. Eur Heart J. 2014;35(10):665–72.
12. Food And Drug Administration US. White paper: initiative to reduce unnecessary radiation exposure from medical imaging. 2010.
13. The 2007 Recommendations of the International Commission on Radiological Protection. ICRP publication 103. Ann ICRP. 2007;37(2–4):1–332.
14. Fetterly KA, Lennon RJ, Bell MR, Holmes DR Jr, Rihal CS. Clinical determinants of radiation dose in percutaneous coronary interventional procedures: influence of patient size, procedure complexity, and performing physician. JACC Cardiovasc Interv. 2011;4(3):336–43.
15. Ryckx N, Goy JJ, Stauffer JC, Verdun FR. Patient dose assessment after interventional cardiology procedures: a multi-centric approach to trigger optimisation. Radiat Prot Dosimetry. 2016;169(1–4):249–52.
16. Kim KP, Miller DL, Balter S, Kleinerman RA, Linet MS, Kwon D, et al. Occupational radiation doses to operators performing cardiac catheterization procedures. Health Phys. 2008;94(3):211–27.
17. Sauren LD, van Garsse L, van Ommen V, Kemerink GJ. Occupational radiation dose during transcatheter

aortic valve implantation. Catheter Cardiovasc Interv. 2011;78(5):770–6.

18. Kallinikou Z, Puricel SG, Ryckx N, Togni M, Baeriswyl G, Stauffer JC, et al. Radiation exposure of the operator during coronary interventions (from the RADIO study). Am J Cardiol. 2016;118(2):188–94.

19. Lange HW, von Boetticher H. Randomized comparison of operator radiation exposure during coronary angiography and intervention by radial or femoral approach. Catheter Cardiovasc Interv. 2006;67(1):12–6.

20. Rehani MM, Srimahachota S. Skin injuries in interventional procedures. Radiat Prot Dosimetry. 2011;147(1–2):8–12.

21. Stewart FA, Akleyev AV, Hauer-Jensen M, Hendry JH, Kleiman NJ, Macvittie TJ, et al. ICRP publication 118: ICRP statement on tissue reactions and early and late effects of radiation in normal tissues and organs—threshold doses for tissue reactions in a radiation protection context. Ann ICRP. 2012;41(1–2):1–322.

22. Abbott JD. Controlling radiation exposure in interventional cardiology. Circ Cardiovasc Interv. 2014;7(4):425–8.

23. Brenner DJ, Hall EJ. Computed tomography—an increasing source of radiation exposure. N Engl J Med. 2007;357(22):2277–84.

24. National Research Council US. Health risks from exposure to low levels of ionizing radiation: BEIR VII phase 2. Washington, DC: The National Academies Press; 2006.

25. Einstein AJ, Weiner SD, Bernheim A, Kulon M, Bokhari S, Johnson LL, et al. Multiple testing, cumulative radiation dose, and clinical indications in patients undergoing myocardial perfusion imaging. JAMA. 2010;304(19):2137–44.

26. Finkelstein MM. Is brain cancer an occupational disease of cardiologists? Can J Cardiol. 1998;14(11):1385–8.

27. Roguin A, Goldstein J, Bar O. Brain tumours among interventional cardiologists: a cause for alarm? Report of four new cases from two cities and a review of the literature. EuroIntervention. 2012;7(9):1081–6.

28. Roguin A, Goldstein J, Bar O, Goldstein JA. Brain and neck tumors among physicians performing interventional procedures. Am J Cardiol. 2013;111(9):1368–72.

29. Reeves RR, Ang L, Bahadorani J, Naghi J, Dominguez A, Palakodeti V, et al. Invasive cardiologists are exposed to greater left sided cranial radiation: the BRAIN study (BRAIN radiation exposure and attenuation during invasive cardiology procedures). JACC Cardiovasc Interv. 2015;8(9):1197–206.

30. Jacob S, Boveda S, Bar O, Brezin A, Maccia C, Laurier D, et al. Interventional cardiologists and risk of radiation-induced cataract: results of a French multicenter observational study. Int J Cardiol. 2013;167(5):1843–7.

31. Miller DL, Vano E, Bartal G, Balter S, Dixon R, Padovani R, et al. Occupational radiation protec-

tion in interventional radiology: a joint guideline of the Cardiovascular and Interventional Radiology Society of Europe and the Society of Interventional Radiology. J Vasc Interv Radiol. 2010;21(5):607–15.

32. Teunen D. The European directive on health protection of individuals against the dangers of ionising radiation in relation to medical exposures (97/43/EURATOM). J Radiol Prot. 1998;18(2):133–7.

33. Hirshfeld JW Jr, Balter S, Brinker JA, Kern MJ, Klein LW, Lindsay BD, et al. ACCF/AHA/HRS/SCAI clinical competence statement on physician knowledge to optimize patient safety and image quality in fluoroscopically guided invasive cardiovascular procedures: a report of the American College of Cardiology Foundation/American Heart Association/American College of Physicians Task Force on Clinical Competence and Training. Circulation. 2005;111(4):511–32.

34. Perisinakis K, Damilakis J, Theocharopoulos N, Manios E, Vardas P, Gourtsoyiannis N. Accurate assessment of patient effective radiation dose and associated detriment risk from radiofrequency catheter ablation procedures. Circulation. 2001;104(1):58–62.

35. Agarwal S, Parashar A, Bajaj NS, Khan I, Ahmad I, Heupler FA Jr, et al. Relationship of beam angulation and radiation exposure in the cardiac catheterization laboratory. JACC Cardiovasc Interv. 2014;7(5):558–66.

36. Pantos I, Patatoukas G, Katritsis DG, Efstathopoulos E. Patient radiation doses in interventional cardiology procedures. Curr Cardiol Rev. 2009;5(1):1–11.

37. Weiss EM, Thabit O. Clinical considerations for allied professionals: radiation safety and protection in the electrophysiology lab. Heart Rhythm. 2007;4(12):1583–7.

38. Limacher MC, Douglas PS, Germano G, Laskey WK, Lindsay BD, McKetty MH, et al. ACC expert consensus document. Radiation safety in the practice of cardiology. American College of Cardiology. J Am Coll Cardiol. 1998;31(4):892–913.

39. Vano E. Radiation exposure to cardiologists: how it could be reduced. Heart. 2003;89(10):1123–4.

40. Klein LW, Tra Y, Garratt KN, Powell W, Lopez-Cruz G, Chambers C, et al. Occupational health hazards of interventional cardiologists in the current decade: results of the 2014 SCAI membership survey. Catheter Cardiovasc Interv. 2015;86(5):913–24.

41. Vano E, Kleiman NJ, Duran A, Romano-Miller M, Rehani MM. Radiation-associated lens opacities in catheterization personnel: results of a survey and direct assessments. J Vasc Interv Radiol. 2013;24(2):197–204.

42. Gilligan P, Lynch J, Eder H, Maguire S, Fox E, Doyle B, et al. Assessment of clinical occupational dose reduction effect of a new interventional cardiology shield for radial access combined with a scatter reducing drape. Catheter Cardiovasc Interv. 2015;86(5):935–40.

Procedure Efficiency in Transcatheter Aortic Valve Implantation

35

Sandeep M. Patel, Yasuhiro Ichibori, Angela Davis, and Guilherme F. Attizzani

35.1 Introduction

Transcatheter aortic valve implantation (TAVI), also called transcatheter aortic valve replacement (TAVR), represents a major advance in the management of native and bioprosthetic aortic stenosis. In its infancy, the procedure was primarily surgically dominated, but as the field evolved, it became clear that a hybrid approach between interventionalists and surgeons was necessary for a safe, effective, and optimal outcome. While the procedure can be daunting to those new to transcatheter valve replacement, the vast majority of experienced operators have been able to tailor and trim the procedure to the essential elements necessary for excellent clinical outcomes. The learning curve of TAVR is one that is based on experience, anxiety, procedural unknowns, and the relative novelty of a such an innovative proce-

dure. It is clear that with increased case-based, practical experience, a "TAVR program" is an inevitable product which ultimately stands to be the basis for all future TAVR procedures. With a "program" the pain points and achievements become notable and are the factors that drive it to either failure or success. From multiple registry data (US and European), there are clear observations that can help mitigate future disappointments and promote best practices. This chapter serves to highlight the most important aspects of TAVR that drive procedural efficiency.

35.2 The Valve Coordinators and the Valve Clinic

The idea that a coordinator for TAVR is a necessary aspect for performing TAVR was a novel concept to the field of interventional cardiology, as many high-risk and complex procedures were being performed on a routine basis with the standard of care being a physician-driven process. It is not the complexity of the TAVR procedure that drives the need for valve coordinators but instead the TAVR process. The process of TAVR does not only involve the procedure, but it begins from the time the patient enters the clinic to the 1-year post-TAVR follow-up and everything in between. Coordinators screen patients, schedule evaluations, collect pre-evaluation testing, ensure appropriate lab work, arrange for the pre-procedural invasive and computed tomographic angiographic evaluations,

S. M. Patel (✉)
Structural Heart Center, St. Rita's Medical Center-Mercy Health, Lima, OH, USA
e-mail: smpatel@mercy.com

Y. Ichibori
Division of Cardiovascular Medicine,
Osaka University Graduate School of Medicine,
Osaka, Japan

A. Davis · G. F. Attizzani
The Valve and Structural Heart Disease Intervention Center, University Hospitals, Cleveland Medical Center, Cleveland, OH, USA
e-mail: angela.davis@uhhospitals.org;
guilherme.attizzani@uhhospitals.org

© Springer Nature Switzerland AG 2019
A. Giordano et al. (eds.), *Transcatheter Aortic Valve Implantation*,
https://doi.org/10.1007/978-3-030-05912-5_35

evaluate nursing, dental, fragility, and psychosocial needs, as well as coordinate procedure scheduling and post-procedure follow-ups [1–5]. Additionally, this person typically takes the lead on presenting patients at the combined heart team meetings and is intimately involved with patients and families to help answer questions and alleviate angst. Thus, the valve coordinator serves as a prime fulcrum for procedural efficiency as they understand all of the cohesive elements necessary for a successful valve implantation and are constantly working toward the goal from the moment of patient referral.

The valve clinic is one that is a multispeciality clinic involving all members of the valve heart team. Typically, interventional cardiologists and cardiothoracic surgeons who perform TAVR should independently evaluate the patients during the same visit and collectively review the necessary data to ensure that the most appropriate management pathway is undertaken. The focus of the valve clinic should not be TAVR vs. SAVR but instead should be AVR or no AVR, and then the work-up is to ensue based on clinical, laboratory, and imaging to provide an optimal replacement strategy. The valve clinic can and should include heart failure specialists, imaging cardiologists, and, if available geriatricians, social workers, palliative care, physiatrists, and psychiatric experts [1–5]. A view from each of these perspectives can provide new insights into the patient and the management pathway that takes a holistic approach to AVR. Depending on the needs of the patient, specialists from other disciplines may be consulted such as nephrology, hematology/oncology, pulmonology, etc. to formulate a well-rounded "game plan" for the patient. Preemptively determining and educating the entire team on the factors that may complicate intraprocedural elements can improve the efficiency of the procedure and reduce complications.

35.3 Pre-procedural CTA Evaluation

Patient selection for TAVR is a major determinant in procedural efficiency. In order to ensure success, the importance of procedural planning in terms of access approach, aortic annulus sizing, choice of prosthesis, preimplantation valvuloplasty, and the anatomy of the iliofemoral arterial system and the aortic arch are key determinants to optimal prosthesis implantation. Multislice, gated, computed tomography provides the most comprehensive noninvasive evaluation of the aortic valve in order to evaluate the anatomic parameters necessary for TAVR [4, 6]. The three-dimensional imaging is the gold standard for pre-TAVR imaging and comprehending the aortic valve, coronary anatomy, peripheral vasculature, and surrounding structures. Dedicated and standardized imaging interpretation is necessary for all TAVR operators and helps improve efficiency by allowing for prediction of access issues, need for specialized sheaths, preimplantation peripheral intervention, and the use of specialized guidewires for valve advancement and for evaluating the type of valve most appropriate for implantation [2, 3, 7–11]. Coronary heights, sino-tubular or left ventricular outflow tract calcification, narrow sinuses of Valsalva, bicuspid aortic leaflets, and abnormal aortoventricular angle all can affect the decision between using a self-expanding and balloon-expandable prosthesis [2–4, 7–11]. Of note, three-dimensional magnetic resonance imaging can provide similar assessment but requires time and may be contraindicated in those with metallic implants, pacemakers, or claustrophobia [12–14]. Review of the imaging can help operators prep their teams with specific approaches, instruct on bailout equipment, and ensure all team members' expectations are set to ensure a smooth, predictable procedure [4].

35.4 Heart Team Approach

Risk assessment represents a pivotal element of TAVR. As TAVR is currently indicated for intermediate-, high-, and prohibitive-risk surgical patients and is currently being studied in low-risk patients, understanding the definition of "risk" is of paramount importance. Multiple risk scores and models have been used for cardiac surgery mortality. In the current era of TAVR, the two most common patient scoring systems include the EuroSCORE and the STS-PROM [1, 4].

The current state of literature suggests that the STS-PROM more closely approximates the operative and long-term mortality for high-risk patients undergoing AVR [15]. Further, certain incremental risk factors including frailty, chronic lung disease, chronic liver disease, and nutritional status may elevate patient's risks as not captured by the standard method of STS-PROM and EuroSCORE. These scores and risk models are not absolutes for determining TAVR criteria and henceforth require contextual understanding of the patient's candidacy for TAVR—heart team approach [1–5]. Input from the various care providers regarding the patient's physical, emotional, and social anatomy in conjunction with risk assessment for operative mortality can help select appropriate patients to benefit from TAVR and thus ensure procedural efficiency.

35.5 Procedure

On the day of the procedure, multiple steps can be taken to improve the overall flow of the patient from pre-procedure admission to post-procedural care. The valve coordinator should be communicating with patients, families, and caregivers to set expectations of pre-procedural lab work and post-discharge care to home or skilled nursing facilities. Once brought to the pre-procedural holding area, a supine transthoracic echocardiogram can provide a baseline study for comparison and ensures that the echocardiographer is familiar with the patient's acoustic windows to be able to repeat imaging on the procedural table. Thereafter, the patient is assessed by the primary implanter and if part of the procedural team, anesthesia services. Avoiding pre-TAVR insertions of central venous catheters, arterial lines, and urinary catheters helps to save time and facilitates "loading" of the patient onto the procedure table, which in turns facilitates sterile prep. Prior research in this area has demonstrated that procedural outcomes are similar without these instruments and does not compromise patient safety [16].

With the current state of TAVR, the majority of procedures are being performed via a transfemoral route [17]. In cases where there is a need

for alternative access (subclavian/axillary, carotid, transcaval, and transapical), the bulk of these procedures require the use of a hybrid operating room, general anesthesia, and surgical access site exposure. However, given that a number of centers are attempting to focus on transfemoral access, the decision for type of anesthesia becomes a major factor in procedural efficiency.

Of note, as transfemoral TAVR has become almost as standard as cardiac catheterization, a trend toward performing the procedure without intubation and general anesthesia has become popular. In certain TAVR centers, the term minimalist approach TAVR (MAT) has become a standard of care [16]. In the MAT setting, the procedure is performed in a standard cardiac catheterization laboratory, using local anesthesia and mild conscious sedation, without transesophageal echocardiography and endotracheal intubation or the need for a perfusion team or a primed heart-lung bypass machine. The study of this approach, although non-randomized data, via the TVT/STS registry has shown that this approach improves efficiency, cost ratios, and resource utilization and maintains patient safety and excellent procedural outcomes [18–20]. The concept of avoiding intraprocedural TEE has also been a point of contention between TAVR operators, but again prior work in this area demonstrates that the avoidance of TEE does not promote poorer outcomes and in fact delivers similar results and prevents the usage of deep sedation which may result in fluctuations in hemodynamics, necessitate intubation, and complicate the overall implantation [21, 22].

If a percutaneous approach is feasible, the anesthetic management with MAT is typically with the use of standard analgesia and anxiolytics administered under physician supervision via procedural nurses. It is important to note that advanced anesthetic management using monitored-anesthesia care (MAC) or general anesthesia (GA) is evaluated on a case-by-case basis during the heart team approach and planned prior to the patient arriving to the procedural suite. Patient-specific factors including severe respiratory disease, severe anxiety, the need for higher doses of medications, hemodynamic status, procedural complexity, and patient preference are typical reasons for requiring advanced anesthetic support. However, typically, a combination of the above and the overall clinical picture along with patient safety drives the need for advanced anesthetic support.

Once in the procedural suite, a team approach for preparation of the patient should be undertaken. Roles should be clearly defined, and only necessary team members should be present in the room to minimize confusion in tasks. We suggest a pre-procedural planning blueprint that is posted in the room for all members of the team to see. This document may be heart team specific and provides the salient points of the patient's key clinical history, CTA measurements, procedural plan, and bailout strategies to prepare all team members prior to access (Fig. 35.1).

Once sterile prep has been completed, typically, we begin with the insertion of a right internal jugular transvenous pacemaker (TVP), followed by the non-primary access site, and then the pre-closed, large bore primary access site. The TVP is typically inserted via 6–7Fr standard sheath that allows for central venous infusion of medications while maintaining access for the TVP. Given that the coplanar angle is pre-calculated from CT imaging, we perform aortic root angiography in this view and then begin the process of crossing the valve. We begin with a standard sequence of using a 6Fr AL1 catheter and a 0.035 in., fixed-core, 150 cm guide wire. We then use the wire and catheter simultaneously to identify the aortic valve jet which is then used as a guide to advance toward the aortic valve opening. Multiple, meticulous, and calculated passes of the wire may be needed; if due to anatomy, calcification, angulation of the aorta, other catheters may be required, such as AR1, JR4, AL2, AL3, etc. Straight 0.035-in. hydrophilic guidewires have been used by many operators; however this can result in difficult tracking of the

TAVR preop checklist

Age:	STS score
Comorbidities:	
Pacemaker/ICD	Allergies
Prohibitive surgical risk: Yes/No	Creatinine Hb/platelet

Coronary artery dis:	
ECHO: EF AV PG/MG AVA	LV size/thickness Other valves
ECG	

CT measurement Annulus Area: Sinus: Coronary Heights Left: LVOT calcium:	Perimeter: STJ: Right: Others:	%Oversize
Peripherals: (Narrowest diameter) Right: Calcification/Tortuosity	Left:	

TAVR Plan Valve (Type/Size): Access: Antiplatelet/Anticoagulation

Intra-procedural details

Date: _____ Time: start _____ ; end _____

Primary access site: **LFA/RFA/** _____

Closure methods for primary access site: Proglides x ___ +/- Angioseal ___ Fr x ___

Secondary access site: LFA/RFA, closure method: _____

ACT: _____ seconds

Blood pressure: _____ (pre); _____ (post)

Peak to peak gradient: _____ (pre); _____ (post)

LVEDP: _____ (pre); _____ (post)

Fluroscopy time: _____ ; contrast volume: _____

Name and size of balloon: _____

Name and size of valve: _____ ; position: low/optimal/high

Sapien valve: fully filled balloon / ___ cc underfilled / ___ cc overfilled

Rate of rapid pacing: during BAV ____ bpm; during valve deployment _____ bpm

Protamine use: y / n; dose of protamine use: _____

Any intraprocedural complications: y / n; if yes please check the box below
- LBBB: ___
- AV block: ___ ; degree of AV block: 1 / 2a / 2b / 3
- Acute pulmonary edema: ___
- VT/VF: ___
- Volume infusion: ___
- Prolong hypotension: ___
- Coronary obstruction: ___
- Stroke: ___
- Annular rupture: ___
- Emergemy surgery: ___
- Pericardial effusion: ___

Any groin complications or special notes (please describ in words):

Fig. 35.1 Sample procedural planning document. Reproduced with permission granted by Medtronic

catheter advancement across the valve; thus we do not typically recommend this approach. Once across the aortic valve, we typically insert a J-tipped 0.035 in., 260 cm wire into the left ventricle. A clockwise turn of the catheter as the guidewire is advanced typically allows the wire to be free of the mitral apparatus and to reach the true left ventricular apex. Once the wire is in the apex, we insert a 6Fr angled pigtail catheter into the left ventricle and measure hemodynamics. Through this pigtail catheter, we insert a pre-shaped stiff guide wire into the left ventricular apex and again ensure that the wire is not entangled in the mitral apparatus. Care must be taken to avoid placing the wire too deep into the apex and not too proximal toward the aortic valve. In the balloon-expandable prosthesis, standard balloon valvuloplasty is now performed, while in self-expanding prostheses, balloon valvuloplasty is performed on a case-by-case basis as determined by the pre-procedural planning. We then advance a valve over this guidewire and deploy the valve according to manufacturer recommendations for each system. Typically only 1–2 more contrast injections are taken to ensure appropriate valve implantation depth, position, and stability. Once the valve is implanted, post-procedure hemodynamics are taken, and supine transthoracic echocardiography is performed to evaluate for implantation success. Only if there is discordance between the hemodynamics and the echocardiogram is a contrast aortography performed. With each step, the operator is to be meticulous to prevent any untoward complications and follow best practices (Tables 35.1 and 35.2) from the point of access to vascular closure. Due to the nature of the procedure, there is a learning curve that can be overcome for the various valve replacement systems when taking these approaches, and it is clear that fluoroscopy time, contrast usage, procedure time, and complication rates are all optimized and minimized [23, 24].

Vascular closure represents the final step in the TAVR procedure. Multiple techniques have been described including manual pressure, pre-closure, "crossover" wire technique, and primary surgical closure. The authors' preference is CTA-based, fluoroscopically guided anterior wall, single stick puncture with two orthogonally placed incomplete Perclose sutures that are closed over a

Table 35.1 Designation and differences in the multidisciplinary heart team and the procedural heart team

The multidisciplinary heart team	Procedural heart team
Primary team	*Primary implantation team*
Referring physician	Interventional cardiologist
Valve clinic coordinator	Cardiothoracic surgeon
Interventional cardiologist	Catheterization technologist
Cardiothoracic surgeon	Procedural nurse
Imaging cardiologist	Circulating/pharmacologic nurse
General cardiologist	Valve system preparation technologist
	Device representative
	Transthoracic echocardiography technologist
Supporting specialists	
Electrophysiology	
Heart failure cardiologist	
Geriatrician	
Psychiatry	
Pulmonologist	
Vascular surgery	
Ancillary services	*Supporting specialists*
Social work	Cardiac anesthesiologist
Case manager	Transesophageal physician echocardiographer
Home health services	Operating room staff
Physiatry/rehabilitation	Perfusionist

Table 35.2 Best practices for self-expanding and balloon-expandable prosthesis

Intraprocedural best practices: self-expanding prosthesis

1. Single, anterior wall puncture
2. Pre-closure method, preferably double, orthogonal Perclose
3. Adequate subcutaneous tissue dissection to prevent wire/valve kinking
4. Use of a dedicated, manufacturer pre-shaped aortic valve guidewire for placement in left ventricular apex
5. Sheathless valve insertion
6. Continuous left anterior oblique fluoroscopic guidance of valve advancement across the aortic arch
7. Place marker pigtail in the NCC and ensure it is at the very bottom of the cusp
8. Remove parallax from the valve prior to beginning deployment (further LAO and minimal CAU)
9. Three-operator deployment working in concert
   Operator #1—Valve positioner
   Operator #2—Valve deployer
   Operator #3—Wire manager
10. Extremely slow valve deployment; a quarter turn every 5–10 s
11. As the valve flares, the use of pacing at 100–120 bpm to minimize extrasystoles and avoid valve pop-out
12. Intermittent angiography to ensure appropriate valve trajectory toward the LCC
13. Once 80% of the valve has flared, remove the parallax and perform angiography to confirm valve position
14. Center the nose cone by withdrawing the guidewire
15. Very slow release of each paddle, one at a time, till the valve is fully released
16. Recapture of the nose cone in the straightest portion of the descending aorta

Intraprocedural best practices: balloon-expandable prosthesis

1. Single, anterior wall puncture
2. Pre-closure method, preferably double, orthogonal Perclose
3. Adequate subcutaneous tissue dissection to prevent wire/valve kinking
4. Insertion of the manufacturer sheath over stiff guide wire
5. Suture the sheath to the skin
6. Use of a dedicated, manufacturer pre-shaped aortic valve guidewire for placement in left ventricular apex
7. Valvuloplasty during rapid, short (5–10 s) pacing run (180–200 bpm) once MAP <40–50 mmHg
8. Place marker pigtail in the NCC and ensure it is at the very bottom of the cusp
9. Insert valve delivery system and remove parallax from the valve in CRA view prior to loading on the balloon
10. Turn the knob of the flex catheter at least 50% to ensure a smooth transition across the aortic arch
11. Advance the valve in the LAO projection around the arch to aortic valve
12. Pull back to the valve pusher system once the valve is across the native aortic valve
13. Establish roles of contrast injector, pigtail puller, valve positioner, and valve inflator
14. Initiate rapid pacing, taking contrast angiogram to ensure appropriate position, pull pigtail, and being to inflate the valve
15. Inflate the balloon completely and hold the inflation for 3–5 s, and then rapidly deflate
16. Stop pacing once the balloon is completely deflated
17. Unturn the flex catheter and remove all equipment from the patient

standard 0.035 in. guidewire in sequential fashion after removal of the large sheath or valve delivery system [25]. Closure of the large bore access first is key as to ensure that the secondary access is available for possible crossover access and vascular bailout if there is a complication. Although no one vascular closure technique has been established as the gold standard for TAVR through randomized trials, the method employed by each team should be one that the operator is most comfortable with, understands different iterations and manipulations necessary for various patient anatomies, and importantly prioritizes patient safety and adequate hemostasis.

35.6 Internal Quality Improvement Program

Undertaking the endeavor of a TAVR program necessitates that the program is providing the highest level of care based on currently accepted success and complication rates. Participation in national (and international) registries is a requirement for TAVR programs and is linked to reimbursement for US-based TAVR programs. However, a team effort involving coordinators, implanters, registry assistants, and researchers should be expected to internally organize and document center-specific patient data in order to comprehensively understand the program's strengths and weaknesses. Data analyses should be performed quarterly and reported to all team members. The heart team should meet regularly to discuss the results and address issues that prohibit positive outcomes. Implementation of changes should be evidence-based, and time periods for improvement should be outlined to all members of the team and ancillary staff to achieve goals. With constant and active reassessment of various program elements, identification of the needs, resources, and fundamentals necessary for a successful and efficient program become evident and a primary goal of all those involved.

35.7 Conclusion

TAVR promises to become the standard of care for aortic valve disease management. As with all new procedures, as comfort is developed by operators, procedural efficiency becomes a norm. Standard best practices have been established and the Heart Team/implanters should be trained and well-versed in these methods. A TAVR center should recognize that the procedural efficiency is determined prior to the start of procedure and relies on procedural planning from identifying patient rehab needs, determining valve prostheses, understanding CTA imaging, and being competent in vascular access/closure management. As a TAVR program grows, the team should constantly re-evaluate processes outside and inside the procedural suite to identify problems and successes to help continually improve the overall quality of the patient experience and clinical outcomes.

References

1. Holmes DR Jr, Rich JB, Zoghbi WA, Mack MJ. The heart team of cardiovascular care. J Am Coll Cardiol. 2013;61:903–7.
2. Nishimura RA, Otto CM, Bonow RO, et al. 2017 AHA/ACC focused update of the 2014 AHA/ACC guideline for the management of patients with valvular heart disease: a report of the American College of Cardiology/American Heart Association Task Force on Clinical Practice Guidelines. J Am Coll Cardiol. 2017;70:252–89.
3. Nishimura RA, Otto CM, Bonow RO, et al. 2014 AHA/ACC guideline for the management of patients with valvular heart disease: executive summary: a report of the American College of Cardiology/American Heart Association Task Force on Practice Guidelines. J Am Coll Cardiol. 2014;63:2438–88.
4. Otto CM, Kumbhani DJ, Alexander KP, et al. 2017 ACC expert consensus decision pathway for transcatheter aortic valve replacement in the management of adults with aortic stenosis: a report of the American College of Cardiology Task Force on Clinical Expert Consensus Documents. J Am Coll Cardiol. 2017;69:1313–46.
5. Passeri JJ, Melnitchouk S, Palacios IF, Sundt TM. Continued expansion of the heart team concept. Futur Cardiol. 2015;11:219–28.
6. Tops LF, Wood DA, Delgado V, et al. Noninvasive evaluation of the aortic root with multislice computed tomography implications for transcatheter aortic valve replacement. JACC Cardiovasc Imaging. 2008;1:321–30.
7. Jilaihawi H, Kashif M, Fontana G, et al. Cross-sectional computed tomographic assessment improves accuracy of aortic annular sizing for transcatheter aortic valve replacement and reduces the incidence of paravalvular aortic regurgitation. J Am Coll Cardiol. 2012;59:1275–86.
8. Khalique OK, Hahn RT, Gada H, et al. Quantity and location of aortic valve complex calcification predicts severity and location of paravalvular regurgitation and frequency of post-dilation after balloon-expandable transcatheter aortic valve replacement. JACC Cardiovasc Interv. 2014;7:885–94.
9. Schultz CJ, Tzikas A, Moelker A, et al. Correlates on MSCT of paravalvular aortic regurgitation after transcatheter aortic valve implantation using the Medtronic CoreValve prosthesis. Catheter Cardiovasc Interv. 2011;78:446–55.
10. Shavelle DM, Budoff MJ, Buljubasic N, et al. Usefulness of aortic valve calcium scores by electron beam computed tomography as a marker for aortic stenosis. Am J Cardiol. 2003;92:349–53.
11. Willson AB, Webb JG, Labounty TM, et al. 3-dimensional aortic annular assessment by multidetector computed tomography predicts moderate or severe paravalvular regurgitation after transcatheter

aortic valve replacement: a multicenter retrospective analysis. J Am Coll Cardiol. 2012;59:1287–94.

12. Caruthers SD, Lin SJ, Brown P, et al. Practical value of cardiac magnetic resonance imaging for clinical quantification of aortic valve stenosis: comparison with echocardiography. Circulation. 2003;108:2236–43.

13. Gleeson TG, Mwangi I, Horgan SJ, Cradock A, Fitzpatrick P, Murray JG. Steady-state free-precession (SSFP) cine MRI in distinguishing normal and bicuspid aortic valves. J Magn Reson Imaging. 2008;28:873–8.

14. Pouleur AC, le Polain de Waroux JB, Pasquet A, Vancraeynest D, Vanoverschelde JL, Gerber BL. Planimetric and continuity equation assessment of aortic valve area: head to head comparison between cardiac magnetic resonance and echocardiography. J Magn Reson Imaging. 2007;26:1436–43.

15. Dewey TM, Brown D, Ryan WH, Herbert MA, Prince SL, Mack MJ. Reliability of risk algorithms in predicting early and late operative outcomes in high-risk patients undergoing aortic valve replacement. J Thorac Cardiovasc Surg. 2008;135:180–7.

16. Attizzani GF, Alkhalil A, Padaliya B, et al. Comparison of outcomes of transfemoral transcatheter aortic valve implantation using a minimally invasive versus conventional strategy. Am J Cardiol. 2015;116:1731–6.

17. Grover FL, Vemulapalli S, Carroll JD, et al. 2016 Annual Report of The Society of Thoracic Surgeons/American College of Cardiology Transcatheter Valve Therapy Registry. J Am Coll Cardiol. 2017;69:1215–30.

18. Hyman MC, Vemulapalli S, Szeto WY, et al. Conscious sedation versus general anesthesia for transcatheter aortic valve replacement: insights from the National Cardiovascular Data Registry Society of Thoracic Surgeons/American College of Cardiology Transcatheter Valve Therapy Registry. Circulation. 2017;136:2132–40.

19. Babaliaros V, Devireddy C, Lerakis S, et al. Comparison of transfemoral transcatheter aortic valve replacement performed in the catheterization laboratory (minimalist approach) versus hybrid operating room (standard approach): outcomes and cost analysis. JACC Cardiovasc Interv. 2014;7:898–904.

20. Frohlich GM, Lansky AJ, Webb J, et al. Local versus general anesthesia for transcatheter aortic valve implantation (TAVR)—systematic review and meta-analysis. BMC Med. 2014;12:41.

21. Attizzani GF, Ohno Y, Latib A, et al. Transcatheter aortic valve implantation under angiographic guidance with and without adjunctive transesophageal echocardiography. Am J Cardiol. 2015;116:604–11.

22. Goncalves A, Nyman C, Okada DR, et al. Transthoracic echocardiography to assess aortic regurgitation after TAVR: a comparison with peri-procedural transesophageal echocardiography. Cardiology. 2016;137:1–8.

23. Minha S, Waksman R, Satler LP, et al. Learning curves for transfemoral transcatheter aortic valve replacement in the PARTNER-I trial: success and safety. Catheter Cardiovasc Interv. 2016;87:165–75.

24. Alli O, Rihal CS, Suri RM, et al. Learning curves for transfemoral transcatheter aortic valve replacement in the PARTNER-I trial: technical performance. Catheter Cardiovasc Interv. 2016;87:154–62.

25. Griese DP, Reents W, Diegeler A, Kerber S, Babin-Ebell J. Simple, effective and safe vascular access site closure with the double-ProGlide preclose technique in 162 patients receiving transfemoral transcatheter aortic valve implantation. Catheter Cardiovasc Interv. 2013;82:E734–41.

Predictors of Success of Transcatheter Aortic Valve Implantation

36

Alessandro Maloberti, Domenico Sirico, Andrea Buono, and Giannattasio Cristina

36.1 Introduction

The role of transcatheter aortic valve implantation (TAVI), also called transcatheter aortic valve replacement (TAVR), as an alternative to surgical aortic valve replacement (SAVR) is established in patient with symptomatic severe aortic stenosis (AS) who are at high surgical risk [1]. Furthermore, recent evidence shows promising clinical outcomes for TAVR compared to SAVR for intermediate surgical risk patients [2]. However, current selection of patients undergoing TAVR relies on risk stratification models derived from surgical patient population (EuroSCORE and Society of Thoracic Surgery score), and many concerns regarding the suitability of these models in predicting TAVR mortality or complications risks have been raised. In fact, the evaluation of survival, as well as the incidence of major or minor complications, is of paramount importance and contributes to decision-making in interventions for severe AS. Nevertheless, the assessment of individual patient's prognosis after TAVR is challenging because heart valve team should take into consideration a variety of predictors, which could be divided into three main groups: pre-procedural, procedural, and post-procedural (Fig. 36.1). The former ones are patient-related including clinical history, comorbidities, and cardiovascular morphological and functional variables; procedural predictors are represented by technique-related issues (i.e., vascular access, type of implanted valve, pre- and post-dilation, etc.); and the latter ones could represent, on the one hand, minor or major complications and on the other being predictors of major events such as mortality (i.e., conduction disturbance, paravalvular leaks, etc.). Finally, TAVR success predictors have been extensively evaluated by several studies with some heterogeneity in results probably dependent from differences in population size and characteristics.

36.2 Predictors of Mortality

Mortality is considered the principal clinical outcome and is frequently assessed as all-cause mortality in the primary endpoint and as cardiovascular mortality in the secondary endpoints. Moreover, it is commonly divided in early-term (in-hospital and 30-day), mid-term (1-year), and late-term mortality. Its principal predictors are showed in Fig. 36.2.

A. Maloberti · D. Sirico · A. Buono · G. Cristina (✉)
"A. De Gasperis" Department,
Niguarda Ca Granda Hospital, Milan, Italy

School of Medicine and Surgery,
Milano-Bicocca University, Milan, Italy
e-mail: Alessandro.maloberti@ospedaleniguarda.it;
domenico.sirico@ospedaleniguarda.it;
andrea.buono@ospedaleniguarda.it;
cristina.giannattasio@ospedaleniguarda.it

© Springer Nature Switzerland AG 2019
A. Giordano et al. (eds.), *Transcatheter Aortic Valve Implantation*,
https://doi.org/10.1007/978-3-030-05912-5_36

Fig. 36.1 Pre-procedural, procedural and post-procedural predictors of TAVI success

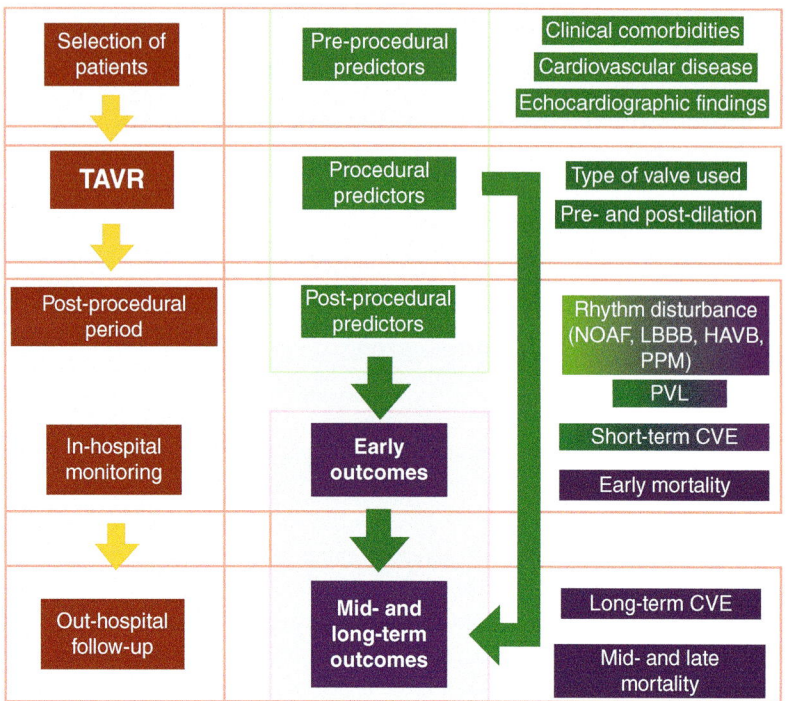

Fig. 36.2 Pre-procedural, procedural and post-procedural predictors of post-TAVI mortality

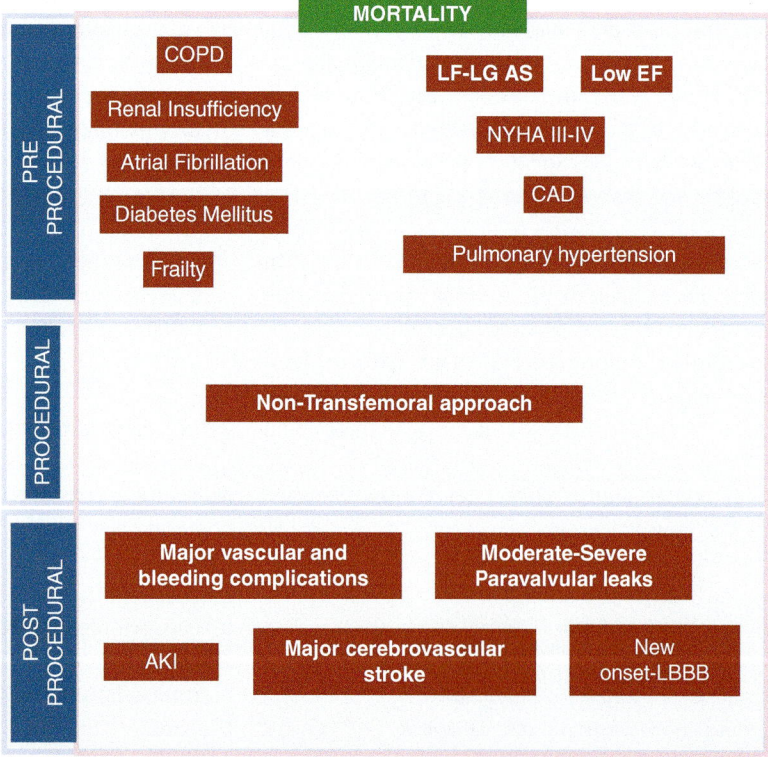

36.2.1 Pre-procedural Predictors

Among pre-procedural predictors echocardiographic and patient baseline characteristics need to be discussed.

In the first group, reduced ejection fraction (EF), low flow-low gradient (LF-LG) stenosis, and reduced stroke volume index (SVI) have been found to be important predictors of mortality. Contrasting data on the impact of left ventricular EF (LVEF) before TAVR have been reported. In the Placement of Aortic Transcatheter Valves (PARTNER) trial, reduced LVEF has not been related to worse outcomes [3]. In contrast, two recent meta-analyses showed that in patients with low EF, both all-cause and cardiovascular mortalities were significantly higher when compared with patients with normal EF [4, 5].

The condition of LF-LG, represented by low mean trans-aortic gradient (<40 mmHg), is an independent factor related to a poorer prognosis in patients with severe AS as it reflects an advanced stage of the natural history of the disease [6]. Furthermore, in TAVR patients, a significant higher mortality was found only in patients with LF-LG and low LVEF (also called classical LF-LG) but not in patients with LF-LG and normal LVEF (also called paradoxical LF-LG) [7]. Recently, Conrotto et al. showed that the combination of low LVEF with LF-LG is the strongest independent negative prognostic predictor in TAVR patients (both LVEF and mean trans-aortic gradient are not independently related to prognosis if considered separately). The authors (using a cutoff value of 40 for both parameters) showed that having at least one value (LVEF or mean transvalvular gradient) over 40 leads to a similar good prognosis, whereas the combination of the two confers 2.4 times the risk of mortality at 3 years [8]. Conversely, Baron et al. showed that LF-LG alone, independently from LVEF, was associated with higher mortality (HR 1.21; 95% CI 1.11–1.32; $p < 0.001$) and higher rates of heart failure (HF) with a HR of 1.52 (95% CI 1.36–1.69; $p < 0.001$) [9].

Recent data suggest that reduced SVI (<35 mL/m^2) alone may be an independent predictor of mortality after TAVR [10]. Finally, a meta-analysis enrolling 7673 patients evaluated the association between low SVI, LF-LG (<40 mm Hg), and low EF (<50% and <30%) on 1-year all-cause mortality: each factor was associated with increased 1-year mortality after TAVR with similar prognostic impact (HR 1.52–1.60) [11].

Preoperative patients' characteristics represent a paradoxical issue. In fact, the presence of multiple comorbidities raises the surgical risk leading, with higher probability, to the choice of a transcatheter approach. On the other hand, the same comorbidities act as factor that are able to predict all causes and cardiovascular mortality.

Among them, the following has been found to be important predictors of all-cause mortality.

1. Chronic obstructive pulmonary disease (COPD): it is a recognized strong and independent risk factor for mid-term mortality after TAVR (HR 3.14; 95% CI 1.05–9.40; $p = 0.04$) [12]. Moreover, among COPD patients, a higher degree of airway obstruction and a lower exercise capacity were responsible of a higher risk of pulmonary complications and mortality, respectively. Interestingly, TAVR treatment was not beneficial in more than one-third of the COPD patients, and a shorter distance walked at the 6MWT (<170 meters) helped to predict the lack of benefit after TAVR [12]. Furthermore, chronic obstructive pulmonary disease represents a predictor of late hospital readmissions, which is also an independent predictor of mid- and late-term mortality after TAVR (HR 1.56; 95% CI 1.02–2.39; $p = 0.043$) [13].

2. Chronic kidney disease (CKD): preoperative CKD and dialysis have shown to predict independently mid- and late-term mortality after TAVR [14]. In particular, a pre-TAVR estimated glomerular filtration rate (eGFR) <30 mL/min was associated with increased risk of death (with a OR of 3), and for each 10 mL/min decrease in eGFR, there was a further relative increase in the risk of all-cause death (35%; $p < 0.001$) and cardiovascular death (14%; $p = 0.018$) [15]. Moreover,

patients with CKD or end-stage renal disease (ESRD) have worse in-hospital outcomes after TAVR [16]. Finally, CKD increases the risk of acute kidney injury (AKI) after TAVR, which is associated with an elevated risk of mortality (see below in post-procedural predictors) [17].

3. New York Heart Association (NYHA) functional class: a NYHA class of III or IV was associated with higher mortality in patients undergoing SAVR for severe AS [18]. Similarly, in TAVR patients baseline NYHA functional class III to IV is associated with higher late mortality [14]. Furthermore, all-cause and cardiac mortality were significantly higher in those with residual impairment of functional capacity than in those in NYHA I class after TAVR [19].

4. Body mass index (BMI): The Valve Academic Research Consortium-2 has defined a BMI <20 kg/m^2 as indicative of frailty. In fact, an higher BMI was associated with a lower risk of mortality at 30 days after TAVR [20], while low BMI was associated with increased late mortality after both SAVR and TAVR (HR 2.45, $p = 0.01$) [21].

5. Atrial fibrillation (AF): like the presence of AF has been associated with higher mortality after SAVR [22], it has been reported as a prominent predictor also after TAVR [23]. As an example, in the German registries, chronic AF was significantly associated with adverse outcomes at 1 year [24] and was an independent cardiovascular and all-cause mortality predictor (HR 2.33 and 1.88, respectively) [25].

6. Pulmonary hypertension: baseline high pulmonary arterial systolic pressure (PASP) >60 mm Hg was an independent echocardiographic predictor of death from HF and other causes in TAVR patients (HR 1.99 and 1.90, respectively) [25].

7. Diabetes mellitus (DM): the presence of this comorbidity has been extensively evaluated with heterogeneous results in literature. In a subgroup analysis of the PARTNER trial, diabetics had favorable outcomes when compared to nondiabetics [26]. However, other studies showed DM had either adverse or no

significant impact on TAVR outcomes [27, 28]. In a large meta-analysis evaluating the impact of DM on outcomes of patients undergoing TAVR, it was associated with increased 1-year all-cause mortality (OR 1.14) but not with early mortality. Interestingly, DM had no impact on early mortality, major bleeding, or major vascular complications, while diabetic patients had a higher risk of AKI after TAVR when compared to nondiabetics [29].

8. Frailty: it plays a pivotal role in defining older patient's capability to recover after a TAVR or SAVR procedure [30]. However, its evaluation in clinical practice has been limited by a lack of consensus on how to measure. In fact many TAVR-centric frailty scales have been derived [31] with different results. In a multivariable analysis, the four-item Essential Frailty Toolset (EFT) demonstrated the strongest association with 1-year mortality (OR 3.72; 95% CI 2.54–5.45) and outperformed other frailty scales to identify vulnerable older adults who are at higher risk of poor outcomes after TAVR [32].

9. Coronary artery disease (CAD): prevalence of coexisting CAD is high (about 50%) in patients with severe AS referred for TAVR [33]. Furthermore, most of the surgical risk scores (EuroSCORE, STS), which are used also for selecting candidates to TAVR, consider CAD an item. However, previous evidence has shown that CAD was not associated with an increased risk of adverse events after TAVR and that complete revascularization may not constitute a prerequisite [34]. Furthermore, a meta-analysis of adjusted observational studies enrolling 2472 patients revealed that CAD did not affect mid-term outcome [35].

36.2.2 Procedural Predictors

1. Type of implanted valve: it seems that no differences regarding mortality could be related to the type of valve. In fact, Tarantini et al. compared long-term clinical outcome data and hemodynamic performance of TAVR with

either self-expandable CoreValve or the balloon-expandable Edwards SAPIEN XT. The authors showed that clinical outcomes and long-term hemodynamic performance (i.e., mean trans-prosthetic gradient, effective orifice area, and incidence of aortic regurgitation) were favorable regardless of prostheses type [36]. Similarly, in the UK TAVR registry, there was no difference in survival between the two main valve types on multivariate analysis [23]. Despite these results type of implanted valve represents an important predictor of other TAVR-related complication such as for conduction disturbances (see later).

2. Vascular approaches: non-transfemoral approaches have been associated with a marked increase in early and late mortality after TAVR. In particular, the transapical approach was associated on multivariate analysis with increased early- and mid-term mortality [37]. Similarly, the use of the transapical route was associated with increased risk of death from advanced HF (HR 2.38; 95% CI 1.60–3.54; $p < 0.001$) [25]. Also the subclavian approach has been associated with increased late mortality [14]. In contrast to these findings, multivariate analysis of a large series of patients undergoing TAVR from the German Aortic Valve Registry (GARY) showed that the transapical approach was not an independent predictor of death [18].

36.2.3 Post-procedural Predictors

1. Paravalvular regurgitation, conduction disturbances, and cerebrovascular events: these types of complication will be treated extensively below also as predictors of mortality.
2. AKI: it is a common complication following TAVR and presents an important prognostic value as it is associated with higher rates of mortality, major bleeding, and vascular complications. Hypertension, COPD, blood transfusion, transapical access, preoperative creatinine values, peripheral vascular disease, and procedural bleeding events were

predictive factors of AKI [38]. In a meta-analysis enrolling almost 9000 TAVR patients, AKI stage >2 was the strongest 30-day mortality predictor (OR 18.0; 95% CI 6.25–52), and AKI stage 3 was an important predictor for cumulative mid-term mortality (OR 6.80; 95% CI 2.55–15.66) [4].

3. Brain natriuretic peptide (BNP): it has been shown to be elevated in patients with symptomatic AS and to decrease after successful SAVR [39]. In TAVR patients, pre-procedural BNP and pro-BNP levels have been identified as independent predictors of both short- and long-term mortality after TAVR [40]. In the same meta-analysis cited regarding AKI, baseline elevated pro-BNP levels (measured 24 h before TAVI) were a strong independent predictor of both 30-day (OR 5.35; 95% CI 1.74–16.5) and mid-term mortality (OR 11; 95% CI 1.51–81) [4]. The unfavorable outcome of valve interventions in patients with high pre-procedural BNP levels is believed to be related to the presence of impaired systolic and/or diastolic left ventricular function [41], suggesting that those patients might benefit from optimization of their hemodynamic status before proceeding to TAVR. We deal with this factor as a post-procedural predictor because it has been showed that BNP level elevation at 30 days after TAVR intervention is a significant independent predictor of 1-year mortality (OR 1.82; 95% CI 1.26–2.62) [42]. The persistence of BNP elevation suggests an incomplete reduction in wall stress in these patients, and the same authors suggest postprocedural paravalvular regurgitation as the potential cause of volume overload.

4. Myocardial injury: it is defined as a postprocedural peak value of cardiac troponin T and/or creatine kinase-MB (CK-MB) >5 times the upper reference limit and is a frequent complication after TAVR. Anyway, the impact on short-term outcomes remains controversial, and the association with long-term prognosis is a matter of debate. Myocardial injury is most likely caused by global myocardial ischemia, resulting from a mismatch in oxygen supply and demand. Approximately

50–60% of patients showed an increase in troponin T and CK-MB, and it emerged as a strong independent predictor of 30-day mortality, while it is less strongly related to mid-term mortality [43]. In contrast, Stundl et al. found no significant correlation between myocardial injury and all-cause mortality at 1 year [44].

36.2.4 Risk Scores

Current indication for TAVR vs. SAVR treatment in patients with severe AS relies on risk assessment models derived from surgical patient population (i.e., STS-PROM, EuroSCORE) in addition to the functional assessment, comorbidities, and procedure-related hurdles. However, risk stratification scores tailored for TAVR population would be better in stratifying patient risks before and after intervention. In the last few years, awareness of the limitations of conventional risk scores is increased, and several TAVR-specific risk models have been proposed.

Debonnaire et al. developed the TAVI2-SCORe, which includes all the variables found to be independent predictors of 1-year mortality post-TAVR on the basis of a retrospective analysis of 511 consecutive patients. It includes porcelain thoracic aorta, anemia, LVEF, recent myocardial infarction, male sex, critical AS, age, and CKD. Patients were stratified in five risk groups according to the number of points assigned in 0 (reference), 1 (HR 2.6 for 1-year mortality), 2 (HR 3.6), 3 (HR 10.5), and ≥4 (HR 17.6). The score showed better discrimination ability compared with logistic EuroSCOREs and STS-PROM scores [45].

Another simple risk score is the OBSERVANT one developed to predict 30-day mortality after TAVR. This score is based on seven variables derived from the homonym study: eGFR <45 mL/min (6 points), critical preoperative state (5 points), NYHA class IV (4 points), pulmonary hypertension (4 points), DM (4 points), previous balloon aortic valvuloplasty (3 points), and LVEF<40% (3 points). Compared to logistic EuroSCORE, the model showed greater discrimination (C statistic

0.71 vs. 0.66) and better global accuracy (Brier score 0.054 vs. 0.073) [46].

A further risk score model for TAVR patients was developed from the FRANCE 2 registry based on a patient cohort of similar size of the STS-PROM model. This nine-variable risk score is aimed to estimate early mortality; however, despite a good concordance between predicted and observed mortality, it achieved only a moderate discrimination in the development and in the validation sample (C-index 0.67 and 0.59, respectively) [37].

Recently, the Transcatheter Valve Therapy (TVT) registry model tool has been developed by the Society of Thoracic Surgeons/American College of Cardiology, as a predictive model of in-hospital mortality for patients undergoing TAVR. The final model included as predictors age, eGFR, hemodialysis, NYHA class IV, severe COPD, non-femoral access, and procedural acuity categories. The model C statistic for discrimination was 0.67 (95% CI 0.65–0.69) in the development group and 0.66 (95% CI 0.62–0.69) in the validation group [47]. Interestingly, the model has been externally validated in an independent data set of consecutively enrolled patients in the Swiss TAVR registry and was found to have moderate discrimination (C-index, 0.66 and 0.67 for in-hospital and 30-day mortality, respectively) and good calibration. Furthermore, when compared with the STS-PROM score, the TVT registry model demonstrated improved calibration for both in-hospital and 30-day mortality [48].

In conclusion, all these scores have shown to represent an alternative to the most commonly used ones; nevertheless, their clinical use in the real-world requires further external validations.

36.3 Predictors of Quality of Life Improvement

Both TAVR and SAVR were found to improve symptoms and health-related quality of life (QoL) over medical therapy in patients affected by severe symptomatic AS. These benefits, assessed by disease-specific Kansas City

Cardiomyopathy Questionnaire (KCCQ), were seen early after valve replacement, continued to improve at 1 year, and were largely sustained also after 3 years of follow-up [49].

However, a considerable number of patients may lack improvement in QoL or functional status after TAVR, and identifying this subgroup of patients could help physician to acknowledge the possibility of futile treatment. In particular, futility has been defined as a lack of medical efficacy or lack of a meaningful survival benefit [50].

To best identify such patients, Arnold et al. have proposed a definition for poor outcome at 6 months after TAVR that combines death, KCCQ<45 (comparable to a NYHA class IV), or a decrease of more than ten points in the KCCQ from baseline. According to this definition, about 35% of patients treated with TAVR in the PARTNER trial had a poor outcome [51].

Data from the TVT registry shows that poor outcome, as defined above, at 1 year was predicted by severe COPD, dialysis, or very poor baseline health status [52].

In a recent analysis of the GARY registry, QoL outcome after TAVR was assessed using the EuroQoL (EQ-5D) questionnaire. Valve replacement leads to mean improvements in QoL, even though a considerable group of patients did not develop any benefits. Independent predictors for less pronounced QoL benefits were age, female sex, BMI, NYHA class III or IV, dialysis, peripheral arterial vascular disease, mitral insufficiency, postoperative transient ischemic attack or stroke, and postoperative hospitalization [53]. However, EuroQoL is a generic health status measure, and it may be not as sensitive as a disease-specific health measure in detecting changes in symptoms, function, and QoL, and consequently, it could underestimate the extent of benefits in patients undergoing TAVR [54].

36.4 Predictors of Cerebrovascular Events

Cerebrovascular events (CVE) are one of the most dreadful complications of TAVR as they are themselves an important cause of increased morbidity and mortality after these procedures. The nature of these events is principally ischemic, while a little proportion of hemorrhagic one is present. In the PARTNER trial, CVE occurred more frequently after TAVR than after SAVR at 30 days and 1 year in high surgical risk patients with severe AS [55]. The risk of CVE has declined over the years down to rates of 2.5–3% largely due to the increasing operator experience and improvement in valve technology and patient selection [18, 23]. For example, in the PARTNER-II trial, the 30-day risk of stroke was 3.2% compared to a 5.5–6.7% in the PARTNER-I [56].

As shown in Fig. 36.3, numerous potential risk factors and independent predictors able to determine CVE have been highlighted [57].

Firstly, CVE could be classified by the time of appearance in two main groups: short-term events, either early (less than 7 days from procedure) or subacute (within 30 days), and long-term CVE (1 year and later). This classification suggests the presence of different risk factors and mechanisms at the basis of CVE incidence, as well as different predictors. In general, early- and mid-term CVE are strongly associated with periprocedural aspects, while long-term events depending on patient- and/or disease-related factors, highlighting a more severe, generalized atherosclerotic burden. Approximately 50–60% of strokes occur within 24 h from TAVR with a second peak within 1 week from the procedure [58]. This could explain the reason why we have more predictors evaluated for short-term CVE than for long-term one.

36.4.1 Predictors of Early CVE

Following the classification of predictors proposed above, among constitutional characteristics that predict early CVE, there are female sex, older age, small aortic annuli, and small aortic valve area, these probably due to the fact that tighter valves present more calcification that could potentially embolize during TAVR [57, 59]. In fact, males present a lower risk of short-term CVE probably due to a larger aortic annuli and left ventricular outflow tract that could

Fig. 36.3 Pre-procedural, procedural and post-procedural predictors of cerebrovascular events after TAVI

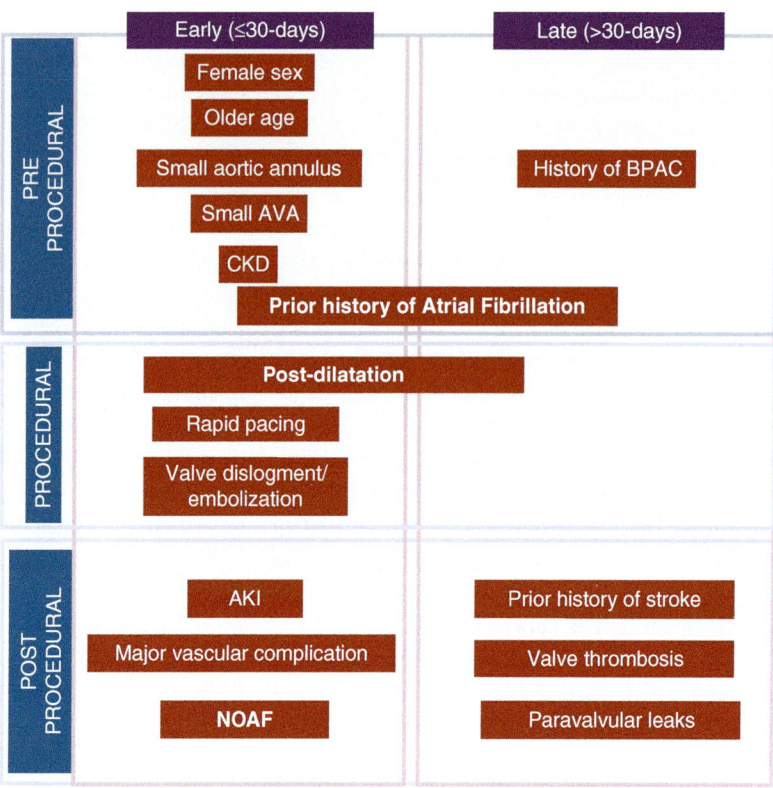

decrease the mechanical interaction between the native and prosthetic aortic valves during positioning and implantation, which represent the two maneuvers associated with the highest risk of cerebral emboli during TAVR procedure [59]. Furthermore, comorbidities such as CKD have been associated with CVE, while the most important pre-procedural predictor is a history of AF, being associated in different studies with both short- and long-term CVE [57, 60].

Procedural aspects have been extensively ameliorated by improvements in valve technology and better operator's experience. Despite heterogeneous results with different type of valves have been reported [61], accordingly to the most recent evidences, valve type and approach (transapical vs. transfemoral) do not seem to influence directly the incidence of CVE [62]. Nevertheless, despite similar stroke risk, there may be an important difference in timing of stroke inherent to each valve. Focusing on the high-risk period of stroke

during positioning and valve deployment, Kahlert et al. showed that the risk with the CoreValve is higher during the slow stepwise implantation, while that with the Edwards valve is maximum during the slow positioning of the device prior to implantation [63].

Another procedural predictor is the balloon post-dilatation (BPD), used to low the risk of paravalvular leaks. In fact, different studies have demonstrated the association between BPD and strokes, making stronger the concept that the manipulation of the aortic root (independently by the TAVR approach) rather than the manipulation of the aortic arch (typical of transfemoral approach) is likely to be the determinant of CVE [64]. Furthermore, one could speculate that BPD-induced leaflet deformation/damage might increase the risk of bioprosthesis thrombosis.

AKI and vascular complications (VC) represent the most strong post-procedural predictors of short-term CVE [57] as well as new-onset AF [59].

36.4.2 Predictors of Late CVE

Predictors of late CVE have been less investigated. The risk appears to be more related to patients' characteristics prior to TAVR than to procedural or post-procedural factors. Particularly, a previous history of aortocoronary bypass and AF are the most powerful predictors of stroke at 1 year [57]. Moreover, in the PARTERN trial, predictors of late strokes were history of stroke from 6 to 12 months before the procedure, non-transfemoral approach (that could be interpreted as a higher burden of atherosclerosis and worse vasculopathy), and higher NYHA class [55].

Another source of thromboembolism might be bioprosthesis incomplete endothelialization. Free space left between prosthesis and native aortic valve, manifested as paravalvular leakage, might increase the risk of abnormal blood flow pattern. However, although suggested by a previous smaller study [64], in subsequent studies there was no association between paravalvular leakage and CVE occurrence.

36.4.3 CVE as Predictor of Mortality

As reported before, CVE are themselves predictors of mortality [61]. The outcome of patients with stroke after TAVR seems to be influenced by the severity of the neurologic event. In patients with stroke and no permanent deficits, data suggest that mortality may not be affected. However, patients with major stroke post-TAVR in the PARTNER trial had significantly increased 1-year mortality rate compared [65].

36.5 Predictors of Conduction Disturbances

TAVR-related conduction disturbances, mainly new-onset left bundle-branch block (LBBB) and advanced atrioventricular block (AAVB) requiring permanent pacemaker (PPM) implantation, remain the most common complication of this procedure. These complications rise over time,

despite the increased experience of operators, the improved repositioning/retrievability capability, and the anti-paravalvular leak properties of the newer valves. A careful electrocardiographic monitoring for at least 48 h is needed in order to rapidly recognize these complications. In fact, most conduction disturbances occur during the TAVR procedure or within hours after that. A significant proportion of conduction disturbances are transient (especially LBBB), particularly with the use of balloon-expandable valves. Development of delayed AAVB ($\geq$48 h after TAVR) is more uncommon than periprocedural one and should be evaluated for the need of PPM.

Furthermore, new-onset LBBB and PPM represent themselves detrimental predictors for patient's prognosis [66]. LBBB is associated with a greater risk of 1-year cardiovascular mortality, probably due to an increased risk of sudden cardiac death and ventricular dyssynchrony with consequent systolic dysfunction [25].

The principal factors able to predict the conduction disturbances are the anatomical ones (Fig. 36.4). In fact, a left-sided or just below endocardium position of atrioventricular bundle, a short membranous septum, the calcium deposition on the conduction system or aortic valve, and the dimension of left ventricular outflow tract are of particular importance in predicting these disturbances [67]. Beyond anatomical aspects, other pre-procedural predictors are the presence of previous conduction abnormalities, female sex, previous coronary artery bypass graft, and DM [68].

Turning to procedural predictors, a central role is determined by the type of valve implanted. In fact, the rate of new-onset LBBB is higher after implantation of the mechanically expanded Lotus valve (Boston Scientific, Natick, MA) [69]. Moreover, the self-expandable CoreValve system (Medtronic Inc., Minneapolis, MN) is more commonly associated with new-onset LBBB compared to the balloon-expandable Edwards SAPIEN valve (Edwards Lifesciences LLC, Irvine, CA), and the self-expandable Portico TAVR system (St. Jude Medical, St. Paul, MN). These association could be explained by the higher depth of the CoreValve prosthesis implantation within the left ventricular outflow

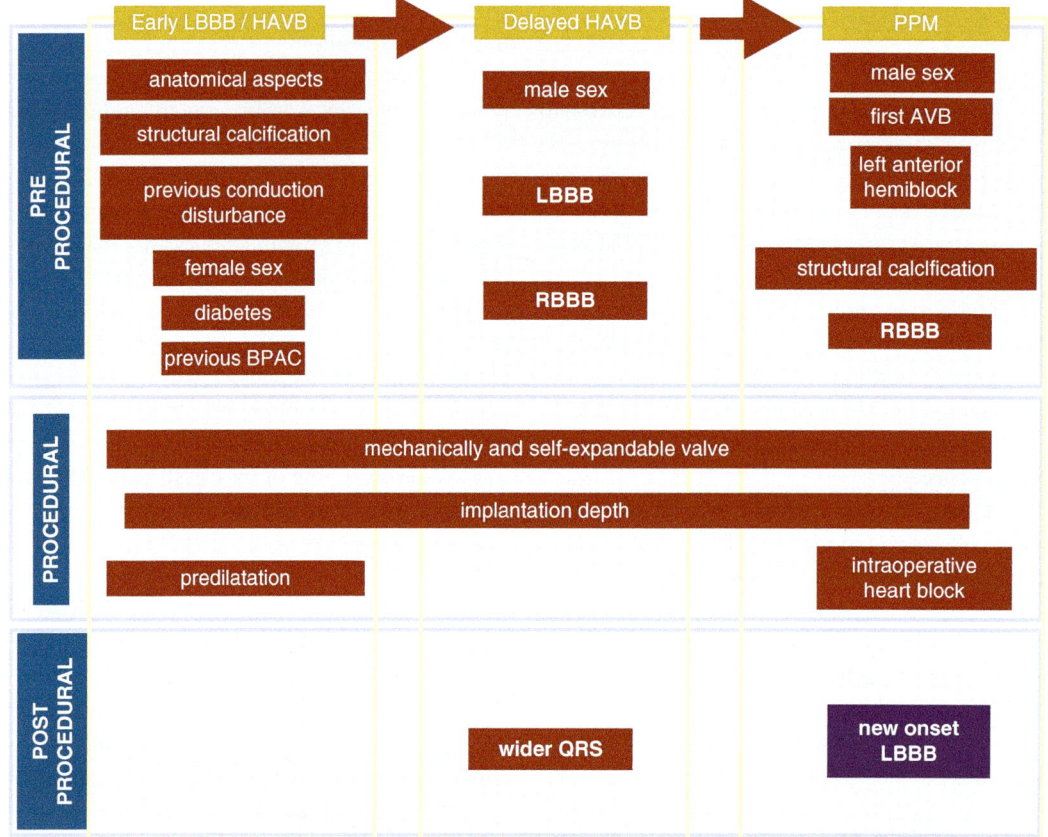

Fig. 36.4 Pre-procedural, procedural and post-procedural predictors of arrhytmic complication after TAVI

tract exerting high radial forces near to the conduction system [70]. Same reason could be found also for the association of predilatation with conduction disturbances [71].

Male sex, the presence of left or right BBB, and a QRS duration >128 ms after TAVR are independent predictors of delayed AAVB [72].

Similar to LBBB, PPM was five times more frequent among self-expandable CoreValve recipients compared with patients who received a balloon-expandable Edwards SAPIEN/SAPIEN XT valve [73]. In a meta-analysis, Siontis et al. identified male sex, first-degree AVB, left anterior hemiblock, and right BBB as pre-procedural predictors of PPM, whereas the presence of intraoperative AAVB and the use of a self-expandable prosthesis were the procedural predictors [74]. As reported for LBBB,

anatomical characteristics such as calcifications of the aortic valve and mitral annulus and the depth of prosthesis implantation have been associated with PPM after TAVR [66].

36.6 Predictors of Paravalvular Regurgitation

One of the most common TAVR complications are paravalvular regurgitations (PVR). PVR are six times more frequent after TAVR than SAVR. Most of the times, PVR are mild, but in 20% of cases, it is possible to observe a regurgitation with a moderate to severe degree, which has been related with a worse prognosis. Figure 36.5 shows the principal predictors of PVR.

Fig. 36.5 Pre-procedural, procedural and post-procedural predictors of paravalvular leaks

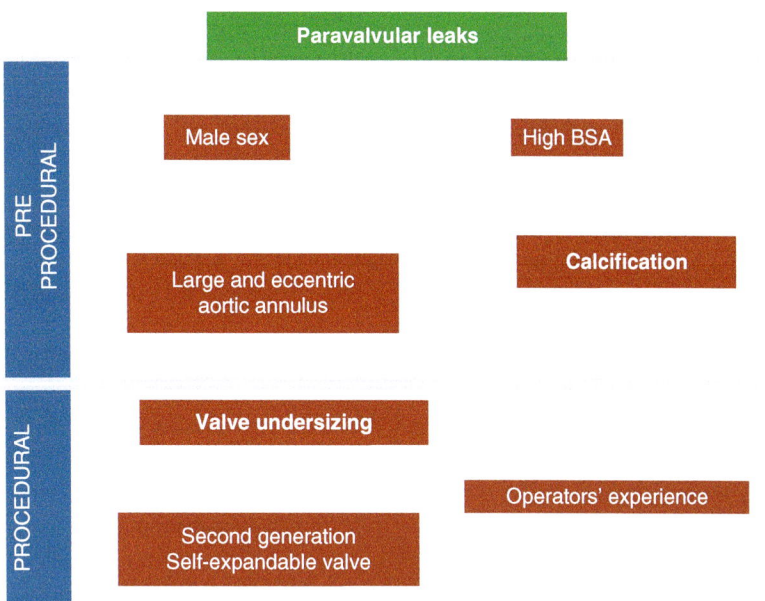

36.6.1 Pre-procedural Predictors

This section deals with all the aspect that could lead to a prosthesis-patient mismatch, reflecting an inadequate sizing of the valve. Among subjects' characteristics, a larger body surface area (BSA) and male sex result as significant predictors of a greater PVR severity [75], because they are associated with a larger aortic annulus. After that, anatomical aspects are the most important pre-procedural predictors. Larger and eccentric annulus were identified as predictors of PVR, and, in fact, PVR higher than moderate has never been detected in patients with aortic annulus <22 mm [76].

In addition, the more the shape veers off the circular one, the more the prosthesis fails to completely cover the valve orifice. All these anatomic features are founded in bicuspid aortic valves, which are indeed at higher risk of PVR development.

Another anatomical factor that has been investigated is the angle between the axis of the ascending aorta (which would represent the landing zone for the upper part of the bioprosthesis) and the axis of the left ventricular outflow tract (i.e., the landing zone of the lower part of the valve): the greater the angle, the higher the PVR

incidence [77]. A wider angle affects the ability of prosthesis to seal the paraprosthetic space, particularly with the longer stent of CoreValve compared to Edwards SAPIEN.

However, the most investigated pre-procedural predictor is aortic valve calcium. Several studies found significant associations between aortic valve calcification and PVR [78]. Obviously, when a significant amount of calcium is present at the circumference of the native valve, it does not allow the perfect juxtaposition between the prosthesis and the aortic wall, resulting in PVR. In particular calcification at any aortic level (from the outflow tract to the valve annulus and leaflets) and their asymmetry or protrusion are predictors of greater than mild PVR. One method to quantify calcification is to calculate the Agatston score by computer tomography (CT), and findings confirmed an increased risk of significant PVR with Agatston scores >3000 HU [79].

In one study, Watanabe et al. have identified two independent predictors of equal or more than moderate PVR in patients undergoing TAVR with Edwards valves, namely, valve diameter/calculated average annulus diameter (CAAD) ratio by CT and the valve calcification index (VCI), defined as aortic root calcification volume/BSA. They developed a predicting score determined by allotting one point when the valve diameter/CAAD ratio was <1.055 and one point when VCI was >418.4 mm³/m². The incidence of significant PVR was 5.3%, 11.8%, and 37.5% when the results of the score were 0, 1, or 2, respectively [80].

In conclusion, incomplete prosthesis juxtaposition to the native annulus due to patterns or extent of calcification or annular eccentricity seems to be the most powerful pre-procedural predictor of PVR, and appropriate pre-procedural planning for TAVR should include careful annulus sizing, quantification of calcium burden, and assessment of left ventricular outflow tract and annulus asymmetry by CT.

36.6.2 Procedural Predictors

Undersizing of the valve and malpositioning of the device are the main procedural mechanisms at the base of PVR. These observations seem to be true for both balloon-expandable and self-expandable valves.

Regardless of the valve type, valve sizing has been shown to be one of the strongest predictors of PVR. Instinctually, greater degrees of oversizing are associated with lower rates of PVR with the lowest rate associated with oversizing >25% [81]. The other face of the coin is that the oversizing is associated to many complication, such as conduction disturbances and cerebrovascular events. To sum up, a certain degree of prosthesis oversizing, but not too much, may be required to prevent PVR.

Two studies have tried to give a measure of annulus-device congruence. Détaint et al. described the "cover index" represented by the formula [100 × (prosthesis diameter-transesophageal echocardiography annulus diameter)/prosthesis diameter] that has been demonstrated an independent predictor of more than moderate PVR [76]. In fact, a low cover index reflects a lower degree of oversizing of the prosthesis and significantly predicts PVR. Conversely, a cover index >8% has not been associated to significant regurgitation. Santos et al. defined a "mismatch index" expressed as annulus area-prosthesis

area using three-dimensional transesophageal echocardiography [67]. Like the previous study, they evaluated only Edwards SAPIEN valve, finding this index to be the only independent predictor of significant PVR.

The best imaging modality to size the aortic annulus is represented by CT. Adherence to CT-based oversizing was associated with a reduced incidence of PVR, while adherence to a bidimensional transesophageal echocardiography-based sizing was not. When CT-based sizing criteria were met, there was a 21% decrease in the incidence of PVR [82].

Type of device used for TAVR procedure may have significant implication on incidence of post-procedural PVR. This can be explained by different prosthesis architecture and implantation techniques. Evidence is almost exclusively related to the second-generation devices and suggests that CoreValve carries a higher risk of PVR when compared to Edwards SAPIEN valve [83, 84]. In contrast, in the PRAGMATIC trial, the rate at 1 year of moderate to severe PVR was not statistically different between patients who received a CoreValve and those who underwent TAVR with a balloon-expandable device [85]. However, the trend was toward a higher incidence of moderate/severe PVR in the CoreValve group compared with the Edwards SAPIEN, and probably this study failed to reach statistical significance because of smaller population compared to the before-mentioned meta-analysis.

The higher incidence with the self-expandable valve is likely due to several reasons. First of all, concerns have been raised over the weaker radial strength of the nitinol frame, especially with highly calcific lesions. In fact, while nitinol stents may exhibit greater ability to withstand stress and manipulation than stainless steel, it lacks the stiffness required to withstand the compressive force of the hard and calcified native valve. Incomplete device expansion and resultant impaired apposition of the CoreValve to the native annulus and the left ventricular outflow tract have been implicated. Also stent length, which is bigger in CoreValve compared to Edwards SAPIEN, plays a central role, in particular if the angulation between the left ventricular outflow tract and the ascending aorta is very acute, which reduces the ability of the self-expanding prosthesis to form a tight seal to close the paravalvular space [68].

Moreover, PVR is influenced significantly by the implantation depth. When misplaced high or low, the skirt of the prosthetic valve does not provide an adequate seal around the annulus. This is particularly true with the use of CoreValve: due to its trapezoid lower segment, its depth of deployment is more challenging. A lower depth of implantation was found to predict PVR, while a 5–10 mm device depth from the non-coronary cusp minimized the risk of significant PVR [77].

However, prevalence of PVR is expected to soon significantly drop as third-generation devices will be largely used. Medtronic Corevalve Evolut R can be fully recaptured and repositioned for obtaining optimal valve positioning and have an extended sealing skirt. The SAPIEN 3 system incorporates a skirt surrounding the bottom of the valve with the objective of reducing PVR. The Portico self-expandable valve (St. Jude) offers full resheathability (the ability to retrieve the valve) and large cells in the annulus section, to minimize the risk of PVR [86]. Those devices lower the rate of PVR below 30% compared to the >50% observed with the older-generation valve. Operators' experience, obviously, is a significant predictor of the incidence of PVR.

36.6.3 PVR as Predictor of Mortality

Strong evidence exists on the negative impact of residual moderate to severe PVR on survival after TAVR while less understood remain the prognostic role of mild PVR. In fact, PVR >2 grade has been defined as device failure according to the Valve Academic Research Consortium-2 (VARC-2) criteria and is one of the strongest predictors of acute and mid-term mortality [84].

Some studies have shown a detrimental effect of even mild PVR. In fact, results from the cohort A of the PARTNER trial demonstrated that with balloon-expandable valve, even mild PVR was associated with a worse survival at 2 years and at 5 years. The presence of greater severity PVR was also associated with reduced improvement in NYHA class and higher rates of rehospitalization [1, 75].

36.7 Predictors of Vascular and Bleeding Complications

Predictors of VC and bleeding complications (BC) are summarized together mainly for two reasons: firstly, BC have to be considered ones of VC accordingly to the VARC-2 classification that includes types 2, 3, and 5 of bleedings defined by the Bleeding Academic Research Consortium (BARC). The other reason is that VC are one of the principal predictors of BC.

Identification of predictors has been evaluated by several studies, and multiple emerged as independent ones, but heterogeneous definition of VC and BC has been used among studies. The VARC-2 criteria allow a more meaningful distinction between major and minor VC and so a stronger association between those and mortality.

36.7.1 Vascular Complications

VC depend on the access site: since the transfemoral approach is the most used one, ileofemoral complications are the most frequent, and we will focus on them.

The rate of vascular access-site complications is influenced by several factors, which include pre-procedural (patient's anatomy) and procedural ones (the size of the devices and the operator's experience/technique in deploying the closure devices) as shown in Fig. 36.6.

Small vessel dimensions and moderate-severe calcification are the most important anatomical predictors, and the combination of these two anatomical aspects was associated with the highest vascular complication rate [87]. Blakeslee-Carter et al. have developed an iliac morphology score (IMS) model to predict VC. IMS comprises iliac artery calcification and iliac artery minimum diameter evaluated by CT. A high IMS (≥5) and femoral artery area were strong predictors of VC [88].

More than the absolute measure of the iliofemoral diameter, it is important the sheath-to-femoral

Fig. 36.6 Pre-procedural, procedural and post-procedural predictors of vascular and bleeding complication after TAVI

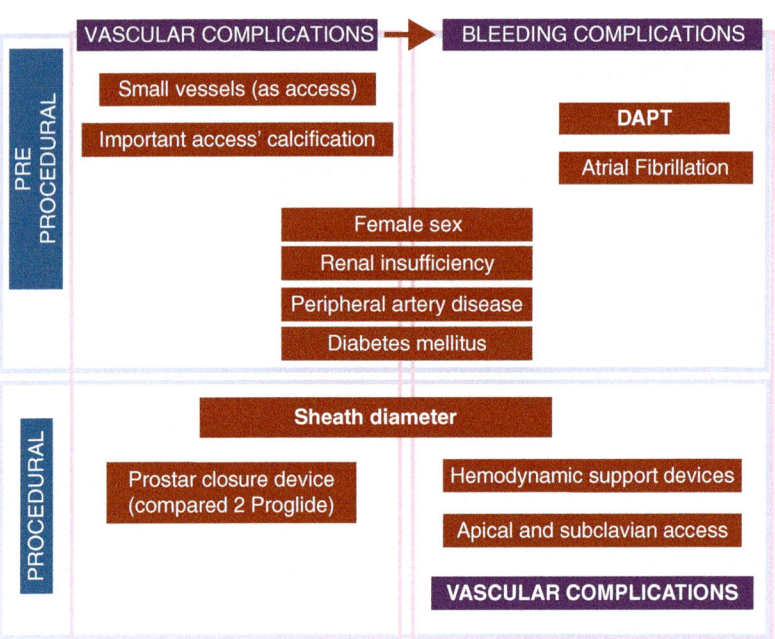

artery ratio, defined as the ratio between the sheath outer diameter and the femoral artery minimal lumen diameter. A ratio > 1.05 is a strong predictor of major VC and 30-day mortality [87].

Among patients' characteristics, female gender, age, height, DM, CKD, and peripheral artery disease have been correlated with VC [89]. In fact, all these factors are associated with smaller arterial diameter or calcification of the arterial wall. As previously reported for other types of complications, also in this case, operator's experience plays a pivotal role [90].

The most important procedural predictor is the sheath diameter. Recent data from the STS/ACC Transcatheter Valve Therapy Registry suggest that the frequency of VC is declining over time. In fact, major VC are significantly lowered by newer-generation TAVR devices that require smaller delivery sheaths, reducing complication from 8% (using 22–24 Fr sheaths) to 1% (using 18–19 Fr sheaths) [91].

The type of valve does not seem to influence primarily the rate of VC, except for some rare complication such as annular rupture that appears more frequently with balloon-expandable valves

with an extreme oversizing. The main difference compels again the required sheath: the Medtronic CoreValve has been associated with a lower risk of vascular complications compared to the older-generation Edwards SAPIEN devices that required sheaths with an inner diameter of 22–24 F. However, the newer-generation SAPIEN XT valves (18 or 19 F delivery systems) and Edwards SAPIEN valve 3 systems (with even smaller delivery systems) present lower VC compared to the first-generation valves. A large European multicenter registry compared the two newer-generation types of valve and found no difference in the rate of vascular complications from Medtronic CoreValve vs. Edwards SAPIEN XT valves [92]. With the recent approval of Medtronic CoreValve Evolut R systems, which use 14 F sheath, and Edwards SAPIEN valve 3 systems, which use a 14 F expandable sheath (allowing transient sheath expansion during valve delivery and returning to a low-profile diameter immediately after), the real-world incidence of vascular complications is expected to decline.

Finally, the type of vascular closure devices needs to be discussed. In fact, a lower incidence of VC and BC has been found with the double Preclose Proglide system, especially when compared to Prostar XL system (both by Abbott Vascular, Abbott Park, IL, USA) [93]. In the CONTROL multicenter study, Prostar use has been independently associated with both VC and BC with a sixfold increased risk of major complications when compared to Proglide [90].

36.7.2 Bleeding Complications

The temporal pattern of BC development permits to distinguish early bleeding (periprocedural period) and the late one. The former is an access-site bleeding originating from the puncture site or adjacent areas and is related mainly to procedural or technical factors. The latter, generally non-access-site bleeding, seems to be the expression of patient bleeding susceptibility.

As shown in Fig. 36.5, female gender, age, peripheral artery disease, CKD, AF, lower BMI, a high surgical risk, and DM have resulted to be the strongest predictor of BC, both early and late [94].

A major aspect of BC regards the therapeutic regimen. A strategy using mono vs. dual anti-platelet therapy (DAPT) during the pre-procedural phase in patients undergoing TAVR reduces life-threatening and major BC. The result of the recent OCEAN-TAVI registry, comparing DAPT vs. single antiplatelet therapy (SAPT) showed a twofold increase of any BC with the second approach [95].

More confusion exists about the role of anti-platelet regimen after TAVR in predicting BC. A meta-analysis suggests that at 30 days following TAVR, DAPT may have a higher bleeding risk vs. SAPT [96]; however, another recent meta-analysis found higher rate of BC with DAPT only when non-randomized trials were considered, losing significance with only randomized trial [97].

Once again, among procedural factors, the diameter of delivery system represents a major issue, and transapical and trans-subclavian vascular accesses have emerged as predictors [94].

36.8 Perspectives

Recently, novel variables have been assessed in predicting outcome after TAVR. Sinning et al. showed that the elevation of growth differentiation factor-15, a stress-responsive cytokine produced in response to inflammation and tissue injury, and interleukin-8, involved in innate immune responses, was associated with an increased risk of 1-year mortality. Moreover, the combination of these biomarkers with the EuroSCORE II added prognostic information to risk score alone [98].

Interestingly, patients undergoing TAVR who presented a worsening of pre-existing thrombocytopenia (TP) showed poorer in-hospital clinical outcomes with a 2.8-fold and three-fold increased risk of developing major VC and BC [99].

Furthermore, in patients with severe AS, arterial stiffness evaluated by pulse wave velocity (PWV) was correlated with transvalvular gradient and, in patients undergoing TAVR, was able to predict the echocardiographic procedure response. Therefore, baseline evaluation of PWV before TAVR could help in the selection of patients [100].

Finally, patients with severe AS undergoing TAVR and an invasive intraprocedural measurement of cardiac index (CI) <1.9 L/min/m^2 had significantly higher mortality at 30 days and 1 year, and those with lower CI at baseline without post-valve implantation improvement had the worst survival at 1-year follow-up [101].

The definitive role of these new factors need further study to be confirmed, but it could be that in the next future new variables will be added to predictive model to increase the sensibility to predict TAVR-related mortality and complications.

36.9 Conclusions

In this chapter, we have reviewed the principal predictors of mortality and complications of TAVR. Although many patients present an optimal response to TAVR with no complication and an improvement in mortality and QoL, a considerable number of patients don't answer this way. Understanding the predictors behind mortality, lack of improvement in QoL, or functional status as well as complications after TAVR could help in identifying a subgroup of patients in which the treatment could be defined as futile and so avoided. New variables are under study, and in the next future, they could be added to the predictive model in order to increase the sensibility to predict TAVR-related mortality and complications.

Conflict of Interest and Funding None to be declared.

References

1. Mack MJ, Leon MB, Smith CR, Miller DC, Moses JW, Tuzcu EM, et al. 5-year outcomes of transcatheter aortic valve replacement or surgical aortic valve replacement for high surgical risk patients with aortic stenosis (PARTNER 1): a randomised controlled trial. Lancet. 2015;385:2477–84.
2. Reardon MJ, Van Mieghem NM, Popma JJ, Kleiman NS, Søndergaard L, Mumtaz M, et al. Surgical or transcatheter aortic-valve replacement in intermediate-risk patients. N Engl J Med. 2017;376:1321–31.
3. Elmariah S, Palacios IF, McAndrew T, Hueter I, Inglessis I, Baker JN, et al. Outcomes of transcatheter and surgical aortic valve replacement in high-risk patients with aortic stenosis and left ventricular dysfunction: results from the placement of aortic transcatheter valves (PARTNER) trial (cohort A). Circ Cardiovasc Interv. 2013;6:604–14.
4. Giordana F, D'Ascenzo F, Nijhoff F, Moretti C, D'Amico M, Biondi Zoccai G, et al. Meta-analysis of predictors of all-cause mortality after transcatheter aortic valve implantation. Am J Cardiol. 2014;114:1447–55.
5. Sannino A, Gargiulo G, Schiattarella GG, Brevetti L, Perrino C, Stabile E, et al. Increased mortality after transcatheter aortic valve implantation (TAVI) in patients with severe aortic stenosis and low ejection fraction: a meta-analysis of 6898 patients. Int J Cardiol. 2014;176:32–9.
6. Amabile N, Agostini H, Gilard M, Eltchaninoff H, Iung B, Donzeau-Gouge P, et al. Impact of low preprocedural transvalvular gradient on cardiovascular mortality following TAVI: an analysis from the FRANCE 2 registry. EuroIntervention. 2014;10:842–9.
7. Lauten A, Figulla HR, Möllmann H, Holzhey D, Kötting J, Beckmann A, et al. TAVI for low-flow, low-gradient severe aortic stenosis with preserved

or reduced ejection fraction: a subgroup analysis from the German aortic valve registry (GARY). EuroIntervention. 2014;10:850–9.
8. Conrotto F, D'Ascenzo F, Stella P, Pavani M, Rossi ML, Brambilla N, et al. Transcatheter aortic valve implantation in low ejection fraction/low transvalvular gradient patients: the rule of 40. J Cardiovasc Med. 2017;18:103–8.
9. Baron SJ, Arnold SV, Herrmann HC, Holmes DR, Szeto WY, Allen KB, et al. Impact of ejection fraction and aortic valve gradient on outcomes of transcatheter aortic valve replacement. J Am Coll Cardiol. 2016;67:2349–58.
10. Le Ven F, Freeman M, Webb J, Clavel M-A, Wheeler M, Dumont É, et al. Impact of low flow on the outcome of high-risk patients undergoing transcatheter aortic valve replacement. J Am Coll Cardiol. 2013;62:782–8.
11. Eleid MF, Goel K, Murad MH, Erwin PJ, Suri RM, Greason KL, et al. Meta-analysis of the prognostic impact of stroke volume, gradient, and ejection fraction after transcatheter aortic valve implantation. Am J Cardiol. 2015;116:989–94.
12. Mok M, Nombela-Franco L, Dumont E, Urena M, DeLarochellière R, Doyle D, et al. Chronic obstructive pulmonary disease in patients undergoing transcatheter aortic valve implantation: insights on clinical outcomes, prognostic markers, and functional status changes. JACC Cardiovasc Interv. 2013;6:1072–84.
13. Nombela-Franco L, del Trigo M, Morrison-Polo G, Veiga G, Jimenez-Quevedo P, Abdul-Jawad Altisent O, et al. Incidence, causes, and predictors of early (≤30 days) and late unplanned hospital readmissions after transcatheter aortic valve replacement. JACC Cardiovasc Interv. 2015;8:1748–57.
14. Gilard M, Eltchaninoff H, Donzeau-Gouge P, Chevreul K, Fajadet J, Leprince P, et al. Late outcomes of transcatheter aortic valve replacement in high-risk patients. J Am Coll Cardiol. 2016;68:1637–47.
15. Codner P, Levi A, Gargiulo G, Praz F, Hayashida K, Watanabe Y, et al. Impact of renal dysfunction on results of transcatheter aortic valve replacement outcomes in a large multicenter cohort. Am J Cardiol. 2016;118:1888–96.
16. Gupta T, Goel K, Kolte D, Khera S, Villablanca PA, Aronow WS, et al. Association of chronic kidney disease with in-hospital outcomes of transcatheter aortic valve replacement. JACC Cardiovasc Interv. 2017;10:2050–60.
17. Goebel N, Baumbach H, Ahad S, Voehringer M, Hill S, Albert M, et al. Transcatheter aortic valve replacement: does kidney function affect outcome? Ann Thorac Surg. 2013;96:507–12.
18. Walther T, Hamm CW, Schuler G, Berkowitsch A, Kötting J, Mangner N, et al. Perioperative results and complications in 15,964 transcatheter aortic valve replacements. J Am Coll Cardiol. 2015;65:2173–80.

19. Abdelghani M, Cavalcante R, Miyazaki Y, de Winter RJ, Sarmento-Leite R, Mangione JA, et al. Prevalence, predictors, and prognostic implications of residual impairment of functional capacity after transcatheter aortic valve implantation. Clin Res Cardiol. 2017;106:752–9.

20. van der Boon RMA, Chieffo A, Dumonteil N, Tchetche D, Van Mieghem NM, Buchanan GL, et al. Effect of body mass index on short- and long-term outcomes after transcatheter aortic valve implantation. Am J Cardiol. 2013;111:231–6.

21. Koifman E, Kiramijyan S, Negi SI, Didier R, Escarcega RO, Minha S, et al. Body mass index association with survival in severe aortic stenosis patients undergoing transcatheter aortic valve replacement. Catheter Cardiovasc Interv. 2016;88:118–24.

22. Schulenberg R, Antonitsis P, Stroebel A, Westaby S. Chronic atrial fibrillation is associated with reduced survival after aortic and double valve replacement. Ann Thorac Surg. 2010;89:738–44.

23. Ludman PF, Moat N, de Belder MA, Blackman DJ, Duncan A, Banya W, et al. Transcatheter aortic valve implantation in the United Kingdom clinical perspective: temporal trends, predictors of outcome, and 6-year follow-up: a report from the UK transcatheter aortic valve implantation (TAVI) registry, 2007 to 2012. Circulation. 2015;131:1181–90.

24. Zahn R, Gerckens U, Linke A, Sievert H, Kahlert P, Hambrecht R, et al. Predictors of one-year mortality after transcatheter aortic valve implantation for severe symptomatic aortic stenosis. Am J Cardiol. 2013;112:272–9.

25. Urena M, Webb JG, Eltchaninoff H, Muñoz-García AJ, Bouleti C, Tamburino C, et al. Late cardiac death in patients undergoing transcatheter aortic valve replacement. J Am Coll Cardiol. 2015;65:437–48.

26. Lindman BR, Pibarot P, Arnold SV, Suri RM, McAndrew TC, Maniar HS, et al. Transcatheter versus surgical aortic valve replacement in patients with diabetes and severe aortic stenosis at high risk for surgery: an analysis of the PARTNER trial (placement of aortic transcatheter valve). J Am Coll Cardiol. 2014;63:1090–9.

27. Abramowitz Y, Jilaihawi H, Chakravarty T, Mangat G, Maeno Y, Kazuno Y, et al. Impact of diabetes mellitus on outcomes after transcatheter aortic valve implantation. Am J Cardiol. 2016;117:1636–42.

28. Abramowitz Y, Kazuno Y, Chakravarty T, Kawamori H, Maeno Y, Anderson D, et al. Concomitant mitral annular calcification and severe aortic stenosis: prevalence, characteristics and outcome following transcatheter aortic valve replacement. Eur Heart J. 2017;38:1194–203.

29. Mina GS, Gill P, Soliman D, Reddy P, Dominic P. Diabetes mellitus is associated with increased acute kidney injury and 1-year mortality after transcatheter aortic valve replacement: a meta-analysis. Clin Cardiol. 2017;40:726–31.

30. Talbot-Hamon C, Afilalo J. Transcatheter aortic valve replacement in the care of older persons with aortic stenosis. J Am Geriatr Soc. 2017;65:693–8.

31. Afilalo J, Alexander KP, Mack MJ, Maurer MS, Green P, Allen LA, et al. Frailty assessment in the cardiovascular care of older adults. J Am Coll Cardiol. 2014;63:747–62.

32. Afilalo J, Lauck S, Kim DH, Lefèvre T, Piazza N, Lachapelle K, et al. Frailty in older adults undergoing aortic valve replacement: the FRAILTY-AVR study. J Am Coll Cardiol. 2017;70:689–700.

33. Lombard JT, Selzer A. Valvular aortic stenosis. A clinical and hemodynamic profile of patients. Ann Intern Med. 1987;106:292–8.

34. Gautier M, Pepin M, Himbert D, Ducrocq G, Iung B, Dilly M-P, et al. Impact of coronary artery disease on indications for transcatheter aortic valve implantation and on procedural outcomes. EuroIntervention. 2011;7:549–55.

35. D'Ascenzo F, Conrotto F, Giordana F, Moretti C, D'Amico M, Salizzoni S, et al. Mid-term prognostic value of coronary artery disease in patients undergoing transcatheter aortic valve implantation: a meta-analysis of adjusted observational results. Int J Cardiol. 2013;168:2528–32.

36. Tarantini G, Purita PAM, D'Onofrio A, Fraccaro C, Frigo AC, D'Amico G, et al. Long-term outcomes and prosthesis performance after transcatheter aortic valve replacement: results of self-expandable and balloon-expandable transcatheter heart valves. Ann Cardiothorac Surg. 2017;6:473–83.

37. Iung B, Laouénan C, Himbert D, Eltchaninoff H, Chevreul K, Donzeau-Gouge P, et al. Predictive factors of early mortality after transcatheter aortic valve implantation: individual risk assessment using a simple score. Heart. 2014;100:1016–23.

38. Elhmidi Y, Bleiziffer S, Deutsch M-A, Krane M, Mazzitelli D, Lange R, et al. Acute kidney injury after transcatheter aortic valve implantation: incidence, predictors and impact on mortality. Arch Cardiovasc Dis. 2014;107:133–9.

39. Neverdal NO, Knudsen CW, Husebye T, Vengen OA, Pepper J, Lie M, et al. The effect of aortic valve replacement on plasma B-type natriuretic peptide in patients with severe aortic stenosis—one year follow-up. Eur J Heart Fail. 2006;8:257–62.

40. O'Sullivan CJ, Stortecky S, Heg D, Jüni P, Windecker S, Wenaweser P. Impact of B-type natriuretic peptide on short-term clinical outcomes following transcatheter aortic valve implantation. EuroIntervention. 2015;10:e1–8.

41. Bergler-Klein J, Klaar U, Heger M, Rosenhek R, Mundigler G, Gabriel H, et al. Natriuretic peptides predict symptom-free survival and postoperative outcome in severe aortic stenosis. Circulation. 2004;109:2302–8.

42. O'Neill BP, Guerrero M, Thourani VH, Kodali S, Heldman A, Williams M, et al. Prognostic value of serial B-type natriuretic peptide measurement

in transcatheter aortic valve replacement (from the PARTNER trial). Am J Cardiol. 2015;115:1265–72.

43. Koskinas KC, Stortecky S, Franzone A, O'Sullivan CJ, Praz F, Zuk K, et al. Post-procedural troponin elevation and clinical outcomes following transcatheter aortic valve implantation. J Am Heart Assoc. 2016;5:e002430.

44. Stundl A, Schulte R, Lucht H, Weber M, Sedaghat A, Shamekhi J, et al. Periprocedural myocardial injury depends on transcatheter heart valve type but does not predict mortality in patients after transcatheter aortic valve replacement. JACC Cardiovasc Interv. 2017;10:1550–60.

45. Debonnaire P, Fusini L, Wolterbeek R, Kamperidis V, van Rosendael P, van der Kley F, et al. Value of the "TAVI2-SCORe" versus surgical risk scores for prediction of one year mortality in 511 patients who underwent transcatheter aortic valve implantation. Am J Cardiol. 2015;115:234–42.

46. Capodanno D, Barbanti M, Tamburino C, D'Errigo P, Ranucci M, Santoro G, et al. A simple risk tool (the OBSERVANT score) for prediction of 30-day mortality after transcatheter aortic valve replacement. Am J Cardiol. 2014;113:1851–8.

47. Edwards FH, Cohen DJ, O'Brien SM, Peterson ED, Mack MJ, Shahian DM, et al. Development and validation of a risk prediction model for in-hospital mortality after transcatheter aortic valve replacement. JAMA Cardiol. 2016;1:46.

48. Pilgrim T, Franzone A, Stortecky S, Nietlispach F, Haynes AG, Tueller D, et al. Predicting mortality after transcatheter aortic valve replacement: external validation of the transcatheter valve therapy registry model. Circ Cardiovasc Interv. 2017;10:e005481.

49. Baron SJ, Arnold SV, Reynolds MR, Wang K, Deeb M, Reardon MJ, et al. Durability of quality of life benefits of transcatheter aortic valve replacement: long-term results from the CoreValve US extreme risk trial. Am Heart J. 2017;194:39–48.

50. American Thoracic Society. Withholding and withdrawing life-sustaining therapy. Ann Intern Med. 1991;115:478–85.

51. Arnold SV, Spertus JA, Lei Y, Green P, Kirtane AJ, Kapadia S, et al. How to define a poor outcome after transcatheter aortic valve replacement: conceptual framework and empirical observations from the placement of aortic transcatheter valve (PARTNER) trial. Circ Cardiovasc Qual Outcomes. 2013;6:591–7.

52. Arnold SV, Spertus JA, Vemulapalli S, Li Z, Matsouaka RA, Baron SJ, et al. Quality-of-life outcomes after transcatheter aortic valve replacement in an unselected population: a report from the STS/ACC transcatheter valve therapy registry. JAMA Cardiol. 2017;2:409.

53. Lange R, Beckmann A, Neumann T, Krane M, Deutsch M-A, Landwehr S, et al. Quality of life after transcatheter aortic valve replacement. JACC Cardiovasc Interv. 2016;9:2541–54.

54. Spertus J, Peterson E, Conard MW, Heidenreich PA, Krumholz HM, Jones P, et al. Monitoring clinical

changes in patients with heart failure: a comparison of methods. Am Heart J. 2005;150:707–15.

55. Leon MB, Smith CR, Mack M, Miller DC, Moses JW, Svensson LG, et al. Transcatheter aortic-valve implantation for aortic stenosis in patients who cannot undergo surgery. N Engl J Med. 2010;363:1597–607.

56. Leon MB, Smith CR, Mack MJ, Makkar RR, Svensson LG, Kodali SK, et al. Transcatheter or surgical aortic-valve replacement in intermediate-risk patients. N Engl J Med. 2016;374:1609–20.

57. Bosmans J, Bleiziffer S, Gerckens U, Wenaweser P, Brecker S, Tamburino C, et al. The incidence and predictors of early- and mid-term clinically relevant neurological events after transcatheter aortic valve replacement in real-world patients. J Am Coll Cardiol. 2015;66:209–17.

58. Stortecky S, Windecker S, Pilgrim T, Heg D, Buellesfeld L, Khattab AA, et al. Cerebrovascular accidents complicating transcatheter aortic valve implantation: frequency, timing and impact on outcomes. EuroIntervention. 2012;8:62–70.

59. Auffret V, Regueiro A, Del Trigo M, Abdul-Jawad Altisent O, Campelo-Parada F, Chiche O, et al. Predictors of early cerebrovascular events in patients with aortic stenosis undergoing transcatheter aortic valve replacement. J Am Coll Cardiol. 2016;68:673–84.

60. Yankelson L, Steinvil A, Gershovitz L, Leshem-Rubinow E, Furer A, Viskin S, et al. Atrial fibrillation, stroke, and mortality rates after transcatheter aortic valve implantation. Am J Cardiol. 2014;114:1861–6.

61. Eggebrecht H, Schmermund A, Voigtländer T, Kahlert P, Erbel R, Mehta RH. Risk of stroke after transcatheter aortic valve implantation (TAVI): a meta-analysis of 10,037 published patients. EuroIntervention. 2012;8:129–38.

62. Athappan G, Gajulapalli RD, Sengodan P, Bhardwaj A, Ellis SG, Svensson L, et al. Influence of transcatheter aortic valve replacement strategy and valve design on stroke after transcatheter aortic valve replacement: a meta-analysis and systematic review of literature. J Am Coll Cardiol. 2014;63:2101–10.

63. Kahlert P, Al-Rashid F, Döttger P, Mori K, Plicht B, Wendt D, et al. Cerebral embolization during transcatheter aortic valve implantation: a transcranial Doppler study. Circulation. 2012;126:1245–55.

64. Hahn RT, Pibarot P, Webb J, Rodes-Cabau J, Herrmann HC, Williams M, et al. Outcomes with post-dilation following transcatheter aortic valve replacement: the PARTNER I trial (placement of aortic transcatheter valve). JACC Cardiovasc Interv. 2014;7:781–9.

65. Daneault B, Kirtane AJ, Kodali SK, Williams MR, Genereux P, Reiss GR, et al. Stroke associated with surgical and transcatheter treatment of aortic stenosis: a comprehensive review. J Am Coll Cardiol. 2011;58:2143–50.

66. Auffret V, Puri R, Urena M, Chamandi C, Rodriguez-Gabella T, Philippon F, et al. Conduction

disturbances after transcatheter aortic valve replacement: current status and future perspectives. Circulation. 2017;136:1049–69.

67. Santos N, de Agustín JA, Almería C, Gonçalves A, Marcos-Alberca P, Fernández-Golfín C, et al. Prosthesis/annulus discongruence assessed by three-dimensional transoesophageal echocardiography: a predictor of significant paravalvular aortic regurgitation after transcatheter aortic valve implantation. Eur Heart J Cardiovasc Imaging. 2012;13:931–7.

68. O'Sullivan KE, Gough A, Segurado R, Barry M, Sugrue D, Hurley J. Is valve choice a significant determinant of paravalular leak post-transcatheter aortic valve implantation? A systematic review and meta-analysis. Eur J Cardiothorac. 2014;45:826–33.

69. Zaman S, McCormick L, Gooley R, Rashid H, Ramkumar S, Jackson D, et al. Incidence and predictors of permanent pacemaker implantation following treatment with the repositionable Lotus™ transcatheter aortic valve. Catheter Cardiovasc Interv. 2017;90:147–54.

70. Franzoni I, Latib A, Maisano F, Costopoulos C, Testa L, Figini F, et al. Comparison of incidence and predictors of left bundle branch block after transcatheter aortic valve implantation using the CoreValve versus the Edwards valve. Am J Cardiol. 2013;112:554–9.

71. Lange P, Greif M, Vogel A, Thaumann A, Helbig S, Schwarz F, et al. Reduction of pacemaker implantation rates after CoreValve® implantation by moderate predilatation. EuroIntervention. 2014;9:1151–7.

72. Toggweiler S, Stortecky S, Holy E, Zuk K, Cuculi F, Nietlispach F, et al. The electrocardiogram after transcatheter aortic valve replacement determines the risk for post-procedural high-degree AV block and the need for telemetry monitoring. JACC Cardiovasc Interv. 2016;9:1269–76.

73. Abdel-Wahab M, Mehilli J, Frerker C, Neumann F-J, Kurz T, Tölg R, et al. Comparison of balloon-expandable vs self-expandable valves in patients undergoing transcatheter aortic valve replacement: the CHOICE randomized clinical trial. JAMA. 2014;311:1503–14.

74. Siontis GCM, Jüni P, Pilgrim T, Stortecky S, Büllesfeld L, Meier B, et al. Predictors of permanent pacemaker implantation in patients with severe aortic stenosis undergoing TAVR: a meta-analysis. J Am Coll Cardiol. 2014;64:129–40.

75. Kodali S, Pibarot P, Douglas PS, Williams M, Xu K, Thourani V, et al. Paravalvular regurgitation after transcatheter aortic valve replacement with the Edwards sapien valve in the PARTNER trial: characterizing patients and impact on outcomes. Eur Heart J. 2015;36:449–56.

76. Détaint D, Lepage L, Himbert D, Brochet E, Messika-Zeitoun D, Iung B, et al. Determinants of significant paravalvular regurgitation after transcatheter aortic valve: implantation impact of device and annulus discongruence. JACC Cardiovasc Interv. 2009;2:821–7.

77. Sherif MA, Abdel-Wahab M, Stöcker B, Geist V, Richardt D, Tölg R, et al. Anatomic and procedural predictors of paravalvular aortic regurgitation after implantation of the Medtronic CoreValve bioprosthesis. J Am Coll Cardiol. 2010;56:1623–9.

78. Khalique OK, Hahn RT, Gada H, Nazif TM, Vahl TP, George I, et al. Quantity and location of aortic valve complex calcification predicts severity and location of paravalvular regurgitation and frequency of post-dilation after balloon-expandable transcatheter aortic valve replacement. JACC Cardiovasc Interv. 2014;7:885–94.

79. Koos R, Mahnken AH, Dohmen G, Brehmer K, Günther RW, Autschbach R, et al. Association of aortic valve calcification severity with the degree of aortic regurgitation after transcatheter aortic valve implantation. Int J Cardiol. 2011;150:142–5.

80. Watanabe Y, Lefèvre T, Arai T, Hayashida K, Bouvier E, Hovasse T, et al. Can we predict postprocedural paravalvular leak after Edwards SAPIEN transcatheter aortic valve implantation? Catheter Cardiovasc Interv. 2015;86:144–51.

81. Leber AW, Eichinger W, Rieber J, Lieber M, Schleger S, Ebersberger U, et al. MSCT guided sizing of the Edwards Sapien XT TAVI device: impact of different degrees of oversizing on clinical outcome. Int J Cardiol. 2013;168:2658–64.

82. Mylotte D, Dorfmeister M, Elhmidi Y, Mazzitelli D, Bleiziffer S, Wagner A, et al. Erroneous measurement of the aortic annular diameter using 2-dimensional echocardiography resulting in inappropriate CoreValve size selection: a retrospective comparison with multislice computed tomography. JACC Cardiovasc Interv. 2014;7:652–61.

83. Moat NE, Ludman P, de Belder MA, Bridgewater B, Cunningham AD, Young CP, et al. Long-term outcomes after transcatheter aortic valve implantation in high-risk patients with severe aortic stenosis: the U.K. TAVI (United Kingdom Transcatheter Aortic Valve Implantation) Registry. J Am Coll Cardiol. 2011;58:2130–8.

84. Athappan G, Patvardhan E, Tuzcu EM, Svensson LG, Lemos PA, Fraccaro C, et al. Incidence, predictors, and outcomes of aortic regurgitation after transcatheter aortic valve replacement. J Am Coll Cardiol. 2013;61:1585–95.

85. Chieffo A, Buchanan GL, Van Mieghem NM, Tchetche D, Dumonteil N, Latib A, et al. Transcatheter aortic valve implantation with the Edwards SAPIEN versus the Medtronic CoreValve Revalving system devices: a multicenter collaborative study: the PRAGMATIC Plus Initiative (Pooled-RotterdAm-Milano-Toulouse In Collaboration). J Am Coll Cardiol. 2013;61:830–6.

86. Paradis J-M, Altisent OA-J, RodÉs-Cabau J. Reducing periprocedural complications in transcatheter aortic valve replacement: review of paravalvular leaks, stroke and vascular complications. Expert Rev Cardiovasc Ther. 2015;13:1251–62.

87. Hayashida K, Lefèvre T, Chevalier B, Hovasse T, Romano M, Garot P, et al. Transfemoral aortic valve implantation new criteria to predict vascular complications. JACC Cardiovasc Interv. 2011;4:851–8.

88. Blakeslee-Carter J, Dexter D, Mahoney P, Ahanchi S, Steerman S, Larion S, et al. A novel iliac morphology score predicts procedural mortality and major vascular complications in transfemoral aortic valve replacement. Ann Vasc Surg. 2018;46:208–17.

89. Sardar MR, Goldsweig AM, Abbott JD, Sharaf BL, Gordon PC, Ehsan A, et al. Vascular complications associated with transcatheter aortic valve replacement. Vasc Med. 2017;22:234–44.

90. Barbash IM, Barbanti M, Webb J, Molina-Martin De Nicolas J, Abramowitz Y, Latib A, et al. Comparison of vascular closure devices for access site closure after transfemoral aortic valve implantation. Eur Heart J. 2015;36:3370–9.

91. Holmes DR, Nishimura RA, Grover FL, Brindis RG, Carroll JD, Edwards FH, et al. Annual outcomes with transcatheter valve therapy: from the STS/ACC TVT registry. J Am Coll Cardiol. 2015;66:2813–23.

92. Di Mario C, Eltchaninoff H, Moat N, Goicolea J, Ussia GP, Kala P, et al. The 2011-12 pilot European sentinel registry of transcatheter aortic valve implantation: in-hospital results in 4,571 patients. EuroIntervention. 2013;8:1362–71.

93. Mehilli J, Jochheim D, Abdel-Wahab M, Rizas KD, Theiss H, Spenkuch N, et al. One-year outcomes with two suture-mediated closure devices to achieve access-site haemostasis following transfemoral transcatheter aortic valve implantation. EuroIntervention. 2016;12:1298–304.

94. Piccolo R, Pilgrim T, Franzone A, Valgimigli M, Haynes A, Asami M, et al. Frequency, timing, and impact of access-site and non-access-site bleeding on mortality among patients undergoing transcatheter

aortic valve replacement. JACC Cardiovasc Interv. 2017;10:1436–46.

95. Hioki H, Watanabe Y, Kozuma K, Nara Y, Kawashima H, Kataoka A, et al. Pre-procedural dual antiplatelet therapy in patients undergoing transcatheter aortic valve implantation increases risk of bleeding. Heart. 2017;103:361–7.

96. Aryal MR, Karmacharya P, Pandit A, Hakim F, Pathak R, Mainali NR, et al. Dual versus single antiplatelet therapy in patients undergoing transcatheter aortic valve replacement: a systematic review and meta-analysis. Heart Lung Circ. 2015;24:185–92.

97. Gandhi S, Schwalm J-DR, Velianou JL, Natarajan MK, Farkouh ME. Comparison of dual-antiplatelet therapy to mono-antiplatelet therapy after transcatheter aortic valve implantation: systematic review and meta-analysis. Can J Cardiol. 2015;31:775–84.

98. Sinning J-M, Wollert KC, Sedaghat A, Widera C, Radermacher M-C, Descoups C, et al. Risk scores and biomarkers for the prediction of 1-year outcome after transcatheter aortic valve replacement. Am Heart J. 2015;170:821–9.

99. Flaherty MP, Mohsen A, Moore JB, Bartoli CR, Schneibel E, Rawasia W, et al. Predictors and clinical impact of pre-existing and acquired thrombocytopenia following transcatheter aortic valve replacement. Catheter Cardiovasc Interv. 2015;85:118–29.

100. Bruschi G, Maloberti A, Sormani P, Colombo G, Nava S, Vallerio P, et al. Arterial stiffness in aortic stenosis: relationship with severity and echocardiographic procedures response. High Blood Press Cardiovasc Prev. 2017;24:19–27.

101. Kiramijyan S, Koifman E, Magalhaes MA, Ben-Dor I, Didier R, Jerusalem ZD, et al. Intraprocedural invasive hemodynamic parameters as predictors of short- and long-term outcomes in patients undergoing transcatheter aortic valve replacement. Cardiovasc Revasc Med. 2018;19:257–62.

Learning Curve Characteristics and Relationship of Procedural Volumes with Clinical Outcomes for Transcatheter Aortic Valve Implantation

37

Anthony Wassef and Asim N. Cheema

Transcatheter aortic valve implantation (TAVI), also called transcatheter aortic valve replacement (TAVR), has experienced marked growth in utilization after successful outcome of large randomized trails confirming clinical utility of TAVR for patients at high [1–3] and intermediate risk for surgical aortic valve replacement (SAVR) [4, 5]. With the expanding indications for TAVR [6], there has been a significant increase in the number of centers performing TAVR as well as the number of procedures being performed at each center. Compared to 2012, when 4627 procedures were performed at 198 centers in the United States, greater than 24000 procedures were performed at more than 400 centers in 2015 [7]. An increasing proportion of elderly population in the Western society over the next decades [8, 9] will require a greater demand for TAVR procedures with a concomitant increase in the need of new operators and centers [10]. However, TAVR is a technically challenging procedure requiring a unique skill set that is distinct from conventional learning in interventional cardiology and cardiac surgery [11]. Therefore, ongoing quality assurance is highly desirable to optimize clinical outcomes and maintain excellence for operators and sites performing TAVR.

The phenomenon of procedural learning curve has been well described for technically difficult or complex procedures [12, 13]. In addition, the effects of operator and institutional volumes on procedural success rates and patient outcomes are well documented in the surgical literature [14]. However, limited information is available regarding the learning curve and annual volume relationship with clinical outcome for TAVR procedures.

In this chapter, we will review the general principles associated with the learning curve phenomenon and the relationship between institutional or operator volumes with clinical outcomes. In addition we will discuss the evidence for TAVR learning curve and data examining the effect of annual institutional volumes on patient outcomes as well as identify areas that require further research to answer outstanding questions.

A. Wassef
Cardiac Catheterization Laboratory, St. Mary's General Hospital, Kitchener, ON, Canada

A. N. Cheema (✉)
Division of Cardiology, St. Michael's Hospital, Toronto, ON, Canada
e-mail: Cheemaa@smh.ca

37.1 General Principles for Learning Curve Analysis

The concept of the learning curve was first introduced in aircraft manufacturing in 1936, where Wright described how the cost of aircraft

© Springer Nature Switzerland AG 2019
A. Giordano et al. (eds.), *Transcatheter Aortic Valve Implantation*,
https://doi.org/10.1007/978-3-030-05912-5_37

manufacturing decreased with increasing time and experience [15]. This has since been applied to other industries including the medical profession supporting the principle that people and organizations would become better at performing specific tasks with increasing exposure and experience [16]. In contrast to pharmacological treatments, both surgical and interventional procedures including TAVR are difficult to investigate due to their complex and multifaceted nature including need for specific training and continued experience for satisfactory results [16–18]. Cook et al. [19] described a conceptual approach to learning curve analysis where incremental improvement in outcomes finally reaches a plateau. It is important to note that "surgical skill" is not a quantity or variable that can be measured directly; instead the two quantities that are assessed in the learning curve analysis include measures of process (operative time, contrast volume, etc.) and measures of clinical outcome (e.g., death, stroke, bleeding, etc.) [17].

37.2 Learning Curve Phenomenon in Clinical Medicine

The learning curve has been assessed in multiple studies, primarily related to surgical specialties and medical education [18]. In terms of clinical implications, the most notable case is related to the excessive rates of death among pediatric patients undergoing cardiac surgery in Bristol, UK, when the poor outcomes were identified to be related to the limited experience of the surgeon [20]. In cardiovascular medicine, the presence of a learning curve has been documented for both interventional and cardiac surgery procedures. For coronary artery bypass grafting (CABG), Bridgewater et al. showed that patient mortality rates consistently declined from 2.2% for surgeons in the first year of practice after completion of residency training to 1.2% for the fourth year of practice post training [21]. Similarly, operative time for CABG has been shown to decrease by over 17 min when comparing new with experienced surgeons [22]. In

interventional cardiology, the phenomenon of learning curve has been demonstrated for transradial cardiac catheterization and coronary interventions (PCI). Ball et al. [13] studied 1672 patients undergoing transradial PCI by 28 operators and found that failure rates and contrast use were significantly higher for the first 50 cases compared to experienced radial operators and the odds of radial failure reduced by 32% for every 50 case increase in the operator experience. Similar results were reported from the much larger CathPCI registry confirming that a minimum of 50 case volume was required to achieve technical proficiency for transradial PCI [23].

37.3 Learning Curve for Transcatheter Aortic Valve Implantation (TAVR)

37.3.1 TAVR Learning Curve: Measures of Process

Multiple studies have demonstrated that with increasing procedural experience, measures of process for TAVR including procedure time, fluoroscopy time, and contrast use will improve (Table 37.1). Early single center trials focusing on transapical TAVR (TA-TAVR) [24] showed that fluoroscopy time (7.1 min vs. 6.2 min) and contrast volume (104 mL vs. 93 mL) significantly decreased after the initial 150 cases. Similarly, D'Anconna et al. [25] showed a 5% decrease in operative time and 15% lowering of radiation exposure for every 100 TAVR procedures performed. A similar analysis from the PARTNER trial was reported by Suri et al. and included 1100 patients undergoing TA-TAVR showing significant reductions in fluoroscopy time (14–12 min) and contrast volume (114–90 mL) after the initial 60 cases [26]. A similar trend for transfemoral TAVR (TF-TAVR) cohort from PARTNER study ($n = 1521$) was reported with a decrease in procedure time from 154 to 85 min and reduced fluoroscopy time from 28 to 20 min over the course of the study duration [27].

Table 37.1 Summary of studies examining the learning curve for transcatheter aortic valve implantation

Study	Year	Source data/ population	N	Access	Principle comparison/ analysis	Principle findings
Gurvitch et al. [30]	2011	Single center	270	TF and TA	First half (135) vs. second half (135)	Significant increase in overall procedural success (92.6% vs. 97.8%), significant decrease in overall mortality (13.3% vs. 5.9%)
Kempfert et al. [24]	2011	Single center	299	TA	First half (150) vs. second half (149)	Significantly reduced contrast load (104 mL vs. 93 mL), balloon re-dilation and reduced 30-day mortality (11.3–6.0%)
Alli et al. [47]	2012	Single center	44	TF and TA	1st to 3rd tertile	Significant decrease in median contrast volume (180 to 160 to 130 mL), valvuloplasty to valve time, fluoroscopy time (26.1 to 17.2 to 14.3 min) and radiation dose
D'Ancona et al. [25, 48, 49]	2014	Single center	500	TA	Linear and nonparametric correlation	5% reduction in operating time and 15% reduction in contrast dose per 100 cases performed
Lundardi et al. [50]	2016	Single center	177	TF	Cumulative Sum (CUSUM)	54 cases for plateau of primary composite end point of major complications; 32 cases for plateau of device success
Arai et al. [31]	2016	3 centers	312	TF	Cumulative Sum (CUSUM) early experience Edwards valve (86 procedures), CoreValve (40 cases)	Edwards valve: 30-day mortality (17% to 7%) and 1 year mortality (34–21%) improved. CoreValve: 30-day mortality (20–6%) and 1 year mortality (38–15%) improved.
Arai et al. [51]	2016	3 centers	257	TAo	Cumulative Sum (CUSUM) early experience 128 cases vs. later experience	30-day mortality was not significantly different, the incidence of life-threatening bleeding (9% vs. 1%), stroke (5% vs. 0%,) and AKI (16% vs. 6%) decreased in the late phase group
Suri et al. [26]	2016	Multicenter— PARTNER	1100	TA	Nonlinear mixed modeling 30–45 cases	30 cases: Procedure time decreased from 131 to 116 min; 45 cases: Device success increased to 90%
Minha et al. [32]	2016	Multicenter— PARTNER	1521	TF	Plateau of effect – clinical	22 cases: 80% device success; 70 cases: major bleeding below 10%; 25 cases: major vascular complications below 5%; 28 cases: consistently low 30-day mortality.
Alli et al. [27]	2016	Multicenter— PARTNER	1521	TF	Plateau of effect – technical	Procedure time decreased from 154 to 85 min; fluoroscopy time from 28 to 20 min. Plateau achieved at 25 cases for centers entering late

(continued)

Table 37.1 (continued)

Study	Year	Source data/ population	N	Access	Principle comparison/ analysis	Principle findings
D'Anconna et al. [52]	2017	Single center	133	TF	Early learning (20 cases) phase vs. consolidation	Statistically significant reduction in catheterization time after first 20 cases
Henn et al. [53]	2017	Single center	400	TF, TA, and TAo	Case sequence	Technical proficiency begins to develop by the 25th case, and achieved by 50th case
Gurevitch et al. [44]	2017	Single center— recent initiation with mentorship	269	TF and alternative	Mentorship between experienced center and novice center	After 1 year and 50 cases: No difference in outcomes (procedural safety, procedure times, length of stay) between experienced center and novice center
Wassef et al. [28]	2017	International Multicenter Registry	1953	TF and alternative	Case sequence quantiles Q1:0–62, Q2:63–133, Q2:134–242, Q4: >243	Q4 vs. Q1: All-cause mortality decreased (4% vs. 8%), improved device success (89% vs. 78%), reduced combined safety end point (10% vs. 19%)
Carrol et al. [29]	2017	STS/TVT Registry	42998	TF and alternative	Case sequence quartiles, linear and nonlinear modeling	Increasing site volume associated with lower mortality, bleeding, vascular access complications but not stroke. High risk of adverse vascular and bleeding outcomes in the first 100 cases

We have previously examined the learning curve phenomenon in a large cohort of patients from an international TAVR registry comprising 1953 patients [28]. Data for all TAVR cases was collected from the start of the respective TAVR programs and stratified into chronological quantiles. We observed a consistent decrease in procedure time with increasing case volume. The TAVR performed in the fourth quantile (>243 procedures) showed a procedure time >120 min for only 2.3% of cases compared to 13.3% in the first quantile (<62 procedures). Similarly, <5% of cases in the fourth quantile utilized contrast volume of >100 mL compared to 15% of cases in the first quantile. These findings were later confirmed in a publication from the TVT registry from the United States for 42,988 TAVR patients also showing a comparable decrease in contrast use, air kerma radiation dose, and fluoroscopy time with increasing experience [29].

37.3.2 TAVR Learning Curve: Clinical Outcomes

As with measures of process examining procedural outcomes, multiple studies have studied and reported an improvement in clinical outcomes for TAVR with increasing procedural experience (Table 37.1). The initial report of a learning curve from the Vancouver group [30] divided their initial 270 cases into first and second half and showed improved 30-day mortality that decreased from 13.3% among the first half to 5.9% among the second half of procedures. A three-center study from France and Japan examined early learning curve for TA- and TF-TAVR [31]. The authors observed that 1-year mortality significantly improved after the initial 86 cases for the Sapien valve (34% vs. 21%) and after the initial 40 cases for the CoreValve (38–14%) for TF-TAVR. However, there was no significant difference in mortality with higher volume for TA-TAVR, though life-threatening bleeding (9% vs. 1%), stroke (5% vs. 0%), and acute kidney injury (16% vs. 6%) decreased only after the first 128 cases.

Three large multicenter studies have examined relationship of procedural volumes with clinical outcomes among TAVR populations. Minha et al. [32] used data from 1521 patients undergoing TF-TAVR from the PARTNER trial and found that 80% device success was achieved by 22 cases, major vascular complications fell below 5% after 70 cases, and major bleeding was <10% after the 25 case volume. Wassef et al. [28] (Fig. 37.1) used data from the international TAVR registry from nine centers with 1953 patients and stratified all cases in chronological case quantiles (Q1 ≤ 62 cases, Q2 63–133, Q3 134–233, Q4 ≥ 234). The authors reported a significant increase in device success (78% for Q1 to 89% for Q4), decreased incidence of moderate to severe paravalvular leak (19% for Q1 to 11% for Q4), and lower rates of valve embolization (3.8% for Q1 to 0.2% for Q4) with greater TAVR vol-

ume. The overall rate of the early safety end point improved from 19% for patients in Q1 to 10% for patients in Q4, with a significant decrease from Q1 to Q 4 for the rate of major vascular complications (9% vs. 4%), major bleeding (4.4% vs. 1.6%), and all-cause mortality (8.3% vs. 3.7%). Multivariate correction for baseline and procedural variables demonstrated that Q2 (OR 2.18), Q3 (OR 3.82), and Q4 (OR 13.5) were independently associated with higher device success, while Q3 (OR 0.67) and Q4 (OR 0.41) were associated with higher early safety end point. Q4 was also independently associated with a lower mortality (OR 0.36). Using data from the TVT registry, Carrol et al. also demonstrated a similar learning curve (Fig. 37.2) [29]. In their analysis of 42,988 TAVR procedures at 395 hospitals in the United States performed between 2011 and 2015, the modeled rates of mortality, vascular complications, and bleeding complications for the first case versus the 400th case reduced from 3.6% vs. 2.6%, 6.1% vs. 4.2%, and 9.6% vs. 5.1%, respectively. The differences in outcomes were most pronounced for the first 100 cases.

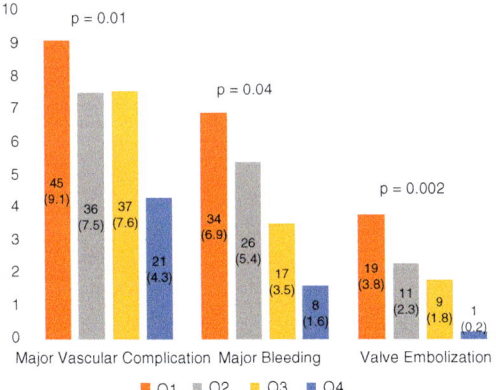
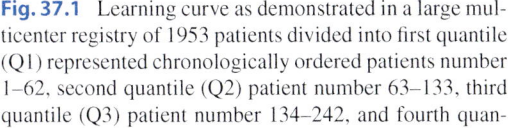
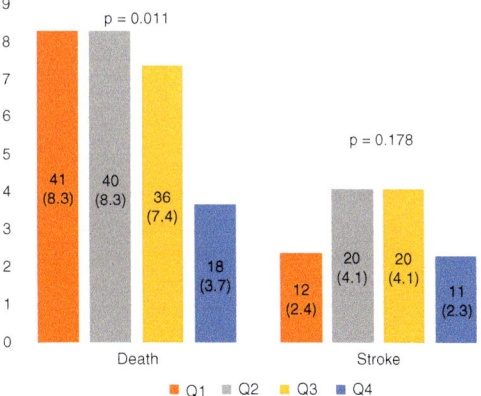

Fig. 37.1 Learning curve as demonstrated in a large multicenter registry of 1953 patients divided into first quantile (Q1) represented chronologically ordered patients number 1–62, second quantile (Q2) patient number 63–133, third quantile (Q3) patient number 134–242, and fourth quantile (Q4) patient number 243–476. With increasing procedural experience, major vascular complications, major bleeding, valve embolization, and death all improved. Reproduced from Wassef et al. 2017 [28]

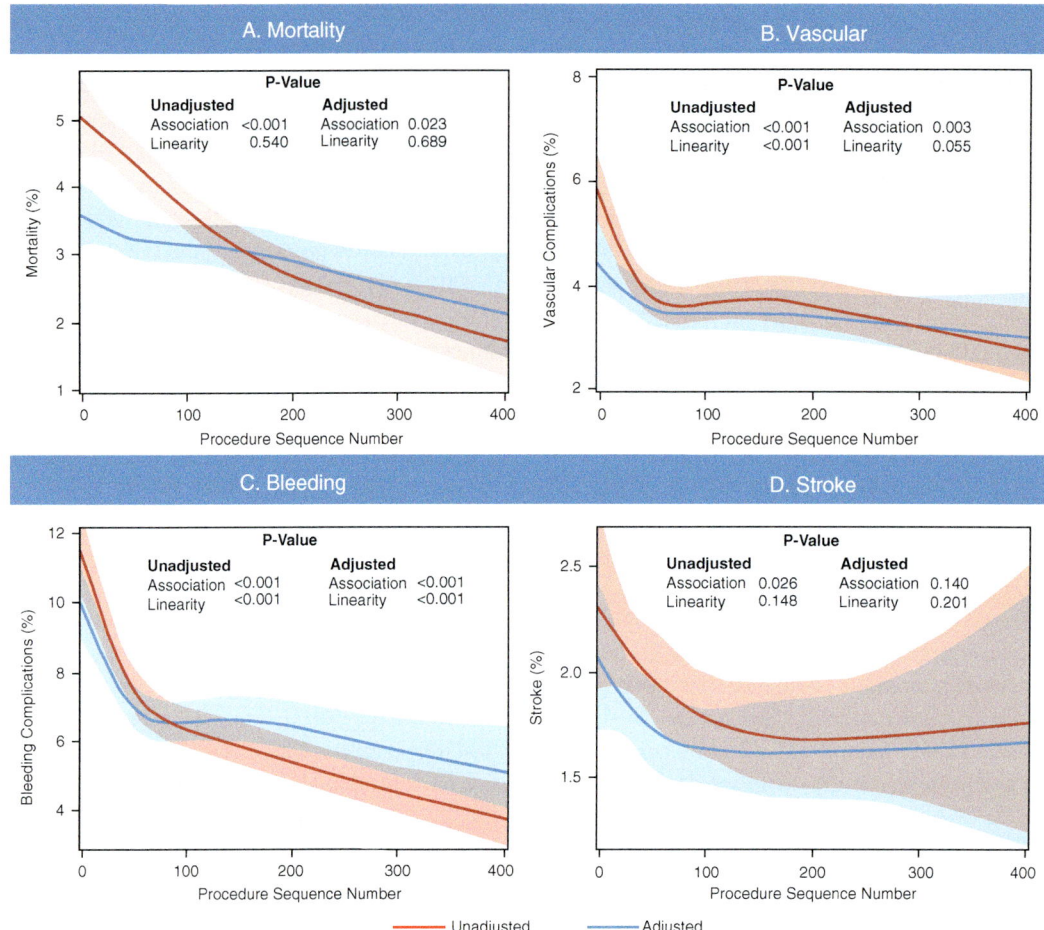

Fig. 37.2 Association of (**a**) mortality, (**b**) vascular complications, (**c**) bleeding, and (**d**) stroke with procedure sequence number, with the most marked improvement in outcomes being in the first 100 cases. Reproduced with permission from Carrol et al. 2017 [29]

37.4 Procedural Volume and Outcome Relationship for TAVR

37.4.1 Procedural Volume and Outcomes in Clinical Medicine

The relationship between hospital and operator volumes and adverse outcomes for surgical procedures has been well described, with the first large report published by Luft et al. in 1979 reporting improved mortality for a variety of surgical procedures in high-volume compared to low-volume hospitals [33]. Factors that may influence improved surgical outcome in higher-volume hospital include more skilled surgeons, referral bias to surgeons with better outcomes, increased familiarity with and ability to anticipate and manage postoperative complications, greater resources to manage complex patients, and better communication between the healthcare team [33, 34]. The role of postoperative management and "failure to rescue" from a complication has also been identified as another important factor for adverse outcomes seen among low-volume centers. Results from a series of >100,000 US Medicare patients undergoing cardiovascular surgery procedures showed that there was a 12% higher rate of major complications, but 57% were more likely to die from the complications when procedures were performed at centers in the lowest compared to the highest annual volume quintile [34]. Although studies have examined volume–outcome relationships for both individual operators and institutions, a recent systematic review suggests that institutional volumes are more predictive of adverse outcomes for complex procedures, while operator volumes are reasonable predictor for outcomes of less complex procedures [35]. Birkmeyer et al. reported from a large series of nearly half a million patients undergoing a variety of common surgical procedures showing a strong relationship between hospital surgical volume and adjusted operative mortality for CABG (5.5% for >162 procedures/year vs. 3.5% for <101 procedures/year), aortic valve replacement (10% for >42 procedures/year vs. 6% for <22 procedures/year), and repair of abdominal aortic aneurysm (6% for >18% procedures/year vs. 4% for <8 procedures/year) [36]. In interventional cardiology, several studies have reported on the important relationship between annual procedure volume and clinical outcomes. A widely known study by Hannan et al. analyzed data from the New York PCI registry and found a significantly higher rate of mortality (0.96% vs. 0.90%) and same-stay CABG (3.9% vs. 3.4%) for hospitals performing <600 procedures and operators performing <75 PCI procedures per year [14]. With the multitude of studies and meta-analyses demonstrating improved outcomes with higher operator and hospital volumes, a public initiative is suggested to limit complex surgical procedures to specific operators and institutions [37].

37.5 Procedure Volume and Outcome Relationship for TAVR

TAVR is a complex procedure that requires involvement of specialists from multiple specialties including interventional cardiology, cardiovascular surgery, cardiac imaging, and anesthesia for appropriate patient selection, procedure performance, and postoperative management. In view of the heart team approach for TAVR,

examination of operator volume and clinical outcome relationship has limited application, and most investigators have focused on delineating the influence of hospital volumes on clinical outcome of TAVR as summarized in Table 37.2. Recognizing the importance of hospital volumes on clinical excellence in a variety of medical procedures, the Centers for Medicare and Medicaid Services in the United States requires a hospital to perform at least 50 SAVR, employ 2 or more cardiac surgeons, and perform ≥ 1000 coronary angiograms and ≥ 400 PCI prior to be approved as a TAVR site [38].

With regard to clinical end points of interest, Kim et al. [39] using the US National Inpatient Sample (256 hospitals, 7660 patients) found a correlation between clinical outcome and hospital volumes. Low-volume TF-TAVR centers (<20 TAVR/year) had higher rates of all-cause death (OR 1.55), bleeding (OR 1.53), and pacemaker implantation (OR 1.39) with no significant difference in stroke when compared to high-volume centers (>20 TAVR/year). Similarly, low-volume TA-TAVR centers (<10 TAVR/year) had higher rates of death (OR 3.1), pacemaker implantation (OR 6.0), and myocardial infarction (OR 5.4) compared to high-volume TA-TAVR (>20 TAVR/year) centers. Similarly, Badheka et al. [40] using the US National Inpatient Sample ($n = 1481$) divided the population into hospital volume quartiles (<5 TAVR/year for lowest and >20 TAVR/year for highest) and found in-hospital mortality rates decreased with increasing hospital volume with 6.4% (first quartile), 5.9% (second quartile), 5.2% (third quartile), and 2.8% (fourth quartile). In addition, length of stay and index hospital costs were significantly lower for the fourth quartile hospitals. However, contrary to the above findings, de Baisi et al. [41] also used the US National Inpatient Sample, but did not find a linear inverse relationship between hospital volume and mortality for TAVR, with comparable mortality at both very high- and very low-volume centers. Khera et al. [42] reported from the 2014 Nationwide Readmissions Database representing 49% of all US hospitalizations and found a significant inverse relationship between hospital TAVR volume and rates of readmission after the

Table 37.2 Summary of studies examining the volume-outcome relationship for transcatheter aortic valve replacement

Study	Year	Source data/population	N	Access	Principle comparison	Principle findings
Kim et al. (40)	2015	USA: National Inpatient Sample	7660 in 256 hospitals	TF and TA	Low vs. high volume (TF—20 cases/year, TA—10 cases/year)	TF: Significantly higher mortality, renal failure, vascular complications, pacemaker implantation at low-volume centers. TA: Significantly higher mortality (3.6% vs. 2.3%,), renal failure, pacemaker implantation low-volume center
Badheka et al. [40]	2015	USA: National Inpatient Sample	1418	TF and alternative	Annual volume quartiles first (<5 / year), second (6–10/year), third (11–20/year), and fourth (>20/year)	With multivariate analysis, statistically significantly lower risk of death (2.4% lowest vs. 6.4% highest quartile), death and morbidity, hospital stay >6 days in hospitals with the highest volume quartile
De Biasi et al. [41]	2016	USA: National Inpatient Sample	7,635	TF and alternative	TAVR distributed <20, 20–40, 40–60, >60	Hospital volume did not predict in-hospital morbidity and mortality
Verma et al. [43]	2016	USA: 3 Center	3 hospitals, 181 cases	NR	Correlation of CT site reported annulus sizing to independent review	Higher rate of correlation between site reported annulus size and re-reviewed annulus size in high-volume center; mismatch predicted higher composite end point
Khera et al. [42]	2017	USA: National Readmissions Database	129 hospitals, 16,252 TAVR	TF and alternative	Hospitals were classified as low (<50), medium (≥50 to <100), and high (≥100) volume	Significantly lower rates of readmission in the high-volume hospitals, with no difference in index length of stay, procedural cost
Bestehorn et al. [54]	2017	Germany	87 hospitals, 9924 patients	TF and alternative		Continuous decrease in mortality with increasing hospital volume, statistically higher mortality in hospitals performing < 50 TAVR vs. > 200 TAVR/year

index procedures. The 30-day readmission rates were lowest in high-volume (≥100 procedures/year) compared with medium-volume (50–100 procedures/year) (OR 0.76) and low-volume (≤50 procedures/year) (OR 0.75) hospitals. These observations suggest that technical excellence and possibly superior post procedure care may be large contributors to the differences in clinical outcomes. It is interesting to note that the volume-outcome relation for TAVR may also be applicable for TAVR quality measures. A recent study by Verma et al. [43] examined CT reports performed at multiple institutions and reported that CT performed at high-volume sites (>75 TAVR/year) had excellent correlation with independent reporting of annular size and transcatheter valve size ($r = 0.96$), a finding that was not reproduced for lower annual volume centers.

37.6 Implications for Clinical Practice

TAVR is a complex procedure with cognitive and technical aspects that are unique and different than those of cardiac surgery and interventional cardiology [11]. These include understanding of the underlying pathophysiology, comprehension, and analysis of diagnostic workup including cardiac hemodynamics, noninvasive imaging, as well as technical expertise including large bore access, implantation of the prosthesis, and management of potential operative and postoperative complications with appropriate clinical follow-up schedule. With this complexity, there is little doubt that experience gained from prior similar procedures (i.e., learning curve) will further improve procedural success, and concentration of services in high-volume centers will result in superior outcomes. The available data consistently shows that both a learning curve phenomenon and a volume-outcome relationship exist for TAVR procedures.

However, there are important limitations with regard to methodology used and patient population studied. In addition, TAVR is an advancing field with major modification in available devices with significant decrease in size of catheters, improved valve designs, and incorporation of features (retrievability) that allow bail out in case of procedural challenges. Furthermore, improved clinical knowledge with incorporation of CT findings, better anticipation of potential complications, and advances in care algorithm (percutaneous access, conscious sedation) greatly impact the procedural success rates and clinical outcomes. Defining learning curve thresholds and institutional volume criteria is inherently difficult for any evolving field including TAVR.

In addition, most published studies were done at early adopting centers that used first- and second-generation devices. Whether recent improvement is TAVR technology translates into a shorter learning curve remains uncertain. In addition, the role of a formal mentorship arrangement is poorly understood. In a recent study, a formal mentorship agreement between a new program and an established program in Minnesota, USA, greatly improved technical proficiency as measured by procedural time, device success, and safety with comparable results demonstrated for the new and the established program after 50 cases and at 1 year [44]. Another approach has been adopted by the province of British Columbia in Canada that has enacted a regionalization policy for TAVR programs with a central medical director with a TF-TAVR as the default strategy for all sites. All non-TF-TAVR, valve in valve, and non-aortic valve intervention can only be performed at a center of excellence [45]. In the most recent 2017 AATS/ACC/SCAI/STS Expert Consensus Systems of Care document, specific recommendations have been made for new TAVR programs [46]. These include interventional cardiologist to have ≥100 TAVR experience with 50 as a primary operator and the surgeon with ≥100 SAVR career cases or 25 SAVR during the prior year or 50 SAVR over the last 2 years, along with the hospital performing ≥ 300 PCI and ≥40 SAVR per year.

There are important implications for the learning curve threshold as well as annual procedural volume criteria for maintaining necessary skill set, hospital credentialing, as well as for the medicolegal area. Furthermore, it is increasingly important to rationally allocate resources in the era of constantly rising healthcare costs. TAVR is a pioneering procedure for transcatheter structural heart intervention, and the lessons learned are likely applicable to future similar systems of care in this field.

Finally, as TAVR transitions to the mainstream interventional cardiology, a robust understanding of the learning curve thresholds and procedural volume-outcome relationship is needed for the development of competency-based training programs for structural interventional fellowship to produce the next generation of TAVR operators.

37.7 Conclusions

Transcatheter aortic valve replacement is a maturing technology with a marked increase in the number of procedures performed and centers offering TAVR. TAVR is also a technically complex procedure, with a characteristic learning curve and clinically important relationship between institutional volume and patient outcomes. The operator excellence in TAVR procedures continues to improve for a case volume

>240 procedures. In addition, available evidence suggest improved clinical outcomes for institutions with an annual TAVR volume >50 procedures.

However, it is important to note that these thresholds are devised by data from early adopting centers that included first- and second-generation TAVR devices. It remains unclear whether new centers implanting contemporary TAVR devices with formal mentorship arrangements can achieve proficiency with a shorter learning curve and achieve comparable clinical outcomes to high-volume centers. Further research will be required to refine the above thresholds as advances in technology, formal physician training, and evolving indications change the landscape of TAVR.

TF Transfemoral, *TA* Transapical, *TAo* Transaortic, *AKI*, Acute kidney injury, *STS/TVT* Society of thoracic surgeons/transcatheter valve therapy

TF Transfemoral, *TA* Transapical

References

1. Leon MB, Smith CR, Mack M, et al. Transcatheter aortic-valve implantation for aortic stenosis in patients who cannot undergo surgery. N Engl J Med. 2010;363(17):1597–607.
2. Smith CR, Leon MB, Mack MJ, et al. Transcatheter versus surgical aortic-valve replacement in high-risk patients. N Engl J Med. 2011;364(23):2187–98.
3. Adams DH, Popma JJ, Reardon MJ, et al. Transcatheter aortic-valve replacement with a self-expanding prosthesis. N Engl J Med. 2014;370(19):1790–8.
4. Reardon MJ, Van Mieghem NM, Popma JJ, et al. Surgical or transcatheter aortic-valve replacement in intermediate-risk patients. N Engl J Med. 2017;376(14):1321–31.
5. Leon MB, Smith CR, Mack MJ, et al. Transcatheter or surgical aortic-valve replacement in intermediate-risk patients. N Engl J Med. 2016;374(17):1609–20.
6. Nishimura RA, Otto CM, Bonow RO, et al. 2017 AHA/ACC focused update of the 2014 AHA/ACC guideline for the management of patients with valvular heart disease: a report of the American College of Cardiology/American Heart Association Task Force on Clinical Practice Guidelines. J Am Coll Cardiol. 2017;70(2):252–89.
7. Grover FL, Vemulapalli S, Carroll JD, et al. 2016 annual report of The Society of Thoracic Surgeons/American College of Cardiology Transcatheter Valve Therapy Registry. J Am Coll Cardiol. 2017;69(10):1215–30.
8. Stewart BF, Siscovick D, Lind BK, et al. Clinical factors associated with calcific aortic valve disease. Cardiovascular Health Study. J Am Coll Cardiol. 1997;29(3):630–4.
9. Wan He DG, Paul Kowal An aging world: 2015 International Population Reports. US Census Bureau, International Population Reports, P95/16-1, 2016.
10. Osnabrugge RL, Mylotte D, Head SJ, et al. Aortic stenosis in the elderly: disease prevalence and number of candidates for transcatheter aortic valve replacement: a meta-analysis and modeling study. J Am Coll Cardiol. 2013;62(11):1002–12.
11. Tommaso CL, Bolman RM 3rd, Feldman T, et al. Multisociety (AATS, ACCF, SCAI, and STS) expert consensus statement: operator and institutional requirements for transcatheter valve repair and replacement, part 1: transcatheter aortic valve replacement. J Thorac Cardiovasc Surg. 2012;143(6):1254–63.
12. Sanchez PL, Harrell LC, Salas RE, et al. Learning curve of the Inoue technique of percutaneous mitral balloon valvuloplasty. Am J Cardiol. 2001;88(6):662–7.
13. Ball WT, Sharieff W, Jolly SS, et al. Characterization of operator learning curve for transradial coronary interventions. Circ Cardiovasc Interv. 2011;4(4):336–41.
14. Hannan EL, Racz M, Ryan TJ, et al. Coronary angioplasty volume-outcome relationships for hospitals and cardiologists. JAMA. 1997;277(11):892–8.
15. Wright TP. Factors Affecting the Cost of Airplanes. J Aeronaut Sci. 1936;3(4):122–8.
16. Craig P, Dieppe P, Macintyre S, et al. Developing and evaluating complex interventions: the new Medical Research Council guidance. BMJ. 2008;337:a1655.. (Clinical research ed)
17. Subramonian K, Muir G. The 'learning curve' in surgery: what is it, how do we measure it and can we influence it? BJU Int. 2004;93(9):1173–4.
18. Hopper AN, Jamison MH, Lewis WG. Learning curves in surgical practice. Postgrad Med J. 2007;83(986):777–9.
19. Cook JA, Ramsay CR, Fayers P. Statistical evaluation of learning curve effects in surgical trials. Clin Trials. 2004;1(5):421–7.
20. The Report of the Public Inquiry into children's heart surgery at the Bristol Royal Infirmary 1984–1995, 2001.
21. Bridgewater B, Grayson AD, Au J, et al. Improving mortality of coronary surgery over first four years of independent practice: retrospective examination of prospectively collected data from 15 surgeons. BMJ. 2004;329(7463):421.. (Clinical research ed)
22. Maruthappu M, Duclos A, Lipsitz SR, et al. Surgical learning curves and operative efficiency: a cross-specialty observational study. BMJ Open. 2015;5(3):e006679.
23. Hess CN, Peterson ED, Neely ML, et al. The learning curve for transradial percutaneous coronary intervention among operators in the United States: a study

from the National Cardiovascular Data Registry. Circulation. 2014;129(22):2277–86.

24. Kempfert J, Rastan A, Holzhey D, et al. Transapical aortic valve implantation: analysis of risk factors and learning experience in 299 patients. Circulation. 2011;124(11 Suppl):S124–9.

25. D'Ancona G, Pasic M, Unbehaun A, et al. Transapical aortic valve implantation: learning curve with reduced operating time and radiation exposure. Ann Thorac Surg. 2014;97(1):43–7.

26. Suri RM, Minha S, Alli O, et al. Learning curves for transapical transcatheter aortic valve replacement in the PARTNER-I trial: technical performance, success, and safety. J Thorac Cardiovasc Surg. 2016;152(3):773–80.e14.

27. Alli O, Rihal CS, Suri RM, et al. Learning curves for transfemoral transcatheter aortic valve replacement in the PARTNER-I trial: technical performance. Catheter Cardiovasc Interv. 2016;87(1):154–62.

28. Wassef AWA, Alnasser S, Rodes-Cabau J, et al. Institutional experience and outcomes of transcatheter aortic valve replacement: results from an international multicentre registry. Int J Cardiol. 2017;245:222–7.

29. Carroll JD, Vemulapalli S, Dai D, et al. Procedural experience for transcatheter aortic valve replacement and relation to outcomes: The STS/ACC TVT registry. J Am Coll Cardiol. 2017;70(1):29–41.

30. Gurvitch R, Tay EL, Wijesinghe N, et al. Transcatheter aortic valve implantation: lessons from the learning curve of the first 270 high-risk patients. Catheter Cardiovasc Interv. 2011;78(7):977–84.

31. Arai T, Lefevre T, Hovasse T, et al. Evaluation of the learning curve for transcatheter aortic valve implantation via the transfemoral approach. Int J Cardiol. 2016;203:491–7.

32. Minha S, Waksman R, Satler LP, et al. Learning curves for transfemoral transcatheter aortic valve replacement in the PARTNER-I trial: Success and safety. Catheter Cardiovasc Interv. 2016;87(1):165–75.

33. Luft HS, Bunker JP, Enthoven AC. Should operations be regionalized? The empirical relation between surgical volume and mortality. N Engl J Med. 1979;301(25):1364–9.

34. Gonzalez AA, Dimick JB, Birkmeyer JD, et al. Understanding the volume-outcome effect in cardiovascular surgery: the role of failure to rescue. JAMA Surg. 2014;149(2):119–23.

35. McAteer JP, LaRiviere CA, Drugas GT, et al. Influence of surgeon experience, hospital volume, and specialty designation on outcomes in pediatric surgery: a systematic review. JAMA Pediatr. 2013;167(5):468–75.

36. Birkmeyer JD, Stukel TA, Siewers AE, et al. Surgeon volume and operative mortality in the United States. N Engl J Med. 2003;349(22):2117–27.

37. Urbach DR. Pledging to eliminate low-volume surgery. N Engl J Med. 2015;373(15):1388–90.

38. US Department of Health and Human Services, Centers for Medicare and Medicaid Services.

Transcatheter Aortic Valve Replacement (TAVR) hospital program volume requirements.

39. Kim LK, Minutello RM, Feldman DN, et al. Association between transcatheter aortic valve implantation volume and outcomes in the United States. Am J Cardiol. 2015;116(12):1910–5.

40. Badheka AO, Patel NJ, Panaich SS, et al. Effect of hospital volume on outcomes of transcatheter aortic valve implantation. Am J Cardiol. 2015;116(4):587–94.

41. de Biasi AR, Paul S, Nasar A, et al. National analysis of short-term outcomes and volume-outcome relationships for transcatheter aortic valve replacement in the era of commercialization. Cardiology. 2016;133(1):58–68.

42. Khera S, Kolte D, Gupta T, et al. Association between hospital volume and 30-day readmissions following transcatheter aortic valve replacement. JAMA Cardiol. 2017;2(7):732–41.

43. Verma DR, Pershad Y, Pershad A, et al. Impact of institutional volume and experience with CT interpretation on sizing of transcatheter aortic valves: a multicenter retrospective study. Cardiovasc Revasc Med. 2016;17(8):566–70.

44. Gurevich S, John R, Kelly RF, et al. Avoiding the learning curve for transcatheter aortic valve replacement. Cardiol Res Pract. 2017;2017:7524925.

45. Stub D, Lauck S, Lee M, et al. Regional systems of care to optimize outcomes in patients undergoing transcatheter aortic valve replacement. JACC Cardiovasc Interv. 2015;8(15):1944–51.

46. Bavaria JETC, Carroll JD, Deeb GM, Feldman TE, Gleason TG, Horlick EM, Kavinsky CJ, Kumbhani DJ, Miller DC, Seals AA, Shemin RJ, Sundt TM, Thourani VH. 2018 AATS/ACC/SCAI/STS Expert Consensus Systems of Care Document: Operator and Institutional Requirements for Transcatheter Aortic Valve Replacement. J Am Coll Cardiol. 2019;73:340–74.

47. Alli OO, Booker JD, Lennon RJ, et al. Transcatheter aortic valve implantation: assessing the learning curve. JACC Cardiovasc Interv. 2012;5(1):72–9.

48. Pasic M, Unbehaun A, Dreysse S, et al. Introducing transapical aortic valve implantation (part 1): effect of a structured training program on clinical outcome in a series of 500 procedures. J Thorac Cardiovasc Surg. 2013;145(4):911–8.

49. Pasic M, Unbehaun A, Dreysse S, et al. Introducing transapical aortic valve implantation (part 2): institutional structured training program. J Thorac Cardiovasc Surg. 2013;145(4):919–25.

50. Lunardi M, Pesarini G, Zivelonghi C, et al. Clinical outcomes of transcatheter aortic valve implantation: from learning curve to proficiency. Open Heart. 2016;3(2):e000420.

51. Arai T, Romano M, Lefevre T, et al. Impact of procedural volume on outcome optimization in transaortic transcatheter aortic valve implantation. Int J Cardiol. 2016;223:292–6.

52. D'Ancona G, Agma HU, Kische S, et al. Introducing transcatheter aortic valve implantation with a

new generation prosthesis: Institutional learning curve and effects on acute outcomes. Neth Hear J. 2017;25(2):106–15.

53. Henn MC, Percival T, Zajarias A, et al. Learning alternative access approaches for transcatheter aortic valve replacement: implications for new transcatheter aortic valve replacement centers. Ann Thorac Surg. 2017;103(5):1399–405.

54. Bestehorn K, Eggebrecht H, Fleck E, et al. Volume-outcome relationship with transfemoral transcatheter aortic valve implantation (TAVI)—insights from the compulsory German quality assurance registry on aortic valve replacement (AQUA). EuroIntervention. 2017;13:914–20.

Role of Balloon Aortic Valvuloplasty in the Transcatheter Aortic Valve Implantation Era

38

Laura Gatto, Enrico Romagnoli, Vito Ramazzotti, and Francesco Prati

38.1 Introduction

Calcific aortic stenosis is the most frequent aortic valve disease in Western countries, with an increasing prevalence as the population ages and affecting up to 4% of adults more than 85 years of age [1]. Clinical history of aortic stenosis is characterized by a long latent evolution, but after symptoms onset, patients show a significantly reduced survival, mostly due to the absence of a definitive therapy [2]. O'Keefe et al. in a retrospective study reported that in subjects with untreated severe aortic stenosis, 1-year, 2-year, and 3-year survival rates were 57%, 37%, and 25%, respectively [3].

Surgical aortic valve replacement represents the best treatment option of severe calcific aortic stenosis as recommended in the most recent guidelines by European Society of Cardiology and American College of Cardiology/American Heart Association [4, 5]. The relief of outflow obstruction ameliorates both hypertrophy and function of the left ventricle with a persistent symptomatic improvement. However many patients don't undergo surgery because of their high-risk surgical profile (e.g., comorbidities) and patient/physician refusal. Indeed, the Euro Heart Survey reported that about 32% of patients with severe valvular heart disease were excluded from surgical treatment for cardiac causes and for other comorbidities, such as advanced age, chronic obstructive pulmonary disease, renal failure, and short life expectancy [6].

Balloon aortic valvuloplasty (BAV), which increases the aortic valve orifice through percutaneous balloon dilatation, is a historical nonsurgical option that provides temporary symptomatic and hemodynamic improvement (i.e., bridging therapy) in selected patients with severe aortic stenosis and offers an alternative treatment for inoperable patients.

With the recent introduction of transcatheter aortic valve implantation (TAVI), also called transcatheter aortic valve replacement (TAVR), the incidence of BAV has been increasing, as this has been performed as a part of the TAVI procedure or as a bridge to elective TAVI procedure [7].

38.2 Balloon Aortic Valvuloplasty: Historical and Technical Aspects

The first adult BAV was performed by Alain Cribier in France in 1985 and nowadays still represents a suitable therapeutic alternative in selected conditions [8].

L. Gatto (✉) · E. Romagnoli · V. Ramazzotti
F. Prati
Division of Cardiology, San Giovanni Addolorata Hospital, Via Dell'Amba Aradam 8, Rome, Italy

Centro Per la Lotta Contro l'Infarto Foundation, Rome, Italy

The effects of BAV on diseased valve have been studied extensively, but no single mechanism of action has been definitively proven. The most common hypothesis is that the fracture of intraleaflet calcific nodules, increasing the flexibility within the calcified aortic valve, improves thereby the valve opening. Other mechanisms proposed include annular stretching and the separation of fused leaflets, as well as the scattering of leaflet micro-fractures and cleavage planes along collagenized stroma [9].

The BAV procedure, which has not changed much in the last 20 years, has been significantly improved by constant advances in balloon design, guide wires, and newer imaging modalities, such as transesophageal echocardiography, intracardiac echocardiography, and aortic computer tomography. Moreover, the introduction of vascular closure devices has also recently reduced the rate of access-site vascular complications [10].

BAV is generally performed using a retrograde approach: during the procedure, a wire passes through the stenotic valve, and then a procedural balloon is advanced, positioned, and inflated across the valve (Fig. 38.1). The balloon may be inflated many times, and after its removal, an aortography is generally performed to define the presence and the severity of acute aortic regurgitation, a potentially fatal complication. The retrograde technique necessarily requires vascular anatomy suitable for large-caliber sheaths, and the femoral artery is the most common site of vascular puncture. The requirement of an arterial access is associated with a risk of bleeding complications, and it could be an important concern in elderly patients with peripheral arterial disease or in patients with previous vascular surgery or documented iliac-femoral vessel tortuosity. Indeed, a problematic retrograde approach may limit the guide wire in crossing a stenotic valve [11].

As alternative, BAV may be performed through an anterograde way using the femoral vein as entry site. This technique is more technically challenging, because it supposes the transseptal puncture and the balloon delivery across the left ventricular apex. A possible complication of this approach is the creation of a permanent atrial septal defect (5% of patients) with a left-to-right shunt that increases the cardiac output conditioning a fallacious computing of post-procedural valve area improvement [12]. The anterograde

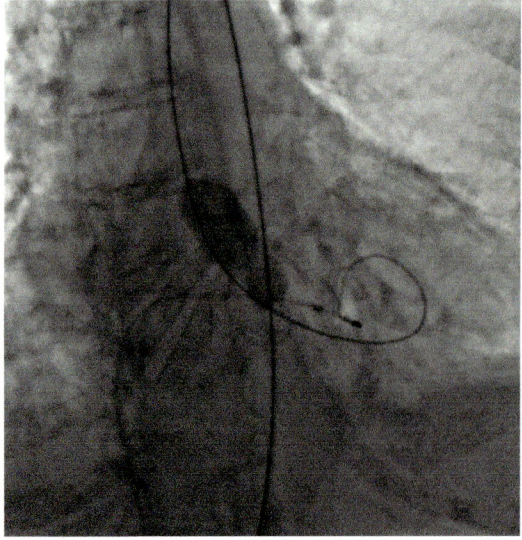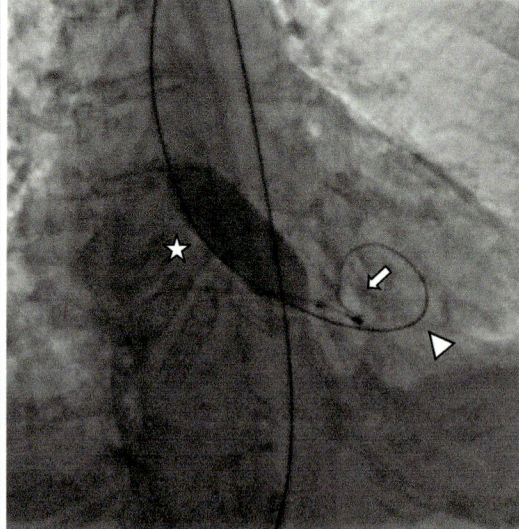

Fig. 38.1 Case study of balloon aortic valvuloplasty. The left panel shows the initial phase of dilation with the valve leaflets indenting the balloon. The right panel shows the fully inflated balloon. Star, arrowhead, and arrow highlight, respectively, the inflated balloon (Valver Ag, Balton), the guidewire (Amplatz SuperStiff, Boston Scientific), and the right ventricular pacing catheter (Spike Flow, FIAB)

technique uses the Inoue balloon, which is typically used for mitral valvuloplasty but has been shown to improve the post-procedural aortic valve area (AVA) compared with the conventional aortic balloon (used in the retrograde approach) with a decreased inflation and deflation time [13].

There are no randomized comparisons of the two techniques, but observational data show comparable results. Already in 1987, Block demonstrated a similar reduction in aortic gradient and comparable increase in AVA, but vascular complications were more common with the retrograde approach [14]. More recently, Cubeddu et al. published a retrospective single-center registry including 157 patients with severe aortic stenosis treated with either anterograde or retrograde BAV. No differences in hemodynamic parameters and in clinical outcomes at 2 years were reported in the two groups, despite a significantly higher incidence of peripheral arterial disease and higher rate of vascular complications in patients treated with retrograde technique [15].

Several technical aspects of BAV have never been standardized and are currently left to the operator's discretion. Variability includes, among others, balloon sizing, definition of procedural success, use of rapid ventricular pacing, vascular sheath size, and hemostasis.

The sizing of the balloon for the valvuloplasty was generally performed according to the aortic valve annulus diameter measured at echocardiography and taken from a long axis view which measures the shorter axis of the elliptical aortic annulus [16]. In most of cases, the balloon size was 1 mm smaller than echo measured aortic annulus: balloon diameter 18 mm for annulus ≤19 mm, balloon diameter 20 mm for annulus >20<23 mm, and balloon diameter 23 mm for annulus ≥24 mm. Patients with bulky leaflet calcifications may be preferred a balloon with a diameter 2 mm smaller than echo measured aortic annulus. This represents a conservative but systematic sizing; it is reasonable to speculate that a more aggressive choice of balloon size would achieve great improvements in gradient and valve area at the expense of more complications [17].

In the past, BAV balloons were inflated manually with large syringes, but the fully inflation of these large balloons by hand was very difficult: simple hand inflation usually results in under-inflation to 1 or 2 mm under the nominal diameter. In current practice, inflation devices are often used, or a smaller side syringe is employed to "boost" the final part of the inflation. These new techniques result in full balloon inflation to nominal diameter [18].

Successful BAV was traditionally defined as a reduction >40% in the mean gradient and/or increase in AVA >40%. At the end of the procedure, pressures were recorded during pullback across the aortic valve; peak and mean gradients, together with thermo-dilution cardiac outputs, were measured, and AVA was calculated using the Gorlin equation [10]. Alternatively, the AVA and the mean trans-aortic gradient may also be assessed by echocardiography early after BAV. These parameters collected shortly after valvuloplasty may be more reliable than the procedural success evaluated through hemodynamic measurements immediately after balloon inflation. In fact, BAV generates short phase of hypotension and stress in patients which can lead to a reaction characterized by a release of catecholamines, tachycardia, and increased contractility, and for these reasons the mean trans-aortic gradient can be acutely overestimated. Thirty minutes should be a reasonable time frame to allow full hemodynamic stabilization after procedural stress or transient complications [19].

Rapid ventricular pacing is commonly used during balloon inflation to obtain temporary circulatory arrest and to stabilize the balloon at the valve orifice, increasing the success procedural rate by preventing the balloon migration. Ventricular pacing at 180–200 bpm rate was generally started just before balloon inflation and stopped at the time of deflation, for a maximum duration of 10 s [10]. Yet, in expert hands, BAV can be performed without rapid pacing with an overall less invasive and possibly better tolerated approach. In fact, fast ventricular stimulation sometimes may be the cause of a respiratory arrest, or it can be poorly hemodynamically accepted in fragile patients with scarce coronary reserve [20]. Registry data suggest similar procedural safety with the two techniques, but less efficacy in the rapid pacing technique, in terms of a smaller post-procedural AVA, despite easier balloon stabilization [21]. More recently Dall'Ara and colleagues conducted a randomized study to compare the effectiveness and safety of BAV performed with or without rapid ventricular pacing in 100 patients, 70 years of age or older, with severe degenerative aortic stenosis. No significant differences, between the two groups, were observed in achievement of both primary efficacy endpoint (defined as 50% reduction in the mean echocardiographic trans-aortic gradient) and safety endpoint (composite of death, myocardial infarction, stroke, acute aortic regurgitation, and BARC bleeding $\geq$3 at 30-day). However, the no-pacing group showed a better procedural tolerance (16% vs. 41%), requiring significantly fewer bailout temporary pacemakers ($P = 0.048$) and showing lower incidence of moderate/severe post-procedural renal function worsening ($P = 0.052$) [19].

A mini-invasive approach with rapid pacing through the 0.035-inch left ventricular support wire could be a new strategy, extremely appealing, recently introduced by Hilling-Smith and colleagues. The authors described a case series of 132 cases of TAVI and 76 of BAV done using ventricular pacing via the left ventricular lead by simply connecting one electrode to the patient's skin and one electrode through the left ventricular wire. They reported that all procedures have been successfully performed and no BAV patients required temporary pacing wire or permanent pacemaker insertion [22].

38.3 Balloon Aortic Valvuloplasty: Complications

Balancing symptomatic improvement and procedural risk is a crucial point in the selection of patients undergoing BAV, because complications are not infrequent including death, ischemic stroke, bleeding, and acute severe aortic regurgitation. In the National Heart, Lung, and Blood Institute Balloon Valvuloplasty Registry, the incidence of transfusion, cerebrovascular accident, and mortality were 23%, 3%, and 3%, respectively [23].

38.3.1 Bleeding

The requirement of large-bore arterial sheath is associated with a reported incidence of periprocedural vascular injury between 10% and 15% [24, 25]. However, in the last 20 years, technical improvements, such as the use of vascular closure devices (VCD) and novel anticoagulants, considerably decreased the complication rates of the access site. Ben-Dor et al. in a case series of 333 patients with severe aortic stenosis undergoing BAV reported a cumulative vascular complication rate of 8.4% including perforation, limb ischemia, arteriovenous fistula, pseudoaneurysm requiring intervention, and access-site infection. However, the use of VCD (suture-mediated closure devices, and recently reported collagen-based closure devices) with respect to manual compression was related with a significantly reduced risk of access-site events (7% vs. 17%, $P < 0.001$), with a lower incidence of transfusion and shorter hospital length of stay [26]. Similar results have been recently reported in another multicenter retrospective study comparing suture-mediated versus manual compression access site showing that the first technique was associated with significant reductions in major bleeding, major adverse cardiovascular events, and net adverse clinical events (10.0% vs. 24.5%, $P < 0.001$) [27].

Indeed, major bleeding and blood transfusion occur in approximately 20% of patients underwent BAV. During this percutaneous procedure, traditionally, a proper anticoagulant is achieved using intravenous unfractionated heparin, but recent data suggest that bivalirudin may be a valid and safer option. Kini and colleagues compared the outcomes of consecutive patients who underwent elective or urgent BAV with intraprocedural use of bivalirudin or heparin at two high-volume centers, in the BRAVO (The Effect of Bivalirudin on Aortic Valve Intervention Outcomes) registry. Of 427 patients, 223 patients received bivalirudin and 204 received heparin. Respect to patients treated with heparin, patients treated with bivalirudin had significantly less major bleeding (4.9% vs. 13.2%, $P = 0.003$). There was no significant difference in the rates of major adverse cardiovascular events (MACE) defined as a composite of mortality, myocardial infarction, or stroke (6.7% vs. 11.3%, $P = 0.1$) and in the rate of vascular complications (major, 2.7% vs. 2.0%; minor, 4.5% vs. 4.9%; $P = 0.83$); but cumulatively the net adverse clinical events (NACE) including major bleeding and MACE were reduced in the bivalirudin group (11.2% vs. 20.1%, $P = 0.01$) [28].

38.3.2 Acute Aortic Regurgitation

About 60% of patients had baseline aortic regurgitation of any grade, but BAV has been proved relatively safe in patients with combined aortic stenosis and significant aortic regurgitation, because the pathogenesis of both valvular defects is the reduced mobility of the leaflets due to severe calcifications [29].

Conversely, acute aortic regurgitation is a rare but fearsome complication of BAV and is correlated with a grim prognosis. It is generally defined as the sudden onset of severe valve insufficiency after BAV, associated with hemodynamic instability or overt cardiogenic shock, irrespective of the pre-procedural grade of valvular regurgitation. During acute aortic regurgitation, continuous pressure monitoring typically shows a combination of the following features: a sudden drop of the systolic and diastolic pressure values; a "ventricularization" of the aortic pressure curve; a sharp increase of ventricular diastolic pressure with end-diastolic pressure equivalent to the aortic diastolic pressure; and, less frequently, a widening of the QRS complex at the electrocardiogram with severe bradycardia and high-degree AV block. The occurrence of such a complication deserves immediate interruption of the scheduled balloon inflations in order to try to correct both the hemodynamic imbalance and eventually the responsible structural problem of the valve. However, no further valve dilatations are recommended, even after acute aortic regurgitation resolution [30]. A recent paper by Eltchaninoff et al. reported an incidence of severe aortic regurgitation of 1.5% and showed this complication to be an independent predictor of long-term mortal-ity [31]. Dall'Ara and colleagues, out of 1517 consecutive patient undergoing BAV, identified 26 cases (1.7%) of acute aortic regurgitation with overt hemodynamic instability. This complication occurred in 80% of cases after one or two balloon inflation and in 8 patients out 26 (30.8%) spontaneously resolved within few minutes. For persisting aortic regurgitation, the authors reported a rescue maneuver, called the "reinforced pigtail" maneuver, attempted in the cases with a fluoroscopic evidence or suspicion of one or more cusps stuck in the open position. This maneuver was successful in 13 out of 18 patients in which has been performed and consists in the retrograde insertion of a 6 Fr pigtail into the ascending aorta until it reaches the valve plane. A 0.035-inch J wire or, more often, the proximal tip of a 0.035-inch extra-stiff wire is left inside the pigtail. The tip of the wire should be preferably angulated manually before the insertion within the pigtail to help the operator directing the distal end of the catheter selectively toward each of the Valsalva's sinuses, between the sinus wall and the displaced open cusp. A moderate pressure over the valve cusps associated with clockwise or counter-clockwise rotation of the pigtail catheter might be able to actually reposition (and "close") the displaced aortic valve [32].

38.4 Balloon Aortic Valvuloplasty: Early and Long-Term Results

38.4.1 Early Results

Most studies have documented modest but significant improvements in various hemodynamic parameters including trans-aortic gradient, cardiac output, and AVA following BAV (Table 38.1). Although results vary according to severity of underlying aortic stenosis and technique, reductions in peak gradient range between 30% and 40% with similar improvements in AVA [23–25, 33–36]. These favorable changes in post-procedure hemodynamic parameters result in early symptomatic benefit generally reported as a reductions in New York Heart Association (NYHA) functional class.

Table 38.1 Early improvements in hemodynamic parameters and complication rate in balloon aortic valvuloplasty registries

	Patients	Age (years)	Increase in AVA (cm²)	Decrease in mean AV gradient (mmHg)	Decrease in peak to peak AV gradient	Periprocedural complication rate (%)
Otto CM [23]	674	78 ± 9	From 0.50 ± 0.20 to 0.80 ± 0.30	From 55 ± 21 to 29 ± 13	–	25
McKay R [24]	492	79±8.4	From 0.50±0.18 to 0.82 ± 0.30	From 60 ± 23 to 30 ± 13	–	20.5
Klein A [25]	78	78 ± 11	From 0.63 ± 0.21 to 1.01 ± 0.36	From 50 ± 16 to 29 ± 14	–	22
Agarwal A [33]	212	82 ± 8	From 0.6 ± 0.2 to 1.2 ± 0.3	From 44 ± 18 to 18 ± 9	From 55 ± 22 to 20 ± 11	25.8
Elmariah S [34]	281	83.0 ± 9.4	From 0.64 ± 1.8 to 1.23 ± 0.3	From 45 ± 18 to 16 ± 9	–	12.7 of death at 30 days
Kuntz RE [35]	205	78 ± 10	From 0.60 ± 0.2 to 0.90 ± 0.30	From 55 ± 19 to 30 ± 12	From 67 ± 28 to 33 ± 15	17
Lieberman E [36]	165	78 ± 11	From 0.50 ± 0.20 to 0.70 ± 0.30	–	From 68 ± 38 to 38 ± 28	–

In the National Heart, Lung, and Blood Institute Registry, including 674 patients mainly considered inoperable due to age or other comorbidities, BAV was associated with a significant reduction in peak aortic gradient from 65 to 31 mmHg (*P* < 0.001), with a concordant increase in AVA from 0.5 to 0.8 cm² (*P* < 0.001), and at 1 month all surviving patients experienced significant symptom improvement. However, complication rate was high (31% prior to discharge) with a significant mortality risk at 30 days (14%) [23].

In the Mansfield Scientific Aortic Valvuloplasty Registry enrolling 492 patients, with advance age, severe aortic stenosis, and high surgical risk, aortic valvuloplasty resulted in a significant improvement in AVA (from 0.50 ± 0.18 to 0.82 ± 0.30 cm²), in the mean aortic valve gradient (from 60 ± 23 to 30 ± 13 mmHg), and in cardiac output (from 3.86 ± 1.26 to 4.05 ± 1.31 L/min). Procedural success rate, defined as at least 25% increase in AVA or at least 50% decrease in mean aortic valve gradient in the absence of death or conversion to surgery in the first 7 days post-procedure, has been achieved in 87% of patients. Serial aortography demonstrated a moderate or severe increase in aortic insufficiency in only 2.1% of patients, but the overall complication rate was 20.5%, including vascular injury (11%), embolic phenomenon (2.2%), ventricular perforation resulting in tamponade (1.8%), and nonfatal arrhythmia (0.8%). Death occurred within 24 h of the procedure in 4.9% of patients and within 7 days in an additional 2.6%, but at 1 year of follow-up, a 20% decrease in the incidence of symptoms of heart failure was observed [24].

Agarwal and colleagues, in a series of 212 patients with severe AS undergoing BAV, in the same way, found a significant decrease in peak trans-aortic gradient (from 55 ± 22 to 20 ± 11 mmHg) and an increase in AVA (from 0.6 ± 0.2 to 1.2 ±0.3 cm²) [33].

38.4.2 Long-Term Results

Regardless of immediate improvements in clinical and hemodynamic parameters, benefits are not persistent: mid-term and long-term outcomes following BAV are poor for the high incidence of restenosis and comorbidities in this population. Serial echocardiographic and clinical follow-up of patients after BAV procedure showed a restenosis rate of 60% at 6 months. Otto and colleagues compared echocardiographic findings in 187 patients before and 6 months after BAV. Despite an immediate increase in AVA from 0.57 to 0.78 cm², at 6 months mean AVA was reduced to 0.65 cm² [23].

Also survival, following BAV, is expectedly reduced. Agarwal et al. found 1-year, 3-year, and 5-year survival rates of 64%, 28%, and 14%, respectively [33]. These results are slightly better with respect to survival rates of 55% at 1-year and 23% at 3-year reported by Otto and colleagues [37]. Differences in survival rates in these two experiences could be attributable to the impact on outcome of repeat BAV. In the study of Agarwal, 24% of patients underwent an additional BAV, which emerged as an independent factor of lower mortality.

Nevertheless, such poor outcome is not homogeneous in all patients, and most studies have correlated long-term survival, not only to procedural variables but also to baseline patient morbidity and left ventricular function. Agarwal and colleagues reported that female gender (HR 0.80, 95% CI 0.68–0.94, $P = 0.016$) and multiple BAV procedures (HR 0.88, 95% CI 0.80–0.95, $P = 0.021$) were associated with lower mortality risk after BAV, while chronic renal insufficiency (HR 1.30, 95% CI 1.11–1.56, $P = 0.009$) and Charlson comorbidity index (HR 1.12, 955 CI 1.03–1.21, $P = 0.006$), described in Table 38.2, increased mortality risk [33]. Otto et al. equally found the following clinical, echocardiographic, and catheterization predictors of survival: functional status, left ventricular systolic function, cardiac output, cachexia, renal function, mitral regurgitation, and female gender [37].

Klein and colleagues found that the strongest predictor of mortality was age: each 10-year increment in age was associated with a twofold increase in mortality (relative risk 2.0, 95% CI 1.2–3.3, $P = 0.005$), and there was a considerable difference in median survival in patients older than 70 years of age (5.7 months vs. 29.3 months, $P = 0.013$) [25].

Elmariah et al. retrospectively reviewed data of 281 consecutive patients with severe aortic stenosis undergoing BAV at the Mount Sinai Medical Center from January 2001 to July 2007. Predictors of worse clinical outcome following BAV included poor pre-procedural clinical status, renal dysfunction, high pre-procedural right atrial pressure, and low cardiac output. These four variables were used to derive a specific risk

Table 38.2 Parameters considered in the Charlson comorbidity index, a score predicting 10-year survival in patients with multiple comorbidities

Age	<50 years: 0 50–59 years: +1 60–69 years: +2 70–79 years: +3 >80 years: +4
Diabetes mellitus	None: 0 Uncomplicated: +1 End organ damage: +2
Liver disease	None: 0 Mild: +1 Moderate to severe: +3
Malignancy	None: 0 Leukemia, lymphoma, or localized solid tumor: +2 Metastatic solid tumor: +6
AIDS	No: 0 Yes: +6
Moderate to severe chronic kidney disease	No: 0 Yes: +2
Chronic heart failure	No: 0 Yes: +1
Myocardial infarction	No: 0 Yes: +1
Chronic obstructive pulmonary disease	No: 0 Yes: +1
Peripheral vascular disease	No: 0 Yes: +1
Cerebrovascular accident or transient ischemic attack	No: 0 Yes: +1
Dementia	No: 0 Yes: +1
Hemiplegia	No: 0 Yes: +2
Connective tissue disease	No: 0 Yes: +1
Peptic ulcer disease	No: 0 Yes: +1

score, the CRRAC the AV score (critical status, renal dysfunction, right atrial pressure, cardiac output), that identifies patients at higher risk of 30-day mortality after BAV [34]. Compared with the logistic European System for Cardiac Operative Risk Evaluation (Euro-SCORE), this risk model was associated with improved discrimination for short-term mortality. In aggregate, these data suggest that, although outcomes following BAV remain poor, improved patient selection might identify patients with more favorable and sustained benefit.

38.5   Balloon Aortic Valvuloplasty as Bridge Therapy

TAVI has nowadays emerged as a viable and effective therapeutic alternative to surgical aortic valve replacement (SAVR) [4, 5]. The Placement of Aortic Transcatheter Valves (PARTNER) trial, enrolling 358 patients with severe aortic stenosis not suitable candidates for surgery, demonstrated that TAVI is associated with a marked reduction in mortality respect standard treatment (including medical therapy alone or in association with BAV). In this study BAV was performed in all patients before TAVI and in 84% of patients receiving standard therapy.

Although the clear benefits and the great amount of subjects potentially eligible for TAVI, many patients are initially excluded from this procedure for clinical, anatomical reasons. In the study of Ben-Dor, among 469 patients with severe aortic stenosis screened for TAVI, 363 (77.1%) did not meet the inclusion/exclusion criteria. These patients, treated medically or with BAV, had significantly stronger clinical risk (higher NYHA class, higher incidence of renal failure and lower ejection fraction) compared with the TAVI group, with significantly higher Society of Thoracic Surgeons score and EuroSCORE [38].

Generally, TAVI exclusions may be due to permanent (i.e., lack of suitable vascular access) or temporary (i.e., low cardiac output, hemodynamic instability) causes. It is within this latter context that BAV may assume a novel and therapeutic role in the treatment of patients with severe aortic stenosis, namely, as a bridge to TAVI or SAVR [11]. The decrease in aortic valve gradient and the associated increase in cardiac output after BAV can provide an important time-window during which better forward flow improves peripheral perfusion and decreased outflow obstruction reduces pulmonary congestion, with associated benefits in clinical status. Such stabilization offers the opportunity to complete the investigations in order to assess patient suitability for TAVI or SAVR, as well as a period of hemodynamic improvement that can reduce the procedural risk of more definitive and invasive procedures [39].

Supporting this emerging role for BAV, numerous studies demonstrated that patients initially considered too high risk for aortic valve replacement can successfully undergo TAVI or surgery after performing BAV as a bridging procedure. Although the frequency varies, approximately 20–30% of all BAV procedures are today performed as a bridge indication. Saia and colleagues reported that, among 210 consecutive patients referred for BAV, 78 (37%) underwent BAV as a bridge before TAVI. This group comprised patients with low left ventricular ejection fraction, frailty or enfeebled status, symptoms of uncertain origin, critical conditions, moderate-to-severe mitral valve regurgitation, and need of major non-cardiac surgery. Following BAV, 36 patients (46%) underwent TAVI, whereas 22 (28%) improved sufficiently to receive SAVR. The remaining surviving patients, not experiencing any symptomatic improvement despite significant reduction in mean aortic valve gradient after the procedure, were treated medically, because the cause of their symptoms was attributed to other factors [40].

BAV as a bridge to TAVR or SAVR is associated with markedly improved outcomes compared with BAV alone. For example, Ben-Dor and colleagues reported significant and large reductions in mortality among patients with severe aortic stenosis undergoing BAV as a bridge versus BAV alone (22.3% vs. 55.2%, $P = <0.001$) [41].

Similar results have been showed by Kapadia et al. in 99 patients undergoing BAV for severe aortic stenosis from 1990 to 2005. BAV was attempted to temporarily improve hemodynamics, with a goal to improve general health and to achieve aortic valve replacement, performed, ultimately, in 27 patients. The 6-month and 1-year survival rates in patients who underwent valve replacement were 81% and 78%, respectively, versus 57% and 44% in patients treated only with BAV ($P = 0.024$) [42].

It is important to note that when BAV is performed as a bridge to more definitive therapies, the latter must be performed early. Some data suggest that success rate for BAV as a bridging for SAVR or TAVI decrease from 74% with a timelapse of 8 weeks to 26% with a delay up to

7 months. Saia et al. described, in their series, that up to 40% of patients selected to undergo TAVI or SAVR after BAV, did not have these procedures within the following 2 years. They reported that while most of these patients were excluded for objective clinical reasons, such as terminal disease/malignancy or other persistent contraindication, some patients refused definitive treatment, and others died on the waiting list [43]. The excessive delay in destination therapy is one of the strongest predictors for poor mid-term outcome and should be avoided [44].

Malkin et al. suggested the use of BAV to screen the possibility of coronary ostial occlusion by native leaflets during TAVI and also to assess whether a patient might improve from definitive aortic valve treatment, particularly in those patients with left ventricular dysfunction or chronic obstructive pulmonary disease where concern remains about symptom reversibility [45].

Therefore, in these patients, where the main goal is symptom relief, BAV can act as a gate-keeper to more aggressive therapeutic strategy, sparing patients from the higher-risk procedures as well as healthcare systems from the associated costs.

Lastly, BAV can be a useful palliative "destination therapy" in patients with severe aortic stenosis but poor prognosis due to other comorbidities, such as malignancy, as it often leads to significant clinical improvement often allowing hospital discharge [39].

38.6 The Role of Balloon Aortic Valvuloplasty During Transcatheter Aortic Valve Implantation

BAV, especially, during the first TAVI era, has been represented a necessary step before device placement, allowing easier valve delivery and helps to achieve the complete valve expansion. On the other hand, predilation might be responsible in part for distal embolization as well as of atrioventricular conduction disturbances seen during TAVI procedures. Therefore, more recently, after the introduction of self-expanding valves, TAVI is often performed without predilatation. In a pilot study enrolled only 60 patients, Grube et al. showed that TAVI performed with the self-expanding Medtronic CoreValve bioprosthesis (Medtronic, Minneapolis, MN, USA) is a feasible procedure, resulting in similar acute safety and efficacy as the standard TAVI approach with predilation [46].

Comparable results were reported with the balloon expandable Edwards Sapien XT (Edwards Lifescience, Irvine, CA, USA) implanted in 26 patients enrolled in a retrospective study and compared with 30 patients previously treated with predilatation [47].

A prospective, two-armed, multicenter registry (EASE-IT TA) on patients undergoing transapical TAVI with or without BAV, using the Edwards SAPIEN 3 valve (Edwards Lifescience, Irvine, CA, USA), was recently published. The 61 patients receiving preliminary BAV showed similar reductions in peak and mean transvalvular gradients when compared to 137 patients treated without BAV. Moreover, there was a significant reduction of fluoroscopy time without BAV (4.7 vs. 7.9 min; $P = 0.039$) and significantly decreased odds of catecholamine administration (17.5% vs. 32.8%; $P = 0.017$), but no differences were observed in the composite end point at 6 months even after multivariable adjustment [48].

Irrespective of these results, BAV will continue to have a role in TAVI as a predilatation tool, especially in cases where valve area is particularly small and leaflet calcification is extensive and in cases where "direct" valve crossing is not possible [49]. Finally, in cases of valve underexpansion or poor apposition to the annulus, BAV is often required for post-dilatation to decrease paravalvular leak that has been demonstrated to worsen the long-term outcome. Valve underexpansion is visible on fluoroscopy, whereas paravalvular aortic regurgitation is usually evident either on transesophageal echocardiography or on aortography. BAV in these cases is usually performed using a balloon of a smaller size as compared with that of the implanted valve to minimize the risks of annular rupture [50].

38.7   Conclusion

Although provides only a temporary solution for patients with severe aortic stenosis, BAV continues to have an important role in the treatment of this valvular disease. It can be a stabilizing measure in high-risk symptomatic patients and can represent a "bridging therapy" to more definitive treatments, as TAVI and SAVR. Finally, BAV will continue to be an essential step of the TAVI procedure where required either as a pre- or post-dilatation tool. Ongoing studies will further define the role of BAV in the TAVI era and future improvements as well as the development of drug-coated balloons could be improve the mid-term results in term of restenosis.

Acknowledgments
Conflicts of Interest
Prof. Prati has consulted for Abbott Vascular and Amgen. The other authors have no conflicts of interest to declare.
Funding
None.

References

1. Lindroos M, Kupari M, Heikkila J, Tilvis R. Prevalence of aortic valve abnormalities in the elderly: an echocardiographic study of a random population sample. J Am Coll Cardiol. 1993;21:1220–5.
2. Ross J Jr, Braunwald E. Aortic stenosis. Circulation. 1968;38:61–7.
3. O'Keefe JH Jr, Vlietstra RE, Bailey KR, Holmes DR Jr. Natural history of candidates for balloon aortic valvuloplasty. Mayo Clin Proc. 1987;62:986–91.
4. Baumgartner H, Falk V, Bax JJ, De Bonis M, Hamm C, Holm PJ, Iung B, Lancellotti P, Lansac E, Rodriguez Muñoz D, Rosenhek R, Sjögren J, Tornos Mas P, Vahanian A, Walther T, Wendler O, Windecker S, Zamorano JL, ESC Scientific Document Group. 2017 ESC/EACTS Guidelines for the management of valvular heart disease. Eur Heart J. 2017;38:2739–91.
5. Nishimura RA, Otto CM, Bonow RO, Carabello BA, Erwin JP 3rd, Fleisher LA, Jneid H, Mack MJ, McLeod CJ, O'Gara PT, Rigolin VH, Sundt TM 3rd, Thompson A. 2017 AHA/ACC focused update of the 2014 AHA/ACC guideline for the management of patients with valvular heart disease: a report of the American College of Cardiology/American Heart Association Task Force on clinical practice guidelines. Circulation. 2017;135:e1159–95.
6. Iung B, Baron G, Butchart EG, Delahaye F, Gohlke-Bärwolf C, Levang OW, Tornos P, Vanoverschelde JL, Vermeer F, Boersma E, Ravaud P, Vahanian A. A prospective survey of patients with valvular heart disease in Europe: the Euro heart survey on valvular heart disease. Eur Heart J. 2003;24:1231–43.
7. Leon MB, Smith CR, Mack M, Miller DC, Moses JW, Svensson LG, Tuzcu EM, Webb JG, Fontana GP, Makkar RR, Brown DL, Block PC, Guyton RA, Pichard AD, Bavaria JE, Herrmann HC, Douglas PS, Petersen JL, Akin JJ, Anderson WN, Wang D, Pocock S, PARTNER Trial Investigators. Transcatheter aortic-valve implantation for aortic stenosis in patients who cannot undergo surgery. N Engl J Med. 2010;363:1597–607.
8. Cribier A, Savin T, Saoudi N, Behar P, Rocha P, Mechmèche R, Berland J, Letac B. Percutaneous transluminal aortic valvuloplasty using a balloon catheter. A new therapeutic option in aortic stenosis in the elderly. Arch Mal Coeur Vaiss. 1986;79:1678–86.
9. Jabbour RJ, Dick R, Walton AS. Aortic balloon valvuloplasty—review and case series. Heart Lung Circ. 2008;17(Suppl 4):S73–81.
10. Ji DM, Si BD. Percutaneous aortic valve intervention. In: Cohn L, editor. Cardiac surgery in the adult. New York: McGraw-Hill; 2008. p. 963–71.
11. Baber U, Kini AS, Moreno PR, Sharma SK. Aortic stenosis: role of balloon aortic valvuloplasty. Cardiol Clin. 2013;31:327–36.
12. Feldman T. Transseptal antegrade access for aortic valvuloplasty. Catheter Cardiovasc Interv. 2000;50:492–4.
13. Eisenhauer AC, Hadjipetrou P, Piemonte TC. Balloon aortic valvuloplasty revisited: the role of the inoue balloon and transseptal antegrade approach. Catheter Cardiovasc Interv. 2000;50:484–91.
14. Block PC, Palacios IF. Comparison of hemodynamic results of anterograde versus retrograde percutaneous balloon aortic valvuloplasty. Am J Cardiol. 1987;60:659–62.
15. Cubeddu RJ, Jneid H, Don CW, Witzke CF, Cruz-Gonzalez I, Gupta R, Rengifo-Moreno P, Maree AO, Inglessis I, Palacios IF. Retrograde versus antegrade percutaneous aortic balloon valvuloplasty: immediate, short- and long-term outcome at 2 years. Catheter Cardiovasc Interv. 2009;74:225–31.
16. Lang RM, Badano LP, Mor-Avi V, Afilalo J, Armstrong A, Ernande L, Flachskampf FA, Foster E, Goldstein SA, Kuznetsova T, Lancellotti P, Muraru D, Picard MH, Rietzschel ER, Rudski L, Spencer KT, Tsang W, Voigt JU. Recommendations for cardiac chamber quantification by echocardiography in adults: an update from the American Society of Echocardiography and the European Association of Cardiovascular Imaging. J Am Soc Echocardiogr. 2015;28:1–39.e14.
17. Feldman T, Guerrero M. Balloon aortic valvuloplasty in the TAVR era: not so new but definitely improved. Catheter Cardiovasc Interv. 2017;90:311–2.

18. Feldman T, Chiu YC, Carroll JD. Single balloon aortic valvuloplasty: increased valve areas with improved technique. J Invasive Cardiol. 1989;1:295–300.

19. Dall'Ara G, Marzocchi A, Taglieri N, Moretti C, Rodinò G, Chiarabelli M, Bottoni P, Marrozzini C, Sabattini MR, Bacchi-Reggiani ML, Rapezzi C, Saia F. Randomized comparison of balloon aortic valvuloplasty performed with or without rapid cardiac pacing: the pacing versus no pacing (PNP) study. J Interv Cardiol. 2018;31:51–9.

20. Gupta SD, Das S, Ghose T, Sarkar A, Goswami A, Kundu S. Controlled transient respiratory arrest along with rapid right ventricular pacing for improving balloon stability during balloon valvuloplasty in pediatric patients with congenital aortic stenosis—a retrospective case series analysis. Ann Card Anaesth. 2010;13:236–40.

21. Witzke C, Don CW, Cubeddu RJ, Herrero-Garibi J, Pomerantsev E, Caldera A, McCarty D, Inglessis I, Palacios IF. Impact rapid ventricular pacing during percutaneous balloon aortic valvuloplasty in patients with critical aortic stenosis: should we be using it? Catheter Cardiovasc Interv. 2010;75:444–52.

22. Hilling-Smith R, Cockburn J, Dooley M, Parker J, Newton A, Hill A, Trivedi U, de Belder A, Hildick-Smith D. Rapid pacing using the 0.035-in. Retrograde left ventricular support wire in 208 cases of transcatheter aortic valve implantation and balloon aortic valvuloplasty. Catheter Cardiovasc Interv. 2017;89:783–6.

23. Percutaneous balloon aortic valvuloplasty. Acute and 30-day follow-up results in 674 patients from the NHLBI Balloon Valvuloplasty Registry. Circulation. 1991;84:2383–97.

24. McKay RG. The Mansfield Scientific Aortic Valvuloplasty Registry: overview of acute hemodynamic results and procedural complications. J Am Coll Cardiol. 1991;17:485–91.

25. Klein A, Lee K, Gera A, Ports TA, Michaels AD. Long-term mortality, cause of death, and temporal trends in complications after percutaneous aortic balloon valvuloplasty for calcific aortic stenosis. J Interv Cardiol. 2006;19:269–75.

26. Ben-Dor I, Looser P, Bernardo N, Maluenda G, Torguson R, Xue Z, Lindsay J, Pichard AD, Satler LF, Waksman R. Comparison of closure strategies after balloon aortic valvuloplasty: suture mediated versus collagen based versus manual. Catheter Cardiovasc Interv. 2011;78:119–24.

27. O'Neill B, Singh V, Kini A, Mehran R, Jacobs E, Knopf D, Alfonso CE, Martinez CA, Martinezclark P, O'Neill W, Heldman AW, Yu J, Baber U, Kovacic JC, Dangas G, Sharma S, Sartori S, Cohen MG. The use of vascular closure devices and impact on major bleeding and net adverse clinical events (NACEs) in balloon aortic valvuloplasty: a sub-analysis of the BRAVO study. Catheter Cardiovasc Interv. 2014;83:148–53.

28. Kini A, Yu J, Cohen MG, Mehran R, Baber U, Sartori S, Vlachojannis GJ, Kovacic JC, Pyo R, O'Neill B, Singh V, Jacobs E, Poludasu S, Moreno P, Kim MC, Krishnan P, Sharma SK, Dangas GD. Effect of bivalirudin on aortic valve intervention outcomes study: a two-centre registry study comparing bivalirudin and unfractionated heparin in balloon aortic valvuloplasty. EuroIntervention. 2014;10:312–9.

29. Saia F, Marrozzini C, Ciuca C, Bordoni B, Dall'Ara G, Moretti C, Taglieri N, Palmerini T, Branzi A, Marzocchi A. Is balloon aortic valvuloplasty safe in patients with significant aortic valve regurgitation? Catheter Cardiovasc Interv. 2012;79:315–21.

30. Gotzmann M, Lindstaedt M, Mügge A. From pressure overload to volume overload: aortic regurgitation after transcatheter aortic valve implantation. Am Heart J. 2012;163:903–11.

31. Eltchaninoff H, Durand E, Borz B, Furuta A, Bejar K, Canville A, Farhat A, Fraccaro C, Godin M, Tron C, Sakhuja R, Cribier A. Balloon aortic valvuloplasty in the era of transcatheter aortic valve replacement: acute and long-term outcomes. Am Heart J. 2014;167:235–40.

32. Dall'Ara G, Saia F, Moretti C, Marrozzini C, Taglieri N, Bordoni B, Chiarabelli M, Ciuca C, Rapezzi C, Marzocchi A. Incidence, treatment, and outcome of acute aortic valve regurgitation complicating percutaneous balloon aortic valvuloplasty. Catheter Cardiovasc Interv. 2017;89:E145–52.

33. Agarwal A, Kini AS, Attanti S, Lee PC, Ashtiani R, Steinheimer AM, Moreno PR, Sharma SK. Results of repeat balloon valvuloplasty for treatment of aortic stenosis in patients aged 59 to 104 years. Am J Cardiol. 2005;95:43–7.

34. Elmariah S, Lubitz SA, Shah AM, Miller MA, Kaplish D, Kothari S, Moreno PR, Kini AS, Sharma SK. A novel clinical prediction rule for 30-day mortality following balloon aortic valuloplasty: the CRRAC the AV score. Catheter Cardiovasc Interv. 2011;78:112–8.

35. Kuntz RE, Tosteson AN, Berman AD, Goldman L, Gordon PC, Leonard BM, McKay RG, Diver DJ, Safian RD. Predictors of event-free survival after balloon aortic valvuloplasty. N Engl J Med. 1991;325:17–23.

36. Lieberman EB, Bashore TM, Hermiller JB, Wilson JS, Pieper KS, Keeler GP, Pierce CH, Kisslo KB, Harrison JK, Davidson CJ. Balloon aortic valvuloplasty in adults: failure of procedure to improve long-term survival. J Am Coll Cardiol. 1995;26:1522–8.

37. Otto CM, Mickel MC, Kennedy JW, Alderman EL, Bashore TM, Block PC, Brinker JA, Diver D, Ferguson J, Holmes DR Jr. Three-year outcome after balloon aortic valvuloplasty. Insights into prognosis of valvular aortic stenosis. Circulation. 1994;89:642–50.

38. Ben-Dor I, Pichard AD, Gonzalez MA, Weissman G, Li Y, Goldstein SA, Okubagzi P, Syed AI, Maluenda G, Collins SD, Delhaye C, Wakabayashi K, Gaglia MA Jr, Torguson R, Xue Z, Satler LF, Suddath WO, Kent KM, Lindsay J, Waksman R. Correlates and causes of death in patients with severe symptomatic aortic stenosis who are not eligible to participate in a clinical trial of transcatheter aortic valve implantation. Circulation. 2010;122:S37–42.

39. Costopoulos C, Sutaria N, Ariff B, Fertleman M, Malik I, Mikhail GW. Balloon aortic valvuloplasty as a treatment option in the era of transcatheter aortic valve implantation. Expert Rev Cardiovasc Ther. 2015;13:457–60.

40. Saia F, Marrozzini C, Moretti C, Ciuca C, Taglieri N, Bordoni B, Dall'ara G, Alessi L, Lanzillotti V, Bacchi-Reggiani ML, Branzi A, Marzocchi A. The role of percutaneous balloon aortic valvuloplasty as a bridge for transcatheter aortic valve implantation. EuroIntervention. 2011;7:723–9.

41. Ben-Dor I, Maluenda G, Dvir D, Barbash IM, Okubagzi P, Torguson R, Lindsay J, Satler LF, Pichard AD, Waksman R. Balloon aortic valvuloplasty for severe aortic stenosis as a bridge to transcatheter/surgical aortic valve replacement. Catheter Cardiovasc Interv. 2013;82:632–7.

42. Kapadia SR, Goel SS, Yuksel U, Agarwal S, Pettersson G, Svensson LG, Smedira NG, Whitlow PL, Lytle BW, Tuzcu EM. Lessons learned from balloon aortic valvuloplasty experience from the pre-transcatheter aortic valve implantation era. J Interv Cardiol. 2010;23:499–508.

43. Saia F, Marrozzini C, Ciuca C, Guastaroba P, Taglieri N, Palmerini T, Bordoni B, Moretti C, Dall'ara G, Branzi A, Marzocchi A. Emerging indications, in-hospital and long-term outcome of balloon aortic valvuloplasty in the transcatheter aortic valve implantation era. EuroIntervention. 2013;8:1388–97.

44. Nwaejike N, Mills K, Stables R, Field M. Balloon aortic valvuloplasty as a bridge to aortic valve surgery for severe aortic stenosis. Interact Cardiovasc Thorac Surg. 2015;20:429–35.

45. Malkin CJ, Judd J, Chew DP, Sinhal A. Balloon aortic valvuloplasty to bridge and triage patients in the era of trans-catheter aortic valve implantation. Catheter Cardiovasc Interv. 2013;8:358–63.

46. Grube E, Naber C, Abizaid A, Sousa E, Mendiz O, Lemos P, Kalil Filho R, Mangione J, Buellesfeld L. Feasibility of transcatheter aortic valve implantation without balloon pre-dilation: a pilot study. JACC Cardiovasc Interv. 2011;4:751–7.

47. Möllmann H, Kim WK, Kempfert J, Blumenstein J, Liebetrau C, Nef H, Van Linden A, Walther T, Hamm C. Transfemoral aortic valve implantation of Edwards SAPIEN XT without predilatation is feasible. Clin Cardiol. 2014;37:667–71.

48. Strauch J, Wendt D, Diegeler A, Heimeshoff M, Hofmann S, Holzhey D, Oertel F, Wahlers T, Kurucova J, Thoenes M, Deutsch C, Bramlage P, Schröfel H. Balloon-expandable transapical transcatheter aortic valve implantation with or without predilation of the aortic valve: results of a multicentre registry. Eur J Cardiothorac Surg. 2018;53:771–7.

49. Chan PH, Mario CD, Moat N. Transcatheter aortic valve implantation without balloon predilatation: not always feasible. Catheter Cardiovasc Interv. 2013;82:328–32.

50. Van Belle E, Juthier F, Susen S, Vincentelli A, Iung B, Dallongeville J, Eltchaninoff H, Laskar M, Leprince P, Lievre M, Banfi C, Auffray JL, Delhaye C, Donzeau-Gouge P, Chevreul K, Fajadet J, Leguerrier A, Prat A, Gilard M, Teiger E, FRANCE 2 Investigators. Postprocedural aortic regurgitation in balloon-expandable and self-expandable transcatheter aortic valve replacement procedures: analysis of predictors and impact on long-term mortality: insights from the FRANCE2 Registry. Circulation. 2014;129:1415–27.

Part IV

Surgical Perspectives

Role of the Heart Team in Decision-Making for Transcatheter Aortic Valve Implantation

39

Carlo Savini and Roberto Di Bartolomeo

39.1 Introduction

The advent of transcatheter aortic valve prosthetic implantation (TAVI), also called transcatheter aortic valve replacement (TAVR), has been a factor in substantial changes in the clinical and organizational practice of all the cardiology and cardiac surgery centers where the TAVI program has been carried out. The TAVI have the merit of having given dignity to the figure of the Heart Team, originally born as a proposal for the evaluation of the treatment of coronary pathology simultaneously with the advent of drug-eluting stents. In decision-making processes for aortic valve pathologies, the Heart Team has assumed a decisive relevance, so much so that it can be extended to other areas wherever an interventional option is envisaged as an alternative to surgery for the treatment of cardiac structural diseases. In this chapter we will deal with the main aspects regarding the establishment of the Heart Team and its decisional and procedural responsibilities.

C. Savini (✉)
Azienda Ospedaliero-Universitaria Policlinico S. Orsola di Bologna, Bologna, Italy
e-mail: carlo.savini@aosp.bo.it

R. Di Bartolomeo
Department of Experimental, Diagnostic and Specialty Medicine—DIMES, University of Bologna, Bologna, Italy
e-mail: roberto.dibartolomeo@unibo.it

39.2 Heart Team

39.2.1 Theoretical Assumptions and Practical Considerations

The theoretical basis of the modern concept of Heart Team has ancient roots that can find a formal description in the statistical theory of Venn diagrams [1]. Originally described by John Venn in the 1880s to teach elementary set theory, these diagrams are most often used to illustrate set relationships in such fields as probability, statistics, and computer science. Venn diagrams are illustrations composed of overlapping circles that demonstrate the relations between finite collections of things and are most useful in defining areas of commonality among different aggregations.

Venn diagrams can be useful for understanding the roles of various stakeholders in the management of cardiovascular disease from its diagnosis through its treatment [2]. As the field progresses, the area of overlap of the cardiovascular disease Venn diagram continues to expand. This is evident in many aspects of cardiovascular disease management, including individual diagnosticians and treatment specialists, diseases, technologies, institutions, payers, and regulators. The overlap of the Venn diagrams for interventional cardiology and cardiovascular surgery has grown larger since the promulgation of the multidisciplinary Heart Team concept. Specialty

© Springer Nature Switzerland AG 2019
A. Giordano et al. (eds.), *Transcatheter Aortic Valve Implantation*,
https://doi.org/10.1007/978-3-030-05912-5_39

team-based care is not a concept new to medicine; for example, tumor boards make multispecialty disease management decisions in oncology [3, 4]. The use of the specific term "Heart Team" is more recent and was only incorporated in guidelines subsequent to the presentation of the results of the pivotal SYNTAX trial [5]. SYNTAX evaluated the two randomized strategies of coronary bypass graft surgery and percutaneous coronary intervention in patients with complex multivessel or left main coronary artery disease. Working together, a team composed of a surgeon, an interventional cardiologist, a primary cardiologist, and the patient agreed upon the optimal revascularization strategy [6, 7]. This Heart Team approach has been codified in the European Society of Cardiology/European Association for Cardio-Thoracic Surgery (ESC/EACTS) guidelines on myocardial revascularization, which recommend that patients with complex coronary artery disease be seen by a Heart Team, which includes cardiovascular surgeons and interventional cardiologists. Using a Heart Team approach is a Class I-C recommendation of the 2011 ACC/AHA guidelines for coronary artery bypass graft surgery [8].

This concept finally arrived to the field of structural heart disease, specifically aortic stenosis and transcatheter aortic valve replacement (TAVR) [9, 10]. In this setting, the Venn diagrams of cardiovascular surgeons and interventional cardiologists coalesce to form the core of the team responsible for planning and implementing the chosen strategy for aortic valve replacement (see Fig. 39.1). This convergence has now been mandated for reimbursement by federal regulatory agencies.

It is interesting to note how the concept of Heart Team for heart structural diseases and, mainly, for aortic stenosis has taken on more and more body in recent years. This phenomenon has become necessary not only for the evident clinical decision-making needs but also for the obligation to share the same work environment for the execution of the procedure. The coronary pathology, in fact, provides a multidisciplinary approach only in the decision-making phase, and then the patient follows different paths (surgery vs. PCI vs. medical therapy). The aortic pathology, on the other hand, if carried out to a transcatheter treatment, leads to subject the patient to a procedure where, theoretically, the presence of both operative figures is required: the interventional cardiologist and the cardiac surgeon. The hybrid operating theater, in this way, physically represents the Heart Team in its full expression. Real-time image fusion technology requires the concurrent multidisciplinary presence of industry specialists who collaborate on the success of the procedure. At the same time, any procedural complexities (surgical access, protection of coronary ostia, management of complications, etc.) require the availability of both figures at the operating table. Local Heart Teams in this way, for a patient with aortic valvular stenosis who must undergo transcatheter treatment, share a joint path that goes from the initial decision-making process to the implant procedure.

The TAVI gave a great contribution to create the conditions for an epochal change in the management of cardiological and cardiac surgery patients. In real life things are not so idyllic: cardiologists and cardiac surgeons are often still antagonistic rather than friends. However, there are two main aspects, in my opinion, which must predominate: the first is the patient, but the social and health policies with the relative economic implications are also of considerable importance.

In this sense, the Heart Team has a huge responsibility role, as it has full decision-making powers on a patient who has the right to be treated at best, but also on the use of devices that have a significant economic impact. It is no coincidence that the main European and North American guidelines remain quite general in defining TAVI plant indications. The most recent update of the American guidelines [11], for example, states, in level of evidence I, that: "For patients in whom TAVR or high-risk surgical AVR is being considered, a heart valve team consisting of an integrated, multidisciplinary group of healthcare professionals with expertise in VHD, cardiac imaging, interventional cardiology, cardiac anesthesia, and cardiac surgery should collaborate to provide optimal patient care." The ESC guidelines follow approximately the same policy, as well as

Fig. 39.1 Venn's diagram for TAVI Heart Team

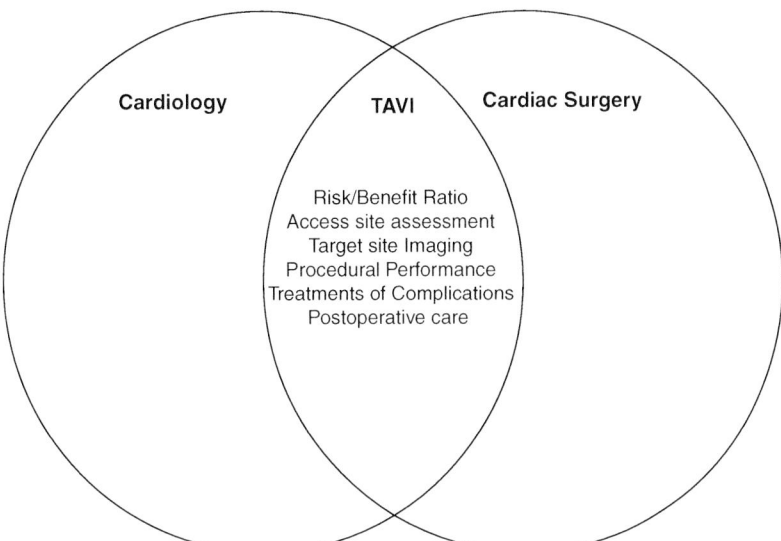

giving more specific indications on the composition and responsibilities of the Heart Team [12]. The responsibility delegated to the local Heart Team is, therefore, mainly due to the fact that to date the path that leads the patient to the implant of a TAVI is not yet universally standardizable: the specialists that make up the Heart Teams of each single center are the only ones, beyond the purely clinical aspect, to know the potential of their center in terms of professional skills, logistical capabilities, and availability of resources.

This background of increasing convergence among cardiovascular disciplines contrasts starkly with our silo-bound professional societies: the American College of Cardiology (ACC), American Heart Association (AHA), Society of Thoracic Surgeons (STS), American Association for Thoracic Surgery (AATS), Society for Cardiovascular Angiography and Interventions (SCAI), American Society of Echocardiography (ASE), and American Society of Nuclear Cardiology (ASNC) or, respectively, in Europe, the ESC and EACTS. Each silo touches the others competitively, sometimes antagonistically, and, at other times, collaboratively. Each silo has many similar discrete components—executive committees; volunteer and paid staff; advocacy; and scientific, educational, and regulatory groups, to name but a few. In addition, the core mission of each silo may be very similar. While each profes-

sional society serves its core constituency well, there are many disadvantages to such a situation, including overlapping efforts that are inefficient; conflicting aims that confuse patients, payers, and regulators alike; and diffusion of efforts to obtain increasingly scarce industry and government funding. Other disadvantages specific to cardiology and cardiovascular surgery are these: competing outpatient registries (e.g., ACC and AHA); confusing messaging for procedural reimbursement (e.g., carotid stenting); redundant grants for disease-specific approaches (e.g., Heart Rhythm Society, ACC, STS for atrial fibrillation); and a plethora of requirements for credentialing and certification (e.g., ASE and ASNC).

But the spirit that wants to change, and improve, things is very present. The current Heart Teams are for the most part still represented by specialists who have had a very compartmentalized "old style" training. Today it is necessary to set the conditions for creating specialists with transversal skills able to manage what is required by technological development. STS and ACC have begun an unprecedented collaboration with federal regulatory and reimbursement agencies and industry around TAVR, addressing its optimal utilization and developing a national registry, educational programs, requirements for credentialing, and metrics for procedural performance [10, 13]. There have been several examples of close relationships between surgery and cardiology: among others, these include the fact that the third president of the American College of Cardiology, Robert Glover (from 1953 to 1954), was a surgeon from Philadelphia. Our task should be to create a single professional society which would include all segments of the cardiovascular team: surgeons, cardiologists, vascular radiologists, anesthesiologists, cardiovascular nurses, educational and scientific groups, and advocacy under one administrative umbrella. The goal would be to have the administrative umbrella of a single professional society that coordinate the educational and scientific initiatives, the disease management registries and outcomes analyses, the advocacy approach toward reimbursement, and the training, education, and credentialing of physicians and allied health professionals.

At the same time, at university level in specialty training schools, it is necessary to establish educational programs aimed at encouraging the learning of both surgical and cardiological interventional bases. A heart valve center should have structured training programs. Surgeons and cardiologists performing any valve intervention should undergo focused training as part of their basic local board certification training. Learning new techniques should take place through mentoring to minimize the effects of the "learning curve." Only in this way can we think that the various components of a future Heart Team can be able to sustain the weight of responsibility that is attributed to it. Experience in the full spectrum of surgical procedures—including valve replacement; aortic root surgery; mitral, tricuspid, and aortic valve repair; repair of complicated valve endocarditis such as root abscess; treatment of atrial fibrillation; as well as surgical myocardial revascularization—must be available. The spectrum of interventional procedures in addition to TAVI should include mitral valvuloplasty, mitral valve repair (edge to edge), closure of atrial septal defects, closure of paravalvular leaks, and left atrial (LA) appendage closure as well as percutaneous coronary intervention (PCI). Expertise in interventional and surgical management of vascular diseases and complications must be available.

Now is the time to make a more practical cut to the chapter: who should the Heart Team be composed of, and how should it act?

Chambers et al. [14] have well defined the essential requirements that must have a center that deals with the treatment of structural heart diseases (SHVD):

1. Multidisciplinary teams with competencies in valve replacement; aortic root surgery; mitral, tricuspid, and aortic valve repair; as well as transcatheter aortic and mitral valve techniques including reinterventions. The Heart Team must meet on a regular basis and work with standard operating procedures.
2. Imaging, including three-dimensional (3D) and stress echocardiographic techniques, perioperative transesophageal echocardiography (TEE), cardiac computed tomography (CT), magnetic resonance imaging (MRI), and positron emission tomography-CT.
3. Regular consultation with community, other hospitals, and extra cardiac departments and between noninvasive cardiologists and surgeons and interventional cardiologists.
4. Backup services including other cardiologists, cardiac surgeons, Internist care, and other medical specialties.
5. Data review:
   • Robust internal audit processes including mortality and complications, reoperation rate with a minimum of 1-year follow-up
   • Results available for review internally and externally
   • Participation in national or international quality databases

The path of a patient who goes to TAVI is made of different steps that involve different professional figures: the Heart Team must be conceived, therefore, as a dynamic entity where it is important that the right people are at the right time of the path. Figure 39.2 represents a flow diagram of the patient with the corresponding specialists for each moment. Of course heart surgeons and interventional cardiologists have a key position in the main decision-making hubs, but all the professional figures are necessary for the process to be successful.

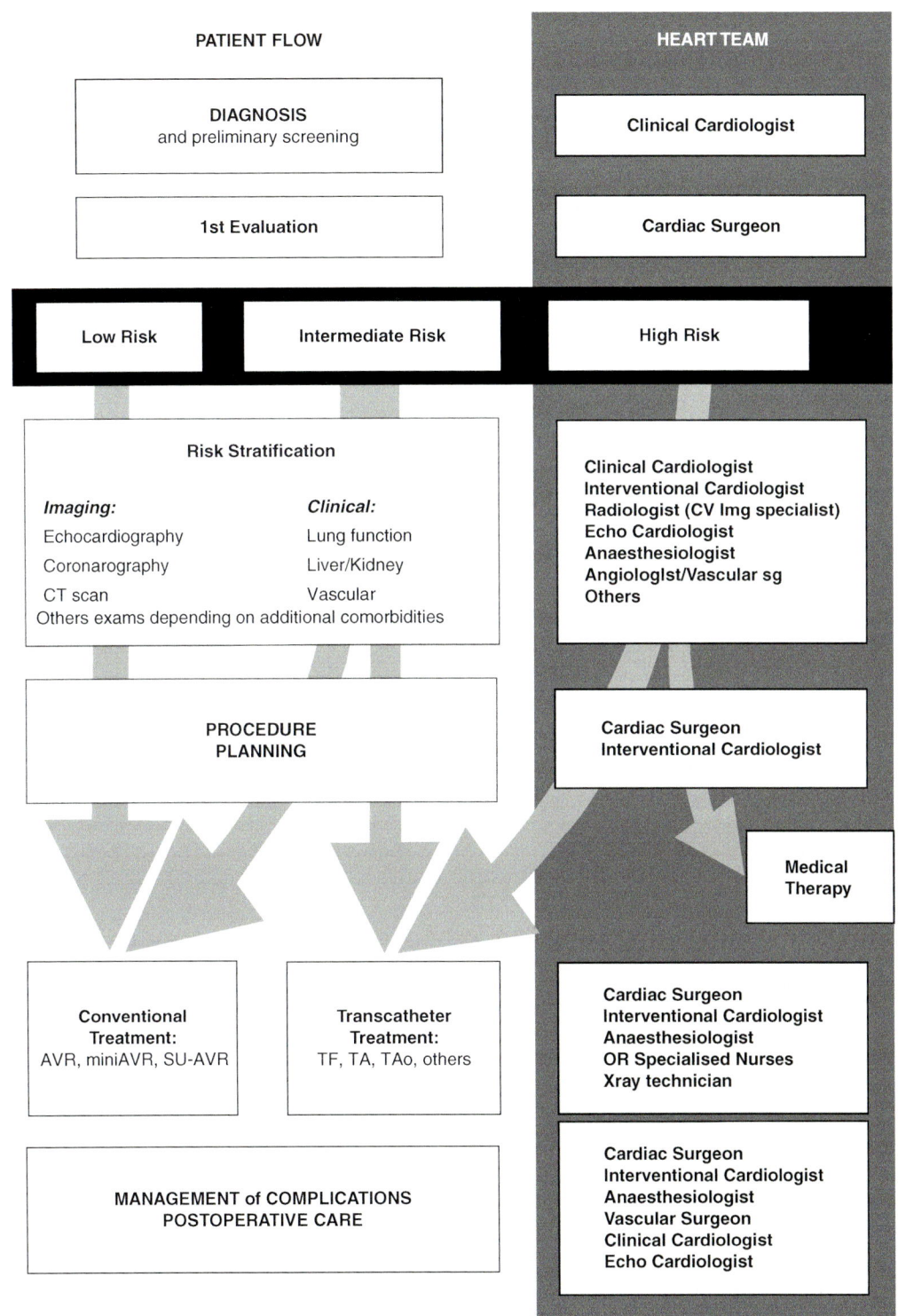

Fig. 39.2 Scheme of multidisciplinary involvement within the path for a patient with aortic valvular aortic stenosis *CV* Cardiovascular, *sg* Surgeon, *CT* Computed tomography, *AVR* Aortic valve replacement, *SU-AVR* Sutureless aortic valve replacement, *TF* Transfemoral, *TA* Transapical, *TAo* Transaortic, *OR* Operating room

39.3 Conclusion

The Heart Team is a concept that in recent years has gained a position of absolute importance.

Its functions are to guarantee the appropriateness of indications during the decisional phase and safety during the procedural phase. Patients with aortic valvular stenosis arriving at a transcatheter implant (TAVI) are currently already placed within well-established pathways, shaped by the characteristics of local Heart Teams. The new frontiers in the treatment of structural heart diseases will see the Heart Teams engaged in different situations on which to adapt their professional skills. This is why it is important that in hospitals where an advanced treatment program for structural heart diseases is being developed or planned, there are the conditions for always having a pool of professionals used to working in a multidisciplinary manner.

Conflict of Interest
None declared.

References

1. Chen H, Boutros PC. Venn diagram: a package for the generation of highly customizable Venn and Euler diagrams in R. BMC Bioinformatics. 2011;12:35.
2. Holmes DR Jr, Mohr F, Hamm CW, Mack MJ. Venn diagrams in cardiovascular disease: the Heart Team concept. Eur Heart J. 2014;35:66–8.
3. Taylor C, Munro AJ, Glynne-Jones R. Multidisciplinary team working in cancer: what is the evidence? Br Med J. 2010;340:c951.
4. Gabel M, Hilton NE, Nathanson SD. Multidisciplinary breast cancer clinics. Do they work? Cancer. 1997;79:2380–4.
5. Serruys PW, Morice MC, Kappetein AP, Colombo A, Holmes DR, Mack MJ, Stahle E, Feldman TE, van den Brand M, Bass EJ, Van Dyck N, Leadley K, Dawkins KD, Mohr FW, SYNTAX Investigators. Percutaneous coronary intervention versus coronary artery bypass grafting for severe coronary artery disease. N Engl J Med. 2009;360:961–72.
6. Rothberg MB, Sivalingam SK, Ashraf J, Visintainer P, Joelson J, Kleppel R, Vallurupalli N, Schweiger MJ. Patients' and cardiologists' perceptions of the benefits of percutaneous coronary intervention for stable coronary disease. Ann Intern Med. 2010;153:307–13.
7. Brownlee S, Wennberg J, Barry M, Fisher E, Goodman D, Bynum J. Improving Patient Decision-Making in Health Care: A 2011 Dartmouth Atlas Report Highlighting Minnesota. The Dartmouth Institute for Health Policy and Clinical Practice, 2011.
8. Hillis LD, Smith PK, Anderson JL, Bittl JA, Bridges CR, Byrne JG, Cigarroa JE, Disesa VJ, Hiratzka LF, Jr Hutter AM, Jessen ME, Keeley EC, Lahey SJ, Lange RA, London MJ, Mack MJ, Patel MR, Puskas JD, Sabik JF, Selnes O, Shahian DM, Trost JC, Winniford MD. 2011 ACCF/AHA Guideline for Coronary Artery Bypass Graft Surgery: executive summary: a report of the American College of Cardiology Foundation/American Heart Association Task Force on Practice Guidelines. Circulation. 2011;124:2610–42.
9. Holmes DR Jr, Mack MJ. Transcatheter valve therapy. J Am Coll Cardiol. 2011;58:445–55.
10. Holmes DR Jr, Mack MJ, Kaul S, Agnihotri A, Alexander KP, Bailey SR, Calhoon JH, Carabello BA, Desai MY, Edwards FH, Francis GS, Gardner TJ, Kappetein AP, Linderbaum JA, Mukherjee C, Mukherjee D, Otto CM, Ruiz CE, Sacco RL, Smith D, Thomas JD, American College of Cardiology Foundation, American Association for Thoracic Surgery, Society for Cardiovascular Angiography and Interventions, Society for Thoracic Surgeons, American Heart Association, American Society of Echocardiography, European Association for Cardio-Thoracic Surgery, Heart Failure Society of America, Mended Hearts, Society of Cardiovascular Anesthesiologists, Society of Cardiovascular Computed Tomography, Society for Cardiovascular Magnetic Resonance. 2012 ACCF/AATS/SCAI/STS expert consensus document on transcatheter aortic valve replacement. Ann Thorac Surg. 2012;93:1340–95.
11. 2017 AHA/ACC Focused Update of the 2014 AHA/ACC Guideline for the Management of Patients With Valvular Heart Disease. A Report of the American College of Cardiology/American Heart Association Task Force on Clinical Practice Guidelines. JACC. 2017;70(2):252–89.
12. Baumgartner H, Falk V, Bax JJ, De Bonis M, Hamm C, Holm PJ, Iung B, Lancellotti P, Lansac E, Muñoz DR, Rosenhek R, Sjögren J, Mas PT, Vahanian A, Walther T, Wendler O, Windecker S, Zamorano JL, ESC Scientific Document Group. 2017 ESC/EACTS Guidelines for the management of valvular heart disease. The Task Force for the Management of Valvular Heart Disease of the European Society of Cardiology (ESC) and the European Association for Cardio-Thoracic Surgery (EACTS). Eur Heart J. 2017;38:2739–91.
13. Carroll JD, Edwards FH, Marinac-Dabic D, Brindis RG, Grover FL, Peterson ED, Tuzcu M, Shahian DM, Rumsfeld JS, Shewan CM, Hewitt K, Holmes DR Jr, Mack MJ, On behalf of the STS/ACC TVT Registry Steering Committee. The STS-ACC transcatheter

valve therapy national registry. A new partnership and infrastructure for the introduction and surveillance of medical devices and therapies. J Am Coll Cardiol. 2013;62:1026–34.

14. Chambers J, Prendergast B, Iung B, Rosenhek R, Zamorano JL, Pierard LA, Modine T, Falk V, Kappetein AP, Pibarot P, Sundt T, Bamgartner H, Bax JJ, Lancellotti P. Standards defining a "heart valve centre": ESC Working Group on Valvular Heart Disease and European Association for Cardiothoracic Surgery viewpoint. Eur Heart J. 2017;38:2177–82.

Comparison of Transcatheter Aortic Valve Implantation to Surgical Aortic Valve Replacement in Intermediate-Risk Patients

40

Anita W. Asgar and Nathan Messas

40.1 Introduction

Transcatheter aortic valve implantation (TAVI), also called transcatheter aortic valve replacement (TAVR), is first-line therapy for patients with severe symptomatic aortic stenosis (AS) and a prohibitive risk for standard surgical aortic valve replacement (SAVR) [1]. Accumulating clinical experience of TAVR operators and technological advances in transcatheter valve systems have led to a massive expansion of TAVR interventions worldwide. TAVR is now available in more than 65 countries around the world with over 250,000 procedures performed to date. As a result, there is now an interest to expand TAVR indications to patients at lower surgical risk such as those at intermediate or low risk. At present, SAVR remains the gold standard treatment for aortic stenosis patients at low or intermediate surgical risk; however recent evidence from observational studies and randomized trials are shifting this treatment paradigm from surgery closer to TAVR.

40.2 Defining Risk for Patients with Aortic Stenosis

Aortic stenosis (AS) is now the most common indication for valve replacement in Europe and North America, with an ever-increasing disease prevalence due to the aging population. Decision making in valvular heart disease necessitates a careful evaluation of the risk-to-benefit ratio, considering both the results of intervention and the severity-adjusted risk of adverse outcomes without intervention. Appropriate risk stratification is therefore crucial to select the optimal treatment strategy for patients with symptomatic severe AS. Factors associated with adverse clinical outcomes include poor functional capacity, advanced age, and concomitant coronary disease [2].

Evaluation of risk in AS is often focused on risk of surgical intervention or operative mortality. There are numerous clinical factors that are associated with increased operative risk including the need for emergency intervention, left ventricular dysfunction, pulmonary hypertension, advanced age, previous cardiac surgery, and comorbidities such as renal insufficiency and severe chronic obstructive pulmonary disease (COPD). To facilitate risk evaluation, multivariate risk scores have become commonplace to stratify patients into risk categories. The most commonly used scores include the Society for Thoracic Surgeons score (STS score) which calculates the predicted risk of mortality (STS-

A. W. Asgar (✉) · N. Messas
Department of Medicine, Montreal Heart Institute,
Université de Montréal, Montreal, QC, Canada
e-mail: anita.asgar@umontreal.ca

© Springer Nature Switzerland AG 2019
A. Giordano et al. (eds.), *Transcatheter Aortic Valve Implantation*,
https://doi.org/10.1007/978-3-030-05912-5_40

Table 40.1 Definition of operative risk

	Low risk	Intermediate risk	High risk	Prohibitive risk
Clinical characteristics	No frailty No comorbidities	No more than mild frailty Or 1 major organ system compromise not to be improved postoperatively	Moderate-severe frailty or >2 major organ system compromises not to be improved postoperatively	Severe frailty Or ≥3 major organ system compromises not to be improved postoperatively
STS-PROM	<4%	4–8%	>8%	PROM >50% at 1 year
EuroSCORE II	<10%	10–20%	>20%	

PROM) and the EuroSCORE. Both scores utilize a numeric scoring system based on clinical parameters to calculate risk using an algorithmic risk model. It should be noted that surgical risk scores share several limitations by insufficiently considering multiple factors that may increase the risk related to surgery; patient frailty, cognitive impairment, the risk of delirium, anatomical characteristics such as a porcelain aorta, and social support post-discharge are some of the factors that are not evaluated in the traditional risk scores. Finally, they do not take into account the local surgical results in a given institution, which may potentially have a lower operative risk.

Definition of risk categories in aortic stenosis has been driven by randomized control trials of TAVR which have created four risk groups: low, intermediate, high, and prohibitive risk as shown in Table 40.1. The first three groups are defined by the STS-PROM score as follows: low risk [<4%], intermediate risk [4–8%], or high risk [>8%]. Prohibitive risk is defined as risk of mortality and morbidity at 1 year >50%, compromise of ≥3 major organ systems, severe frailty, or severe procedure-specific impediments [3].

There is consensus, according to North American and European guidelines, that TAVR is a class IA recommendation for inoperable or prohibitive-risk patients with severe symptomatic AS but a life expectancy of at least 12 months [1, 4]. TAVR is an acceptable treatment option (class IA) in those patients with a high operative risk provided a multidisciplinary heart team has confirmed the TAVI indication, and there is a sufficient life expectancy. As of this writing, TAVR is also now deemed a reasonable alternative (class IIA) to SAVR in symptomatic AS patients at intermediate surgical risk [1].

Despite what has been published in the literature, the spectrum of patients with symptomatic severe aortic stenosis who require aortic valve replacement is much larger than that of patients previously studied in TAVI trials [5–9]. In fact, the high-risk population studied in the TAVI trials represents a small percentage of the total patient population needing aortic valve replacement. The Society of Thoracic Surgeons database of aortic valve disease cases during 2002–2010 ($N = 141,905$) shows that just 6.2% were ranked as high risk, whereas most patients (79.9%) were low risk, and 13.9% were intermediate risk [10]. In light of this distribution of patients and the focus on expanding indications for TAVR, there is increased interest to push the boundaries of the technology into the lower-risk cohorts.

40.3 Comparison of TAVR to SAVR in Intermediate-Risk Patients: Clinical Evidence

TAVR is established therapy for symptomatic severe AS in both inoperable/prohibitive-risk and high-risk patients. The journey to establishing an indication in intermediate risk began with data from cohort studies and prospective matched studies (see Table 40.2) finally culminating in data from prospective randomized trials of both balloon expandable and self-expandable transcatheter heart valves.

Table 40.2 Cohort studies (propensity match analysis) of TAVR vs. SAVR in intermediate-risk patients

Reference	# patients	Mean risk score	30-day mortality (%)	Vascular complications (%)	Permanent pacemaker (%)
Latib et al.	222	4.6 (STS)	1.8 vs. 1.8 (p = NS)	33.3 vs. 0.9 ($p < 0.001$)	11.7 vs. 2.7 ($p = 0.009$)
Fraccaro et al.	830	9.9 (EuroSCORE)	2.7 vs. 3.6 (p = NS)	6.0 vs. 0.5 ($p < 0.0001$)	13.4 vs. 3.7 ($p < 0.0001$)
Schymik et al.	432	8.7 (EuroSCORE)	1.4 vs. 4.2 (p = NS)	10.6 vs. 0.0 ($p < 0.001$)	13.9 vs. 4.6 ($p < 0.0001$)
Piazza et al.	510	17.4 (EuroSCORE)	7.8 vs. 7.1 (p = NS)	*	*
Thourani et al.	2021	5.3 (STS)	1.1 vs. 4	6.1 vs. 5.4	10.2 vs. 7.3

*Not reported

40.4 Prospective Nonrandomized Cohort Studies

Early insights into outcomes of TAVR in intermediate-risk patients were published in 2012 in a small propensity matched study of patients undergoing TAVR using either the Edwards SAPIEN XT or Medtronic CoreValve device. Latib et al. compared clinical outcomes of transfemoral TAVR vs. SAVR in 111 patients, propensity matched for clinical characteristics and risk scores, with a mean STS score of 4.6 ± 2.3 (TAVR) vs. 4.6 ± 2.6 (SAVR). There were no significant differences in all-cause mortality at 1 year (6.4% for TF-TAVR and 8.1% for SAVR; p = 1.0). Transfemoral TAVI was associated with a higher rate of vascular complications (33.3% vs. 0.9%, $p < 0.001$) and permanent pacemaker (11.7% vs. 2.7%, $p = 0.009$), while acute kidney injury was more frequent in the SAVR group (26.1% vs. 8.1%, $p < 0.001$) [11].

Additional prospective cohort data was available from the single-nation, multicenter cohort of patients treated with either SAVR or TAVR in Italy. The OBservational Study of Effectiveness of SAVR-TAVR procedures for severe Aortic stenosis Treatment (OBSERVANT) study enrolled 7618 consecutive patients with symptomatic severe AS who underwent SAVR or TAVI from December 2010 to June 2012 in 93 Italian participating hospitals. After excluding those patients felt to be inoperable or higher risk, due to concomitant coronary artery bypass, patients that underwent TAVR and SAVR were propensity matched. The authors found no significant difference in early mortality or myocardial infarction between TAVI and SAVR with a 30-day death of 3.6% for SAVR and 2.7% for TAVR ($p = 0.4328$). The incidence of stroke (3.0% SAVR and 0.0% TAVR; $p = 0.0455$) was slightly higher in those undergoing SAVR. There were higher rates of acute renal failure (9.6% vs. 3.6%, $p = 0.001$) and blood transfusions in the SAVR cohort (63.2% vs. 34.5%; $p < 0.001$). TAVR was however associated with increased vascular complications (6.0% vs. 0.5%; $p < 0.0001$) and new permanent pacemaker implantation (13.4% vs. 3.7%; $p < 0.0001$) [12].

More recent comparisons of intermediate-risk patients have compared newer-generation transcatheter valves with surgical aortic valve replacement. The propensity matched study of Thourani et al. compared intermediate-risk TAVR patients from the PARTNER 2 SAPIEN 3 observational study [13] with intermediate-risk SAVR patients from the PARTNER 2A randomized study using a pre-specified propensity score analysis to account for between-trial differences in baseline characteristics [14]. The primary endpoint for the propensity score analysis was the 1-year nonhierarchical composite event of death from any cause, all strokes, and posttreatment aortic regurgitation. The mean age was 81 years, and 88% underwent transfemoral

TAVR with a mean STS score of 5.3%. Compared with previously published data, the use of the SAPIEN 3 was associated with lower rates of all-cause mortality of 1.1%, disabling stroke of 1.0%, moderate or severe PVL of 4.2%, major vascular complications of 6.1%, life-threatening bleeding of 4.6%, and new permanent pacemaker implantation of 10%. Furthermore, the authors found a significant superiority of TAVR for the composite endpoint of mortality, strokes, and moderate or severe aortic regurgitation (weighted difference of proportions -9.2%, 95% CI -13.0 to -5.4; $p < 0.0001$) to surgical valve replacement.

40.5 Randomized Controlled Trial Data

To date, there have been three randomized controlled trials (RCTs) examining TAVR in intermediate surgical risk patients as shown in Table 40.3.

The Nordic Aortic Valve Intervention (NOTION) trial, a multicenter all-comers study, compared TAVR using a self-expanding prosthesis with SAVR in low- to intermediate-risk patients with severe aortic valve stenosis. A total of 280 patients were included, to be followed up for 5 years. Patients' clinical risk was estimated using both the Society of STS-PROM and EuroSCORE I and II. Around 80% of participants were considered low-risk patients. In the intention-to-treat analysis, no differences were found in the primary endpoint, a composite of death from any cause, stroke, or myocardial infarction (MI) at 1 year (13.1% for TAVI vs. 16.3% for SAVR; $p = 0.43$) [15].

In the prospective, randomized, non-inferiority PARTNER 2A trial, TAVR with the balloon-expandable SAPIEN XT valve (Edwards Lifesciences, USA) was compared with SAVR in 2032 patients with severe AS deemed to be at intermediate surgical risk, defined by a STS score of 4–8% (mean 5.8%). The primary endpoint, a composite of death from any cause or disabling stroke at 2-year follow-up, was similar between the TAVR and SAVR groups ($P = 0.001$ for meeting the non-inferiority criteria), and the 2-year survival curve event rates were not significantly different in the TAVR and SAVR cohorts (16.7% and 18.0%, respectively). Interestingly, among the 76% of patients who underwent TAVR with the use of TF access, all-cause death and disabling stroke rates were 21% lower ($P = 0.05$) than in the SAVR group. Moreover, the improvements in aortic valve areas and gradients at all time points after the procedure were significantly better with TAVR than with SAVR. Conversely, a higher rate of mild or worse paravalvular leaks was observed in the TAVR group [8].

Finally, in the prospective randomized non-inferiority SURTAVI trial of the Medtronic CoreValve, 1746 patients at intermediate surgical risk (mean STS 4.5%) were enrolled to evaluate the safety and efficacy of the self-expanding bioprosthesis CoreValve or Evolut R (Medtronic, USA) versus SAVR. At 2 years, the incidence of all-cause death or disabling stroke (the primary endpoint) was similar in the TAVR and SAVR groups, as assessed with a Bayesian analytical approach (12.6% and 14.0%, respectively). TAVR patients had lower mean transaortic gradients and larger aortic valve areas than patients who underwent SAVR, whereas TAVR was associated with a 26% rate of permanent pacemaker implantation and higher rates of moderate or severe residual paravalvular AR [9].

Taken together, these randomized trials with a non-inferiority design strongly support the safety and efficacy of TAVR for patients with severe AS whose operative risk of death is intermediate and have thus resulted in an updated indication of IIA [1].

Table 40.3 Randomized control trial data of TAVR vs. SAVR in intermediate-risk patients

Reference	# patients	Mean risk score	30-day mortality (%)	Vascular complications (%)	Permanent pacemaker (%)
PARTNER 2A	2032	5.8 (STS)	3.9 vs. 4.1 ($p = 0.78$)	7.9 vs. 5.0 ($p = 0.008$)	8.5 vs. 6.9 ($p = 0.17$)
SURTAVI	1746	4.5 (STS)	2.2 vs. 1.7	6 vs. 1.1	25.9 vs. 6.6

40.6   Meta-Analysis of Current Data

A meta-analysis by Singh et al. evaluated the results of aortic valve replacement in 2375 and 2377 intermediate-risk patients undergoing TAVI and SAVR, respectively. This analysis found similar 30-day all-cause mortality ($p = 0.07$), 30-day cardiac mortality ($p = 0.53$), and 12-month all-cause mortality ($p = 0.34$) between the two groups. However, TAVR via transfemoral access had a significantly lower mortality than SAVR (OR 0.58, $p = 0.006$). The incidence of moderate or greater aortic insufficiency ($p < 0.00001$) and new permanent pacemaker implantation ($p < 0.0001$) was higher in the TAVR group [16].

In the largest meta-analysis to date of patients with severe aortic stenosis, Gargiulo et al. compared mortality after TAVR or SAVR in 16,638 patients. Overall, there was no statistically significant difference between TAVI and SAVR in early (odds ratio [OR], 1.01 [95% CI, 0.81–1.26]) or midterm (OR, 0.96 [CI, 0.81–1.14]) all-cause mortality; however the analysis combined patients at all risk levels from prohibitive to intermediate risk. Analysis of the patient subgroup of low to intermediate risk showed statistically non-significant reductions in early (OR, 0.67 [CI, 0.42–1.07]) and midterm (OR, 0.91 [CI, 0.67–1.23]) mortality with TAVI. TAVR was associated with significant reductions in rates of major bleeding, acute kidney injury, and new-onset atrial fibrillation however was also associated with an increased need for permanent pacemaker implantation, vascular complications, and paravalvular leak which were significantly lower in the SAVR group. Interestingly, a significant long-term mortality benefit was found for TAVR in randomized trials within the transfemoral subgroup, $p = 0.001$ [17].

40.7   Remaining Questions

TAVR is the standard of care for high-risk or inoperable patients with symptomatic severe aortic stenosis and is now recommended in intermediate-risk patients as well. As indications widen to the lower-risk populations, remaining questions become ever more important to clarify.

Vascular complications, once the Achilles heel of the technology, are steadily decreasing with advances in transcatheter valve technology. They are however associated with significant morbidity and mortality as well as increased cost [18, 19]. The increased rates of new permanent pacemakers with TAVR vary according to the technology used but are a source of increased healthcare costs and clinical concern. Recent published work suggests that new pacemakers, although not associated with increased mortality do have an impact on increased incidence of heart failure hospitalizations and lack of improvement in left ventricular function post-intervention. Chanandi et al. performed a retrospective multicenter study to evaluate the incidence and outcomes of new permanent pacemaker implantation. In a population of over 1600 patients, approximately 20% required a new pacemaker within 30 days and up to 86% of these patients did require pacing. At follow-up, patients with new pacemaker had higher rates of rehospitalization due to heart failure (22.4% vs. 16.1%; adjusted HR 1.42; 95% CI 1.06–1.89; p 1/4 0.019) and the combined endpoint of mortality or heart failure rehospitalization (59.6% vs. 51.9%; adjusted HR 1.25; 95% CI 1.05 to 1.48; p 1/4 0.011). In addition, new pacemaker was associated with lesser improvement in LVEF over time (p 1/4 0.051 for changes in LVEF between groups), particularly in patients with reduced LVEF before TAVR (p 1/4 0.005 for changes in LVEF between groups) [20]. Further work will be required to determine whether in those patients that become pacemaker dependent if cardiac resynchronization therapy would be of potential benefit to reduce the incidence of heart failure.

The durability of transcatheter heart valves remains a question as experience is limited to the past 5–7 years. Issues regarding structural valve deterioration of both transcatheter and surgical valves are under scrutiny, and new definitions promise to create a more standardized approach to evaluation and follow-up [21]. It remains an important issue that will require rigorous follow-up however in the years to come.

40.8   Conclusions

Transcatheter aortic valve replacement has changed the treatment of aortic stenosis in those at high surgical risk, providing a less invasive treatment option with superior results. For those patients at intermediate surgical risk, TAVR is also now a non-inferior option. The pendulum is now swinging in the direction of the low-risk patient, and we anxiously await data in this population to fully comprehend the potential of this technology. Questions remain, and we must be vigilant to answer them in order to provide the best possible care for our patients.

References

1. Nishimura RA, Otto CM, Bonow RO, Carabello BA, Erwin JP 3rd, Fleisher LA, et al. 2017 AHA/ACC focused update of the 2014 AHA/ACC guideline for the management of patients with valvular heart disease: a report of the American College of Cardiology/American Heart Association Task Force on clinical practice guidelines. J Am Coll Cardiol. 2017;70(2):252–89.
2. Vahanian A, Otto CM. Risk stratification of patients with aortic stenosis. Eur Heart J. 2010;31(4):416–23.
3. Otto CM, Kumbhani DJ, Alexander KP, Calhoon JH, Desai MY, Kaul S, et al. 2017 ACC expert consensus decision pathway for transcatheter aortic valve replacement in the management of adults with aortic stenosis: a report of the American College of Cardiology Task Force on clinical expert consensus documents. J Am Coll Cardiol. 2017;69(10):1313–46.
4. Baumgartner H, Falk V, Bax JJ, De Bonis M, Hamm C, Holm PJ, et al. 2017 ESC/EACTS Guidelines for the management of valvular heart disease. Eur Heart J. 2017;38(36):2739–91.
5. Makkar RR, Fontana GP, Jilaihawi H, Kapadia S, Pichard AD, Douglas PS, et al. Transcatheter aortic-valve replacement for inoperable severe aortic stenosis. N Engl J Med. 2012;366(18):1696–704.
6. Popma JJ, Adams DH, Reardon MJ, Yakubov SJ, Kleiman NS, Heimansohn D, et al. Transcatheter aortic valve replacement using a self-expanding bioprosthesis in patients with severe aortic stenosis at extreme risk for surgery. J Am Coll Cardiol. 2014;63(19):1972–81.
7. Reardon MJ, Adams DH, Coselli JS, Deeb GM, Kleiman NS, Chetcuti S, et al. Self-expanding transcatheter aortic valve replacement using alternative access sites in symptomatic patients with severe aortic stenosis deemed extreme risk of surgery. J Thorac Cardiovasc Surg. 2014;148(6):2869–76 e1-7.
8. Leon MB, Smith CR, Mack MJ, Makkar RR, Svensson LG, Kodali SK, et al. Transcatheter or surgical aortic-valve replacement in intermediate-risk patients. N Engl J Med. 2016;374(17):1609–20.
9. Reardon MJ, Van Mieghem NM, Popma JJ, Kleiman NS, Sondergaard L, Mumtaz M, et al. Surgical or transcatheter aortic-valve replacement in intermediate-risk patients. N Engl J Med. 2017;376(14):1321–31.
10. Thourani VH, Suri RM, Gunter RL, Sheng S, O'Brien SM, Ailawadi G, et al. Contemporary real-world outcomes of surgical aortic valve replacement in 141,905 low-risk, intermediate-risk, and high-risk patients. Ann Thorac Surg. 2015;99(1):55–61.
11. Latib A, Maisano F, Bertoldi L, Giacomini A, Shannon J, Cioni M, et al. Transcatheter vs surgical aortic valve replacement in intermediate-surgical-risk patients with aortic stenosis: a propensity score-matched case-control study. Am Heart J. 2012;164(6):910–7.
12. Fraccaro C, Tarantini G, Rosato S, Tellaroli P, D'Errigo P, Tamburino C, et al. Early and midterm outcome of propensity-matched intermediate-risk patients aged >/=80 years with aortic stenosis undergoing surgical or transcatheter aortic valve replacement (from the Italian Multicenter OBSERVANT Study). Am J Cardiol. 2016;117(9):1494–501.
13. Kodali S, Thourani VH, White J, Malaisrie SC, Lim S, Greason KL, et al. Early clinical and echocardiographic outcomes after SAPIEN 3 transcatheter aortic valve replacement in inoperable, high-risk and intermediate-risk patients with aortic stenosis. Eur Heart J. 2016;37(28):2252–62.
14. Thourani VH, Kodali S, Makkar RR, Herrmann HC, Williams M, Babaliaros V, et al. Transcatheter aortic valve replacement versus surgical valve replacement in intermediate-risk patients: a propensity score analysis. Lancet. 2016;387(10034):2218–25.
15. Sondergaard L, Steinbruchel DA, Ihlemann N, Nissen H, Kjeldsen BJ, Petursson P, et al. Two-year outcomes in patients with severe aortic valve stenosis randomized to transcatheter versus surgical aortic valve replacement: the all-comers nordic aortic valve intervention randomized clinical trial. Circ Cardiovasc Interv. 2016;9(6):e003665.
16. Singh K, Carson K, Rashid MK, Jayasinghe R, AlQahtani A, Dick A, et al. Transcatheter aortic valve implantation in intermediate surgical risk patients with severe aortic stenosis: a systematic review and meta-analysis. Heart Lung Circ. 2018;27(2):227–34.
17. Gargiulo G, Sannino A, Capodanno D, Barbanti M, Buccheri S, Perrino C, et al. Transcatheter aortic valve implantation versus surgical aortic valve replacement: a systematic review and meta-analysis. Ann Intern Med. 2016;165(5):334–44.
18. Genereux P, Cohen DJ, Mack M, Rodes-Cabau J, Yadav M, Xu K, et al. Incidence, predictors, and prognostic impact of late bleeding complications after transcatheter aortic valve replacement. J Am Coll Cardiol. 2014;64(24):2605–15.
19. Redfors B, Watson BM, McAndrew T, Palisaitis E, Francese DP, Razavi M, et al. Mortality, length of

stay, and cost implications of procedural bleeding after percutaneous interventions using large-bore catheters. JAMA Cardiol. 2017;2(7):798–802.

20. Chamandi C, Barbanti M, Munoz-Garcia A, Latib A, Nombela-Franco L, Gutierrez-Ibanez E, et al. Long-term outcomes in patients with new permanent pacemaker implantation following transcatheter aortic valve replacement. JACC Cardiovasc Interv. 2018;11(3):301–10.

21. Dvir D, Bourguignon T, Otto CM, Hahn RT, Rosenhek R, Webb JG, et al. Standardized definition of structural valve degeneration for surgical and transcatheter bioprosthetic aortic valves. Circulation. 2018;137(4):388–99.

New Approaches for Aortic Valve Disease: From Transcatheter Aortic Valve Implantation to Sutureless Aortic Valves

41

Giuseppe Santarpino, Renato Gregorini, and Theodor Fischlein

The conventional aortic valve replacement (AVR) has a relatively high success rate associated with a perioperative mortality risk of approximately 1–3% in patients younger than 70 years undergoing isolated AVR increasing to 4–8% when combined with coronary artery bypass grafting. However, not all patients are suitable for surgery, with several factors affecting a patient's suitability for surgery.

In the early 2000s, aortic valve surgery was approaching a stalemate, as only two types of primary prosthetic aortic valves – mechanical and biological – were available. In addition, many patients were deemed inoperable with conventional surgery by the attending cardiologist or practitioner because of comorbidities or advanced age per se. Older age, left ventricle dysfunction or neurological dysfunction due to their high operative risk, and a late outcome after surgery were listed in a 2005 European Heart Survey on valvular heart study which found that 33% of patients with severe aortic stenosis did not undergo surgery.

The most appropriate treatment strategy for old "intermediate- and high-risk" patients with aortic valve stenosis is still a matter of debate. According to the recent guidelines of the European Society of Cardiology on the management of valvular heart disease, AVR is recommended as first-line therapy in patients with severe symptomatic aortic valve stenosis to improve both symptoms and survival [1].

Transcatheter aortic valve implantation has emerged as an alternative treatment to conventional surgery for patients of advanced age who are deemed inoperable [2, 3].

The advent of transcatheter aortic valve implantation (TAVI), also called transcatheter aortic valve replacement (TAVR), which does not require cardiopulmonary bypass (CPB), has produced a real revolution in the management of valvular heart disease, providing new hope and an alternative treatment option to patients who were previously considered too high risk for conventional surgery.

The introduction of the TAVI technology has gained widespread enthusiasm, such that nowadays, several cardiologists expect to perform TAVI in "every patient with aortic valve disease," leading to complete abandonment of the surgical approach. In a more collaborative environment, TAVI has brought cardiology and cardiac surgery

G. Santarpino (✉)
Città di Lecce Hospital, GVM Care & Research, Lecce, Italy

Klinikum Nürnberg, Paracelsus Medical University Nuremberg, Nuremberg, Germany

R. Gregorini
Città di Lecce Hospital, GVM Care & Research, Lecce, Italy

T. Fischlein
Klinikum Nürnberg, Paracelsus Medical University Nuremberg, Nuremberg, Germany
e-mail: theodor.fischlein@klinikum-nuernberg.de

© Springer Nature Switzerland AG 2019
A. Giordano et al. (eds.), *Transcatheter Aortic Valve Implantation*,
https://doi.org/10.1007/978-3-030-05912-5_41

closer together, and therapeutic options are tapered to the needs of the single patients. Therefore, physicians can carefully consider the strengths and weaknesses of each management strategy so as to identify the most appropriate treatment option for their individual patients.

In particular after the publication of the Cohort A results of the PARTNER (Placement of AoRTic TraNscathetER Valve) trial, there has been great debate regarding alternative therapeutic strategies such as TAVI for high-risk patients with symptomatic severe aortic valve stenosis [4].

Catheter-based techniques have found widespread acceptance among patients needing an aortic valve intervention. The perception of having done the procedure through "a little whole in the groin" as compared to having the "whole chest cracked" by a surgeon depicts a patients' likewise choice of TAVI over open surgery.

It is worth noting that, in the most important multicenter clinical studies conducted up to date, the TAVI approach has always been compared with surgical AVR using conventional prosthetic aortic valves through a full sternotomy. Basically, it means that the greatest innovation in cardiology (TAVI) has been compared with an "ancient" or otherwise "remote" surgical procedure (sutured AVR, full sternotomy) considered as the standard treatment in experienced centers that are at the forefront of cardiac surgery. Moreover, studies comparing TAVI with conventional surgical aortic valve replacement in elderly patients showed that isolated advanced age per se should not be considered an indication for TAVI [5]. On the other hand, transcatheter aortic valve implantation has become clinical routine in most centers worldwide for the treatment of severe symptomatic aortic stenosis in inoperable or high-risk patients, with number of procedures surpassing conventional aortic valve surgery [6].

From the dualism between the surgical and transcatheter approaches, a new option has emerged: recent studies have demonstrated better clinical and cosmetic results with minimally invasive techniques for AVR versus conventional surgery [7].

The use of minimally invasive techniques for aortic valve replacement is a matter of continuing debate as well as a surgical goal since many years. Available data from recent systematic reviews and meta-analyses do not provide strong evidence of a significant improvement in patient outcome to support the abandonment of conventional AVR through a full sternotomy. The drawback of minimally invasive surgery is that it generally requires longer cross-clamp and operative times. This may expose patients to potential additive risks, especially if the procedure is performed by surgeons who are not experts or are still on the learning curve. Although there are no data supporting this observation, a high level of surgical skills is required for these procedures because of the increasing use of technology, and a learning curve is unavoidable. More recently, sutureless AVR devices have been developed that enable short procedural times and also easy implantation of the aortic valve prosthesis when using a minimally invasive surgical approach [8–11]. In addition, the use of new sutureless aortic bioprostheses that allow shorter cardiopulmonary bypass (CPB) and cross-clamp times [12] has proved to be associated with good outcome in octogenarians [13]. The lack of prospective randomized trials comparing sutureless versus stented aortic bioprostheses is a major factor accounting for the exclusion of these devices from the therapeutic armamentarium recommended by current guidelines for the management of aortic valve disease.

These devices are mounted on a stent and are self-anchoring within the aortic annulus with no need for sutures, resulting in shorter operative and, hence, ischemic times. The use of these devices makes therefore valve implantation easier and faster, which seems to improve postoperative outcomes. At present, there are two commercially available sutureless aortic valves: the Perceval S (LivaNova Group, Milan, Italy) (Fig. 41.1) and the Intuity (Edwards Lifesciences, Irvine, CA) (Fig. 41.2).

As for the other two types of sutureless valves, the Perceval bioprosthesis has a collapsible design that allows easier implantation in the aortic annulus. This special feature does not pertain also to Intuity, which is anchored to a rigid frame as in conventional prosthetic valves.

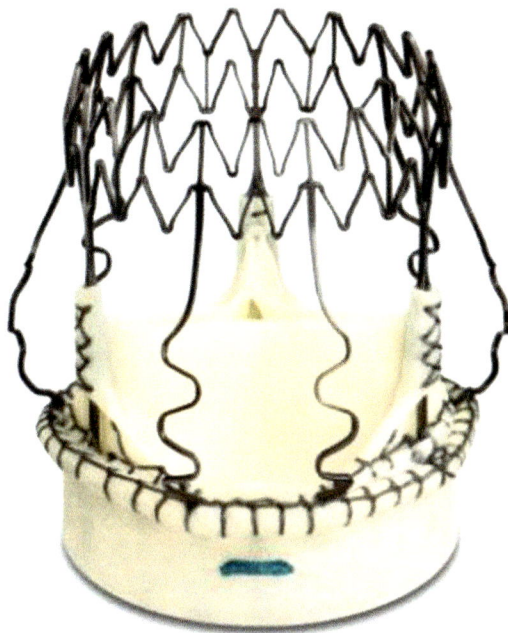

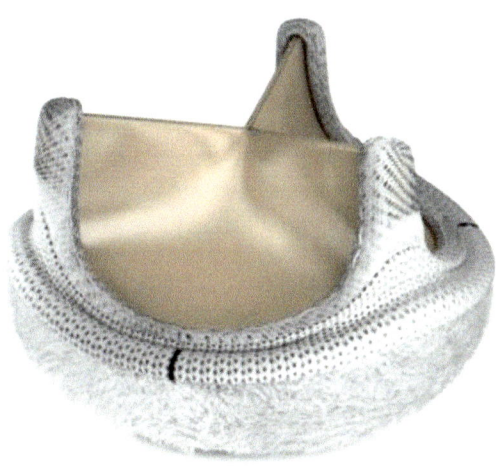

The earliest experience with the sutureless Perceval aortic bioprosthesis was aimed at establishing the safety of the device. At the time of the first implants in humans (2007), the primary question was whether a sutureless aortic valve would result in increased risk of device migration or dislodgement in patients, for example, with high blood pressure and abnormal heart rhythm, though the results from in vitro and animal studies were largely reassuring. Later observations confirmed the safety of the implant in terms of no risk of prosthesis migration even at long term and also suggested the possibility of short operative times, with less than 20 min of aortic cross-clamping using full sternotomy. Definitive evidence of shorter operative times was then provided by a study that included 100 patients undergoing minimally invasive isolated AVR using the sutureless Perceval aortic valve ($n = 50$) or a conventional stented bioprosthesis ($n = 50$). All procedures were performed by the same senior surgeon. Aortic cross-clamp and CPB times were 39.4% and 34% shorter, respectively, in the Perceval group than in the stented group.

The development of sutureless devices for use in clinical practice was aimed at making minimally invasive surgical procedures easier. In particular, sutureless AVR with the Perceval valve is most commonly performed via mini J-sternotomy and right lateral minithoracotomy, showing optimal performance with both approaches.

The Perceval device also proved to be a useful tool in the armamentarium of cardiac surgeons, allowing for shorter cross-clamp times. The main contribution of sutureless AVR through right lateral minithoracotomy consists in making implantation feasible also when the anatomical position of the aorta is unfavorable to the use of conventional prostheses that would be difficult to suture.

Ease of implantation with a minimally invasive approach has been confirmed also in a European multicenter study that evaluated 267 consecutive patients undergoing isolated AVR with the sutureless Perceval bioprosthesis through ministernotomy or full sternotomy. No differences were found between groups in aortic cross-clamp and CPB times.

Sutureless and rapid deployment bioprostheses could alleviate these concerns by improving ease of implantation. Since their introduction in clinical practice for aortic valve replacement, they appeared to provide enhanced implantability and favorable hemodynamics, particularly advisable in minimally invasive surgery, in difficult anatomical situations or elderly patients. Implants of sutureless bioprosthesis are increasingly performed, and the first meaningful findings have been released and herewith analyzed.

The stent fits the anatomy of the aorta and follows its movement during the entire cardiac cycle. It is designed to distribute the stresses in order to minimize the risk of damage to the aortic root. No sutures are required to fix the valve in place. This potentially reduces the risk damage to the aorta, reduces the operation time, and facilitates patients' faster recovery. The reduced profile of the valve, when mounted in its dedicated holder, enhances visibility and control for the surgeon.

In the Nuremberg University Hospital, from January 2010 to March 2012, 122 patients underwent minimally invasive Perceval sutureless aortic valve replacement, and 122 underwent TAVI. After propensity matching, 37 matched pairs were available for a clinical and echocardiographic analysis [14]. Predischarge echocardiographic data showed higher paravalvular leak rate in the TAVI group. At mean follow-up, survival was significantly differed between groups (sutureless 97.3% vs. TAVI 86.5%; $P = 0.015$). In the TAVI group, a significant difference in mortality was observed between patients with and without paravalvular leak. In other words, in our opinion, removal of the diseased native valve may enhance procedural quality by avoiding paravalvular leak.

However, these findings together suggest that recently developed surgical and interventional techniques may also be adopted in high-risk elderly patients. This issue has a significant economic relevance for healthcare systems, given the high costs of the new devices and the limited life expectancy of this patient population.

Keeping this goal in mind, we made a new analysis with a total of 626 patients were distributed between transcatheter aortic valve implantation (364) and sutureless (262) groups. Patients of both groups were not comparable for clinical and surgical characteristics, but many patients were in a "gray zone"; therefore, a new retrospective propensity score analysis was possible and

performed. For the 102 matched pair samples, postoperative, follow-up clinical data and costs data were obtained [15]. Also in this second analysis with more patients and a longer follow-up, paravalvular leakage occurred more frequently in patients in TAVI group (34% vs. 6.9%; $p < 0.001$) with an impact on the survival rate. But the most interesting part of the results of this study is the costs: these costs associated with the two procedures are similar when the cost of the device was excluded. When included, the sutureless approach resulted in a cost saving (22,451 Euro vs. 33,877 Euro, $p < 0.001$).

Although several unanswered questions remain over the clinical outcomes and the cost-effectiveness of TAVI, there has been a change in access route choice over the years, which has resulted in the rapid rise in transfemoral (TF) procedures with respect to the transapical (TA) approach. The latter is generally perceived to be less invasive and associated with more complications and usually tends to be performed in patients with significant comorbid conditions (e.g., vasculopathy) who cannot receive TF-TAVI [16, 17].

Given the increasing trend toward using the TF route and the ongoing debate regarding patients considered in the "gray zone" between TAVI and conventional surgery, in a third study, we aimed at comparing TF-TAVI vs. elective isolated AVR with the sutureless Perceval S aortic valve bioprosthesis [18]. Our results demonstrate that both minimally invasive AVR with the sutureless Perceval aortic valve and TF-TAVI are safe and effective in this cohort of the study. However, several differences emerged between the two techniques that deserve discussion: paravalvular leakage at discharge was present in 3.8% of the sutureless group and in 32.9% of the TF-TAVI ($p < 0.001$). Consequently, survival rates were 97.5% and 84.8% in the sutureless vs. TF-TAVI group, respectively ($p = 0.001$). We could conclude that both TF-TAVI and sutureless AVR are well-standardized, safe, and effective procedures for the treatment of patients with symptomatic severe aortic stenosis. However, TF-TAVI seems to be a valuable alternative to surgical AVR for frail patients. In patients with no concurrent disease (e.g., malignancy) and a favorable long-term survival outcome, minimally invasive AVR remains the procedure of choice in this cohort of the study population, as it is associated with better long-term results.

In our opinion, in the TAVI era, AVR still has to be considered as the true curative treatment alternative: TAVI does not allow for decalcification of the aortic annulus and removal of the diseased native valve; therefore it can be used as a "palliative procedure," which however is associated with a high risk of postoperative cerebral embolism and a higher incidence of paravalvular leakage significantly affecting survival. TAVI represents an extremely effective treatment option for high-risk patients who cannot undergo surgery, but its use remains questionable in low- and intermediate-risk patients because of the very limited evidence available.

At present, the sutureless Perceval aortic valve is a helpful addition to the surgeon's armamentarium and proved to be the first-choice bioprosthesis in particular clinical and anatomical situations. Since its clinical introduction and CE mark, experienced groups have further expanded the original indication for Perceval implantation, proving feasibility for the sake of patient safety. A prospective randomized clinical trial (PERSIST-AVR) is going to evaluate whether shorter operative times are associated with improved clinical outcomes. If this will be the case and good long-term durability will be confirmed, the sutureless technology will likely become the new gold standard in the surgical treatment of aortic valve disease, supporting its inclusion in future guidelines.

In conclusion, the most appropriate treatment strategy for this patient population remains to be clearly established and should include a multidisciplinary heart team approach. We believe that sutureless aortic valve prostheses have the potential to shorten the surgical time, and future research will determine whether this advantage will also translate into better outcomes in high-risk patients. Sutureless aortic valve replacement has been shown to be associated with improved survival compared with transcatheter aortic valve implantation, owing to the lower or no rates of residual aortic regurgitation. Only randomized prospective studies comparing the two surgical techniques will allow definite conclusions to be drawn regarding this issue.

References

1. Vahanian A, Alfieri O, Andreotti F, Antunes MJ, Baron-Esquivias G, Baumgartner H, et al. Guidelines on the management of valvular heart disease (version 2012): the Joint Task Force on the Management of Valvular Heart Disease of the European Society of Cardiology (ESC) and the European Association for Cardio-Thoracic Surgery (EACTS). Eur J Cardiothorac Surg. 2012;42:S1–44.
2. Leon MB, Smith CR, Mack M, Miller DC, Moses JW, Svensson LG, Tuzcu EM, Webb JG, Fontana GP, Makkar RR, Brown DL, Block PC, Guyton RA, Pichard AD, Bavaria JE, Herrmann HC, Douglas PS, Petersen JL, Akin JJ, Anderson WN, Wang D, Pocock S, PARTNER Trial Investigators. Transcatheter aortic-valve implantation for aortic stenosis in patients who cannot undergo surgery. N Engl J Med. 2010;363:1597e1607.
3. Popma JJ, Adams DH, Reardon MJ, Yakubov SJ, Kleiman NS, Heimansohn D, Hermiller J Jr, Hughes GC, Harrison JK, Coselli J, Diez J, Kafi A, Schreiber T, Gleason TG, Conte J, Buchbinder M, Deeb GM, Carabello B, Serruys PW, Chenoweth S, Oh JK, CoreValve United States Clinical Investigators. Transcatheter aortic valve replacement using a self-expanding bioprosthesis in patients with severe aortic stenosis at extreme risk for surgery. J Am Coll Cardiol. 2014;63:1972e1981.
4. Reynolds MR, Magnuson EA, Wang K, Thourani VH, Williams M, Zajarias A, Rihal CS, Brown DL, Smith CR, Leon MB, Cohen DJ, PARTNER Trial Investigators. Health-related quality of life after transcatheter or surgical aortic valve replacement in high-risk patients with severe aortic stenosis: results from the PARTNER (Placement of AoRTic TraNscathetER Valve) Trial (Cohort A). J Am Coll Cardiol. 2012;60:548–58.
5. Strauch JT, Scherner M, Haldenwang PL, Madershahian N, Pfister R, Kuhn EW, Liakopoulos OJ, Wippermann J, Wahlers T. Transapical minimally invasive aortic valve implantation and conventional aortic valve replacement in octogenarians. Thorac Cardiovasc Surg. 2012;60:335e342.
6. Beckmann A, Funkat AK, Lewandowski J, et al. Cardiac surgery in Germany during 2014: a report on behalf of the German Society for Thoracic and Cardiovascular Surgery. Thorac Cardiovasc Surg. 2015;63:258–69.

7. Johnston DR, Atik FA, Rajeswaran J, Blackstone EH, Nowicki ER, Sabik JF III, et al. Outcomes of less invasive J-incision approach to aortic valve surgery. J Thorac Cardiovasc Surg. 2012;144:852–8.e3.

8. Martens S, Sadowski J, Eckstein FS, Bartus K, Kapelak B, Sievers HH, et al. Clinical experience with the ATS 3f Enable Sutureless Bioprosthesis. Eur J Cardiothorac Surg. 2011;40:749–55.

9. Kocher AA, Laufer G, Haverich A, Shrestha M, Walther T, Misfeld M, et al. One-year outcomes of the Surgical Treatment of Aortic Stenosis With a Next Generation Surgical Aortic Valve (TRITON) trial: a prospective multicenter study of rapid-deployment aortic valve replacement with the EDWARDS INTUITY Valve System. J Thorac Cardiovasc Surg. 2013;145:110–5.. discussion 115-6

10. Folliguet TA, Laborde F, Zannis K, Ghorayeb G, Haverich A, Shrestha M. Sutureless Perceval aortic valve replacement: results of two European centers. Ann Thorac Surg. 2012;93:1483–8.

11. Santarpino G, Pfeiffer S, Schmidt J, Concistre G, Fischlein T. Sutureless aortic valve replacement: first-year single-center experience. Ann Thorac Surg. 2012;94:504–8.. discussion 508-9

12. Santarpino G, Pfeiffer S, Concistré G, Grossmann I, Hinzmann M, Fischlein T. The Perceval S aortic valve has the potential of shortening surgical time: does it also result in improved outcome? Ann Thorac Surg. 2013;96:77e81.

13. Santarpino G, Pfeiffer S, Vogt F, Hinzmann M, Concistrè G, Fischlein T. Advanced age per se should not be an exclusion criterion for minimally invasive aortic valve replacement. J Heart Valve Dis. 2013;22:455e459.

14. Santarpino G, Pfeiffer S, Jessl J, Dell'Aquila AM, Pollari F, Pauschinger M, Fischlein T. Sutureless replacement versus transcatheter valve implantation in aortic valve stenosis: a propensity-matched analysis of 2 strategies in high-risk patients. J Thorac Cardiovasc Surg. 2014;147(2):561–7.

15. Santarpino G, Pfeiffer S, Jessl J, Dell'Aquila A, Vogt F, von Wardenburg C, Schwab J, Sirch J, Pauschinger M, Fischlein T. Clinical outcome and cost analysis of sutureless versus transcatheter aortic valve implantation with propensity score matching analysis. Am J Cardiol. 2015;116(11):1737–43.

16. Biancari F, Rosato S, D'Errigo P, et al. Immediate and intermediate outcome after transapical versus trans-femoral transcatheter aortic valve replacement. Am J Cardiol. 2016;117:245–51.

17. Blackstone EH, Suri RM, Rajeswaran J, et al. Propensity-matched comparisons of clinical outcomes after transapical or transfemoral transcatheter aortic valve replacement: a placement of aortic transcatheter valves (PARTNER)-I trial substudy. Circulation. 2015;131:1989–2000.

18. Santarpino G, Vogt F, Pfeiffer S, Dell'Aquila AM, Jessl J, Cuomo F, von Wardenburg C, Fischlein T, Pauschinger M, Schwab J. Sutureless vs transfemoral transcatheter aortic valve implant: a propensity score matching study. J Heart Valve Dis. 2017;26:255–61.

Hybrid Procedures for Aortic Valve Disease: Transapical Aortic Valve Implantation Through Lower Left Anterior Mini-thoracotomy Versus Sutureless Valve Implantation Through Upper Right Anterior Mini-thoracotomy

42

Terézia B. Andrási

42.1 Introduction

At present, there is no consensus regarding the optimal management of aortic valve stenosis in multimorbid elderly patients with respect to type of less-invasive approaches.

Transapical (TA) transcatheter aortic valve implantation (TAVI), also called transcatheter aortic valve replacement (TAVR), over mini left anterior thoracotomy and sutureless aortic valve implantation over mini right anterior thoracotomy (RAMT-AVR) are considered indicated in a narrow range of high-risk patients not eligible for mini-sternotomy or for transfemoral endovascular procedures.

This chapter will review the preoperative decision-making, procedural characteristics, and postoperative outcomes of transapical transcatheter aortic valve implantation through left anterior mini-thoracotomy and sutureless aortic valve implantation through right anterior mini-thoracotomy.

T. B. Andrási (✉)
Department of Thoracic, Cardiac and Vascular Surgery, Georg August University of Göttingen, Göttingen, Germany
e-mail: terezia.andrasi@med.uni-goettingen.de

A better understanding of these emerging minimal-invasive techniques may ease the indication for these approaches in a wider range of high-risk patients.

42.2 Preprocedural Evaluation and Patient Enrollment

A small synopsis of preoperative inclusion and exclusion criteria for TA-TAVI and RAMT-AVR are presented in Table 42.1. Although enhanced design modifications of TA-TAVI transcatheter aortic valve implantation increased effective orifice area and reduced strut height leading to superior hemodynamics [1–3], this therapy is currently reserved for patients who are ineligible for traditional aortic valve replacement because of advanced age, poor left ventricular systolic function, severe comorbidities, and high-risk anatomic characteristics [4, 5]. Previous studies [1–5] revealed that the mean Log EUROSCORE I values for the TA-TAVI patients were significantly higher than that for the transfemoral TAVI ($p = 0.008$) as was the STS score ($p < 0.001$).

Rapid deployment aortic valve replacement was developed to lessen the duration of myocardial ischemia and cardiopulmonary bypass and

© Springer Nature Switzerland AG 2019
A. Giordano et al. (eds.), *Transcatheter Aortic Valve Implantation*,
https://doi.org/10.1007/978-3-030-05912-5_42

Table 42.1 Inclusion and exclusion criteria for RAMT-AVR and TA-TAVI

RAMT-AVR	TA-TAVI
Inclusion criteria	Inclusion criteria
• Calcified native aortic valve stenosis • Stenosis-based insufficiency • Previously implanted aortic valve • Aortic valve in transverse position • Age older than 70 years	• Severe symptomatic aortic stenosis • Symmetric valve cusps calcification • Aortic valve in transverse position • Aortic annulus <25 mm • Advanced peripheral disease • Severly calcified thoracic aorta • Age older than 75 years • High-risk patients • Log EuroScore >20%
Exclusion criteria	Exclusion criteria
• Noncalcified valve pathology • Bicuspid aortic valve • Aortic annulus >27 mm • Narrow sinotubular junction • Progressed calcification of the aorta and/or the sinotubular junction • Pure aortic insufficiency • Aneurysm of Ao. Root/Ao. asc. • Endocarditis within 3 months • LV-EF <25% • Reoperation (after sternotomy) • Associated cardiac procedures	• Noncalcified aortic stenosis • Bicuspid aortic valve • Aortic annulus >25 mm • Subvalvular aortic stenosis • HOCM • Intracardiac thrombus or vegetation • Untreated coronary artery disease • Myocardial infarction <1 month • Endocarditis • LV-EF <20% • Recent stroke

facilitates aortic valve replacement through smaller incisions. To be considered successful, however, it must meet or exceed attributes of conventionally implanted valves with regard to hemodynamic performance, adaptability to patient anatomy (sizes and shapes), long-term durability, and absence of incremental risk [6].

Patients with a bicuspid aortic valve or non-spherical aortic annulus may not be good candidates for either RAMT-AVR or TA-AVI.

The TRANSFORM trial [6] put forward anomalous coronary artery or coronary ostial position, extensive annular root calcification, and significant calcification of the anterior mitral leaflet or interventricular septum – as important intraoperative exclusion criteria for sutureless valve implantation. In addition, patients after sternotomy, mini-sternotomy, TAVI, associated cardiac procedures (except atrial fibrillation ablation), and reoperation cases were initially excluded from RAMT-AVR in many trials. Nonetheless, sutureless valves have been used also in combination with other valvular or coronary surgical repair [7].

A computed tomography of the chest and abdomen should always be performed previous to RAMT-AVR and TA-TAVI in order to assess (1) the degree of aortic and arterial calcification, (2) the position of the ascending aorta in relation to the sternum, and (3) the position of the aortic valve in relation to the ascending aorta (horizontal root).

The CT scan of the chest should ensure a midline position of the aortic annulus and evaluate the distance between the aortic annulus and the right second intercostal space and the distance between the aortic annulus and the sternum [8]. RAMT-AVR preferred if the aorta is on the right side and close to the rib cage, whereas mini-sternotomy would be preferred if the aorta is in the midline or deeper [9, 10]. Approaching the aortic valve directly facilitates the correct placing particularly in a horizontal root.

Accurate sizing of the annulus is key to success of both RAMT-AVR and TA-TAVI procedures. Whereas in RAMT-AVR direct sizing is performed, in TA-TAVI an indirect preoperative calculation of the annulus size and the angulation of the aortic root is determined based on the CT scan.

42.3 Surgical Procedure for RAMT-AVR and TA-AVI

The TA-TAVI was initially described by Ye et al. [11] in 2006 and represents an alternative access route of cases with nonviable femoral access (Table 42.2). The procedure requires general anesthesia and is optimally performed in a hybrid surgery room. After left anterolateral mini-thoracotomy in the fifth or sixth intercostal space (ICS), the pericardium is opened and left ventricular apex exposed. A double purse-string suture with Teflon or pericardium is placed around the puncture site. Direct puncture is followed by direct left ventricular apex sheet insertion. The aortic valve is crossed with a guide-wire and the valve deployed as described for transfemoral approach. Once the valve has been deployed, sheath is withdrawn, and sutures are tied under rapid ventricular pacing to keep low pressure until repair completion.

Laufer and colleagues [12] were the first to use the Intuity valve system in a right anterior thoracotomy setting and showed the suitability for this access (Table 42.2). RAMT-AVR is performed in the second to fourth right intercostal space; no rib resection but only spreading is required to obtain surgical access to the lateral mediastinum. After longitudinal incision and suspension of the pericardium, the ascending aorta was cannulated distally [7] in standard fashion. The venous cannulation may be performed either directly through the right atrial appendage (RAA) or femoral venous when the appendage is difficult to visualize. An external cross-clamp was applied directly to the aorta, just before the origin of the brachiocephalic arterial trunk.

Antegrade cardioplegia is delivered via the aortic root or directly into the coronary arteries. After transverse aortotomy and inspection, the calcified aortic valve is removed in the standard manner. Excessive debridement of annular calcification should be avoided in order to prevent large annular defects. After direct sizing, three braided sutures are placed at the nadir of each aortic valve sinus and then separately placed on the sewing ring of the prosthesis, which are then deployed at the target location following the manufacturer's instructions. By the closure of the transverse aortotomy, intracardiac air is aspirated either through aortic root or left ventricular venting. Transesophageal echocardiography is routinely performed after both procedures to verify correct prosthesis positioning, identify paravalvular leakage, and determine pressure gradients.

Edwards Sapien and CoreValve prosthesis were predominantly used for TA-TAVI procedures [13, 14], whereas mainly Perceval S and Edwards Intuity bioprosthesis were used as sutureless valves.

42.4 Procedural Characteristics

It has been shown that aortic cross-clamp time >60 min and prolonged CPB time are independent predictors of mortality and morbidity in low- and high-risk cardiac patients [15, 16]. A 20 to 30 min reduction in ischemic time would lower the risk of serious perioperative cardiac morbidity or mortality [7].

The TRANSFORM study [6] showed a relative reduction in aortic cross-clamp time and cardiopulmonary bypass time and an excellent hemodynamic performance. Bening et al. [17] demonstrated a markedly reduced aortic cross-clamp time with RAMT, whereas Schlömicher

Table 42.2 Procedural details

	RAMT-AVR	TA-TAVI
Pre-OP CT scan	Sternum-aorta relation	Aortic valve characteristics
Surgical incisions	5–7 cm incision right second, third, fourth ICS without rib resection aortic incision	5–7 cm incision left fifth, sixth ICS without rib resection left ventricular puncture
Cannulation sites	Venous—groin or RAA Arterial—Asc. Ao. or groin	Venous—groin Arterial—groin
Aortic valve	Aortic valve excision annulus decalcification	With/without pre-dilatation Balloon valvuloplasty
Operation time (min)	120–180	60–160

et al. [18] with hemithoracotomy. Glauber et al. [19] were able to reduce aortic cross-clamp time for mini-thoracotomy AVR by 28 min when using a sutureless Perceval S prosthesis.

Similarly, Wendler et al. [20] reported significant reduction of procedural times for TA-TAVI when the balloon aortic valvuloplasty step was omitted (75 min vs. 122 min, $p < 0.001$).

Compared to conventional TAVI with balloon aortic valvuloplasty, Strauch et al. [21] revealed that the approach without valvuloplasty is at least comparable, with several potential safety advantages, including considerable reduction in the need for procedural catecholamine use.

Although associated with aortic cross-clamp, sutureless valve implantation offers valuable valve fixation. Whereas the braided sutures secure fixation of the valve in the annulus during RAMT-AVR, TA-AVI remains associated with a higher risk for dislocation and migration. Nonetheless, Gilmanov [7] emphasizes that bigger size prosthesis could be implanted with sutureless method, which is in line with no pledget and sutures present inside the aortic root. Less surgical manipulation on the aortic root and reduced quantity of foreign material left around the aortic annulus might be a real advantage of the sutureless technology [7].

Oppositely, many physicians are concerned about potential injury to the left ventricle by the apical surgical manipulation performed during TA-TAVI [22, 23]. However, Imnaze et al. [24] conclude that cannulation of the apex did not cause significant damage to the cardiac tissue, although biomarker levels were not assessed.

Moreover, vascular complications and need for circulatory support after TAVI were shown to be associated with threefold risk for severe bleeding [25] with sheet diameter remaining a week predictor of postoperative bleeding after TAVI. Importantly, transapical approach was only moderate predictor associated with twofold bleeding risk [25].

Taken together, complications during TA-TAVI procedure might be related to left ventricular pricking by direct myocardial or mitral injury, bleeding, hemodynamic or respiratory compromise, and thoracotomy pain [14], whereas bleeding and laceration of the right ventricle or atrium by the percutaneous venous cannula were also described during RAMT-AVR procedures [17].

Last, but not least, patients with low preoperative LV-EF as well as old patients at risk for postoperative pleural effusion require pleural drainage. Since RAMT consists of left pleural opening, whereas TA-TAVI a right pleural opening, both techniques permit intraoperative pleural drainage placement.

42.5   Postoperative Outcomes

Sutureless AVR in RAMT approach significantly reduces operative and mechanically assisted ventilation times compared with sutured prostheses and is associated with low mortality and morbidity, leading to excellent surgical and hemodynamic results [7] and, thus, becoming highly competitive alternative for TA-TAVI.

Transesophageal echocardiography is routinely performed at the end of both procedures to assess left ventricular function, to rule out paravalvular leak, and to confirm valve function by measuring the effective opening area and the pressure gradients of the aortic valve (Table 42.3).

Table 42.3 Postoperative valve function and cardiac rhythm

At discharge	RAMT-AVR		TA-TAVI
	Edwards Intuity	Perceval S	Edwards Sapien
Mean gradient (mmHg)	9–12	11–15	8–12
Peak gradient (mmHg)	10–22	19	16–22
Incidence PPM > 2 (%)	3–10	0–2	0–3
Incidence PVL (%)	0.7–2.2	0–8	0.5–4
NOAF (%)	12	4–7	14.5
Permanent pacemaker (%)	4–12	2–6	7–9

42.5.1 Left Ventricular Function

Preoperative poor left ventricular ejection fraction (LV-EF) is a risk factor for poor outcomes after both TA-TAVI and RAMT-AVR [26, 27]. For patients with severe LV dysfunction, any further damage to the cardiac muscle during TAVI could greatly worsen the outcome, and many physicians are concerned about potential injury to the left ventricle by the apical surgical manipulation performed during TA-TAVI [22, 23, 28].

TA-TAVI has been reported to increase biomarkers of cardiac tissue injury and to cause more LV damage compared with TF-TAVI; however, these studies did not specifically concern patients with low EF [28, 29].

The data of Imnadze et al. [24] suggest that, for patients with a reduced EF, TA-TAVI is not associated with a poorer outcome compared with transfemoral TAVI. Transapical access should not be discounted based on the presence of left ventricular dysfunction alone, since the access route has little or no effect on recovery of the LV function. Furthermore it remains unclear how left ventricular dysfunction affects cardiac remodeling and EF recovery after TAVI.

Higher enzyme release has been shown after TA-TAVI when compared to transfemoral TAVI [26]. However, this enzyme release may be reflected by a transient segmental apical dysfunction that does not affect mortality [28]. D'Onofrio et al. [27] pointed out that it is likely that even if some degree of myocardial dysfunction arises after TA-TAVI, this is far outweighed by the afterload reduction that ultimately yields beneficial final results. Global longitudinal myocardial strain improved in all TAVI patients, independently of approach [30], suggesting that it is the preprocedural strain impairment, and not the method of approach, that dictates postoperative functional recovery [31].

Logstrup et al. [32] found similar improvement in EF after 1 year for patients who had undergone TA or transfemoral TAVI. Other studies have assessed LV remodeling after TAVI and found no differences between the TA and transfemoral procedures in terms of LV mass decrease [33]. This is of particular interest, as a reduction in LV mass index has been shown to be independently associated with a lower risk of rehospitalization after TAVI [34].

Haverich et al. [35] showed that at 3 years, the Intuity valve was associated with significant LV mass regression accompanied by significant improvements in patient functional status after sutureless AVR.

42.5.2 Patient-Prosthesis Mismatch

Indexed effective orifice area (iEOA) <0.65 cm^2/m^2 was considered severe patient-prosthesis mismatch (PPM), whereas iEOA <0.85 cm^2/m^2 as moderate PPM [36].

Sutureless valves had significantly lower transvalvular gradients and a lower proportion of patient-prosthesis mismatch when compared to those who received a conventional bioprosthesis [35, 37, 38].

Mohty et al. [39] found that severe PPM (EOA $<$ 0.65 cm^2/m^2) was associated with decreased 5- and 10-year survival (74% and 40%, respectively), significantly worse than for patients with mild or no PPM (5- and 10-year survival rate, 84% and 61%, respectively).

In the study of Haverich et al. [35], the indexed EOA and rate of severe PPM calculated by echographic core lab was 0.9 cm^2/m^2 and 3% at 1 year, whereas Hahn at al. [40] reported in the PARTNER trial a rate of 30% severe PPM at 1 year. Although the PARTNER trial included a higher risk population with features predictive of postoperative PPM, such as advanced age, coronary artery disease, diabetes, and renal failure [41], it is unlikely that these differences alone sufficiently explain the 10-fold increase in severe PPM.

According to Pibarot und Dumesnil [38], annular calcification and fibrosis might restrict the diameter of the bioprosthetic implant and the structural support of the bioprosthesis, which occupies space within the aortic root and may reduce the EOA available for blood flow and cause PPM.

The very low rate of PPM observed in the study of Haverich et al. [35] may also suggest that the subannular positioning of the cloth-covered stent frame optimize the flow characteristics through the valve inlet by widening and reshaping the LV outflow tract.

The unique design of the Intuity valve may lessen the risk for prosthesis-patient mismatch, particularly in patients with a small aortic root [42].

42.5.3 Paravalvular Leakage

Paravalvular leakage (PVL) has a major impact on patient outcome. The PARTNER trial revealed that even mild paravalvular leakage is strongly associated with late mortality [2]. Kodali et al. [43] reported 7% and 6.9% PVL after TAVI at 1 and 2 years, respectively, whereas the surgical AVR was associated with 1.9% and 0.9% PVL at 1 and 2 years, respectively. Haverich et al. [35] observed 1.2% moderate and severe PVL rate at 1 year after Edwards Intuity valve implantation, comparable to that after surgical AVR.

The results of the TRITON trial [44] have confirmed the safety and efficacy of the rapid deployment AVR using the sutureless Edwards Intuity. Removal of calcifications during RAMT-AVR allows better sealing of the valve and less PVL.

Moreover, when compared with standard surgical bioprostheses, the Edwards Intuity might be associated with larger EOAs in smaller valve sizes, a lower risk of PPM owing to the structural valve design, and a low rate of significant postoperative PVL [35].

42.5.4 Valvular Pressure Gradients

Elevated transvalvular gradients can contribute to persistent left ventricular hypertrophy and diastolic dysfunction after aortic valve replacement, which can raise the patient-prosthesis mismatch and decreased survival [45]. In a study of 2576 patients who survived AVR,

Borger [46] found that Edwards Intuity patients had significantly lower transvalvular gradients and a lower proportion of patient-prosthesis mismatch when compared to those who received a conventional bioprosthesis.

The results of Bening et al. [16] and Borger et al. [47] showed lower mean gradients after 3 months for the Edwards Intuity valve compared to standard stented valves, although the implanted valve size revealed no differences.

The improved transvalvular gradient is probably related to the flared subvalvular stent in the left ventricular outflow tract which appears to optimize laminar flow across the valve prosthesis. Accola [48] points out that the emphasis of RAMT-AVR technology is not necessarily "speed" of implantation but rather ease of implantation and superb transvalvular gradients, specifically in the smaller valve sizes.

However, the present scientific data (Table 42.3) reveals no significant pressure gradient differences after TA-TAVI and RAMT-AVR, suggesting appropriate clinical indication for the procedures.

42.5.5 Atrial Fibrillation

The prognostic implications of preexisting atrial fibrillation (AF) and new-onset AF (NOAF) after TA-TAVI and RAMT-AVR remain uncertain. Whereas preexisting AF was present in 30.9% of the study population, NOAF was observed in 9.3% of the patients after TAVI, with preexisting AF known to be an independent predictor of mortality at 1 year [49].

42.5.6 Permanent Pacemaker Implantation

Whether balloons expansion of the subvalvular skirt frame has a negative impact on the conduction system was not yet evaluated, however, previous studies showed that preoperative rhythm disturbances correlate with postoperative PM implantation after RAMT-AVR and TA-TAVI

[50, 51]. Patients with permanent pacemaker before TAVI have higher risk profile, with notable differences [52] with higher incidence of preoperative cardiac arrhythmias.

Whereas in the TRANSFORM study, the overall rate of new permanent pacemaker implantation in patients with isolated AVR was 11.9%, in contrast to the observed rate of 5% as reported in the European Intuity studies for isolated AVR, whereas the remaining end point were similar overall [50]. This may be related to the high prevalence of preoperative induction abnormalities observed in the current study. Dawkins et al. [51] observed that patients with preoperative conduction abnormalities were significantly more likely to require a new permanent pacemaker compared with those without 16% vs. 6% ($p = 0.004$). Likewise in the sutured valves, a greater rate of pacemaker implantation (11-fold) has been observed in the presence of preoperative right bundle branch block [53]. Of note, the new permanent pacemaker implantation rate of 2% and 4% observed for the Intuity valve was lower than that reported with Perceval S valve of 7% [54, 55].

Whether Intuity's balloon-expandable frame imparts greater radial force within LVOT compared with a conventional valve and, therefore, predisposes to a greater likelihood of pacemaker implantation in patients with baseline conduction abnormalities warrants additional study.

42.5.7 Survival

Survival benefit can be obtained in elderly patients with both RAMT-AVR and TA-TAVI (Table 42.4). Noteworthy, the learning curve and procedural volume have no impact on patient survival after TA-TAVI [56]. Heart failure, pneumonia, and bleeding complications are etiologies of readmission in patients after TAVI. Although patients who undergone TA-TAVI are more likely to be resubmitted to the hospital [57], TA-TAVI was not a predictor of in-hospital mortality during primary admission, but during the readmission. Therefore, it seems that the higher mortality assessed in the TA-TAVI studies (Table 42.4) is due to the worse preoperative status. In consent,

Table 42.4 Morbidity and mortality

At 30 days	RAMT-AVR	TA-TAVI
Conversion rate (%)	0.1–4.6	0.6–3
Revision for bleeding (%)	0.2–7	2–8
New atrial fibrillation (%)	4–12	14.5
Pacemaker implantation (%)	1.7–9.9	1.5–10.2
Stroke (%)	1.5–4	1.5–4
Endocarditis (%)	0	0
ICU stay (days)	1–2	0–2
Hospital stay (days)	3–10	2–7
Mortality at 30 days (%)	0–5	0–11.3–35.1
Mortality at 1 year (%)	1.9–6	4.7–20

in low-risk patients with aortic valve stenosis undergoing TA-TAVI, no differences appeared on health-related quality of life compared with surgical aortic valve replacement during 5-year follow-up period [58].

Although, the TRANSFORM trial [6] on RAMT-AVR revealed that the rate of surgical complications at 30 days was exceptionally low with all-cause mortality of 0.8%, in studies that applied unadjusted analysis [17, 19], longer cross-clamping times were associated with increased mortality and morbidity after sutureless valve implantation. Nissinen and colleagues [59] proposed a critical threshold value for aortic cross-clamp of 150 min, where observed mortality was 1.8% versus 12.2%. However, numerous confounding factors account for increases in both cross-clamp time and operative mortality, such as high predicted operative risk, technical complexity, and intraoperative complications.

Nevertheless, Edwards Intuity valve implantation was associated with lower cross-clamp times and CPB times compared with unadjusted data from the STS database. Miceli et al. [60] showed excellent results with an early mortality rate of 0.7% in a high-risk patient collective using this technique in combination with the Perceval S valve. Distinct advantages in postoperative atrial fibrillation, ventilation time, and hospital length of stay compared with partial sternotomy were shown by the same group [61].

A 1-year mortality was significantly higher in both preexisting AF (16.3%) and NOAF (14.6%)

patients when compared with the sinus rhythm (6.5%, $p = 0.007$) patients. Preexisting AF is associated with a twofold increased risk of 1-year mortality. This negative effect is most pronounced in patients discharged with single antiplatelet therapy compared with other antithrombotic regimens [49]. Postoperative anticoagulation should be performed in accordance with the recent Guidelines for Management of Patients with Valvular Disease [62].

A Bayesian network meta-analysis comparing mini-sternotomy or mini-thoracotomy for minimally invasive classic aortic valve replacement revealed longer aortic cross-clamp and CPB times for mini-thoracotomy AVR with similar outcomes compared to mini-sternotomy [63].

Barnhard et al. [6] emphasizes that if the casual relationship between aortic cross-clamp time and adverse events becomes stronger as the cross-clamp time excess the critical values, then it may be reasonable to assume the benefit of Intuity will be greater as the degree of surgical complexity rises.

42.6 Conclusion

Sutureless RAMT-AVR approach becomes highly competitive alternative for TA-TAVI, in particular for the treatment of elderly patients who present a higher surgical risk profile and frailty. Rapid deployment, considerable reduction in implantation time, and the surgical precision of the implantation on a decalcified aortic annulus are the main advantages of the sutureless aortic valve prostheses.

Sutureless technology may enhance the use of minimally invasive approaches. Not only the surgical incision but also the manipulation inside of the aortic root is reduced compared to the conventional aortic valve replacement, offering a synergic reduction of the surgical trauma.

Nonetheless, patients requiring complex multivalve or combined procedures, as well as those with a low preoperative ejection fraction, would also benefit from rapid deployment valves, however without benefiting from the minimally invasive approaches.

TA-TAVI is particularly recommended in cases with high risk of stroke or other embolic events, such as patients with advanced peripheral artery disease or severely calcified thoracic and ascending aorta.

Conflict of Interest None

References

1. Leon MB, Smith CR, Mack M, Miller DC, Moses JW, Svensson LG, Tuzcu EM, Webb JG, Fontana GP, Makkar RR, Brown DL, Block PC, Guyton RA, Pichard AD, Bavaria JE, Herrmann HC, Douglas PS, Petersen JL, Akin JJ, Anderson WN, Wang D, Pocock S, PARTNER Trial Investigators. Transcatheter aortic-valve implantation for aortic stenosis in patients who cannot undergo surgery. N Engl J Med. 2010;363:1597–607.
2. Smith CR, Leon MB, Mack MJ, Miller DC, Moses JW, Svensson LG, Tuzcu EM, Webb JG, Fontana GP, Makkar RR, Williams M, Dewey T, Kapadia S, Babaliaros V, Thourani VH, Corso P, Pichard AD, Bavaria JE, Herrmann HC, Akin JJ, Anderson WN, Wang D, Pocock SJ, PARTNER Trial Investigators. Transcatheter versus surgical aortic-valve replacement in high-risk patients. N Engl J Med. 2011;364:2187–98.
3. Mack MJ, Leon MB, Smith CR, Miller DC, Moses JW, Tuzcu EM, Webb JG, Douglas PS, Anderson WN, Blackstone EH, Kodali SK, Makkar RR, Fontana GP, Kapadia S, Bavaria J, Hahn RT, Thourani VH, Babaliaros V, Pichard A, Herrmann HC, Brown DL, Williams M, Akin J, Davidson MJ, Svensson LG, PARTNER 1 trial investigators. 5-year outcomes of transcatheter aortic valve replacement or surgical aortic valve replacement for high surgical risk patients with aortic stenosis (PARTNER 1): a randomised controlled trial. Lancet. 2015;385:2477–84.
4. Miller DC, Blackstone EH, Mack MJ, Svensson LG, Kodali SK, Kapadia S, Rajeswaran J, Anderson WN, Moses JW, Tuzcu EM, Webb JG, Leon MB, Smith CR, PARTNER Trial Investigators and Patients, PARTNER Stroke Substudy Writing Group and Executive Committee. Transcatheter (TAVR) versus surgical (AVR) aortic valve replacement: occurrence, hazard, risk factors, and consequences of neurologic events in the PARTNER trial. J Thorac Cardiovasc Surg. 2012;143:832–43.
5. Al-Attar N, Himbert D, Descoutures F, Iung B, Raffoul R, Messika-Zeitoun D, Brochet E, Francis F, Ibrahim H, Vahanian A, Nataf P. Transcatheter aortic valve implantation: selection strategy is crucial for outcome. Ann Thorac Surg. 2009;87:1757–62.
6. Barnhart GR, Accola KD, Grossi EA, Woo YJ, Mumtaz MA, Sabik JF, Slachman FN, Patel HJ, Borger MA, Garrett HE Jr, Rodriguez E, McCarthy

PM, Ryan WH, Duhay FG, Mack MJ, Chitwood WR Jr, TRANSFORM Trial Investigators. TRANSFORM (Multicenter Experience With Rapid Deployment Edwards INTUITY Valve System for Aortic Valve Replacement) US clinical trial: performance of a rapid deployment aortic valve. J Thorac Cardiovasc Surg. 2017;153:241–51.

7. Gilmanov D, Miceli A, Ferrarini M, Farneti P, Murzi M, Solinas M, Glauber M. Aortic valve replacement through right anterior minithoracotomy: can suture-less technology improve clinical outcomes? Ann Thorac Surg. 2014;98:1585–92.

8. Lenos A, Diegeler A. Minimally invasive implantation of the EDWARDS INTUITY rapid deployment aortic valve via a right minithoracotomy. Innovations (Phila). 2015;10:215–7.

9. Bapat VN, Bruschi G. Transaortic access is the key to success. EuroIntervention. 2013;9(Suppl):S25–32.

10. Bruschi G, de Marco F, Botta L, Cannata A, Oreglia J, Colombo P, Barosi A, Colombo T, Nonini S, Paino R, Klugmann S, Martinelli L. Direct aortic access for transcatheter self-expanding aortic bio-prosthetic valves implantation. Ann Thorac Surg. 2012;94:497–503.

11. Ye J, Cheung A, Lichtenstein SV, Carere RG, Thompson CR, Pasupati S, Webb JG. Transapical aortic valve implantation in humans. J Thorac Cardiovasc Surg. 2006;131(5):1194–6.

12. Laufer G, Wiedemann D, Vadehra A, Rosenhek R, Binder T, Kocher A. CMP27 mini-thoracotomy for sutureless-rapid-deployment aortic valve replacement: Initial single-center experience. Innovations (Phila). 2013;8:86–109.

13. Lichtenstein SV, Cheung A, Ye J, Thompson CR, Carere RG, Pasupati S, Webb JG. Transapical transcatheter aortic valve implantation in humans: initial clinical experience. Circulation. 2006;114(6):591–6.

14. Pascual I, Carro A, Avanzas P, Hernández-Vaquero D, Díaz R, Rozado J, Lorca R, Martín M, Silva J, Morís C. Vascular approaches for transcatheter aortic valve implantation. J Thorac Dis. 2017;9(Suppl 6):S478–87.

15. Salis S, Mazzanti VV, Merli G, Salvi L, Tedesco CC, Veglia F, Sisillo E. Cardiopulmonary bypass duration is an independent predictor of morbidity and mortality after cardiac surgery. J Cardiothorac Vasc Anesth. 2008;22(6):814–22.

16. Al-Sarraf N, Thalib L, Hughes A, Houlihan M, Tolan M, Young V, McGovern E. Cross-clamp time is an independent predictor of mortality and morbidity in low- and high-risk cardiac patients. Int J Surg. 2011;9(1):104–9.

17. Bening C, Hamouda K, Oezkur M, Schimmer C, Schade I, Gorski A, Aleksic I, Leyh R. Rapid deployment valve system shortens operative times for aortic valve replacement through right anterior minithoracotomy. J Cardiothorac Surg. 2017;12:27. https://doi.org/10.1186/s13019.

18. Schlömicher M, Haldenwang PL, Moustafine V, Bechtel M, Strauch JT. Minimal access rapid deployment aortic valve replacement: initial single-center experience and 12-month outcomes. J Thorac Cardiovasc Surg. 2015;149:434–40.

19. Glauber M, Miceli A, Gilmanov D, Ferrarini M, Bevilacqua S, Farneti PA, Solinas M. Right anterior minithoracotomy versus conventional aortic valve replacement: a propensity score matched study. J Thorac Cardiovasc Surg. 2013;145:1222–6.

20. Wendler O, Dworakowski R, Monaghan M, MacCarthy PA. Direct transapical aortic valve implantation: a modified transcatheter approach avoiding balloon predilatation. Eur J Cardiothorac Surg. 2012;42:734–6.

21. Strauch J, Wendt D, Diegeler A, Heimeshoff M, Hofmann S, Holzhey D, Oertel F, Wahlers T, Kurucova J, Thoenes M, Deutsch C, Bramlage P, Schröfel H. Balloon-expandable transapical transcatheter aortic valve implantation with or without predilation of the aortic valve: results of a multicentre registry. Eur J Cardiothorac Surg. 2017; https://doi.org/10.1093/ejcts/ezx397.

22. Bleiziffer S, Ruge H, Mazzitelli D, Hutter A, Opitz A, Bauernschmitt R, Lange R. Survival after transapi-cal and transfemoral aortic valve implantation: talking about two different patient populations. J Thorac Cardiovasc Surg. 2009;138:1073–80.

23. D'Onofrio A, Bizzotto E, Rubino M, Gerosa G. Left ventricular pseudoaneurysm after transapical aortic valve-in-valve implantation. Eur J Cardiothorac Surg. 2016;49:1010–1.

24. Imnadze G, Hofmann S, Billion M, Ferdosi A, Kowalski M, Smith KH, Deutsch C, Bramlage P, Warnecke H, Franz N. Transapical transcath-eter aortic valve implantation in patients with a low ejection fraction. Interact Cardiovasc Thorac Surg. 2018;26:224–9.

25. Sun Y, Liu X, Chen Z, Fan J, Jiang J, He Y, Zhu Q, Hu P, Wang L, Xu Q, Lin X, Wang J. Meta-analysis of predictors of early severe bleeding in patients who underwent transcatheter aortic valve implantation. Am J Cardiol. 2017;120:655–61.

26. Rodés-Cabau J, Gutiérrez M, Bagur R, De Larochellière R, Doyle D, Côté M, Villeneuve J, Bertrand OF, Larose E, Manazzoni J, Pibarot P, Dumont E. Incidence, predictive factors, and prognostic value of myocardial injury following uncomplicated transcatheter aortic valve implantation. J Am Coll Cardiol. 2011;57:1988–99.

27. D'Onofrio A, Salizzoni S, Filippini C, Agrifoglio M, Alfieri O, Chieffo A, Tarantini G, Gabbieri D, Savini C, Immè S, Ribichini F, Cugola D, Raviola E, Loi B, Pompei E, Cappai A, Cassese M, Luzi G, Aiello M, Santini F, Rinaldi M, Gerosa G. Transapical aortic valve replacement is a safe option in patients with poor left ventricular ejection fraction: results from the Italian Transcatheter Balloon-Expandable Registry (ITER). Eur J Cardiothorac Surg. 2017;52:874–80.

28. Barbash IM, Dvir D, Ben-Dor I, Badr S, Okubagzi P, Torguson R, Corso PJ, Xue Z, Satler LF, Pichard AD, Waksman R. Prevalence and effect of myocardial injury after transcatheter aortic valve replacement. Am J Cardiol. 2013;111:1337–43.

29. Meyer CG, Frick M, Lotfi S, Altiok E, Koos R, Kirschfink A, Lehrke M, Autschbach R, Hoffmann R. Regional left ventricular function after transapical vs. transfemoral transcatheter aortic valve implantation analysed by cardiac magnetic resonance feature tracking. Eur Heart J Cardiovasc Imaging. 2014;15:1168–76.

30. Trenkwalder T, Pellegrini C, Holzamer A, Philipp A, Rheude T, Michel J, Reinhard W, Joner M, Kasel AM, Kastrati A, Schunkert H, Endemann D, Debl K, Mayr NP, Hilker M, Hengstenberg C, Husser O. Emergency extracorporeal membrane oxygenation in transcatheter aortic valve implantation: a two-center experience of incidence, outcome and temporal trends from 2010 to 2015. Catheter Cardiovasc Interv. 2017; https://doi.org/10.1002/ccd.27385.

31. Ando T, Takagi H, Grines CL. Transfemoral, transapical and transcatheter aortic valve implantation and surgical aortic valve replacement: a meta-analysis of direct and adjusted indirect comparisons of early and mid-term deaths. Interact Cardiovasc Thorac Surg. 2017;25:484–92.

32. Løgstrup BB, Andersen HR, Thuesen L, Christiansen EH, Terp K, Klaaborg KE, Poulsen SH. Left ventricular global systolic longitudinal deformation and prognosis 1 year after femoral and apical transcatheter aortic valve implantation. J Am Soc Echocardiogr. 2013;26:246–54.

33. Ewe SH, Delgado V, Ng AC, Antoni ML, van der Kley F, Marsan NA, de Weger A, Tavilla G, Holman ER, Schalij MJ, Bax JJ. Outcomes after transcatheter aortic valve implantation: transfemoral versus transapical approach. Ann Thorac Surg. 2011;92:1244–51.

34. Lindman BR, Stewart WJ, Pibarot P, Hahn RT, Otto CM, Xu K, Devereux RB, Weissman NJ, Enriquez-Sarano M, Szeto WY, Makkar R, Miller DC, Lerakis S, Kapadia S, Bowers B, Greason KL, McAndrew TC, Lei Y, Leon MB, Douglas PS. Early regression of severe left ventricular hypertrophy after transcatheter aortic valve replacement is associated with decreased hospitalizations. JACC Cardiovasc Interv. 2014;7:662–73.

35. Haverich A, Wahlers TC, Borger MA, Shrestha M, Kocher AA, Walther T, Roth M, Misfeld M, Mohr FW, Kempfert J, Dohmen PM, Schmitz C, Rahmanian P, Wiedemann D, Duhay FG, Laufer G. Three-year hemodynamic performance, left ventricular mass regression, and prosthetic-patient mismatch after rapid deployment aortic valve replacement in 287 patients. J Thorac Cardiovasc Surg. 2014;148:2854–60.

36. Zoghbi WA, Chambers JB, Dumesnil JG, Foster E, Gottdiener JS, Grayburn PA, Khandheria BK, Levine RA, Marx GR, Miller FA Jr, Nakatani S, Quiñones MA, Rakowski H, Rodriguez LL, Swaminathan M, Waggoner AD, Weissman NJ. Zabalgoitia MRecommendations for evaluation of prosthetic valves with echocardiography and doppler ultrasound. J Am Soc Echocardiogr. 2009;22:975–1014.

37. Bleiziffer S, Ali A, Hettich IM, Akdere D, Laubender RP, Ruzicka D, Boehm J, Lange R, Eichinger W. Impact of the indexed effective orifice area on mid-term cardiac-related mortality after aortic valve replacement. Heart. 2010;96:865–71.

38. Pibarot P, Dumesnil JG. Hemodynamic and clinical impact of prosthesis-patient mismatch in the aortic valve position and its prevention. J Am Coll Cardiol. 2000;36:1131–41.

39. Mohty D, Dumesnil JG, Echahidi N, Mathieu P, Dagenais F, Voisine P, Pibarot P. Impact of prosthesis-patient mismatch on long-term survival after aortic valve replacement: influence of age, obesity, and left ventricular dysfunction. J Am Coll Cardiol. 2009;53:39–47.

40. Hahn RT, Pibarot P, Stewart WJ, Weissman NJ, Gopalakrishnan D, Keane MG, Anwaruddin S, Wang Z, Bilsker M, Lindman BR, Herrmann HC, Kodali SK, Makkar R, Thourani VH, Svensson LG, Akin JJ, Anderson WN, Leon MB, Douglas PS. Comparison of transcatheter and surgical aortic valve replacement in severe aortic stenosis: a longitudinal study of echocardiography parameters in cohort A of the PARTNER trial (placement of aortic transcatheter valves). J Am Coll Cardiol. 2013;1:2514–21.

41. Tasca G, Brunelli F, Cirillo M, Dalla Tomba M, Mhagna Z, Troise G, Quaini E. Impact of the improvement of valve area achieved with aortic valve replacement on the regression of left ventricular hypertrophy in patients with pure aortic stenosis. Ann Thorac Surg. 2005;79:1291–6.

42. Theron A, Gariboldi V, Grisoli D, Jaussaud N, Morera P, Lagier D, Leroux S, Amanatiou C, Guidon C, Riberi A, Collart F. Rapid deployment of aortic bioprosthesis in elderly patients with small aortic annulus. Ann Thorac Surg. 2016;101:1434–41.

43. Kodali SK, Williams MR, Smith CR, Svensson LG, Webb JG, Makkar RR, Fontana GP, Dewey TM, Thourani VH, Pichard AD, Fischbein M, Szeto WY, Lim S, Greason KL, Teirstein PS, Malaisrie SC, Douglas PS, Hahn RT, Whisenant B, Zajarias A, Wang D, Akin JJ, Anderson WN, Leon MB, PARTNER Trial Investigators. Two-year outcomes after transcatheter or surgical aortic-valve replacement. N Engl J Med. 2012;366(18):1686–95.

44. Kocher AA, Laufer G, Haverich A, Shrestha M, Walther T, Misfeld M, Kempfert J, Gillam L, Schmitz C, Wahlers TC, Wippermann J, Mohr FW, Roth M, Skwara A, Rahmanian P, Wiedemann D, Borger MA. One-year outcomes of the Surgical Treatment of Aortic Stenosis With a Next Generation Surgical Aortic Valve (TRITON) trial: a prospective multicenter study of rapid-deployment aortic valve replacement with the EDWARDS INTUITY Valve System. J Thorac Cardiovasc Surg. 2013;145:110–5.

45. Head SJ, Mokhles MM, Osnabrugge RL, Pibarot P, Mack MJ, Takkenberg JJ, Bogers AJ, Kappetein

AP. The impact of prosthesis-patient mismatch on long-term survival after aortic valve replacement: a systematic review and meta-analysis of 34 observational studies comprising 27 186 patients with 133 141 patient-years. Eur Heart J. 2012;33:1518–29.

46. Borger MA. Minimally invasive rapid deployment Edwards Intuity aortic valve implantation. Ann Cardiothorac Surg. 2015;4:193–5.

47. Borger MA, Moustafine V, Conradi L, Knosalla C, Richter M, Merk DR, Doenst T, Hammerschmidt R, Treede H, Dohmen P, Strauch JT. A randomized multicenter trial of minimally invasive rapid deployment versus conventional full sternotomy aortic valve replacement. Ann Thorac Surg. 2015;99:17–25.

48. Accola KD. The Edwards Intuity Elite valve: not to repeal nor replace, but rather additive to surgical aortic valve replacement options. J Thorac Cardiovasc Surg. 2017;154:1903.

49. Sannino A, Stoler RC, Lima B, Szerlip M, Henry AC, Vallabhan R, Kowal RC, Brown DL, Mack MJ, Grayburn PA. Frequency of and prognostic significance of atrial fibrillation in patients undergoing transcatheter aortic valve implantation. Am J Cardiol. 2016;118:1527–32.

50. Borger MA, Dohmen PM, Knosalla C, Hammerschmidt R, Merk DR, Richter M, Doenst T, Conradi L, Treede H, Moustafine V, Holzhey DM, Duhay F, Strauch J. Haemodynamic benefits of rapid deployment aortic valve replacement via a minimally invasive approach: 1-year results of a prospective multicentre randomized controlled trial. Eur J Cardiothorac Surg. 2016;50(4):713–20.

51. Dawkins S, Hobson AR, Kalra PR, Tang AT, Monro JL, Dawkins KD. Permanent pacemaker implantation after isolated aortic valve replacement: incidence, indications, and predictors. Ann Thorac Surg. 2008;85:108–12.

52. Santarpino G, Pfeiffer S, Schmidt J, Concistrè G, Fischlein T. Sutureless aortic valve replacement: first-year single-center experience. Ann Thorac Surg. 2012;94:504–8.

53. Vogt F, Pfeiffer S, Dell'Aquila AM, Fischlein T, Santarpino G. Sutureless aortic valve replacement with Perceval bioprosthesis: are there predicting factors for postoperative pacemaker implantation? Interact Cardiovasc Thorac Surg. 2016;22:253–8.

54. Folliguet TA, Laborde F, Zannis K, Ghorayeb G, Haverich A, Shrestha M. Sutureless perceval aortic valve replacement: results of two European centers. Ann Thorac Surg. 2012;93:1483–8.

55. Martens S, Sadowski J, Eckstein FS, Bartus K, Kapelak B, Sievers HH, Schlensak C, Carrel T. Clinical experience with the ATS 3f Enable® Sutureless Bioprosthesis. Eur J Cardiothorac Surg. 2011;40:749–55.

56. D'Onofrio A, Rubino P, Fusari M, Salvador L, Musumeci F, Rinaldi M, Vitali EO, Glauber M, Di Bartolomeo R, Alfieri OR, Polesel E, Aiello M, Casabona R, Livi U, Grossi C, Cassese M, Pappalardo A, Gherli T, Stefanelli G, Faggian GG, Gerosa G. Clinical and hemodynamic outcomes of "all-comers" undergoing transapical aortic valve implantation: results from the Italian Registry of Trans-Apical Aortic Valve Implantation (I-TA). J Thorac Cardiovasc Surg. 2011;142:768–75.

57. Panaich SS, Arora S, Patel N, Lahewala S, Agrawal Y, Patel NJ, Shah H, Patel V, Deshmukh A, Schreiber T, Grines CL, Badheka AO. Etiologies and predictors of 30-day readmission and in-hospital mortality during primary and readmission after transcatheter aortic valve implantation. Am J Cardiol. 2016;118:1705–11.

58. Rex CE, Heiberg J, Klaaborg KE, Hjortdal VE. Health-related quality-of-life after transapical transcatheter aortic valve implantation. Scand Cardiovasc J. 2016;50:377–82.

59. Nissinen J, Biancari F, Wistbacka JO, Peltola T, Loponen P, Tarkiainen P, Virkkilä M, Tarkka M. Safe time limits of aortic cross-clamping and cardiopulmonary bypass in adult cardiac surgery. Perfusion. 2009;24:297–305.

60. Miceli A, Santarpino G, Pfeiffer S, Murzi M, Gilmanov D, Concistré G, Quaini E, Solinas M, Fischlein T, Glauber M. Minimally invasive aortic valve replacement with Perceval S sutureless valve: early outcomes and one-year survival from two European centers. J Thorac Cardiovasc Surg. 2014;148:2838–43.

61. Miceli A, Murzi M, Gilmanov D, Fugà R, Ferrarini M, Solinas M, Glauber M. Minimally invasive aortic valve replacement using right minithoracotomy is associated with better outcomes than ministernotomy. J Thorac Cardiovasc Surg. 2014;148:133–7.

62. Butchart EG, Gohlke-Bärwolf C, Antunes MJ, Tornos P, De Caterina R, Cormier B, Prendergast B, Iung B, Bjornstad H, Leport C, Hall RJ, Vahanian A, Working Groups on Valvular Heart Disease, Thrombosis, and Cardiac Rehabilitation and Exercise Physiology, European Society of Cardiology. Recommendations for the management of patients after heart valve surgery. Eur Heart J. 2005;26:2463–71.

63. Phan K, Xie A, Tsai YC, Black D, Di Eusanio M, Yan TD. Ministernotomy or minithoracotomy for minimally invasive aortic valve replacement: a Bayesian network meta-analysis. Ann Cardiothorac Surg. 2015;4:3–14.

Part V

Future Perspectives

Medical Treatment for Aortic Valve Disease

43

Aydin Huseynov, Michael Behnes, and Ibrahim Akin

43.1 Atherosclerosis in Aortic Stenosis

Calcific aortic stenosis (AS) is the most frequent heart valve disease with a prevalence of 3–9% and the main cause for valve replacement in patients over 60 years of age [1]. The natural history of AS includes an asymptomatic latency period followed by a pronounced progression. The trials of angina, dyspnoea and syncope represent typical symptoms of AS. The onset of symptoms is a prognostic unfavourable sign, being associated with a rapid decrease of survival. Therefore, the development of symptoms in conjunction with third degree of AS requires the replacement of the valve [2].

It is traditionally accepted that aortic valve sclerosis and fibrosis are the major reasons for valve obstruction. Despite wide dissemination of the AS, not all mechanisms of the disease are well investigated. Several underlying mechanisms may alleviate disease progression, including chronic inflammation such as atherosclerosis, representing the leading disease mechanism of the development of AS. Moreover, there is a strong association between severe AS and coronary artery disease (CAD). The histological investigation of severe AS reveals significant amount of calcification, fibrosis and lipid deposition comparable to atherosclerosis [3]. Since both AS and CAD are degenerative processes associated with cell proliferation and calcification of endothelial structures, ageing process and atherosclerotic inflammation appear to be leading aetiologies of both conditions. Hypercholesterinaemia and other CAD risk factors predispose the aortic valve to calcify especially in the elderly population [4]. Based on this knowledge, the hypothesis was elaborated that conservative medical treatment of CAD may attenuate the development and progression AS. It has been suggested that statin therapy may inhibit or reduce the progression, or even induce regression, of calcific AS.

The animal model with rabbits demonstrated that hypercholesterolemia alleviates the development of hyperlipidaemic lesion. Hypercholesterolemia induced both cellular proliferation and calcification of the aortic valve. Moreover, statins show to be able to reduce the extent of atherosclerosis in the in vivo AS rabbit model [5]. This data suggested that such therapy reveals the potential role, especially at the early disease stages of this disease potentially attenuating

A. Huseynov · M. Behnes · I. Akin (✉)
Faculty of Medicine Mannheim, First Department of Medicine, University Medical Centre Mannheim (UMM), University of Heidelberg, Mannheim, Germany

European Center for AngioScience (ECAS) and DZHK (German Center for Cardiovascular Research) Partner Site Heidelberg/Mannheim, Mannheim, Germany
e-mail: ibrahim.akin@umm.de

© Springer Nature Switzerland AG 2019
A. Giordano et al. (eds.), *Transcatheter Aortic Valve Implantation*,
https://doi.org/10.1007/978-3-030-05912-5_43

the time until severe AS occurs and surgical aortic valve replacement becomes necessary. Accordingly, the effect of statins was investigated in the several studies including patients, suffering from AS.

Several retrospective studies suggested a benefit of statins by reducing the progression of AS. Bellamy et al. showed that AS progression was significantly slower in patients taking statins over treatment period [6].

The Navaro et al. study demonstrated that patients without statin treatment showed an annual mean reduction of aortic valve area of 0.11 cm^2; the rate is comparable to the average overall AS patient population. However, the statin-treated group revealed a significant 45% reduction of stenosis progression with an annual stenosis rate of 0.06 cm^2 [7]. Another study showed the impact of combined therapy angiotensin-converting enzymes (ACE) and statin on the delay of valve stenosis. Here, statins could significantly attenuate hemodynamic progression mild-to-moderate as well as in severe AS, whereas ACEs failed to attenuate AS development. The authors supposed that the pleiotropic or anti-inflammatory properties of statins may be more important rather than their cholesterol-lowering effect [8].

In all of these studies, statin therapy slowed the rate of progression as compared to the rate in those patients not receiving statins. Most studies included patients suffering from mild-to-moderate AS. In contrast, there has so far been only one study demonstrating beneficial effect of statins therapy in patients with severely stenosed AS. Generally the above-said studies did not prove any association in between attenuate of AS reduction and reduction of low-density lipoproteins (LDL) [8, 9].

However, already the first randomized trial disproved the hype of statins. The first study was the Scottish Aortic Stenosis and Lipid Lowering Trial, Impact on Regression (SALTIRE). It was designed to clarify whether intensive lipid-lowering therapy with 80 mg of atorvastatin daily would attenuate the progression or induce regression of aortic-jet velocity being assessed by Doppler echocardiography and of aortic valve calcium score being assessed by cardiac computed tomography in patients with calcific aortic stenosis [10]. The study was randomized, double-blinded and placebo-controlled, including a parallel-group trial of lipid-lowering therapy. The results could clearly show that high-dose atorvastatin reduces serum LDL cholesterol concentrations. Surprisingly no evidence of atorvastatin of AS disease could have been demonstrated. Moreover, there was neither a relation between serum LDL cholesterol concentrations and the progression of AS nor was any reduction of clinical endpoints demonstrated. Another randomized, double-blinded trial including 1873 patients with mild-to-moderate, asymptomatic AS investigated simvastatin plus ezetimibe versus placebo on the primary or secondary outcomes (SAES Study) [11]. No beneficial effect of statin/ezetimibe therapy was detected for primary outcome.

Furthermore, the ASTROMER trial, another randomized clinical trial (RCT), investigated the effect of rosuvastatin on progression of AS in patients with mild-to-moderate AS [12].

Until today, no RCT was ever able to demonstrate that extensive lipid-lowering therapy being induced by statins was associated with any improvement of AS.

Several mechanisms explaining the therapeutic lack of statins in AS have been discussed. The plausible one is that atherosclerosis may be an important part of the pathogenesis of AS. However, atherosclerosis predominates in the early stages of AS development, whereas at late stages, morphological features are relevant [7]. Pathophysiology of the AS differs significantly from classical atherosclerosis being present in CAD. Atherosclerosis in AS is characterized by continuous mechanical stress, high blood velocities and loss of valve tissue plasticity. Therefore, atherosclerosis represents only a trigger for AS development without any further role. These hypotheses may explain why statins failed to attenuate mechanical degeneration and valvular calcification.

Another important aspect of AS is the absence of smooth-muscle-cell proliferation and lipid-laden macrophages, which leads to an earlier and more extensive calcification [10]. Decreasing lipid levels and stabilizing coronary plaques represent the basis of statins in CAD, which may affect AS development even less.

In contrast, due to the strong association between AS and CAD, statins may be able to reduce overall mortality due to secondary prevention in order to reduce cardiovascular adverse events such as myocardial infarction [13].

43.2   Aortic Stenosis and CAD

The association between AS and CAD is well known. About 40% of patients with previous aortic valve replacement suffer from severe CAD and do require additional coronary bypass grafting [14]. Statins are recommended in confirmed CAD and elevated levels of plasma LDL-C being causal for atherosclerosis. Statins at doses that effectively reduce LDL-C by at least 50% also seem to halt progression or even contribute to regression of coronary atherosclerosis [13]. The degree of AS progression is influenced by LDL cholesterol level and develops even faster in patients with progredient CAD [15]. Secondary prophylaxis of CAD could improve the prognosis of patients with AS. However, no study was statistically powered to clarify these coincidences reliably question. For example, during the SEAS trial, patients with known diabetes mellitus and atherosclerosis (both coronary and peripheral), two major risk factors of AS, were excluded. This fact should be considered when interpreting the negative results of this study. On the contrary, most trials with a favourable outcome for statin therapy enrolled patients with significantly more risk factors for AS. This perhaps underlines the hypothesis that comorbidities are an underestimated factor for AS disease progression. Therefore, statin therapy may probably be more effective in AS patients with comorbidities [16]. Importantly about two-third of AS patients in real world are suffering from hypercholesterolemia, CAD or diabetes mellitus [17]. Therefore, results of the RCTs should be transferred towards patients without atherosclerotic comorbidities.

The pathophysiology of AS is supposed to be a very complex. Hypercholesterolemia represents a multiplying factor for progression of AS. This was confirmed in the prospective but non-randomized rosuvastatin affecting aortic valve endothelium (RAAVE) study, where only patients with hypercholesterolemia and treated with rosuvastatin were shown to benefit from statin therapy. The progression in aortic valve area in the control group was -0.10 ± 0.09 cm^{2}per year versus -0.05 ± 0.12 cm^{2}per year in the rosuvastatin group ($p = 0.041$) [18].

According to the current guideline, it is strongly recommended to prescribe statins in patients with AS and further risk factors [13, 16]. Especially older patients with moderate-to-severe AS benefit more effectively from the reduction of cardiovascular mortality; thus the prevalence of future adverse coronary events and prior myocardial infarction is higher in patients without mild AS [19]. It is not well understood whether statins may be able to improve prognosis of aortic sclerosis or mild AS, since these patients are usually excluded from large trials. SEAS and ASTRONOMER trials were designed with adequate and realistic study power, however enrolled only patients with mild-to-moderate AS, and may therefore lack any effect despite adequate reduction of LDL cholesterol levels [18].

Therefore, more prospective, randomized trials are needed to investigate the influence of statins particularly at early stages of AS.

43.3   Statins and Heart Surgery

Statins reveal several beneficial effects in patients undergoing cardiothoracic surgery. It was shown recently that statins might reduce the rate of atrial fibrillation coronary bypass surgery (CABG) [20]. Additional studies showed that statin treatment is beneficial in patients undergoing CABG surgery due to reduction of postoperative adverse cardiovascular outcomes [21]. Possible explantation may consist in the reduction of inflammation and oxidative stress, improvement of vascular endothelial function and postoperative hyperlipidaemia and dyslipidemia [22, 23]. Statin effects after CABG surgery may lead to reduction of rates of stroke, atrial fibrillation rates, risk of postoperative thrombocytosis and thrombotic complications. There is a 33% reduction for developing postoperative infection and a 20% reduction of a prolonged postoperative hospitalization. Moreover, preoperative statin therapy might be renoprotective in patients undergoing CABG, reducing the development of atherosclerotic changes in vein grafts [21].

The positive effects of statins were also observed in patients undergoing valvular heart surgery [24]. The problem of early calcification of bioprosthetic valves is well known. Lipid insudation and monocyte infiltrates occur in the cuspidal tissue of porcine bioprostheses similar to early atherosclerosis. These alterations can precipitate structural valve deterioration at longterm, even in the absence of mineralization [25, 26]. Hypercholesterolemia may be considered as a risk factor for calcification for bioprosthetic valve and may even the necessity for an explantation. In a study with 144 patients with revealed bioprosthetic aortic or mitral valves removed, the mean serum cholesterol level in the explanted valve group was significantly higher (189 vs. 163 mg/dL, $p < 0.0001$) than that of the group of patients without valve explantation [27]. This supports the role of hypercholesterolemia as a risk factor for bioprosthetic valve calcification potentially requiring explantation [25]. Hypercholesterolemia seems to be an independent predictor for bioprosthetic aortic or mitral valve calcification [28].

It was reported that statins were able to reduce degeneration of biologic prosthetic aortic valves. Patients treated with statins revealed significantly lower rates of bioprosthetic degeneration compared treated without statins [17]. The authors suggested that the beneficial effect of statins in slowing bioprosthetic valve degeneration is not due to their lipid-lowering effects but rather to their pleiotropic effects over and above lipid lowering, including anti-inflammatory effects [17]. However, some retrospective studies demonstrated that only young age but not hyperlipidaemia revealed to be a significant predictor for reoperation [29].

Moreover, bicuspid aortic valve is investigated in further studies. Bicuspid aortic valve represents the most common congenital cardiac malformation, occurring in 1–2% of the population. Improving management in these patients may avoid the development of AS and other complications such as aortic root dilation, aortic regurgitation and aortic aneurysm [28]. With regard to these complications, some beneficial effects of statins are not worthy. As already described, statins can reduce LDL cholesterol representing a significant factor for AS progression. They are also able to attenuate the calcification of the aortic valve assuming a key mechanism for the development of bicuspid AS. Furthermore, statins were shown limit of the production of matrix metalloproteinases, endogenous enzymes that degrade matrix components, which have been implicated in atherosclerotic aortic aneurysm formation [30].

43.4 Aortic Calcification in Familial Hypercholesterolemia

Familial hypercholesterolemia (FH) is an autosomal inherited disorder caused by mutations in the LDL receptor (*LDLR*) gene, the apolipoprotein B (*APOB*) gene or the proprotein convertase subtilisin/kexin type 9 (*PCSK9*) gene. As a consequence high levels of LDL may arise [31]. Untreated total cholesterol concentrations in homozygous FH can be extremely high (up to 1277 mg/dL (33.2 mmol/L), while the prevalence of aortic valve calcification here may reach up to 100% and is often symptomatic [32]. A strong association was found between calcification scores and age but not with total cholesterol. Hence, the clinical observation suggests that calcification may proceed independently of increasing cholesterol levels once sub-endothelial damage had occurred [33]. Data is lacking whether early treatment with statins in FH may prevent calcific AS. As statins failed to decrease the rate of progression of AS, further studies are urgently needed to find out therapeutic alternatives inhibiting valvular calcification.

43.5 Modern Approaches for Medical Therapy

The outcomes of three major RCTs showed a lack of significant benefit for lipid-lowering therapy on progression or clinical outcomes in AS. According to this evidence, more research was investigated to identify other risk factors besides LDL that could be modified by conservative therapy.

Lipoprotein (a) (Lp(a)) is a lipoprotein subclass, which is a risk factor for atherosclerotic diseases such as CAD and stroke. Lp (a) promotes atherosclerotic stenosis and thrombosis. It has been hypothesized that Lp(a) contributes to wound healing [34]. Plasma levels of Lp(a) are genetically determined by gene variations and gene polymorphisms affecting significantly the expression of Lp(a) levels [35].

The role of Lp (a) in atherosclerosis and coronary artery disease is well investigated [36], whereas the role in the AS was investigated only recently. A large genome-wide association study discovered that the SNP rs10455872 in the gene *LPA* was strongly associated with the presence of aortic valve calcification in European population with replication in independent cohorts from multiple ethnic groups [37]. Lifelong elevations of Lp(a) levels lead to a markedly increased prevalence of aortic valve calcification in adulthood and implicate Lp(a) in the development of aortic valve disease. The determination of Lp(a) levels seem to be a warranted method to assess the risk of AS. However, whether lowering Lp(a) levels can reduce the incidence or progression of AS remains unknown. Lp(a) targeting therapies will be a focus of future investigation trials.

Lp(a) is not significantly modified by statin therapy and therefore depicts an emerging interest in targeted reduction of Lp(a) with novel therapeutic agents such as PCSK9 inhibitors and antisense oligonucleotides [38]. The mutations in PCSK9 are associated with less degradation of the LDL receptor, leading to increasing uptake of LDL cholesterol in hepatocytes. Thereby to levels of LDL cholesterol are lowered in the circulation and may be a cardioprotective. In a study including 103,083 individuals, it was observed that the PCSK9 R46L loss-of-function mutation was associated with lower levels of Lp(a) and consequently with lower levels of LDL cholesterol leading to reduced risk of AS [39]. This data indirectly indicates that patients with AS may have a benefit from treatment with novel PCSK9 inhibitors, which has so far not been investigated yet.

Besides PCSK9 inhibitors, some other drugs may reveal the potential to lower Lp(a) levels. For example, niacin and the cholesteryl ester transfer protein inhibitor anacetrapib were shown to reduce Lp(a) levels. Niacin is known to decrease Lp(a) by up to 40. Even though niacin failed to reduce to LDL levels, niacin may potentially influence Lp(a) levels [40].

Cholesteryl ester transfer protein (CETP) facilitates exchange of cholesteryl esters and triglycerides between HDL particles and atherogenic apolipoprotein B-containing particles in the plasma. Anacetrapib is an orally active CETP inhibitor which is currently investigated in the REVEAL trial. Results of the clinical efficacy and safety by adding anacetrapib to statins are awaited [41].

Other novel therapeutic targets are valvular specific signalling pathways. They comprise a completely different therapy strategy. It aimed to achieve a desirable biomechanical outcome that restores normal aortic valve function. The modification of key proteins could be a potential option for novel pharmacological agents. For example, the inhibition of sodium-dependent phosphate transporters was shown to reverse the osteogenic function of LDL. Peroxisome proliferator-activated receptor γ agonists were shown to reveal a potential in mitigating lipid deposition in calcific aortic valve disease of hypercholesterolaemic mice, etc. [42]. However, no such therapeutic strategy has reached clinical stages so far.

In conclusion, molecular and genetic studies demonstrated that AS is not just the result of an ageing but rather an active pathobiological disorder with several potential therapeutic targets. A number of candidate genes, such as VDR, APOE, APOB, IL10 and ESR1, have been identified however need to be confirmed in larger samples [43]. Genetic research of valvular heart disease may provide a major step forward in disease prevention and treatment.

References

1. Liebe V, Brueckmann M, Borggrefe M, Kaden JJ. Statin therapy of calcific aortic stenosis: hype or hope? Eur Heart J. 2006;27(7):773–8.
2. Baumgartner H, Falk V, Bax JJ, De Bonis M, Hamm C, Holm PJ, et al. 2017 ESC/EACTS Guidelines for the management of valvular heart disease. Eur Heart J. 2017;38(36):2739–91.
3. Otto CM, Kuusisto J, Reichenbach DD, Gown AM, O'Brien KD. Characterization of the early lesion of 'degenerative' valvular aortic stenosis. Histological and immunohistochemical studies. Circulation. 1994;90(2):844–53.
4. Peltier M, Trojette F, Sarano ME, Grigioni F, Slama MA, Tribouilloy CM. Relation between cardiovascular risk factors and nonrheumatic severe calcific aortic stenosis among patients with a three-cuspid aortic valve. Am J Cardiol. 2003;91(1):97–9.
5. Rajamannan NM, Subramaniam M, Springett M, Sebo TC, Niekrasz M, McConnell JP, et al. Atorvastatin inhibits hypercholesterolemia-induced cellular proliferation and bone matrix production in the rabbit aortic valve. Circulation. 2002;105(22):2660–5.
6. Bellamy MF, Pellikka PA, Klarich KW, Tajik AJ, Enriquez-Sarano M. Association of cholesterol levels, hydroxymethylglutaryl coenzyme-A reductase inhibitor treatment, and progression of aortic stenosis in the community. J Am Coll Cardiol. 2002;40(10):1723–30.
7. Novaro GM, Tiong IY, Pearce GL, Lauer MS, Sprecher DL, Griffin BP. Effect of hydroxymethylglutaryl coenzyme a reductase inhibitors on the progression of calcific aortic stenosis. Circulation. 2001;104(18):2205–9.
8. Rosenhek R, Rader F, Loho N, Gabriel H, Heger M, Klaar U, et al. Statins but not angiotensin-converting enzyme inhibitors delay progression of aortic stenosis. Circulation. 2004;110(10):1291–5.
9. Griffin BP. Statins in aortic stenosis: new data from a prospective clinical trial. J Am Coll Cardiol. 2007;49(5):562–4.
10. Cowell SJ, Newby DE, Prescott RJ, Bloomfield P, Reid J, Northridge DB, et al. A randomized trial of intensive lipid-lowering therapy in calcific aortic stenosis. N Engl J Med. 2005;352(23):2389–97.
11. Rossebo AB, Pedersen TR, Boman K, Brudi P, Chambers JB, Egstrup K, et al. Intensive lipid lowering with simvastatin and ezetimibe in aortic stenosis. N Engl J Med. 2008;359(13):1343–56.
12. Chan KL, Teo K, Dumesnil JG, Ni A, Tam J, Investigators A. Effect of Lipid lowering with rosuvastatin on progression of aortic stenosis: results of the aortic stenosis progression observation: measuring effects of rosuvastatin (ASTRONOMER) trial. Circulation. 2010;121(2):306–14.
13. Piepoli MF, Hoes AW, Agewall S, Albus C, Brotons C, Catapano AL, et al. 2016 European guidelines on cardiovascular disease prevention in clinical practice: The Sixth Joint Task Force of the European Society of Cardiology and Other Societies on Cardiovascular Disease Prevention in Clinical Practice (constituted by representatives of 10 societies and by invited experts) developed with the special contribution of the European Association for Cardiovascular Prevention & Rehabilitation (EACPR). Eur Heart J. 2016;37(29):2315–81.
14. Ramaraj R, Sorrell VL. Degenerative aortic stenosis. BMJ. 2008;336(7643):550–5.
15. Pohle K, Maffert R, Ropers D, Moshage W, Stilianakis N, Daniel WG, et al. Progression of aortic valve calcification: association with coronary atherosclerosis and cardiovascular risk factors. Circulation. 2001;104(16):1927–32.
16. Ge H, Zhang Q, Wang BY, He B. Therapeutic effect of statin on aortic stenosis: a review with meta-analysis. J Clin Pharm Ther. 2010;35(4):385–93.
17. Antonini-Canterin F, Hirsu M, Popescu BA, Leiballi E, Piazza R, Pavan D, et al. Stage-related effect of statin treatment on the progression of aortic valve sclerosis and stenosis. Am J Cardiol. 2008;102(6):738–42.
18. Teo KK, Corsi DJ, Tam JW, Dumesnil JG, Chan KL. Lipid lowering on progression of mild to moderate aortic stenosis: meta-analysis of the randomized placebo-controlled clinical trials on 2344 patients. Canadian J Cardiol. 2011;27(6):800–8.
19. Aronow WS, Ahn C, Shirani J, Kronzon I. Comparison of frequency of new coronary events in older persons with mild, moderate, and severe valvular aortic stenosis with those without aortic stenosis. Am J Cardiol. 1998;81(5):647–9.
20. Elgendy IY, Mahmoud A, Huo T, Beaver TM, Bavry AA. Meta-analysis of 12 trials evaluating the effects of statins on decreasing atrial fibrillation after coronary artery bypass grafting. Am J Cardiol. 2015;115(11):1523–8.
21. Paraskevas KI. Applications of statins in cardiothoracic surgery: more than just lipid-lowering. Eur J Cardiothorac Surg. 2008;33(3):377–90.
22. Werba JP, Tremoli E, Massironi P, Camera M, Cannata A, Alamanni F, et al. Statins in coronary bypass surgery: rationale and clinical use. Ann Thorac Surg. 2003;76(6):2132–40.
23. Merla R, Daher IN, Ye Y, Uretsky BF, Birnbaum Y. Pretreatment with statins may reduce cardiovascular morbidity and mortality after elective surgery and percutaneous coronary intervention: clinical evidence and possible underlying mechanisms. Am Heart J. 2007;154(2):391–402.
24. Borger MA, Seeburger J, Walther T, Borger F, Rastan A, Doenst T, et al. Effect of preoperative statin therapy on patients undergoing isolated and combined valvular heart surgery. Ann Thorac Surg. 2010;89(3):773–9; discussion 9-80

25. Antonini-Canterin F, Zuppiroli A, Baldessin F, Popescu BA, Nicolosi GL. Is there a role of statins in the prevention of aortic biological prostheses degeneration. Cardiovasc Ultrasound. 2006;4:26.

26. Ferrans VJ, McManus B, Roberts WC. Cholesteryl ester crystals in a porcine aortic valvular bioprosthesis implanted for eight years. Chest. 1983;83(4):698–701.

27. Farivar RS, Cohn LH. Hypercholesterolemia is a risk factor for bioprosthetic valve calcification and explantation. J Thorac Cardiovasc Surg. 2003;126(4):969–75.

28. Verma S, Szmitko PE, Fedak PW, Errett L, Latter DA, David TE. Can statin therapy alter the natural history of bicuspid aortic valves? Am J Physiol Heart Circ Physiol. 2005;288(6):H2547–9.

29. David TE, Ivanov J. Is degenerative calcification of the native aortic valve similar to calcification of bioprosthetic heart valves? J Thorac Cardiovasc Surg. 2003;126(4):939–41.

30. Thompson RW, Parks WC. Role of matrix metalloproteinases in abdominal aortic aneurysms. Ann N Y Acad Sci. 1996;800:157–74.

31. Brown MS, Goldstein JL. A receptor-mediated pathway for cholesterol homeostasis. Science. 1986;232(4746):34–47.

32. Ten Kate GR, Bos S, Dedic A, Neefjes LA, Kurata A, Langendonk JG, et al. Increased aortic valve calcification in familial hypercholesterolemia: prevalence, extent, and associated risk factors. J Am Coll Cardiol. 2015;66(24):2687–95.

33. Fantus D, Awan Z, Seidah NG, Genest J. Aortic calcification: novel insights from familial hypercholesterolemia and potential role for the low-density lipoprotein receptor. Atherosclerosis. 2013;226(1):9–15.

34. Kamstrup PR, Tybjaerg-Hansen A, Nordestgaard BG. Elevated lipoprotein(a) and risk of aortic valve stenosis in the general population. J Am Coll Cardiol. 2014;63(5):470–7.

35. Clarke R, Peden JF, Hopewell JC, Kyriakou T, Goel A, Heath SC, et al. Genetic variants associated with Lp(a) lipoprotein level and coronary disease. N Engl J Med. 2009;361(26):2518–28.

36. Kamstrup PR, Tybjaerg-Hansen A, Steffensen R, Nordestgaard BG. Genetically elevated lipoprotein(a) and increased risk of myocardial infarction. JAMA. 2009;301(22):2331–9.

37. Thanassoulis G, Campbell CY, Owens DS, Smith JG, Smith AV, Peloso GM, et al. Genetic associations with valvular calcification and aortic stenosis. N Engl J Med. 2013;368(6):503–12.

38. Norrington K, Androulakis E, Oikonomou E, Vogiatzi G. Tousoulis D. Curr Pharm Des: Statins in Aortic Stenosis; 2017.

39. Langsted A, Nordestgaard BG, Benn M, Tybjaerg-Hansen A, Kamstrup PR. PCSK9 R46L loss-of-function mutation reduces lipoprotein(a), LDL cholesterol, and risk of aortic valve stenosis. J Clin Endocrinol Metab. 2016;101(9):3281–7.

40. Khera AV, Everett BM, Caulfield MP, Hantash FM, Wohlgemuth J, Ridker PM, et al. Lipoprotein(a) concentrations, rosuvastatin therapy, and residual vascular risk: an analysis from the JUPITER Trial (Justification for the Use of Statins in Prevention: an Intervention Trial Evaluating Rosuvastatin). Circulation. 2014;129(6):635–42.

41. Group RC, Bowman L, Chen F, Sammons E, Hopewell JC, Wallendszus K, et al. Randomized Evaluation of the Effects of Anacetrapib through Lipid-modification (REVEAL)-A large-scale, randomized, placebo-controlled trial of the clinical effects of anacetrapib among people with established vascular disease: Trial design, recruitment, and baseline characteristics. Am Heart J. 2017;187:182–90.

42. Hutcheson JD, Aikawa E, Merryman WD. Potential drug targets for calcific aortic valve disease. Nat Rev Cardiol. 2014;11(4):218–31.

43. Bosse Y, Mathieu P, Pibarot P. Genomics: the next step to elucidate the etiology of calcific aortic valve stenosis. J Am Coll Cardiol. 2008;51(14):1327–36.

Transcatheter Aortic Valve Implantation for Pure Aortic Regurgitation

44

Luca Testa, Matteo Casenghi, and Francesco Bedogni

Transcatheter aortic valve implantations (TAVI), also called transcatheter aortic valve replacement (TAVR), have been introduced in 2002 as an experimental procedure on a 57-year-old male with severe calcific aortic stenosis and cardiogenic shock [1]. Nowadays, this procedure represents a valid alternative to traditional surgery in intermediate and high-risk patients with aortic stenosis. Paralleled to the development of improved valve prostheses and delivery systems, operators start exploring the feasibility of this technique in off-label indication such as degenerated surgical bioprosthesis, in both mitral and aortic position, bicuspid valvular anatomy, and, in selected case, pulmonary valve disease. Among off-label applications of TAVI, of particular interest is the possibility of treating patients with aortic regurgitation via transcatheter implantation of aortic valve bioprosthesis.

Aortic regurgitation (AR) is caused by disease of the aortic valve cusp and/or abnormalities of the aortic root or ascending aorta and represents a unique form of valvulopathy characterized by both left ventricular volume and pressure overload. The overall prevalence of AR in the general population vary from 4.9% to 10%, with preva-

lence of moderate or greater severity of valvular disease ranging from 0.5% to 2.7% [2, 3]. The prevalence of AR increase with age, and severe form are more often observed in man than in women [4]. Severe AR is associated with higher mortality than the general population with heart failure occurring in almost 50% of patients in 10 years [5]. Once symptoms of decompensated heart failure appear, mortality without surgical treatment can be as high as 10–20% per year [6].

AR can be classified in mild, moderate, or severe, based on echocardiography parameters, or in acute (endocarditis or aortic dissection) and chronic, based on time of onset. In western countries, given that rheumatic disease is now rare, severe chronic AR is frequently due to a congenital disease, such as bicuspid aortic valve or degenerative disease (anulo-aortic ectasia). Chronic AR can also be classified in (1) aortic steno-insufficiency with prevalent regurgitation, (2) pure native aortic valve regurgitation (NAVR) with no calcium, and (3) aortic regurgitation in degenerated bioprosthesis. In all the form of chronic AR, the progressive enlargement of left ventricle (LV) compensates the regurgitant fraction by maintaining a low LV end-diastolic pressure and normal total LV stroke volume, while the eccentric hypertrophy counterweighs the augmented afterload. After a long latent period, elevation of LV end-diastolic pressure, decreasing myocardial perfusion pressure, and increasing

L. Testa (✉) · M. Casenghi · F. Bedogni
IRCCS Policlinico San Donato,
San Donato Milanese, Milan, Italy
e-mail: Francesco.Bedogni@grupposandonato.it

© Springer Nature Switzerland AG 2019
A. Giordano et al. (eds.), *Transcatheter Aortic Valve Implantation*,
https://doi.org/10.1007/978-3-030-05912-5_44

oxygen demands lead to developing of symptoms such as dyspnea and angina.

44.1 Diagnosis

Physical examination, electrocardiography (ECG), and chest X-ray may show signs that are not always specific for severe AR. Clinically, a holodiastolic murmur, a third heart sound, bounding arterial pressure and a widened arterial pressure may be identified. LV hypertrophy is the main feature of severe AR at ECG, while chest X-ray may display cardiomegaly.

Echocardiography has become the mainstay to describe the valve anatomy, evaluate regurgitation mechanism, and assess the severity of aortic regurgitation. Essential aspects that must be evaluated during echocardiography are (1) valve morphology (tricuspid, bicuspid, unicuspid, or quadricuspid), (2) determination of the direction of aortic regurgitation jet, (3) identification of mechanism (insufficient coaptation, cusps prolapse, or cusps retraction), (4) LV function and dimension, and (5) aortic root and ascending aorta dimension. When echocardiography measurements are equivocal, magnetic resonance imaging (MRI) can be used to quantify regurgitant fraction. In case of aortic dilatation, patients should undergo gated multislice computed tomography (CT) before surgery.

44.2 Treatment

44.2.1 Medical Therapy

Vasodilator therapy (i.e., nifedipine or angiotensin-converting-enzyme inhibitors) may be considered for patients with severe aortic regurgitation who are not candidates for surgery to relieve symptoms. It has been demonstrated that beta-blockers and losartan reduce rate of aortic dilatation in patients with Marfan syndrome [7]. However, bradycardia resulting from beta-blockade, prolonging diastole and increasing regurgitant volume, may raise concerns about use of this class of drugs in patients with severe

AR. Physicians have to keep in mind that, if a conservative management is reasonable in asymptomatic patients with severe AR, appearance of symptoms is a definite indication for aortic valve surgery.

44.2.2 Surgery

In patients with acute AR, urgent/emergent surgical intervention is indicated. In patients with chronic severe AR, surgery is indicated in order to relieve symptoms, prevent progression toward heart failure, prevent death, and avoid complication in patients with aortic aneurysm. Although there are no data from randomized trial comparing surgical management of severe AR with nonsurgical treatment, robust observational evidence suggests the benefits of surgery over medical therapy alone. Aortic valve replacement, the usual intervention for AR, is associated with a mortality of 4% when performed in isolation and of 6.8% when performed with coronary by-pass surgery [8]. Aortic valve repair is performed only in selected patients (i.e., prolapsing bicuspid aortic valve), but outcomes have generally been less favorable than mitral valve repair. In case of ascending aortic aneurysm, composite graft replacement is associated with a mortality of 1–10%, depending on severity of aortic regurgitation and LV dysfunction [9]. Last guidelines of the European Society of Cardiology/European Association for Cardio-Thoracic Surgery indicate surgical intervention in symptomatic patients with severe AR and non-prohibitive surgical risk, irrespective of left ventricular ejection fraction (LVEF) (class I LOE B) [10]. On the other hand, surgery is indicated in asymptomatic patients with LV function impaired (LVEF ≤ 50%) (class I LOE B) or in patients with severe LV dilatation (LV end-diastolic diameter >70 mm or LV end-systolic diameter >50 mm) %) (class IIa LOE B). Irrespective of the severity of aortic regurgitation, surgery is indicated in patients with Marfan syndrome and maximal ascending aortic diameter > 50 mm %) (class I LOE C) and should be considered (class

II LOE C) in patients with maximal aortic diameter: (1) ≥45 mm in the presence of Marfan syndrome and additional risk factors or patients with a *TGFBR1* or *TGFBR2* gene mutation (including Loeys-Dietz syndrome), (2) ≥50 mm in the presence of a bicuspid valve with additional risk factors or coarctation, and (3) ≥55 mm for all other patients [10]. If patients have an indication for aortic valve surgery, concomitant replacement of aortic root or tubular ascending aorta should be considered when maximal aortic diameter is ≥45 mm (class IIa LOE C).

44.2.3 Transcatheter Aortic Valve Implantation

Despite surgical aortic valve replacement is considered the therapeutic standard for patients with severe AR, a survey showed that only one in five patients with severe AR and moderate LV systolic dysfunction has undergone surgery. The proportion of patients with severe AR and a LV ejection fraction below 30% referred to surgery was even lower, equal to 3% [11]. Encouraged by the increased experience and excellent outcomes seen in the treatment of aortic stenosis, many patients with mixed aortic disease or AR due to degenerated bioprosthesis have been successfully treated with transcatheter aortic valve implantation [12, 13]. Treatment of pure severe NAVR with TAVI, despite improvement in new-generation device and delivery system, is still considered relatively contraindicated and reserved for patients symptomatic despite optimal medical therapy in which surgical aortic valve replacement is deemed prohibitive.

Transcatheter devices currently available on market are designed for treatment of calcific aortic stenosis. In this setting the devices, thanks to three levels of anchoring (ascending aorta, valve leaflets, annulus and LV outflow tract) and the friction force between metallic stent frame and calcium of native leaflets, remain stable during positioning and delivery phases. Patients with pure NAVR often present dilated aortic root, dilated ascending aorta, and elliptic annulus that may exceed commercially available transcatheter prosthesis size range. Moreover, lack of valvular calcification, suboptimal fluoroscopic visualization of native valve, hypercontractility of the left ventricle, and the regurgitant jet may limit devices' control of proper positioning during implantation.

Data from registries and reports on inoperable patients with severe NAVR has been published, demonstrating that TAVI in this subtype of patients is challenging but potentially feasible. With respect to patients with aortic stenosis or mixed aortic disease, patients with NAVR showed a significantly worse prognosis and tend to be younger, in a higher NYHA class and more frequently with severe pulmonary hypertension [6]. Notably, common risk scores (STS and logistic EuroSCORE) did not differ between patients with aortic stenosis and patients with aortic regurgitation meaning that their performance is inadequate in the latter group [6]. Data from the meta-analysis published by Franzone et al. showed that self-expandable prosthesis were used in 79% of cases while balloon-expandable device in 21% [11]. Procedural success, according to Valve Academic Research Consortium definition, ranged from 74% to almost 100% with post-procedural moderate-to-severe AR and need of a valve-in-valve implantation representing the two most common complications [11]. Of interest, a strong correlation between a need for a second valve and lack of aortic valve calcification has been found [14]. Initial report on use of early-generation self-expandable prosthesis for treatment of pure NAVR showed high rates of procedural complications with a need for a second valve in 18.6% of patients and post-procedural AR ≥ moderate in 21% of patients [14]. Yoon et al., in the largest study published evaluating TAVI in patients with NAVR, reported a substantial incidence of complication with procedure-related death occurred in 3.0%, conversion to open surgery in 3.6%, coronary obstruction in 1.2%, aortic root injury in 1.5%, re-intervention in 4.2%, need for a second valve implantation in 16.6%, and new pacemaker in 18.2% [15]. Residual AR ≥ moderate compared with post-procedural AR ≤ mild was significantly associated with an increased all-cause mortality (46.1% vs. 21.8%) and rehospitalization (66.0% vs. 27.1%). Predictors of all-cause mortality on multivariable analysis included post-procedural AR ≥ moderate, mitral regurgitation ≥ moderate at baseline, LV ejection fraction ≤ 45%, and STS score. Intriguingly, over the 10 years of study enrollment, the overall device success improved from 61.3% to 81.2%. The authors attributed this success to the development of new-generation devices that, with their retrievability, repositioning capacity, and external sealing cuff, were associated with a lower incidence of second valve implantation (12.2% vs. 24.4%) and lower incidence of post-procedural AR ≥ moderate (4.2% vs. 18.8%). These results entailed a lower 1-year cardiovascular mortality (9.6% vs. 23.6%) but not a reduction in 1-year all-cause mortality (20.6% vs. 28.8%). Moreover, compared with the early-generation device, new-generation devices tended to be associated with a higher risk of

stroke (1.7% vs. 5.7%) (Fig. 44.1). This result may be explained by a more frequent use of trans-apical access for prosthesis that are no longer commercially available, such as JenaValve (JenaValve Technology, Munich, Germany) and DirectFlow (Direct Flow Medical, Santa Rosa, California) [15].

Other factors that contribute, over the development of new-generation prosthesis, to improve outcomes were an optimized imaging technique, an increased operator experience, and a more frequent use of general anesthesia. Pre-procedure transthoracic or transesophageal echocardiography and 3D multislice CT should be considered mandatory for a careful examination of annulus and surrounding anatomy. Size of the valve should be chosen according to measurement of annulus perimeter and area, reminding that a 10–20% oversizing is recommended. When using self-expandable

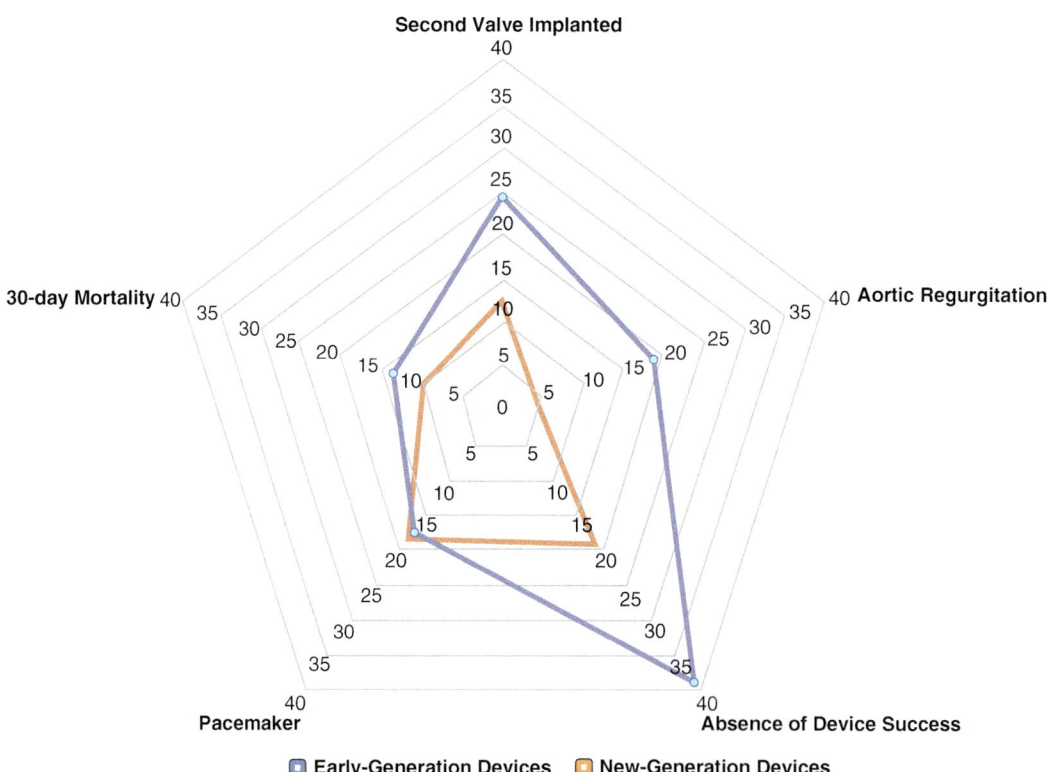

Fig. 44.1 Incidence of second valve implanted, post-procedural aortic regurgitation ≥ moderate, device success, new permanent pacemaker implantation, 30-day mortality following TAVI with early- and new-generation devices [15]

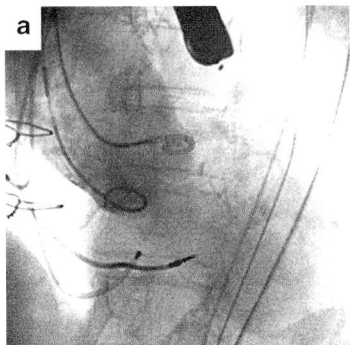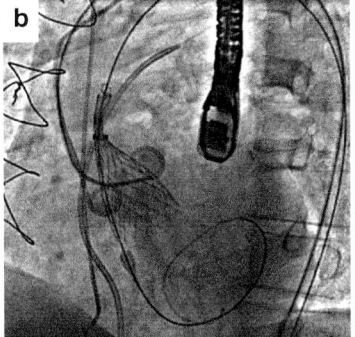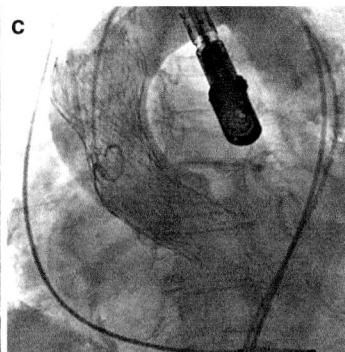

Fig. 44.2 (**a**, **b**) Examples of two pigtail technique with catheters placed in left and non-coronary sinus; (**c**) a second valve implanted due to severe post-procedural AR; a goose neck snare was used to fix the first valve implanted in position

prosthesis, a higher degree of perimeter oversizing ($\geq 15\%$) is recommended since it has been demonstrated that is associated to a less frequent post-procedural AR $\geq$ moderate [15].

During device deployment, to overcome the lack of fluoroscopic markers and device's stability, operators should use some expedients. Placing two pigtail catheters, one in the non-coronary sinus and the other in left sinus, may ensure accurate positioning and reduce contrast doses (Fig. 44.2a, b). When using a self-expandable prosthesis, use of rapid pacing is strongly recommended since it decreases the systolic blood pressure and the regurgitant volume and thus increases device stability. In patients in whom severe paravalvular regurgitation is present after prosthesis placement, a second valve implantation should be taken into account. Indeed, in this subtype of patients in whom the device is expanded, the regurgitation may result from incorrect valve positioning or sizing. For these reasons, valvuloplasty is unlikely to be of any benefits and may be associated to valve embolization. A second valve-in-valve deployment should be performed snaring the first valve implanted in order to fix it in position and prevent ventricular embolization (Fig. 44.2c). In selected case, a "two-valve technique" may be a priori taken into account using the first valve as an anchor for a second valve positioned in proper position. However, cost aside, this technique is associated with an augmented risk of coronary ostia obstruction.

44.3   Conclusive Remarks

Pure aortic regurgitation is characterized by a broad spectrum of clinical and anatomical situations. Notwithstanding surgical aortic valve replacement is considered the therapeutic standard, given the poor prognosis of patients treated conservatively, TAVI may play a role in selected patients in whom the risk of surgery is considered prohibitive. A pre-procedural multimodality imaging evaluation is fundamental in order to assess the proper annuls dimension and choose the correct prosthesis size. At the present time, despite use of new-generation device, outcomes for patients undergoing off-label TAVI for native aortic regurgitation are worse compared to patients treated for on-label indication. New transcatheter valves, specifically designed for treatment of AR, are needed. Future research should focus on anchoring mechanism, sealing cuff, complete retrievability, and additional prosthesis size. It also appears that the high rate of cardiac and all-cause mortality described in recent published registries may be improved by a better patients' selection. Undeniably, too many patients arrive in the cath lab with an end-stage disease when the clinical benefit of TAVI could even be questionable. More effort should be committed to identify patients before they reach a stage of the disease when cardiac mortality is too high to be improved by any form of intervention.

References

1. Cribier A, Eltchaninoff H, Bash A, et al. Percutaneous transcatheter implantation of an aortic valve prosthesis for calcific aortic stenosis: first human case description. Circulation. 2002;106(24):3006–8.

2. Singh JP, Evans JC, Levy D, et al. Prevalence and clinical determinants of mitral, tricuspid, and aortic regurgitation (the Framingham Heart Study). Am J Cardiol. 1999;83(6):897–902.

3. Lebowitz NE, Bella JN, Roman MJ, et al. Prevalence and correlates of aortic regurgitation in American Indians: the Strong Heart Study. J Am Coll Cardiol. 2000;36(2):461–7.

4. Dujardin KS, Enriquez-Sarano M, Schaff HV, Bailey KR, Seward JB, Tajik AJ. Mortality and morbidity of aortic regurgitation in clinical practice. A long-term follow-up study. Circulation. 1999;99(14):1851–7.

5. Enriquez-Sarano M, Tajik AJ. Clinical practice. Aortic regurgitation. N Engl J Med. 2004;351(15):1539–46.

6. Testa L, Latib A, Rossi ML, et al. CoreValve implantation for severe aortic regurgitation: a multicentre registry. EuroIntervention. 2014;10(6):739–45.

7. Jondeau G, Detaint D, Tubach F, et al. Aortic event rate in the Marfan population: a cohort study. Circulation. 2012;125(2):226–32.

8. Edwards FH, Peterson ED, Coombs LP, et al. Prediction of operative mortality after valve replacement surgery. J Am Coll Cardiol. 2001;37(3):885–92.

9. Chaliki HP, Mohty D, Avierinos JF, et al. Outcomes after aortic valve replacement in patients with severe aortic regurgitation and markedly reduced left ventricular function. Circulation. 2002;106(21):2687–93.

10. Baumgartner H, Falk V, Bax JJ, et al. 2017 ESC/EACTS Guidelines for the management of valvular heart disease. Eur Heart J. 2017;38(36):2739–91.

11. Franzone A, Piccolo R, Siontis GC, et al. Transcatheter aortic valve replacement for the treatment of pure native aortic valve regurgitation: a systematic review. JACC Cardiovasc Interv. 2016;9(22):2308–17.

12. Abdelghani M, Cavalcante R, Miyazaki Y, et al. Transcatheter aortic valve implantation for mixed versus pure stenotic aortic valve disease. EuroIntervention. 2017;13(10):1157–65.

13. Bedogni F, Laudisa ML, Pizzocri S, et al. Transcatheter valve-in-valve implantation using Corevalve Revalving System for failed surgical aortic bioprostheses. JACC Cardiovasc Interv. 2011;4(11):1228–34.

14. Roy DA, Schaefer U, Guetta V, et al. Transcatheter aortic valve implantation for pure severe native aortic valve regurgitation. J Am Coll Cardiol. 2013;61(15):1577–84.

15. Yoon SH, Schmidt T, Bleiziffer S, et al. Transcatheter Aortic Valve Replacement in Pure Native Aortic Valve Regurgitation. J Am Coll Cardiol. 2017;70(22):2752–63.

New Generation Devices for Transcatheter Aortic Valve Implantation

45

Iop Laura and Gerosa Gino

45.1 Introduction

The very beginning of the twenty-first century has been marked by the introduction of an extraordinary technical advancement in the fields of cardiac surgery and cardiology: Cribier et al. pioneered the implantation of a valve substitute without the need of open-chest intervention and extracorporeal circulation, but only by the use of a catheter and imaging guidance (fluoroscopy and echocardiography) in beating heart conditions [1]. Transcatheter aortic valve implantation (TAVI), also called transcatheter aortic valve replacement (TAVR), was born in 2002, becoming a common technique for the treatment of high-risk patients and, nowadays, with the potential to be applied also for less hazardous valve replacements.

The scientific excitement around this discovery was particularly high in those years. In fact, catheter-based methodologies were already applied in cardiology (cath lab) for diagnostic purposes but also for balloon aortic valvuloplasty [2]. Few years in advance to Cribier and Leon, namely the fathers of clinical TAVR, Bonhoeffer et al. demonstrated in the lamb animal model, as well as in humans [3, 4], the feasibility to implant

I. Laura (✉) · G. Gino
Cardiovascular Regenerative Medicine, Department of Cardiac, Thoracic and Vascular Sciences, University of Padua and Veneto Institute of Molecular Medicine, Padua, Italy
e-mail: laura.iop@unipd.it; gino.gerosa@unipd.it

a pulmonary heart valve replacement by percutaneously delivering a bovine jugular vein valve mounted into a stent. Earlier, the percutaneous route to treat aortic valve disease was extensively challenged, however without success [5, 6]. Andersen et al. proved in 1992 that a stented porcine valve could be deployed in both sub- and supracoronary aortic positions of nine allogenic animals without major signs of stenosis and/or regurgitation [7].

It was just a matter of time, hence, to realize in humans the aortic valve replacement by means of a similar percutaneous approach, and Cribier and colleagues crossed the finish line beforehand, by conceiving and implanting the first clinical TAVR prototype in a patient with degenerative aortic stenosis [1].

As previously reported in this book, the first TAVR device was realized with a stainless steel stent and pericardial material. This prototype represented already an improvement on to the devices formerly conceived by Andersen et al. and Bonhoeffer et al. In particular, in respect to the model proposed by Andersen and colleagues, the stent maintained the balloon-expandable modality and material composition (stainless steel [1, 7]), but different tubular design (slotted [1] instead of two wires [7]), leaflet composition (changed from porcine aortic valve [7] to bovine pericardium [8]), and, importantly, crimping size (41F [7] versus 24F [1]). The percutaneous modality was distinctive, too: Cribier et al. performed TAVI through an antegrade-transseptal approach from the right femoral vein [1], while Andersen and colleagues used a retrograde one [7].

Initially produced by Percutaneous Valve Technologies Inc. (New Jersey, US), the original TAVR clinical prototype was further developed by Edwards Lifesciences (Irvine, California, US), acquiring the registered name of both its first and newer developers, i.e., Cribier-Edwards® [1]. This valve replacement underwent further optimizations. As first, the Edwards Sapien® model was realized with leaflets in bovine pericardium, opportunely submitted to the Thermafix® treatment to prevent calcification, and with a cuff in polyethylene terephthalate, to cover the TAVR inflow tract [8]. The results of several clinical trials, as REVIVE and PARTNER, conducted in Europe, as well as in the USA, demonstrated the validity of this interventional cardiology approach in a population for which the classic cardiosurgical intervention had very high mortality statistics. After the *Conformité Européenne* (CE) in 2007, this valve prototype received the Food and Drug Administration (FDA) approval in 2011, becoming the first TAVR device with permitted application in the USA [9]. Two other models of Sapien were subsequently generated, i.e., XT and 3, formulated with novel stent designs to reduce the delivery dimension and to ameliorate coronary access, and with improved materials as cobalt chromium to increase the resistance, as well as more efficient delivery systems to ease deployment [10]. Sapien 3 has also an external polymeric skirt in order to prevent paravalvular leakage.

Starting from 2004, Sapien TAVR devices found a competitor in CoreValve (Medtronic, Minneapolis, Minnesota, US), based on a completely different crimping-decrimping modality for both transfemoral and subclavian access. The use of a nickel-titanium alloy, commonly renowned as nitinol, demonstrated to be suitable for the generation of self-expanding stents. An alternative to balloons was hence developed, since the stent could be inflated and deflated by increasing nitinol malleability with a temperature drop; the original conformational and strength state could be restored once at the physiologic temperature of the body. The leaflet composition was also different (por-

cine pericardium, processed with glutaraldehyde and alpha-amino oleic acid (AOA™), as antimineralization treatment). The CE mark arrived in 2007 (as for Edwards Sapien), while the FDA conformity was obtained 10 years later [11, 12]. After the CoreValve, Medtronic advanced the Evolut R by adjusting the design into a scalloped shape and increasing the skirt coverage with the aim to reduce paravalvular leakage (PVL).

More recently, other devices were introduced in the market. Symetis (formerly Symetis, Ecublens, Switzerland; now, Boston Scientific, Marlborough, Massachusetts, US) developed the Acurate devices: the TA™ model was initially envisioned for transapical delivery, while the newer neo™ can be deployed via transfemoral approach. For both TAVI replacements, nitinol is used to fabricate the stents, while the tissue material is realized with porcine pericardium for neo TF and porcine non-coronary aortic leaflets for TA. The Lotus™ valve, a TAVI device produced by the same company, is based on a controlled, mechanically expandable stent design able to sensibly reduce PVL, especially in its Edge version [13]. Another self-expanding TAVI option indicated also for the treatment of aortic regurgitation is the JenaValve™ system (JenaValve Technology GmbH, Munich, Germany), thanks to its unique anchoring modality. In fact, JenaValve™, initially for transapical application, received two CE approvals: in 2011 for aortic stenosis and in 2013 for aortic regurgitation [14]. The first model was manufactured with nitinol stent, porcine aortic valve (leaflets), and pericardium (skirt). It has recently been improved in the JenaValve TAVR system by modifying both stent design and tissue composition (entirely porcine pericardial biomaterial) in order to overcome the 32F lower limit of the delivery catheter imposed by the use of a whole aortic root. The system is now under clinical trial worldwide [14].

Currently, TAVR is a transvascular procedure not only indicated for the treatment of aortic stenosis but also in the case when no calcification is diagnosed, i.e., in aortic regurgitation.

This chapter aims to offer a comprehensive overview of the important challenges still to be faced in terms of actual and possible drawbacks of the existing devices, as well as of the yet unmet clinical and socioeconomical demands. This continuously improving technology is accelerating the path toward a next generation of superior TAVR devices.

45.2   New (and Old) Challenges for a Novel Technology

Despite the incredible advancement, the widespread application of TAVR technique has initially met several resistances, as described by the same Cribier in 2012 in the occasion of the twentieth anniversary of this endeavor [10].

Limitations arose already during the first clinical trials performed: the scarce experience with the transseptal approach appeared to be the earliest bottleneck in the success of the treatment in several centers. Hence, the possibility to use the more common transfemoral, retrograde route rendered TAVR simpler to perform, soon after the improvements introduced through the technology acquisition by Edwards Lifesciences [10]. As a result, TAVR showed its treatment superiority in respect to the classic cardiosurgical approach for the care especially of high-risk patients, further spreading globally the technique.

Apart from the suitability in the treatment of high-risk patients, the introduction of TAVR has not, however, overcome many of the restrictions encountered with the surgical valve substitution, even with the improved generations after the first devices.

45.2.1   Tissue Composition and Valve Degeneration

The performance of bioprosthetic valve substitutes has been widely demonstrated to be reduced overtime by several factors. In particular, valve degeneration occurs after mineralization of the glutaraldehyde-treated animal biological tissue (e.g., porcine aortic roots, as well as porcine, bovine, and equine pericardia) composing the prosthesis in a chronic and often silent process until severe functional impairment. Factors as

young age, highly active calcium metabolism, mechanical stress, glutaraldehyde cytotoxicity (free aldehydes released in the blood, bioprosthetic tissue death, and resulting exposure of calcification triggers, as DNA and phospholipids), and/or immunological responses to incompletely shielded xenoantigens (e.g., alpha-gal) of animal derivation have been identified as crucial in the development of the bioprosthetic valve disease [15–17]. Several treatments have been introduced to prevent or delay the onset of calcification and, hence, increase the durability of the bioprosthetic heart valve replacements over the current 10–15 year clinical duration. During the industrial manufacturing, glutaraldehyde-treated valve substitutes are submitted, for instance, to the application of 2-amino oleic acid, following specific proprietary modalities, as AOA™, aiming at neutralizing the glutaraldehyde-free aldehyde groups, or thermal heating, in order to induce protein denaturation [18–20]. As previously indicated, the same treatments have been applied to the animal tissues used to construct TAVR devices. There are still insufficient clinical data to evaluate the long-term impact of these treatments, and, therefore, no information on TAVR valve durability is available yet. Nevertheless, no other tissue-related causes of valve degeneration have been counteracted so far. It remains to be elucidated throughout a long-term clinical follow-up whether TAVR devices might show a similar durability to classic valve substitutes. It is noteworthy to consider that the mechanical stress at which the replacement is submitted during the crimping/decrimping phase and after implantation might create fenestrations in the glutaraldehyde shield with consequent exposure of xenoantigens. Such a hypothesis is, in fact, valid also for the classic substitutes with a prevalent occurrence during the post-implantation period characterized by an increase of anti-alpha-gal immune response [16, 17]. First-generation TAVR devices were, in fact, reported to show proneness to degeneration already after a midterm follow-up, as revealed in the recent literature. Deutsch et al. disclosed that after 7 years, above 20% of Edwards Sapien and 10% of CoreValve devices, i.e., the first-generation

TAVRs, suffered deterioration [21]. A recent meta-analysis including six observational studies on the performance of several TAVR devices [22–27] evidenced the association between reduced leaflet motion (RLM), detected at 1 year by computed tomography, and increased risk of structural valve degeneration. The very high frequency of RLM observed after TAVR is comparable to the one evaluated for surgical valves [28]. RLM is likely to be provoked by thrombotic events, as documented by echocardiography in non-subclinical cases. Although thrombosis may be triggered by several factors (e.g., mechanical stress during and after deployment [29]), the occurrence of pannus formation, leaflet tear, and mineralization suggests a direct link between tissue composition/treatment and TAVR valve durability, as already demonstrated for the devices implanted in classic surgery. It could also be likely that these observations would not match the case of younger patients, since, so far, TAVR devices have been mainly implanted in elderly, inoperable patients. The age factor has, in fact, not been taken into account as regards the influence it can exert on the progression of the TAVR bioprosthetic disease.

45.2.2 Costs and Availability for a Larger Cohort of Patients

The current estimate on the number of heart valve interventions to be performed each year, i.e., nearly 300,000, is going to tremendously increase in the next decades not only for prolonged life expectancies in the industrialized countries but also for the not yet driven away ghost of rheumatic disease, which is raging in developing globe regions, as Africa, Asia, and South America [30, 31]. Especially for patients affected by this pathology, i.e., mostly young adults, a replacement with a surgical heart valve bioprosthesis is an unaffordable treatment option. In these countries, in fact, TAVR or other interventions are not funded by the health government institutions, and medical expenses have to be sustained by the same private citizens in need. Due to the current costs of TAVR technology [31], it is nowadays

economically unsustainable to transfer it to nations with emerging economies, even if they could much more benefit from such a relatively easy-to-perform and less invasive treatment in respect to cardiac valve surgery.

In Western countries, TAVR has started to be applied also to less risk-prone and/or young patients. The observational studies performed so far are not sufficiently long to gain information on actual TAVR durability in this population. Since the strong effect of age on valve bioprothesis's fate [32], the main clinical preference is, though, to perform as first a classic surgery, by keeping TAVR as a secondary option in case of need for re-treatment due to degeneration (valve-in-valve procedure (ViV)).

45.2.3 Paravalvular Leakage

Apart from the high costs and limited treatable population, which remain unsolved or, in some extents, even worsened restrictions with respect to classic surgery, novel complications have been generated after the introduction of TAVR technology. PVL has represented the first clinical complication in TAVR-treated patients [33–36]. According to the Transcatheter Valve Therapy Registry of the Society of Thoracic Surgeons and the American College of Cardiology [36], moderate or severe aortic regurgitation was diagnosed in 2012 in about 35% of the TAVR patients at 30 days or at discharge. This percentage slightly decreased by substantially 2% in 2015. Despite the addition of skirts in the device design for PVL prevention, the inability to create a perfect adherence between the TAVR annulus and the patient's valve root geometry may remain, especially when the latter is deformed by mineralized deposits.

45.2.4 Permanent Pacemaker

About 10% of the patients submitted to TAVR require the implantation of a pacemaker since the intervention compromised the performance of the electrical impulse propagation in the delicate region of the aortic annulus. This percentage has remained unaltered over time [36], despite the enormous evolution of TAVR devices in terms of encumbrance/outflow tract interaction and the reduction of cases of intervention-related atrial fibrillation [37, 38].

45.2.5 Comorbidities and Complications (Neurological, Valve Thrombosis, and Procedure-Related Complications)

Besides the eventual need of pacemaker implantation due to damages of the conduction system, other complications might be generated during/after TAVR procedure. As previously specified, thrombotic events but also stroke and/or adverse events correlated to the used procedure might verify.

The incidence of neurological disorders decreased in 2015 by 0.4% in respect to 2012, persisting around 1.9% of the clinical strokes at 30 days and with 77% subclinical cases of cerebral microembolization [36, 39].

Less frequently reported (1%), clinical thrombosis interesting the implanted TAVR prosthesis can be effectively treated with oral anticoagulants. It is likely retained to be a complication leading to RLM: it might develop as triggered by the metallic struts of the stent and/or in patients with a pre-existing pro-thrombotic state. Inadequate deployment of the TAVR device and inefficient containment of the native leaflets might also create the opportune conditions for thrombotic complications.

Obstruction of the coronary ostia might have a 1% occurrence with fatal results [40–42].

While the transfemoral approach demonstrated to be superior to the transseptal modality in operational terms, this access is not ideal in case of disseminated calcifications or patient-specific anatomical variabilities (tortuosity, narrowness) of the ileo-femoral arteries, which increase the risks for vascular dissection and/or structural ruptures. For patients with these anatomic or pathologic characteristics, other vascular accesses must be utilized for TAVR. Transapical, transcarotid, transaxillary, and transsubclavian routes might be used for valve percutaneous delivery in these cases, as well as transcaval and transaortic accesses have also been operated [43–47]. The optional preference to the transfemoral approach must be chosen through the specific indications given by a careful analysis of the patient's anatomical features.

Even in conditions of optimal access, damages might rarely occur as a result of operator inexperience. The use of larger delivery systems (19–24F) has been proposed as further, but not always associated cause [48, 49].

45.2.6 Stent Deployment, Repositioning, and Resistance

For the first-generation devices depending on stainless steel stents and balloon-expandable delivery systems, the imaging guide and operator expertise were essential for an efficient deployment and prevention from the onset of paravalvular regurgitation. Cases of stent fracture were reported only for specific TAVR devices [50]. In addition, migration events have been disclosed immediately and after TAVR procedure as a consequence of insufficient anchorage (inadequate expansion depending or not from pre-existing calcifications, valve mismatch, and/or unsatisfactory deployment) [51–53]. With the evolution of the technology, the access to self-expandable, repositionable, and/or retrievable stents and the introduction of sealing skirts and further anchorage modalities have lowered the risk of PVL occurrence.

45.3 The Everlasting Search for the Ideal TAVR Device

So far, the identification of the ideal TAVR device is still an enduring mission for engineers, cardiologists, and cardiac surgeons. From the examination of the benefits and shortcomings of all developed generation devices, the characteristics to incorporate in the optimal system are numerous and still do not take into account possible needs, probably clearer only after a long-term clinical follow-up. Most of these features are well summarized in the ten principles proposed by Harken in 1989 to describe the adequate replacement intended for heart valve surgical substitution (biocompatible and long-lasting composing materials and design, satisfactory hemodynamic performance, the absence of embolization, collateral effects and complications, easy deployment, and effective anchorage) [54]. Following the several advantages presented by TAVR technology, the improvements constantly introduced are aiming at further decreasing the invasive nature of the procedure. Local anesthesia and no need for transesophageal imaging are currently desired plus. Other not yet met requirements are particularly relevant for the full clinical translation of TAVR technology as unique valve replacement modality: cost-effectiveness and successful long-term application for all ages and clinical indications of end-stage valve disease. In order to reply to these clinical demands, several novel devices are currently under testing or are in the research and developmental phase (Table 45.1).

45.3.1 Sapien and CENTERA TAVR Devices

Sapien 3 is one of the last evolutions of Edwards Lifesciences devices. This valve replacement has been evaluated in humans since 2013 for the treatment of aortic stenosis [55]. Sapien 3 stent is formulated in cobalt chromium for balloon-mediated expansion. Glutaraldehyde-treated bovine pericardium is used to recreate the valve leaflets. Apart from these characteristics, the Sapien 3 device is distinctive in respect to its precursor XT, thanks to a superior radial stent, an improved stent geometry (low frame height and open cells to avoid any obstruction and ease the access to the coronary arteries), a PVL-preventing skirt in polyethylene terephthalate at the ventricular side, and, finally, a reduced crimping profile compatible with inferior sheath diameters (14–16F for the transfemoral approach and 18–21F

for the transaortic and transapical modalities). The device is available in four sizes (20, 23, 26, and 29 mm) for application as an aortic or mitral valve replacement, receiving CE and FDA approvals in the biennium 2014–2016 for both high-risk and intermediate-risk stenotic patients. It is also uniquely approved for ViV procedures on degenerated classic substitutes [56]. Nowadays, Sapien 3 has been implanted in more than thousands of patients with generally low mortality rates and reduced PVL but slightly increased occurrence of pacemaker implantation in respect to its predecessor [43, 57–60]. Moreover, the procedure based on Sapien 3 has demonstrated its cost-effectiveness in respect to the classic surgery by reduction of post-intervention hospitalization expenses [61].

On March 2018, Edwards Lifesciences launched a new prospective, single-arm clinical trial for the assessment of the Sapien 3 Ultra [62]. Intended to be evaluated in intermediate-risk patients with severe calcific aortic stenosis, the new device of the Sapien family has been conceived to further reduce PVL, thanks to a higher polymeric sealing skirt, as well as a unique 14F-delivery system facilitating deployment without the need for valve alignment [63].

The outcomes with the Edwards Lifesciences's response to self-expandable TAVR devices, i.e., the CENTERA valve, have been recently disclosed. Realized in nitinol, CENTERA displays leaflets in glutaraldehyde-treated bovine pericardium, is available in three sizes (18, 21, and 23 mm), and is fully retrievable and repositionable through a motorized 14F-sheath delivery system [63]. The clinical studies, realized prevalently in Europe but also in Australia and New Zealand, have revealed very low mortality rate and occurrence of vascular complications, as well as moderate PVL and need for pacemaker implantation [64–66].

45.3.2 CoreValve TAVR Devices

Medtronic has introduced several adjustments to the CoreValve system, the first self-expandable TAVR valve to have received FDA approval.

Table 45.1 The evolution of TAVR devices

TAVR device	Stent features	Leaflet material	Transvascular access	Sealing skirt	Size availability	CE approval	FDA approval	Selected references
Edwards Sapien	Balloon-expansion, stainless steel, no reposition, no recapture	Thermafix/ glutaraldehyde -treated bovine pericardium	TS	No	20, 23, 26, and 29 mm	2007	2011	[1, 8, 9]
Edwards Sapien XT	Balloon-expansion, cobalt chromium, no reposition, no recapture	Thermafix/ glutaraldehyde-treated bovine pericardium	TF, TA	No	20, 23, 26, and 29 mm	2010	2015	[10]
Edwards Sapien 3	Balloon-expansion, cobalt chromium, no reposition, no recapture	Thermafix/ glutaraldehyde-treated bovine pericardium	TF, TA, TA o	Yes (PET)	20, 23, 26, and 29 mm	2014-16	2016	[10, 43, 55–61]
Edwards Centera	Self-expansion, nitinol, reposition, recapture	Thermafix/ glutaraldehyde-treated bovine pericardium	TF	Yes (polyester)	18, 21, and 23 mm	2018	Not yet	[63–66]
Medtronic CoreValve	Self-expansion, nitinol, no reposition, no recapture	AOA/glutaraldehyde-treated porcine pericardium	All, except TA	No	23, 26, 29, and 31 mm	2007	2017	[11, 12, 33, 34, 37]
Medtronic Evolut R	Self-expansion, nitinol, reposition, recapture, resheatability	AOA/glutaraldehyde-treated porcine pericardium	All, except TA	Yes (AOA/glutaraldehyde-treated porcine pericardium)	23, 26, 29, and 34 mm	2014–2016	2017	[67, 68]
Medtronic Evolut PRO	Self-expansion, nitinol, reposition, recapture, resheatability	AOA/glutaraldehyde-treated porcine pericardium	All, except TA	Yes (AOA/glutaraldehyde-treated porcine pericardium)	23, 26, and 29 mm	2017	2017	[69, 70]
Medtronic Engager	Self-expansion, nitinol, anchoring system, reposition, no recapture	AOA/glutaraldehyde-treated bovine pericardium	TA	Yes (polyester)	23 and 26 mm	2013	Not yet	[71–73]
Symetis-Boston Scient. Acurate TA	Self-expansion, nitinol, reposition, no recapture, sheathless	Glutaraldehyde-treated porcine non-coronary aortic leaflets	TA	Yes (glutaraldehyde-treated porcine pericardium)	S, M, and L	2011	Not yet	[74, 75]

(continued)

Table 45.1 (continued)

TAVR device	Stent features	Leaflet material	Transvascular access	Sealing skirt	Size availability	CE approval	FDA approval	Selected references
Symetis-Boston Scient. Acurate neo TF	Self-expansion, nitinol, no reposition, no recapture, sheathless	Biofix/glutaraldehyde-treated porcine pericardium	TF, TA	Yes (glutaraldehyde-treated porcine pericardium)	S, M, and L	2014	Not yet	[74–76]
Symetis-Boston Scient. Acurate neo2	Self-expansion, nitinol, reposition, recapture, sheathless	Biofix/glutaraldehyde-treated porcine pericardium	TF	Yes (inner and outer skirts in glutaraldehyde-treated porcine pericardium)	S, M, and L	Not yet	Not yet	[78, 79]
JenaValve	Self-expansion, nitinol, anchoring system, reposition, recapture, sheathless	Glutaraldehyde-treated porcine aortic valve	TA	Yes (glutaraldehyde-treated porcine pericardium)	23, 25, and 27 mm	2012–2013 for both AS and AR	Not yet	[14, 80–82]
JenaValve iteration	Self-expansion, nitinol, anchoring system, reposition, recapture, sheathless	Glutaraldehyde-treated porcine pericardium	TF	Yes (glutaraldehyde-treated porcine pericardium)	23, 25, and 27 mm	Not yet	Not yet	[80–82]
St. Jude Medical-Abbott Portico TAVR	Self-expansion, nitinol, reposition, recapture, resheatability	Linx/glutaraldehyde-treated bovine pericardium	TF, TAo, TAx	Yes (Linx/glutaraldehyde-treated porcine pericardium)	23, 25, 27, and 29 mm	2012	Not yet	[83, 84]
Boston Scientific Lotus	Mechanical expansion, braded nitinol, reposition, recapture, no resheatability	Glutaraldehyde-treated bovine pericardium	TF, TAx, TAo	Yes (adaptive seal skirt in polyurethane/polycarbonate)	23, 25, and 27 mm	2013 (dismissed in 2016)	Not yet	[86–91]
Boston Scientific Lotus Edge	Mechanical expansion, braded nitinol (Depth Guard), reposition, recapture, no resheatability	Glutaraldehyde-treated bovine pericardium	TF	Yes (adaptive seal skirt in polyurethane/polycarbonate)	21, 23, 25, 27, and 29 mm	2016	Not yet	[13, 92, 93]
Direct Flow valve	Medium-induced expansion (inflation), Dacron-polyester, reposition, recapture, no resheatability	Glutaralde hyde-treated bovine pericardium	TF	Yes (polyester)	23, 25, 27, and 29 mm	2013	Not yet	[94, 95]

Venus A-valve	Self-expansion, nitinol, no reposition, no recapture, no resheatability	Glutaraldehyde-treated porcine pericardium	TF	No	23, 26, 29, and 32 mm	Not yet	Not yet	[31, 96, 97]
Venibri I	Self-expansion, nitinol, reposition, recapture, use also without sheath	Dry, glutaraldehyde-treated porcine pericardium	TF	No	23, 26, 29, and 32 mm	Not yet	Not yet	[98–100]
Venibri II	Self-expansion, nitinol, reposition, recapture, use also without sheath	Dry, glutaraldehyde-treated porcine pericardium	TF	Yes (dry, glutaraldehyde-treated porcine pericardium)	23, 26, 29, and 32 mm	Not yet	Not yet	[98–100]

TAVR transcatheter aortic valve replacement, *TS* transseptal, *TF* transfemoral, *TA* transapical, *PET* polyethylene terephthalate, *TAo* transaortic, *TAx* transaxillary, *AS* aortic stenosis, *AR* aortic regurgitation

Its clinical application was disadvantaged by cerebrovascular complications and PVL, as for other first-generation devices [10, 12, 33, 34, 37]. Although the CoreValve replacement was already possessing a pericardial sealing skirt, it was definitely improved in its iteration Evolut R, smaller in height, deliverable through a 14F sheath and with redesigned outflow to minimize PVL [67, 68]. To further decrease the entity of paravalvular regurgitation, Medtronic conceived the Evolut PRO characterized by a more sealing wrap again realized in pericardium, able to increase the adherence between the replacement and the native valve root. Available in different sizes (23, 26, and 29 mm) with a 16F delivery system, it received the FDA and CE approvals in 2017, but no conformity for clinical application in Canada [69]. After implantation in 60 patients with aortic stenosis distributed in eight US centers, the 30-day results of the clinical trial indicated satisfactory hemodynamics, low mortality rates, moderate PVL in less than 30% of the treated patients, and need for pacemaker implantation in 10% of the cases [70].

Apart from the CoreValve system, Medtronic developed another second-generation TAVR, i.e., the Engager device, based on nitinol self-expanding technology, bovine pericardial leaflets, and a skirt in polyester. The valve has been CE marked in 2013. As per the suggestive commercial name of this TAVR valve, it displays a three-arm anchoring system able to ease efficient deployment through a transapical access. Falk et al. performed the first investigational study of this device in 30 patients. Despite the positive outcomes observed in terms of performance, PVL, and pacemaker implantation, four patients had to be submitted to surgical treatment due to dissections provoked by the delivery system [71]. In the pivotal trial based on 61 patients, 26% were submitted to pacemaker implantation [72]. The 23 mm size was dismissed from the market due to unsatisfactory performance of the replacement in terms of particularly high residual gradients [73].

45.3.3 Acurate TAVR Replacements

Analogously to the newer-generation CoreValve devices, also Acurate ones display a self-expanding nitinol stent and a PVL-preventing skirt in pericardium. Both Acurate TA and neo are available in S, M, and L sizes and depend on a 18F delivery system. Even if slightly different, the stents of Acurate TA and neo valves possess a particular design guaranteeing advanced anchorage and stabilization at the site of deployment. Borgermann et al. recently published the outcomes of the SAVI-1 and SAVI-2 registries on the implantation of Acurate TA in 500 patients. Moderate PVL was documented at 1 year only in 2.6% of the patients [74]. Among 89 patients treated with Acurate neo for 1 year by Moellmann et al., 22.5% died, and 4.5% presented moderate PVL [75]. At 4 years of comparison between the two devices in a total of nearly 200 patients, Hamm et al. observed PVL in 1.9% of the cases. For these patients, 30-day mortality was slightly higher for Acurate neo, as reduced was the 1-year survival in respect to the TA counterpart [76]. When compared with other TAVR valves, as CoreValve, Acurate neo replacements show better performance with reduced rates of pacemaker implantation, as well as of PVL [77].

After acquisition of Symetis by Boston Scientific Corporation, a novel iteration of Acurate, i.e., Acurate neo2™, has been evaluated in patients with aortic valve stenosis. Still not available for sale, this new TAVR replacement, with improved delivery system, as well as inner and outer sealing skirts to more efficiently prevent PVL generation, is awaiting CE conformity in Europe and continuing its IDE trial for FDA approval in the USA [78, 79].

45.3.4 JenaValve TAVR Replacements

The peculiarity of JenaValve is given by the introduction of a clipping system to fasten the diseased native valve, besides a locator engagement, in order to increase the probability of correct anatomical positioning. Available sizes of the first JenaValve device were 23, 25, and 27 mm, and the catheter delivery was operated through 32F [14]. The results obtained with the application of JenaValve with the transapical approach demonstrated the safety and efficacy of the system in both stenosis and regurgitation conditions of the aortic valve [80, 81], as marked by CE. The dismissal of the device was operated due to the sole insertion modality available.

A more advanced prototype intended for transfemoral application has substituted this replacement, proving its suitability for the treatment of pure aortic regurgitation in the first in-human experience [82].

45.3.5 Portico TAVR Valves

Portico TAVR has been developed by St. Jude Medical, now acquired by Abbott Vascular (Abbott Park, IL, US). This replacement has been conceived with the anti-calcification technology Linx™ applied to bovine pericardium, used to realize leaflets and paravalvular skirt. The self-expandable stent in large nitinol cells guarantees to the Portico TAVR full recapture and repositioning, before deployment has been completed. To minimize the need of pacemaker implantation, the TAVR height has been designed low. This replacement for transfemoral, transaortic, and transaxillary implantation is available in four sizes: the two smallest ones (23 and 25 mm) to be inserted with 18F delivery and the others (27 and 29 mm) to be deployed with 19F sheath [83].

The clinical study for the assessment of safety and performance of Portico TAVR with the lower diameters has been performed by Manoharan et al. by enrolling nearly 200 patients. Thirty-day mortality was low (3.9%), with pacemaker implantation in 10% of the cases, similar to other commercial replacements. Severe PVL was absent at 30 days and at 6 months of evaluation, reaching 3% at 1 year [83, 84]. Portico TAVR is now CE approved for clinical use in Europe.

45.3.6 Lotus TAVR Valve

Before acquiring Symetis Acurate devices, Boston Scientific was already investing in another TAVR program, i.e., Lotus Valve system. The predecessor of this valve, i.e., Sadra™ (Sadra Lotus Medical, Campbell, CA, US), was implanted for the first time in 2007 [85]. As an improved iteration, Lotus Valve system has the

peculiarity to possess a mechanically expandable stent, enabling retrieval and repositioning even at deployment occurred. Moreover, the braded nitinol stent displays a thick cell network and reduced height in order to prevent any interaction with the left ventricular outflow tract (LVOT). The leaflets are realized in bovine pericardium. The technology Adaptive Seal™ has been conceived to diminish the risk for paravalvular regurgitation, thanks to a polyurethane/polycarbonate outer skirt able to adapt to the irregular surfaces of the calcific native valve. This replacement has been under investigation in several clinical trials to assess possible non-inferiority in comparison to other approved devices [86–91] and received the CE mark in 2013. Since 2016, it is no longer available in the market due to particularly high post-procedural pacemaker implantation rates. In order to prevent such difficulties and associated complications, Boston Scientific released Lotus Edge™, characterized by the same concept of its first TAVR system improved by the Depth Guard™ technology intended to further minimize the device interactions with the LVOT [13]. Despite these improvements, Lotus Edge encountered technical problems during the deployment phase, causing the withdrawal of all devices [92, 93].

45.3.7 Direct Flow TAVR Devices

A completely innovative TAVR design has been conceived by Direct Flow Medical (Santa Rosa, US) with its homonymous replacement. Fully retrievable and repositionable, this device possesses no metallic frame but an intelligent polymeric material stent. In fact, the composing polymer can be clearly visualized by infusion of physiologic contrast solution and molded by exchange with a solidifier, allowing the rapid curing of the stent material to the desired tridimensional geometry. At complete deployment, the replacement results to be precisely positioned and safely anchored to the native valve of the treated patient [94, 95]. Although the TAVR device received CE approval for its 23 and 25 mm sizes, it is no longer available on the market due to the producer's extinguishment.

45.3.8 Venus A-Valve and Venibri Devices: The Eastern World Response for TAVR

The unique transfemoral TAVR replacement to be available in China is the Venus A-valve (Venus Medtech Inc., Hangzhou, China), which received the conformity by the Chinese FDA in 2017 [96]. Manufactured with porcine pericardium, this self-expandable device was initially lacking of the possibility to be fully retrieved and repositioned during deployment, which now has been implemented in its iteration. With a similar design to CoreValve, it distinguishes itself for a higher radial force, rendering it more suitable in the case of severely calcified and/or bicuspid aortic valves [31, 97].

Venibri is another device to have reached clinical attention not only in the East. It is born from the joint venture of the same Venus Medtech Inc. and Colibri Heart Valve LLC (Broomfield, CO, USA), leader in the dry tissue technology [98]. The first Venibri device was, in fact, characterized by a reinforced nitinol stent and dehydrated porcine pericardial leaflets [99]. Its improved version, Venibri II, presents a sealing skirt and is under testing also in European centers [100].

45.3.9 Polymers and Decellularized Pericardium as New Advanced Biomaterials for TAVR Realization

The TAVR industry has proposed so far several new devices with improved features to minimize paravalvular regurgitation and post-procedural complications. Among the problems still unsolved, the manufacture of more biocompatible, functional TAVR solutions is still to be achieved. As discussed previously, the fabrication of more viable alternatives is urgently needed to prolong the efficacy of available treatments at more reasonable direct and indirect costs.

Similar to the classic valve surgery, the search for new alternatives in TAVR technology is now passing through the use of biomaterials featuring more biocompatible properties and possibly transforming the replacement into a living, functional tissue. In order to bypass the limitations of the glutaraldehyde-treated pericardial leaflets, TAVR replacements have been realized in polymeric materials, as Dacron/styrene-isobutylene-styrene, polyhedral oligomeric silsesquioxane, and polycarbonate urethane [101–104]. In particular, the TRISKELE valve, composed with the latter mixture of polymers, demonstrated a hydrodynamic performance non-inferior or equal to other approved TAVR devices, as Sapien XT and CoreValve, when challenged in an in vitro study [104].

Another interesting concept based on polymeric materials is the JetValve, a fibrous heart valve replacement obtained by a spinning-based manufacturing. The biohybrid scaffold is obtained by the deposition of a mix of poly-4-hydroxybutyrate and gelatin, which can be opportunely tuned with the intent to reproduce valve matrix properties. Once implanted via transapical access into the right ventricle outflow tract, the JetValve demonstrated stable performance in sheep for 15 h [105]. Longer follow-up and evaluation in the LVOT are mandatory to fully understand the potential of this technology for TAVR application.

Currently at the clinical testing is Xeltis (Xeltis BV, Eindhoven, the Netherlands), another bioengineering concept based on electrospinning and endogenous tissue restoration but also on Nobel prize-winning supramolecular polymers [106, 107]. Implantable transapically, this device does not present any metallic component, but it is completely manufactured in polyurethane with the ureidopyrimidinone supramolecular binding motif [107]. By comparison of the data observed in the clinics for Sapien, CoreValve, and Lotus TAVR devices with the ones generated in the preclinical evaluation of Xeltis in an ovine model, the hemodynamic profile in the aortic valve position of the latter appears comparable. In particular, the PVL was equal or inferior to the one described for the commercial replacements [108]. These positive outcomes in the preclinical model need to be confirmed in a first in-human application, which for the moment is only limited to the right ventricular outflow tract [106].

At the latest Heart Valve Society Meeting held in New York [109], Peter Zilla presented a provocative lecture intended to once again shake the Western World medicine focused on a high economical cost system, not affordable for the unprivileged countries. In this occasion, as well as previously [110], he presented a new nonocclusive, self-homing TAVR valve in heparinized polyurethane, developed with Strait Access Technologies (Cape Town, South Africa). This relatively inexpensive solution is intended for the treatment of non-calcific, aortic regurgitation and can be positioned with a self-locating, retractable balloon without the need of fluoroscopy.

Despite the clear advantages of increased crimpability and possible lower costs of fabrication, the use of polymers might be limited by partial endothelialization and/or low repopulation, as well as unsuccessful valve tissue reconstruction, specifically pitfalls already evidenced in the regenerative medicine of classic heart valve substitutes. A more effective solution could be the use of decellularized cardiovascular tissues. By excluding glutaraldehyde treatment from the manufacturing process, this approach could enable the generation of tissue scaffolds devoid of inflammatory, immunogenic, and calcific triggers, prone to be colonized by patient's cells and hence giving life effectively to a self-like, repairing and adapting replacement with long-lasting performances [111]. Decellularized pericardium has been recently demonstrated to be a cytocompatible biomaterial for the construction of TAVR replacements. Ghodsizad et al. developed a TAVR device in decellularized pericardium and nitinol stent, which was stimulated magnetically in a bioreactor to promote repopulation with human mesenchymal cord blood cells [112].

In Padua, in collaboration with the TECAS consortium partners, we also started a TAVR program based on decellularized pericardium-based replacements. Preliminary in vitro analyses revealed a hemodynamic non-inferiority of obtained devices with respect to the ones commercially available, even at high back pressure conditions (unpublished data).

45.4 Conclusions

Despite the great advances realized so far in the worldwide acceptance of TAVR as treatment for aortic stenosis and regurgitation, several issues still hamper the clinical application of this procedure for all indications and ages. The search for the ideal replacement remains therefore an open task. Nevertheless, the continuous refinement operated in all of the main components of this technology will hopefully lead soon to develop a superior generation of TAVR replacements for both stenotic and insufficient aortic valves.

References

1. Cribier A, Eltchaninoff H, Bash A, Borenstein N, Tron C, Bauer F, et al. Percutaneous transcatheter implantation of an aortic valve prosthesis for calcific aortic stenosis: first human case description. Circulation. 2002;106:3006–8.
2. Cribier A, Savin T, Saoudi N, Rocha P, Berland J, Letac B. Percutaneous transluminal valvuloplasty of acquired aortic stenosis in elderly patients: an alternative to valve replacement? Lancet. 1986;1:63–7.
3. Bonhoeffer P, Boudjemline Y, Saliba Z, Hausse AO, Aggoun Y, Bonnet D, et al. Transcatheter implantation of a bovine valve in pulmonary position: a lamb study. Circulation. 2000;102:813–6.
4. Bonhoeffer P, Boudjemline Y, Saliba Z, Merckx J, Aggoun Y, Bonnet D, et al. Percutaneous replacement of pulmonary valve in a right-ventricle to pulmonary-artery prosthetic conduit with valve dysfunction. Lancet. 2000;356:1403–5.
5. Davies H. Catheter-mounted valve for temporary relief of aortic insufficiency. Lancet. 1965;285:250.
6. Moulopoulos SD, Anthopoulos L, Stamatelopoulos S, Stefadouros M. Catheter-mounted aortic valves. Ann Thorac Surg. 1971;11:423–30.
7. Andersen HR, Knudsen LL, Hasenkam JM. Transluminal implantation of artificial heart valves. Description of a new expandable aortic valve and initial results with implantation by catheter technique in closed chest pigs. Eur Heart J. 1992;13:704–8.
8. Cribier A, Litzler P-Y, Eltchaninoff H, Godin M, Tron C, Bauer F, et al. Technique of transcatheter aortic valve implantation with the Edwards-Sapien heart valve using the transfemoral approach. Herz. 2009;34:347–56.
9. Innovation at FDA: reports and fact sheets. https://www.fda.gov/AboutFDA/Innovation/ucm454720.htm.

10. Cribier A. Development of transcatheter aortic valve implantation (TAVI): a 20-year odyssey. Arch Cardiovasc Dis. 2012;105:146–52.

11. CoreValve™ system transcatheter aortic valve delivery catheter system compression loading system. https://www.accessdata.fda.gov/cdrh_docs/pdf13/P130021S033C.pdf.

12. Laborde J, Borenstein N, Behr L, Farah B, Fajadet J. Percutaneous implantation of the corevalve aortic valve prosthesis for patients presenting high risk for surgical valve replacement. EuroIntervention. 2006;1:472–4.

13. TAVI System Clinical Program—LOTUS Edge—Boston Scientific. http://www.bostonscientific.com/en-EU/products/transcatheter-heart-valve/lotus-tavi-valve-system/tavi-system-clinical-trials.html.

14. JenaValve. http://www.jenavalve.com/about/

15. Valente M, Bortolotti U, Thiene G. Ultrastructural substrates of dystrophic calcification in porcine bioprosthetic valve failure. Am J Pathol. 1985;119:12–21.

16. Manji RA, Zhu LF, Nijjar NK, Rayner DC, Korbutt GS, Churchill TA, et al. Glutaraldehyde-fixed bioprosthetic heart valve conduits calcify and fail from xenograft rejection. Circulation. 2006;114:318–27.

17. Naso F, Gandaglia A, Bottio T, Tarzia V, Nottle MB, D'Apice AJF, et al. First quantification of alpha-Gal epitope in current glutaraldehyde-fixed heart valve bioprostheses. Xenotransplantation. 2013;20:252–61.

18. Chen W, Schoen FJ, Levy RJ. Mechanism of efficacy of 2-amino oleic acid for inhibition of calcification of glutaraldehyde-pretreated porcine bioprosthetic heart valves. Circulation. 1994;90:323–9.

19. Padala M. A heart valve is no stronger than its weakest link: The need to improve durability of pericardial leaflets. J Thorac Cardiovasc Surg. 2018;156:207–8.

20. Heart Valve Therapies—Surgical Valve Replacement|Medtronic. http://www.medtronic.com/us-en/healthcare-professionals/therapies-procedures/cardiovascular/heart-valve-replacement.html.

21. Deutsch M-A, Erlebach M, Burri M, Hapfelmeier A, Witt OG, Ziegelmueller JA, et al. Beyond the five-year horizon: long-term outcome of high-risk and inoperable patients undergoing TAVR with first-generation devices. EuroIntervention. 2018;14:41–9.

22. Pache G, Blanke P, Zeh W, Jander N. Cusp thrombosis after transcatheter aortic valve replacement detected by computed tomography and echocardiography. Eur Heart J. 2013;34:3546.

23. Makkar RR, Fontana G, Jilaihawi H, Chakravarty T, Kofoed KF, De Backer O, et al. Possible subclinical leaflet thrombosis in bioprosthetic aortic valves. N Engl J Med. 2015;373:2015–24.

24. Hansson NC, Grove EL, Andersen HR, Leipsic J, Mathiassen ON, Jensen JM, et al. Transcatheter aortic valve thrombosis incidence, predisposing factors, and clinical implications. J Am Coll Cardiol. 2016;68:2059–69.

25. Yanagisawa R, Hayashida K, Yamada Y, Tanaka M, Yashima F, Inohara T, et al. Incidence, predictors, and mid-term outcomes of possible leaflet thrombosis after TAVR. JACC Cardiovasc Imaging. 2017;10:1–11.

26. Vollema EM, Kong WKF, Katsanos S, Kamperidis V, van Rosendael PJ, van der Kley F, et al. Transcatheter aortic valve thrombosis: the relation between hypo-attenuated leaflet thickening, abnormal valve haemodynamics, and stroke. Eur Heart J. 2017;38:1207–17.

27. Chakravarty T, Søndergaard L, Friedman J, De Backer O, Berman D, Kofoed KF, et al. Subclinical leaflet thrombosis in surgical and transcatheter bioprosthetic aortic valves: an observational study. Lancet. 2017;389:2383–92.

28. Makki N, Shreenivas S, Kereiakes D, Lilly S. A meta-analysis of reduced leaflet motion for surgical and transcatheter aortic valves: relationship to cerebrovascular events and valve degeneration. Cardiovasc Revasc Med. 2018;19(7. Pt B):868–73.

29. Sun W, Li K, Sirois E. Simulated elliptical bioprosthetic valve deformation: Implications for asymmetric transcatheter valve deployment. J Biomech. 2010;43:3085–90.

30. Bezuidenhout D, Williams DF, Zilla P. Polymeric heart valves for surgical implantation, catheter-based technologies and heart assist devices. Biomaterials. 2015;36:6–25.

31. Hon JKF, Tay E. Transcatheter aortic valve implantation in Asia. Ann Cardiothorac Surg. 2017;6:504–9.

32. Arsalan M, Walther T. Durability of prostheses for transcatheter aortic valve implantation. Nat Rev Cardiol. 2016;13:360–7.

33. Sherif MA, Abdel-Wahab M, Stöcker B, Geist V, Richardt D, Tölg R, et al. Anatomic and procedural predictors of paravalvular aortic regurgitation after implantation of the Medtronic CoreValve bioprosthesis. J Am Coll Cardiol. 2010;56:1623–9.

34. Athappan G, Patvardhan E, Tuzcu EM, Svensson LG, Lemos PA, Fraccaro C, et al. Incidence, predictors, and outcomes of aortic regurgitation after transcatheter aortic valve replacement: meta-analysis and systematic review of literature. J Am Coll Cardiol. 2013;61:1585–95.

35. Holmes DR, Nishimura RA, Grover FL, Brindis RG, Carroll JD, Edwards FH, et al. Annual outcomes with transcatheter valve therapy: from the STS/ACC TVT Registry. Ann Thorac Surg. 2016;101:789–800.

36. Grover FL, Vemulapalli S, Carroll JD, Edwards FH, Mack MJ, Thourani VH, et al. 2016 Annual Report of The Society of Thoracic Surgeons/American College of Cardiology Transcatheter Valve Therapy Registry. J Am Coll Cardiol. 2017;69:1215–30.

37. Piazza N, Onuma Y, Jesserun E, Kint PP, Maugenest A-M, Anderson RH, et al. Early and persistent intraventricular conduction abnormalities and requirements for pacemaking after percutaneous replacement of the aortic valve. JACC Cardiovasc Interv. 2008;1:310–6.

38. De Torres-Alba F, Kaleschke G, Diller GP, Vormbrock J, Orwat S, Radke R, et al. Changes in the pacemaker rate after transition from Edwards SAPIEN XT to SAPIEN 3 transcatheter aortic valve implantation: the critical role of valve implantation height. JACC Cardiovasc Interv. 2016;9:805–13.

39. Uddin A, Fairbairn TA, Djoukhader IK, Igra M, Kidambi A, Motwani M, et al. Consequence of cerebral embolism after transcatheter aortic valve implantation compared with contemporary surgical aortic valve replacement: effect on health-related quality of life. Circ Cardiovasc Interv. 2015;8:e001913.

40. Drexel T, Helmer G, Garcia S, Raveendran G. Management of left main coronary artery obstruction after transcatheter aortic valve replacement utilizing a periscope approach. Catheter Cardiovasc Interv. 2017;92(7):1444–8.

41. Ramirez R, Ovakimyan O, Lasam G, Lafferty K. A very late presentation of a right coronary artery occlusion after transcatheter aortic valve replacement. Cardiol Res. 2017;8:131–3.

42. Sultan I, Siki M, Wallen T, Szeto W, Vallabhajosyula P. Management of coronary obstruction following transcatheter aortic valve replacement. J Card Surg. 2017;32:777–81.

43. Herrmann HC, Thourani VH, Kodali SK, Makkar RR, Szeto WY, Anwaruddin S, et al. One-year clinical outcomes with SAPIEN 3 transcatheter aortic valve replacement in high-risk and inoperable patients with severe aortic stenosisclinical perspective. Circulation. 2016;134:130–40.

44. Bapat V, Frank D, Cocchieri R, Jagielak D, Bonaros N, Aiello M, et al. Transcatheter aortic valve replacement using transaortic access: experience from the multicenter, multinational, prospective ROUTE registry. JACC Cardiovasc Interv. 2016;9:1815–22.

45. Debry N, Delhaye C, Azmoun A, Ramadan R, Fradi S, Brenot P, et al. Transcarotid transcatheter aortic valve replacement: general or local anesthesia. JACC Cardiovasc Interv. 2016;9:2113–20.

46. Deuschl F, Schofer N, Seiffert M, Mizote I, Schaefer A, et al. Direct percutaneous transaxillary implantation of a novel selfexpandable transcatheter heart valve for aortic stenosis. Catheter Cardiovasc Interv. 2017;90:1167–74.

47. Greenbaum AB, Babaliaros VC, Chen MY, Stine AM, Rogers T, O'Neill WW, et al. Transcaval access and closure for transcatheter aortic valve replacement. J Am Coll Cardiol. 2017;69:511–21.

48. Hines G, Jaspan V, Kelly B, Calixte R. Vascular complications associated with transfemoral aortic valve replacement. Int J Angiol. 2015;25:099–103.

49. Dimitriadis Z, Scholtz W, Ensminger SM, Piper C, Bitter T, Wiemer M, et al. Impact of sheath diameter of different sheath types on vascular complications and mortality in transfemoral TAVI approaches using the Proglide closure device. PLoS One. 2017;12:e0183658.

50. Cools B, Brown S, Budts W, Heying R, Troost E, Boshoff D, et al. Up to 11 years of experience with the Melody® valved stent in right ventricular outflow tract. EuroIntervention. 2018;14(9):e988–94.

51. Maroto LC, Rodríguez JE, Cobiella J, Silva J. Delayed dislocation of a transapically implanted aortic bioprosthesis. Eur J Cardio-Thoracic Surg. 2009;36:935–7.

52. Nijhoff F, Agostoni P, Samim M, Ramjankhan FZ, Kluin J, Doevendans PA, et al. Optimisation of transcatheter aortic balloon-expandable valve deployment: the two-step inflation technique. EuroIntervention. 2013;9:555–63.

53. Leon MB, Smith CR, Mack MJ, Makkar RR, Svensson LG, Kodali SK, et al. Transcatheter or surgical aortic-valve replacement in intermediate-risk patients. N Engl J Med. 2016;374:1609–20.

54. Harken DE. Heart valves: ten commandments and still counting. Ann Thorac Surg. 1989;48:S18–9.

55. Binder RK, Rodés-Cabau J, Wood DA, Mok M, Leipsic J, De Larochellière R, et al. Transcatheter aortic valve replacement with the SAPIEN 3. JACC Cardiovasc Interv. 2013;6:293–300.

56. Edwards SAPIEN 3 transcatheter heart valve|Edwards Lifesciences, https://www.edwards.com/devices/heart-valves/transcatheter-Sapien-3.

57. Webb J, Gerosa G, Lefèvre T, Leipsic J, Spence M, Thomas M, et al. Multicenter evaluation of a next-generation balloon-expandable transcatheter aortic valve. J Am Coll Cardiol. 2014;64:2235–43.

58. Husser O, Pellegrini C, Kessler T, Burgdorf C, Thaller H, Mayr NP, et al. Outcomes after transcatheter aortic valve replacement using a novel balloon-expandable transcatheter heart valve. JACC Cardiovasc Interv. 2015;8:1809–16.

59. Kodali S, Thourani VH, White J, Malaisrie SC, Lim S, Greason KL, et al. Early clinical and echocardiographic outcomes after SAPIEN 3 transcatheter aortic valve replacement in inoperable, high-risk and intermediate-risk patients with aortic stenosis. Eur Heart J. 2016;37:2252–62.

60. Thourani VH, Kodali S, Makkar RR, Herrmann HC, Williams M, Babaliaros V, et al. Transcatheter aortic valve replacement versus surgical valve replacement in intermediate-risk patients: a propensity score analysis. Lancet. 2016;387:2218–25.

61. Edwards SAPIEN 3 transcatheter valve demonstrates significant cost savings over surgery in intermediate risk patients | Edwards Lifesciences. https://www.edwards.com/ns20171031.

62. The SAPIEN 3 Ultra system in intermediate risk patients with symptomatic severe aortic stenosis, ClinicalTrials.gov. https://clinicaltrials.gov/ct2/show/NCT03471065.

63. Edwards announces key events for PCR London valves 2017. https://www.edwards.com/ch-en/ns20170924.

64. Ribeiro H, Urena M, Kuck K-H, Webb JG, Rodés-Cabau J. Edwards CENTERA valve. EuroIntervention. 2012;8:Q79–82.

65. Binder RK, Schäfer U, Kuck K-H, Wood DA, Moss R, Leipsic J, et al. Transcatheter aortic valve replacement with a new self-expanding transcatheter heart valve and motorized delivery system. JACC Cardiovasc Interv. 2013;6:301–7.

66. Kim U, Blanke P, Windecker S, Kasel AM, Schäfer U, Walters D, et al. Computed tomography-based oversizing and incidence of paravalvular aortic regurgitation and permanent pacemaker implantation with a new generation self-expanding transcatheter heart valve. EuroIntervention. 2018;14(5):e511–8.

67. Schulz E, Jabs A, Gori T, von Bardeleben S, Hink U, Kasper-König W, et al. Transcatheter aortic valve implantation with the new-generation Evolut R™: comparison with CoreValve® in a single center cohort. IJC Heart Vasc. 2016;12:52–6.

68. Landes U, Bental T, Barsheshet A, Assali A, Vaknin Assa H, Levi A, et al. Comparative matched outcome of Evolut-R vs CoreValve transcatheter aortic valve implantation. J Invasive Cardiol. 2017;29:69–74.

69. Medtronic Expands TAVR Access to More Patients With Symptomatic, Severe Aortic Stenosis Upon Intermediate Risk FDA Approval. http://newsroom.medtronic.com/phoenix.zhtml?c=251324&p=irol-newsArticle&ID=2285395.

70. Forrest JK, Mangi AA, Popma JJ, Khabbaz K, Reardon MJ, Kleiman NS, et al. Early outcomes with the Evolut PRO repositionable selfexpanding transcatheter aortic valve with pericardial wrap. JACC Cardiovasc Interv. 2018;11:160–8.

71. Falk V, Walther T, Schwammenthal E, Strauch J, Aicher D, Wahlers T, et al. Transapical aortic valve implantation with a self-expanding anatomically oriented valve. Eur Heart J. 2011;32:878–87.

72. Sundermann SH, Holzhey D, Bleiziffer S, Treede H, Jacobs S, Falk V. Second-generation transapical valves: the Medtronic Engager system. Multimed Man Cardio-Thoracic Surg. 2014;2014:mmu001.

73. Del Valle R, Pascual I, Silva J, Avanzas P, Fernández-Suárez F, Moris C. Transapical implantation in the catheterization laboratory of the second generation engager aortic valve. Rev Esp Cardiol. 2016;69:442–54.

74. Börgermann J, Holzhey DM, Thielmann M, Girdauskas E, Schroefel H, Hofmann S, et al. Transcatheter aortic valve implantation using the ACURATE TA system: 1-year outcomes and comparison of 500 patients from the SAVI registries. Eur J Cardio-Thoracic Surg. 2017;51:936–42.

75. Möllmann H, Walther T, Siqueira D, Diemert P, Treede H, Grube E, et al. Transfemoral TAVI using the self-expanding ACURATE neoprosthesis: one-year outcomes of the multicentre "CE-approval cohort". EuroIntervention. 2017;13:e1040–6.

76. Hamm K, Reents W, Zacher M, Kerber S, Diegeler A, Schieffer B, et al. Transcatheter aortic valve implantation using the ACURATE TA and ACURATE neo valves: a four-year single-centre experience. EuroIntervention. 2017;13:53–9.

77. Schaefer A, Treede H, Schoen G, Deuschl F, Schofer N, Schneeberger Y, et al. Improving outcomes: case-matched comparison of novel second-generation versus first-generation self-expandable transcatheter heart valves. Eur J Cardio-Thoracic Surg. 2016;50:368–73.

78. Boston Scientific Next Generation Acurate Neo2™ Aortic Valve System Demonstrates Favorable Outcomes In Clinical Practice. https://www.bostonscientific.com/en-EU/news/newsroom-uk/aortic-valve-disease/press-releases-2018/boston-next-generation-acurate-neo2-aortic-valve-system-demonstrates-favorable-outcomes-in-clinical-practice.html.

79. PCR LV 2018: Favourable outcomes for next-generation Acurate neo2 TAVI system. https://cardiovascularnews.com/pcr-lv-2018-favourable-outcomes-for-next-generation-acurate-neo2-tavi-system/.

80. Treede H, Mohr F-W, Baldus S, Rastan A, Ensminger S, Arnold M, et al. Transapical transcatheter aortic valve implantation using the JenaValve system: acute and 30-day results of the multicentre CE-mark study. Eur J Cardiothorac Surg. 2012;41:e131–8.

81. Seiffert M, Bader R, Kappert U, Rastan A, Krapf S, Bleiziffer S, et al. Initial German experience with transapical implantation of a secondgeneration transcatheter heart valve for the treatment of aortic regurgitation. JACC Cardiovasc Interv. 2014;7:1168–74.

82. Schäfer U, Schirmer J, Niklas S, Harmel E, Deuschl F, Conradi L. First-in-human implantation of a novel transfemoral selfexpanding transcatheter heart valve to treat pure aortic regurgitation. EuroIntervention. 2017;13:1296–9.

83. Portico™ Transcatheter Aortic Heart Valve | St. Jude Medical. https://www.cardiovascular.abbott/int/en/hcp/products/structural-heart/porticoaortic-valve.html.

84. Manoharan G, Linke A, Moellmann H, Redwood S, Frerker C, Kovac J, et al. Multicentre clinical study evaluating a novel resheathable annular functioning self-expanding transcatheter aortic valve system: safety and performance results at 30 days with the Portico system. EuroIntervention. 2016;12:768–74.

85. Wendt D, Thielmann M, Shehada SE, Tsagakis K, Jakob H, El Gabry M. Editorial comment on the RESPOND study. J Thorac Dis. 2017;9:3587–9.

86. Meredith I, Hood K, Haratani N, Allocco D, Dawkins K. Boston Scientific Lotus valve. EuroIntervention. 2012;8:Q70–4.

87. Meredith IT, Worthley SG, Whitbourn RJ, Antonis P, Montarello JK, Newcomb AE, et al. Transfemoral aortic valve replacement with the repositionable Lotus Valve System in high surgical risk patients: the REPRISE I study. EuroIntervention. 2014;9:1264–70.

88. Meredith IT, Walters DL, Dumonteil N, Worthley SG, Tchétché D, Manoharan G, et al. 1-Year outcomes with the fully repositionable and retrievable lotus transcatheter aortic replacement valve in 120 high-risk surgical patients with severe aortic stenosis. JACC Cardiovasc Interv. 2016;9:376–84.

89. De Backer O, Götberg M, Ihlberg L, Packer E, Savontaus M, Nielsen NE, et al. Efficacy and safety of the Lotus Valve System for treatment of patients with severe aortic valve stenosis and intermediate surgical risk: Results from the Nordic Lotus-TAVR registry. Int J Cardiol. 2016;219:92–7.

90. Zaman S, McCormick L, Gooley R, Rashid H, Ramkumar S, Jackson D, et al. Incidence and predictors of permanent pacemaker implantation following treatment with the repositionable Lotus transcatheter aortic valve. Catheter Cardiovasc Interv. 2017;90:147–54.

91. Soliman OII, El Faquir N, Ren B, Spitzer E, van Gils L, Jonker H, et al. Comparison of valve performance of the mechanically expanding Lotus and the balloon-expanded SAPIEN3 transcatheter heart valves: an observational study with independent core laboratory analysis. Eur Heart J Cardiovasc Imaging. 2018;19:157–67.

92. Boston Scientific recalls all lotus valves, including lotus with depth guard. https://www.tctmd.com/news/boston-scientific-recalls-all-lotus-valves-including-lotus-depth-guard.

93. Hahn RT. The Lotus valve: can it float above the muddy waters? Circulation. 2018;137:2568–71.

94. Latib A, Maisano F, Colombo A, Klugmann S, Low R, Smith T, et al. Transcatheter aortic valve implantation of the direct flow medical aortic valve with minimal or no contrast. Cardiovasc Revasc Med. 2014;15:252–7.

95. Bushnaq H, Raspé C, Öner A, Yücel S, Ince H, Sommer S-P. A new technique to implant a transcatheter inflatable, fully repositionable prosthesis in aortic stenosis with severe asymmetric calcification†. Interact Cardiovasc Thorac Surg. 2017;25:679–82.

96. Song G, Jilaihawi H, Wang M, Chen M, Wang J, Wang W, et al. Severe symptomatic bicuspid and tricuspid aortic stenosis in China: characteristics and outcomes of transcatheter aortic valve replacement with the Venus-A valve. Struct Hear. 2018;2:60–8.

97. Liu X-B, He Y-X, Liu C-H, Wang L-H, Gao F, Yu L, et al. First-in-man implantation of the retrievable and repositionable VenusA-Plus valve. World J Emerg Med. 2018;9:64–6.

98. Venibri valve. https://www.colibrihv.com/technology.

99. Feng Y, Zhao Z-G, Baccaro J, Zeng MF, Fish RD, Chen M. First-in-man implantation of a pre-packaged self-expandable dry-tissue transcatheter aortic valve. Eur Heart J. 2018;39:713.

100. Sievert H, Hofmann I, Vaskelyte L, Gafoor S, Bertog S, Matić P, Reinartz M, et al. Venibri: a new TAVI valve with dry leaflet technology. ICI Meeting 2017, Tel Aviv (Israel). https://events.eventact.com/dan/28605/103520.pdf.

101. Claiborne TE, Bluestein D, Schoephoerster RT. Development and evaluation of a novel arti-ficial catheter-deliverable prosthetic heart valve and method for in vitro testing. Int J Artif Organs. 2009;32:262–71.

102. Rahmani B, Tzamtzis S, Ghanbari H, Burriesci G, Seifalian AM. Manufacturing and hydrodynamic assessment of a novel aortic valve made of a new nanocomposite polymer. J Biomech. 2012;45:1205–11.

103. Rahmani B, Tzamtzis S, Sheridan R, Mullen MJ, Yap J, Seifalian AM, et al. A new transcatheter heart valve concept (the TRISKELE): feasibility in an acute preclinical model. EuroIntervention. 2016;12:901–8.

104. Rahmani B, Tzamtzis S, Sheridan R, Mullen MJ, Yap J, Seifalian AM, et al. In vitro hydrodynamic assessment of a new transcatheter heart valve concept (the TRISKELE). J Cardiovasc Transl Res. 2017;10:104–15.

105. Capulli AK, Emmert MY, Pasqualini FS, Kehl D, Caliskan E, Lind JU, et al. JetValve: rapid manufacturing of biohybrid scaffolds for biomimetic heart valve replacement. Biomaterials. 2017;133:229–41.

106. Restorative Heart Valve Therapy: Xeltis' restorative approach. http://www.xeltis.com/restorative-heart-valve-therapy/.

107. Sijbesma RP, Beijer FH, Brunsveld L, Folmer BJ, Hirschberg JH, Lange RF, et al. Reversible polymers formed from self-complementary monomers using quadruple hydrogen bonding. Science. 1997;278:1601–4.

108. Miyazaki Y, Soliman M, Abdelghani A, Katsikis CN, Naz C, Lopes SP, et al. Acute performance of a novel restorative transcatheter aortic valve: preclinical results. EuroIntervention. 2017;13(12):e1410–7.

109. Heart Valve Society, 2018 Scientific Meeting Program, http://heartvalvesociety.org/meeting/abstracts/2018-program.cgi.

110. Scherman J, van Breda B, Appa H, van Heerden C, Ofoegbu C, Bezuidenhout D, et al. Transcatheter valve with a hollow balloon for aortic valve insufficiency. Multimed Man Cardio-Thoracic Surg. 2018;2018

111. Iop L, Gerosa G. Guided tissue regeneration in heart valve replacement: from preclinical research to first-in-human trials. Biomed Res Int. 2015;2015:432901.

112. Ghodsizad A, Bordel V, Wiedensohler H, Elbanayosy A, Koerner MM, Gonzalez Berjon JM, et al. Magnetically guided recellularization of decellularized stented porcine pericardium-derived aortic valve for TAVI. ASAIO J. 2014;60:582–6.

Biorestorative Valve for Transcatheter Aortic Valve Implantation: Tomorrow's World from Preclinical to Clinical

46

Rodrigo Modolo, Yosuke Miyazaki,
Yoshinobu Onuma, Osama I. Soliman,
and Patrick W. Serruys

46.1 Introduction (Rationale of Biorestorative Valve)

The long-term durability of transcatheter heart valves (THV) is becoming an important issue since the selection of patients for transcatheter aortic valve implantation (TAVI), also called transcatheter aortic valve replacement (TAVR),

R. Modolo
Department of Cardiology, Academic Medical Center, University of Amsterdam, Amsterdam, The Netherlands

Department of Internal Medicine, Cardiology Division, University of Campinas, UNICAMP, Campinas, Brazil

Y. Miyazaki
Department of Cardiology, Thoraxcenter, Erasmus Medical Center Rotterdam, Rotterdam, The Netherlands

Y. Onuma · O. I. Soliman
Department of Cardiology, Thoraxcenter, Erasmus Medical Center Rotterdam, Rotterdam, The Netherlands

Cardialysis Core Laboratories and Clinical Trial Management, Rotterdam, The Netherlands
e-mail: osoliman@cardialysis.nl

P. W. Serruys (✉)
Cardiovascular Science Division of the NHLI, Imperial College of Science, Technology and Medicine, London, UK
e-mail: patrick.w.j.c.serruys@pwserruys.com

has been expanded to lower-risk patients, thus younger [1]. A series of clinical trials have tested the implantation of transcatheter aortic valves in patients with high risk for surgical replacement and even below the high-risk stratum, achieving satisfactory results when comparing to the surgical aortic valve replacement (SAVR) [1–3]. Initially patients who were candidates for TAVI were elderly at high surgical risk. Due to the limited life expectancy, there was very little concern regarding to the long-term durability of the device compared to the safety of the TAVI procedure [4]. Thus, the evidence on long-term durability in the field of THV is limited. However for the surgical valves, it is known that the devices derived from animal origin (e.g., bovine, porcine, equine leaflets) tend to degenerate and become calcified with time, suggesting that reintervention is needed one or two decades after the implantation of the bioprosthesis valves [5]. In the field of paediatric cardiac surgery and of not fully grown patients, not only durability of the valve but also the growth process with the need for repaired intervention is considered a problem to overcome. Data derived from long-term cohorts of patients undergoing SAVR with a pericardial bioprosthesis show that younger patients (from 50 to 65 years) are more likely to have valve deterioration than those operated on the eighth decade of life [6].

Current bioprosthetic valves are made from animal-derived glutaraldehyde-fixed pericardial

© Springer Nature Switzerland AG 2019
A. Giordano et al. (eds.), *Transcatheter Aortic Valve Implantation*,
https://doi.org/10.1007/978-3-030-05912-5_46

tissue, which are known to cause biocompatibility concerns and chronic inflammatory responses [7]. The chronic inflammation could lead to calcification through secretion of cytokines by macrophages, such as osteopontin [8–10]. Also, this foreign material could be a major concern for thromboembolism, infection and valve dysfunction such as stenosis or insufficiency.

In order to overcome these issues, a valve with biocompatible material, which could diminish the inherent risk of heterologous material to provoke thrombosis, inflammation, calcification and rapid deterioration, has been conceptualized—a restorative cardiac valve. In order for the material of the valve to restore itself, a technology called the endogenous tissue restoration (ETR) was developed.

With the endogenous tissue restoration approach—better described throughout this chapter—a bioabsorbable material will progressively be replaced by endogenous tissue. Therefore, the heart valve with ETR technology has the potential to improve biocompatibility and overcome the inflammation problem of the current valve provoked by the use of a foreign material. This way, theoretically, the main issue of durability of the valve could be overcome.

Throughout this chapter we will discuss the perspectives on this technology and the preliminary results so far adapting the concept of ETR for the circulatory system.

46.2 Endogenous Tissue Restoration

The endogenous tissue restoration rationale is based upon the fact that a bioabsorbable material could be gradually absorbed and progressively replaced by the body's own tissue. This technology has been extensively studied over the last decades and is the result of scientific research of mainly three disciplines: the field of supramolecular chemistry, the domain of electrospinning and the knowledge about regenerative medicine.

Jean-Marie Lehn, a French chemist, has a key role in the development of this technique. Together with Donald Cram and Charles

Pedersen, in 1987, he received the Nobel Prize for his synthesis of cryptands (a family of synthetic bi- and polycyclic multidentate ligands for a variety of cations) [11] and has innovated in the field of supramolecular chemistry [12, 13]. His findings and effort lead the way to the development of novel polymer material platforms. Based on this technology, tunable material platforms have been developed, from which a full library of material with different parameters can be selected—different degrees of mechanical strength and rates of bioabsorption.

The second component of this new technology is electrospinning, which is a fibre production method which uses electric force to draw charged threads of polymer solutions or polymer melts up to fibre diameters in the order of some hundred nanometres.

Assembling supramolecular polymers in a random fashion and using the electrospinning technique, one can create matrices with somewhat porous structure that can be easily penetrated by endogenous cells, such as red cells, fibroblasts, myofibroblasts, platelets, macrophages and so on (Fig. 46.1).

The third component is the regenerative medicine. In summary, there are basically three phases for a tissue to regenerate itself: phase 1, implantation of the prosthesis; phase 2, neo-tissue formation; and phase 3, functional restoration.

From a physiopathological point of view, ETR is defined as replacement of the absorbable material by the patient's own native cells. This happens through infiltration of these cells into the polymeric matrix, triggering a cascade of events with gradual replacement by native tissue. As absorption begins, the leaflets and conduit are infiltrated by inflammatory cells, releasing growth factors, promoting smooth muscle cell infiltration and matrix production (proteoglycans, collagen with focal elastic tissue). The critical balance between the tissue formation and the implant absorption is the key to success of this technology (Fig. 46.2).

The primary results regarding the use of this technology in a prosthesis that had leaflets in the in vivo setting came from the implant of a pulmonary valved conduit in an ovine model.

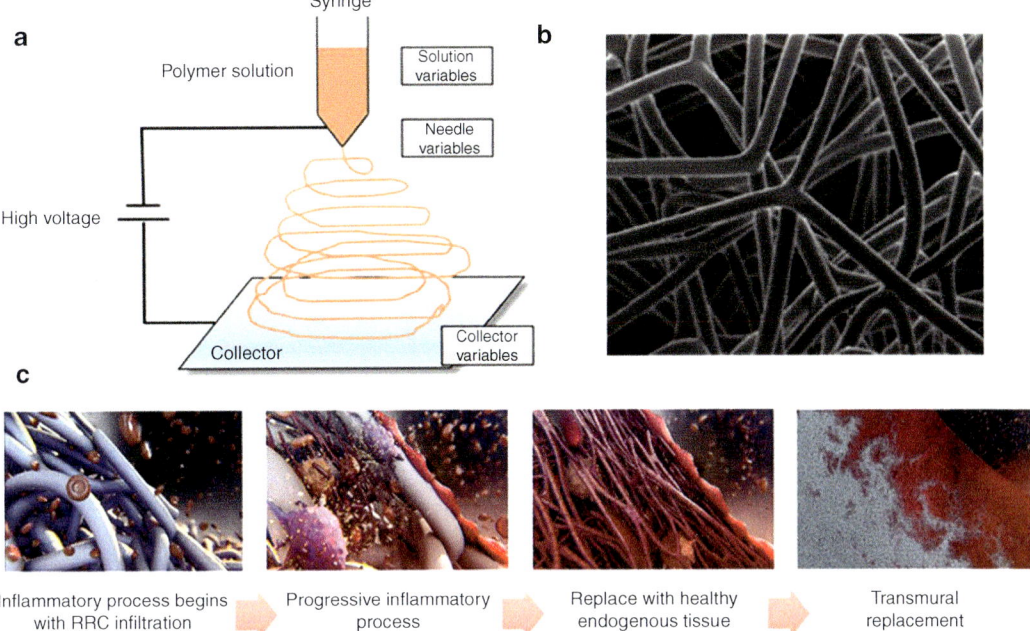

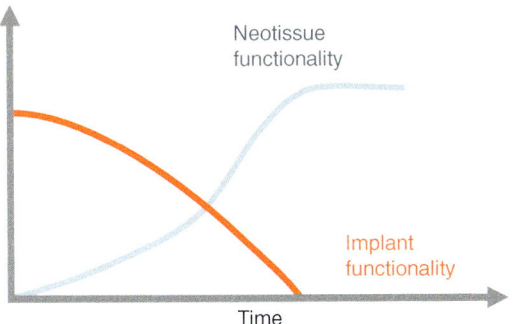

Fig. 46.1 The principle of electrospinning and ETR of the Xeltis aortic valve. (**a**) The principle of electrospinning: electrospinning is a widely used technique for the electrostatic production of nanofibres, during which an electric potential is used to make polymer fibres with diameters ranging from 2 nm to several micrometres from polymer solutions. This process is a major focus of attention because of its versatility and ability to continuously produce fibres on a scale of nanometres, which is difficult to achieve using other standard technologies. Electrospinning is a relatively simple way of creating nanofibre materials, but there are several parameters that can significantly influence the formation and structure of produced nanofibres. These parameters such as solution variables, needle variables or collector variables could be manipulated to produce the desired material. (**b**) Electron microscopic images of the product of electrospinning. (**c**) The principle of ETR: the implant is gradually infiltrated by blood elements (red cells, platelets, macrophages), myoblasts and fibroblasts with subsequent enzymatic and oxidative bioabsorption of the fibres and gradually replaced by endogenous tissue. Reprinted from EuroIntervention Vol 13, number 12, Miyazaki Y, Soliman OII, Abdelghani M, Katsikis A, Naz C, Lopes S, et al. Acute performance of a novel restorative transcatheter aortic valve: preclinical results, pages e1410–e7, Copyright (2017), with permission from Europa Digital & Publishing [17]

Fig. 46.2 Schematic representation of endogenous tissue restoration: the neo-tissue formation (red line) at the same time of the integrity loss of the implanted material (blue line)

46.3 Preclinical Results: Pulmonary Valved Conduit

To test the feasibility of this technology, Soliman et al. reported the performance of the pulmonary valved conduit (Xeltis BV, Eindhoven, the Netherlands), which carries this ETR technology, in the preclinical setting. For that the investigators used 23 adult sheep (ranging from 60 to 90 kg) comparing the new device with the ETR technology to the widely known Hancock® bioprosthetic valved conduit (Medtronic Heart Valve Division, Irvine, CA, USA).

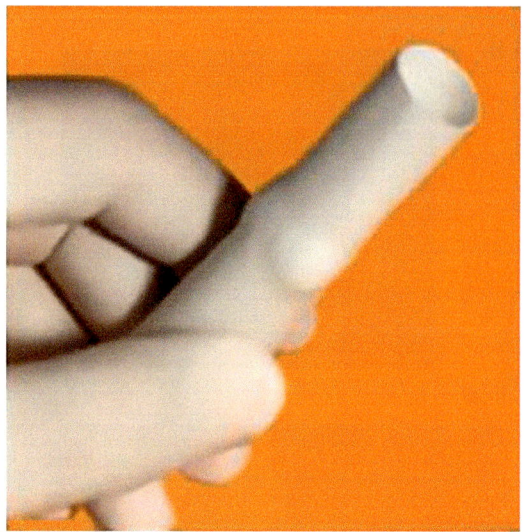
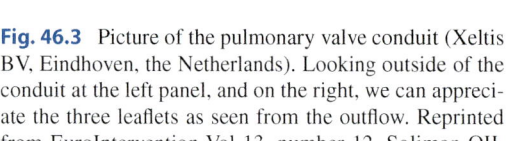
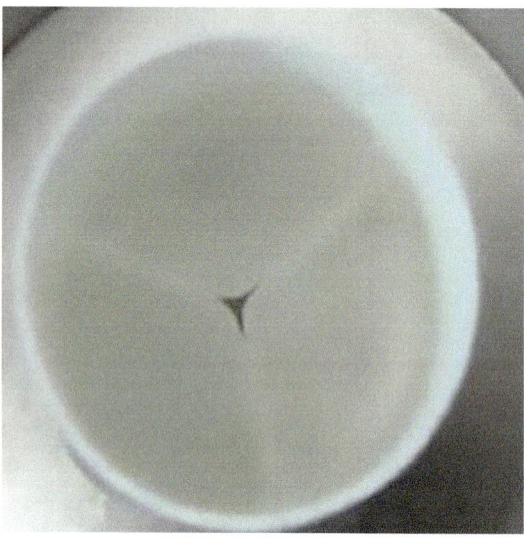

Fig. 46.3 Picture of the pulmonary valve conduit (Xeltis BV, Eindhoven, the Netherlands). Looking outside of the conduit at the left panel, and on the right, we can appreciate the three leaflets as seen from the outflow. Reprinted from EuroIntervention Vol 13, number 12, Soliman OII, Miyazaki Y, Abdelghani M, Brugmans M, Witsenburg M, Onuma Y, et al. Mid-term performance of a novel restorative pulmonary valved-conduit: preclinical results, pages e1418–e1427, Copyright (2017), with permission from Europa Digital & Publishing [14]

The pulmonary valved conduit is a 5-cm-long conduit with three leaflets and an inner diameter of 21 mm (Fig. 46.3). The devices were implanted via a thoracotomy under general anaesthesia as an interposition pulmonary artery vascular graft approximately 1 cm above the native pulmonary valve (which leaflets have been surgically removed). Haemodynamic data were as follows: valvular peak systolic pressure gradient (mmHg) was 25.6 ± 9.7 (3 months), 19.6 ± 7.1 (6 months) and 10.0 ± 9.2 (24 months), which were comparable to the Hancock valve (standard without ETR) as a control group. The investigators concluded that "the XELTIS pulmonary valved conduit showed a favourable and durable hemodynamic performance (up to 2-years after implantation), without conduit narrowing/obstruction or severe regurgitation" [14].

Bennink et al. confirmed these data with histological assessment of the material. Histological demonstration of the replacement of the conduit material by endogenous newly formed tissue can be seen in Fig. 46.4—where endogenous tissue restoration is observed in a chronological evolution (3, 6 and 12 months) [15]. The authors reported data from 18 animals, and only 1 animal with the Xeltis pulmonary valved conduit had significant calcification at 6 months. No significant narrowing of the conduit was observed, while a peak of neo-intimal thickness was seen at 6 months. Inflammatory process reached a peak at 6 months, and a peak of degradation process was observed at 12 months; this contrasted with the outcome of the Hancock prosthesis, where the calcification was much more prominent [15].

These primary results in the preclinical setting paved the way to testing in the clinical setting and also to expand the technology to the aortic valve.

46.4 Preclinical Results: Aortic Valve

For the aortic position, the technology used on the leaflets is the same as the ETR already described [16]. The leaflets, which were synthesized by electrospinning process, were mounted on a self-expandable nitinol frame (Fig. 46.5).

In a recent report, investigators showed the acute performance of this aortic valve implanted in sheep. For this given experiment, the Xeltis aortic valve was implanted through a transapical approach, under general anaesthesia in 33 adult sheep. The procedure was guided by

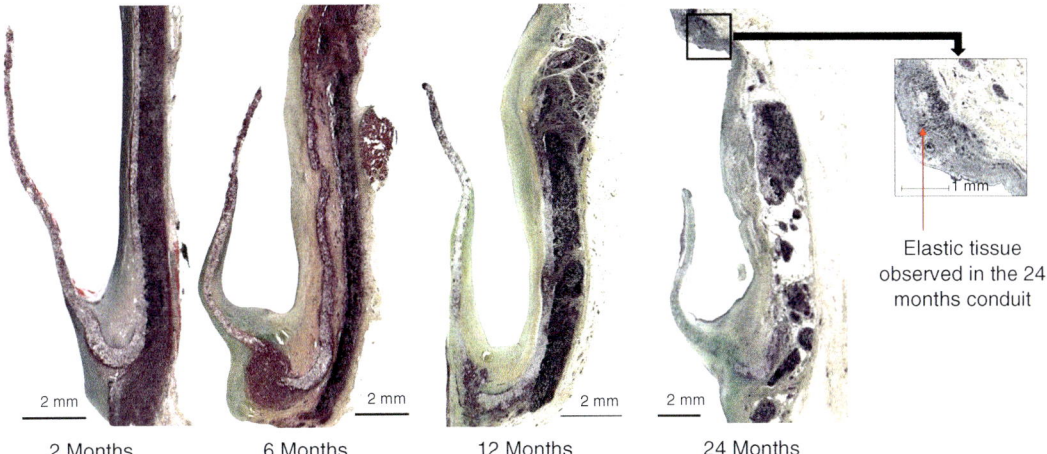

Fig. 46.4 Histology of a Xeltis pulmonary valved conduit gradually replaced over time by newly formed tissue. Histological images in Movat stains. The nuclei are stained in blue/black, elastic tissue in black, collagen in yellow, proteoglycan in green and muscle in dark red. In this image presented by Virmani, R, in EuroPCR Congress 2017 in Paris, France, we can see at 24 months the presence of elastic tissue formation (in details on the right panel). Reproduced with permission from the author

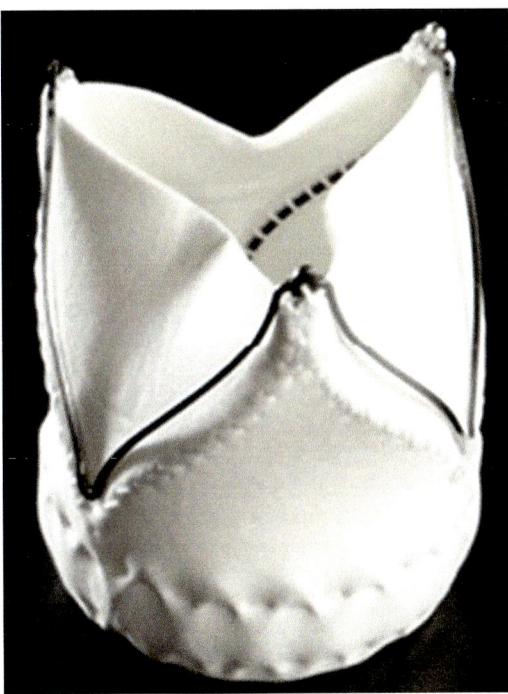

Fig. 46.5 Leaflets with a porous microstructure made through electrospinning process mounted on a self-expandable nitinol frame that included three feelers and a native leaflet clipping mechanism. Adapted and reprinted from EuroIntervention Vol 13, number 12, Miyazaki Y, Soliman OII, Abdelghani M, Katsikis A, Naz C, Lopes S, et al. Acute performance of a novel restorative transcatheter aortic valve: preclinical results, pages e1410–e7, Copyright (2017), with permission from Europa Digital & Publishing [17]

echocardiography, fluoroscopy and the execution of aortograms. The procedure of the implantation is represented in Fig. 46.6 following the steps: (1) positioning, a pigtail catheter was placed in the native aortic valve cusp as reference, and (2) the valve was delivered transapically under fluoroscopic guidance. The distal end of the valve was deployed, after which the delivery system was pulled gently to anchor the three device arms ("the feelers") into the cusps, prior to full deployment ("clipping process") and release of the device. In this report, no major complications related to the TAVI procedure were reported [17]. Assessment of haemodynamic parameters and regurgitation of the prosthesis after implantation was performed with the use of echocardiogram and videodensitomery technique [17]. The quantitative assessment of aortic regurgitation using videodensitometry is a novel, accurate, well-validated tool that uses the image of the aortogram to compare the density of contrast in the aortic root with the density of the regurgitated contrast to the left ventricle outflow tract. This technology has been validated in vitro and in vivo compared with echocardiography and cardiac magnetic resonance. Also, it has shown to have a prognostic value—related to clinical outcomes and mortality [18, 19]. Briefly, the dedicated software (CAAS A-Valve, Pie Medical Imaging, the

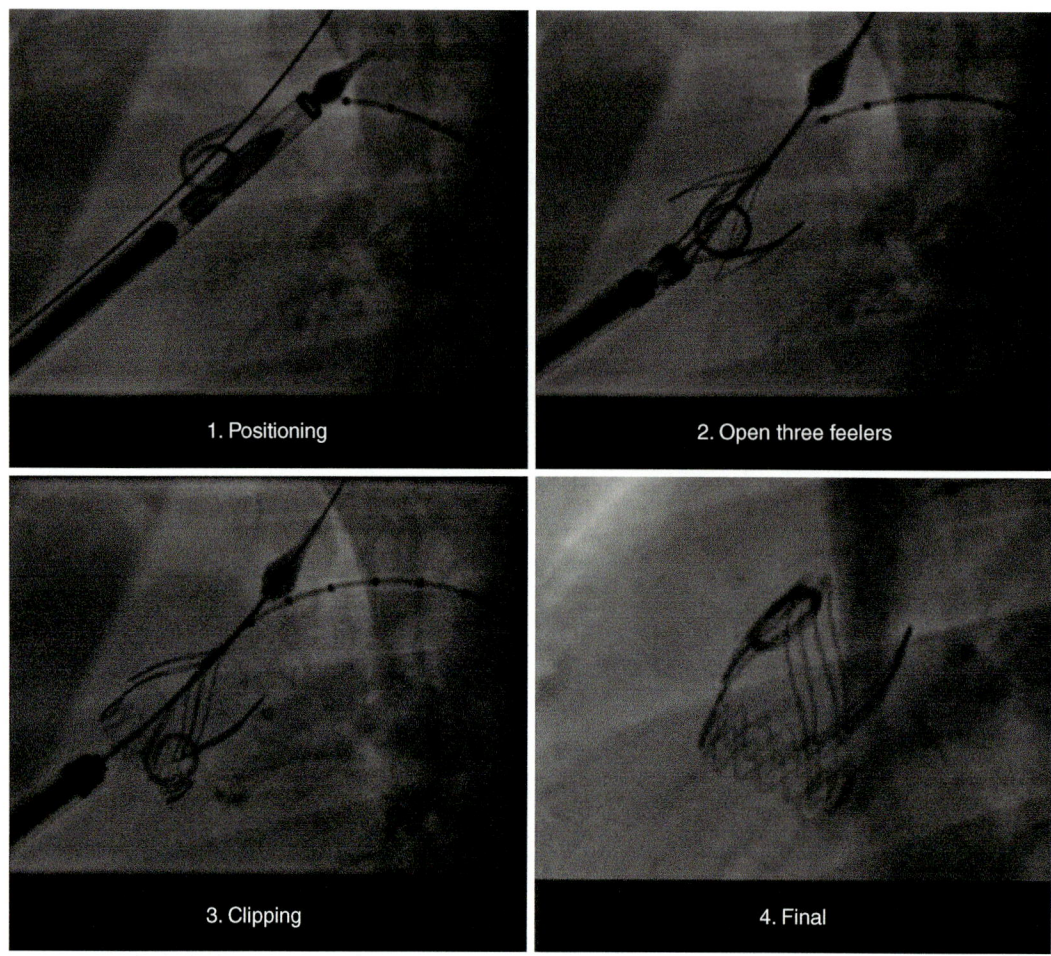

Fig. 46.6 Implantation of the Xeltis aortic valve. Reprinted from EuroIntervention Vol 13, number 12, Miyazaki Y, Soliman OII, Abdelghani M, Katsikis A, Naz C, Lopes S, et al. Acute performance of a novel restorative transcatheter aortic valve: preclinical results, pages e1410–e7, Copyright (2017), with permission from Europa Digital & Publishing [17]

Netherlands) provides the area under the time density curves (AUC) of the reference area (aortic root) and region of interest (left ventricle outflow tract). Simultaneously, the ratio of the area under the time density curve of the region of interest to the area under the time density curve of the reference area was calculated, which corresponds to the fraction of regurgitation. Theoretically, the quantitative videodensitometric assessment ranges from 0% to 100% [18–23]. Figure 46.7 shows the cumulative curve of VD-AR on 28 sheep immediately after TAVI [17]. Three cases showed a regurgitation superior to 17% (0.17), which is the predetermined cutoff value to show significant vital prognostic outcome in clinical situation [18, 19]. The mechanism of the significant regurgitation on these three cases was (1) transvalvular regurgitation determined by echocardiography and (2) inappropriate clipping of the leaflets.

Since the leaflets of the Xeltis aortic valve are made with electrospinning technology, the leaflet has a porous structure with randomly assembled microfibres. Although the concern had been raised that transvalvular (trans-leaflet) AR could be present, no transvalvular regurgitation more than mild was observed acutely in the preclinical study. This is because red blood cells, fibrin and other proteins permeate the leaflet material, sealing the pores and reducing its permeability. This could be

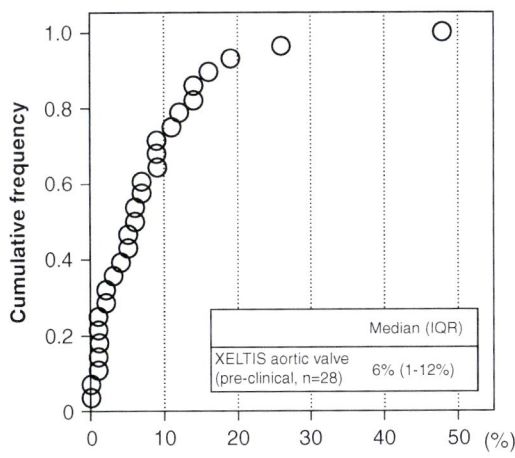

Fig. 46.7 Cumulative frequency distribution of quantitative regurgitation assessment with videodensitometry after implantation of the Xeltis aortic valve. Reprinted from EuroIntervention Vol 13, number 12, Miyazaki Y, Soliman OII, Abdelghani M, Katsikis A, Naz C, Lopes S, et al. Acute performance of a novel restorative transcatheter aortic valve: preclinical results, pages e1410–e7, Copyright (2017), with permission from Europa Digital & Publishing [17]

visually observed in surgical reconstruction of RVOT in clinical cases using this technology on pulmonary conduits. The surgical operator looked at the oozing of the blood through the wall of the conduit, which typically resolves within a few minutes, resulting in haemostasis (Fig. 46.8).

Haemodynamic performance was assessed immediately after implantation of the Xeltis aortic valve in 20 cases. Transvalvular peak pressure gradient (PG) was 7.4 [6.0–8.9] mmHg, mean PG was 4.0 [3.0–5.0] mmHg, and effective orifice area was 2.2 [1.6–2.5] cm^2. These data are comparable with the ones from clinical trials [1–3]. Although the current study is performed in a preclinical setting, and compared to the haemodynamic parameters reported in a clinical setting, the acute haemodynamic performance was excellent [24, 25] (Table 46.1). The study to assess the chronic performance of the Xeltis aortic valve is currently ongoing. Aortographic, echocardiographic and pathological assessment will help to better understand this technology.

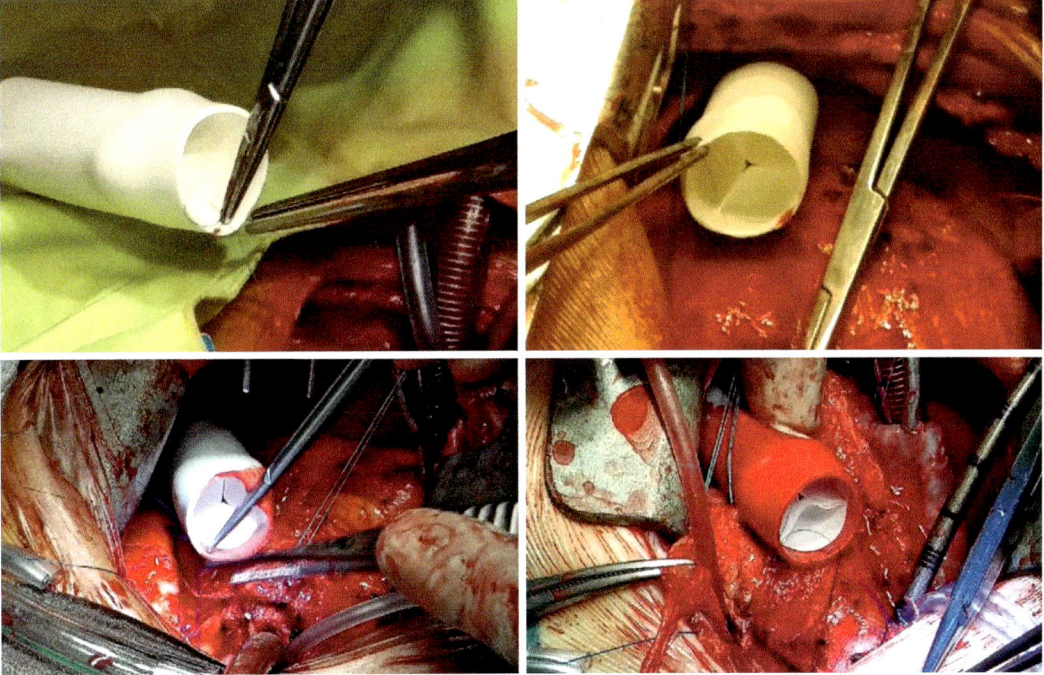

Fig. 46.8 Xeltis pulmonary valved conduit implantation in the right outflow tract of a patient. Reprinted from EuroIntervention Vol 13, number AA, Serruys PW, Miyazaki Y, Katsikis A, Abdelghani M, Leon MB, Virmani R, et al. Restorative valve therapy by endogenous tissue restoration: tomorrow's world? Reflection on the EuroPCR 2017 session on endogenous tissue restoration, pages AA68–AA77, Copyright (2017), with permission from Europa Digital & Publishing [7]

Table 46.1 Comparison of haemodynamic data between current commercially available valve and Xeltis aortic valve

	Human data from clinical trial				Preclinical data from normal sheep
	Edwards SAPIEN (26 mm) [24]	CoreValve (26mm) [24]	Lotus [25]	Sapien3 [25]	Xeltis
Peak pressure gradient (mmHg)	15.8	15.5	20	18	7.4
Mean pressure gradient (mmHg)	8.5	8.4	11	10	4.0
THV EOA (cm^2)	1.82	1.78	1.84	1.99	2.2

Reprinted from EuroIntervention Vol 13, number 12, Miyazaki Y, Soliman OII, Abdelghani M, Katsikis A, Naz C, Lopes S, et al. Acute performance of a novel restorative transcatheter aortic valve: preclinical results, pages e1410–e7, Copyright (2017), with permission from Europa Digital & Publishing [17]

46.5 From Preclinical to Clinical

For valves with the ETR technology in the aortic position, clinical trials have not yet been initiated. However, paediatric conduit (*Fontan*) and pulmonary valved conduit have ongoing follow-up in the clinical setting. Bockeria et al. reported the first clinical experience with five patients (aged 4–12 years old) and demonstrated the assessment by echocardiography, CT scan and MRI including 4D flow. They concluded that "Initial clinical experience with a novel absorbable graft underlines the potential of this new material to improve cardiac and vascular surgical procedures". Indeed these results are the primary data found in human, and longer follow-up and increase in sample is necessary. However, the observation of the longer follow-up in children is crucial in order to check the "growth" of the material with the endogenous tissue, thus confirming the concept of this technology. This better biocompatibility could reduce permanent implant-related complications.

XPLORE-I study is the first clinical feasibility study in patients who underwent right ventricular outflow tract (RVOT) reconstruction with the pulmonary valved conduit using the Xeltis technology (www.clinicaltrials.gov, NCT02700100). XPLORE-II trial (www.clinicaltrials.gov, NCT03022708) will test the early feasibility in the United States, in which ten patients will be enrolled.

46.6 Conclusions

The novel biorestorative valve has been developed based on the ETR concept: a technology combining three scientific disciplines which are supramolecular chemistry, electrospinning and regenerative medicine. A pulmonary valved conduit has been tested in preclinical setting, and clinical testing is ongoing. The aortic valve has been tested in preclinical setting and is expected to be tested in the clinical setting in a later stage.

This is a novel concept that seems appealing for the replacement of vascular structures and valves, due to its potential of being reconstituted by endogenous tissue. This technology might be responsible for the prolonged life duration of an aortic valve bioprosthesis. Ongoing research and clinical trials may be expected to overcome the issues of the current devices.

References

1. Reardon MJ, Van Mieghem NM, Popma JJ, Kleiman NS, Sondergaard L, Mumtaz M, et al. Surgical or transcatheter aortic-valve replacement in intermediate-risk patients. N Engl J Med. 2017;376(14):1321–31.
2. Leon MB, Smith CR, Mack MJ, Makkar RR, Svensson LG, Kodali SK, et al. Transcatheter or surgical aortic-valve replacement in intermediate-risk patients. N Engl J Med. 2016;374(17):1609–20.
3. Thyregod HG, Sondergaard L, Ihlemann N, Franzen O, Andersen LW, Hansen PB, et al. The Nordic aortic valve intervention (NOTION) trial comparing

transcatheter versus surgical valve implantation: study protocol for a randomised controlled trial. Trials. 2013;14:11.

4. Arsalan M, Walther T. Durability of prostheses for transcatheter aortic valve implantation. Nat Rev Cardiol. 2016;13(6):360–7.

5. Bourguignon T, Bouquiaux-Stablo AL, Candolfi P, Mirza A, Loardi C, May MA, et al. Very long-term outcomes of the Carpentier-Edwards Perimount valve in aortic position. Ann Thorac Surg. 2015;99(3):831–7.

6. Bourguignon T, Lhommet P, El Khoury R, Candolfi P, Loardi C, Mirza A, et al. Very long-term outcomes of the Carpentier-Edwards Perimount aortic valve in patients aged 50-65 years. Eur J Cardiothorac Surg. 2016;49(5):1462–8.

7. Serruys PW, Miyazaki Y, Katsikis A, Abdelghani M, Leon MB, Virmani R, et al. Restorative valve therapy by endogenous tissue restoration: tomorrow's world? Reflection on the EuroPCR 2017 session on endogenous tissue restoration. EuroIntervention. 2017;13(AA):AA68–77.

8. Cho HJ, Cho HJ, Kim HS. Osteopontin: a multifunctional protein at the crossroads of inflammation, atherosclerosis, and vascular calcification. Curr Atheroscler Rep. 2009;11(3):206–13.

9. Scatena M, Liaw L, Giachelli CM. Osteopontin: a multifunctional molecule regulating chronic inflammation and vascular disease. Arterioscler Thromb Vasc Biol. 2007;27(11):2302–9.

10. Manji RA, Ekser B, Menkis AH, Cooper DK. Bioprosthetic heart valves of the future. Xenotransplantation. 2014;21(1):1–10.

11. von Zelewsky A. Stereochemistry of coordination compounds. From alfred werner to the 21st century. Chimia (Aarau). 2014;68(5):297–8.

12. Lehninger AL. Supramolecular organization of enzyme and membrane systems. Naturwissenschaften. 1966;53(3):57–63.

13. Lehn J-M. Supramolecular chemistry. Japan: VCH; 1995. isbn:3-527-29311-6.

14. Soliman OI, Miyazaki Y, Abdelghani M, Brugmans M, Witsenburg M, Onuma Y, et al. Midterm performance of a novel restorative pulmonary valved conduit: preclinical results. EuroIntervention. 2017;13(12):e1418–e27.

15. Bennink G, Torii S, Brugmans M, Cox M, Svanidze O, Ladich E, et al. A novel restorative pulmonary valved conduit in a chronic sheep model: mid-term hemodynamic function and histologic assessment. J Thorac Cardiovasc Surg. 2017;155:2591–601.

16. Sijbesma RP, Beijer FH, Brunsveld L, Folmer BJ, Hirschberg JH, Lange RF, et al. Reversible polymers formed from self-complementary monomers using quadruple hydrogen bonding. Science (New York, NY). 1997;278(5343):1601–4.

17. Miyazaki Y, Soliman OII, Abdelghani M, Katsikis A, Naz C, Lopes S, et al. Acute performance of a novel restorative transcatheter aortic valve: preclinical results. EuroIntervention. 2017;13(12):e1410–e7.

18. Tateishi H, Campos CM, Abdelghani M, Leite RS, Mangione JA, Bary L, et al. Video densitometric assessment of aortic regurgitation after transcatheter aortic valve implantation: results from the Brazilian TAVI registry. EuroIntervention. 2016;11(12):1409–18.

19. Tateishi H, Abdelghani M, Cavalcante R, Miyazaki Y, Campos CM, Collet C, et al. The interaction of de novo and pre-existing aortic regurgitation after TAVI: insights from a new quantitative aortographic technique. EuroIntervention. 2017;13(1):60–8.

20. Abdelghani M, Miyazaki Y, de Boer ES, Aben JP, van Sloun M, Suchecki T, et al. Videodensitometric quantification of paravalvular regurgitation of a transcatheter aortic valve: in vitro validation. EuroIntervention. 2018;13(13):1527–35.

21. Miyazaki Y, Abdelghani M, de Boer ES, Aben JP, van Sloun M, Suchecki T, et al. A novel synchronised diastolic injection method to reduce contrast volume during aortography for aortic regurgitation assessment: in vitro experiment of a transcatheter heart valve model. EuroIntervention. 2017;13(11):1288–95.

22. Abdel-Wahab M, Abdelghani M, Miyazaki Y, Holy EW, Merten C, Zachow D, et al. A novel angiographic quantification of aortic regurgitation after TAVR provides an accurate estimation of regurgitation fraction derived from cardiac magnetic resonance imaging. JACC Cardiovasc Interv. 2018;11:287–97.

23. Abdelghani M, Tateishi H, Miyazaki Y, Cavalcante R, Soliman OII, Tijssen JG, et al. Angiographic assessment of aortic regurgitation by video-densitometry in the setting of TAVI: Echocardiographic and clinical correlates. Catheter Cardiovasc Interv. 2017;90(4):650–9.

24. Spethmann S, Dreger H, Schattke S, Baldenhofer G, Saghabalyan D, Stangl V, et al. Doppler haemodynamics and effective orifice areas of Edwards SAPIEN and CoreValve transcatheter aortic valves. Eur Heart J Cardiovasc Imaging. 2012;13(8):690–6.

25. Soliman OI, El Faquir N, Ren B, Spitzer E, van Gils L, Jonker H, et al. Comparison of valve performance of the mechanically expanding Lotus and the balloon-expanded SAPIEN3 transcatheter heart valves: an observational study with independent core laboratory analysis. Eur Heart J Cardiovasc Imaging. 2017;19:157–67.

Focus on Transcatheter Aortic Valve Implantation in Low-Risk Patients

47

A. K. Roy and B. Prendergast

47.1 Introduction

In just more than a decade since the first patients were enrolled in the PARTNER I trial, transcatheter aortic valve implantation (TAVI), also called transcatheter aortic valve replacement (TAVR), has become the treatment of choice for elderly high-risk patients with severe aortic stenosis and those who are deemed unsuitable for conventional surgical aortic valve replacement (SAVR) [1]. Similarly, robust randomized trial data from intermediate-risk patient cohorts support the net superiority of TAVI when undertaken via femoral approach [2, 3]. Furthermore, in clinical practice, contemporary registries from Europe and the USA show that a significant proportion of intermediate to low-risk patients are already being successfully treated with TAVI [4].

As the focus moves to evidence-based treatment of low-risk patients, ongoing trials must address a number of key differentiating features that uniquely define this group of often-younger patients with improved exercise tolerance, longer life expectancy, less comorbidities, and differing anatomical features. This chapter focuses on clinical, procedural, risk score, and patient characteristics that characterize the challenges faced in

treating the large low-risk cohort of patients with severe aortic stenosis.

47.2 Definition of Low Risk

The definition of low-risk patients is complex but, for practical and guideline purposes, has largely been determined by the inclusion criteria of completed or ongoing randomized trials and large-scale registries. Three factors are key: (i) operative mortality scores, (ii) age, and (iii) the agreed impact that other comorbidities may have upon periprocedural risk (as determined by formal Heart Team assessment). Using Society of Thoracic Surgery Predicted Risk of Mortality (STS-PROM) risk scores as the standard for research purposes, high risk for TAVI perioperative mortality is usually defined as an STS score >8% (6% of patients), intermediate risk as STS score 4–8% (14% of patients), and low risk as STS score <4% (80% of patients). The low-risk PARTNER 3 randomized controlled trial (Safety and Effectiveness of the SAPIEN 3 Transcatheter Heart Valve in Low Risk Patients With Aortic Stenosis, ClinicalTrials.gov NCT02675114) defines low risk as STS <4%, with operative mortality <2% and a Heart Team agreement that operative mortality is <4%, using an Edwards Sapien 3 valve via transfemoral approach. Similarly, inclusion criteria for the Medtronic Evolut R Transcatheter Aortic Valve Replacement

A. K. Roy
Mater Private Hospital, Dublin, Ireland

B. Prendergast (✉)
St Thomas' Hospital, London, UK
e-mail: bernard.prendergast@gstt.nhs.uk

© Springer Nature Switzerland AG 2019
A. Giordano et al. (eds.), *Transcatheter Aortic Valve Implantation*,
https://doi.org/10.1007/978-3-030-05912-5_47

in Low Risk Patients Trial (ClinicalTrials.gov NCT02701283) specify the need for "documented Heart Team agreement of low risk for SAVR, where low risk is defined as predicted risk of mortality for SAVR <3% at 30 days per multidisciplinary local Heart Team assessment." The NOTION-2 trial (Comparison of Transcatheter Versus Surgical Aortic Valve Replacement in Younger Low Surgical Risk Patients With Severe Aortic Stenosis, ClinicalTrials.gov Identifier: NCT02825134) also uses an STS score <4% for low-risk inclusion, using any CE mark valve via transfemoral approach.

In this context, it is important to understand that any of the commonly used surgical risk scores (STS-PROM, EuroSCORE, EuroSCORE II, Logistic EuroSCORE) remain imperfect and suboptimally validate measures of risk for the majority of TAVI populations. Furthermore, current TAVI-specific risk models lack significant comparative prospective validation. In general terms (albeit with limitations), EuroSCORE grossly overestimates operative mortality, whereas EuroSCORE II and STS more closely approximate TAVI outcomes. Risk score assessments in low-risk groups must take account of other features that impact upon mortality outcomes and long-term morbidity (Table 47.1).

Regardless of risk score, the average age of patients undergoing TAVI has remained similar (ranging from extreme risk to intermediate-/low-risk groups) across the major randomized trials published to date. For extreme risk, the average ages of patients in the PARTNER IB and US CoreValve Extreme Risk trials were 83.1 years and 81.3 years, respectively [5, 6]. Similarly, average ages in the high-risk PARTNER 1A and US CoreValve High Risk trials were 83.6 and 83.2 years, respectively [1, 7] (Table 47.2). In the intermediate-risk PARTNER 2A and SURTAVI trials, the average age was 81.5 and 79.9 years, respectively [3, 8]. Even in the NOTION study, a randomized all-comers trial that enrolled patients aged 70 years or above, the average age was still 79.2 years [9]. With this in mind, lower TAVI risk does not simply mean younger patients, since an 88-year-old man with severe aortic stenosis and no other comorbidities may have an STS score

Table 47.1 Clinical, procedural, and device-related factors that influence outcomes of TAVI in low-risk patients

Surgical risk score	STS-PROM
	EuroSCORE II
	Logistic EuroSCORE
Clinical factors	Anatomy of the aortic valve and its environment—bicuspid vs. tricuspid, degree and symmetry of calcification
	Complexity of iliofemoral access or need for alternative access
	Porcelain aorta
	Underlying conduction abnormalities
	Presence of coronary artery disease and need for revascularization
	Bleeding vs. stroke risk and choice of antiplatelet/anticoagulant regime post-procedure
Procedural factors	Conscious sedation vs. general anesthesia
	Transfemoral vs. alternative access (carotid, subclavian, axillary, transcaval, transaortic, or transapical)
	Need for pre-/post-dilatation
Device factors	Choice of valve—balloon expandable, self-expanding, or repositionable
	Implant technique

<2% (though surgical data from the large STS databases suggest that lower mortality is observed in lower-risk patients from younger age groups). Whether this trend applies to TAVI patients remains to be seen. NOTION 2 is the only low-risk trial enrolling patients ≤75 years, alongside the MEDTRONIC Registry (ClinicalTrials.gov NCT02628899) that is specifically examining a subgroup aged ≤65 years.

As studies from intermediate groups have shown, SAVR is associated with increased risk of life-threatening/disabling bleeding, stage 3 acute kidney injury, and new atrial fibrillation, whereas TAVI increases the risk of paravalvular leak (PVL), pacemaker requirement, and major vascular complications [8–11]. Given that many low-risk patients are excellent surgical candidates, major improvements must be clearly and robustly demonstrated across all the key comparators of SAVR and TAVI before percutaneous technology can truly evolve toward lower-risk patients. Even more provocatively, as TAVI mortality rates fall (30-day all-cause mortality PARTNER 2A S3 1.1%, to NOTION 2.1%, and PARTNER 2A transfemoral subgroup 3.0%) to levels equivalent

Table 47.2 Age and risk scores for defined risk groups in the major TAVI randomized trials

Risk category	Age (years)	Supporting evidence	Actual trial STS PROM (%)
Extreme risk (STS > 8%, Log EuroSCORE > 20%)	83.1 ± 8.6 83.2 ± 8.7	PARTNER IB US CoreValve Extreme Risk	11.2 ± 5.8 10.3 ± 5.5
High risk	83.6 ± 6.8 83.2 ± 7.1	PARTNER 1A US CoreValve High Risk	11.8 ± 3.3 7.3 ± 3.0
Intermediate risk (STS 4–8%, Log EuroSCORE 10–20%)	81.5 ± 6.7 79.9 ± 6.2	PARTNER 2A (Sapien XT) SURTAVI (CoreValve or Evolut R)	5.8 ± 2.1 4.5 ± 1.5
Intermediate–low risk	79.2 ± 4.9	NOTION	2.9 ± 1.6
Low risk (STS < 4%, Log EuroSCORE <10%)	No specified age limit No specified age limit ≤75 years	PARTNER 3 MEDTRONIC NOTION 2	– – –

to the natural history of severe aortic stenosis (sudden death 1–2% per annum), pre-emptive intervention in asymptomatic patients becomes a serious consideration.

47.3   Paravalvular Leak

Moderate to severe PVL after TAVI remains an important concern, with a prevalence of 23.6% in the CoreValve registry and an associated increase in late mortality (63% vs. 51%; $p = 0.034$). Newer-generation devices that are fully retrievable or incorporate skirts or modified frame designs have significantly reduced rates of PVL, ranging from 5.3% to 7.7% for the CoreValve Evolut R, 0–1.0% for the Evolut PRO, and 3.8% for the Sapien 3 device. While preprocedural planning and accurate annular sizing using multislice CT have evolved considerably, further reduction in the rates of PVL is required for lower-risk cohorts with longer life expectancy or bicuspid valve anatomy.

47.4   Permanent Pacemaker Implantation

As TAVI implantation rates grow exponentially year on year, understanding of the key features that drive conduction disorders and need for permanent pacemaker (PPM) implantation has also progressed significantly. Nevertheless, PPM implantation rates remain high with certain devices. Patient-level predictors of PPM include bicuspid valve anatomy, pre-existing right bundle branch block, heavy calcification of the noncoronary cusp, and a high membranous septum [12]. In the initial PARTNER Registry, PPM was required in 8.8% of patients without prior PPM who underwent TAVI with a balloon-expandable valve. In addition to pre-existing right bundle branch block, the prosthesis:outflow tract diameter ratio and LV end-diastolic diameter were also identified as predictors of PPM requirement.

Device-specific features, such as skirt thickness or frame height, may also dictate PPM implantation rates, with some studies also suggesting that PPM implantation is associated with poorer outcomes. New PPM requirement was associated with a longer duration of hospitalization and higher rates of repeat hospitalization at 1 year in the initial PARTNER trial [5, 13, 14]. Similarly, early postoperative pacemaker implantation increased the risk of late all-cause mortality (HR 1.49; 95% C.I 1.20, 1.84; $p < 0.001$) analyzing long-term in 5842 patients undergoing SAVR over 11 year mean follow-up (range 5.8–16.5 years) [14]. Conversely, a more recent meta-analysis including 11 studies and 7032 patients showed no significant association between PPM and 1-year all-cause mortality (risk ratio, 1.03; 95% CI, 0.90–1.18; $P = 0.64$, $I2 = 0\%$), highlighting the controversies surrounding PPM implantation, particularly in the absence of standardized indications for implantation [15].

Whether these outcomes translate to lower-risk cohorts remains to be seen. These patients may have less underlying conduction disease while improved understanding of the importance of valve implant depth and clearer guidelines for the management of transient bundle branch block may lead to a reduction in rates of PPM implantation after TAVI. Of particular interest are longer-term data from a series of 1629 intermediate-risk patients undergoing TAVI [16] with a total PPM rate of 19.8% (CoreValve 26.9%, Sapien 10.9%)—mostly implanted within 72 h of the procedure—but no differences in total or cardiovascular mortality between PPM and non-PPM groups at 4-year follow-up. Importantly, however, rates of re-hospitalization due to heart failure (22.4% vs. 16.1%, adjusted HR: 1; 42; 95%CI: 1.06–1.89; $p = 0.019$) and lack of improvement in left ventricular function were higher in the PPM implant group, possibly resulting from myocardial dyssynchrony.

Higher implant positioning (and lower rates of PPM implantation) may theoretically be achieved with repositionable valves, although this has not been demonstrated with the LOTUS system to date. Indeed, PPM rates remain markedly higher with most self-expanding valve systems. For example, PPM implantation rates in SURTAVI were significantly greater after TAVI (Evolut R 26.7%, CoreValve 25.5%) compared with SAVR (6.6%). In comparison, PPM rates associated with balloon expandable valves are relatively lower (PARTNER 2A [Sapien XT] 8.5% at 30 days, 9.9% at 1 year, and 11.8% at 2 years; [Sapien 3] 10.2% at 30 days, 12.4% at 1 year) [2]. Nevertheless, many would argue that these rates remain unacceptably high for lower-risk patients, while also driving up the length of hospital stay and overall procedural costs.

New-onset left bundle branch block (LBBB) during or after TAVI is a further important factor to consider in low-risk patients. While commonly occurring as a transient phenomenon during the TAVI procedure, persistent LBBB affects approximately 55% [16] and may be associated with higher degrees of AV block and sick sinus syndrome. New-onset LBBB predicts a twofold higher risk of need for PPM implantation and

Table 47.3 Principal predictors of the need for permanent pacemaker implantation after TAVI[a]

Variable	Multivariable odds ratio
Baseline right bundle-branch block	2.8–46.7
Implantation of a Medtronic CoreValve (vs. Edwards SAPIEN valves)	2.6–25.7
Oversizing/stretching of the aortic annulus/left ventricular outflow tract	1.02–1.5/1%
First-degree atrioventricular block	4.0–11.4

[a]Adapted with permission from Auffret et al. Circulation 2017 [16]

some studies suggest that LBBB or new QRS duration >160 ms following TAVI may increase the rate of sudden cardiac death (1.6–3.3%, log-rank $p = 0.007$; 3.0–9.9%, log-rank $p = 0.010$, respectively) [17]. Several questions therefore arise. Will these subgroups become more apparent as overall mortality rates differ for low-risk populations? What is the optimal management for low-risk patients who will live longer? Is there a role for prophylactic PPM implantation in patients with "at-risk" LBBB conduction disturbances? If so, what clinical impact will it have for those with heart failure or dyssynchrony? Careful observational studies will be of fundamental importance as clinical experience accumulates (Table 47.3).

47.5   Anatomical Considerations

The frequency of bicuspid aortic valve (BAV) stenosis is typically higher in younger patients, with bicuspid valve disease routinely excluded from low- and intermediate-risk TAVI trials due to the uncertainties of unpredictable anatomy and valve performance. Nevertheless, bicuspid aortic stenosis may also occur in up to 20% of octogenarians [18]. Particular hazards include the presence of asymmetric, bulky calcification of the native valve apparatus, elliptical valve orifices, low coronary ostia, and associated aortopathy—all of which make valve selection and sizing more challenging. Sub-annular calcification below the noncoronary cusp may unpredictably influence prosthesis position, and heavy left coronary cusp calcification predicts the need for

PPM implantation. Altered valve frame expansion with resulting asymmetric leaflet expansion and potential for subclinical leaflet thrombosis raises further concerns regarding longer-term valve durability. Nevertheless, early registry data are promising, with no severe PVL, 23.5% PPM rate, and reasonable 30-day mortality in a small series of 51 patients with BAV undergoing TAVI using the Sapien 3 valve [18]. Larger scale trials are ongoing and sorely needed.

47.6 Stroke

Reported rates of stroke after TAVI vary widely (0.4–5%), partly as a result of operator and center proficiency, but also in part due to the lack (until recently) of standardized definitions for periprocedural cerebrovascular events [19]. Rates of disabling stroke in intermediate-risk patients in PARTNER 2A were 3.2% vs. 4.3% for TAVI and SAVR at 30 days ($p = 0.20$), 5.0% vs. 5.8% at 1 year ($p = 0.46$), and 6.2% vs. 6.4% at 2 years ($p = 0.83$) [3]. Moreover, SURTAVI data indicate that stroke rates were lower after TAVI than SAVR, both at 30 days (3.3% vs. 5.4%, log rank $p = 0.031$) and 2 years (6.3% vs. 8.0%, log rank $p = 0.0143$) [8]. Importantly, quality of life measures suggested that SF-36 physical summary assessed improvements after stroke were faster in the TAVI group than the SAVR group at 30 days [8].

The distinction between periprocedural and medium- to long-term event rates is important, since mechanisms for the latter may be very different and are often driven by atrial fibrillation or coexistent vascular disease, or rarely as a consequence of valve thrombosis or endocarditis associated with structural valve degeneration (SVD). Lower profile devices, smaller delivery systems, and improved steerability minimize unnecessary contact with the aorta during device delivery and deployment. Similarly, preliminary balloon valvuloplasty is no longer routine practice during the TAVI procedure, and generally reserved for the small proportion of cases (<10%) where severe calcification or complex valve anatomy is predicted to impair valve crossing or frame expansion [20].

Further distinctions address the differences between clinically manifest stroke and silent cerebral lesions arising as a consequence of device deployment or manipulation, and their potential impact upon neurocognition. The CLEAN TAVI and SENTINEL trials were the first to specifically address the role of cerebral embolic protection devices and both demonstrated safety and efficacy with reduction in the volume of ischemic lesions (but no clear impact on rates of disabling or non-disabling stroke) [21, 22]. Benefits for long-term neurocognitive function in lower-risk patients remain unclear, since neurological impairment (as assessed using mental health and quality of life assessments) does not necessarily correlate directly with diffusion-weighted MRI-detectable cerebral lesions. As the focus turns to younger, lower-risk patients, the utility of cerebral embolic protection devices may be more specifically defined for patients with specific risk markers for embolization, such as left atrial thrombus, premature cerebrovascular/carotid disease, bulky valve leaflets, and aortic arch atheroma.

47.7 Durability, Leaflet Thrombosis, and Valve Failure

The questions of long-term durability and risk of structural valve degeneration (SVD) are of utmost importance in determining the extent of application of TAVI in lower-risk patients with longer life expectancies than those studied so far. Durability data describing the surgical experience with bioprosthetic valves provide the reference standard for rates of SVD and associated interventions, with longer follow-up than currently available for TAVI patients. A systematic review of observational studies demonstrated prolonged median survival after SAVR with bioprosthetic valves (<65 years, 16 years; 65–75 years, 12 years; 75–85 years, 7 years; >85 years, 6 years) and equivalent freedom from SVD (10 years, 94.0%; 15 years, 81.7%; 20 years, 52%) [23]. SVD may arise as a result of degeneration, calcification, thrombosis, infection, and

Table 47.4 Definitions of TAVI structural valve degeneration[a]

Structural valve degeneration (SVD)	Definition
Moderate hemodynamic SVD (any of the following)	Mean transprosthetic gradient ≥20 mmHg and <40 mmHg Mean transprosthetic gradient ≥10 and <20 mmHg change from baseline Moderate intraprosthetic aortic regurgitation, new or worsening (>1+/4+) from baseline
Severe hemodynamic SVD (any of the following)	Mean gradient ≥40 mmHg Mean gradient ≥20 mmHg change from baseline Severe intraprosthetic aortic incompetence, new or worsening (>2+/4+) from baseline
Morphological SVD (any of the following)	Leaflet integrity abnormality (i.e., torn or flail causing intra-frame regurgitation) Leaflet structure abnormality (i.e., pathological thickening and/or calcification causing valvular stenosis or central regurgitation) Leaflet function abnormality (i.e., impaired mobility resulting in stenosis and/or central regurgitation) Strut/frame abnormality (i.e., fracture) Hemodynamic and morphological SVD

[a]Adapted from Capodanno, Petronio, Prendergast et al. [28]

pannus formation and lead to valve-related death or the need for re-intervention. Recently agreed international definitions for clinical and research purposes are summarized in Table 47.4.

Failure of transcatheter valves is usually the result of SVD, infective endocarditis, late embolization, compression, or thrombosis, all of which require different treatment approaches that are undergoing large-scale prospective validation [24]. Nevertheless, 5-year follow-up data from PARTNER 1 are reassuring, demonstrating similar mortality and low rates of re-intervention for SVD after both SAVR and TAVI. Importantly, rates of SVD were significantly lower after TAVI than SAVR at 5-year follow-up of the NOTION study cohort (3.6% vs. 21.5%, $p < 0.0001$), as presented at ACC 2018.

Long-term echocardiographic evaluation has confirmed that aortic valve area remains stable in TAVI recipients at 3–5 years and is superior to SAVR controls [25, 26]. However, given the experience with surgical valve degeneration, more time is needed to understand the potential mechanisms of TAVI failure (and possible preventive strategies), and to ensure there is no precipitous drop in function or durability up to 10 years (and beyond). Reported rates of structural TAVR deterioration range from 0% to 9.7%, depending on the definition and type of valve used [26, 27]. Factors such as the expansion capacity of the valve frame (determined by the underlying stent design) and its influence on the valve leaflets and their symmetry may also play a role in reduced leaflet motion. However, current long-term follow-up studies are small and limited to first generation devices—larger multicenter observational studies are underway.

Subclinical leaflet thrombosis, characterized by hypoattenuated leaflet thickening with or without restricted leaflet motion, is observed using 4-D contrast-enhanced computed tomography in up to 13% of patients with surgical bioprostheses and TAVI devices [29]. However, the clinical significance of this observation and its relationship to SVD remains unclear. Dual antiplatelet therapy offers no protective effects, whereas anticoagulation does (although the proportion of thromboembolic events that could be prevented by long-term anticoagulation remains unclear) [30]. Periprocedural atrial fibrillation is also relatively common after TAVI, easily overlooked and a likely source of thromboembolic events [31]. Ongoing studies will help to determine the optimal regimes of antiplatelet and antithrombotic therapy in specific clinical scenarios and the possible role of concomitant left atrial appendage occlusion for TAVI patients in atrial fibrillation and at high bleeding risk.

47.8   Conclusion

So, how do these considerations translate into practical recommendations for individual patient care? The contemporary Heart Team have a number of procedural and device-related issues to consider when determining the optimal choice of therapy for low-risk patients—and these decisions will soon be underpinned by the outcomes of ongoing large-scale randomized studies. While careful case selection, routine preprocedural planning using MSCT, and increased efficiency of patient care pathways will doubtless impact on overall outcomes, clinicians must nevertheless understand the limits of technology, valve performance, and durability for lower-risk or younger patients. Only when key outstanding questions concerning durability and the elimination of major complications have been addressed will TAVI be accepted as the gold standard treatment of aortic stenosis. Until then, individualized decisions made by informed, evidence-based Heart Teams guided by the needs and expectations of individual patients remain essential.

Conflict of Interest AR—no disclosures to declare. BP—Unrestricted research grants from Edwards Lifesciences; speaker fees from Edwards Lifesciences and Boston Scientific Corporation.

References

1. Smith CR, Leon MB, Mack MJ, et al. Transcatheter versus surgical aortic-valve replacement in high-risk patients. N Engl J Med. 2011;364(23):2187–98.
2. Thourani VH, Kodali S, Makkar RR, et al. Transcatheter aortic valve replacement versus surgical valve replacement in intermediate-risk patients: a propensity score analysis. Lancet. 2016;387(10034):2218–25.
3. Leon MB, Smith CR, Mack MJ, et al. Transcatheter or surgical aortic-valve replacement in intermediate-risk patients. N Engl J Med. 2016;374(17):1609–20.
4. Sawaya FJ, Spaziano M, Lefevre T, et al. Comparison between the SAPIEN S3 and the SAPIEN XT transcatheter heart valves: a single-center experience. World J Cardiol. 2016;8(12):735–45.
5. Leon MB, Smith CR, Mack M, et al. Transcatheter aortic-valve implantation for aortic stenosis in patients who cannot undergo surgery. N Engl J Med. 2010;363(17):1597–607.
6. Popma JJ, Adams DH, Reardon MJ, et al. Transcatheter aortic valve replacement using a self-expanding bioprosthesis in patients with severe aortic stenosis at extreme risk for surgery. J Am Coll Cardiol. 2014;63(19):1972–81.
7. Adams DH, Popma JJ, Reardon MJ. Transcatheter aortic-valve replacement with a self-expanding prosthesis. N Engl J Med. 2014;371(10):967–8.
8. Reardon MJ, Kleiman NS, Adams DH, et al. Outcomes in the randomized CoreValve US pivotal high risk trial in patients with a society of thoracic surgeons risk score of 7% or less. JAMA Cardiol. 2016;1(8):945–9.
9. Thyregod HG, Steinbruchel DA, Ihlemann N, et al. Transcatheter versus surgical aortic valve replacement in patients with severe aortic valve stenosis: 1-year results from the all-comers NOTION randomized clinical trial. J Am Coll Cardiol. 2015;65(20):2184–94.
10. Sondergaard L, Steinbruchel DA, Ihlemann N, et al. Two-year outcomes in patients with severe aortic valve stenosis randomized to transcatheter versus surgical aortic valve replacement: the all-comers nordic aortic valve intervention randomized clinical trial. Circ Cardiovasc Interv. 2016;9(6)
11. Popma JJ, Reardon MJ, Khabbaz K, et al. Early clinical outcomes after transcatheter aortic valve replacement using a novel self-expanding bioprosthesis in patients with severe aortic stenosis who are suboptimal for surgery: results of the Evolut R U.S. study. JACC Cardiovasc Interv. 2017;10(3):268–75.
12. Maeno Y, Abramowitz Y, Kawamori H, et al. A highly predictive risk model for pacemaker implantation after TAVR. J Am Coll Cardiol Img. 2017;10(10 Pt A):1139–47.
13. Nazif TM, Dizon JM, Hahn RT, et al. Predictors and clinical outcomes of permanent pacemaker implantation after transcatheter aortic valve replacement: the PARTNER (Placement of AoRtic TraNscathetER Valves) trial and registry. JACC Cardiovasc Interv. 2015;8(1 Pt A):60–9.
14. Greason KL, Lahr BD, Stulak JM, et al. Long-term mortality effect of early pacemaker implantation after surgical aortic valve replacement. Ann Thorac Surg. 2017;104(4):1259–64.
15. Meredith IT, Walton A, Walters DL, et al. Mid-term outcomes in patients following transcatheter aortic valve implantation in the CoreValve Australia and New Zealand Study. Heart Lung Circ. 2015;24(3):281–90.
16. Auffret V, Puri R, Urena M, et al. Conduction disturbances after transcatheter aortic valve replacement: current status and future perspectives. Circulation. 2017;136(11):1049–69.
17. Urena M, Webb JG, Eltchaninoff H, et al. Late cardiac death in patients undergoing transcatheter aortic valve replacement: incidence and predictors of advanced heart failure and sudden cardiac death. J Am Coll Cardiol. 2015;65(5):437–48.

18. Frangieh AH, Kasel AM. TAVI in bicuspid aortic valves 'made easy'. Eur Heart J. 2017;38(16):1177–81.

19. Lansky AJ, Messe SR, Brickman AM, et al. Proposed standardized neurological endpoints for cardiovascular clinical trials: an academic research consortium initiative. J Am Coll Cardiol. 2017;69(6):679–91.

20. Spaziano M, Sawaya F, Chevalier B, et al. Comparison of systematic predilation, selective predilation, and direct transcatheter aortic valve implantation with the SAPIEN S3 valve. Can J Cardiol. 2017;33(2):260–8.

21. Haussig S, Mangner N, Dwyer MG, et al. Effect of a cerebral protection device on brain lesions following transcatheter aortic valve implantation in patients with severe aortic stenosis: the CLEAN-TAVI randomized clinical trial. JAMA. 2016;316(6):592–601.

22. Kapadia SR, Kodali S, Makkar R, et al. Protection against cerebral embolism during transcatheter aortic valve replacement. J Am Coll Cardiol. 2017;69(4):367–77.

23. Foroutan F, Guyatt GH, O'Brien K, et al. Prognosis after surgical replacement with a bioprosthetic aortic valve in patients with severe symptomatic aortic stenosis: systematic review of observational studies. BMJ. 2016;354:i5065.

24. Mylotte D, Andalib A, Theriault-Lauzier P, et al. Transcatheter heart valve failure: a systematic review. Eur Heart J. 2015;36(21):1306–27.

25. Mack MJ, Leon MB, Smith CR, et al. 5-year outcomes of transcatheter aortic valve replacement or surgical aortic valve replacement for high surgical risk patients with aortic stenosis (PARTNER 1): a randomised controlled trial. Lancet. 2015;385(9986):2477–84.

26. Barbanti M, Petronio AS, Ettori F, et al. 5-Year outcomes after transcatheter aortic valve implantation with CoreValve prosthesis. JACC Cardiovasc Interv. 2015;8(8):1084–91.

27. Foroutan F, Guyatt GH, Otto CM, et al. Structural valve deterioration after transcatheter aortic valve implantation. Heart. 2017;103(23):1899–905.

28. Capodanno D, Petronio AS, Prendergast B, et al. Standardized definitions of structural deterioration and valve failure in assessing long-term durability of transcatheter and surgical aortic bioprosthetic valves: a consensus statement from the European Association of Percutaneous Cardiovascular Interventions (EAPCI) endorsed by the European Society of Cardiology (ESC) and the European Association for Cardio-Thoracic Surgery (EACTS). Eur Heart J. 2017;38(45):3382–90.

29. Chakravarty T, Sondergaard L, Friedman J, et al. Subclinical leaflet thrombosis in surgical and transcatheter bioprosthetic aortic valves: an observational study. Lancet. 2017;389(10087):2383–92.

30. Makkar RR, Fontana G, Jilaihawi H, et al. Possible subclinical leaflet thrombosis in bioprosthetic aortic valves. N Engl J Med. 2015;373(21):2015–24.

31. Jorgensen TH, Thyregod HG, Tarp JB, et al. Temporal changes of new-onset atrial fibrillation in patients randomized to surgical or transcatheter aortic valve replacement. Int J Cardiol. 2017;234:16–21.

Conclusion

48

Arturo Giordano, Giuseppe Biondi-Zoccai,
and Giacomo Frati

*Every new beginning comes from some other
beginning's end*

Seneca

As a new child is born when a couple reaches
its maturity, physically and spiritually, a scientific and technical discipline sees light when
related disciplines have come to adulthood and
prove a solid foundation for further breakthroughs, by also showing their limitations.

The field of transcatheter aortic valve implantation (TAVI), also called transcatheter aortic
valve replacement (TAVR), fulfills precisely
these premises, as it borrowed since inception
from developments in noninvasive cardiology
(mainly pathophysiology and imaging insights),
interventional cardiology (mainly miniaturiza-
tion and other engineering refinements), and cardiac surgery (mainly improvements in biologic
prostheses and minimally invasive surgical techniques). Accordingly, the first transcatheter aortic

valve implantation procedure performed by Alain
Cribier recapitulated all the above advancements,
while representing a true paradigm shift in terms
of science and medical practice [1]. From those
baby steps, pioneering results were achieved with
first-generation transcatheter aortic valve implantation devices in comparison to medical therapy
for inoperable patients, to surgery in high-risk
subjects, in intermediate-risk patients, and, most
recently, in low-risk patients [2–6].

Despite such breakthroughs, the field of transcatheter aortic valve implantation continues to
move forward at a sustained pace. As shown by
glancing at the table of contents of this book, or
reading any of its authoritative chapters, transcatheter aortic valve implantation will hopefully
move from aortic stenosis and degenerated bioprosthesis to also embrace the management of
pure aortic regurgitation, recognizing the importance of addressing the common pathophysio-
logic milieu of cardiovascular inflammation
while maintaining a pragmatic focus on hemodynamics. Moving to individualized decision making, we expect important refinements in scoring
approaches, encompassing different dimensions
of patient risk and suitability to transcatheter aortic valve implantation. In addition, multifaceted,
hybrid and fusion imaging will likely overcome
the limitations inherent to any single imaging
modality. Further insights will also come from

A. Giordano
Unità Operativa di Interventistica Cardiovascolare,
Pineta Grande Hospital, Castel Volturno, Italy

G. Biondi-Zoccai (✉) · G. Frati
Department of Medico-Surgical Sciences
and Biotechnologies, Sapienza University of Rome,
Latina, Italy
e-mail: giuseppe.biondizoccai@uniroma1.it

© Springer Nature Switzerland AG 2019
A. Giordano et al. (eds.), *Transcatheter Aortic Valve Implantation*,
https://doi.org/10.1007/978-3-030-05912-5_48

several niche but key topics stemming from concomitant coronary artery disease to prohibitive risk and biomarker fingerprinting.

The conundrum of choosing the right device for the right patient will need dedicated trials and their formal and explicit synthesis[7, 8], but individualized decision making, capitalizing on each device strengths and weaknesses, as well as local expertise, will most likely continue to dominate clinical practice. Similarly, ancillary devices and techniques will need to be formally tested for comparative clinical effectiveness and economic appeal. Irrespective of the competence of clinical cardiologists and interventional cardiologists, surgeons will continue to play a key role in the future of transcatheter aortic valve implantation. Indeed, their role of allies in patient selection, management, and follow-up, as well as in innovation and research, cannot be overemphasized. Focusing on the future finally brings forward several appealing new developments, spanning from new-generation devices to bioresorbable valves and low-risk patients.

We hope indeed that the present work will provide careful and sound guidance for all practitioners and researchers involved in the present as well as in the future of transcatheter aortic valve implantation, ensuring past and present successes will be hopefully matched and overcome by future ones.

Conflicts of Interest Dr. A. Giordano has consulted for Abbott Vascular and Medtronic. Prof. Biondi-Zoccai has consulted for Abbott Vascular and Bayer.

Funding None.

References

1. Cribier A, Eltchaninoff H, Bash A, Borenstein N, Tron C, Bauer F, Derumeaux G, Anselme F, Laborde F, Leon MB. Percutaneous transcatheter implantation of an aortic valve prosthesis for calcific aortic stenosis: first human case description. Circulation. 2002;106:3006–8.

2. Leon MB, Smith CR, Mack M, Miller DC, Moses JW, Svensson LG, Tuzcu EM, Webb JG, Fontana GP, Makkar RR, Brown DL, Block PC, Guyton RA, Pichard AD, Bavaria JE, Herrmann HC, Douglas PS, Petersen JL, Akin JJ, Anderson WN, Wang D, Pocock S, PARTNER Trial Investigators. Transcatheter aortic-valve implantation for aortic stenosis in patients who cannot undergo surgery. N Engl J Med. 2010;363:1597–607.

3. Gilard M, Eltchaninoff H, Iung B, Donzeau-Gouge P, Chevreul K, Fajadet J, Leprince P, Leguerrier A, Lievre M, Prat A, Teiger E, Lefevre T, Himbert D, Tchetche D, Carrié D, Albat B, Cribier A, Rioufol G, Sudre A, Blanchard D, Collet F, Dos Santos P, Meneveau N, Tirouvanziam A, Caussin C, Guyon P, Boschat J, Le Breton H, Collart F, Houel R, Delpine S, Souteyrand G, Favereau X, Ohlmann P, Doisy V, Grollier G, Gommeaux A, Claudel JP, Bourlon F, Bertrand B, Van Belle E, Laskar M, FRANCE 2 Investigators. Registry of transcatheter aortic-valve implantation in high-risk patients. N Engl J Med. 2012;366:1705–15.

4. Leon MB, Smith CR, Mack MJ, Makkar RR, Svensson LG, Kodali SK, Thourani VH, Tuzcu EM, Miller DC, Herrmann HC, Doshi D, Cohen DJ, Pichard AD, Kapadia S, Dewey T, Babaliaros V, Szeto WY, Williams MR, Kereiakes D, Zajarias A, Greason KL, Whisenant BK, Hodson RW, Moses JW, Trento A, Brown DL, Fearon WF, Pibarot P, Hahn RT, Jaber WA, Anderson WN, Alu MC, Webb JG, PARTNER 2 Investigators. Transcatheter or surgical aortic-valve replacement in intermediate-risk patients. N Engl J Med. 2016;374:1609–20.

5. Reardon MJ, Van Mieghem NM, Popma JJ, Kleiman NS, Søndergaard L, Mumtaz M, Adams DH, Deeb GM, Maini B, Gada H, Chetcuti S, Gleason T, Heiser J, Lange R, Merhi W, Oh JK, Olsen PS, Piazza N, Williams M, Windecker S, Yakubov SJ, Grube E, Makkar R, Lee JS, Conte J, Vang E, Nguyen H, Chang Y, Mugglin AS, Serruys PW, Kappetein AP, SURTAVI Investigators. Surgical or transcatheter aortic-valve replacement in intermediate-risk patients. N Engl J Med. 2017;376:1321–31.

6. Feldman TE, Reardon MJ, Rajagopal V, Makkar RR, Bajwa TK, Kleiman NS, Linke A, Kereiakes DJ, Waksman R, Thourani VH, Stoler RC, Mishkel GJ, Rizik DG, Iyer VS, Gleason TG, Tchétché D, Rovin JD, Buchbinder M, Meredith IT, Götberg M, Bjursten H, Meduri C, Salinger MH, Allocco DJ, Dawkins KD. Effect of mechanically expanded vs self-expanding transcatheter aortic valve replacement on mortality and major adverse clinical events in high-risk patients with aortic stenosis: The REPRISE III randomized clinical trial. JAMA. 2018;319:27–37.

7. Biondi-Zoccai G, editor. Network meta-analysis: evidence synthesis with mixed treatment comparison. Hauppauge, NY: Nova Science Publishers; 2014.

8. Biondi-Zoccai G, editor. Umbrella reviews. Evidence synthesis with overviews of reviews and meta-epidemiologic studies. Cham, Switzerland: Springer International; 2016.